Practice of Geriatrics

Practice of Geriatrics

Third Edition

Edmund H. Duthie, Jr., M.D.

Professor of Medicine and Chief of Geriatrics/Gerontology
Medical College of Wisconsin
Chief of Geriatrics
C. J. Zablocki Veterans Affairs Medical Center—Milwaukee
and Froedtert Memorial Lutheran Hospital
Milwaukee, Wisconsin

Paul R. Katz, M.D.

Associate Professor of Medicine and Director
Finger Lakes Geriatric Education Center
University of Rochester School of Medicine and Dentistry
Medical Director
Monroe Community Hospital
Rochester, New York

W.B. SAUNDERS COMPANY
A Division of Harcourt Brace & Company

Philadelphia   London   Toronto   Montreal   Sydney   Tokyo

W.B. SAUNDERS COMPANY
A Division of Harcourt Brace & Company

The Curtis Center
Independence Square West
Philadelphia, Pennsylvania 19106

Library of Congress Cataloging-in-Publication Data

Practice of geriatrics.—3rd ed. / [edited by] Edmund H. Duthie, Jr., Paul R. Katz.

p.   cm.

Includes bibliographical references and index.

ISBN 0–7216–6599–3

1. Geriatrics.   I. Duthie, Edmund H.   II. Katz, Paul R. (Paul Richard)
    [DNLM: 1. Geriatrics.   WT 100 P8957 1998]

RC952.P64   1998   618.97—dc21

DNLM/DLC   97-22941

PRACTICE OF GERIATRICS   ISBN 0–7216–6599–3

Printed in the United States of America.

Last digit is the print number: 9   8   7   6   5   4   3   2   1

*This text is dedicated to
the men and women who have chosen
to serve the geriatric patient.*

CONTRIBUTORS

Adil Abbasi, M.D.
Clinical Assistant Professor of Medicine, Medical College of Wisconsin, Milwaukee, Wisconsin; Geriatrician/Internist, Harwood Medical Associates, Wauwatosa, Wisconsin
Nutrition

Wendy Adams, M.D., M.P.H.
Assistant Professor of Medicine, University of Nebraska Medical Center, Omaha, Nebraska
Alcohol and Substance Abuse

Judith C. Ahronheim, M.D.
Chief, Section of Geriatric Medicine, St. Vincent's Hospital and Medical Center, New York, New York
Palliative Care

Richard M. Allman, M.D.
Professor of Medicine, Center for Aging, School of Medicine, University of Alabama at Birmingham, Birmingham, Alabama; Chief, Geriatrics Section, Birmingham Veterans Affairs Medical Center, Birmingham, Alabama
Pressure Ulcers

Sonia Ancoli-Israel, Ph.D.
Professor, University of California, San Diego, La Jolla, California; Director, Sleep Disorders Clinic, Veterans Affairs Medical Center, La Jolla, California
Sleep and Aging

Raymond J. Baddour, M.D.
Chief Resident, Department of Neurology, University of Connecticut School of Medicine, Farmington, Connecticut
Nervous System Disease

Randy Berger, M.D.
Clinical Instructor in Dermatology, Boston University School of Medicine, Boston, Massachusetts
Skin Disorders

Rebecca J. Beyth, M.D.
Assistant Professor of Medicine, Case Western Reserve University School of Medicine, Cleveland, Ohio; Staff Physician, University Hospitals of Cleveland, Cleveland, Ohio
Medication Use

Gabriel H. Brandeis, M.D.
Assistant Professor in Medicine, Boston University School of Medicine, Boston, Massachusetts; Chief Medical Officer, Health Drive, Newton, Massachusetts
Urinary Incontinence

Evan Calkins, M.D., M.A.C.P.
Emeritus Professor of Medicine, State University of New York at Buffalo, Buffalo, New York; Attending Physician, Buffalo General Hospital; Partner and Consultant in Geriatrics and Rheumatology, Medical Partners of Western New York, Buffalo, New York
Musculoskeletal Disorders

Mira Cantrell, M.D.
Associate Clinical Professor of Medicine/Geriatrics, University of California, Los Angeles, California; Clinical Director, Nursing Home Care Unit, VA Medical Center, West Los Angeles, California
Infections

Paul P. Carbone, M.D., M.A.C.P., D.Sc.(Hon.)
Professor of Medicine Emeritus, University of Wisconsin Medical School. University of Wisconsin Hospital and Clinics, Madison, Wisconsin
Oncologic Disorders

Julie Chandler, Ph.D., P.T.
Senior Epidemiologist, Merck Research Laboratories, Blue Bell, Pennsylvania
Exercise

James F. Cleary, M.B., B.S., F.R.A.C.P.
Assistant Professor of Medicine (Medical Oncology), University of Wisconsin Medical School, Madison, Wisconsin; Medical Director, Palliative Medicine Service, University of Wisconsin Hospital and Clinics, Madison, Wisconsin
Oncologic Disorders

Harvey Jay Cohen, M.D.
Professor of Medicine, Duke University Medical Center, Durham, North Carolina; Director, Center for the Study of Aging and Human Development, Associate Chief of Staff for Geriatrics and Extended Care, and Director, Geriatric Research, Education and Clinical Center, Duke University and Veterans Affairs Medical Centers, Durham, North Carolina
Hematologic Disorders

Jeffrey Crawford, M.D.

Associate Professor of Medicine, Duke University Medical Center, Durham, North Carolina; Director, Clinical Research, Duke Comprehensive Cancer Center, Durham, North Carolina

Hematologic Disorders

Jeffrey L. Cummings, M.D.

Augustus S. Rose Professor of Neurology and Professor of Psychiatry and Biobehavioral Science, University of California, Los Angeles, School of Medicine; Director, Alzheimer's Disease Center, University of California, Los Angeles, Department of Neurology and Medical Center, Los Angeles, California

Dementia

Faith B. Davis, M.D.

Professor of Medicine, Albany Medical College, Albany, New York; Attending Physician, Endocrinology, Albany Medical Center, Albany, New York

Endocrine Disorders

Paul J. Davis, M.D.

Professor of Medicine, Albany Medical College, Albany, New York; Chairman, Department of Medicine, and Physician-in-Chief, Albany Medical Center, Albany, New York

Endocrine Disorders

Ananias C. Diokno, M.D.

Associate Professor, University of Michigan School of Medicine, Ann Arbor, Michigan; Chief, Department of Urology, William Beaumont Hospital, Royal Oak, Michigan

Prostate Gland Disease

Kulwinder S. Dua, M.D., M.B., B.S., M.R.C.P., DNB

Assistant Professor, Medical College of Wisconsin, Milwaukee, Wisconsin; Chief, G.I. Diagnostic Unit, Veterans Affairs Medical Center; Staff Physician, Froedtert Memorial Lutheran Hospital, Milwaukee, Wisconsin

Gastroenterologic Disorders

Edmund H. Duthie, Jr., M.D.

Professor of Medicine and Chief of Geriatrics/ Gerontology, Medical College of Wisconsin, Milwaukee, Wisconsin; Chief of Geriatrics, C. J. Zablocki Veterans Affairs Medical Center and Froedtert Memorial Lutheran Hospital, Milwaukee, Wisconsin

History and Physical Examination

Joseph Francis, Jr., M.D., M.P.H.

Clinical Assistant Professor of Medicine, Vanderbilt University School of Medicine, Nashville, Tennessee; Clinical Services Manager, Veterans Affairs Mid South Health Care Network, Nashville, Tennessee

Delirium

Kari L. Franson, Pharm. D.

Assistant Professor, Department of Psychiatry, St. Louis University School of Medicine, St. Louis, Missouri

Depression

Marc Gautier, M.D.

Assistant Professor, Department of Medicine, Duke University Medical Center, Durham, North Carolina

Hematologic Disorders

Barbara A. Gilchrest, M.D.

Professor of Dermatology, Boston University School of Medicine, Boston, Massachusetts

Skin Disorders

Patricia S. Goode, M.D., M.S.N., E.T.

Assistant Professor of Medicine, Center for Aging, School of Medicine, University of Alabama at Birmingham, Birmingham, Alabama

Pressure Ulcers

George T. Grossberg, M.D.

Samuel W. Fordyce Professor and Chair, Department of Psychiatry; Director, Division of Geriatric Psychiatry, St. Louis University School of Medicine, St. Louis, Missouri

Depression

William John Hall, M.D., F.A.C.P.

Professor of Medicine and Pediatrics, University of Rochester School of Medicine and Dentistry, Rochester, New York; Vice-Chairman, Department of Medicine, Strong Memorial Hospital, Rochester, New York

Pulmonary Disorders

Donald P. Hay, M.D.

Associate Professor, Department of Psychiatry and Vice Chair for Clinical Programs, St. Louis University School of Medicine, St. Louis, Missouri; Attending, St. Louis University Hospital, St. Louis, Missouri

Depression

Linda Hay, Ph.D.

Assistant Professor, Department of Psychiatry, St. Louis University School of Medicine, St. Louis, Missouri

Depression

Linda Ann Hershey, M.D., Ph.D.

Professor of Neurology, State University of New York at Buffalo, Buffalo, New York; Chief of Neurology Service, VA Western New York Healthcare System, Buffalo, New York

Cerebrovascular Disease

Calvin H. Hirsch, M.D.

Associate Professor of Medicine, Epidemiology, and Preventive Medicine, School of Medicine and Medical Center, University of California, Davis, Davis, California

Hypothermia and Hyperthermia

Helen M. Hoenig, M.D.

Assistant Professor of Medicine, Duke University Medical Center, Durham, North Carolina; Chief, Physical Medicine and Rehabilitation Service, Veterans Affairs Medical Center, Durham, North Carolina

Rehabilitation

Jay B. Hollander, M.D.

Director, Urologic Education, William Beaumont Hospital, Royal Oak, Michigan

Prostate Gland Disease

Timothy Howell, M.D., M.A.

Associate Professor (CHS), Department of Psychiatry, University of Wisconsin School of Medicine, Madison, Wisconsin; Director, Mental Health Clinic, Madison Veterans Affairs Hospital, Madison, Wisconsin

Emotional and Behavioral Problems

Iyad Jamali, M.D.

Cardiology Fellow, Medical College of Wisconsin, Milwaukee, Wisconsin

Cardiac Disorders

Fran E. Kaiser, M.D.

Professor of Medicine, Division of Geriatric Medicine, St. Louis University School of Medicine, St. Louis, Missouri; Director, Sexual Dysfunction Clinic, and Director, Menopause Clinic, St. Louis University, St. Louis, Missouri

Sexuality

Marshall B. Kapp, J.D., M.P.H.

Professor, Department of Community Health, Psychiatry; Director, Office of Geriatric Medicine and Gerontology, Wright State University School of Medicine, Dayton, Ohio; Adjunct Faculty Member, University of Dayton School of Law, Dayton, Ohio

Ethical and Legal Issues

Jurgis Karuza, Ph.D.

Visiting Professor of Medicine, Finger Lakes Geriatric Education Center, University of Rochester, Rochester, New York; Professor of Psychology, State University of New York at Buffalo, Buffalo, New York

Social Support

Paul R. Katz, M.D.

Associate Professor of Medicine and Director, Finger Lakes Geriatric Education Center, University of Rochester School of Medicine and Dentistry, Rochester, New York; Medical Director, Monroe Community Hospital, Rochester, New York

Nursing Home Care

Timothy J. Keay, M.D., M.A.-Th.

Associate Professor, Family Medicine, University of Maryland School of Medicine, Baltimore, Maryland; Soros Faculty Scholar, Project on Death in America, Open Society, New York, New York

Home Care

Timothy R. Koch, M.D.

Professor of Medicine, West Virginia University School of Medicine, Morgantown, West Virginia; Chief, Section of Gastroenterology, Byrd Health Sciences Center, West Virginia University, Morgantown, West Virginia

Gastroenterologic Disorders

Carol R. Kollarits, M.D.

Clinical Professor of Ophthalmology, Medical College of Ohio, Toledo, Ohio; Medical Director, Eye Institute of Northwestern Ohio, Toledo, Ohio

Ophthalmologic Disorders

Daniel F. Kripke, M.D.

Professor of Psychiatry, University of California, San Diego, La Jolla, California

Sleep and Aging

David Gordon Lichter, M.B., Ch.B., F.R.A.C.P.

Associate Professor, Department of Neurology, School of Medicine and Biomedical Sciences, State University of New York at Buffalo, Buffalo, New York; Attending Neurologist, VA Western New York Healthcare System; Director, Movement Disorders Clinic, Buffalo General Hospital, Buffalo, New York

Parkinson's Disease and Parkinsonian Syndromes

Robert D. Lindeman, M.D.

Professor of Medicine, University of New Mexico School of Medicine, Albuquerque, New Mexico; Chief, Division of Gerontology, University of New Mexico Health Sciences Center, Albuquerque, New Mexico

Renal and Electrolyte Disorders

Kenneth W. Lyles, M.D.

Associate Professor of Medicine and Director, Sarah
Stedman Nutrition Center, Duke University Medical
Center, Durham, North Carolina; Clinical Director,
Veterans Affairs Medical Center, Durham, North
Carolina

Osteoporosis

Scott L. Mader, M.D.

Associate Professor of Medicine, Oregon Health
Sciences University, Portland, Oregon; Clinical
Director, Rehabilitation and Long-Term Care
Division, Veterans Affairs Medical Center, Portland,
Oregon

Orthostatic Hypotension, Dizziness, and Syncope

Mark Joseph Magenheim, M.D., M.P.H.

Adjunct Professor of Epidemiology, College of Public
Health, University of South Florida, Tampa, Florida;
Medical Director, Hospice of Southwest Florida,
Inc., and Consulting Physician, Columbia Doctors
Hospital, Sarasota, Florida

Preventive Health Maintenance

Diane E. Meier, M.D.

Associate Professor of Geriatrics and Medicine,
Mount Sinai School of Medicine, New York, New
York; Co-Director, Osteoporosis and Metabolic Bone
Disease Program, and Chief of Geriatrics,
Departments of Geriatrics and Medicine, Mount
Sinai Medical Center, New York, New York

Palliative Care

R. Sean Morrison, M.D.

Assistant Professor of Geriatrics and Medicine,
Mount Sinai School of Medicine, New York, New
York; Co-Director, ACE Unit, Mount Sinai Medical
Center, New York, New York

Palliative Care

Luis R. Navas, M.D.

Geriatrics Fellow, Department of Medicine, Division
of Geriatrics, Duke University Medical Center, and
Geriatrics Research, Education, and Clinical Center;
Veterans Affairs Medical Center, Durham, North
Carolina

Osteoporosis

Dean C. Norman, M.D.

Professor of Medicine/Geriatrics, University of
California, Los Angeles, California; VA Medical
Center, West Los Angeles, California

Infections

Robert Marshall Palmer, M.D., M.P.H.

Head, Section of Geriatric Medicine, Cleveland
Clinic Foundation, Cleveland, Ohio

Acute Care

Bradford S. Patt, M.D., F.A.C.S.

Assistant Clinical Professor, Department of
Otolaryngology–Head and Neck Surgery, University
of Texas Southwestern Medical Center, Dallas, Texas;
Private Practice, Houston ENT Clinic, Houston,
Texas

Otologic Disorders

John Burdett Redford, M.D.

Distinguished Professor (Emeritus), Department of
Rehabilitation Medicine, Kansas University Medical
Center, Kansas City, Kansas

Assistive Devices

William E. Reichman, M.D.

Associate Professor of Clinical Psychiatry, University
of Medicine and Dentistry of New Jersey—Robert
Wood Johnson Medical School, Piscataway, New
Jersey; Director, Brief Treatment Services, University
Behavioral Health Care, Piscataway, New Jersey

Dementia

Neil M. Resnick, M.D.

Associate Professor of Medicine, Harvard Medical
School, Boston, Massachusetts; Chief of Geriatrics,
Brigham and Women's Hospital, Boston,
Massachusetts

Urinary Incontinence

David B. Reuben, M.D.

Professor of Medicine, University of California, Los
Angeles, School of Medicine, Los Angeles, California;
Chief, Division of Geriatrics, and Director,
Multicampus Program in Geriatric Medicine and
Gerontology, UCLA Medical Center, Los Angeles,
California

Driving

Thomas P. Sculco, M.D.

Clinical Professor of Orthopedic Surgery, Cornell
Medical College, New York, New York; Director of
Orthopedic Surgery and Chief, Surgical Arthritis
Service, Hospital for Spinal Surgery, New York, New
York

Orthopedic Disorders

Reza Shaker, M.D.

Professor of Medicine, Radiology, and Surgery
(Otolaryngology), and Director, Digestive Disease
Research Center, Medical College of Wisconsin,
Milwaukee, Wisconsin; Chief, Division of
Gastroenterology and Hepatology, Froedtert
Memorial Lutheran Hospital; Acting Chief,
Gastroenterology, Veterans Affairs Medical Center,
Milwaukee, Wisconsin

Gastroenterologic Disorders

Kenneth Shay, D.D.S., M.S.

Adjunct Associate Professor of Hospital Dentistry, Department of Oral Medicine, Pathology, and Surgery, University of Michigan School of Dentistry, Ann Arbor, Michigan; Chief, Dental Service, Ann Arbor Veterans Affairs Medical Center, Ann Arbor, Michigan

Dental and Oral Disorders

Ronald I. Shorr, M.D., M.S.

Associate Professor of Preventive Medicine, University of Tennessee School of Medicine, Memphis, Tennessee; Associate Director, Internal Medicine and Transitional Residency Program, Methodist Hospitals of Memphis, Memphis, Tennessee

Medication Use

Marsha Smith, M.D.

Private Practice, Princeton, New Jersey

Gynecologic Disorders

Stephanie Studenski, M.D., M.P.H.

Associate Professor, Department of Internal Medicine, University of Kansas School of Medicine, Kansas City, Kansas; Director, Center on Aging, University of Kansas Medical Center, Kansas City, Kansas

Exercise; Instability and Falls

Mark Andrew Supiano, M.D.

Associate Professor of Internal Medicine, University of Michigan School of Medicine, Ann Arbor, Michigan; Associate Director for Research, Geriatric Research Education and Clinical Center, Ann Arbor Veterans Affairs Medical Center, Ann Arbor, Michigan

Hypertension

George Taler, M.D.

Associate Professor, Family Medicine and Internal Medicine, University of Maryland School of Medicine, Baltimore, Maryland

Home Care

Eric G. Tangalos, M.D., C.M.D.

Associate Professor of Medicine, Mayo Medical School, Rochester, Minnesota; Head, Section of Geriatrics, and Chair, Division of Community Internal Medicine, Mayo Clinic, Rochester, Minnesota

Office Practice

Donald D. Tresch, M.D.

Professor of Medicine, Cardiology, and Geriatric Medicine, and Director of Cardiology Fellowship Program, Medical College of Wisconsin, Milwaukee, Wisconsin

Cardiac Disorders

Roy B. Verdery, Ph.D., M.D.

Associate Professor of Medicine, Arizona Center on Aging, University of Arizona School of Medicine, Tucson, Arizona

Failure to Thrive

Adrian O. Vladutiu, M.D., Ph.D., F.A.C.P.

Professor of Pathology, Microbiology, and Medicine, State University of New York at Buffalo, Buffalo, New York; Director of Clinical Laboratories, Buffalo General Hospital, Buffalo, New York

Musculoskeletal Disorders

T. Franklin Williams, M.D.

Professor of Medicine Emeritus, University of Rochester School of Medicine, Rochester, New York; Physician, Monroe Community Hospital, Rochester, New York; VA Distinguished Physician, Veterans Affairs Medical Center, Canandaigua, New York

Comprehensive Geriatric Assessment

Leslie Wolfson, M.D.

Professor and Chair, Department of Neurology, University of Connecticut School of Medicine, Farmington, Connecticut; Chief of Neurology, Hartford Hospital, Hartford, Connecticut

Nervous System Disease

Lynda Wolter, M.D.

Staff Geriatrician, Santa Fe Senior Health Center, Raytown, Missouri; Staff, Columbia Independence Regional Medical Center, Independence, Missouri

Instability and Falls

PREFACE

In 1984, Evan Calkins, M.D., conceived the idea for this textbook of geriatric medicine. His vision, enthusiasm, and hard work culminated in the publication of the first two editions of the *Practice of Geriatrics*. Now, over a decade later, Dr. Calkins has "passed the torch" to one previous editor (Paul Katz, M.D.), who participated in the editing and writing of the second edition, and to a new editor (Edmund Duthie, Jr., M.D.). This transition represents a maturation of the field of geriatrics, since both editors are fellowship trained and certified in geriatrics and both have spent their entire careers practicing and teaching geriatric medicine.

The need for this text now is no different from the need for it at the time of its inception. Clinicians caring for adults continue to be challenged by the increasing numbers of older persons in their practices. This text has been assembled to assist clinicians in their care of elderly persons. As physicians, the editors are most familiar with the medical care of older persons. The editors believe that their orientation will benefit not only readers who are physicians, medical students, or residents-in-training but also other clinical providers such as nurses, nurse practitioners, social workers, pharmacists, physical therapists, occupational therapists, dietitians, psychologists, and others who need access to materials to help provide medical care to older adults.

As in past editions, the text is designed to aid practitioners by providing practical information about the care of the elderly. The text is intended to be an easy-to-read source of information that will assist clinicians who care for elderly patients in ambulatory, acute, and long-term care settings. This book is divided into sections to help the reader conceptualize an approach to geriatric care. The initial section—general issues in geriatric practice—sets the stage for the clinical encounter and reviews the approach to the patient, the concept of functional assessment, the milieu of practice (family issues, ethical and legal issues), and other issues that are common and, on occasion, overlooked (e.g., medication use, sexuality, driving). The second section emphasizes that geriatric care is not simply "internal medicine in the elderly patient" but rather is a system of care in varying sites spanning hospital, nursing home, home, office, and hospice. The third section focuses on prevention and health maintenance or optimization of function. Prevention is viewed in its broadest context to include "tertiary prevention" or restoration of function in the face of established illness (i.e., rehabilitation).

As the text proceeds, the fourth section addresses areas of practice that challenge clinicians in geriatric practice but are often not well covered in traditional texts of medical practice. Topics included here are urinary incontinence, falls, osteoporosis, pressure ulcers, and sleep disorders. New to this edition is a discussion of the entity of "failure to thrive." In the fifth section, special attention is paid to neuropsychiatric disorders, which are so prevalent, disabling, and time consuming in the practice of geriatrics. Also new to this edition are chapters on problem behaviors, alcohol and substance abuse, and the neurologic evaluation. The final section addresses medical and surgical disorders seen in geriatric practice. This section incorporates age-related changes in organ system function as well as how disease presentation, evaluation, and management are affected by aging.

The team of editors and authors for this third edition represents a significant change from past editions. Forty-one new authors have been recruited to write portions of this text. Eight new topic areas have been included.

All authors writing for this text have distinguished themselves by their training, expertise, interest, and experience in geriatric practice. Authors were chosen particularly for their abilities as clinicians actively engaged in geriatric practice. An attempt was made to choose authors from all regions of the United States, emphasizing diverse approaches to geriatric care around the country. Chapters that are entirely new to this text are concerned with acute care, exercise, failure to thrive, problem behavior, alcohol and substance abuse, neurologic evaluation, hypertension, and orthopedic disorders. Authors have tried to condense topic areas so that practitioners find key areas emphasized in a succinct fashion. Extensive referencing has been discouraged. Authors have highlighted recent contributions to the literature since the last edition.

This text is, therefore, intended for primary care practitioners who regularly see elderly patients in their daily practice. These practitioners may be primary care physicians (e.g., internists, family physicians, gynecologists), specialist physicians (e.g., psychiatrists, neurologists, physiatrists, surgeons), or subspecialist physicians (e.g., cardiologists or oncologists). Other practitioners who will find this text useful are nurses, nurse practitioners, physician assistants, social workers, dietitians, rehabilitation therapists, pharmacists, dentists, and psychologists who participate in geriatric care and work as members of the interdisciplinary health care team that serves elderly patients. Also, practitioner trainees (e.g., medical/nursing students; residents in internal medicine, family medicine, gynecology, psychiatry, neurology, and physiatry) will find this text to be helpful during clinical geriatric rotations as well as in the study/care of elderly patients during their training programs. Finally, geriatricians will find this text a helpful adjunct in training/teaching practitioners, students, and postgraduate trainees about the management precepts for geriatric patients who seek primary medical services.

In summary, this text is intended to be a concise current reference for primary care clinicians caring for elderly persons. The ultimate goal is to aid busy practitioners so that the care they render to their elderly patients is of the highest quality, affording the patient maximal function in the least restrictive environment.

EDMUND H. DUTHIE, JR., M.D.
Milwaukee, Wisconsin

PAUL R. KATZ, M.D.
Rochester, New York

ACKNOWLEDGMENTS

The authors wish to thank their mentors and colleagues at the Medical College of Wisconsin, the University of Rochester Medical Center School of Medicine and Dentistry, and their respective affiliated medical facilities (Clement J. Zablocki VAMC and Froedtert Memorial Lutheran Hospital, Milwaukee, Wisconsin; and Monroe Community Hospital, Rochester, New York) for inspiration, support, and encouragement during the preparation of this text. We also owe thanks to the contributors for meeting deadlines, revising manuscripts, and enduring our editorial critique. A particular debt is due to Karen Hartzell and Karen McDowell for the support and organization they provided during the entire editorial process. Together they have left an indelible mark on this text.

In preparing this work, the guidance and patience of the team at W.B. Saunders (Ray Kersey, Senior Editor Medical Books; David Kilmer, Senior Developmental Editor; and Catherine Stamato, Senior Editorial Assistant) have been essential in moving this project forward. Thanks are also due to Barbara (Bobbie) B. Reitt, Ph.D., who helped launch this project during its inception and the critical initial organizational phase. Her knowledge, pleasant manner, and attention to detail were invaluable.

We must make special mention of our predecessor editors who conceived this text at an earlier time when geriatrics in the United States was emerging as an organized discipline. These pioneers include Paul Davis, M.D. (first edition), and Amasa Ford, M.D. (first and second editions). Perhaps most noteworthy in this regard is Evan Calkins, M.D. Dr. Calkins has been the driving force for this text since its inception. His energy, vision, and enthusiasm know no bounds. He has profoundly influenced the careers of both of us. He continues to cast a long shadow, not only on this text but upon the entire field of geriatric medicine.

Finally, to the Duthies (Ann, John, Elizabeth, and Laura) and the Katzs (Laurie, Abigail, and Jonathan), we say "thank you" for the unconditional love and support you provided the editors: your husbands and fathers. You provide meaning for this work and our careers and lives.

CONTENTS

SECTION V

NEUROPSYCHIATRIC DISORDERS IN GERIATRIC PRACTICE

SECTION VI

MEDICAL AND SURGICAL DISORDERS IN GERIATRIC PRACTICE

SECTION

I

General Issues in Geriatric Practice

1

History and Physical Examination

Edmund H. Duthie, Jr., M.D.

GERIATRICS AND GERIATRICIANS

Geriatric medicine has been defined as a branch of medicine that concerns itself with the aging process; the prevention, diagnosis, and treatment of health care problems in the aged; and the social and economic conditions that affect the health care of the elderly.[1] Arbitrarily, the aged or elderly population is defined as persons aged 65 years or older. The 1990 U.S. Census estimated the elderly population as 13% of the total population of the United States. Although this is an impressive number, even more noteworthy is the amount of health care resources used by elderly patients, including the amount of time spent by primary care physicians with older persons (e.g., internists, 30% of time), the percentage of total health care expenditures (25%), the percentage of visits to office-based physicians (24%), and the percentage of prescription drug use (25%). Given this use of resources, it is essential that any physician who cares for adult patients be conversant with the principles of geriatric medicine.

Geriatricians (physicians who specialize in the care of elderly patients) are typically physicians who are certified in internal or family medicine and who have either completed fellowship training in geriatrics or have successfully passed the certificate of added qualifications examination offered by the American Board of Internal Medicine or the American Board of Family Practice. Geriatricians frequently find themselves caring for the oldest old (arbitrarily defined as people aged 85 and over, the "old old" being those aged 75 to 85). These patients are often frail, require an interdisciplinary team approach, and are receiving long-term care services in the home, community, or nursing home. A major goal of geriatric medicine is to educate students and physicians about the principles of geriatric medicine and to discover new knowledge about aging and the diseases that disable elderly patients through research. As a result, geriatricians have achieved high visibility in medical schools and academic medical centers.

Working in concert, geriatricians and other clinician colleagues strive to optimize the health and function of older persons. Fundamental to geriatric practice is the fact that there is tremendous heterogeneity among elderly people. Clinicians recognize that chronologic age is a poor descriptor of a patient's functional status. Therefore, basing treatment or management decisions on a patient's age may be fraught with error. Better determinants of outcome may be the natural history of illnesses and comorbidities within a patient, the patient's functional status, or the social context (e.g., economic resources, family support) of the patient's life. This is the paradox of geriatrics—the study and practice of medicine in the elderly population, which is considered a group and yet is so diverse.

With this brief introduction, the remainder of this chapter will describe the clinical encounter with the elderly patient, emphasizing the medical interview and history, the physical examination, and the formulation of a treatment plan.

GOALS OF GERIATRIC MEDICINE

The goals of geriatric care are listed in Table 1–1. These goals occur in the context of a high prevalence of chronic illness in geriatric patients and focus on detecting and managing disease rather than on curing disease. Also paramount in geriatric practice is an emphasis on the measurement and promotion of function. For decades, medical practice has emphasized the diagnosis of illness and associated therapy. This approach remains essential to geriatric practice but must be complemented by an assessment of the im-

TABLE 1–1 **GOALS OF GERIATRIC CARE**

Care versus cure
Improvement or maintenance of function and
quality of life
Prevention
Comfort for the terminally ill

TABLE 1–3 **DEATHS BY AGE AND LEADING CAUSE**

Age 45 to 64	Age 65 and Over
1. Cancer	1. Heart disease
2. Heart disease	2. Cancer
3. Stroke	3. Stroke
4. Accidents	4. Chronic obstructive pulmonary disease
5. Chronic obstructive pulmonary disease	5. Pneumonia/ influenza

U.S. Bureau of the Census: Statistical Abstracts of the
United States: 1996, 116th ed. Washington, DC, U.S.
Government Printing Office, 1996, p. 96 (No. 131: Deaths
by Age and Leading Cause: 1993).

pact of illness on the patient's life. Table 1–2 lists
the common chronic conditions that occur in
later life.

In the young and middle-aged patient, disability resulting from illness is fairly obvious from
the diagnosis. The aged patient frequently has
multiple complex illnesses, and loss of function
is the net effect of these interacting disease processes. Functional assessment must be part of the
evaluation of any geriatric patient. When caring
for older patients, clinicians must recognize that
preventive practice is still necessary and can have
an important impact on the quality of life in the
later years. Finally, there is the inescapable finality of life in geriatric practice. No other age
group has the mortality rates seen in the geriatric
population. Issues germane to death and terminal illness (e.g., advanced directives or palliative
care) must be addressed by the practitioner. Table 1–3 lists the primary cause of death for populations of varying ages. Many of these illnesses
not only cause death but are associated with
attendant suffering.

In summary, practitioners caring for adults are
heavily involved with the care of persons over
the age of 65. Geriatric practice is not simply the
practice of internal medicine, surgery, psychiatry,

or radiology in the old. Rather, geriatric practice
is a comprehensive system of care of older patients that embodies the principles of adult medicine, modifies these principles to accommodate
changes related to aging (Table 1–4), and employs an interdisciplinary approach when needed.
Care for patients should occur in the least restrictive environment possible that optimizes independence, function, and autonomy.

PRELUDE TO THE EXAMINATION

Geriatric patients are cared for in a variety of
settings: office, home, nursing home, adult day
center, subacute unit, or acute care hospital.
General principles of medical history-taking
should be incorporated into each of these settings. Before seeing the patient, the physician

TABLE 1–2 **COMMON CHRONIC CONDITIONS IN OLDER PERSONS (AGE 75 AND OVER)**

Men	Women
1. Hearing impairment (447.1)	1. Arthritis (604.4)
2. Heart condition (429.9)	2. Hypertension (417.5)
3. Arthritis (424.9)	3. Heart condition (361.4)
4. Hypertension (339.2)	4. Hearing impairment (307.8)
5. Cataracts (214.7)	5. Cataracts (259.2)

Parentheses indicate prevalence per 1000 persons.
U.S. Bureau of the Census: Statistical Abstract of the
United States: 1996, 116th ed. Washington, DC, U.S.
Government Printing Office, 1996, p. 143 (No. 219:
Prevalence of Selected Chronic Conditions by Age and Sex:
1994).

TABLE 1–4 **UNIQUE FEATURES OF GERIATRIC PATIENTS**

Multiplicity and complexity of disease
Altered functional response of many organ
systems
Chronicity of illness
Greater severity of acute illnesses and slower
recovery
Functional impairments limiting the ability to live
independently
Fragility of response to illness, intervention, and
stress whether physical, emotional, or
socioeconomic
Unstable economic and social supports
Limitation in reversibility of impairments makes
cure less likely and maintenance of
rehabilitation the main treatment focus

From Federated Council for Internal Medicine: Geriatric
Medicine: A statement from the Federated Council for
Internal Medicine. Ann Intern Med 1981;95:372–376.

should not be biased by the patient's age or location. It must be reemphasized that the patient's chronologic age provides little or no information. Every practitioner should examine his or her own views about aging and the aged. Negative prejudicial stereotypes of aging (ageism) are rampant. Years of training and clinical encounters with sick or frail elders may lead to the development of biases about elderly patients. Personal life experiences with aged relatives may also be a strong influence. The clinician must put aside prejudices about aging or certain aged patients and approach each patient with an open mind, focusing on the goals of geriatric care.

On learning that an elderly patient resides in a nursing home or lives at home, the practitioner may begin to make assumptions about the patient. Given the rapidly changing health care scene, it is erroneous to draw conclusions about patients in any setting. Nursing home residents may be recuperating from an acute illness (e.g., hip fracture) and may be capable of a high level of functioning in a community setting once they are rehabilitated. Alternatively, patients at home may be very debilitated and capable of home residence only through family support with the aid of home health agencies, which can provide intense monitoring and assistance with modalities such as intravenous support or even ventilator management.

In approaching the elderly patient, the practitioner should be aware that patients have their own biases and prejudices about their own aging. Patients may assume that their symptoms are simply a normal part of aging and therefore do not seek medical attention. Alternatively, they may fear aging and seek out alternative medicine practitioners or therapies to maintain youthfulness. Clinicians should also keep in mind that old age or functional decline is not necessarily accompanied by a disinterest in life or medical treatments. Other issues that may influence the interview include the age gap between the patient and physician, which may make it difficult to establish rapport. This can be a particular problem for inexperienced young interviewers who become insecure when patients comment, "You seem too young to be a doctor" or when recounting the medical history remark, "You're too young to remember that."

Additionally, there are issues that affect the psychologic interplay between the patient and physician, such as the physician assuming the role of a child or grandchild in relation to the senior patient. Gender differences between patients and practitioners can also influence the patient-practitioner relationship in late life. Clinicians may have a tendency to infantilize older ill patients by assuming a paternal or maternal stance, thereby jeopardizing the therapeutic relationship.

Third Party Interview

Clinical encounters with geriatric patients often occur with family present. Frail elderly persons may rely on children or others for transportation. Children often take the time to accompany a parent to a medical visit to support the patient, to assist with the treatment plan, and to obtain information so that the optimum living situation can be determined and plans for the future can be made. Some research suggests that a third party is present as often as 15% to 20% of the time when the geriatric patient sees a physician.

The practitioner should consider the role played by the family member in the encounter.[2] The family presents a challenge and on opportunity in caring for the patient. The challenge is to maintain the patient's autonomy and keep the focus of the encounter on the practitioner-patient relationship. The patient should play the key role in determining what he or she wishes the family's involvement to be. Every visit should allow some private time for the clinician and patient to discuss the patient's condition. Sensitive issues such as failing cognition, urinary incontinence, sexual dysfunction, or elder abuse or neglect may be overlooked unless provision is made for private clinician-patient contact. However, care must be taken not to overtly exclude the family or caregivers because they are important allies of both patient and practitioner.

When families are involved in the clinical encounter it is important that the patient not feel that any confidence or trust is being betrayed. Care should be exercised to avoid allowing the interview to proceed between the clinician and family to the exclusion of the patient. If during the interview the patient is spoken of in the third person, a lack of proper patient involvement in the interview exists. Families provide the opportunity to reinforce information about the patient's illness, provide corroboration of the medical history, assist with the treatment plan, and help to set and achieve the goals of medical care.

To summarize, the clinician is often faced with a geriatric patient accompanied by his or her family. Family involvement should be negotiated with the patient, individualized according to the clinical circumstances, and reflect a balance between patient autonomy and the dependence caused by illness.

THE MEDICAL HISTORY

Traditionally, the medical history is thought to be the cornerstone of the clinical encounter. This remains true in geriatric medicine. There are, however, challenges in geriatric medical history-taking that must be anticipated and overcome.

The history begins in the usual fashion with introductions and an explanation of the manner of the examination. The interviewer should assume that the patient is cogent. Unless directed otherwise by the patient, the patient should be referred to by his or her surname. There is a very real tendency for health providers to address elderly persons by their first name, particularly sick or frail elderly patients. This is probably a manifestation of the tendency toward infantilization referred to previously. As is customary in medical interviews, the clinician should anticipate immediate patient needs such as the patient's comfort, the need to urinate or defecate, or the pressure of competing activities such as meals, therapeutic programs, or diagnostic studies.

Communication Issues

The setting of the interview should be quiet and undisturbed and should ensure privacy. Hospitals, nursing homes, and day care centers may lack this proper environment, impeding the interview. Sensory loss (eyesight and hearing) is ubiquitous in late life and should be anticipated. Quiet rooms that reduce extraneous noise (e.g., music, conversation, machine or appliance noise, overhead pages, and so on) will greatly facilitate history-taking. Patients who use eyeglasses, hearing aids, or dentures should be instructed beforehand to bring these to the interview so that optimal communication can occur.

If communication appears to be problematic during the initial stages of the interview, a solution should be sought before one proceeds further. Some geriatric clinics have office staff who screen patients for these problems and take action, such as inspecting the ear canals and removing cerumen impactions before the clinician meets the patient. Some practitioners own pocket amplifiers and provide these to hearing-impaired patients to facilitate the interview. Hearing aids should be tested by the office staff and batteries replaced if they are no longer working.

Generally, it is a good idea for the examiner to be on the same level as the patient. Lighting should be adequate to highlight the interviewer's face. Indirect light that avoids both glare and shadow is best. Turning away from the patient when speaking or leaving the patient's visual field may reduce visual cues used by the patient to assist with communication. When speaking, slow clear enunciation is helpful. The pace of speech

should not be modified excessively, and shouting should be avoided, particularly into one ear (which is often out of the patient's visual field).

Geriatric patients may have other special communication problems. Patients who are edentulous may articulate poorly and should be advised to wear dentures to the interview or, in hospitals or nursing homes, to insert them. Patients with aphasia need further analysis of the type of aphasia to determine the future conduct of the interview. Some of these patients are able to answer simple yes or no questions adequately. Patients with delirium or dementia need to have another person present to corroborate the history.

Reliability of Historian

Assessment of a historian's reliability is important in geriatrics. As noted previously, the assumption is that the patient is reliable. It is generally assumed that mental status testing is part of any medical interview, and this is particularly true in geriatrics. Such testing can be done early in the interview and should be tactfully and appropriately introduced. This approach will assist in assessing the reliability of the patient's history and in detecting subclinical cognitive deficits. If found, such deficits will also alert the practitioner to the need to reinforce to relatives or caregivers instructions about the patient's condition or therapy.

History-Taking Issues

It does appear that more skill is needed to extract a medical history from the aged patient than from other adults. Table 1–5 summarizes some

---

TABLE 1–5 **ISSUES IN GERIATRIC HISTORY-TAKING**

Underreporting of illness
    Illness accepted as inevitable
    Illness is confused with normal aging
    Patient intimidated by busy practitioner
    Denial of illness
    Patient cannot afford to see the physician
    Patient fears consequences of reporting
      symptoms (tests, medicines)
Atypical presentation of illness
    Painless dental caries
    Dyspnea as an angina equivalent
    Apathetic thyrotoxicosis
    Nonspecific presentation of acute illness (e.g.,
      delirium or falls)
Communication barriers
Extensive history with multiple problems

of the reasons why more skill may be required in taking a geriatric history. The implications are that more time is invariably required to extract and record a medical history from a geriatric patient.

CHIEF COMPLAINT AND HISTORY OF PRESENT ILLNESS

There is general agreement that the concept of a "chief complaint" is often not applicable to geriatric patients. These patients frequently have multiple complex problems that are interacting. The patient may emphasize issues that seem trivial to the practitioner and unrelated to the manifest disease processes, but the clinician must address the patient's concerns or risk losing his or her confidence and adherence to the treatment plan.

The history of the present illness should develop chronologically the sequence of events that have led to the patient's current condition. Each medical condition has its own chronology. The interviewer must recognize the problems of underreporting of illness and the atypical nature of some symptoms when interpreting the history (see Table 1–5).

It may be useful for the clinician to prioritize complaints by asking questions like, "If we could do one thing for you, what would it be?" to focus the priorities of the patient with multiple complex problems. Another strategy might be to ask for a description of a typical day to get a sense of the impact of the medical condition on daily life and the social support available to the patient.

Medication use deserves special mention. Patients should be encouraged to bring their medications to each visit for review. This allows the physician to review the therapy and helps to emphasize the importance of adherence to the regimen. Specific inquiry about over-the-counter medicine usage is mandatory.

Functional Assessment as Part of the History

Functional assessment should to be part of the evaluation of the geriatric patient. Often this assessment is accomplished through the history and could occur as part of the history of the present illness. Table 1–6 is an example of one instrument that measures function; many others have been used and are advocated for use among geriatric patients. At a minimum, the activities of daily living (see Table 2–1) should be assessed. Assessment of the instrumental activities of daily living (see Table 2–2) provides further insight

into the patient's abilities and the effects of illness. Functional assessment also serves as a benchmark that allows the effects of illness or intervention to be monitored. In certain long-term care settings, functional assessment may be available as part of an admission data base (e.g., the Minimum Data Set in nursing homes). In some cases, the clinician may believe that observation of function is needed and request occupational therapy, speech therapy, physical therapy, or nursing assistance to help make an accurate determination.

Past Medical History

Obtaining the past medical history may be a particular challenge in geriatric patients. The use of forms that are completed prior to the encounter may expedite this process and enhance reliability. An effort should be made to obtain primary sources of data such as office records from prior practitioners, clinic notes, hospital or nursing home notes, and discharge summaries. These data may be voluminous and may take considerable time to read, but they can be essential for patient management and to avoid repeat testing or evaluation. Special efforts should be made to review data on prior hospitalizations, nursing home stays, and surgical procedures.

The relevance of childhood illnesses to geriatric patients has been questioned. A history of exposure to tuberculosis or a diagnosis of tuberculosis remains important into late life. Since rheumatic heart disease may become manifest initially in geriatric patients, a history of rheumatic or scarlet fever could be important.

Family History

Like childhood illness, the family history may have little relevance to the management of patients in their seventies and beyond. One suggestion has been that, rather than focusing on ancestors, the family history should "go forward" to review the health of subsequent generations. Germane to geriatric practice are issues relating to neurodegenerative disorders or mood disorders.

Social History

This portion of the history is particularly important in the practice of geriatrics. It serves as a focal point through which the clinician can get to know the patient better as a person. Through the occupational history the patient's exposure to health hazards (noise, toxins, and so on) can be uncovered. Living arrangements and depen-

TABLE 1–6 BARTHEL SELF-CARE INDEX (BI)—DEFINITION AND DISCUSSION OF SCORING

A patient scoring BI 100 is continent, feeds himself, dresses himself, gets out of bed and chairs, bathes himself, walks at least one block, and can ascend and descend stairs. Patients who score 70 and below need significant physical or supervisory assistance of a caregiver or attendant and often begin to consider nursing home care.

A score of 0 is given in all of the activities of daily living when the patient cannot meet the criteria as defined below.

Feeding

10 = Independent. The patient can feed himself a meal from a tray or table when someone puts the food within reach. He must put on an assistive device if this is needed, cut the food, use salt and pepper, pour liquids, spread butter, and so forth.

5 = Some help is necessary or patient unable to feed himself in a reasonable time.

Moving from Wheelchair to Bed and Return or on and off Bed and Chair Without Wheelchair

15 = Independent in all phases of this activity. (Patient can safely approach the bed in his wheelchair, lock brakes, lift footrests, move safely to bed, lie down, come to a sitting position on the side of the bed, change the position of the wheelchair [if necessary] to transfer back into it safely, and return to the wheelchair).

10 = Either some minimal help is needed in some step of this activity or the patient needs physical assistance to transfer.

5 = Patient can come in a sitting position without help of a second person but needs physical assistance to transfer.

Personal Hygiene

5 = Patient can wash hands and face, comb hair, clean teeth, and shave. He may use any kind of razor but must put in blade or plug in razor without help as well as get it from place of storage. Female patients must put on make-up but not style hair.

Toileting

10 = Patient is able to get on and off toilet, fasten and unfasten clothes, prevent soiling of clothes, and use toilet paper without help. He may use grab bar or other stable object for support. (If it is necessary to use a bed pan instead of a toilet, he must be able to place it on a chair, empty it, and clean it.)

5 = Patient needs help with balance, handling clothing, or using toilet paper.

Bathing

5 = Patient may use a bath tub or shower or take a complete sponge bath. He must be able to do all the steps involved in whichever method is employed without another person being present.

Walking

15 = Patient can walk without help or supervision. He may wear braces or prostheses and use crutches, canes or a walkerette, but not a rolling walker. He must be able to lock and unlock braces if used, assume the standing position and sit down, get the necessary mechanical aids into position for use, and dispose of them when he sits. (Putting on and removing braces is scored under *Dressing*.)

10 = Patient needs help or supervision in any of the above but can walk at least 50 yards with a little help.

5 = Patient can walk for short distances (less than 50 yards) with physical assistance or supervision.

5 = *Propelling a wheelchair* if a person cannot ambulate independently. He must be able to go around corners, turn around, maneuver the wheelchair to a table, bed, toilet, etc. He must be able to push manual wheelchair 50 yards or use electric wheelchair. Do not score this item if the patient gets a score for *Walking*.

Ascending and Descending Stairs

10 = Patient is able to go up and down a flight of stairs safely without help or supervision. He may and should use handrails, canes, or crutches, when needed. He must be able to carry canes or crutches as he ascends or descends stairs.

5 = Patient needs help with or supervision of any one of the above items.

Dressing and Undressing

10 = Patient is able to put on and remove all clothing, doing all fasteners or using adaptive methods or equipment, and tie shoe laces. The activity includes putting on and removing special garments or braces when these are prescribed. Such special clothing as suspenders, loafer shoes, or dresses that open down the front may be used when necessary.

5 = Patient needs help in putting on and removing or fastening any clothing. He must do at least half the work himself. He must accomplish this in a reasonable time. Women need not be scored on use of a brassiere or girdle unless these are prescribed garments.

TABLE 1–6 **BARTHEL SELF-CARE INDEX (BI)—DEFINITION AND DISCUSSION OF SCORING**
(*Continued*)

Continence of Bowels

10 = Patient is able to control his bowels or independently manage his bowel program and have no accidents.

 5 = Patient has occasional accidents or needs help in managing his bowel program.

Controlling Bladder

10 = Patient is able to control his bladder day and night. Patients who wear an external device and leg bag must put them on independently, clean and empty bag, and stay dry day and night.

 5 = Patient has occasional accidents or cannot wait for the bed pan or get to the toilet in time or needs help with external device.

Adapted from Mahoney FI, Barthel DW: Functional evaluation: The Barthel Index. Md State Med J 1965;14(Feb):61–65.

dence on family or others for assistance should be identified. Issues of abuse or neglect, caregiver stress, and advance directives merit review at this time. Generally, it will become apparent that losses are ubiquitous in late life, and loss of job, spouse, friends, adult children, income, domicile, and recreational opportunities may be recounted. How the patient has coped with these losses provides important insights into patient management.

As part of this assessment, issues centering on transportation and driving should be addressed. This section of the history is also where questions about alcohol use, tobacco use, and, on occasion, illicit drug use can be raised. Social workers may be needed to assist with further assessment and implementation of a plan when the situation is complex, and they are frequently involved in the management of patients in hospitals or nursing homes.

Review of Systems

Though often a tedious portion of the history, some key issues in geriatrics merit special attention and may not arise in caring for other groups of adult patients. These are listed in Table 1–7.

Summary of Medical History

In summary, the medical history remains the foundation of medical care for the geriatric patient. The history may be extensive and may require multiple visits before it can be completed. Previsit questionnaires; records from health care providers, agencies, hospitals, nursing homes, and pharmacies; auxiliary historians (family, friends, caregivers); and a "hands on" medication review can all assist in the collection of a complete and reliable data base. Computers and facsimile machines should help with data collec-

tion. The principles of sound medical history taking, augmented by an emphasis on some unique features of geriatrics discussed earlier, should ensure optimal medical assessment.

THE PHYSICAL EXAMINATION

After completing the medical history, the clinician proceeds to the examination of the patient. An astute clinician will have already made observations such as grip strength when shaking hands, skin pallor, obvious tremor, speech disturbances, obvious sensory deficits, or neuromuscular deformities.

Age-related changes and commonly found abnormalities should be recognized and distinguished from other pathologies. Frail, ill geriatric patients who are bedbound present a special challenge because they may not be able to cooperate fully with an examination. This requires the examiner to be resourceful in finding ways to complete the examination. On occasion, compro-

TABLE 1–7 **SPECIAL CONSIDERATIONS IN GERIATRIC SYSTEMS REVIEW**

Cognitive impairment
Dental status
Falls
Foot disorders
Gait abnormalities or use of adaptive equipment
Hearing loss
Incontinence (fecal and urinary)
Nutrition or feeding impairment
Osteoporosis
Pressure ulcers
Psychiatric illness (depression, paranoia, anxiety, grief)
Sexual history
Sleep disorders
Vision loss

mise may be necessary, for example, examining the patient in a wheelchair rather than on a table or in bed. Limited examinations are better than no examination, but the examiner must be mindful of missing important findings such as decubitus ulcers or dependent edema.

Patient comfort must be anticipated. Cool examining rooms are a source of patient tension, and the availability of blankets may help. Spinal deformities from arthritis or osteoporosis may require the adjustment of pillows so that the examination can proceed comfortably. Adaptive devices to assist with ambulation (e.g., canes, walkers, wheelchairs, and so on) should be available during the examination. This permits the examiner to inventory these devices (many of which are obtained or used without medical input) and to see how the patient functions with their help. Adequate space to accommodate these devices and to perform a gait evaluation can be a problem in some practice settings.

Vital Signs

The examination begins with assessment of the patient's weight, pulse, temperature, respiration, and blood pressure. Problems of overweight and underweight are common among older patients, requiring weight measurement with each visit. Weight appears to plateau in middle life and then decline slightly in the later years. It is important to remember that with aging, there is a relative increase in body fat and a decrease in lean body mass. Therefore, even a "stable" weight does not imply the presence of similar body composition from the middle years into late life.

Pulse rate should not be significantly affected by age. Arteriosclerotic changes of the blood vessel walls may tend to make the arterial pulse more forceful or "bounding" in geriatric patients. This tendency toward a forceful pulse may mask such classic findings as the "pulsus parvus et tardus" seen in aortic stenosis. Careful detection of all pulses is important because atherosclerotic blockages can lead to significant pathology in elderly patients such as peripheral vascular disease with amputation, subclavian steal syndrome with dizziness and falls, or cerebrovascular disease with ischemia or stroke.

Stiffened blood vessels also have implications for blood pressure determination in late life. Systolic blood pressure rises throughout life in Western populations, whereas diastolic pressure peaks and plateaus in middle age and later life. "Normal" blood pressure has been defined by determining the cardiovascular risk associated with a given blood pressure (see Chapter 35).

The presence of an isolated rise in the systolic pressure without a diastolic rise (isolated systolic hypertension) is fairly unique to older patients and, unlike younger patients, does not necessarily imply anemia, thyrotoxicosis, or aortic insufficiency, which can cause a bounding pulse and wide pulse pressure in the young.

Determination of orthostatic blood pressure should be routinely performed in geriatric patients. Although a number of factors, such as declining baroreceptor sensitivity, diminished arterial compliance, increased venous tortuosity, decreased renal sodium conservation, and diminished plasma volume, could combine to cause a drop in orthostatic blood pressure among older patients, there is no clear evidence that the pressure drops solely as a function of age. However, a blood pressure drop when changing from the supine to the upright position is common among geriatric patients (possibly as many as 30% of unselected patients may experience a 20-mmHg or more drop in systolic pressure). Diseases and medications that cause the problem should be sought (see Chapter 5).

Stiff and noncompressible blood vessels in older patients have been thought to contribute to the entity called pseudohypertension. This condition is an elevated blood pressure detected by sphygmomanometer with little target organ damage, sensitivity to antihypertensive medications, and normal intra-arterial pressure. Attempts to distinguish patients with pseudohypertension from true hypertensives using bedside clinical maneuvers have not been particularly reproducible.

Temperature determination in the aged is the same as it is in other patients. Norms for fever or hypothermia have not been adjusted for age. Elderly people do have a tendency toward disturbances of temperature regulation (hypothermia or hyperthermia). It is possible that some elderly patients, like others, may present with serious infections that do not produce much temperature rise. It is difficult to generalize too much about this observation.

Respiratory rate and patterns do not change significantly with age. A raised respiratory rate may be a subtle clue to a serious medical illness (e.g., acidosis, hypoxia, central nervous system disturbance) and should be detected and pursued as in any other patient.

Head and Neck Examination

The head of the geriatric patient should be inspected for gross deformities that might give a clue to Paget's disease, a condition that has a higher prevalence in older adults. Hair loss and graying of the hair occur with aging. The temporal arteries should be palpated routinely, since temporal arteritis is another condition that has a predilection for older people. Facial skin may be wrinkled and lax, lack turgor, and appear pale because of diminished vascularity. Lesions such as lentigines, seborrheic keratoses, actinic keratoses, seborrheic dermatitis, and carcinomas are all common and should be noted (see Chapter 43).

Associated with facial skin changes is a change in the appearance of the eyes in older patients. The eye tends to recede into the orbit, and the lids become lax and may bulge. Lid laxity may give the appearance of ptosis. In advanced situations, frank lid ectropion (eversion) or entropion (inversion) may be seen. The hair of the eyebrows does become thinner, but this does not necessarily represent any pathology. The pupillary orifice becomes smaller over the years and does not dilate to the same degree in geriatric patients as in younger persons. This may be due to structural changes in the iris and autonomic receptors in the eye. A graying of the limbus where the outer cornea meets the sclera has been termed arcus senilis. This finding is common in older patients and has no special significance. Cataract surgery is very common among older patients, and evidence of this surgery (e.g., the presence of implants, subcapsular contacts, iridectomies) should be noted.

The lens of the eye becomes thicker and yellower with age. Accommodation can be affected. Some evaluation of visual acuity is worthwhile among geriatric patients. Cataracts occur in as many as one third of patients in their eighties and should be recognized. On funduscopic examination, the arterioles of geriatric patients appear narrow, pale, straight, and less brilliant than the vessels of the young. The fundus should be inspected for evidence of macular degeneration, the most common cause of irreversible eyesight loss in late life (see Chapter 42).

The clinician should specifically ask the geriatric patient about eye care. He or she should not assume that eyeglass use means that an eye specialist has seen the patient. Patients may use spectacles that they obtain from relatives or friends, or they may purchase clear lenses over the counter that have little therapeutic benefit.

Examination of the ears should include some screening of hearing ability. Bedside maneuvers such as whispering, giving the Weber-Rinne test, and giving commands outside the patient's visual field (e.g., behind the patient) can be used. More formal screening procedures including the use of questionnaires, the audioscope, and bedside measures may be more sensitive in detecting the hearing deficits that are so common in late life

(see Chapter 41). Cerumen impactions are common in older patients and require treatment.

When examining the mouth, it is important to remove dentures so that the mucosa can be properly inspected. This is especially important for patients with a history of tobacco use or significant alcohol intake. Inspection of dental appliances can give the examiner some idea of the patient's oral hygiene. Dry mouth should not be attributed to normal aging (see Chapter 44). Dilated veins beneath the tongue, termed a "caviar" tongue, are seen more frequently in geriatric patients than in younger patients. The mechanism for the development of these varicosities has not been established. Inexperienced examiners can mistake this finding for petechiae or the lesions of Kaposi's sarcoma. With aging of the immune system, lymphatic atrophy develops. Tonsillar tissue frequently recedes in geriatric patients. Palpable nodes in the neck or an enlarged tonsil should raise a suspicion of some underlying pathology. Ptotic submandibular salivary glands can sometimes be easily felt in geriatric patients and may be mistaken for masses.

Geriatric patients may have limited mobility during examination of the neck owing to degenerative changes of the disks and facet joints. Palpation of the thyroid gland is important, as it is in any age group, but it can be challenging in older adults. With aortic uncoiling and tortuosity, arterial pulsations can be seen on inspection and felt on palpation; they must to be distinguished from arterial aneurysms. Neck vein inspection may be more reliable on the right side of the neck because venous inflow may be impeded on the left side because of dilated, tortuous large arteries. With advancing age, atherosclerosis increases in prevalence; it may result in a carotid bruit. Since systolic heart murmurs are so common in older patients (see later section, Cardiovascular Examination), particularly at the base, a bruit in the neck must be distinguished from a transmitted heart murmur.

Chest Examination

The chest should be inspected for evidence of kyphosis, which may be a clue to the presence of osteoporosis. Although a number of changes in pulmonary function occur with age, these generally do not influence the clinical lung examination. In older women, an increasing incidence of breast cancer has been documented through the ninth decade. Therefore, detection of breast cancer remains an important issue for elderly women. Glandular atrophy occurs after menopause, and some elongation of the breast or a pendulous appearance may be seen. Palpable masses need an explanation.

Cardiovascular Examination

Examination of the blood pressure, pulse, neck veins, and carotid pulse has already been reviewed. Frequently, the apical impulse and point of maximal intensity are difficult to locate in a geriatric patient. Palpable thrills, especially over the aortic area, should be sought because of the frequency of systolic murmurs. Splitting of the second heart sound may be difficult to detect in older patients. The presence of a third heart sound is not physiologic in elderly patients, as it is in young adults. Debate exists about whether a fourth heart sound may be accepted as normal in aged patients. My own view is that because heart disease is so common in older persons, it is not surprising that fourth heart sounds are frequently reported. This does not mean, however, that a fourth sound is the inevitable consequence of aging; rather, it reflects the high prevalence of cardiac disease in the geriatric population.

Systolic heart murmurs have been reported in as many as a third to a half of octogenarians. These murmurs may be due to aortic sclerosis, aortic stenosis, mitral regurgitation from numerous causes, mitral valve prolapse, idiopathic hypertrophic subaortic stenosis, tricuspid regurgitation, or atrial septal defect. Clinicians examining geriatric patients should, therefore, expect to hear systolic heart murmurs often and be prepared to assess patients further through maneuvers and associated findings to determine the cause of the murmurs. "Innocent" murmurs, described in children or young adults, are not found in the geriatric age group. Valvular pathology and cardiac dysfunction are the likely explanations of a murmur in a geriatric patient.

Abdominal Examination

There is no great difference between the abdominal examination of a geriatric patient and that of a younger patient. In geriatric patients with severe scoliosis or kyphosis, the abdominal examination can be difficult owing to compression of the visceral contents by the musculoskeletal deformities. Skin atrophy and wrinkling can mask prior surgical scars; therefore, the examiner must be alert in looking for these and should query patients about scars that are located. Patients who are inactive can develop marked wasting of the abdominal musculature. As a result, palpation can detect viscera, vessels, or masses that would not otherwise be palpable in younger patients.

For example, palpation of a normal aorta may be mistaken for an aneurysm, or stool in the colon may raise a suspicion of a mass. These palpable findings require serial examinations and sometimes adjunctive radiologic testing to make a precise diagnosis.

The "acute" surgical abdomen in the geriatric patient can be a diagnostic challenge. Inexperienced examiners who expect to find the textbook characteristics of tenderness or rigidity that occur in young patients with ischemic viscera, an inflamed or perforated viscus, or peritonitis may dismiss a geriatric patient with minimal tenderness and a soft abdomen. As a result, diagnosis in the geriatric patient with serious surgical intraabdominal disease may be delayed, and significant morbidity may ensue.

Genitourinary Examination

In aged men and women pubic hair decreases in amount and becomes gray. Prostate assessment is important in elderly men with urinary complaints. The digital rectal examination has significant limitations in both sensitivity and specificity for conditions such as cancer or hyperplasia. In women, estrogen loss results in atrophy of the labia and vaginal mucus. Mild eversion of the urethral mucosa (caruncle) is common in older women and may be present in as many as 50% of patients. Inspection of the vulva for skin abnormalities, especially squamous cell carcinoma, is important. The cervix can be difficult to identify on speculum examination. On palpation, uterine and ovarian atrophy can make palpation of these organs difficult. In fact, the presence of a palpable ovary in an elderly women should raise a suspicion of some pathology, especially malignancy. Elderly women with urinary incontinence need to undergo a gynecologic examination as part of their assessment.

The examiner requires an appropriate examination table, space, light, and equipment to perform a pelvic examination successfully. Orthopedic or neurologic deformities can make the examination difficult. A small speculum may be needed for women with significant atrophy and a small introitus. Proper preparation of the patient, allowance of adequate time, and the presence of an experienced attendant who can assist with the examination increase the likelihood of success in performing a gynecologic examination that will assist with patient management.

Musculoskeletal Examination

Since arthritis is a leading chronic illness among elderly people (see Table 1–2), a careful musculoskeletal examination is required. Findings of osteoarthritis should be sought and documented. Evidence of arthritis other than osteoarthritis (e.g., gout, pseudogout, rheumatoid arthritis), periarticular problems (e.g., tendonitis or bursitis), or neural dysfunction (e.g., neuropathy or radiculopathy) can be commonly found and should be distinguished from osteoarthritis. Careful inspection of the feet is especially important. Deformities resulting from degenerative disease are common. Pulses should be routinely palpated. Evidence of neuropathy or ischemia should alert the examiner to the need for special footwear, care, and vigilance so that amputation can be avoided.

Neurologic Examination

Testing of higher cortical functions (mental status) should be done formally and routinely in every geriatric patient. Healthy older people should be cognitively intact. Failure to test mental status formally will result in missed diagnoses and failed patient management.

In examination of the cranial nerves, testing of sensory function (especially eyesight and hearing) must be reemphasized. Olfactory acuity, though rarely formally tested, does decline with advancing age. As a result, detection of flavors, which depends on olfaction, may also be affected. On testing extraocular muscle movements, clinicians often find that geriatric patients can have difficulty in raising their eyes upward to the same degree as younger patients. Testing of the gag reflex is appropriate but has limited value in predicting speech or swallowing function.

In motor testing, orthopedic deformity, neural disease, and disuse may all combine to result in atrophy. Interosseous wasting is commonly described and may be related to any number of the just-mentioned abnormalities. Muscle does atrophy as a function of age, even with sustained use. Bedside testing of strength should be normal in healthy older patients, although some sophisticated laboratory measures are more sensitive in detecting age-related decrements of strength. Deep tendon reflexes at the ankle are absent in a "significant minority" of elderly persons. Con-

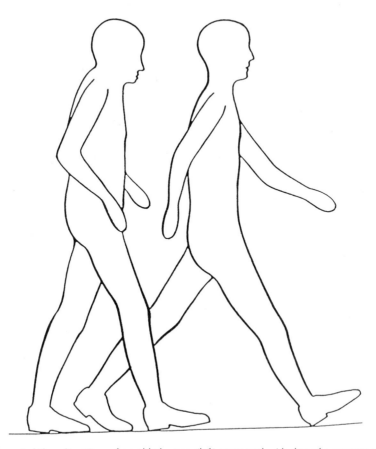

Figure 1–1 The characteristic gait pattern of an elderly man *(left)* compared with that of a younger man *(right)*. (From: Murray MP, Kory RC, Clarkson BH: Walking patterns in healthy old men. J Gerontol 24:176, 1969.)

troversy exists about whether this reflects common neural pathology in late life or is a normal variant.

On examination the sense of touch should be intact to pin prick, light touch, and position. Like absent ankle reflexes, lost vibratory sensation is frequently encountered in older people in the distal lower extremities. Once again, this may reflect some subclinical pathology.

Gait testing should be performed in every geriatric patient. Office space frequently limits the ability to assess the gait properly. A simple screening test could include having the patient arise from a chair without using his or her arms, walking normally, standing with the feet together with the eyes open and then closed, supporting body weight on the heels and then the toes, and then sitting back down. With aging, the gait changes. Patients have more flexion at the elbows, waist, and hips. There is diminished arm swing. Step length is shorter, and foot lift is less than that seen in the young (Fig. 1–1).

Assessment of function has been previously emphasized. Historical data can be supplemented by asking the patient to raise the arms over the head and undress or dress without assistance but under observation to check for fine motor abilities.

THE ASSESSMENT

After performing a detailed history and physical examination, the clinician formulates a problem list together with the appropriate diagnostic and therapeutic strategies. Since a multitude of problems is likely, prioritization is frequently needed. The problems that contribute most to the patient's dysfunction should be given highest priority. Readily reversible or treatable problems also merit prompt attention. Serial determination

of functional assessment can help to gauge the impact of therapies.

The benefits and risks of intervention need careful attention. Geriatric patients are often more prone to the complications accompanying invasive diagnostic procedures and surgical interventions. Pharmacotherapy also is more problematic in elderly patients than in young patients, and adverse drug reactions are more likely as the number of drugs taken by a patient increases. Clinical judgment is the key in knowing when patients can tolerate an intervention and are likely to benefit and when complications and serious morbidity are a significant reality. The clinician should not deny effective treatment when it can benefit a patient nor initiate an evaluation or treatment when it will not result in a significantly improved outcome for the patient. Balancing these priorities requires experience and an in-depth knowledge of the literature on clinical trials in aged patients. This is the challenge presented by geriatric practice for the practitioner.

References

1. Federated Council for Internal Medicine: Geriatric medicine: A statement from the Federated Council for Internal Medicine. Ann Intern Med 1981;95:372–376.
2. Green MG, Majerouitz SD, Adelman RO, Rizzo C: The effects of the presence of a third person on the physician-older patient medical interview. J Am Geriatr Soc 1994;42:413–419.

Additional Readings

Gastel B: Working with Your Older Patient: A Clinician's Handbook. Bethesda, MD, National Institute on Aging, National Institutes of Health, 1994.
Schneiderman H: Physical examination of the aged patient. Conn Med 1993;57(5):3–10.
Schwartz MH: The geriatric patient. *In* Schwartz MH (ed): Textbook of Physical Diagnosis. Philadelphia, WB Saunders, 1994, pp. 584–597.

2 Comprehensive Geriatric Assessment

T. Franklin Williams, M.D.

Comprehensive geriatric assessment has been well defined as a "multidimensional—usually interdisciplinary—diagnostic process designed to quantify an elderly individual's medical, psychosocial, and functional capabilities and problems with the intention of arriving at a comprehensive plan for therapy and long-term follow-up."[1, 2] This approach to decision making and developing plans for the care of older patients with complex problems at critical points in their lives has developed from the experience and observations of clinicians who have been deeply involved in the care of older persons during the past 60 years. This approach has been examined and refined in a number of studies in both inpatient and outpatient settings.

The Consensus Development Conference at the National Institutes of Health concluded that such an approach, when appropriately targeted, is effective in achieving the goals of improved diagnostic accuracy, guidance in selection of interventions to restore or preserve health, and aid both in choosing an optimal environment for care and in predicting outcomes and monitoring clinical change over time.[3, 4] Recent meta-analysis of controlled trials of comprehensive geriatric assessment has provided convincing evidence that these programs can decrease the use of institutional services, improve physical and mental functioning, and increase survival, particularly when the comprehensive assessment team continues to take primary responsibility for management and accomplishment of the goals determined.[5, 6] The value of such an assessment process is recognized in many countries.[7–9]

THE CONCEPT OF COMPREHENSIVE ASSESSMENT

As is well documented in other chapters in this text, many older people acquire chronic diseases that in turn result in varying degrees of disability. This is clearly not true for all elderly people. Some in their eighties and nineties continue to be vigorous in all aspects of life. However, the number of older people who have some degree of impairment in carrying out their usual functions does increase in the later years, with over 70% of those aged 80 and older reporting some limitation in activity.[10] Such older people may be referred to as frail elderly and they are the ones who are likely to need some form of long-term assistance or care to continue to maintain as much independence in living as possible.

To determine the types of assistance needed by frail elderly people and to help make arrangements for their care, the physician and other health professionals must conduct a comprehensive diagnostic evaluation or assessment that is fully analogous to the careful diagnosis that must precede any type of treatment decision. The medical conditions that underlie and contribute to the functional losses must be identified and appropriately treated, but this is only a part of the necessary effort. The types and degrees of functional losses themselves must be carefully addressed as well as the extent of family and other social supports available to help meet the older person's needs.

Unfortunately, careful functional and social assessments as steps in decision making for long-term care are often neglected, resulting in the provision of inappropriate types of long-term care. Without a careful diagnostic evaluation, frail elderly people may end up in nursing homes when they might be able to live in less confining settings or at home with support services. Conversely, the patient with unassessed needs may not be provided with the type or degree of long-term care that he or she requires, resulting in increased disability or accelerated burnout on the part of family caregivers.

In contrast, careful use of comprehensive assessment and recommendations for long-term care result both in care that is more appropriate for the needs of the person and in less use of institutional care such as nursing homes. Functional assessment is also essential as a basis for the choice of rehabilitative therapies and for following the progress of patients with chronic disabilities.

In this chapter the following aspects of assessment are addressed:

- Situations in which assessments may be or should be carried out.
- Special features of the diagnostic assessment that are relevant to long-term decisions (i.e., the multiple domains that must be assessed, the need for comprehensive multidisciplinary efforts, and the need for consistency).
- Comprehensive assessment instruments.
- Translation of the identified needs into appropriate services and appropriate settings for care.
- The need for continuing review of assessment findings.

SITUATIONS IN WHICH ASSESSMENT MAY BE REQUIRED

Assessment of frail elderly people may be needed for a variety of purposes: (1) screening for early detection of potential disabilities, (2) case finding to offer relevant care to those who need it, (3) comprehensive diagnostic work-up as part of developing a plan of therapy, (4) monitoring progress, (5) determining the level or setting of long-term care required, and (6) determining the appropriateness of use of long-term care services and facilities.

The approach to assessment and the methods used must be modified according to which purpose is relevant. Unfortunately, there is a tendency to attempt to apply a method or protocol developed for one purpose to another use or in different circumstances, and this leads to unsatisfactory results. This chapter deals primarily with comprehensive assessment as a necessary part of the diagnostic work-up of individual frail elderly people; reference to the other purposes served by assessments is made simply to remind the reader that caution must be exercised in considering the use of guides or protocols developed for other purposes.

The most important use of comprehensive assessment as part of the diagnostic work-up of a frail elderly person is to evaluate a patient whose physical, mental, or social condition is changing, most likely in the direction of an increased need for long-term services. Such a person may be seen in one of the following ways: He or she may (1) present to a physician in his or her office; (2) be referred to a health or social agency, which in turn recommends a comprehensive diagnostic assessment; (3) be seen on geriatric consultation in a hospital; or (4) be referred to a geriatric evaluation clinic or inpatient unit. These people are reaching or have reached a critical point because of changes in their functional status or changes in the family support system available, and they are often facing a decision about whether to continue to live at home with increased support services or to enter a long-term care institution.

In the presence of such complex and relatively urgent problems it is difficult for a physician to conduct an adequate assessment in his or her office. Both the constraints of time and the limited immediate availability of a range of professionals from other disciplines usually require the physician to conduct or arrange for a comprehensive multidisciplinary assessment in a clinic or hospital or nursing care unit established to serve this need.

The essential components of such specialized geriatric units and clinics include (1) regular participation in the diagnostic evaluation by physicians, nurses, and social workers with special competence in this area; (2) accessibility of consultants in other specialties such as psychiatry, neurology, and rehabilitation medicine, and occasionally in other fields such as arthritis, endocrinology, physical therapy, occupational therapy, and speech therapy; (3) ready availability and appropriate use of diagnostic radiologic and laboratory procedures; (4) development of consistent data bases; and (5) establishment of regular team conferences to review all information and an effective system for transmission of findings and recommendations to other professionals for follow-up.

DOMAINS OF ASSESSMENT

Comprehensive geriatric assessment should begin with a careful thorough general medical evaluation (see Chapter 1 and also the detailed summary by Applegate[11]). The most important domains or areas that must be considered when making decisions about long-term care include (1) the need for chronic medical treatment, (2) the level of physical functioning, (3) the level of mental functioning, (4) the availability of family and social supports, and (5) environmental features. These areas of assessment are discussed next in relation to the approaches and methods that may be used in clinical practice; more detailed analyses, including critical comparisons of different methods and discussion of other uses of assessment, are available elsewhere.[7, 12, 13]

Need for Chronic Medical Treatment

A patient's need for certain modalities of chronic treatment may call for very specific equipment and specialized personnel, which in turn have a major impact on the care plan, including who will provide the care and where the care can be given. For example, a patient may need help in managing a tracheostomy or other type of ostomy; he may need oxygen, intravenous fluids or medications, traction, or frequent treatments by a respiratory therapist, physical therapist, occupational therapist, or speech therapist; or he may need specialized nursing care, for example, for care of a major pressure ulcer. In some instances it may be possible to train family caregivers to provide such care. In other instances it is important to recognize when family members are not capable of carrying out these services, which then must be provided by professional home support services or in an institution. In any event, these treatment needs must be fully identified in the assessment process.

Assessment of Physical Function

Limitations in a person's ability to carry out ordinary daily physical activities are the most common cause of a need for long-term care assistance. It may appear to be tautologic to say that a person who cannot carry out an ordinary daily activity that is necessary for independent living must have some assistance or service; however, diagnostic assessment of such functional characteristics has been neglected so often that the need for it must be emphasized. The therapeutic goal is to provide assistance to compensate for the identified functional disability or disabilities, thus ensuring continued independent living to the maximum extent possible.

Assessment of physical and mental function is part of the diagnostic work-up of a frail older patient and is distinct from and only secondarily related to the diagnosis of specific disease entities that may cause the loss of such function. That is, it is necessary to determine the functional characteristics of a patient and address them specifically in the therapeutic plan no matter what the underlying causes are. Proper treatment of the latter may contribute to improved function, but some degree of functional loss may continue even with optimal treatment of disease.

TABLE 2–1 ASSESSMENT OF ACTIVITIES OF DAILY LIVING

Assess whether the person can accomplish each activity independently, whether he or she needs partial supervision or assistance, and whether he or she is fully dependent on others.

Personal self-care

Feeding oneself
Bathing
Toileting

Mobility

Able to move from bed to a standing position or to a chair
Able to walk (with or without assistive devices) or use a wheelchair

Continence

Continent of urine: always or rarely incontinent, or frequently or usually continent
Continent of feces

The development of consistent useful approaches to the assessment of physical function owes much to the original work of Katz and his colleagues[14] in defining activities of daily living (ADL) and to Lawton and Brody[15, 16] in defining the so-called instrumental activities of daily living (IADL). Tables 2–1 and 2–2 list the key elements in these assessments.

The ordinary activities of daily living can be categorized as personal self-care activities (e.g., feeding oneself, bathing, dressing, toileting), activities involving moving around independently (e.g., moving from bed to a walking position

TABLE 2–2 ASSESSMENT OF INSTRUMENTAL ACTIVITIES OF DAILY LIVING

Assess whether the person can accomplish each activity necessary to manage his or her living environment independently or whether he or she is dependent on others.

Within the home

Cooking
Housecleaning
Laundry
Management of medications
Management of telephone
Management of personal accounts

Outside the home

Shopping for food, clothing, drugs, etc.
Use of transportation to travel to necessary and desired activities (e.g., physician's appointments, religious and social events)

or wheelchair, and achieving locomotion), and maintaining control of bladder and bowel function. A person who can carry out all these functions independently does not need the assistance of anyone else. Conversely, the lack of ability to perform any of these activities does mean that some external assistance must be provided. Some help with bathing and dressing, if this is all that is required, can usually be provided by a family member or staff of a minimum-care domiciliary facility once or twice a day. On the other hand, a person who needs regular help with ambulation or feeding or who is incontinent obviously requires almost constant attendance.

The IADL involve the ability of a person to manage his or her living environment—that is, to procure and prepare food, manage the laundry and clean the house, and travel to necessary or desirable activities outside the home. Any lack of ability to carry out these functions for oneself means that some type of assistance or service is needed; such services may be more varied and may not have to be as personal as those required to address ADL needs.

In assessing all of these characteristics of daily functioning it is essential to determine not only what the person *can* do but also what she or he *does* do based on direct observations or reports by a reliable observer (family member or professional). Also, in persons with a cognitive impairment (who often have normal physical function), it is essential to assess and record how much supervision, cueing, and reminding is required by caregivers. Such needs can be at least as burdensome as actually providing care to compensate for a physical impairment.

To document the ADL and IADL status of patients, a number of protocols and scales have been developed to provide consistency in the information obtained so that it can be communicated more easily between health care providers and may also be useful in documenting changes that take place over time. Such protocols are also useful as decision-making tools by those who provide and pay for services. The most widely used assessment forms and guides have recently been reviewed.[12, 17]

In regular medical practice it is highly desirable to select a format in which to record the functional assessment information routinely and consistently as part of the medical record. A good example is the procedure outlined by Lachs and colleagues.[18] The precise details of any functional limitation should be noted because such details serve as a basis for planning recommendations for specific supportive services. A total score or scale, made in an attempt to summarize an overall impression of degree of disability, serves no

useful purpose in guiding specific therapeutic plans.

Assessment of Mental, Emotional, and Psychobehavioral Function

Limitations in mental function can result in losses of autonomy that are just as severe as losses due to problems in physical function, and they can, of course, also contribute to limitations in ADL and IADL. Losses of mental function often require types of assistance that differ from the assistance needed to compensate for physical needs.

Methods of assessing the mental, emotional, and psychobehavioral status of frail elderly people in ways that are useful in determining the need for long-term care services are not as adequately developed as is desirable. Several relatively short tests of mental or cognitive function have been developed and are widely used. Each of them includes questions that test the individual's orientation, short-term and longer-term memory, ability to do arithmetic, and ability to reproduce a geometric design. The most commonly used tests are described by Applegate and colleagues[12] and Gurland and associates.[19, 20] These tests can identify the presence of a significant degree of decline in mental or cognitive function. However, they do not correlate well with how well a person can actually perform his or her daily living activities. For example, a patient with considerable loss of memory (typically the first sign of dementia) may perform very poorly on such tests (e.g., the patient may be oriented only to people and have no ability to answer the other questions correctly) and yet may still function satisfactorily and independently in his or her familiar home environment. Conversely, a person may score well on a number of items, such as the arithmetic and geometry questions, and may show some features of retained memory, yet he may be quite confused when carrying out ordinary daily activities and need almost constant supervision. Furthermore, we do not yet know enough to relate specific segments of such cognitive tests to specific anatomic or physiologic abnormalities in the central nervous system.

Despite such limitations, it is probably still helpful to employ one of the commonly used tests as a regular part of the work-up of an elderly frail patient to identify any gross evidence of dementia and to provide a baseline for future comparisons to detect evidence of change. The identification of any evidence of dementia by such tests should call for a thorough work-up to determine the extent and nature of the dementia and to identify potentially modifiable functional disorders of whatever cause. More refined and useful techniques for measuring and following mental status are under development.

Other mental disorders in older persons that may have major effects on mental function include depression, delirium, and paranoid psychotic states. Depression occurs so commonly and is so often either not recognized or passed off as dementia that special attention should be paid to detecting its presence. In the regular work-up of the patient, the observations of the physician, nurse, or social worker should provide clues to this problem. In addition, one of the standardized short depression tests may be used as a screening test to identify the need for a more intensive work-up and possible treatment (see Chapter 28). However, as with the mental status tests, the results of these depression tests cannot be used as a quantitative reflection of the degree of loss of daily functional ability due to depression.[21]

In a patient with any features that suggest delirium, including hallucinations and paranoid tendencies, one should always look for possible causes, such as the side effects of medications, the use of drugs or alcohol, or the presence of metabolic disorders (see Chapter 27).

Symptoms of unusual or difficult behavior in confused or depressed patients can impose severe burdens on those who are providing care, whether at home or in an institution, and the presence or absence of such symptoms should be ascertained from the caregivers. Questions should be asked about wandering, agitation, abusive or assaultive behavior, fluctuating emotional state, bizarre actions (e.g., hoarding, undressing), hallucinations, impaired judgment, or depressive and suicidal tendencies. It is very important to learn what may be worrying the patient or triggering her or his symptoms. Knowledge of the lifetime patterns of daily practices and preferences can help caregivers understand and respond usefully to these symptoms. Approaches to addressing these challenges are further discussed in Chapter 29.

Assessment of Social Function and Social Supports

The characteristics of the environment in which the frail elderly person is currently living, including both the social and physical environments, often contribute, positively or negatively, to the clinical condition for which the patient is being seen and are always important in making plans for long-term care. The degree of social function and the degree of support that the patient receives and can expect to receive from family and friends are often deciding factors in determining whether institutional care is necessary. The capabilities and desires of family members must be assessed as well as the presence or extent of burnout from their current care burdens. Information is also needed about the present and potential availability of services from supportive agencies. The social worker on the assessment team should be involved with the family, social agencies, and patient and should play a role from the earliest stage of the assessment consultation in obtaining essential information.[22, 23]

As discussed by Kane[22] and others, other social dimensions that should be assessed include the presence of social networks and resources, the patient's subjective well-being, values, and preferences, the burden on the caregiver and any evidence of elder abuse.

Assessment of Environmental Characteristics

The physical environment of the patient's home and surroundings should be assessed by a visiting or community health nurse or by a member of the assessment team. This is an essential step in determining whether the patient can continue to function safely and effectively in that setting, given his or her functional limitations. This assessment can also identify measures that might be taken to modify the home to make it more suitable to the patient's limitations, such as the installation of handrails, raised toilet seats, or widened doors for wheelchair use. To make precise recommendations, it is often necessary for an occupational therapist or a specially trained community health or visiting nurse to visit the home. Guidelines for assessing the home environment have recently been presented in practical detail.[24]

COMPREHENSIVE ASSESSMENT INSTRUMENTS

Because most of the elements of assessment described in the preceding section are essential parts of the diagnostic work-up and the decision-making process for determining what types of long-term supportive services are needed, a number of comprehensive multidisciplinary assessment guides or protocols have been developed. These have been used primarily by community-based agencies in their role as decision makers—that is, in determining the types of services needed. However, the information collected in this way can also be very helpful to the physician and other members of the assessment team during their diagnostic work-up of a patient and in following the course of the patient. Examples are the Philadelphia Geriatric Center multilevel assessment instrument of Lawton and associates,[25] the Older American Resources and Services (OARS) instrument used at Duke University,[26] and the comprehensive assessment and referral evaluation (CARE) instrument.[27]

One major development is the use of a national resident assessment instrument for nursing homes, the Minimum Data Set (MDS), which is now required for admission of all persons to nursing homes as part of the Omnibus Budget Reconciliation Act of 1987. This portion of the Act in turn was a response by Congress to the Institute of Medicine report on the quality of care in nursing homes.[28] The development of the MDS has been described[29] and commented upon.[30] Its contents have been carefully developed to assist the staffs of nursing homes in developing comprehensive individual approaches to the care of each new resident. It is likely (and desirable) that the newly revised MDS 2 will become a routine part of guiding the care of older people in organized home care services as well as nursing homes and will be found useful in all comprehensive geriatric assessment settings as well.

Although the information that may be made available to the assessment team from the use of such instruments can be helpful, it does not take the place of careful review and, when indicated, further exploration of each of the areas of assessment described previously.

TRANSLATING IDENTIFIED NEEDS INTO APPROPRIATE LONG-TERM CARE SERVICES AND SETTINGS

Once the information described previously has been gathered, the physician and other health professionals must work with the patient, family members, and any relevant agency personnel to develop a plan of care that is appropriate for the identified needs of the patient. This plan should identify the specific types of services required and the options for settings in which these services may be appropriately provided.

Development of such a plan of care usually requires the expert knowledge and participation of others on the health care team—that is, a community health or visiting nurse, a social worker, and often others as well, such as an occupational or physical therapist. In other words, a true team effort, involving the patient and family as well as professionals, is usually necessary to establish a sound care plan. Although members of such a team may be dis-

persed in various community agencies, the goals of formulating a care plan can be accomplished through consulting relationships.

It should be kept in mind that the entire process of assessment and decision making about long-term care is in itself a stressful experience for the frail older person. A trusted personal advocate who is a source of personal support should always accompany and help sustain the older person through this process. This person can be a family member, a close friend, or a representative of a social agency.[31]

It is useful to organize one's thinking about this translation of identified needs into service plans around some form of decision sequence.[32] The following series of questions may serve the same purpose. These questions, which are based on assessment data, should be considered in developing long-term care plans:

1. Does this person need further specialized diagnostic work-up or intensive rehabilitation treatment before a long-term care plan can be developed?

   If so, such steps should be taken first on an outpatient or inpatient basis.

2. Is this person physically and mentally capable of managing independently all activities of daily living and instrumental activities of daily living?

   If so, no special long-term care plans or living arrangements are needed. However, the person should undergo appropriate periodic checkups for chronic conditions, and arrangements should be made to ensure that he or she is in regular contact with a supportive network.

3. Can this person manage all personal and instrumental activities of daily living within his or her home? That is, does he or she simply need assistance in traveling to and from necessary or desirable activities outside the home, such as shopping, visits to physicians, or social and religious activities?

   If so, assistance with transportation or provision of shopping services should suffice. However, such a person is at high risk for social isolation, and positive attention should be paid to maintaining or adding social activities, including day programs.

4. Can this person prepare regular and adequate meals and perform other household chores (e.g., cleaning, laundry) by himself or herself, or are these functions performed by a spouse or other

housemate?

If not, these housekeeping functions must be provided by nearby family members, meals-on-wheels or housekeeper services, or staff members of a domiciliary facility in which the person may live.

5. Can this person maintain adequate personal hygiene (e.g., bathe himself or herself) and dress and undress adequately?

   If not, some help or supervision is needed, probably twice daily, from a family member, home health aide, or similar staff member of a congregate living institution, such as those in an assisted living or intermediate care facility.

6. Can this person ambulate independently, with or without mechanical assistive devices such as canes or walkers, and manage any necessary stairs in his or her dwelling?

   If not, can the person transfer to and operate a wheelchair without assistance? Any limitation in locomotion or transfer may require a different living environment (e.g., a one-floor dwelling or a congregate living facility) or personal assistance several times daily by a family member or health aide for toileting, coming to meals, and so forth.

7. Is this person sufficiently oriented and mentally and emotionally competent to manage being alone all day or for hours at a time?

   If not, constant or almost constant supervision by a family member, companion, or health aide is necessary in the home; alternatively, residence in a facility that has a restricted environment or a constantly supervising staff may be needed. Regular attendance in a highly supportive day center may help meet this need as well as adding variety and social involvement to the person's life.

8. Is this person usually continent of urine and feces?

   If not, thorough evaluation and an effort to treat any identifiable causes are indicated. If these are not successful, frequent daily personal care by family members or personal care aides in the home or an institution is necessary.

9. Can this person feed himself?

   If not, assistance with eating at every meal by family or personal care aides at home or in an institution is necessary.

10. Does this person have some disability that requires regular nursing or rehabilitative therapy, such as care of pressure ulcers, ostomy care, respiratory treatment, or physical or occupational therapy?

    If so, this care must be provided by visiting home health care services or in an institution staffed to provide these services.

THE NEED FOR CONTINUING REVIEW OF ASSESSMENT FINDINGS

This chapter has focused on the importance of developing an approach to functional assessment as an essential part of making an initial decision about long-term care. The findings must be incorporated into the ongoing care activities of the primary physician, the other professionals involved in the care of the patient, and family members, and must be reviewed regularly because further changes in the functional status of the patient are likely.

References

1. Rubenstein LZ: Geriatric assessment: An overview of its impacts. Clin Geriatr Med 1987;3:1–15.
2. Rubenstein LZ: An overview of comprehensive geriatric asessment. *In* Rubenstein LZ, Wieland D, Bernabei R (eds): Geriatric Assessment Technology: The State of the Art. Milan, Editrice Kurtis, 1995, pp. 1–9.
3. National Institutes of Health, Consensus Development Conference Series: Geriatric Assessment Methods for Clinical Decision Making, vol. 6. National Institutes of Health, October 19–27, 1987, p. 13.
4. Solomon DH: Geriatric assessment: Methods for clinical decision making. JAMA 1988;259:2450–2452.
5. Stuck AE, Siu AL, Wieland GD, et al: Effects of comprehensive geriatric assessment on survival, residence, and function: A meta-analysis of controlled trials. Lancet 1993;342:1032–1036.
6. Stuck AE, Wieland D, Rubenstein LZ, et al: Comprehensive geriatric assessment: Meta-analysis of main effects and elements enhancing effectiveness. *In* Rubenstein LZ, Wieland D, Bernabei R (eds): Geriatric Assessment Technology: The State of the Art. Milan, Editrice Kurtis, 1995, pp. 11–26.
7. Brocklehurst JC, Williams TF (eds): Multidisciplinary health assessment of the elderly. Dan Med Bull 1989;7.
8. Wieland GD: Geriatric assessment: A review and guide to the literature. *In* Brocklehurst JC, Williams TF (eds): Multidisciplinary health assessment of the elderly. Dan Med Bull 1989;7:7–23.
9. Kane RL: The role of geriatric assessment in different countries. *In* Rubenstein LZ, Wieland D, Bernabei R (eds): Geriatric Assessment Technology: The State of the Art. Milan, Editrice Kurtis, 1995, pp. 297–304.
10. Guralnick JM, LaCroix AZ, Everett DF, et al: Aging in the eighties: The prevalence of co-morbidity and its association with disability. National Center for Health Statistics, Advance Data, Number 170, 1989, p. 3.

11. Applegate WB: The medical evaluation. *In* Rubenstein LZ, Wieland D, Bernabei R (eds): Geriatric Assessment Technology: The State of the Art. Milan, Editrice Kurtis, 1995, pp. 41–50.

12. Applegate WB, Blass JP, Williams TF: Instruments for the functional assessment of older patients. N Engl J Med 1990;322:1207–1214.

13. Hedrick SO: Comprehensive geriatric assessment: Assessment techniques. *In* Rubenstein LZ, Wieland D, Bernabei R (eds): Geriatric Assessment Technology: The State of the Art. Milan, Editrice Kurtis, 1995, pp. 27–39.

14. Katz S, Ford AB, Moskowitz RW, et al: Studies of illness in the aged. The index of ADL: A standardized measure of biological and psychosocial function. JAMA 1963;185:94.

15. Lawton MP, Brody E: Assessment of older people: Self-maintaining and instrumental activities of daily living. Gerontologist 1969;9:179–186.

16. Lawton MP: Assessing the competence of older people. *In* Kent D, Kastenbaum R, Sherwood J (eds): Research, Planning and Action for the Elderly. New York, Behavioral Publications, 1972.

17. Hedrick SO: Assessment of functional status: Activities of daily living. *In* Rubenstein LZ, Wieland D, Bernabei R (eds): Geriatric Assessment Technology: The State of the Art. Milan, Editrice Kurtis, 1995, pp. 51–58.

18. Lachs MS, Feinstein AR, Coohey LM Jr, et al: A simple procedure for general screening for functional disability in elderly patients. Ann Intern Med 1990;112:699–706.

19. Gurland BJ, Côté LJ, Cross PS, et al: The assessment of cognitive function in the elderly. Clin Geriatr Med 1987;3:53–63.

20. Gurland BJ, Wilder D: Detection and assessment of cognitive impairment and depressed mood in primary care of older adults: A systems approach to the uses of brief scales. *In* Rubenstein LZ, Wieland D, Bernabei R

(eds): Geriatric Assessment Technology: The State of the Art. Milan, Editrice Kurtis, 1995, pp. 111–134.

21. Gallagher D: Assessing affect in the elderly. Clin Geriatr Med 1987;3:65–85.

22. Kane RA: Assessing social function in the elderly. Clin Geriatr Med 1987;3:87–98.

23. Kane RA: Assessment of social functioning: Recommendations for comprehensive geriatric assessment. *In* Rubenstein LZ, Wieland D, Bernabei R (eds): Geriatric Assessment Technology: The State of the Art. Milan, Editrice Kurtis, 1995, pp. 91–110.

24. Steel K, Musliner M, Berg K: Assessment of the home environment. *In* Rubenstein LZ, Wieland D, Bernabei R (eds): Geriatric Assessment Technology: The State of the Art. Milan, Editrice Kurtis, 1995, pp. 135–145.

25. Lawton MP, Moss M, Fulcomer M, et al: A research and service oriented multi-level assessment instrument. J Gerontol 1982;37:91–99.

26. Duke University Center for the Study of Aging and Human Development: Multi-dimensional functional assessment. The OARS Methodology. Durham, NC, Duke University, 1978.

27. Gurland BJ, Kuriansky J, Sharpe L, et al: The comprehensive assessment and referral evaluation (CARE)—Rationale, development and reliability. Part II. A factor analysis. Int J Aging Hum Dev 1977;8:9–42.

28. Institute of Medicine, Committee on Regulation of Nursing Homes: Improving the Quality of Care in Nursing Homes. Washington, DC, National Academy Press, 1986.

29. Morris JN, Hawes C, Fries BE, et al: Designing the national resident assessment instrument for nursing homes. Gerontologist 1990;30:293–307.

30. Kane RL: Standardized assessment as a means rather than an end. Gerontologist 1990;30:291–292.

31. Silverstone B, Furack-Weiss A: The social work function in nursing homes and home care. J Gerontol Soc Work 1982;5:7.

32. Williams ME, Williams TF: Assessment of the elderly for long term care. J Am Geriatr Soc 1982; 30: 71–77.

3 Social Support

Jurgis Karuza, Ph.D.

The purpose of this chapter is to discuss the importance of social support in the lives of older adults and its relevance to the delivery of geriatric care. First, a brief literature review documents the nature of social relationships in later life. Second, the link between social support and the well-being of older adults is explored. Third, the informal caregiving network is examined, highlighting the impact of caregiving on the caregiver. Finally, the significance of social support and family issues in the assessment and delivery of clinical care is considered.

DEMOGRAPHY OF SOCIAL RELATIONSHIPS

Several reviews document the current and projected future demographic landscape.[1-5] Salient changes in marital and childrearing patterns, longevity, and women's labor force participation are expected to contribute to a more diverse pattern of family and social relationships among older adults. Currently, 77% of older adult men and 41% of older adult women are married. Older women are more likely to be widowed than men, and the prevalence of widowhood increases with age. Thirty-four percent of women and 7% of men aged 65 to 69 are widowed, whereas 82% of women and 43% of men aged 85 and above are widowed. Slightly over 3% of older adults are divorced; however, in view of the current divorce rate, the number of divorced older adults is expected to increase in the future. Remarriage rates have been pegged at 2% for older adult women and 20% for older adult men.[2] About 5% of older adults have never married. Over 80% of older adults have living siblings, but the number of surviving siblings decreases with age.[4]

Because of the sharp increases in fertility following World War II, the number of childless older adults will drop during the next few years. However, because of reduced fertility, high rates of divorce, and low rates of remarriage, the availability of spouses or children to provide care for the aging "baby boomers" will decline precipitously later in the twenty-first century.[5] Several demographers comment that the future family structure will resemble a "bean pole" as the number of living generations increases and the number of individuals within each family generation decreases owing to lower fertility rates.[1] This pattern has implications for the structure of future family relationships, with family members having more vertical relationships across generations and fewer horizontal relationships with same-aged siblings and extended kin. Given the trends in life expectancy, a significant overlap in the life spans of great grandparents, grandparents, parents, and children will result. Four- and five-generational families will be more common. Already, the number of adult years a woman spends with one or both of her parents over age 65 has increased to 18 years. Increasingly, older adults will be more likely to have a surviving older parent.

The prevailing trend is toward intergenerational solidarity and contact among older adults and their children. Intergenerational relationships can best be described as "intimacy at a distance." Older adults typically live apart from their children, either with a spouse or alone. But over 80% of older adults report regular weekly face-to-face or telephone contact with their children.[1] Daughters, compared to sons, tend to have more frequent contact with their parents. Widowed parents have higher rates of contact with their children than married parents. Social class and ethnic differences in the extent of contact have been found, lower classes and families from Hispanic backgrounds having the highest levels of interaction.[1, 3]

The norm of filial responsibility remains strong, and 80% of frail older adults' care needs are provided by the family.[6] It is not correct to assume that all older adults are dependent recipients of assistance within their families. Among well elderly, a pattern of reciprocity describes the patterns of intergenerational social exchange, in which older adults give as well as receive help. An important psychosocial byproduct of this pattern is the improved self-concept, sense of autonomy, and sense of well-being that is found among older adults who engage in altruistic behavior.[7]

Another major trend has been the changing role of grandparents. Currently, 3.3 million children live with grandparents, a figure that reflects a 44% increase since 1980. In 1991, 12.3% of African-American children, 5.6% of children of Hispanic ancestry, and 3.7% of white children lived in their grandparents' home, a prevalence that reflects increases of 24%, 40%, and 54%, respectively.[8] This increase has been a response to the instabilities of contemporary family life that are created by divorce, unemployment, and drug and alcohol abuse.[9] Initial studies indicate that parenting grandparents may face a series of problems including stress-related illnesses, social isolation, and economic problems.[10] But the grandchildren may be at no greater risk for health and school adjustment problems.[11] Often, because they lack legal custody or guardianship, parenting grandparents experience difficulty in obtaining financial, medical, or educational services for their grandchildren.[12] Custodial grandparents may struggle with ambivalent feelings. On the one hand, they may desire to keep the nuclear family together, but they fear that the child may not be cared for by the parent and dread the loss of the newly formed attachment to the grandchild.[9]

As older adults' social networks become smaller owing to the death or relocation of friends and relatives, their families increasingly become important elements in their social support system.[13] A major social policy question looming for the twenty-first century is the effect of a smaller family size and an increased number of single heads of household on the social support network, quality of life, and health care utilization of older adults. Family relations involving older adults should be seen as dynamic and interactive, reflecting changes in the individual, the family life cycle, and larger demographic and societal trends. Monitoring these trends becomes even more important in light of the powerful relationship between well-being and the adequacy of the social support network.

SOCIAL SUPPORT

In a general sense, social support is defined as resources provided by others. Several reviewers have noted a strong association between social relationships and health.[14, 15] Attenuated social support has been found to be consistently related to a variety of negative outcomes including higher mortality rates, depression, physical illness, poorer recovery from surgery, stress, and impaired immunologic functioning.[5, 16–18] The importance of the older adult's social support network is further underscored by the evidence that family supports are related to reduced health resource use by and delayed institutionalization of frail older adults.[19]

Social support, along with retention of a sense of personal autonomy and control, is mentioned specifically as one of the key ingredients in successful aging.[20] Preliminary results from the MacArthur Studies on Successful Aging showed, for example, that maintenance of better physical performance in older adults was influenced by the amount of emotional support available.[21]

Current conceptualizations of social support underscore the importance of distinguishing among its *functional content* (i.e., focusing on emotional concerns or provision of instrumental aid),[14, 15] its *structure* (e.g., who provides social support), the *density* of the social support network, and its *quantity*.

Several researchers have outlined the manifold active ingredients in social support relationships including *emotional support*, such as expressing feelings of liking, trust, esteem, or concern or providing opportunities for venting or openly expressing feelings; *appraisal support*, such as affirming the values and beliefs of others and providing opportunities for social comparison; *informational support*, such as providing relevant advice or information; and *instrumental support*, such as offering aid in kind, labor, money, and so on.[15]

The person who provides the social support appears to moderate its impact in complex ways. Emotional support from spouses seems to be especially important in recovery from surgery[17] and depression in chronically ill women. In fact, Mutran and colleagues[17] found that depression in older adult women following hip replacement surgery was associated with a child (not a husband) assuming the role of confidant. Among widows, higher morale was associated with support received from friends, neighbors, and siblings rather than from children. Presumably this is true because of the difficulties associated with being in a position of growing dependency on one's children.[1]

Research indicates that the association between the size of a person's social support network and health outcomes is not a simple linear one. Those who are isolated and have relatively few or no social relationships are especially at risk for mortality. But above a threshold level, increases in the number of social relationships seem to produce diminishing returns in regard to improved health.[14]

Subjective perceptions of the adequacy and satisfaction with social support influence the effectiveness of the social support.[13, 17, 22] Social support relationships can have a negative side if significant others become critical and de-manding. These negative interactions may be more likely among more intimate family members than among friends.[22]

Significant others must be careful in *how* and *when* they provide support. Help given to an older adult may send an undercutting message of dependency rather than conveying the sense that the older adult is valued and respected.[23] This message of dependency is amplified when the older adult does not have a choice in what help to get, when to get it, or when to stop getting it.

To maximize the positive impact of social support strategically, it may be as important to minimize any negative interactions among family and friends of older adults as it is to encourage the amount and frequency of supportive behaviors. Encouraging reciprocity of help within families, respecting the older adult's sense of personal control and autonomy, and promoting a sense of volunteerism among older adults may be effective strategies to minimize the risks associated with poor social support.[7, 13]

A considerable variety of social support measures are used in research.[15] Given that a lack of social support is a risk factor for the well-being of older adults, clinicians may find it valuable to include questions about the extent and quality of older adults' social support relationships in the clinical assessment of their patients.

FAMILY AND THE CAREGIVING ROLE

Eighty percent of the caregiving assistance given to the 1.3 million frail older adults in the United States comes from families. Of the 2.2 million family members who provide care, most (two thirds) are women.[24] One third of the women caregivers are employed. The typical caregiving workload is 4 to 8 hours per day. The length of time spent in the caregiving role usually is 1 to 4 years, but a substantial number of families (20%) provide care for more than 4 years.[25] The annual cost of caregiving provided by families with demented relatives has been estimated at $18,256, with 29% of costs paid in cash and 71% in unpaid labor.[26]

Trends toward minimizing hospital stays have resulted in discharge of older adults with more complex medical problems and more complicated care needs.[27] This result only intensifies and complicates the caregiving demands in families.

In general, families are not quick to institutionalize their older adult relative. Lack of a social support network remains a major risk fac-tor for institutionalization. Within families, behavioral problems and incontinence are salient factors that predict the decision to institutionalize an older adult relative (see Chapter 29).

Caregivers and the caregiving context are marked by diversity, and no single generic caregiver role can be defined. The process of dividing caregiving responsibilities within a family is best understood as a product of mutual negotiation among family members. However, the literature points to several demographic and geographic factors that may make a family member more likely to assume the caregiving role.

Typically, in the United States, the primary caregiving responsibility falls on women: wives, daughters, and daughters-in-law.[28] Depending on availability, a caregiving "line of succession" is often followed in families; spouses are most likely to assume the caregiver role, followed by children and then other relatives and friends or neighbors.[28] Among children, the oldest child or only daughter is most likely to assume the principal caregiving role.[29] Interestingly, Matthews[29] found that although in families with only one daughter the siblings made every effort to divide caregiving responsibilities, the lone daughter was perceived to be "in charge" and the caregiving contributions of the brothers tended to be discounted by all the siblings. Those who live closer to the older adult care recipient are also more likely to assume the caregiving role.

Gender differences in the quality of caregiving have been noted. Men are less likely to help with household tasks and personal care tasks such as bathing or dressing and are more likely to enlist the assistance of other helpers while women are more likely to be solo caregivers.[30] Consequently, there is a potential risk that older women may have more unmet care needs when their primary caregiver is their husband. Men tend to be more comfortable in offering assistance related to administrative and financial issues or providing transportation and running errands.[30] In general, sons are more likely to perform less intense help while daughters are more likely to provide personal care assistance, although the size and gender composition of the sibling network has been found to moderate the caregiving patterns.[29]

With demographic changes, the likelihood that a woman will assume a caregiving role at some point in her life is *increasing* compared to that in previous generations.[31] Also increasing is the probability that multiple caregiving roles will be adopted, with 10% of women's caregiving time involving care for two or more individuals.[32] There is evidence that women from more traditional lifestyles (e.g., those who married earlier or had more children) are more likely to become caregivers, but employment *does not decrease* the likelihood of a woman adopting the caregiver role.[32] Women who are employed seem to provide the same number of hours of care as those who are not in the workforce, but the types of care may shift (i.e., the caregiving burden for food preparation and personal care is more likely to be shared). The increased presence of women in the workforce, coupled with the finding that women do not "trade off" employment roles for caregiving roles, is resulting in more women juggling work and caregiving roles. Recent legislative initiatives such as the Family Leave Act can provide some short-term relief for caregivers who face acute problems but do little to address the long-term burden of caregiving.

Given the central role of the family in providing long-term care in the United States, caregiver burden and its impact on families should be a major concern for clinicians. There is strong evidence that caregiving may be associated with a variety of negative *psychological* effects for caregivers, including increased depression and anxiety.[33] Major risk factors for negative psychological effects include family income level, caregiver's perceived quality of life, including things such as self-rated health, perceived stress, and satisfaction with life, and a pattern of behavioral problems in the care recipient.[33]

Far less clear is the unique impact of caregiving on the *physical* health of the caregiver; studies have shown a weak, mixed, or absent relationship between caregiving and measures of physical morbidity such as symptomatology, health care utilization, and self-reports of health.[33] Although many characteristics of the care recipient, such as age and gender, do not seem to be related consistently to health outcomes, demented care recipients' behavior problems do appear to be a source of distress to caregivers. This is especially noteworthy because disruptive care recipient behavior has been linked to an increased likelihood of institutionalization.

In response to the burdens of caregiving, a variety of interventions such as family respite, caregiver support groups, and individual counseling have been developed.[34] Despite a disappointing mixed pattern of success, limits in the research methods make it difficult to draw definitive conclusions about the efficacy of these interventions.[35] Educational interventions that teach problem-solving or stress management skills appear to show promise.[36]

Considerable attention has been paid to the interplay between informal family-based caregiving and help received from formal community-based organizations. A major concern is whether formal community-based care "substitutes" for or "supplements" the family care given to older adults. Evidence is mixed, with some research suggesting that racial differences exist. Among African-Americans, families receiving formal services did not decrease the amount of informal supports they provided.[37] Some research has found that use of formal health care services offsets the negative effects of caregiving for caregivers of impaired older adults.[38]

FAMILY CAREGIVERS AND MEDICAL CARE

In recognition of the major role played by families in the health care of older adults and the burdens of caregiving, there have been calls for the development of more effective physician-caregiver relationships that consider the caregiver and patient as a single unit.[39, 40] Building on a biopsychosocial model, this approach enlists the family as a partner with the physician in the care of the patient. Families are recognized as important resources that can help the physician with health promotion, assessment, and care management. By specifically focusing on the patient-caregiver unit, the physician is better able to make care decisions, taking into account the unique pattern of interdependencies within the family, the available caregiver resources, and the level of caregiving stress and burden. At the same time, the physician is able to address the needs of the "hidden patient," the caregiver. The physician is in a unique position to support the caregiver and provide help for the psychosocial and health problems created by the caregiving burden.

Although the model holds much potential, the few studies that have been done in this area indicate that a minority of caregivers receive help from physicians on psychosocial problems or are involved in the clinical decision-making process.[39] Major barriers to development of a caregiver-physician partnership include the resistance of caregivers, patients, and physicians to acceptance of a more egalitarian approach to the physician-patient interaction, and inadequate communication between physicians and family members.[39] It is important to realize that many family members, although "quick studies," do not have the specific skills or information necessary to be maximally effective as caregivers. Physicians should recognize their own potential as role models who can teach family members skills through the behavior they model, such as participating in a "team approach" to care.

To promote the caregiver-patient-physician

partnership model the following components of practice are encouraged:[40]

- Formation of a patient-caregiver unit.
- Comprehensive home-based approach, including home visits.
- Caregiver and patient reassessment (e.g., charting changes in physical function, functional health, and quality of life).
- Provision of training to caregivers either directly or through referrals to help families cope with the caregiving situation. This training includes diagnostic monitoring, behavior management, case management, and self-care behaviors.
- Offers of specific help for controlling or managing patient behavior problems.
- Validation of the caregiving role.
- Acting as a case manager.

Finally, three important areas of concern are highlighted that may be relevant to the caregiver-physician partnership model.

Alcohol Abuse

The prevalence of alcoholism or problem drinking in persons aged 60 and older has been estimated as 2% to 10% (see Chapter 30). The Council of Scientific Affairs of the American Medical Association (AMA) states that "attitudes toward alcoholism and the elderly on the part of the patient, the physician and the family can be formidable obstacles to the identification, diagnosis and treatment."[41] Given the structure and focus of the bulk of the programs aimed at alcohol prevention and treatment, it is not surprising that older adults frequently "fall through the cracks." The physician is one of the few people who can recognize the early warning signs in older patients and can intervene early in those with late-onset alcoholism. Treatment recommendations stress the importance of involving the older adult's family and friends. The prognosis is by no means hopeless, and evidence suggests that both late-onset and lifelong older adult alcoholics respond well to treatment.

Elder Abuse

In a large-scale random sample survey the prevalence of physical violence, verbal aggression, and neglect was estimated as 32 older adults per 1000.[42] Underreporting of this form of abuse is a problem in that only 1 in 14 cases is estimated to reach public attention. Abuse victims are equally likely to be male or female, and spouses are the most likely abusers. Barriers to identification of elder abuse in the physician's office include lack

of awareness by physician of regulations, lack of training in identifying signs of abuse, and inadequate information from the older adult and the family. Mandatory abuse reporting requirements for professionals differ from state to state. To assist with identification of elder abuse, the AMA has issued a set of guidelines, which are summarized in Table 3–1.[43]

As with other cases of domestic abuse, both the abused older adult and the abusive family member need treatment. It is often the case that neglect of older adults may be unintentional; the caregiver may not know how to give proper care or may be ill or depressed.

Advance Medical Directives

Although living wills and medical proxies are becoming more familiar to the lay public, a major

TABLE 3–1 **GUIDELINES FOR ELDER ABUSE**

Type of Abuse	Indicator
Physical abuse	Punching, hitting, pinching
	Force feeding
	Improper use of restraints
	Improper use of medication
Physical neglect	Failure to provide necessities (e.g., food, drink, eyeglasses, hearing aid)
Psychological abuse	Causing mental anguish through berating, intimidating, or threats of punishment or isolation
Psychological neglect	Failure to provide social stimulation
	Prolonged isolation
	Ignoring or giving silent treatment
Financial or material abuse	Stealing money or possessions
	Coercing signature on contracts
Financial or material neglect	Failure to use available funds and resources to sustain health and well-being
Violating personal rights	Denying right to privacy
	Denying right to make own personal and health decisions
	Forcible eviction or forcible placement in nursing home

Adapted from American Medical Association: Diagnosis and Treatment Guidelines on Elder Abuse and Neglect. Chicago, American Medical Association, 1992.

problem is the failure of the physician to engage caregivers and their older adult relatives in a discussion of end-of-life treatment options and wishes (see Chapter 4 for a discussion of legal-ethical issues). One complication is the frequently found incongruence between a surrogate's judgments and the older adult's expressed preferences.[44] One solution is to ask surrogates specifically to make a substituted judgment rather than to "make their best recommendation." Additional evidence suggests that surrogates are not very accurate in interpreting or expressing the patient's satisfaction with care or the quality of life.[45, 46] Finally, there may be important ethnic differences in the acceptance of advance directives and the choice of health care wishes.[47] These concerns make it even more important for the physician to facilitate a dialogue among family members on end-of-life issues early, before loss of function and medical crises complicate the discussions.

SUMMARY

In summary, social relationships and social supports of older adults are pivotal in the maintenance of older adults' well-being and health. At the very least, physicians must be sensitive to social support issues in geriatric assessment and in developing care plans. Further, the physician should not lose sight of the fact that she or he is in a unique position to strengthen the older adults' social support network and thereby enhance the function, health, and quality of life of older adults and their families.

References

1. Bengston V, Rosenthal C, Burton L: Families and aging: Diversity and heterogeneity. *In* Birren J, Schaie KW (eds): Handbook of the Psychology of Aging. Orlando, FL, Academic Press, 1990, pp. 263–287.
2. Glick P: Fifty years of family demography: A record of social change. J Marriage Family 1988; 50:861.
3. Lopata HZ: Current Widowhood: Myths and Realities. Thousand Oaks, CA, Sage, 1996.
4. Hays J: Aging and family resources: Availability and proximity of kin. Gerontologist 1984; 24:149.
5. Freedman VA: Family structure and the risk of nursing home admission. J Gerontol 1996; 51B: S61.
6. Brody E: Women in the middle and family help to older people. Gerontologist 1981; 21:327.
7. Midlarsky E: The generous elderly: Naturalistic studies of donations across the life span. Psychol Aging 1991; 4:346.
8. Saluter AF: Marital Status and Living Arrangements: March 1991. Current Population Reports, Population Characteristics. Series P-20, No. 467. Washington, DC, U.S. Government Printing Office, 1991.
9. Jendrek MP: Grandparents who parent their grandchildren: Circumstances and decisions. Gerontologist 1994; 34:206.
10. Minkler M, Roe KM: Grandparents as surrogate parents. Generations 1996; 20:34.
11. Solomon JC, Marx J: To grandmothers house we go: Health and school adjustment of children raised solely by grandparents. Gerontologist 1995; 35:386.
12. Karp N: Legal problems of grandparents and other kinship caregivers. Generations 1996; 20:57.
13. Krause N: Negative interaction and satisfaction with social support among older adults. J Gerontol 1995; 50B:P59.
14. House JS, Landis KR, Umberson D: Social relationships and health. Science 1988; 241:540.
15. House JS, Kahn RL: Measures and concepts of social support. In Cohen S, Syme SL (eds): Social Support and Health. Orlando, FL, Academic Press, 1985, pp. 83–108.
16. Blazer DG: Social support and mortality in an elderly community population. Am J Epidemiol 1982; 115:684.
17. Mutran EJ, Reitzes DC, Mossey J, Fernandez ME: Social support, depression and recovery of walking ability following hip fracture surgery. J Gerontol 1995; 50B:S354.
18. Magaziner J, Simonsick EM, Kashner M, Hebel JR, Kenzora JE: Predictors of functional recovery following hospital discharge for hip fracture: A prospective study. J Gerontol 1990; 45:M101.
19. Penning MJ: Health social support and the utilization of health services among older adults. J Gerontol 1995; 50B:S330.
20. Rowe J, Kahn RL: Human aging: Usual and successful. Science 1987; 237:143.
21. Seeman TE, Berkman LF, Charpentier PA, Blazer DG, Albert MS, Tinetti ME: Behavioral and psychosocial predictors of physical performance: MacArthur Studies of Successful Aging. J Gerontol 1995; 50A:M177.
22. Rook KS: Stressful aspect of older adults' social relationships: Current theory and research. In Stephens MAP, Crowther JH, Hobfoll SE, Tennenbaum DL (eds): Stress and Coping in Later Life Families. New York, Hemisphere, 1990, pp. 173–192.
23. Brickman P, Rabinowitz VC, Karuza J, Coates D, Cohn E, Kidder L: Models of helping and coping. Am Psychol 1982; 37:368.
24. Finely NJ: Theories of family labor as applied to gender differences in caregiving for elderly persons. J Marriage Family 1989; 51:79.
25. Stone R, Cafferata GL, Sangl R: Caregivers of the frail elderly: A national profile. Gerontologist 1987; 27: 616.
26. Stommel M, Collins C, Given B: The cost of family contributions to the care of persons with dementia. Gerontologist 1994; 34:199.
27. Shaughnessy PW, Kramer AM: The increased needs of patients in nursing homes and patients receiving home care. N Engl J Med 1990; 322:21.
28. Stoller EP: Parental caregiving by adult children. J Marriage Family 1983; 45:851.
29. Matthews SH: Gender and division of filial responsibility between lone sisters and their brothers. J Gerontol 1995; 50B:S312.
30. Allen SM: Gender differences in spousal caregiving and unmet need for care. J Gerontol 1994; 49:S187.
31. Moen P, Robison J, Fiels V: Women's work and caregiving roles: A life course approach. J Gerontol 1994; 49:S176.
32. Robison J, Moen P, Dempster-McClain D: Women's caregiving: Changing profiles and pathways. J Gerontol 1995; 50B:S362.
33. Schulz R, O'Brien AT, Bookwala J, Fleissner K: Psychiatric and physical morbidity effects of dementia

caregiving: Prevalence, correlates and causes. Gerontologist 1995; 35:771.

34. Toseland RW, Rossiter CM: Group interventions to support family caregivers: A review and analysis. Gerontologist 1989; 29:438.

35. Knight BG, Lutzky SM, Macofsky-Urban F: A meta-analytic review of interventions for caregiver distress: Recommendations for future research. Gerontologist 1993; 33:240.

36. Lovett S, Gallagher D: Psychoeducational interventions for family caregivers: Preliminary efficacy data. Behav Ther 1988; 19:321.

37. Miner S: Racial differences in family support and formal service utilization among older persons: A nonrecursive model. J Gerontol 1995; 50B:S143.

38. Bass DM, Noelker LS, Rechlin LR: The moderating influence of service use on negative caregiving consequences. J Gerontol 1996; 51B:S121.

39. Haug M: Elderly patients, caregivers, and physicians: Theory and research on health care triads. J Health Soc Behav 1994; 35:1.

40. Council on Scientific Affairs: Physicians and family caregivers: A model for partnership. JAMA 1993; 269:1282.

41. Council of Scientific Affairs: Alcohol in the elderly. JAMA 1996; 275:797.

42. Pillemer K, Finkelhor D: The prevalence of elder abuse: A random survey. Gerontologist 1988; 28:51.

43. American Medical Association: Diagnosis and treatment guidelines on elder abuse and neglect. Chicago, American Medical Association, 1992.

44. Tomlinson T, Howe K, Notman M, Rossmiller D: An empirical study of proxy consent for elderly persons. Gerontologist 1990; 30:54.

45. Epstein AM, Hall JA, Tognetti MA, Son LH, Conant L: Using proxies to evaluate quality of life: Can they provide valid information about patients' health status and satisfaction with medical care? Med Care 1989; 27:S91.

46. Lavizzo-Mourey R, Zinn J, Taylor L: Ability of surrogates to represent satisfaction of nursing home residents with quality of care. J Am Geriatr Soc 1992; 40:39.

47. Eleazer P, Hornung C, Egbert C, Egbert J, Eng C, Hedgepeth J, McCann R, Strothers H, Sapir M, Wei M, Wilson M: The relationship between ethnicity and advance directives in a frail older population. J Am Geriatr Soc 1996; 44:938.

4 Ethical and Legal Issues

Marshall B. Kapp, J.D., M.P.H.

The ethical and legal relationship between a physician and a patient may be characterized in several ways. Establishment of this relationship imposes a variety of obligations on the physician.

First, the physician-patient relationship is a binding contract in which each party has made explicit or implicit promises to each other (e.g., "I will be your physician if you will be my patient"). These promises, both those that have been put into written or spoken words and those that are reasonably understood and relied on by the parties, are supported ethically by the principle of fidelity and also are legally enforceable. Thus, for instance, a physician who has explicitly or impliedly promised to maintain certain patient information as confidential and then reveals that information without proper justification to a third party may be held liable for breach of promise. Even when an older patient is brought to a physician for care by a guardian, legally appointed agent, or other substitute decision-maker (e.g., an adult child), the physician owes contractual responsibilities to the patient; the patient in that situation is considered a "third-party beneficiary" of the contract formed between the physician and the person acting as the patient's representative.

The physician-patient relationship is also fiduciary in nature. A fiduciary or trust relationship is one in which the more powerful partner (such as the knowledgeable and skilled physician) has an obligation to act in the best interests of the less powerful, more dependent partner (such as the sick older patient who needs the physician's services). When fiduciary obligations are violated (e.g., substandard medical care is rendered), a civil wrong called a tort occurs, for which money damages may be awarded by a court.

With the exception of the emergency department context, in which there is an obligation to accept all who appear, the physician-patient relationship is one that is formed voluntarily by the parties. The physician in private practice may legally accept or reject his or her own patients, although strong financial incentives today may impinge on that choice. Even for physicians who work for or are associated with government or private organizations that are obligated to accept particular patients (e.g., Veterans Affairs facilities, health maintenance organizations [HMOs]), the physician-patient relationship is still considered voluntary, because the organization has chosen to obligate itself and the physician has chosen to work for or with the organization.

Unless precluded from doing so by a contract he or she has entered into (e.g., as the medical director in a nursing facility),[1] the physician in private practice may terminate a relationship with a patient. No reasons need be cited. However, the physician who wishes for any reason to discontinue caring for a specific patient must be careful to end the physician-patient relationship in a fashion that does not simply abandon the patient and cause harm. That is, a patient cannot simply be left high and dry, in need of medical attention and deprived of a fair opportunity to secure it because the physician, upon whom the patient had been depending, discontinued his or her services without adequate warning. Abandonment can be particularly dangerous for older, vulnerable patients in need of continuity of medical care, and therefore physicians serving such persons must be especially sensitive to the serious medical and associated legal risks of abandonment. Additionally, the ethical principles of beneficence (i.e., doing good) and nonmaleficence (preventing harm) limit the physician's prerogatives in this area.

To terminate a patient's care without risking a claim of abandonment, the physician should take several steps. The physician should notify the patient or proxy, preferably in writing, that he or she will no longer provide services to that patient. If applicable, this notification should instruct the patient that if he or she continues to need medical attention, the patient should actively seek such attention elsewhere. The physician should make a reasonable effort to help the patient obtain competent medical care elsewhere; usually this obligation is sufficiently discharged by directing the patient to local health care referral systems. The physician should offer a reasonable grace period of medical coverage to enable the patient to secure care elsewhere; in some jurisdictions (e.g., California), a minimum grace period is set by statute. In the nursing home context, in which patients have less ability to shop around, it may be wisest to continue one's relationship with a patient until a successor physician has actually undertaken the patient's care. Finally, a terminating physician should cooperate with the patient's subsequent caregivers by providing requested copies of clinical records and other information and generally should not interfere with the continuity of the patient's care.

In matters pertaining to the initiation, fulfillment, and termination of the physician-patient relationship, ethical considerations of social or distributive justice as well as those pertaining to the principles of beneficence and nonmaleficence (noted earlier) must be taken into account. Justice implies a fair or equitable distribution of resources, or, in other words, that persons in need of certain basic services are not unfairly deprived of access to them. Although no single physician can reasonably be expected to remedy broad social failings of inequitable access to health services, physicians in their individual practices ought not act in ways that unnecessarily exacerbate the lack of justice for particular (and particularly vulnerable) patients.

REGULATING THE QUALITY OF CARE

Fundamental principles embodied in all medical ethics codes command physicians to render the best patient care they are capable of. Legally, the standards for quality of care to which physicians are held in delivering care to older patients emanate from a variety of sources. Violation of these standards may expose the physician to civil liability (i.e., financial damages), statutory and administrative sanctions (i.e., professional discipline), organizational discipline (e.g., loss of practice privileges within an institution), reporting of the physician to the National Practitioner Data Bank mandated by the Health Care Quality Improvement Act,[2] or, in extreme cases (e.g., patient abuse), criminal prosecution and punishment.

Malpractice claims represent a civil law remedy available to patients that allows them to recover financial damages from physicians who deviate from accepted professional standards.[3, 4] Substantive malpractice law has evolved mainly through common or judge-made law—that is,

through the precedents accumulated over time of individual court decisions adjudicating disputes between particular parties. Statutes enacted by legislatures, especially on the state level, also help to define the physician's obligations in terms of malpractice.

For a plaintiff to succeed in proving a malpractice complaint, each of four separate elements of that claim must be established by a preponderance of the evidence (i.e., there is more than a 51% likelihood of truth). First, there must be proof that the physician owed the patient a duty of care, a duty that rests on the existence of a physician-patient relationship. The specific standards that delineate that duty of care are determined by testimony from expert witnesses about the way in which competent, prudent physicians belonging to the defendant's medical specialty would have behaved in similar circumstances. A patient's advanced years may substantially influence that determination. Expert testimony on this matter may be supplemented by pertinent government regulations and voluntary standards.

The second element of proof in a malpractice action is that a breach or violation of the applicable standard of care occurred—in other words, the physician was at fault. Negligence is the unintentional but blameworthy deviation from accepted professional standards. The plaintiff must also convince the trier of fact, ordinarily a jury, that he or she was injured, and that the injury was the proximate or direct result of the physician's violation of his or her standard of care.

Older persons are statistically quite underrepresented as medical malpractice plaintiffs.[5] These last two elements of negligence—injury and proximate causation—are particularly steep stumbling blocks for many older persons. An ill, frail elderly person may have great difficulty in proving that he or she has sustained injuries of the sort that the American malpractice system is designed to compensate, principally lost future wages. Similarly, many older potential plaintiffs are unable to establish that their injuries were directly caused by the negligence of the physician rather than by their underlying medical infirmities.

Particularly in the care of older patients, statutory and administrative law may be as great as or even more potent a force in setting quality of care standards than the fear of malpractice claims. State and federal legislatures enact laws called statutes that exert an impact on medical practice (e.g., professional licensure requirements). Through the enactment of statutes, a legislature may delegate to an administrative or regulatory agency, such as a health or social service department, the authority to create and publish laws called rules or regulations. A pertinent example is the detailed federal and state administrative regulations pertaining to physician treatment of patients in nursing homes that participate in the Medicare and Medicaid programs.[6]

It is imperative to understand that administrative rules and regulations and legislatively enacted statutes as well as judicial decisions creating common law principles are *all* forms of "law." Unless and until any of these types of law have been specifically invalidated by the courts for violating the Constitution or on other grounds, they carry the full force of law and must be obeyed. The commonly encountered attempt by physicians to distinguish between "real" law (i.e., a statute) and "only" or "mere" regulations (or case law) is based on a serious misunderstanding of the legal system.[7]

Thus, violation of administrative regulations may expose a physician as well as an involved health care institution to licensure sanctions, fines, or jeopardy regarding continued Medicare or Medicaid participation. As noted earlier, applicable agency rules may be introduced in addition as evidence in a malpractice trial on the issue of the appropriate standard of care under the circumstances.

Voluntary nongovernment guidelines and ethical codes issued by private organizations like the American Medical Association, state medical societies, medical specialty boards, the American Hospital Association, and nursing home trade associations also help to set standards for medical practice. The standards of the Joint Commission on Accreditation of Healthcare Organizations (JCAHO) are especially influential in this category.

During the past decade, the development and dissemination of these voluntary guidelines (also referred to as clinical practice parameters, among other labels) by a variety of different bodies have accelerated, and the guidelines have often become more formal. The practice parameter movement, which has produced a number of diagnostic and therapeutic documents that are especially relevant to geriatric practitioners,[8] has been driven largely by a desire to address simultaneously the problems of medical quality, costs, and exposure to liability.

The precise legal ramifications of the practice parameter movement are not yet settled.[9] However, although voluntary standards are not set by the government, they are very important in the sense that their violation may expose a physician to sanctions by a private organization in which he or she is a member and may jeopardize desirable private certifications for a health care institution.

Further, voluntary standards and ethical codes are often introduced and accepted in malpractice cases as probative evidence of the standard of care according to which a physician or institution has publicly represented that he or she will practice. Thus, guidelines that are private in origin may become legal in their practical enforcement.

An example of physician practice that is governed by tort (malpractice), statutory, and administrative law as well as by voluntary standards is the prescription of therapeutic drugs and devices, an important aspect of geriatric health care. Improper use of drugs for an older patient, including the prescription of a drug, dosage, or route of administration that is inappropriate, failure to take into account the interaction of a prescribed drug with others the patient is taking, failure to inform the patient adequately about the risks, benefits, and reasonable alternatives to the drug, or failure to monitor the patient's reaction to a prescribed drug may lead to a negligence claim. The federal Food, Drug and Cosmetic Act and the Controlled Substances Act and their implementing regulations as well as state drug statutes and regulations closely control which drugs are available for prescription, information that must be available about those drugs, documentation requirements, and mandates for reporting adverse reactions. Parallel laws set requirements for the use of medical devices such as hearing aids, pacemakers, and artificial hips. Private professional organizations also issue guidelines in this area, especially guidelines concerning the prescription, administration, and documentation of pharmaceutical products in health care institutions such as nursing homes.

PATIENT INCAPACITY AND PROXY DECISION MAKING

Ordinarily, the physician is obligated to discuss all relevant information and negotiate treatment plans directly with the patient. Sometimes, however, the patient is not mentally capable of assimilating pertinent information and engaging in a rational, voluntary decision-making process about the proposed and alternative medical interventions. In cases of decisional incapacity, the physician may not dispense with informed consent but instead must deal with someone else who acts as a surrogate or proxy on the patient's behalf. Assessing decisional capacity in older persons may be a complex and difficult task,[10, 11] and no simple mechanical "capacimeter" exists to make it easier.[12] Nonetheless, certain general guidelines for conducting this type of assessment may be helpful.

The best analyses urge that capacity not be

evaluated on the basis of the patient's clinical diagnosis or category nor on the wisdom of the patient's specific choice of treatment. Rather, the focus should be on the patient's functional ability—that is, on the thought processes used in arriving at the "good" or "bad" decision.

In a functional inquiry, among the basic questions to be asked are: (1) Can the person make and communicate (in any understandable form) decisions? (2) Is the person able to offer reasons for the choices made, such that some degree of reflection and consideration are evident? (3) Are the reasons underlying the choices based on logic and on factually accurate premises? For example, an elderly woman who refused to consent to amputation of her gangrenous leg because she denied the existence of any medical problem other than dirt on her leg which could easily be washed off was properly deemed to be decisionally incapacitated. (4) Can the patient comprehend the ramifications (i.e., the likely risks and benefits) of the options presented and the choices expressed, and the fact that these ramifications apply to that patient? (5) Does the individual in fact understand the implications of the choices for him or her?

Capacity needs to be assessed on a decision-specific basis; in other words, an individual may be capable of rationally making some decisions (e.g., whether or not to follow a low salt diet) but not others (e.g., whether or not to undergo bypass surgery). Thus, capacity should not be treated as a global matter for all decisions. Partial capacity is possible. The patient may be capable "enough" to make the particular decision in question.

In addition, capacity may vary for a specific patient according to factors such as time of day, day of the week, physical location, acute and transient medical problems, other persons available to support or coerce the patient's choice, and medication reactions. In many cases, some of these factors may be susceptible to manipulation by the physician so that discussions with the patient about care can take place in the most lucid circumstances possible. When feasible, physicians should attempt to maximize the patient's ability to participate in medical choices before they turn to a surrogate who acts in place of the patient (see following paragraphs).

The older person may use legal mechanisms of advance planning to take steps while still mentally capable to anticipate and prepare for eventual incapacity by voluntarily delegating or directing future medical decision-making authority. The durable power of attorney is a written document in which an individual (the principal) may appoint an agent, or "attorney-in-fact," to make future decisions. Almost every state has enacted statutes that explicitly permit the use of a durable power of attorney to empower the agent to make medical decisions on the patient's behalf should the patient lose decision-making capacity.

Several ethical principles undergird such legislation. Autonomy is the precept that individuals ought to have control over what happens to their own bodies. To exercise autonomy by making decisions, the patient needs information about alternatives and potential outcomes. In the case of mentally incapacitated patients, the patient's autonomy is best served by informing a surrogate (ideally chosen by the patient) of the patient's own views and then expecting that surrogate to make decisions based on the patient's substituted judgment (i.e., what the patient would have chosen if presently able to make and express personal decisions).

Durable powers of attorney fall into two categories. An immediate power comes into effect when the agent is named. In a springing power, the legal authority transfers ("springs") from the patient to the agent only on the occurrence of some named future event, such as verification of the principal's incapacity by a designated number of examining physicians. The patient should be informed when decision-making authority has sprung to the designated agent, so that he or she can utter a protest, if desired, to the agent's power.

The durable power of attorney, which is a proxy directive, is distinguishable from a living will, which is an instruction directive. In the latter, a competent patient documents in a general way his or her wishes regarding future medical treatment rather than naming an agent to make future treatment decisions in the case of incapacity. These two legal devices are not mutually exclusive, and patients may be encouraged to execute them in tandem because the living will can help an agent named under a durable power of attorney to exercise the patient's substituted judgment more accurately.

A variety of models have been suggested for effectuating the competent patient's right to create a living will or other instruction directive regarding future treatment. Some of the proposed devices focus on specific clinical scenarios and medical interventions (e.g., do not resuscitate me if I suffer cardiac arrest when I am permanently and severely demented),[13, 14] whereas others concentrate more on identifying the patient's key values and objectives[15, 16] (e.g., I want to avoid pain and indignity more than I desire to live forever). Ideally, the physician has discussed these issues previously with the patient and helped her or him to draft the instruction directive in the calm and proactive setting of the physician's office or at least at the time of admission to a health care facility; actually most such discussions (to the extent that they occur at all)[17] take place at the bedside after the patient is already critically ill.

To whom can the physician turn if a patient is decisionally incapable but has not previously executed a living will or appointed a health care decision-making agent? About half the states have enacted legislation empowering family members to make medical decisions for incapacitated persons who have not created a durable power of attorney. In states that have family consent statutes, the approved procedure ordinarily consists of documenting unanimous agreement among the attending physician, specified relatives (usually in a stated order of preference), and sometimes consultant physicians as well. The legislative trend in this direction has been fueled by the United States Supreme Court's decision in *Cruzan*[18] holding that the extent and conditions of proxy (including family) medical decision-making authority is a matter of state legislative rather than federal constitutional policy. In a number of states without family consent statutes, courts recognize as a matter of common law or the state's own constitution the family's authority to exercise the incapacitated patient's decision-making rights on his or her own behalf. Most of these cases establish legal precedent for families to act in other, future cases without the need for prior court approval.

In its *Cruzan* decision, the Supreme Court held that a state could constitutionally require surrogate decision makers to prove the incompetent patient's preference for abating treatment by "clear and convincing" evidence to overcome the legal presumption that treatment should proceed. Several states currently appear to hold to this demanding standard of proof. The Supreme Court left unclear precisely what kind of evidence would be necessary to meet the "clear and convincing" test, although almost certainly some written, witnessed documentation of the patient's wishes made while he or she was still mentally capable would be sufficient. What proof short of a living will type of document may be adequate depends on a case-by-case determination, and the outcome may vary among different jurisdictions.

One of several issues the *Cruzan* decision clarified is the legal status of artificial feeding and hydration. The Supreme Court was almost unanimous in finding that artificial feeding and hydration for patients unable to eat by mouth is a form of medical treatment, and that withholding or withdrawing such treatment is acceptable under the same circumstances that govern abatement of other forms of medical treatment such as ventilators, dialysis, cardiopulmonary resuscitation (CPR), and so on. This position is consistent with the weight of ethical opinion, although some controversy on this point persists.

In situations where there is no durable power of attorney, family consent statute, or judicial precedent empowering the family to act, creation of a guardianship or conservatorship may be advisable to transfer decision-making power officially from an incapacitated patient to a proxy. This process entails appointment by a state probate court of a surrogate (the "guardian" or "conservator") who is empowered to make certain decisions on behalf of a decisionally incapable person (the "ward"), ordinarily in response to a petition filed by the family or a caregiver; this appointment is combined with a review by the probate court of the sworn affidavit or live testimony of a physician who is familiar with the patient.

This form of intervention usually is benevolently inspired, as translated into the state's *parens patriae* power to protect the vulnerable. Nonetheless, because creating total ("plenary") guardianship usually involves extensive deprivation of an individual's basic personal and property rights, the "least restrictive alternative" doctrine makes a limited guardianship preferred when feasible.[19] Probate courts possess the authority to limit the proxy's power to decide only particular types of decisions that the ward personally is incapable of handling rationally.

Traditionally, the guardian has been required to make decisions consistent with the guardian's view of the patient's best interests. Many states still hold guardians to the best interests standard. The modern trend in proxy decision making, though, has been toward a substituted judgment standard. Under this approach, the guardian is obligated to make those decisions that the patient would make, according to the patient's own preferences and values to the extent they can be ascertained, if the patient were presently able to make and express competent decisions.

Congressional enactment of the federal Patient Self-Determination Act (PSDA)[20] in the wake of *Cruzan* has influenced medical practice in this area. Hospitals, nursing facilities, hospices, HMOs, preferred provider organizations, and home health agencies that receive Medicare or Medicaid funds are required by this statute to, among other things, adopt and make available to patients or their surrogates an organizational policy on medical decision making, inquire of patients about the existence of advance directives they might have executed previously, and offer currently competent patients a chance to execute an advance directive if they wish. *Cruzan*, the PSDA, and hospital accreditation standards of the JCAHO have encouraged many health care providers, especially hospitals, to put various forms of institutional ethics committees[21] into place to assist in policymaking, case consultation, and education about difficult ethical questions confronting physicians and other members of the geriatric treatment team.

INVOLUNTARY COMMITMENT

Every state has legislation that permits the involuntary (civil) commitment to a mental health facility of persons who are adjudged mentally ill and dangerous to themselves or others. Older persons are sometimes the subject of involuntary commitment proceedings. In most jurisdictions, anyone may file a petition initiating a commitment proceeding. This proceeding is generally conducted in a state probate court, and in it the state bears the burden of proving by at least clear and convincing evidence (a few states require proof beyond a reasonable doubt, as in criminal prosecutions) the mental illness and dangerousness of the person to be committed. The physician's role in the civil commitment process, once it gets to court, is as a provider of evidence, through a sworn affidavit or live testimony, on the issue of the patient's mental condition. The physician may be instrumental beforehand, however, in helping the patient, family, and other caregivers to explore more reasonable alternatives that thus keep the matter out of the probate court system altogether.

INTERACTING WITH THE LEGAL SYSTEM

Older persons frequently have problems that present initially as medical but in fact prove to be multidimensional and require the active involvement and expertise of professionals from various backgrounds. Often the older patient's needs involve a legal component, such as dealing with public benefits programs or financial planning to shelter assets without jeopardizing the patient's Medicaid eligibility or the economic viability of family members. The physician delivering geriatric care must be able to recognize the overt or disguised presentation of problems commanding an attorney's services, to guide the patient, diplomatically but firmly, toward such services, and to interact with attorneys effectively for the benefit of a patient or client who is being served by both the physician and an attorney.[22]

Many older persons are inhibited from seeking legal counsel. This hesitation may be due to fear of a strange and seemingly incomprehensible legal system and its practitioners or a concern, often realistic, about the costs of legal representation. When legal counsel appears advisable, the physician should try to assist the older patient to overcome these barriers.

In addition to the legal services provided by privately practicing attorneys retained directly by older persons or their surrogates, legal services for the elderly are available from a variety of other sources. These sources include pro bono (donated) services by the private bar, legal aid offices funded through government grants and local charitable contributions, and frequently law school clinical programs. Information on reduced or nonfee legal services for the elderly generally may be obtained from one's local bar association, long-term care ombudsman's office, legal aid office, or area agency on aging. Information on private pro bono services is available from the American Bar Association Commission on Legal Problems of the Elderly in Washington, DC.

Physicians caring for older patients are often contacted by attorneys and asked to provide information about a patient to assist in resolving a legal matter—for example, a guardianship petition or a disability claim. Physician involvement with the legal system (which might be characterized as "medicolegal" services) may take the form of informal discussions with the attorney, writing reports, review of medical records, provision of an affidavit, or sworn testimony given at a deposition or trial. The physician should provide confidential information about a specific patient only on satisfactory documentation of the patient's permission for release of the information or the presentation of a court order compelling release of the information. Information should be provided fully, honestly, and objectively; the physician, regardless of which side of a legal dispute has requested his or her medicolegal services, is a provider of information to the court, not a partisan advocate for one party or the other.

The physician usually is entitled to financial compensation for the time spent in providing these medicolegal services, although this right is waived in some circumstances. Although there is no set fee schedule for such services, a fair rule of thumb is that a physician's charge for medicolegal services should be roughly equivalent to the charge levied for spending a comparable amount of time in providing clinical care. In other words, it seems appropriate that the physician neither suffers financially nor secures a windfall by cooperating with and contributing to the resolution of a patient's legal problem.

CONCLUSION

This chapter has briefly outlined the parameters of the relationship of the physician with an older patient and a few of the ethical and legal obligations and issues for the physician that emanate from that relationship. A variety of other subjects arise at the intersection of ethics, law, medicine, and gerontology (e.g., adult protective services, limiting treatment near the end of life, confidentiality) whose explication is precluded here by space limitations. The ethical and legal implications of geriatric practice present physicians with difficult challenges but also with substantial opportunities to serve the broader interdisciplinary needs of those who turn to them for help.

References

1. Fortinsky RH, Raff L: The changing role of physicians in nursing homes. Generations 1995–1996;19:30–35.
2. 45 Code of Federal Regulations §60.1 et seq.
3. Boumil MM, Elias CE: The Law of Medical Liability. St. Paul, West Publishing Company, 1995.
4. McClellan FM: Medical Malpractice: Law, Tactics, and Ethics. Philadelphia. Temple University Press, 1994.
5. U.S. General Accounting Office: Medical Malpractice: Medicare/Medicaid Beneficiaries Account for a Relatively Small Percentage of Malpractice Losses, GAO/HRD-93-126. Washington, DC, U.S. General Accounting Office, 1993.
6. Kapp MB: Limiting medical interventions for nursing home residents: The role of administrative law. Adv Long-Term Care 1991;1:109–123.
7. Meisel A: Barriers to foregoing nutrition and hydration in nursing homes. Am J Law Med 1995;21:335:–382.
8. U.S. Department of Health and Human Services, Agency for Health Care Policy and Research: Pressure Ulcers in Adults: Prediction and Prevention. AHCPR Publication No. 92-0050. Washington, DC, Agency for Health Care Policy and Research, 1992.
9. National Health Lawyers Association: Colloquium Report on Legal Issues Related to Clinical Practice Guidelines. Washington, DC, National Health Lawyers Association, 1995.
10. Kapp MB: Assessment of competence to make medical decisions. *In* Carstensen L, Edelstein B, Dornbrand L (eds): The Practical Handbook of Clinical Gerontology. Thousand Oaks, CA, SAGE Publications, 1996, pp. 174–187.
11. Smyer M, Schaie KW, Kapp MB (eds): Older Adults' Decision-Making and the Law. New York, Springer, 1996.
12. Kapp MB, Mossman D: Measuring decisional capacity: Cautions on the construction of a "capacimeter." Psychol Publ Policy Law 1996;2:73–95.
13. Cantor NL: My annotated living will. Law Med Health Care 1990;18:114–122.
14. Emanuel L, Emanuel E: The medical directive: A new comprehensive advance care document. JAMA 1989;261:3288–3293.
15. Lambert P, Gibson J, Nathanson P: The values history: An innovation in surrogate medical decision-making. Law Med Health Care 1990;18:202–212.
16. Doukas D, Reichel W: Planning for Uncertainty—A Guide to Living Wills and Other Advance Directives for Health Care. Baltimore, Johns Hopkins University Press, 1993.
17. Moskowitz EH, Nelson JL: Dying well in the hospital: The lessons of SUPPORT. Hastings Center Report (special suppl) 1995;25:S1–S36.
18. *Cruzan v. Director, Missouri Department of Health*, 110 S Ct 2841 (1990).
19. Kapp MB: Ethical aspects of guardianship. Clin Geriatr Med 1994;10:501–512.
20. Kapp MB: Patient Self-Determination in Long-Term Care. New York, Springer, 1994.
21. Minogue B: Bioethics—A Committee Approach. Boston, Jones and Bartlett, 1996.
22. Kapp MB: Legal services. *In* Maddox GL (ed): The Encyclopedia of Gerontology, 2nd ed. New York, Springer, 1995, pp. 543–544.

5 Medication Use

Rebecca J. Beyth, M.D.

Ronald I. Shorr, M.D., M.S.

Persons aged 65 and older compose only about 12% of the United States population, yet one third of all drugs are prescribed for them, and they consume more than 50% of over-the-counter medicines as well.[1] Overall, more than 80% of all older people take at least one medication daily. Because an increasing number of patients are surviving to older ages and now account for such a large proportion of drug use, it is necessary for health care providers to understand the risks, benefits, and consequences of drug therapy in older patients. Several important pharmacologic and nonpharmacologic issues influence the safety and effectiveness of drug therapy in this population. This chapter focuses on these issues and attempts to offer practical suggestions to physicians who prescribe drugs for older patients.

CLINICAL PHARMACOLOGY

Pharmacokinetics

Pharmacokinetics, the study of the action of a drug in the body over a period of time, changes with age. The physiologic changes that accompany aging affect the pharmacologic processes of absorption, distribution, metabolism, and excretion (Table 5–1). The effects of these age-related changes are variable and difficult to predict. Some of these physiologic changes are related solely to aging, whereas others most likely are due to the combined effects of age, disease, and the environment. Although increasing age is often accompanied by reductions in the physiologic reserve of many organ systems independent of the effects of disease, these changes are not uniform. There is substantial variation from individual to individual, making some older patients more vulnerable than others. The alterations in pharmacokinetics and pharmacodynamics that occur with increasing age suggest a pharmacologic basis for concern about the vulnerability of the elderly to the effects of medications. Unfortunately, the results of epidemiologic studies that explore these relationships are unclear, in part

due to the small number of older people included in premarketing studies relative to the patient population most likely to be exposed to the drug. The oldest-old (i.e., those aged 80 years or older) have generally not been included in clinical trials of investigational drugs, and those older subjects who do participate in such trials tend to be healthy "young-old" people. Thus, the results of these trials and the side effects reported often have limited application to the older patient with multiple illnesses who is taking several medications. In general, consideration of the individual patient, his physiologic status (i.e., hydration, nutrition, and cardiac output), and how this status affects the pharmacology of a particular drug is more important in prescribing that drug than any specific age-related changes.

Absorption of drugs, which occurs mainly by passive diffusion, changes little with advancing age. The changes listed in Table 5–1 could potentially affect drug absorption. More important changes result from concurrent administration of several medications. For example, antacids decrease the oral absorption of cimetidine, and alcohol accelerates the absorption of chloral hydrate.

Unlike absorption, drug distribution is affected by age in clinically meaningful ways. In older persons, the relative increase in body fat and the decrease in lean body mass alter drug distribution so that fat-soluble drugs are distributed more widely and water-soluble drugs less widely[2] (Table 5–2). The increased distribution of fat-soluble drugs can delay elimination and may result in prolonged duration of action of a single dose. This effect is especially important for drugs such as hypnotics and analgesics, which are given in single doses on an intermittent basis. For example, the volume of distribution of diazepam is increased almost twofold in older patients, and the elimination half-life is prolonged from 24 hours in young patients to approximately 90 hours in older patients.

In contrast, the volume of distribution of water-soluble compounds, such as digoxin, is decreased in older patients, and thus the dose re-

TABLE 5–1 **AGE-RELATED CHANGES RELEVANT TO DRUG PHARMACOLOGY**

Pharmacologic Process	Physiologic Change	Clinical Significance
Absorption	Decreased absorptive surface Decreased splanchnic blood flow Increased gastric pH Altered gastrointestinal motility	Little change in absorption with age
Distribution	Decreased total body water Decreased lean body mass Increased body fat Decreased serum albumin Altered protein binding	Higher concentration of drugs that distribute in body fluids; increased distribution and often prolonged elimination half-life of fat-soluble drugs Increased free fraction in plasma of some highly protein-bound acidic drugs
Metabolism	Reduced hepatic mass Reduced hepatic blood flow Decreased phase I metabolism	Often decreased first-pass metabolism and decreased rate of biotransformation of some drugs
Elimination	Reduced renal plasma flow Reduced glomerular filtration rate Decreased tubular secretion function	Decreased renal elimination of drugs and metabolites; marked interindividual variation
Tissue sensitivity	Alterations in receptor number Alterations in receptor affinity Alterations in second-messenger function Alteration in cellular and nuclear responses	Patients are "more sensitive" or "less sensitive" to an agent

quired to reach a target plasma concentration is decreased. Likewise, due to the decreased volume of distribution, the loading dose of aminoglycosides is less in older patients.

For drugs that bind to serum proteins, an equilibrium exists between the bound or ineffective portion and the unbound (free) or effective portion. For acidic drugs that are highly bound to albumin, the free plasma concentration may correlate best with pharmacologic effect. Although albumin levels decrease only slightly with age, they tend to decrease during periods of illnesses. This can result in elevated levels of free (unbound) acidic drugs in older persons during episodes of illnesses, and thus in an increased

TABLE 5–2 **VOLUME OF DISTRIBUTION OF COMMONLY PRESCRIBED DRUGS**

Increased Volume°	Decreased Volume°
Acetaminophen	Cimetidine
Chlordiazepoxide	Digoxin
Diazepam	Ethanol
Oxazepam	Gentamicin
Prazosin	Meperidine
Salicylates	Phenytoin
Thiopental	Quinine
Tolbutamide	Theophylline

°If the volume of distribution is decreased, drug levels tend to be higher.

potential for toxicity. These changes can be significant for drugs such as thyroid hormone, digoxin, warfarin, and phenytoin.

On the other hand, some basic drugs such as lidocaine and propranolol bind mainly to alpha-1 acid glycoprotein, an acute phase reactant protein. The concentration of this protein tends to rise as a person ages and is elevated following myocardial infarction and in chronic inflammatory diseases and malignant conditions.[3] The plasma binding of these drugs is increased in older patients, but because these age-related changes are not great, their exact clinical relevance is uncertain.

Overall, changes in protein binding are an important consideration initially when a drug is being started, when the dosage is changed, when serum protein levels change, or when a drug displaces other protein-bound drugs. Because the free portion of the drug is generally smaller than the bound portion, the normal mechanisms of metabolism and excretion ultimately eliminate the free drug. If either hepatic or renal function is impaired due to age or disease, this elimination may be slowed.

Although in vitro studies of drug-metabolizing enzyme activity from human liver biopsy samples have not demonstrated any changes with aging, some investigators speculate that the decline in liver size with age may result in decreased metabolic capacity. A significant decline in liver blood flow occurs with age, reductions of 25% to 47%

being reported in persons between the ages of 25 and 90. This decrease in hepatic blood flow is clinically important because hepatic metabolism is the rate-limiting step that determines the clearance of most metabolized drugs. This change is especially relevant for drugs that undergo rapid hepatic metabolism (e.g., propranolol). Also, drugs that undergo extensive first-pass metabolism are likely to reach higher blood levels if hepatic blood flow is decreased.

The liver metabolizes drugs through two distinct systems. Phase I metabolism involves drug oxidation and reduction and is catalyzed primarily by the cytochrome P450 system in the smooth endoplasmic reticulum of hepatocytes. Phase I metabolism activity decreases substantially with age. Drugs that are metabolized through phase I enzymatic activity have prolonged half-lives. Examples of drugs whose metabolism is slowed because of these age-related changes in hepatic metabolism are listed in Table 5–3. Phase II hepatic metabolism involves the conjugation of drugs or their metabolites to organic substrates. The elimination of drugs that undergo phase II metabolism by conjugation (i.e., acetylation, glucouronidation, sulfation, and glycine conjugation) is generally altered less with age. Thus, drugs that require only phase II metabolism for excretion (e.g., triazolam) do not have a prolonged half-life in older people. These drugs contrast with drugs such as diazepam that undergo both phases of metabolism and have active intermediate metabolites. Although the effect of aging on hepatic drug metabolism is variable, phase I metabolism is the process that is most likely to decrease in older persons.

The apparent variable effect of age on drug metabolism is probably due to the fact that age is only one of many factors that affect drug metabolism. For example, cigarette smoking, alcohol intake, dietary modification, drugs, viral illness, caffeine intake, and other unknown factors also affect the rate of drug metabolism.

TABLE 5–3   COMMONLY PRESCRIBED DRUGS WITH PROLONGED HEPATIC METABOLISM

Acetaminophen	Meperidine
Amitriptyline	Nortriptyline
Barbiturates	Phenytoin
Chlordiazepoxide	Prazosin
Diazepam	Propranolol
Diphenhydramine	Quinidine
Flurazepam	Salicylates
Ibuprofen	Theophylline
Labetalol	Tolbutamide
Lidocaine	Warfarin

TABLE 5–4   DRUGS WITH DECREASED RENAL ELIMINATION IN OLDER PERSONS

Amantadine	Hydrochlorothiazide
Ampicillin	Kanamycin
Atenolol	Lithium
Ceftriaxone	Pancuronium
Cephradine	Penicillin
Cimetidine	Phenobarbital
Digoxin	Procainamide
Doxycycline	Ranitidine
Furosemide	Sotalol
Gentamicin	Triamterene

Induction of drug metabolism can occur in older persons. The rate of elimination of theophylline is increased by smoking and by phenytoin in both young and older persons alike.[4] Thus, this adaptive response is preserved with age. Not all metabolizing isoenzymes are induced equally in the young and the old. For example, antipyrine elimination is increased after pretreatment with dichloralphenazone in younger patients but not in older patients.

An important pharmacokinetic change that occurs in persons of advanced age is that of reduced renal drug elimination (Table 5–4). This change results from the age-related decline in both glomerular filtration rate and tubular function. Drugs that depend on glomerular function (e.g., gentamicin) and drugs that depend on tubular secretion (e.g., penicillin) for elimination both exhibit reduced excretion in older patients. Because drug elimination is correlated with creatinine clearance, measurement of creatinine clearance is helpful in determining the maintenance dose. In the kidney, the average creatinine clearance declines by 50% from age 25 to age 85 despite a serum creatinine level that remains unchanged at approximately 1.0 mg/dL. Because the serum creatinine tends to overestimate the actual creatinine clearance in older persons, the commonly cited formula devised by Cockroft and Gault may be used to estimate creatinine clearance (CrCl) in older adults:

$$CrCl = \frac{(140 - age) \cdot weight\ (kg)}{72 \cdot serum\ Cr}$$

In women, the estimated value is 85% of the calculated value at the same weight and serum creatinine concentration. Although this equation is useful in adjusting for age, weight, and the measured serum creatinine level, it does not account for individual variation. This formula has been validated in ambulatory and hospitalized patients, but some studies suggest that it may not be accurate when applied to frail nursing home patients.[5]

Altered renal clearance leads to two clinically relevant consequences: (1) the half-lives of renally excreted drugs are prolonged, and (2) the serum levels of these drugs are increased. For drugs with large therapeutic indexes (e.g., penicillin), this is of little clinical importance, but for drugs with a narrower therapeutic index (e.g., digoxin, cimetidine, aminoglycosides), side effects may occur in older patients if dose reductions are not made. Thus, it is not surprising that digoxin is the drug that most often causes side effects in the elderly, especially if the dose exceeds 0.125 mg daily.[6] To further define dose requirements, therapeutic drug monitoring should also be performed for drugs with a low therapeutic index.

Pharmacodynamics

In addition to the factors that determine the drug concentration at the site of action (pharmacokinetics), the effect of a drug also depends on the sensitivity of the target organ to the drug. The biochemical and physiologic effects of drugs and their mechanisms of action (pharmacodynamics) and the effects of aging are not clearly known. Pharmacodynamics has been even less extensively studied in older patients than pharmacokinetics. Generalizations are not straightforward, and the effect of age on sensitivity to drugs varies with the drug studied and the response measured. These differences in sensitivity occur in the absence of marked reductions in the metabolism of the drug and its related compounds. Thus, sensitivity to drug effects may either increase or decrease with increasing age.

For example, older patients seem to be more sensitive to the sedative effects of given blood levels of benzodiazepine drugs (e.g., diazepam) but less sensitive to the effects of drugs mediated by beta-adrenergic receptors (e.g., isoproterenol, propranolol). Although an age-related decline in hormone receptor affinity or number (e.g., in beta-adrenergic receptors) is suspected, definitive data demonstrating such an alteration are sparse. Other possible explanations offered for these differences are alterations in second-messenger function and alterations in cellular and nuclear responses.

Since the response of older patients to any given medication is variable and cannot be foreseen, all drugs should be used appropriately but judiciously in older patients, and the physician should resist the temptation to apply protocol medicine. In general, knowledge of the pharmacology of the drugs prescribed, limits on the number of drugs used, determination of the preparation and dosage of the drug based on the patient's general condition and ability to handle the drug combined with downward adjustment of the dose in the presence of known hepatic or renal impairment, and surveillance for untoward effects will minimize the risks of medication use in the elderly.

THERAPEUTIC RISKS: SPECIAL CONSIDERATIONS IN THE ELDERLY

Adherence to Drug Therapy

Despite consideration by the clinician of age-related changes and possible drug-drug and drug-disease interactions, the full benefit of a drug may not be seen if the patient does not take the drug as prescribed. Adherence is the extent to which a patient's behavior concurs with the directions provided by his or her physician. Nonadherence with medication prescriptions is a problem common in patients of all ages and is not unique to older patients. But because older patients use more medications than younger ones, and nonadherence increases in proportion to the number of medications used, nonadherence is more common in older patients.

Nonadherence with drug therapy is reported to occur in one third to one half of older patients.[7] Approximately one in five prescriptions is not filled, and between one third and two thirds of patients who do fill their prescriptions use the medication in a manner different from that intended. Several causes of nonadherence have been identified and are listed in Table 5–5.

The cost of medication and insurance coverage can affect adherence in various ways. Patients may not purchase drugs if they cannot afford the out-of-pocket cost. On the other hand, expensive medications are sometimes perceived as being more powerful and therefore more beneficial. If patients do not pay for their medications because of their insurance benefits, adherence with the more expensive medications may be increased.

Among the causes of adherence, careful explanation by the doctor of the purpose of the medication is especially important for older patients.[8] Poor communication with the prescribing physician, coupled with a decline in cognitive abilities, makes older patients particularly vulnerable to misuse of medications. Persons with mild dementia may forget to take medications even though they are otherwise capable of living in an unsupervised environment. In fact, most or 90% of instances of nonadherence take the form of underadherence or taking too little of a pre-

TABLE 5–5 **FACTORS INFLUENCING ADHERENCE**

Factor	Effect on Adherence
Age	None
Sex	None
Education level	None
Ethnicity	None
Financial status	None
Actual severity of disease	None
Actual effectiveness or toxicity of drug	None
Belief by the patient that the disease being treated is serious	None
Belief by the patient that the medication will treat or prevent the disease or condition	Increase
Careful explanation by the doctor of the purpose of the medication	Increase
Number of drugs used	Decrease
Long duration of therapy	Decrease
Complex scheduling	Decrease
Safety closure bottles	Decrease

scribed medication.[9] Devices that sound a buzzer to remind patients to take a medication, reminder calls from a family member or friend, and the act of laying out medications daily are helpful aids in improving adherence. If possible, it is helpful to prescribe medications that can be taken less frequently. In fact, older patients may attain adherence rates as high as 80% to 90% if they are given clear written and verbal instructions, a simple dosing schedule, and a reduced number of medications.[10]

Serious complications can arise if the prescriber incorrectly assumes that the patient has adhered to the therapy. When a medication appears to be ineffective, the prescriber often increases the dose or prescribes a more powerful drug. A change in circumstance, such as increased supervision from a home nursing agency or family member or hospitalization can then lead to toxicity.

Another kind of problem with adherence is exemplified by the role of diet in the adjustment of diuretics and oral hypoglycemic agents. The dosages of these medications are often prescribed initially in the hospital, where the patient's diet is strictly controlled. However, when the patient is discharged to a less controlled environment where he or she does not adhere to salt or carbohydrate restrictions, readmission for congestive heart failure or hyper-

glycemia may result. This type of adverse outcome might be avoided if the medication were adjusted to a more realistic diet while the patient is still in the hospital.

Knowledge Base of Safety and Efficacy

Drug therapy in elderly persons is complicated by many factors that are unique to this age group. Multiple comorbid conditions, environmental conditions, genetic variations, and the physiologic effects of aging all interact with each other to affect drug disposition in the elderly. Although a judicious use of medications can profoundly affect the mortality and morbidity of many diseases in the elderly, appropriate use of medications is hampered by a lack of data. There are few data on the effects of age at the sites of drug action, and likewise, there is insufficient information about drug disposition and response in the very elderly, those over 85 years of age. These older patients, who are often the intended targets of new drug therapies, are usually not recruited to participate in clinical drug trials, so extrapolations on dosage and possible side effects of drugs may or may not be appropriate.

It is known that older patients experience adverse outcomes about twice as often as younger patients.[6] Older patients experience more adverse reactions than younger patients regardless of the number of drugs they use (Fig. 5–1). Because the proportion of people over 75 years of age is expected to continue to increase, and the prevalence of major chronic diseases such as hypertension, arthritis, stroke, cancer, and diabetes also increases with age, a larger proportion of older patients can be expected to be exposed to therapeutic drugs. Clinicians must be attentive to the goals and consequences of drug therapy in the elderly and must individualize therapy as much as feasible.

Risk of Adverse Drug Reactions

Older patients are at increased risk of incurring adverse reactions from certain classes of drugs. *Primum non nocere* (first do no harm) is a phrase that is especially applicable when prescribing drugs for the elderly. Adverse drug reactions are the most common form of iatrogenic illness. The incidence of adverse drug reactions in hospitalized patients increases from about 10% in 40- to 50-year-old patients to 25% in patients older than 80 years of age. In 1986, 51% of deaths due to adverse drug reactions occurred in elderly patients. Reported rates of drug-related hospital

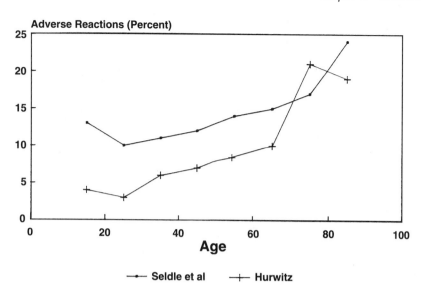

Figure 5–1 Adverse drug reactions by age. (Redrawn from Medication for the Elderly. A Report of the Royal College of Physicians of London, Vol. 18. London, Royal College of Physicians, 1984, pp. 7-17.)

admissions have ranged from 2.3% to 27.3%. An analysis by Johnson and Bootman[11] estimated that drug-related morbidity and mortality cost $76.6 billion in ambulatory patients in the United States, and the largest component of this total cost was associated with drug-related hospitalizations.

Many drugs commonly prescribed for older patients result in potentially life-threatening or disabling adverse reactions (Table 5–6). Cardiovascular and psychotropic drugs are the agents

TABLE 5–6 **EXAMPLES OF ADVERSE DRUG REACTIONS**

Type of Drug	Common Adverse Reaction
Narcotics	Constipation
Aminoglycosides	Renal failure, hearing loss
Anticholinergics	Dry mouth, constipation, urinary retention, delirium
Antiarrhythmics	Diarrhea (quinidine); urinary retention (disopyramide)
Diuretics	Dehydration, hyponatremia, hypokalemia, incontinence
Antipsychotics	Delirium, sedation, hypotension, extrapyramidal movement disorders
Sedative-hypnotics	Excessive sedation, delirium, gait disturbances

most commonly associated with serious adverse reactions in the elderly. This fact results from a combination of their narrow therapeutic-toxic window, age-related changes such as reduced renal excretion, and a prolonged duration of action, which predisposes the older patient to adverse reactions. Because clinical drug trials generally do not require drugs to be tested in the population that will ultimately receive them (i.e., older patients with one or more serious illnesses), the risk-versus-benefit ratio of most drugs is not clearly known for older patients. Adverse drug reactions are often not recognized because the symptoms are nonspecific or mimic the symptoms of other illnesses. Often another drug is prescribed to treat these symptoms, resulting in polypharmacy and further increasing the likelihood of an adverse drug reaction. This effect may be compounded when patients visit multiple physicians who prescribe drugs independently of each other. Drugs that are commonly prescribed for older patients that can interact with each other are described in Table 5–7.

Despite the association of increased adverse drug reactions with older age, many studies have failed to show an effect independent of age. What is known is that polypharmacy correlates strongly with the incidence of adverse drug reactions, and, as noted earlier, older patients are prescribed more drugs than their younger counterparts. Older patients also have other characteristics that further predispose them to adverse drug reactions. These include a greater severity of illness, multiple comorbidities, smaller body size, changes in hepatic and renal metabolism and excretion, and prior drug reactions. The

TABLE 5–7 **EXAMPLES OF POTENTIALLY IMPORTANT DRUG-DRUG INTERACTIONS**

Example	Interaction	Potential Effects
Antacids with digoxin, isoniazid (INH), and antipsychotics	Interference with drug absorption	Decreased drug effectiveness
Warfarin with oral hypoglycemics, aspirin, chloral hydrate	Displacement from binding proteins	Increased effects and risk of toxicity
Cimetidine with propranolol, theophylline, phenytoin (Dilantin)	Altered metabolism	Decreased drug clearance, increased risk of toxicity
Lithium with diuretics	Altered excretion	Increased risk of toxicity and electrolyte imbalance

more common types of potential adverse drug interactions in older patients are drug displacement from protein-binding sites by other highly protein-bound drugs, induction or suppression of the metabolism of other drugs, and the additive effects of different drugs on blood pressure and mental function. Additionally, several drugs also interact adversely with underlying medical conditions in older patients creating "drug-disease" interactions (Table 5–8). Health care providers should not only have a thorough knowledge of the more common drug side effects, adverse drug reactions, and potential drug interactions in older patients, they should also question patients about common side effects when they review drug regimens.

DRUG TREATMENT OF SPECIFIC CONDITIONS

Pain

Older patients use analgesic agents more frequently than any other age group. This is not surprising given the fact that 48% of elderly patients report arthritis as their primary illness. Nonsteroidal anti-inflammatory drugs (NSAIDs) are the drug of choice for many rheumatologic conditions. All NSAIDs inhibit cyclooxygenase, the major enzyme in prostaglandin biosynthesis. Impairment in renal function can occur when NSAIDs suppress the prostaglandin-mediated compensatory mechanisms that maintain renal blood flow and glomerular filtration. A prospec-

TABLE 5–8 **SOME IMPORTANT DRUG-DISEASE INTERACTIONS IN OLDER PATIENTS**

Disease	Drug	Adverse Effects
Dementia	Psychotropic drugs, levodopa, antiepileptic agents	Increased confusion, delirium
Glaucoma	Antimuscarinic drugs	Acute glaucoma
Congestive heart failure	Beta-blockers, verapamil	Acute cardiac decompensation
Cardiac conduction disorders	Tricyclic antidepressants	Heart block
Hypertension	NSAIDs*	Increase in blood pressure
Peripheral vascular disease	Beta-blockers	Intermittent claudication
Chronic obstructive pulmonary disease	Beta-blockers, opiates	Bronchoconstriction, respiratory depression
Chronic renal impairment	NSAIDs,* contrast agents, aminoglycosides	Acute renal failure
Diabetes mellitus	Diuretics, prednisone	Hyperglycemia
Prostatic hyperplasia	Antimuscarinic agents	Urinary retention
Depression	Beta-blockers, centrally acting antihypertensives, alcohol, benzodiazepines, corticosteroids	Precipitation or exacerbation of depression
Hypokalemia	Digoxin	Cardiac arrhythmias
Peptic ulcer disease	NSAIDs,* anticoagulants	Gastrointestinal hemorrhage

*Nonsteroidal anti-inflammatory drugs.

tive study of elderly residents of a large long-term care facility who were newly treated with NSAIDs demonstrated that 13% developed azotemia during a short course of therapy.[12] This adverse effect was associated with higher NSAID dosages and the concomitant use of loop diuretics.

The use of NSAIDs is also related to upper gastrointestinal (UGI) bleeding. A study revealed that older age was associated with a higher risk of gastrointestinal toxicity.[13] Recent or current users of NSAIDs are significantly more likely to suffer from UGI bleeding. This iatrogenic illness is likely to increase in older patients because of the increased availability and use of prescription and nonprescription NSAIDs. The risks associated with NSAID use by elderly persons emphasize the need for careful monitoring of patients who have risk factors for NSAID-associated nephrotoxicity and gastropathy. To limit these adverse effects, NSAID therapy should be limited to clinical situations in which it is absolutely required, and the lowest possible dose should be prescribed for the shortest time necessary. The best treatment for NSAID-associated nephrotoxicity and gastropathy is discontinuation of the offending NSAID. Alternative analgesics like nonacetylated salicylate or acetaminophen may be used safely. No dosage adjustment is needed for acetaminophen because of its wider therapeutic index even though its hepatic metabolism is often impaired in older patients.

Anticoagulation

Long-term oral anticoagulant therapy with warfarin is essential for the optimal management of many thromboembolic and vascular disorders, which are more prevalent among elderly patients. For example, the proportion of strokes associated with atrial fibrillation increases from 6.7% for persons aged 50 to 59 years to 36.2% for those aged 80 to 89 years. Clinical trials have shown that the risks of stroke from atrial fibrillation can be substantially decreased with anticoagulation therapy.[14, 15]

Unfortunately, one drawback of anticoagulant therapy is that it can cause serious bleeding, and the risk of anticoagulant-related bleeding is not clearly defined for older patients, who are likely to benefit the most from this therapy. Older patients may be at increased risk for anticoagulant-related bleeding because of their increased incidence of adverse drug reactions, increased prevalence of comorbidities and polypharmacy, and increased vascular endothelial fragility. Furthermore, older patients may also have an increased sensitivity to warfarin. It has been reported that the anticoagulant response to warfarin is enhanced with age.

Most studies that have examined age as a risk factor for heparin-related bleeding have found that bleeding is more frequent in older patients; patients 60 years and older were approximately three times more likely to develop bleeding during heparin therapy than younger patients.[16] Studies that have examined age as a risk factor for warfarin-related bleeding have reported conflicting results.[16] Seven studies, enrolling a total of 14,388 patients, found that older patients were approximately twice as likely to bleed during warfarin therapy. In contrast, seven different studies enrolling a total of 2940 patients found no increase in the frequency of warfarin-related bleeding in older patients.

The reasons for the discrepancies in warfarin-related bleeding in older patients are not clear. Several factors are likely to have contributed to the different results, including chance, differences in measurement methods, biases inherent in observational studies, especially those enrolling patients who have been treated with anticoagulants for some time (i.e., noninception cohorts), and nonenrollment of selected older patients.

A large number of drugs are known to interact with anticoagulants, and since patients tend to take anticoagulants for several months, there is ample time for an adverse reaction to occur. Some drugs potentiate the anticoagulant effect, resulting in an increased prothrombin time and risk of bleeding. Examples of these drugs include phenylbutazone, cimetidine, metronidazole, phenytoin, erythromycin, and thyroxine. Other drugs, such as barbiturates and rifampin, increase hepatic metabolism, which decreases the anticoagulant effect, thereby increasing the dosage requirements. Discontinuation of these latter drugs can lead to an increased prothrombin time and an increased risk of bleeding.

As more patients are considered candidates for anticoagulant therapy, it becomes increasingly important to define the risk of anticoagulant-related bleeding associated with age. Older patients have more frequent adverse drug reactions in general, and may have a disproportionate number of other risk factors for anticoagulant-related bleeding. These findings also indicate the potential value of methods of decreasing the frequency of anticoagulant-related bleeding in older patients. Such methods include maintaining the anticoagulant effect within the therapeutic range and recognizing other modifiable factors, such as medication use, that may promote bleeding. The probable age-related risk of anticoagulant-related bleeding should be considered in making decisions about the use of anticoagulants. Although this risk may be high enough to avoid anticoagulants in some older patients, it is unlikely that age-related risk alone will outweigh the substantial benefits of anticoagulant therapy in many older patients.

PRESCRIBING IN THE NURSING HOME

More medications are prescribed for residents in nursing homes, the most frail of all elderly persons, than for their noninstitutionalized peers.[1, 17] Nursing home residents are also more vulnerable because they usually have no input in their medical therapy because of either frailty or dementia. This patient population is at increased risk for adverse drug reactions and polypharmacy because of their complex medical conditions and their institutional environment. Also, sufficient data to determine the appropriate use of medications as well as the risk versus the benefits of therapy in these institutionalized persons are lacking.

In 1974, the Health Care Financing Administration mandated that medications must be renewed monthly and that pharmacy consultation must be obtained for all nursing home residents. This monthly review provides a potential opportunity to reassess the need for medications, to discontinue medications, to reduce the dosage of medicines that might be just as effective at a lower dose, and to scan the patient for drug-drug and drug-disease interactions. Often this opportunity falls short when the physician fails to review the drug regimens thoroughly and when communication between the pharmacist and the physician is less than optimal. Nonetheless, this is a unique aspect of nursing homes in that regular involvement of a pharmacist in drug monitoring is required.

More recently, federal legislation has been implemented to limit the use of psychoactive drugs in nursing home residents. The Nursing Home Reform Amendments of the Omnibus Budget Reconciliation Act (OBRA 1987) require regulation of the use of psychoactive medications in Medicare- and Medicaid-certified nursing homes in the form of explicit documentation in the medical record to justify the need for such drugs as well as close monitoring and periodic withdrawal of these antipsychotic medications.[18, 19] Guidelines for antipsychotics, anxiolytics, and sedatives were developed and implemented. Although the effects of these guidelines on the use of anxiolytics and sedatives have not been determined, the use of antipsychotic drugs in nursing homes has been shown to be reduced.[20]

Although these recent regulatory changes have had some impact, studies still indicate that one or more psychoactive drugs are prescribed for about 50% of all nursing home residents. Antipsychotic medications are often used for the treatment of agitation in older patients with dementia, although data supporting their effectiveness are limited.[21] These drugs are known to be associated with extrapyramidal symptoms, gait instability, falls, and hip fractures. Likewise, the use of benzodiazepines to treat agitation, especially agents with long elimination half-lives, is associated with falls, fractures, daytime somnolence, confusion, and ataxia.[22, 23]

Often nonpharmacologic interventions may be just as effective with less risk in managing some of the behaviors seen in elderly nursing home residents.[24, 25] Examples include increased tolerance from staff members for repetitive requests, specially designed facilities to accommodate freedom of movement and supervision, more personal attention and support, avoidance of caffeine at night, regular exercise, and later bedtimes.

SUMMARY

It is important for health care providers to be aware of the issues involved in using drug therapies in older patients because older patients are the ones most vulnerable to the adverse effects of drugs. Although more data are needed to guide clinical decision making in prescribing drugs for older patients, some simple considerations can make drug use safer and more effective. Careful, compassionate attention to these factors can have a profound effect on improving the quality of life, medication use, and the overall cost of health care in this vulnerable population.

References

1. Ostrom JF, Hammarlund ER, Christensen DB, Plein JB, Kethley AJ: Medication usage in an elderly population. Med Care 1985;23:157–164.
2. Vestal RE, Dawson GW: Handbook of the Biology of Aging, 2nd ed. New York, Van Nostrand Reinhold, 1985, pp. 744–819.
3. Abernethy DR, Kerzner L: Age effects on alpha-1-acid glycoprotein concentration and imipramine plasma protein binding. J Am Geriatr Soc 1984;32:705–708.
4. Crowley JJ, Cusak BJ, Jue SG, Koup JR, Park BK, Vestal RE: Aging and drug interactions. II. Effect of phenytoin and smoking on the oxidation of theophylline and cortisol in healthy men. J Pharmacol Exp Ther 1988;245:513–523.
5. Drusano GL, Munice HL, Hoopes JM, Damron DJ, Warren JW: Commonly used methods of estimating creatinine clearance are inadequate for elderly debilitated nursing home patients. J Am Geriatr Soc 1988;36:437–441.

6. Nolan L, O'Malley K: Prescribing for the elderly. Part I. Sensitivity of the elderly to adverse drug reactions. J Am Geriatr Soc 1988;36:142–149.
7. Morrow D, Leirer V, Sheikh J: Adherence and medication instructions: Review and recommendations. J Am Geriatr Soc 1988;36:1147–1160.
8. Becker MH: Patient adherence to prescribed therapies. Med Care 1985;23:539–555.
9. Cooper JK, Love DW, Raffoul PR: Intentional prescription nonadherence (noncompliance) by the elderly. J Am Geriatr Soc 1982;30:329–333.
10. Black DM, Brand RJ, Greenlick M, Hughes G, Smith J: Compliance to treatment for hypertension in elderly patients: The SHEP pilot study. J Gerontol 1987;43:552–557.
11. Johnson JA, Bootman JL: Drug-related morbidity and mortality: A cost-of-illness model. Arch Intern Med 1995;155:1949–1956.
12. Gurwitz JH, Avorn J, Ross-Degnan D, Lipsitz LA: Nonsteroidal anti-inflammatory drug-associated azotemia in the very old. JAMA 1990;264:471–475.
13. Bollini P, Rodriguez LA, Perez Gutthann SP, Walker AM: The impact of research quality and study design on epidemiologic estimates of the effect of nonsteroidal anti-inflammatory drugs on upper gastrointestinal tract disease. Arch Intern Med 1992;152:1289–1295.
14. Stroke Prevention in Atrial Fibrillation Study Group Investigators: Stroke prevention in atrial fibrillation study. Final results. Circulation 1991;84:527–539.
15. Stroke Prevention in Atrial Fibrillation Study Group Investigators: Warfarin versus aspirin for prevention of thromboembolism in atrial fibrillation: Stroke prevention in atrial fibrillation II study. Lancet 1994;343:687–691.
16. Beyth RJ, Landefeld CS: Anticoagulants in older patients: A safety perspective. Drugs Aging 1995;6:45–54.
17. Chrischilles EA, Foley DJ, Wallace RB, et al: Use of medications by persons 65 and over: Data from the established populations for epidemiologic studies of the elderly. J Gerontol 1992;47:137–144.
18. Winograd CH, Pawlson LG: OBRA 87—A commentary. J Am Geriatr Soc 1991;39:724–726.
19. Elon R, Pawlson LG: The impact of OBRA on medical practice within nursing facilities. J Am Geriatr Soc 1992;40:958–963.
20. Shorr RI, Fought RL, Ray WA: Changes in antipsychotic drug use in nursing homes during implementation of OBRA-87 regulations. JAMA 1994;271:358–362.
21. Schneider LS, Pollock VE, Lyness SA: A meta-analysis of controlled trials of neuroleptic treatment in dementia. J Am Geriatr Soc 1990;35:553–563.
22. Ray WA, Griffin MR, Downey W: Benzodiazepines of long and short elimination half-life and the risk of hip fracture. JAMA 1989;262:3303–3307.
23. Cummings SR, Nevitt MC, Browner WS, et al: Risk factors for hip fracture in white women. Study of Osteoporotic Fractures Research Group. N Engl J Med 1995;332:767–776.
24. Avorn J, Gurwitz JH: Drug use in the nursing home. Ann Intern Med 1995;123:195–204.
25. Avorn J, Soumerai SB, Everitt DE, et al: A randomized trial of a program to reduce the use of psychoactive drugs in nursing homes. N Engl J Med 1992;327:168–173.

6 Sexuality

Fran E. Kaiser, M.D.

. . . you and I are old . . .
Though much is taken, much abides;
and though
We are not now that strength which in
the old days
Moved earth and heaven, that which we
are, we are
One equal temper of heroic hearts.

— Alfred, Lord Tennyson 1809–1892

Aging and sexuality (sexual attitudes, behaviors, practice, and activity) are not the two opposite ends of a spectrum. Until the twentieth century, this was a "nonissue" because individuals did not always live beyond their reproductive years. Although our society has often labeled sexual activity in older adults in pejorative terms —inappropriate, bizarre, limited to "dirty" old men and women[1]—these labels are far from reality for many older adults. As the over-65 population doubles, and one of five people in the United States will be over the age of 65 in the year 2030, sexual myths and barriers may be shattered. It also must be recognized that sexual activity is not just intercourse. Masturbation remains a viable alternative for many individuals.[2, 3] The desire for intimacy, affection, and love does not end at any age.[4]

PREVALENCE OF SEXUAL ACTIVITY WITH AGING

Although the frequency of sexual activity tends to decrease with age, an average of approximately 70% of healthy 70-year-olds continue to have sexual intercourse on a regular basis.[5] In a study of men aged 66 to 71, 28% reported having intercourse weekly, and by age 78, 20% of men remained sexually active.[6, 7] Although interest in sex was maintained in 75% to 85% of men in their sixties and seventies, only 32% to 42% of women in the same age group maintained sexual interest.[8] Data from the National Survey of Families and Households, which examined 807 mar-

ried individuals aged 60 and over, showed that 53% of the entire sample and 24% of those over age 76 remained sexually active.[9] Diokno and colleagues[10] found that 73.8% of married older men and 55.8% of married older women were sexually active, but these percentages dropped dramatically in unmarried individuals, with 31.9% of men and 5.3% of women remaining active. More recently, the Janus report noted that among those over 65, 69% of men and 74% of women were sexually active at least weekly.[11] In perhaps the largest sexual survey reported of those over age 65, comprising data on 1604 men and women aged 65 to 95, it was noted that 40% of the respondents were sexually active (52% of men, 30% of women).[12] Among those older adults who were not sexually active, 65% of men and 29% of women said they would like to be. Sixty-five percent of all respondents strongly or partly agreed that sex was "fun."

Other forms of sexual expression remain viable regardless of age. Forty percent of 80- to 102-year-old women masturbated, and 13% acknowledged at least weekly activity, whereas 72% of men practiced masturbation.[4] Another study found that 17% of men and 2% of women over 65 practiced masturbation daily or a few times per week, and 50% of men and 27% of women engaged in this activity at least once a month.[11] Eighty-six percent of older adults enjoy hugging, and when asked what matters most in an intimate relationship, only 5% of survey respondents listed sex, but 87% noted companionship, and 8% said romance was important.[12]

48

TABLE 6–1	**BARRIERS TO SEX AND SEXUALITY: PSYCHOSOCIAL FACTORS**

Lack of partner
Erectile dysfunction
Bereavement
Self or spousal or partner illness
Ageism
Adult children's attitudes
Altered body image
Previous attitude towards sex and sexuality
Depression
Autonomy of choice
Privacy
Marital conflict
Libido "mismatch"

PSYCHOSOCIAL ISSUES

Clearly, data about sexual activity are skewed for those who have no partner or whose partner's (or their own) problems (illness, erectile dysfunction, availability, and so on) decrease the frequency of activity when that activity is measured as intercourse. Because women tend to marry men older than themselves and have a life expectancy that is 7 to 8 years greater than that of men, they face the prospect of surviving to a later age alone. By age 85, there are 39 men for every 100 women. Fifty percent of men over age 85, but only 1 in 12 women over 85 are married. Numerous studies have dissociated the reported decline in sexual activity from aging by linking such declines to disease, medication, or clearly identifiable sociocultural or psychological factors. These factors may include ageist attitudes (old people "don't do this") or the attitude that sex is a procreational "only" activity or a "chore"), depression, altered body image, anxiety, and marital (or partner) strife or conflict. Even the disapproval of adult children of an older adult's search for partnership may occur. Considerations of

health and disease in the patient or partner, availability of a functioning partner, quality of life, sexual quality of life, privacy, and autonomy of choice are also important issues in older adults. All of these factors may act as barriers to sexual activity (Table 6–1).

AGING AND PHYSIOLOGIC ALTERATIONS IN THE SEXUAL CYCLE

Aging has an effect on each of the four stages of the sexual response cycle: excitement, plateau, orgasm, and resolution, which were initially described by Masters and Johnson[13] (Table 6–2). Excitement or arousal is a combination of olfactory, visual, auditory, memory, and other emotional stimuli as well as physical stimuli, all of which merge as sexual stimuli. The exact neurotransmitter (or neurotransmitters) involved in these functions remains unidentified. The plateau phase is marked by maintenance and intensification of arousal. Orgasm—rhythmic muscular contractions producing intense physical tension followed by relaxation—is the release of accumulated sexual tension. It should be noted that in men, ejaculation and orgasm are not identical. Orgasm can occur without ejaculation (or with retrograde ejaculation), for example, in men with prostate disease and following prostatic surgery. Diminished ability or complete lack of ejaculatory capacity has been associated with many medications.[14]

HORMONES, AGING, AND SEXUAL FUNCTION

The loss of estrogen in women with the onset of menopause has a well-recognized impact on sexual function in terms of comfort (Table 6–3). The loss of estrogen can result in a variety of symptoms ranging from hot flashes to loss of sleep

TABLE 6–2 AGING AND PHYSIOLOGIC CHANGES IN THE SEXUAL RESPONSE CYCLE

Stage	Women	Men
Excitement	Slower response, decreased breast and genital vasocongestion, decreased vaginal lubrication	Slower response, decreased scrotal vasocongestion, decreased scrotal tensing, reduced testicular elevation
Plateau	Reduced elevation of uterus and labia majora	Prolonged, decreased pre-ejaculatory secretion
Orgasm	Shorter duration, fewer and weaker uterine contractions, multiorgasmic capacity retained	Shorter duration, decreased prostatic and urethral contractions, decreased ejaculatory force
Resolution	Rapid reversion to prearousal state	Rapid detumescence and testicular descent, prolonged refractory period

TABLE 6–3 **CHANGES IN SEX HORMONES WITH AGING AND THEIR IMPACT ON SEXUAL FUNCTION**

Males	Females
↓ Testosterone	↓ Estrogen
↓ Bioavailable testosterone	↓ Estradiol : testosterone ratio
↑ Estradiol : testosterone ratio	↑ ↑ FSH (FSH > LH)
↑ SHBG	↑ LH
Normal LH > ↑ LH	Hot flashes, irritability
↑ FSH	↓ Vulval tissue, ↓ vaginal lubrication
↓ Libido	↓ Vaginal expansion
↓ Energy	↑ Dyspareunia
+/− Effect on erections	

SHBG, sex hormone–binding globulin; LH, luteinizing hormone; FSH, follicle-stimulating hormone.

and irritability (perhaps secondary to the interruption in sleep). Shortening of the vaginal vault, thinning of the vaginal mucosa, and loss of rugae can occur with estrogen deficiency. Urogenital atrophy can result in vaginitis, loss of vaginal lubrication, thinning and increased friability of vaginal tissue, and problems such as stress incontinence.[15] The loss of lubrication and tissue alterations of estrogen deficiency can lead to dyspareunia, and although this can result from a variety of causes ranging from skin conditions to orthopedic problems, perhaps the most readily treatable are those related to estrogen loss.[16, 17] As many as 30% of postmenopausal women experience dyspareunia.

Estrogen, however, does not have a major effect on libido in women, and testosterone has been known since 1943 to enhance libido in women. Controlled studies of surgically menopausal women have shown that testosterone is important in maintaining libido. However, it is less clear that replacing testosterone in normal postmenopausal women is of benefit. No statistically significant improvement in sexual function was found when administration of estrogen plus testosterone was compared with administration of estrogen alone. However, this area remains controversial, and a study by Davis and colleagues showed that improvement in sexuality (and bone density) occurred in women treated with estrogen and testosterone implants.[18] Nor does topical testosterone seem to offer any benefit. Although topical testosterone has been used to treat conditions such as vulvar lichen sclerosis and atrophic vaginitis, vaseline was just as effective (resulting in 75% improvement) as 2% testosterone propionate-petrolatum ointment (66.6% improvement).[19] Adverse effects of testosterone include worsening cardiovascular risk, hepatic dysfunction with oral use, and, theoretically, a "hyperandrogenic state" possibly associated with insulin resistance.

Testosterone in men has been clearly linked to libido but is less well linked to erectile ability. A study by Schiavi and colleagues noted that non–sex hormone-binding globulin (non-SHBG) bound testosterone, also called bioavailable testosterone (BT), was related to the frequency of sexual thoughts and sexual desire.[20] Testosterone withdrawal results in decreased sexual drive or desire and some decrement in erectile capacity, whereas testosterone administration may, in a small subset of patients, improve erectile function by increasing libido. The decrease in testosterone and BT concentrations that occurs with aging (i.e., in over 60% of men over age 60) is not generally accompanied by a rise in luteinizing hormone (LH) levels[21–23] (see Table 6–3), suggesting that some impairment of the hypothalamic pituitary axis has occurred. In both men and women these altered hormonal states have an impact on the risk of developing other disease states such as cardiovascular disease, osteoporosis, cognitive impairment, and muscular weakness. Clearly, hormonal changes in men and women have effects that go beyond sexual issues, and evaluation of hormone replacement in hormone-deficient individuals should be given serious consideration by the patient and his or her health care provider.

IMPORTANCE OF SEXUAL ASSESSMENT

There is no question that issues of sex and sexuality are difficult for the patient (and often the health care provider) to deal with. Many older adults never broach this subject on their own. Many causes of sexual dysfunction are in fact quite treatable. Both erectile dysfunction and dyspareunia are eminently treatable conditions. Furthermore, sexual function is a quality of life issue that is important to many older adults. Taking a sexual history was deemed an appropriate part of the medical examination by 91% of patients over age 65. An "opening" created by the physician for patients to discuss sexual issues may be the first time they've had an opportunity to discuss the problem.

ERECTILE DYSFUNCTION

The Massachusetts Male Aging study found a prevalence of erectile dysfunction (inability to attain or maintain an erection satisfactory for intercourse) in 52% of the 1290 men surveyed.[24] In individuals with particular disease states, such as diabetes, the prevalence of this disorder increases to as high as 95% in those over age 75, and it occurs in over 50% of patients with diabetes within 10 years of diagnosis. Although the prevalence of erectile problems triples between the ages of 40 and 70, the markedly increased prevalence of erectile problems with diseases such as diabetes, hypertension, and cardiovascular disease reinforces the concept that disease rather than aging per se is responsible for the development of the problem. Just as hypertension is commonly seen with aging but is not considered normal, erectile dysfunction is not considered a "normal" part of aging.

Causes of Erectile Dysfunction

Vascular Problems. Although erectile problems are often multifactorial in the older male, the most common cause of such problems in older men is vascular (Fig. 6–1). On penile Doppler studies, atherosclerotic vascular disease was found to cause approximately 50% of the impotence seen in males over age 50. In men with minor arterial problems, alterations in vascular pressure and flow may be diagnosed only with lower extremity exercise. Even minor vascular changes can be associated with erectile problems. The incidence of both arterial and venous disease increases with age.

The pelvic steal syndrome may redistribute blood flow away from a partially blocked artery. Severe alterations in the penile brachial pressure index can serve as a warning of the presence of vascular disease elsewhere because the occurrence of a myocardial infarction or stroke is five times greater in subjects with abnormal penile brachial Doppler study results than in those impotent men with normal penile indices. Additionally, men with low penile brachial indices are more likely to have abnormal results on an electrocardiographic or dipyridamole thallium stress test than those with normal indices. The probability of erectile dysfunction in men treated for heart disease is 94.2% in smokers and 78.1% in nonsmokers.[24] Among men aged 31 to 86 years of age, 64% had erectile problems.

As previously noted, problems with venous leakage increase with aging, perhaps because of

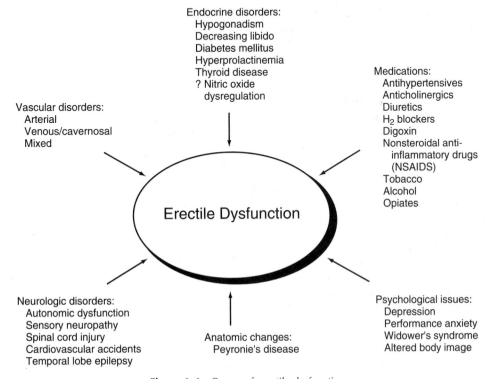

Figure 6–1 Causes of erectile dysfunction.

localized ischemia or increased collagen deposition in the tunica albuginea. Because diagnosis of the venous leak syndrome is invasive and involves the use of cavernosometry and cavernosography to diagnose the loss of intracavernosal pressure and locate the site, its use should be considered only in those patients willing to undergo a surgical procedure for correction. In the best hands, this surgery may result in erectile improvement in 75% of subjects, but the effects rarely last for more than 5 years.

Hormonal Problems. Change in the form of hypogonadism has been previously discussed (see earlier section on hormones and aging). Diabetes, which is associated with vascular changes and accelerated atherosclerosis, is also associated with both autonomic and peripheral neuropathy, which can contribute to further functional loss. In diabetes, changes in neurotransmitters, such as nitric oxide and vasoactive intestinal peptide, may have a negative impact on erectile ability. Because diabetes occurs in almost 18% of those between the ages of 65 and 74 as well as in more than one quarter of African-Americans, this disease is an important issue in men with erectile dysfunction.[25, 26] Elevated prolactin levels, which may be seen in men with uremia, hypothyroidism, or pituitary adenomas, may also be associated with erectile dysfunction and appear to cause this effect independent of any change in testosterone concentration. A prolactinoma is found in 10% or less of those with elevated prolactin concentrations. Other endocrinopathies, such as Cushing's syndrome, hypothyroidism, and hyperthyroidism, may be associated with erectile problems.

Medication and Drug Effects. The compendium of medications that affect erection or arousal and ejaculation is lengthy. Among 1000 medical clinical outpatients, up to 25% had erectile dysfunction that had a medication-related cause. Although diuretics and all classes of antihypertensive agents can cause erectile problems, thiazide diuretics and beta blockers appear to be the drugs causing the most problems. Calcium channel blockers, angiotensin-converting enzyme (ACE) inhibitors, and alpha blockers may all be associated with erectile difficulty but cause fewer problems than beta blockers or thiazide diuretics. Nearly all antidepressants, including many of the selective serotonin reuptake inhibitors, may be associated with erectile failure. Notable exceptions include trazodone and buspirone. Cigarette usage, alcohol use, and "recreational" drugs, including opiates, cause problems. Drugs that are now sold over the counter may be a cause of

some concern. H$_2$ blockers (such as cimetidine) and nonsteroidal anti-inflammatory drugs (NSAIDs) have been associated with erectile disturbances. H$_2$ blockers act as antiandrogens, elevate prolactin levels, and contract the penile smooth musculature, reducing penile arterial dilatation. However, many of the conditions for which patients receive these medications as treatment (such as hypertension, cardiovascular disease, depression, and so on) are also associated with a high prevalence of erectile dysfunction, and therefore, it is difficult always to ascribe the cause of erectile dysfunction to the medication.

Neurologic Changes. Stroke and its related disabilities can cause a marked reduction in sexual activity. Reduced libido, mobility, altered visual perception, fear of incontinence, and erectile dysfunction have been associated with stroke. Temporal lobe epilepsy and multiple sclerosis can be associated with erectile dysfunction; the latter disease often presents (in about 60% of cases) with erectile dysfunction. Both autonomic and peripheral neuropathies may be associated with impotence.

Psychological Issues. Many psychosocial factors have already been noted, but it should be mentioned in addition that depression is not an uncommon cause of erectile dysfunction, and depression can also be a consequence of erectile problems, resulting in not only loss of ability to perform an intimate act but also loss of self-esteem, and this may in turn cause mental discord. Loss of libido and the presence of impotence as well as low testosterone levels may be found in depressed men. Anxiety, which increases the adrenergic response, may guarantee erectile difficulty; fear of failure is an important problem in those with impotence. Widower's syndrome occurs when a man feels pressure or guilt in having intercourse, perhaps because of an unfinished grieving process. Although a reduction in libido may occur with stress or illness, the presence of hypogonadism should be sought because libido can improve with testosterone repletion.

Diagnosis

A careful history of the dysfunction (as well as an especially detailed sexual, medical, and psychosocial history) should be obtained. Often this history can define whether the problem is one of erectile dysfunction, ejaculation or orgasmic factors, or loss of libido. Just creating a milieu in which the patient feels comfortable in responding to queries such as, "Do you have any problems (or concerns or difficulty) with having sex? Are you sexually active now? If not, why not?" can help the patient by showing him that it is all right to discuss these issues. Assessment of the patient for depression using a standard tool such as the Beck Depression Inventory or the Yesavage Geriatric Depression Scale should be performed. The physical examination should include careful evaluation of the penis for bands or plaques (Peyronie's disease). Evidence of hypogonadism (decreased testicular size, decreased axillary, pubic, or facial hair) may be found. A neurologic examination should be performed, including testing of the S_2–S_4 reflex arc using the bulbocavernosus reflex (squeezing gently behind the glans and assessing rectal sphincter tightening) or the cremasteric reflex (stroking the thigh should cause the testicle on the ipsilateral side to rise). Altered penile sensation or evidence of peripheral or autonomic dysfunction should be sought. Sensory or reflex deficits were found in 47% of patients in one study.[27] However, such deficits have a variable contribution to erectile dysfunction. The use of penile Doppler studies with or without beta duplex ultrasonography can detect the presence of vascular disease that can predict the risk of cerebrovascular or cardiovascular disorders in asymptomatic individuals.[17] Intracavernosal injections can be used to assess the vascular response to pharmacologic agents; however, it is important to recognize that there is no standard dose, and the patient's anxiety may result in a poor response.

Because many men over the age of 50 are indeed hypogonadal, a total and bioavailable testosterone (BT) level (non-SHBG [weakly bound] testosterone level) should be measured, as well as LH concentration, glucose level, and thyroid function. It is imperative *not* to rely solely on the total testosterone level because this can be normal in the presence of a low BT. Patients with low BT levels should have the prolactin level measured, and it is important to keep in mind that a low or normal LH level may indicate a need for further diagnostic testing to rule out a pituitary tumor. These tests can range from a gonadotropin-releasing hormone (GnRH) stimulation test to magnetic resonance imaging of the pituitary.

Nocturnal penile tumescence testing has little place in the evaluation of the older male; it cannot reasonably distinguish between organic and psychogenic impotence.[28, 29]

Treatment

In patients with a clear-cut problem such as depression, thyroid problems, or hypogonadism,

the appropriate therapy of these conditions should be undertaken. However, because in most patients the cause is multifactorial, there are at present essentially three types of therapy available.

Therapy with a vacuum device (a device that creates negative pressure that enhances the entry of blood into the penis, the erection being maintained by a band or ring) has been a useful modality for many couples. It can be used on its own, or it can be used synergistically with a penile prosthesis or with intracavernosal (penile) injection therapy. Occasional bruising (ecchymosis) of the penis, a tip that may be cooler than normal, having the scrotal skin drawn up when pumping, removal of the band at the end of 30 minutes, and a perceived lack of spontaneity appear to be the only negative features of the vacuum device.

Penile injection therapy in the form of alprostadil (prostaglandin E) has recently been approved by the Food and Drug Administration (FDA).[30] Intracavernosal therapy with papaverine and phentolamine has not been approved, nor has "tri-mix," the combination of alprostadil, papaverine, and phentolamine, although the three-drug mixture appears to be somewhat more effective. The risks of intracavernosal injection therapy include penile bleeding, bruising, and priapism. Long-term effects may include fibrosis, but at present these effects for alprostadil remain unknown. Intraurethral administration of alprostadil has been approved and offers another therapeutic option.

A penile prosthesis should be considered if more conservative measures have failed. Semirigid and inflatable (also called nonhydraulic and hydraulic) devices are the types available. The simplest device (but the one that is more difficult to conceal in the flaccid state) is the semirigid rod; however, infection, device malfunction, and migration or erosion of the device are some of the adverse effects.

DYSFUNCTION IN WOMEN

In women, far less is known about the impact of medication, vascular changes, and many of the other well-known contributors to sexual dysfunction in men. Additionally, anatomic indicators of dysfunction are not as readily apparent as in men. Dyspareunia and orgasmic changes have many causes (Fig. 6–2).

Hormonal and Vascular Problems

All older women undergo the hormonal changes characteristic of menopause. These result in the

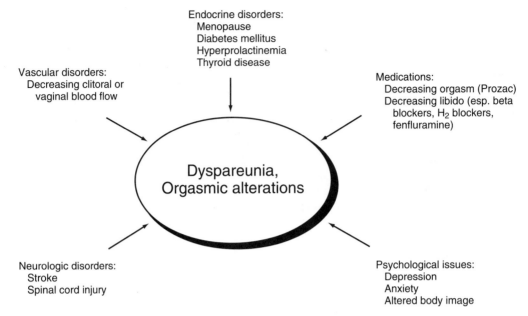

Figure 6–2   Causes of dyspareunia and orgasmic changes.

previously noted changes of decreased lubrication, atrophic vaginitis, and diminished vaginal elasticity. Additionally, reductions in vaginal blood flow and clitoral blood flow occur. Whether these changes are directly attributable to estrogen deficiency or atherosclerosis is not clear. However, because it is also clear that estrogen deficiency carries with it an increased risk of cardiovascular disease and possibly hypertension-accelerating atherosclerosis, a vicious cycle may occur.[31, 32] No data exist on genital neurotransmitter alterations with age or dysfunction. Other hormonal changes may alter libido in women; hyperthyroidism and hypothyroidism, hyperprolactinemia, and Cushing's syndrome may all be associated with impaired sexual function in women. Diabetes has been associated with both orgasmic impairment and decreased vaginal lubrication; however, this appears to be more of a problem in type II diabetes than in type I diabetes. The increased prevalence of vulvovaginal infections in diabetic women may serve as a further deterrent to sexual activity.

Medications

Medication effects on sexual function are barely known in women. Antidepressants such as imipramine may impair orgasmic response, although selective serotonin reuptake inhibitors seem to have little effect with the exception of fluoxetine (Prozac). With fluoxetine, anorgasmia, dysorgasmia, and decreased libido have been noted.[14] Interestingly, trazodone may improve libido (al-

though an improvement in depression usually improves libido as well). Other medications, including beta and H_2 blockers, may diminish libido.[14] Unfortunately, little attention has been paid to the sexual impact on women of the many drugs on the market.

Psychological Problems

Menopause does not increase the occurrence of depression, and the prevalence of major depression may actually decrease with age.[33] Although a variety of diseases, such as Parkinson's disease and stroke, present with depression, and although medications (especially sedative anxiolytics) may cause depression, any chronic illness, stressor, or pain can be associated with depression. Depression may result from lack of sexual activity, including a sense of rejection (whether real or perceived), if the partner's illness or erectile dysfunction makes sexual intimacy a problem, or if the woman is "locked" into an unhappy relationship. Years of accumulated problems may develop gradually into sexual dysfunction. The loss of a partner and the paucity of older men or other available partners may also result in withdrawal from sexual activity.

Neurologic Changes

Diseases such as strokes also affect sexual function in women. Regardless of which hemisphere is involved in a stroke, intercourse frequency diminishes. In women with a left-sided stroke resulting in right-sided paralysis, decreased libido appears to be especially common. Altered body image and continence issues can hamper both sexuality and the emptying of bladder and bowel. A toileting routine can diminish this as a problem.

Multiple sclerosis in women is associated with decreased sexual activity and diminished sensation, loss of vaginal lubrication, and orgasmic dysfunction. Dysfunction was associated with depression and incontinence in this latter study.[34]

Management of Sexual Issues

One of the most important facets of dealing with people with sexual dysfunction is the ability to elicit problems. Unfortunately, there is no validated sexual questionnaire for older women that would enhance this process. Discussion of the physiology of aging and the creation of an "opening" for discussion of sexual issues are vital.

In patients with atrophic vaginitis or loss of lubrication or vaginal elasticity, a frank discussion of a given woman's risks and benefits with hormonal replacement should be undertaken. It should be understood that although topical estrogen is often effective, it may take a year or more for the greatest effect to accrue. Yet it is still associated with many of the same systemic effects characteristic of hormonal therapy. For those who choose not to use estrogen to enhance vaginal lubrication, water-soluble lubricants such as Maxilube, Astroglide, Slick, and Embrace personal lubricant, to name a few, may enhance sexual function. The latter two are less "tenacious," and many women prefer a "closer to natural" lubricant. Different positions can enhance sexual function in those with arthritic or muscular problems. For example, side-by-side spoon fashion can alleviate hip and knee problems.

We must become more accustomed to discussing sexual issues with our patients because therapy for many of their problems is available. The quest for maximizing the quality of life, in which sex and sexuality play so important a role, is one that does not end at any age.

References

1. Covey HC: Perceptions and attitudes toward sexuality of the elderly during the middle ages. Gerontologist 1989;29:93–100.
2. Dodsin B: Sex for one. New York, Crown Publishers, 1987.
3. Starr B, Weiner M: The Starr-Weiner Report on Sex and Sexuality in the Mature Years. New York, Stein and Day, 1981.
4. Bretschneider JG, McCoy NL: Sexual interest and behavior in healthy 80 to 102 year olds. Arch Sex Behav 1988;17:109–129.
5. Kaiser FE: Sexuality in later life. Clin Geriatr Med 1991;7:63–72.
6. Pfeiffer E, Verwoerdt A, Davis GC: Sexual behavior in middle life. Am J Psychiatr 1972;128:1262–1267.
7. Pfeiffer E, Verwoerdt A, Wang HS: Sexual behavior in aged men and women. Arch Gen Psychiatry 1968;19:735–758.
8. Pfeiffer E, Verwoerdt A, Wang HS: The natural history of sexual behavior in a biologically advantaged group of aged individuals. J Gerontol 1969;24:193–198.
9. Marsiglio W, Donnelly D: Sexual relations in later life: A national study of married persons. J Gerontol 1991;46:S38–S44.
10. Diokno AC, Brown MB, Herzog AR: Sexual function in the elderly. Arch Intern Med 1990;150:197–200.
11. Janus SS, Janus CI: The Janus Report on Sexual Behavior. New York, John Wiley, 1993, p. 25.
12. Clements M: Sex after 65—a groundbreaking national survey. Parade March 17, 1996, pp. 4–6.
13. Masters WH, Johnson VE: Human Sexual Response. Boston, Little, Brown, 1966.
14. Anonymous: Drugs that cause sexual dysfunction: An update. Med Lett 1992;34:73–78.
15. Roughan PA, Kaiser FE, Morley JE: Sexuality and the older woman. Clin Geriatr Med 1993;9:87–106.
16. Kaiser FE, Wilson MMG, Morley JE: Menopause and beyond. In Cassel CK, Cohen HJ, Larson EB, et al (eds): Geriatric Medicine, 3rd ed. New York, Springer-Verlag, 1997, pp 527–540.
17. Kaiser FE: Sexuality in the elderly. Urol Clin North Am 1996;23:99–109.
18. Davis SR, McCloud P, Strauss BJG, Burger H: Testosterone enhances estradiol's effects on postmenopausal bone density and sexuality. Maturitas 1995;21:227–236.
19. Sideri M, Origoini M, Spinaci L, Ferrari A: Topical testosterone in the treatment of vulvar lichen sclerosis. Int J Gynecol Obstet 1994;46:53–56.
20. Schiavi RC, Schreiner-Engel P, Mandeli J, et al: Healthy aging and male sexual function. Am J Psychiatr 1990;147:766–771.
21. Korenman SG, Morley JE, Mooradian AD, et al: Secondary hypogonadism in older men: Its relation to impotence. J Clin Endocrinol Metab 1990;71:963–969.
22. Kaiser FE, Morley JE: Gonadotropins, testosterone and the aging male. Neurobiol Aging 1994;15:559–563.
23. Morley JE, Kaiser FE: Hypogonadism in the elderly man. Adv Endocrinol Metab 1993; 4:241–262.
24. Feldman HA, Goldstein I, Hatzichristore DG, et al: Impotence and its medical and psychosocial correlates: Results of the Massachussetts Male Aging study. Urology 1994;151:54–61.
25. Rajfer J, Aronson WJ, Bush PA, et al: Nitric oxide as a mediator of relaxation of the corpus cavernosum in response to nonadrenergic, noncholinergic neurotransmission. N Engl J Med 1992;326:90–94.
26. Lieberman LS: Diabetes and obesity in elderly black Americans. In Jackson JS (ed): The Black American Elderly. New York, Springer, 1988, pp. 130–189.
27. Bemelmans BLH, Meuleman EJH, Antwin BWM, et al: Penile sensory disorders in erectile dysfunction. J Urol 1991;146:777–782.
28. Conra M, Morales A, Surridge D, et al: The unreliability of nocturnal penile tumescence recording as an outcome measurement in the treatment of organic impotence. J Urol 1986;135:280–282.
29. Schiavi RC, Schreiner-Engel P: Nocturnal penile tumescence in healthy aging men. J Gerontol 1988; 43:M146–150.
30. Linet OI, Ogrinc FC: Efficacy and safety of intracavernosal alprostadil in men with erectile

dysfunction. The Alprostadil Study Group. N Engl J Med 1996; 339:873–877.

31. Staessen J, Bulpitt CJ, Fagard R, et al: The influence of menopause on blood pressure. J Human Hypertension 1989;3:427–433.

32. Gordon T, Kannel WB, Hjortland MC, McNamera PM: Menopause and coronary artery disease. The Framingham Study. Ann Intern Med 1978;89:157–161.

33. Musetti L, Perugi G, Soriani A, et al: Depression before and after age 65: A re-examination. Br J Psychiatr 1989;155:330–336.

34. Mattson D, Petrie M, Srivastava DK, McDermott M: Multiple sclerosis, sex dysfunction and its response to medications. Arch Neurol 1995;52:862–868.

Additional Readings

Kaiser FE, Viosca SP, Morley JE, et al: Impotence and aging: Clinical and hormonal factors. J Am Geriatr Soc 1988;36:511–519.

Kaplan HS: Sex, intimacy and the aging process. J Am Acad Psychoanal 1990;3:309–314.

Korenman SG, Viosca SP, Kaiser FE, et al: Use of a vacuum tumescence device in the management of impotence. J Am Geriatr Soc 1990;38:217–220.

Morley JE, Perry HM III, Kaiser FE, et al: Effects of testosterone replacement in old hypogonadal males: A preliminary study. J Am Geriatr Soc 1993;41:149–152.

Myers LS, Dixen J, Morrissett D, et al: Effects of estrogen, androgen, and progestin on sexual psychophysiology and behavior in postmenopausal women. J Clin Endocrinol Metab 1990;40:11124–11131.

National Institutes of Health: Consensus development conference statement: Impotence. Int J Impotence Rep 1993;5:181–199.

Rajfer J, Rosciszewski A, Mehringer M: Prevalence of corporeal venous leakage in impotent men. J Urol 1988;140:69–73.

Tenover JS: Effects of testosterone supplementation in the aging male. J Clin Endocrinol Metab 1992;75:1092–1098.

7 Driving

David B. Reuben, M.D.

The population of older drivers is rapidly increasing. Between 1984 and 1994, the number of licensed drivers 70 years of age or older increased by 45% to 15.7 million.[1] Moreover, the rate of increase will rise dramatically as the "baby boomers" reach age 65 in 2010. Although driving skills appear to be well preserved in healthy older persons,[2] the diseases that accompany aging increase the risk of unsafe driving. As a result, older drivers have the highest crash rate per mile driven of any age group except teenagers. Although older drivers represent only 9% of all licensed drivers, they account for 13% of all traffic fatalities.[1]

Many older drivers, when confronted with the diseases of aging, simply decide to stop driving. Based on several recent studies, the most common factors associated with ceasing to drive include increasing age, female gender, functional impairment, neurologic disease (including dementia, Parkinson's disease, and stroke), and visual impairment.[3-5] Alternatively, older people may change their driving patterns. For example, older persons concentrate their driving during daylight and off-peak hours (9:00 AM to 4:00 PM) and are more likely than younger persons to rely on public transportation for trips more than 75 miles from home. They also tend to drive on surface streets and they avoid freeways, which are safer on a per-mile basis.[6]

Older drivers also tend to be involved in particular types of violations and crashes. Failure to yield the right-of-way or disobedience of signs and signals are major contributors to crashes among older persons.[7] Compared to younger people, they also have a much higher rate of collisions when making left turns but are much less likely to be intoxicated with alcohol when involved in traffic fatalities.

Because licenses to operate a motor vehicle are conferred by the state, it might be argued that the physician has little responsibility in decisions regarding continued driving by his or her patient. However, other than simple tests for gross sensory impairments (e.g., vision testing), state departments of motor vehicles have little insight into age-related physiologic changes and medical conditions that may impair driving ability. Moreover, the physician's relationship to the patient as his or her advocate allows the issue of whether to continue driving to be raised in the context of concern about the well-being of the patient rather than in the administrative setting of a licensing station. This relationship can also extend to assistance by the physician in mobilizing family and social service resources to help maintain the older person's mobility in the community in the absence of driving. Often a frank discussion and careful planning can obviate a stressful and sometimes humiliating experience with state licensing authorities. Thus, the roles of the physician and the state in regard to the older driver are complementary.

The physician can best address the possibility of age-related disabilities that may impair the capacity to drive by knowing the potential risks of physiologic changes and the common diseases that occur with aging, inquiring about the presence or absence of these, and searching for pertinent findings on physical examination. Physicians must also know and follow state guidelines for reporting potentially unsafe drivers.

PATHOPHYSIOLOGY

Age-Related Physiologic Changes that May Affect Driving

There are three general categories of age-related physiologic changes that may affect driving: sensory, cognitive, and psychomotor functioning, including reaction time[8] (Table 7–1). Among sensory changes, those affecting visual function are most important. However, with some exceptions, the data linking these changes to violations and collisions are inconclusive. Constriction of horizontal visual fields, alone or combined with measures of visual acuity and contrast sensitivity,[9] has been predictive of crashes. Among cognitive changes, impaired visual attention as measured by the useful field of view has been associated with crashes during the previous 5-year period.[10]

Diseases and Disorders Commonly Occurring in Older Persons that May Affect Driving

Far more important than age-related physiologic changes in determining the risks of unsafe driv-

TABLE 7–1 **AGE-RELATED PHYSIOLOGIC CHANGES THAT MAY AFFECT DRIVING**

Sensory Changes	Cognitive Changes	Psychomotor Changes
Presbycusis (hearing loss)	Distraction by irrelevant	Slowed speed of behavior
Visual decrements in:	stimuli	Decreased reaction time
Static visual acuity	Memory retrieval impairment	Declines° in
Acuity under low lumination	Decline in spatial orientation	Strength
Resistance to glare	Decreased visual searching	Range of motion
Contrast sensitivity (static	Decreased visuomotor	Trunk and neck mobility
and dynamic)	integration	Proprioception
Visual fields		
Depth perception		

°The contribution of age-related changes versus deconditioning and diseases remains unclear.

ing are diseases that affect older people (Table 7–2). For many of these diseases and disorders, the relationship is only speculative. However, recent epidemiologic studies have clarified the risk for some conditions. The most consistent relationships have been demonstrated for neurologic diseases and diabetes mellitus, and there is lesser support for coronary artery disease, depression, alcohol abuse, falls, and foot disorders.[11, 12]

The cognitive impairments that define dementia—including the hallmark features of memory loss, visual-spatial disturbances, and impaired judgment—place the person with dementia at increased risk for unsafe driving. Other, more subtle impairments that are characteristic of patients with Alzheimer's disease, such as poor ability to engage in divided attention, poor ability to engage in selective focused attention,[13] and visual field limitations,[14] may contribute to or aggravate this risk. The potential risk of unsafe driving by drivers with dementia has been substantiated in most[15–18] though not all[19] retrospective studies that have demonstrated higher rates of motor vehicle crashes and in performance-

based studies that have demonstrated poor driving skills on road tests.[13, 20, 21] Although the precise magnitude of risk incurred by the driver who has dementia cannot be estimated from the existing literature, this risk is likely to be substantial. One study reported that 33% of demented persons who were still driving had had motor vehicle crashes or moving violations within the previous 6 months.[1]

An increased risk of motor vehicle crashes has also been demonstrated for persons with advanced Parkinson's disease[22] and seizures, although the increased risk for the latter is modest.[23] Because of the wide variation in deficits that accompany stroke, the risk associated with this disorder has been particularly difficult to assess.

Despite the presumed risk of crashes due to arrhythmias, sudden death, and ischemia, well-designed studies that substantiate or estimate the magnitude of such risks are lacking. Although a small study demonstrated that persons with severe sleep apnea had higher crash rates than all drivers in Virginia,[24] studies assessing crash risk

TABLE 7–2 **DISEASES AND DISORDERS THAT COMMONLY OCCUR IN OLDER PERSONS AND MAY AFFECT DRIVING**

Neurologic Diseases	Cardiovascular and Pulmonary Diseases	Metabolic Diseases	Arthritis and Functional Impairment	Eye Diseases	Drugs
Dementia	Coronary artery	Diabetes	Osteoarthritis	Age-related	Alcohol
Parkinson's	disease	mellitus	Falls	macular	Antidepressants
disease	Arrhythmias		Functional	degeneration	Antihistamines
Seizures	Sleep apnea		impairment	Cataracts	Antipsychotics
Stroke	Chronic			Diabetic	Benzodiazepines
Neuropathies	obstructive			retinopathy	Hypnotics
	pulmonary			Glaucoma	Muscle
	disease				relaxants
					Narcotics

in drivers with chronic obstructive pulmonary disease have not been conducted.

Diabetes can increase the risk of unsafe driving because of the effects of the disease (e.g., blurred vision due to poor metabolic control, retinopathy, neuropathy) or complications associated with treatment (e.g., hypoglycemia). The risk of collisions resulting in injury to older persons with diabetes has become better defined. The risks were substantially increased among all older diabetic drivers, particularly those taking insulin or oral agents, those with disease of more than 5 years' duration, and those with coexisting coronary heart disease.[11] In contrast, those who had had the disease for a short time and those being treated with diet alone had no increased risk. These findings are consistent with a variety of explanations but certainly raise concern about the increased risk that might be associated with increased efforts to achieve tight blood glucose control.

Although arthritis is the most common self-reported condition among older persons, and the accompanying limitations in range of motion (e.g., difficulty in turning and looking to the rear to change lanes) might affect safe driving, the impact of arthritis on adverse driving events (e.g., violations and crashes) has not been systematically studied. However, foot deformities and impairment in functional status (not walking at least a block a day) have been associated with automobile crashes and moving violations.[12]

Eye diseases, which are common among older persons, probably increase the risk of unsafe driving through the same mechanisms described earlier under age-associated physiologic changes. Although all eye diseases may decrease visual acuity, some produce other characteristic effects (e.g., visual field loss with glaucoma, reduced contrast sensitivity with glaucoma or cataract, decreased resistance to glare with cataract) that may augment the risk beyond that of a simple loss of acuity.

The role of drugs in increasing the risk of unsafe driving may be substantial given the wide use of medications that have psychoactive properties in older persons. Other than alcohol, which remains a contributing factor in fatal crashes among persons 70 years of age or older (albeit less frequently than in younger people), research on the risks associated with prescribed medications has been inconsistent. The most convincing data implicate cyclic antidepressants and benzodiazepines.[25] Nevertheless, the systemic effects, particularly those on cognitive and psychomotor function, of many medications commonly used in treating older persons (see Table 7–2) have

the potential to compromise driving safety in individual patients.

CLINICAL ASSESSMENT

Few clinicians caring for older persons routinely focus specifically on the patient's driving capabilities in the course of giving clinical care. Rather, driving problems usually are brought to the physician's attention by family members or other concerned parties. Nevertheless, the salient points regarding assessment of medical considerations relevant to driving can be integrated into the standard initial and subsequent evaluation and management of the older patient.

For example, the use of a previsit questionnaire that can be completed by patients, family members, or caregivers can identify the medical conditions and medications mentioned earlier[26] and can determine whether the patient currently drives. Patients who are still driving should be asked about crashes, "near misses", or moving violations. If any of these have occurred, the circumstances should be determined. Sometimes simple suggestions may allow the patient to continue to drive safely under designated conditions. For example, if a patient with cataracts and visual acuity that is not severely compromised has had "near misses" at night, such an individual may be able to continue to drive safely by restricting driving to the daytime. Many states have adopted the practice of granting graduated or restricted licenses that permit driving only under specified conditions. If there is a concern about safe driving based on any medical considerations identified, a more detailed history of the person's driving patterns should be determined. Perhaps most important is a determination of the person's need to continue to drive. For example, does the patient need to drive to perform essential errands such as shopping and banking? Are other alternatives (e.g., shopping services, family members, neighbors) available to provide these services should the person cease driving?

The physical examination should focus on vision, mental status, mobility, and possible neurologic conditions. For most older persons, there is no need for a separate "driving-specific" examination. For example, copying a pentagon, which is a component of the commonly employed Mini-Mental State Examination, has been found to be an independent predictor of adverse driving events.[12] Visual acuity, which can be tested by office staff using a Snellen eye chart, is only one component of the visual function necessary for safe driving. More detailed visual testing (e.g., visual field testing) is usually conducted by an optometrist or ophthalmologist, and these records should be requested if there is a question about visual impairment. Gait, balance, and mobility evaluations, including cervical neck motion, are components of the initial physical examination of most older persons. In conducting these examinations the clinician must be aware that impairments discovered on the standard examination may contribute to unsafe driving, and he or she must synthesize the relevant information accordingly.

The physician's ability to assess driving capability adequately is quite limited but can be supplemented by appropriate referral to rehabilitation therapists, particularly occupational therapists, who have developed expertise in assessing and treating physically impaired drivers. Frequently, these assessments include simulators and on-road evaluations. Unfortunately, the quality of driver assessment programs varies widely, and physicians must often learn by word-of-mouth about the availability of reliable programs in their geographic area.

A variety of formal tests of skills and function have been developed in an attempt to identify older drivers who are at increased risk for motor vehicle accidents. Although some of these have shown promise in correctly identifying those at risk, they are still best regarded as research tools that may eventually be incorporated into clinical practice or, more likely, into driver licensing procedures.

MANAGEMENT

Management of the older patient who is at risk for driving unsafely consists of appropriate treatment for any medical conditions and age-associated physiologic changes, careful consideration of the ethical issues involved, and compliance with state laws. In addition, sometimes vehicle modifications and assistive devices can attenuate some of the risk associated with medical impairments.

Once a medical condition has been identified, optimal treatment should be initiated in an attempt to reduce its potential risk. This treatment may be as simple as providing the appropriate refraction to improve visual acuity or discontinuing an inappropriate medication. Unfortunately, in many cases medical management is more complicated with respect to its impact on driving. For example, the goal of treatment of diabetes may be excellent metabolic control to forestall the vascular complications of the disease. Such control may result in hypoglycemic episodes that substantially increase the risk of accidents. Other disorders, such as dementia, are resistant to medical therapy.

With many patients, the physician is faced with the decision of whether to recommend that the patient cease driving. Such decisions are usually difficult, particularly if no alternative methods are available to meet the patient's transportation needs. Some patients may be willing to take the risk of a fatal crash if it means that they can continue to maintain their independence. The physician may feel torn between preserving the independence and autonomy of the patient and protecting society against an unsafe driver. In these cases, the physician must depart from the traditional role of patient advocate in recommending that the patient cease driving. Such decisions are particularly difficult in states that have mandatory reporting requirements (e.g., in California, physicians must report patients who have Alzheimer's disease and related disorders) and are likely to have a negative impact on the physician-patient relationship. Nevertheless, physicians must comply with such regulations or they may be subject to loss of their medical license as well as legal liability should one of their patients who should have been reported be involved in a collision.

State-initiated policies may be effective in reducing fatal accidents. A recent analysis of license renewal policies and fatal crashes involving drivers aged 70 years or older demonstrated that state-mandated tests of visual acuity were associated with lower fatal crash rates.[27] Several states are developing and testing performance-based methods of assessing risk for adverse driving events among older drivers. Such methods will probably be used as screening tests that can be administered quickly to identify those who need more extensive testing, such as on-road driving tests. The National Highway Traffic Safety Administration has also become interested in promoting increased reporting of potentially unsafe driving by family members. As these methods are refined further, the physician will be increasingly relied on to optimize medical treatment and provide information on the severity and prognosis of medical conditions.

References

1. National Highway Traffic Safety Administration: Traffic Safety Facts 1994: Older Population. Washington, DC, U.S. Department of Transportation, 1994.
2. Carr D, Jackson WJ, Madden DJ, Cohen HJ: The effect of age on driving skills. J Am Geriatr Soc 1992;40:567–573.
3. Kington R, Reuben D, Rogowski J, Lillard L: Sociodemographic and health factors in driving patterns after 50 years of age. Am J Pub Hlth 1994; 84:1327–1329.
4. Campbell MK, Bush TL, Hale WE: Medical conditions associated with driving cessation in community-

dwelling, ambulatory elders. J Gerontol Soc Sci 1993;48:S230–S234.

5. Marottoli RA, Ostfeld AM, Merrill SS, Perlman GD, Foley DJ, Cooney LM: Driving cessation and changes in mileage driven among elderly individuals. J Gerontol Soc Sci 1993;48:S255–S260.

6. Janke MK: Age-Related Disabilities that May Impair Driving and Their Assessment (literature review). National Highway Traffic Safety Administration, RSS-94-156. Sacramento, CA, California Department of Motor Vehicles, 1994, pp. 1–379.

7. Gebers MA, Romanowicz PA, McKenzie DM: Teen and Senior Drivers. Sacramento, CA, California Department of Motor Vehicles, 1993.

8. Fozard JL, Vercruyssen M, Reynolds SL, Hancock PA, Quilter RE: Age differences and changes in reaction time: The Baltimore longitudinal study of aging. J Gerontol Psych Sci 1994;49:P179–P189.

9. Decina LE, Staplin L: Retrospective evaluation of alternative vision screening criteria for older and younger drivers. Accid Anal Prev 1993;25:267–275.

10. Ball K, Owsley C, Sloane ME, Roenker DL, Bruni JR: Visual attention problems as a predictor of vehicle crashes in older drivers. Invest Ophthalmol Vis Sci 1993;34:3110–3123.

11. Koepsell TD, Wolf ME, McCloskey L, et al: Medical conditions and motor vehicle collision injuries in older adults. J Am Geriatr Soc 1994;42:695–700.

12. Marottoli RA, Cooney LM Jr, Wagner DR, Doucette J, Tinetti ME: Predictors of automobile crashes and moving violations among elderly drivers. Ann Intern Med 1994;121:842–846.

13. Fitten LJ, Perryman KM, Wilkinson CJ, et al: Alzheimer and vascular dementias and driving: A prospective road and laboratory study. JAMA 1995;273:1360–1365.

14. Steffes R, Thralow J: Visual field limitation in the patient with dementia of the Alzheimer's type. J Am Geriatr Soc 1987;35:198–204.

15. Friedland RP, Koss E, Kumar A, et al: Motor vehicle crashes in dementia of the Alzheimer type. Ann Neurol 1988;24:782–786.

16. Lucas-Blaustein MJ, Filipp L, Dungan C, Tune L: Driving in patients with dementia. J Am Geriatr Soc 1988;36:1087–1091.

17. Gilley DW, Wilson RS, Bennett DA, et al: Cessation of driving and unsafe motor vehicle operation by dementia patients. Arch Intern Med 1991;151:941–946.

18. Dubinsky RM, Williamson A, Gray CS, Glatt SL: Driving in Alzheimer's disease. J Am Geriatric Soc 1992;40:1112–1116.

19. Waller PF, Trobe JD, Olson PL, Teshima S, Cook-Flannagan C: Crash characteristics associated with early Alzheimer's disease. Presented at the 37th Annual Proceedings, Association for the Advancement of Automotive Medicine, San Antonio, Texas, November 1993.

20. Hunt L, Morris JC, Edwards D, Wilson BS: Driving performance in persons with mild senile dementia of the Alzheimer type. J Am Geriatr Soc 1993;41:747–753.

21. Odenheimer G, Albert M, Jette A, Beaudet M, Grande L, Minaker K: Cognitive skills are related to driving performance in the elderly (abstract). J Am Geriatr Soc 1991;39:A9.

22. Dubinsky RM, Gray C, Husted D, et al: Driving in Parkinson's disease. Neurology 1991;41:517–520.

23. Hansotia P, Broste SK: The effect of epilepsy or diabetes mellitus on the risk of automobile accidents. N Engl J Med 1991;324:22–26.

24. Findley LJ, Fabrizio M, Thommi G, Suratt PM: Severity of sleep apnea and automobile crashes (letter). N Engl J Med 1989;320:868–869.

25. Ray WA, Fought RL, Decker MD: Psychoactive drugs and the risk of injurious motor vehicle crashes in elderly drivers. Am J Epidemiol 1992;136:873–883.

26. Reuben DB, Yoshikawa TT, Besdine RB, et al (eds): Geriatrics Review Syllabus: A Core Curriculum. *In* Geriatric Medicine, 3rd ed. New York, American Geriatrics Society, 1997.

27. Levy DT, Vernick JS, Howard KA: Relationship between driver's license renewal policies and fatal crashes involving drivers 70 years or older. JAMA 1995;274:1026–1030.

SECTION

II

Systems of Care in Geriatric Practice

8 Acute Care

Robert Marshall Palmer, M.D., M.P.H.

Whereas hospitalization offers older patients the potential benefits of specialty consultation and advances in medical technology, it also exposes them to the risks of iatrogenic illness and functional decline (a loss of independence in self-care activities). Knowledge of the risks of hospitalization and the management of common geriatric syndromes, however, helps primary physicians optimize their patients' independent self-care and quality of life.

AGING AND HOSPITALIZATION

Patients aged 65 years and older account for 31% of hospital discharges and 42% of inpatient days of care.[1] Rates of hospitalization are higher for the age group 85 years and older compared to the age group of 65 to 74 years. These trends continue despite changes in health care delivery such as that of the prospective payment system and the growth of managed care programs. Compared to younger patients, elderly patients have longer and more frequent hospitalizations, and the severity of illness is greater. Even when older patients recover from acute illnesses they may remain too functionally impaired to return home safely, necessitating discharge to a subacute care or long-term care facility. Early unplanned readmissions from these settings or from home are common for elderly patients, especially those with acute exacerbations of chronic diseases such as congestive heart failure.

Longitudinal studies demonstrate that a small proportion of older adults are consistently extensive users of hospital services. In the Longitudinal Study on Aging, a population-based study of 7527 individuals aged 70 years or older who were followed by interview from 1984 through 1991, 42.6% had no hospital episodes; among those with one or more hospital admissions, hospitalization occurred less than once a year among survivors as a rule, whereas about 20% of survivors and decedents were consistently high users of hospitalizations.[2] These data imply a need for physicians to target their efforts to prevent functional decline in the high-risk patient, many of whom have chronic medical conditions, functional impairments at admission, and inadequate social supports at home.

GERIATRIC SYNDROMES: DETECTION AND MANAGEMENT

Hospitalized elderly patients are likely to show evidence of one or more of the common geriatric syndromes. Among the most important of these are iatrogenic illness, functional dependency (functional decline), cognitive dysfunction, immobility, depression, and undernutrition. Despite their high frequency among hospitalized elderly patients, these syndromes are often unrecognized or are not addressed. A systematic assessment for each of these syndromes, however, is achievable and can be facilitated through interdisciplinary collaboration and the use of common screening instruments. Interventions directed at detection and management of these syndromes will help to optimize patient care and improve the functional outcomes of hospitalization (Table 8–1).

Iatrogenic Illness

Iatrogenic illness is any illness that results from a diagnostic procedure or therapeutic intervention or any harmful occurrence that is not a natural consequence of the patient's underlying illness. Iatrogenic illness may be categorized as cardiopulmonary complications, hospital-acquired infections (for example, urosepsis following insertion of an indwelling catheter), adverse drug events, complications of diagnostic or therapeutic procedures, unintentional injuries, or nonspecific events (e.g. pressure sores).[3] Rates of iatrogenic illness and negligence are higher in elderly patients, in part because of the higher rates of comorbid illness in these patients and their longer lengths of hospitalization.

Iatrogenic illnesses are potentially preventable (see Table 8–1). In particular, careful attention to the prescription of drugs and the rational use of medications will help to lessen the risk of iatrogenic effect. Drugs with psychoactive effects, especially benzodiazepines and narcotic

---

TABLE 8–1   **GERIATRIC SYNDROMES: PREVENTION AND MANAGEMENT**

Iatrogenic Illnesses

- *Practice rational drug prescribing.* Know pharmacology in relation to aging. Avoid psychoactive drugs when alternatives are available. If possible, avoid using two or more drugs affecting phase I (cytochrome P450) hepatic metabolism. Use lower than usual maintenance doses of renally excreted drugs. Consider therapeutic drug monitoring.
- *Avoid nosocomial infection.* Use hygienic handwashing techniques. Narrow the spectrum of empirically selected antibiotics when cultures are completed. Avoid or discontinue continuous urethral catheterization.
- *Minimize the use of risky diagnostic studies.* Avoid contrast studies when equally useful alternatives are available. Maintain patient hydration before and after studies. Avoid duplicative studies (e.g., both barium and endoscopic gastrointestinal studies).

Functional Dependency

- *Modify physical environment.* Unclutter hallways, add handrails and grab bars, add clocks and calendars to patient rooms.
- *Perform functional assessment at admission.* Document changes from baseline in basic activities of daily living, cognition, and ambulation. Observe patient's ability to sit up in bed, transfer to chair, and walk in room.
- *Link functional assessment to interventions.* Prescribe assistive devices (cane, walkers) to promote ambulation. Prescribe toileting schedule. Prescribe food supplements or snacks. Prescribe activity orders.

Cognitive Dysfunction

- *Assess mental status daily.* Establish baseline level of cognition. Identify delirium—acute onset and fluctuating course, inattention, disorganized thinking or altered level of consciousness.
- *Avoid precipitating delirium.* Avoid polypharmacy, iatrogenic illness, use of bladder catheter, and undernutrition.
- *Apply behavioral and environmental interventions* such as reality orientation, quiet room, soft lights, correction of sensory impairments (vision and hearing aids, headphones with amplifier), family members or sitters at bedside.
- *Prescribe psychotropic drugs judiciously.* Low doses of neuroleptics (e.g., haloperidol 0.5 to 1.0 mg IM) for treatment of psychotic symptoms or benzodiazepines (e.g., lorazepam 0.5 to 1.0 mg PO or IM) for associated anxiety.

Depression

- *Assess mood at admission and detect depression.* Use depression screening instruments. Suspect depression in patients who are withdrawn, irritable, or uncooperative, or who present with a "failure to thrive."
- *Apply behavioral, environmental, and physical interventions* such as psychological counseling (e.g., consult a psychiatric clinical nurse specialist), socialization with family or other patients (e.g., in an activity room), occupational and physical therapy.
- *Consider psychiatric consultation.* To clarify diagnosis, initiate antidepressant drug therapy and arrange follow-up care.

Immobility

- *Prescribe activity orders.* For bed-confined patients—range of motion exercises for hips, knees, ankles, and trunk; for unsteady patients—assisted ambulation, use of walker, low-impact resistive exercises of lower extremities.
- *Avoid physical and chemical restraints.* Consider alternatives such as an activity room or family member or bedside sitter. Change treatments to avoid the need to restrain mobility (e.g., intermittent rather than continuous tube feedings).

Undernutrition

- *Assess nutritional status at admission and daily.* Identify patients with low body weight, diminished visceral and somatic proteins, and dehydration, and measure quantities of food and fluids consumed by them daily.
- *Prescribe food supplements* for malnourished patients and for patients with inadequate caloric intake.
- *Consider nutrition support team consultation* for patients needing central or peripheral alimentation or percutaneous endoscopic gastrostomy.
- *Consider swallowing evaluation* for patients at risk for oropharyngeal dysphagia and pulmonary aspiration (e.g., for confused or generally weak patients).

agents, are potential causes of cognitive impairment in elderly hospitalized patients. The risk of cognitive impairment from benzodiazepines is greater in patients who have abnormal cognitive function when they are admitted. These and other psychoactive drugs should be used judiciously in high-risk patients (e.g., patients with dementia or malnutrition). Drug-drug interactions, leading to adverse drug events, may occur when patients receive two or more drugs that undergo biotransformation in the liver by the cytochrome P450 oxidase system (e.g., diazepam and theophylline); act as inducers (e.g., phenobarbital) or inhibitors (e.g., cimetidine) of the microsomal oxidases; or compete for protein binding, especially albumin (e.g., warfarin and sulfa antibiotics), thereby increasing the availability of the unbound portion of the agent at the receptor site. Thus, the risk of adverse drug events can be reduced by prescribing drugs without known drug-drug interactions (e.g., hydrophilic drugs that undergo hepatic conjugation); by cautiously monitoring patients who receive drugs known to have narrow therapeutic windows (e.g., warfarin, gentamicin); and by adjusting the doses of drugs that compete for albumin binding.

Iatrogenic illness may be manifested as a nosocomial infection—e.g., from the use of broad-spectrum antibiotics that eliminate normal flora and lead to infections due to resistant microorganisms. Nosocomial infections can also be transmitted by professional caregivers or hardware (e.g., unclean stethoscopes). Nosocomial urinary tract infections are likely to occur in patients who undergo prolonged urethral catheterization. However, if careful attention is paid to hygienic handwashing techniques, cleaning of medical equipment, and the use of alternatives to continuous catheterization, the risk of iatrogenic illness can be reduced.

Functional Dependency

At the time of hospital admission, over half of patients aged 70 years and older who are admitted for medical illness are dependent in one or more activities of daily living.[4] From admission to discharge, 25% to 35% of elderly patients lose independence in one or more of the basic activities of daily living. The loss of independent functioning during hospitalization is associated with important sequelae including prolonged length of hospital stay, greater risk of institutionalization, and, in some studies, higher mortality rates.[4]

The pathogenesis of functional decline is complex and involves an interaction among aging,

hospitalization, acute illness, and comorbid illnesses. Elderly patients are predisposed to functional decline related to the impact of multiple comorbid conditions, impaired homeostatic reserves, and elements of hospitalization (e.g., physical restraint) that limit mobility and self-care.

Patients at risk of functional decline in the hospital can be identified at the time of hospital admission. Functional decline occurs more often in patients aged 75 years and older, those with cognitive impairment as indicated by correct responses to fewer than 15 of the first 21 items on the mini-mental state examination, and those who are dependent in two or more instrumental activities of daily living prior to admission.[5] Functional decline in hospital may also occur more often in patients who are admitted with a pressure sore, baseline functional dependency, or a history of low social activity level.[6] Symptoms of depression and delirium are consistently associated with functional decline and with poor recovery in both functional and psychosocial status following hospitalization.

Detection of functional impairment is achievable through self-reports of basic activities of daily living (ADL) and bedside observations. During their work rounds, physicians and nurses can observe a patient's ability to bathe, dress, transfer from bed to chair, toilet, and eat independently, and they can monitor the patient's ability to maintain continence. Balance and gait can be assessed simply by observing the patient getting out of bed or up from the chair and walking to the door of the room and back.

Patients with impaired independence in performance of basic ADL, gait, or ambulation often benefit from physical and occupational therapy consultation. Graded bedside exercises, increased physical activity, avoidance of restraints, and the use of assistive devices or aids may help to enhance the patient's independent self-care.

Cognitive Dysfunction

Elderly patients are often admitted with evidence of cognitive dysfunction, commonly attributable to either dementia or delirium. Dementia is the single most important risk factor for the development of delirium or acute confusional state.[7] Delirium is found at admission or during hospitalization in about 25% of elderly patients admitted for acute medical illnesses. Patients with baseline dementia and severe systemic illness are predisposed to delirium. Factors known to precipitate delirium include the use of physical restraints, the addition of more than three medications to the regimen, the use of a bladder catheter, malnutrition, and any iatrogenic event.[3] These precipitating factors are potentially amenable to medical intervention (e.g., alternatives to physical restraint), underscoring the importance of a careful assessment of risk factors in every elderly hospitalized patient.

The diagnosis of delirium is suspected in patients with changes in mental status—impaired alertness, orientation, behavior, and perception. The diagnosis is further confirmed through bedside observations including brief tests of attention (e.g., digit span) and cognition (e.g., mental status examination); through interviews with family members and caregivers to ascertain the baseline level of cognition and the presence of recent changes; and through a review of progress notes and nurses' observations to determine whether patients have had a fluctuating course in hospital, inappropriate behaviors, and delusions or hallucinations. The confusion assessment method (CAM) provides good sensitivity and specificity for the diagnosis of delirium: delirium is likely in patients with a change in mental status characterized by an acute onset and fluctuating course, inattention, and either disorganized thinking or an altered level of consciousness.[7]

The diagnosis of delirium should lead to intensive investigation of its cause and management (see Chapter 27). Both medical treatments and behavioral approaches are effective in alleviating the symptoms of delirium. In selected cases, low doses of anxiolytics or neuroleptics are indicated for treating patients with severe anxiety, delusions, or hallucinations. The symptoms of delirium may persist following hospital discharge. Many of these patients fail to return to their baseline level of cognition, and in their self-care abilities may remain impaired, suggesting the need for careful follow-up of their cognition level following hospital discharge.

Depression

Symptoms of depression are present in 10% to 25% of older patients at hospital admission and may coincide with symptoms of anxiety. In the absence of typical symptoms or a past history of major depression, a diagnosis of depression should be suspected in patients who appear withdrawn, uncooperative, or intermittently agitated. These patients are often functionally impaired and may have cognitive deficits. Detection of depressive symptoms is achievable with case-finding instruments such as the Geriatric Depression Scale or observations of the patient's mood by professional caregivers or family members.

Therapy of patients with depressive symptoms includes environmental, psychosocial, and pharmacologic interventions. Environmental changes, physical and occupational therapy, increased frequency of family visits, and psychological counseling may be of immediate benefit to the depressed patient. Psychiatric consultation is most useful in characterizing the depressive disorder and in initiating antidepressant drug therapy. Therapies begun in the hospital should be continued following discharge to maximize their effectiveness.

Immobility

Aging, decreasing muscle mass and strength, diminished physiologic reserves, and acute illness combine to predispose older patients to immobility and functional decline.[8] During an acute illness, many older patients prefer to remain in bed. However, sustained bedrest has adverse physiologic effects. For example, it leads to cardiac deconditioning, muscle atrophy, and accelerated loss of muscle strength. After several days of prolonged bedrest, many older patients are unable to transfer from bed to chair or to stand without assistance. The deleterious effects of acute illness and immobility are further exacerbated by bedrest, the use of physical or chemical restraints, restrictions on patient mobility imposed by intravenous lines and catheters, and limitations on independent mobility due to environmental conditions, such as absent handrails in hallways or slippery floors.[4, 8]

Patient mobility can be readily evaluated through observations of patient transfers and walking and can be addressed each day during hospital rounds. Activities that maintain joint function and strength of the lower extremities should be prescribed on the first hospital day, particularly for bedbound patients. As patients convalesce from acute illnesses, the intensity of prescribed exercises should increase. Prescribed exercises range in intensity from both passive and active range of motion of joints to resistive exercises of the lower extremities and assisted ambulation and to even more rigorous exercises performed in the physical therapy department. Low-impact resistance exercises are especially recommended for bedbound patients to maintain the strength of the lower extremities until they regain weight-bearing capacity. Gentle resistance or pressure is applied by hand as the patient completes foot circles (pressure is applied to the ankle as each foot moves around in a circle), knee bends (pressure is applied as the patient straightens each leg), leg lifts (pressure is applied as the patient lifts each leg off the bed), and side leg stretches (pressure is applied to each leg during abduction). In many hospitals these exercises are conducted by nursing care assistants or physical therapy technicians with a physician's order. Patients at high risk of falls and those who develop postural instability or gait impairment are evaluated by physical therapy. The value of these exercises is worth underscoring; even the marginal benefits of aerobic and resistive exercises may enable the patient to regain the physical independence needed to return home rather than entering a nursing care facility following hospital discharge.

Patients whose activity is limited to bed or chair are at risk for development of stage II (or greater) pressure ulcers. Ulcers occur more often in patients who have nonblanchable erythema, lymphopenia, immobility, dry skin, and decreased body weight.[9] Patients with these risk factors need aggressive mobilization to avoid developing pressure sores.

Undernutrition

Malnutrition is present in 30% to 40% of elderly hospitalized patients with medical illnesses.[4] Elderly patients are at risk for undernutrition before and during hospitalization. The risks are due to the common concurrence of chronic medical illnesses (e.g., heart failure, chronic obstructive pulmonary disease), cognitive impairment, social isolation, poor dentition, reduced thirst perception, and limited access to food and fluids. Protein-calorie malnutrition is associated with functional dependency and contributes to a higher risk of death from chronic diseases such as congestive heart failure.[10]

Malnutrition is diagnosable on the basis of objective anthropometric measurements such as scapular skin-fold thickness and body mass index and on biochemical measures of nutrition. Malnutrition can be suspected on clinical grounds in patients who report a significant history of weight loss in the previous 6 months and who have physical findings suggestive of malnutrition (loss of subcutaneous fat, muscle wasting, ankle edema, sacral edema, and ascites). Many of these patients also have abnormal biochemical parameters consistent with a diagnosis of protein-calorie malnutrition—e.g., a serum albumin level of below 3.5 g/dL, normocytic anemia, and a serum cholesterol level of less than 160 mg/dL). They may also have anergy to common antigens, a low total lymphocyte count, and depressed levels of transferrin or prealbumin.

Patients who are identified as malnourished at admission or who are at high risk of undernutrition in hospital (e.g., patients who have impaired self-feeding ability or are cognitively impaired) may benefit from consultation with a dietitian and from prescribed and monitored quantities of food and fluids consumed daily. For some of these patients, calorie-dense and nutritious but palatable food supplements or snacks can be offered. Patients with generalized weakness or a history suggestive of aspiration pneumonia should be carefully assessed for oropharyngeal dysphagia. Formal evaluation of swallowing conducted by a speech therapist and complemented by a modified barium swallow examination is useful when patients are at risk for aspiration pneumonia. Patients with dysphagia when swallowing liquids may benefit from a pureed diet or thickened liquids, which enable them to swallow safely and provide sufficient calories and hydration.

Patients with a significant risk of aspiration due to severe oropharyngeal dysphagia or to severe weakness or confusion may require short-term enteral or parenteral alimentation. Enteral dietary supplementation was shown to reduce the rate of complications and mortality in patients with hip fractures who were given a balanced nutritional supplement.[11] The benefits and risks of nasoenteral supplementation should be discussed with the patient and with family members prior to placement of the feeding tube. A percutaneous endoscopic gastrostomy tube should be considered for patients who are severely malnourished or have dysphagia that is unlikely to resolve in the foreseeable future. When enteral alimentation is contraindicated for an indefinite period of time (e.g., due to bowel obstruction or inflammatory bowel disease), total parenteral nutrition should be considered following consultation with the nutrition support team.

PATIENT VALUES AND COMFORT

The patient's personal values and perceptions of the hospital experience should be sought early in the course of hospitalization. Because many acutely ill patients may lose their ability to make medical care decisions, preferences for care and advance directives should be reviewed early in the hospitalization with the patient and family members. The patient's expectations of treatment and attitudes toward cardiopulmonary resuscitation may serve to guide medical treatment. This information can assist the physician in making critical decisions about the aggressiveness of diagnostic evaluation or the management of difficult medical problems (e.g., whether to transfer a patient to an intensive care unit or to undertake invasive diagnostic or therapeutic interventions).

Periodic discussions with the patient and family members also help to allay their fears and anxieties about hospitalization, the patient's illness, the prognosis, and home care requirements. The patient's personal and emotional needs can be further supported through other measures including continuity of nursing care, correction of sensory deficits, reality orientation, and a quiet environment that promotes relaxation and sleep at night.[4]

INTERDISCIPLINARY COLLABORATION

The complex physical, psychosocial, and medical needs of older patients are often best addressed through interdisciplinary collaboration. Physicians work with a variety of health care professionals, each of whom has an important role to play in the complex assessment and management of elderly patients (Table 8–2). Collaboration between the physician and nurses is of paramount importance. This collaboration facilitates early detection of treatable functional impairments that may benefit from interdisciplinary interventions (e.g., physical therapy evaluation for patients with generalized weakness, or dietitian consultation for patients with malnutrition). The physician and nurse may agree on specific care plans for the patient including clinical pathways and the need to include other health professionals in the patient's hospital management.

Interdisciplinary collaboration between physicians and other health professionals has beneficial effects on patient outcomes. The effectiveness of a nurse-directed, multidisciplinary intervention on rates of hospital readmission of elderly patients with congestive heart failure was recently demonstrated.[12] Elderly patients receiving the intervention—comprehensive education

---

TABLE 8–2 **THE INTERDISCIPLINARY TEAM**

Team Member	Roles
Patient's nurse and nurse specialist	Assess functional status (basic and instrumental activities of daily living, risk of falling, cognition, mood, special senses, nutrition, skin condition). Implement guidelines to prevent functional decline. Conduct daily interdisciplinary rounds. Teach patient self-care.
Social worker	Assess patient's social support network, health insurance coverage, caregiving needs. Review advance directives (living will, durable power of attorney for health care). Evaluate family dynamics (potential caregiver stress or elder abuse). Arrange referrals to community agencies (e.g., home care, meals-on-wheels). Arrange transfer to nursing home or rehabilitation hospital.
Physical therapist	Evaluate gait and mobility. Help patient to maintain or improve strength, flexibility, and endurance of muscles and range of motion of joints. Recommend assistive devices for ambulation. Administer treatment modalities.
Occupational therapist	Evaluate patient's ability to perform activities of daily living. Fit splints for upper extremities. Perform environmental assessment (home visit); determine home safety, need for appliances and devices. Teach use of assistive aids and devices.
Dietitian	Assess nutritional status. Recommend nutritional interventions (e.g., special diets and food supplements). Monitor enteral and parenteral alimentation.
Speech pathologist	Evaluate patients with aphasia or dysphagia. Recommend swallowing techniques to prevent pulmonary aspiration.
Home care coordinator	Participate in comprehensive discharge planning. Assure smooth transition of care from the hospital to home. Coordinate patient's care after discharge with physicians and other providers.

Adapted from Palmer RM: Acute hospital care of the elderly: Minimizing the risk of functional decline. Cleve Clin J Med 1995;62:117–128.

of the patient and family, prescribed diet, social service consultation and early plans for discharge, review of medications, and close follow-up after discharge were less likely to be readmitted for the same diagnosis and reported a higher quality of life 90 days later.

The benefits of interdisciplinary collaboration have also been demonstrated in acute care geriatric units.[13] These acute care units typically include a physical environment that fosters independent patient functioning, emphasize expanded roles for nurses and multidisciplinary collaboration, initiate comprehensive discharge planning early in the patient's hospital course, and make provisions for transition of care from hospital to home. In a clinical trial of an acute care of elders (ACE) unit, interdisciplinary collaboration was one of the interventions associated with a decrease in the prevalence of functional decline (loss of independent self-care) in hospitalized, medically ill, elderly patients.[14] ADL function was significantly better at discharge than on admission for patients receiving the ACE intervention than for patients receiving the usual medical care. Fewer patients receiving ACE intervention were discharged for the first time to institutional long-term care (9% compared to 16% of patients receiving usual care), and mean hospital charges and length of stay were similar for both groups of patients.

Ongoing interdisciplinary collaboration throughout the patient's hospitalization may be the key to improving clinical and functional outcomes. When geriatric assessment at the time of admission is performed by a team not involved in the patient's care, no benefit of consultation on hospital outcomes or mortality is demonstrated.[15]

Comprehensive Discharge Planning

The process of discharge planning is most effective when it is initiated shortly after the patient is admitted. Most hospitals employ either a clinical nurse specialist, clinical nurse manager, or other discharge planner to assist physicians with the process of discharge planning. When clinical nurse specialists coordinate the discharge planning of hospitalized elderly patients with common diagnoses such as congestive heart failure and myocardial infarction, patients are less likely to be readmitted to the hospital, have fewer total days of rehospitalization, and to incur lower charges for health care services after discharge.[12, 16] However, the interdisciplinary process of discharge planning is easiest to conduct in ACE units, where all health professionals have an opportunity for daily interaction through team rounds and contact with the nurse specialist.[13]

The pressure on physicians to discharge patients rapidly from the hospital makes the need for early discharge planning more critical. Discharge planning helps physicians estimate a patient's hospital length of stay, create a trajectory of the patient's functional status at hospital discharge, and anticipate the patient's needs for social support and services following discharge. Collaboration with the interdisciplinary team helps the physician decide the best disposition site for patients following discharge.

Hospital Discharge

Most elderly patients return home after hospitalization, but some require rehabilitation or short-term subacute care, whereas others require home care with skilled nursing services or long-term care placement. Patients admitted with a self-limited illness who can perform self-care activities independently may return home, usually without the need for formal (paid) home-care services. Patients with categorical illnesses, such as hip fracture or stroke, who have good rehabilitative potential and adequate informal supports may be accepted for transfer to a rehabilitation hospital. For patients who are unable to tolerate the rigors of extensive physical therapy (e.g., 3 or more hours daily) in a rehabilitation hospital, a subacute care unit (skilled nursing facility) can provide short-term restorative services prior to the patient's return home. Home health care is a reasonable alternative when patients and their families prefer to receive restorative services at home. Patients who are functionally impaired and lack adequate social supports will probably require placement in a long-term care facility. Terminally ill patients can be admitted to pallia-

---

TABLE 8-3 **CLINICAL INSTABILITY: DAY OF PLANNED DISCHARGE**

1. New finding of:

   - Incontinence
   - Chest pain
   - Dyspnea
   - Delirium
   - Tachycardia
   - Hypotension

2. Temperature $\geq 38.3°C$
3. Diastolic blood pressure ≥ 105 mmHg

Data from Kosecoff J, Kahn KL, Rogers WH, et al: Prospective payment system and impairment at discharge. The "quicker and sicker" story revisited. JAMA 1990; 264:1980–1983; and Brook RH, Kahn KL, Kosecoff J: Assessing clinical instability at discharge: The clinician's responsibility. JAMA 1992;268:1321–1322.

tive care (hospice) programs either in a hospital or at home.

Patients should not be discharged from the acute care hospital if there is evidence of clinical instability on the day preceding the planned discharge (Table 8–3). Patients who are discharged to home in an unstable condition have a higher mortality risk after hospitalization compared to patients whose condition is stable.[17, 18]

The loss of functional independence is not an inevitable consequence of acute illness and hospitalization among elderly patients. Interventions—daily assessment linked to treatment, medical care review, and interdisciplinary care with comprehensive discharge planning—may improve the functional outcomes of hospitalization.[14]

References

1. United States Department of Health and Human Services: Vital and Health Statistics: Health Data on Older Americans, 1992. Series III: Analytic and epidemiological studies, No. 27. DHHS Publication No. 93-1411. Hyattsville, MD, U.S. Dept. of Health and Human Services, 1993.
2. Wolinsky FD, Stump TE, Johnson RJ: Hospital utilization profiles among older adults over time: Consistency and volume among survivors and decedents. J Geront Soc Sci 1995;50B:S88–S100.
3. Inouye SK, Charpentier PA: Precipitating factors for delirium in hospitalized elderly persons. Predictive model and inter-relationship with baseline vulnerability. JAMA 1996;275:852–857.
4. Palmer RM: Acute hospital care of the elderly: Minimizing the risk of functional decline. Cleve Clin J Med 1995;62:117–128.
5. Sager MA, Rudberg MA, Jalaluddin M, et al: Hospital admission risk profile (HARP): Identifying older patients at risk for functional decline following acute medical illness and hospitalization. J Am Geriatr Soc 1996;44:251–257.
6. Inouye SK, Wagner DR, Acampora D, et al: A predictive index for functional decline in hospitalized elderly medical patients. J Gen Intern Med 1993;8:645–652.
7. Inouye SK, Viscoli CM, Horwitz RI, Hurst LD, Tinetti ME: A predictive model for delirium in hospitalized elderly medical patients based on admission characteristics. Ann Intern Med 1993;119:474–481.
8. Creditor MC: Hazards of hospitalization of the elderly. Ann Intern Med 1993;118:219–223.
9. Allman RM, Goode PS, Patrick MM, Burst N, Bartolucci AA: Pressure ulcer risk factors among hospitalized patients with activity limitation. JAMA 1995;273:865–870.
10. Cederholm T, Jagren C, Hellstrom K: Outcome of protein-energy malnutrition in elderly medical patients. Am J Med 1995;98:67–74.
11. Delmi M, Rapin C-H, Vengoa J-M, Delmas PD, Vasey H, Bonjour J-P: Dietary supplementation in elderly patients with fractured neck of the femur. Lancet 1990;335:1013–1016.
12. Rich MW, Beckham V, Wittenberg C, Leven CL, Freedland KE, Carney RM: A multidisciplinary intervention to prevent the re-admission of elderly patients with congestive heart failure. N Engl J Med 1995;333:1190–1195.
13. Palmer RM, Landefeld CS, Kresevic D, Kowal J: A medical unit for the acute care of the elderly. J Am Geriatr Soc 1994;42:545–552.
14. Landefeld CS, Palmer RM, Kresevic DM, Fortinsky RH, Kowal J: A randomized trial of care in a hospital medical unit especially designed to improve the functional outcomes of acutely ill older patients. N Engl J Med 1995;332:1338–1344.
15. Reuben DB, Borok GM, Wolde-Tsadik G, et al: A randomized trial of comprehensive geriatric assessment in the care of hospitalized patients. N Engl J Med 1995;332:1345–1350.
16. Naylor M, Brooten D, Jones R, Lavizzo-Mourrey R, Mezey M, Pauly M: Comprehensive discharge planning for the hospitalized elderly. A randomized clinical trial. Ann Intern Med 1994;120:999–1006.
17. Kosecoff J, Kahn KL, Rogers WH, Reinisch EJ, Sherwood MJ, Rubenstein LV, Draper D, Roth CP, Chew C, Brook RH: Prospective payment system and impairment at discharge. The "quicker and sicker" story revisited. JAMA 1990;264:1980–1983.
18. Brook RH, Kahn KL, Kosecoff J: Assessing clinical instability at discharge. The clinician's responsibility. JAMA 1992;268:1321–1322.

9 Nursing Home Care

Paul R. Katz, M.D.

The demand for nursing home (NH) services has increased dramatically during the past several years, reflecting an aging population with its attendant high level of physical and psychosocial disability.[1] Despite the large numbers of elderly people now receiving institutionalized long-term care, the NH, until very recently, was removed from the medical mainstream. Ageism, economic constraints, an overemphasis on cure at the expense of care, and a lack of commitment to geriatrics on the part of medical educators all contributed to the perception of the NH as a place devoid of intellectual challenge and one in which professional fulfillment is rarely achieved. By reviewing the scope of NH services, resident needs, and complexities of care, this chapter strives to correct any lingering misconceptions about the NH. It is hoped that a realistic portrayal of NH care, including the challenges that lie ahead, will serve as a lure for greater professional involvement in and commitment to this sector of health care.

HISTORICAL PERSPECTIVE

The modern NH is, surprisingly, a relatively new phenomenon. Prior to passage of Titles XVIII and XIX of the Social Security Act in 1965 (Medicare and Medicaid), the federal government had a limited role in the provision of long-term care services. Private, often religious-affiliated groups provided many needed services to the frail elderly but were generally limited in scope. Indeed, even at the turn of the century, almshouses for the poor and handicapped were major sources of support for long-term care.[2]

With the enactment of Medicare and Medicaid, the federal government committed itself not only to significant funding for NH care but also to the oversight of such care. To be eligible as a provider of services for Medicare and Medicaid patients and thus receive reimbursement, long-term care facilities must abide by a set of standards established by law. The Health Care Financing Administration (HCFA), under the auspices of the Department of Health and Human Services, has been given the task of ensuring that all standards of care (i.e., conditions or requirements of participation) are adhered to on the state level. Although states must, at the very least, meet the minimum requirements established at the federal level, they may choose to exceed these and establish their own higher standards of care. To ensure compliance, states undertake periodic surveys of all nursing homes that include direct observation and documentation of a facility's operation.

Despite seemingly intense scrutiny, a consensus developed in the early 1980s that quality care in nursing homes was spotty. Although facilities complied with the letter of the law, the benefits to individual residents were often not realized. In response to these concerns, the Institute of Medicine (IOM) in 1983, under the auspices of the National Academy of Sciences, undertook an extensive review of NH practices, culminating in a report entitled *Improving the Quality of Care in Nursing Homes.*[3] The IOM report highlighted significant deficiencies and recommended a number of changes to improve the quality of care given in nursing homes. One of the major recommendations focused on the need to concentrate more on the actual outcomes achieved than on the processes used to achieve them. Less emphasis on "paper compliance" would, it was hoped, free facilities to concentrate on the actual hands-on care of the NH resident.

The majority of the IOM's recommendations were incorporated into law with the passage of the Omnibus Budget Reconciliation Act (OBRA) of 1987. In addition, residents' rights were more clearly articulated, especially those related to freedom from unnecessary medications or restraints. Further, a comprehensive assessment was to be completed on all NH residents within 14 days of admission and periodically thereafter when there was any significant change in condition. This resident assessment instrument, also referred to as the Minimum Data Set (MDS) encompasses a full biopsychosocial overview focusing specifically on 18 target conditions (Table 9–1). If one or more of these conditions is present or the resident has a risk for acquiring such, the care team is referred to resident assessment

TABLE 9–1 **CLINICAL ISSUES HIGHLIGHTED IN MINIMUM DATA SET**

Delirium
Cognitive decline
Visual function
Communication
ADL° functional/rehabilitative potential
Urinary incontinence and indwelling catheter
Psychosocial well-being
Mood state
Behavior problem
Activities
Falls
Nutritional status
Feeding tubes
Dehydration/fluid maintenance
Dental care
Pressure ulcer
Antipsychotic drug use
Physical restraints

°Activities of daily living.
From Elon R, Pawlson LG: The impact of OBRA on medical practice within nursing facilities. J Am Geriatr Soc 1992;40:958–963.

protocols (RAPs), which outline standard diagnostic and therapeutic approaches to the specific problem in question. These RAPs are, in essence, practice guidelines specific to long-term care. Although documentation is not required, clinicians should document the rationale for treatment that may vary from these guidelines.

Although OBRA 87 has, in many respects, revolutionized NH care, its impact on quality has been difficult to measure. Nevertheless, the dramatic reductions in the use of chemical and physical restraints seen in nursing homes during the past several years are, in large measure, a direct result of OBRA.[4] Investigators are currently studying the role that specific questions in the MDS might play in measuring NH quality longitudinally.[5]

Finally, although the current regulatory system no doubt enhances patient care, at times such care is jeopardized by the fear and paranoia engendered by many state health departments. Such fear often distorts the real meaning behind many of the edicts and regulations emanating from the health department and results, unfortunately, in risk management strategies that seek to minimize exposure of the NH whenever possible. To ensure optimum care of each resident, physicians and other professionals in the NH must understand fully the principles of administrative law, particularly as it relates to rights of access to all pertinent regulations and opinions, the interpretation of statutes on the part of health depart-

ment representatives, and the right to contest punitive judgments.[6] Physicians should never lose sight of the fact that they are in a unique position to set medical care priorities in the NH and to ensure the protection of resident rights.

SCOPE OF NURSING HOME CARE

The number of NH beds in the United States currently exceeds those in acute care hospitals, and they have occupancy rates approaching 90%. Presently, there are over 16,000 nursing homes, and the bed capacity exceeds 1.7 million.[7]° The majority of homes are proprietary and have an average of 106 beds. Depending on the assumptions one makes about mortality, the number of NH residents will probably exceed 2 million by the turn of the century and will range from 3.6 to 5.9 million by the year 2040. Indeed, the number of NH residents 85 years old and over in 2040 may be two or three times the number of all residents 65 years old and over who currently reside in nursing homes today![8]

Of the elderly population 65 years of age and over, approximately 5% reside in a NH at any given time (3% males, 6% females). The chances of entering a NH sometime during one's lifetime may approach 40%, and the risk of institutionalization increases with age.[9] Whereas 1% of men and women aged 65 to 74 reside in a NH, 15% of men and 25% of women 85 years and over live in NHs.[7] Minorities remain under-represented in nursing homes, although they are more functionally dependent at the time of admission.[10]

Understandably, the current cohort of NH residents is rather old (average age 86) and dependent, and has limited socioeconomic reserves.[7] For example, compared to individuals residing in the community, NH residents are twice as likely to be widowed. Although over half of NH residents have difficulty with urinary or fecal incontinence, two thirds or more require assistance in performing basic activities of daily living (ADLs) such as bathing, dressing, and toileting. Although the average resident has a substantial level of disability, the NH population is not as homogeneous as one might surmise. The needs of individual residents, and thus the spectrum of NH services required, are extremely variable and range from custodial to short-term rehabilitative care. Because many NHs are reimbursed according to the actual care needs of their residents, a mix of residents is often sought. For

°Since the advent of the Omnibus Budget Reconciliation Act of 1987, nursing homes are referred to as residential health care facilities. The distinction between skilled and intermediate (health-related) facilities is no longer valid.

example, the resource utilization groups (RUGs) system in New York State, a prototype for the rest of the country, has 16 classifications of resident needs, all of which have different levels of reimbursement.[11] Unfortunately, under a prospective payment system such as this, there is often no financial incentive to decrease the care needs of individual residents. Even when monetary incentives have been employed, medical and functional outcomes of residents have not been appreciably affected.[12]

The heterogeneity of the NH population is a consequence not only of the manner in which nursing homes are paid but also of the way in which acute care hospitals are funded. With the advent of the prospective payment system under the guise of diagnosis-related groups (DRGs), many patients have been discharged from hospitals "quicker but sicker." Although the need to avoid lengthy hospital stays is obvious, the prospective payment system places many elderly patients in jeopardy because functional disabilities, as opposed to diagnoses, are often not recognized in determining the allowed length of stay.

There is now ample evidence of the negative impact of hospital-based DRGs on the outcomes of older individuals. Fitzgerald and colleagues[13] compared outcomes in elderly hip fracture patients before and after the advent of DRGs and reported decreases in the number of physical therapy sessions needed, the maximal distance walked in the hospital, and the percentage of patients discharged back to the community after the advent of prospective payment. Tresch and colleagues[14] noted that, among 100 consecutive admissions to a hospital-based NH care unit after the use of DRGs, 27% required readmission to the acute-care hospital within 30 days. This was almost triple the incidence of readmission prior to the advent of DRGs. Indeed, of the 27 patients readmitted to the hospital, approximately two thirds were judged to have been admitted to the NH too early.

Reflecting the trend to discharge hospital patients before their illness has completely resolved, those people now receiving care in nursery homes are sicker and more disabled than those admitted just 5 or 10 years ago. The changing nature of the NH population can also be seen in recent trends that demonstrate an increase in the number of NH deaths across the United States coincident with a decline in hospital deaths.[15] The percentage of NH deaths increased from 18.9% per year in 1982 (pre-DRG) to 21.5% in 1985 (post-DRG), whereas hospital deaths, declined from 65% to 61% in the same period. These figures reflect both an increased mortality rate among long-stay residents and a

trend to transfer terminally ill patients to the NH for final care.[16] Less aggressive care practices have also contributed to this trend.[17] Although demonstration projects have documented the feasibility of treating acute disease in the NH setting when adequate financial incentives are forthcoming, such programs have yet to be applied on a large scale.[18]

WHO PAYS FOR NURSING HOME CARE?

In contrast to acute care, NH care is paid for almost entirely by two sources: "private pay" (the patient's own resources) and Medicaid, the federal program for the poor. In 1993, Medicaid reimbursed nursing facilities almost $29 billion.

For persons who use nursing homes after the age of 65, 44% begin and end their stay as private payers, 27% begin and end as Medicaid recipients, and 14% eventually spend down their assets to qualify for Medicaid. Put another way, 17% of all persons who turn 65 years of age will reside in a NH at some time before they die and will be dependent on Medicaid for support.[19]

Ironically, Medicare,° the federal program specifically designed for the elderly, pays less than 10% of total NH costs.[20] Private insurance for long-term care is growing rapidly, and most major insurance companies now offer coverage for both NH and home care; almost 4 million policies were sold between 1987 and 1994. Although long-term care insurance presently accounts for a very small percentage of NH payments it is likely to figure prominently in new health care reform policies. Interestingly, underwriting practices may reject up to 23% of Americans for long-term care insurance.[21] The total cost of NH care is substantial and is rising rapidly; in 1985 the cost was $35 billion, but this is projected to increase to $139 billion by 2040.[8]

Even with the rapid growth of public contributions to pay for NH care, the burden on the elderly themselves is still great. Approximately 42% of the out-of-pocket costs of older persons goes for NH care, a larger percentage than is required for physician and hospital out-of-pocket expenses combined.[20] Because the average yearly

---

°Most health care professionals are probably familiar with the Medicare system, but for those who are not, the following is a brief overview. Medicare was created in 1965 as Title XVIII of the Social Security Act to assist the elderly and disabled to remain out of poverty by paying for the most expensive portions of health care. Medicare is an entitlement program, and those over 65 years of age and some specific categories of the disabled are eligible. Medicare has two parts: Part A pays mainly for acute hospital care and is free to the beneficiaries; Part B pays mainly for physician and outpatient services, and requires a monthly fee. For an excellent review of the history and current development of both the Medicare and Medicaid programs, see Health Care Financing Review 6 (Suppl), 1985.

cost of a nursing home in 1995 was $30,000, this expense can be considerable.

In recent years, the advent of managed care has heightened interest in the development of more efficient and cost-effective health systems designed to enhance care for the frail elderly. Although managed care organizations are cautious in assuming risk for nursing home residents with their significant burden of chronic illness, it is hoped that more rational incentives will evolve under the rubric of managed care and will lead to innovations whereby the type and intensity of long-term care services will become more person-centered and less dependent on the site of care.

THE DECISION TO INSTITUTIONALIZE

Contrary to popular belief, there is no magic formula that allows a clinician to predict with certainty whether or not a given individual is destined for a NH. Although several variables have been identified as potential predictors of institutionalization (such as cognitive impairment, incontinence, poor socioeconomic supports, and functional incapacity), quantifying the risk has been problematic. Much of this uncertainty can be attributed to variations in availability and accessibility of community-based long-term care services. For many frail elderly, the availability of services such as respite care, transportation, legal or psychological counseling, specialized housing, and in-home medical care are the major factors that determine the need for NH placement. Increasingly, caregiver burden has been identified as a key variable in predicting NH admission. The use of formal community services, interestingly, has been associated with an increased chance of NH use. Informal care, however, may lower the chances of NH admission. When a spouse or child can share caregiving responsibilities, the risk of a long NH stay is lowered by 9.3%; for childless individuals living alone, the risk increases to 18% and rises to 46% for elderly people living alone with adults other than a spouse or children.[22, 23]

Unfortunately, services vary enormously from one locale to another. Even when services are available, they may not be accessible owing to a lack of knowledge about the scope of such services among families and health care professionals. The accessibility of services may also be a factor in personal or public financing (or the lack thereof).[24] Whether innovative case management approaches will be effective in linking patient needs and services in the community, thus cir-

cumventing many of the availability or accessibility issues noted earlier, remains to be seen.[25]

In addition to an individual's physical, mental, and socioeconomic health status and gaps in the continuum of care, other factors may play an important role in the decision to institutionalize an elderly person. These factors include discrimination based on payer status and on race.

Although inappropriate admissions to nursing homes are much less frequent today than they were in years past, physicians must be certain that all alternatives have been thoroughly explored. Notwithstanding the capacity for short-term rehabilitation for acute medical problems, many individuals, once admitted to a NH, become products of the institution. Learned dependency is a particularly difficult problem to overcome. Interestingly, the availability of home care services in itself has not been found to exert an appreciable impact on NH utilization rates.[25]

LENGTH OF STAY

In view of the heterogeneity of the NH population, it is not surprising to find that a sizable number of NH residents have a relatively short length of stay (LOS), particularly those individuals with a terminal illness or those who suffer from acute orthopedic or neurologic deficits amenable to rehabilitation (e.g., stroke, hip fracture). Functional dependency and cognitive impairment may be less predictive of short NH stays than of long stays.[26] Because nursing homes are not subject to the same prospective payment system that drives many acute care hospital-based rehabilitation centers, ample time may be allowed for rehabilitation of the older frail patient, thus facilitating the transition of these individuals back into the community. Although almost half of all NH patients have a LOS of less than 6 months, short stays account for only 5% of all NH days. The average LOS is currently approximately 19 months, and two thirds of discharges from the NH are accounted for by death.[27] Nonetheless, one third of the lifetime NH risk relates to stays of 90 days or less. Although approximately 25% of patients discharged from the NH return home, only 7% remain alive at home at 2-year follow-up.[28] Although this is not surprising in view of the frail nature of the NH population, the reasons for most deaths in the NH usually remain unverified, as demonstrated by a NH autopsy rate of less than 1%.[29]

THE ACUTE CARE–LONG-TERM CARE INTERFACE

Transfer of NH residents between the NH and an acute care hospital occurs frequently. In 1987,

816,000 persons (8.5% of all Medicare hospital admissions) were transferred from nursing homes to hospitals.[30] Similarly, more than half of all NH admissions originate from short-stay hospitals; approximately one third of females 85 years and older discharged from hospitals are transferred to nursing homes.[31] Unfortunately, there are significant problems with the coordination and content of the information that is transferred between acute care and long-term care providers. Recent national surveys have indicated that frustration exists on the part of both hospital discharge planners and NH admission coordinators. Discharge planners often do not clearly understand the services offered by nursing homes or the regulatory framework under which they operate. Many nursing homes believe, rightly or wrongly, that the true condition of patients is often hidden to facilitate a transfer. Not infrequently, discharge summaries are delayed or incomplete, thus jeopardizing the continuity of care; this is an especially important issue when the attending physician in the hospital is not the one attending in the NH. In the future, computerized linkages between hospitals and nursing homes will probably circumvent many of these difficulties as well as managed care practices that seek to establish a seamless flow throughout the continuum of care. The links between hospitals and nursing homes will continue to evolve as nursing facilities assume care for increasingly sick and unstable patients under the rubric of "subacute" care.

Although transfer of residents from the NH to the hospital is usually based on a need to treat an acute illness, most commonly one secondary to infection, a host of other reasons may be implicated. Many of these are administrative and social-structural factors not directly linked to the severity of the underlying illness.[32] Such factors include a lack of adequately trained staff in the NH, an inability or lack of authorization on the part of nursing staff to administer intravenous therapy, a lack of diagnostic services such as radiography, physician convenience, and pressure from both staff and family to transfer difficult cases to a hospital. Nonetheless, many nursing homes remain reluctant to hospitalize residents because of the risk of incurring iatrogenic conditions. One study showed that 30% of patients transferred from a NH to a hospital return with new pressure sores![33]

HEALTH CARE DELIVERY IN THE NURSING HOME: STAFFING ISSUES

The NH is unique among health care institutions in two major ways. First, because the NH func-

tions as a permanent home for many of its residents, it strives to maintain the attributes of a home. At the very least, this entails respect for privacy, self-determination, encouragement of independent functioning, and inclusion of family and friends within the framework of care provided. Second, nursing homes are unique in terms of the comprehensiveness of the medical care services that are required. Residents must be assessed as often as every 30 days but no less often than every 60 days, even when they are medically stable. In addition, dental and podiatry services are routinely offered, whereas ophthalmologic, gynecologic, and other specialty services are provided on an as-needed basis. Balancing the needs of home versus health care facility is often tenuous, particularly because many nursing homes continue to be based on a medical model of care. Although not necessarily desirable, the medical model of care is understandable in view of the more frail and acutely ill nature of the NH population noted earlier.

Although nursing homes resemble hospitals in many respects, their staffing patterns are widely divergent. NH nurses are relatively few in number, accounting for just over 10% of all NH employees. There is an average of only one registered nurse (RN) per 49 patients in the NH compared to one per five patients in acute care hospitals. This ratio results in an average of 7 to 12 minutes of daily contact between each NH resident and a nurse. Although the federal government has mandated minimum requirements for nursing staff (as well as training for nurses' aides), one third of nursing homes have been unable to comply. The fact that both total nursing hours and the ratio of professional to nonprofessional nursing staff have been used as reliable markers of quality care has significant policy and clinical implications.[34]

Most hands-on care in nursing homes is provided by nurses' aides, who constitute the majority of the work force. Only one third of nurses' aides have a high school education, and they have turnover rates that average 70% to 100% per year. Vacancy rates for nurses in nursing homes generally exceed those in acute care hospitals. Salary disparities are significant, and RNs and nurses' aides often earn from 35% to 60% less than their counterparts in acute care hospitals.

Even more than nurses, physicians traditionally have not been attracted to the NH setting. Lack of exposure and firsthand experience in long-term care during training cause many physicians to avoid nursing homes from pure ignorance. Unfortunately, increasing regulations and a demand for greater documentation of all activities that affect the care of residents have had a negative impact on physician recruitment into nursing homes. Currently, only one in five primary care physicians spends more than 2 hours per week in a NH.[35] It is hoped that increasing recognition of the educational and research opportunities inherent in nursing homes as well as exposure of medical residents to physician role models devoted to long-term care issues will attract greater numbers of physicians to the NH. In addition, recognition by managed care organizations of the pivotal role played by professionals who are knowledgeable about long-term care will certainly help promote the cause.[36]

THE ROLE OF THE PHYSICIAN IN THE NURSING HOME

In the NH, care is optimal when all members of the health care team, including nurses' aides, nurses, and physicians, cooperate in the planning and initiation of all treatments. Such a "team" effort ensures that all pertinent information about the rationale and goals of intervention will be effectively shared among all health care providers. Success in the NH depends on the physician's willingness to seek out and listen to the opinions of others, regardless of their professional standing. Rather than feeling threatened by others, the physician must make every attempt to understand each individual's role in the NH as well as the manner in which the NH is governed by state and federal regulations. This is especially important if the physician is to forge a successful constructive relationship with the NH administrator, director of nursing, and pharmacist consultant. Although the medical director is occasionally perceived as a source of aggravation and interference by other physicians, a better appreciation for the role of the medical director will go a long way toward reducing needless friction (Table 9–2).

In the context of the team and through interactions with staff, residents, and family, physicians often serve as role models for NH health care professionals. Skill at communication, clear and concise documentation in the medical record, and an overriding respect for individual rights and dignity are cornerstones of medical practice in the NH. The various roles of the attending physician in the NH are further outlined in Table 9–3.

As one might expect in a very frail and elderly population, much of the illness that becomes manifest in the NH presents atypically. Although the underlying pathophysiology remains the same no matter where care is being delivered, many of the problems encountered in the NH,

TABLE 9–2 **ROLE OF THE MEDICAL DIRECTOR**
1. Participate in administrative decision making and recommend and approve policies and procedures.
2. Participate in the development and conduct of education programs.
3. Organize and coordinate physician services and services of other professionals as they relate to resident care.
4. Participate in the process to ensure the appropriateness and quality of medical and medically related care.
5. Help articulate the facility's mission to the community and represent the facility in the community.
6. Participate in the surveillance and promotion of the health, welfare, and safety of employees.
7. Acquire, maintain, and apply knowledge of social, regulatory, political, and economic factors that relate to resident care services.
8. Provide medical leadership for research and development activities in geriatrics and long-term care.
9. Participate in establishing policies and procedures for assuring that the rights of individuals are respected.

From Levenson SA: Medical Policies and Procedures for Long-Term Care. Clinical and Administrative Guidelines. Owings Mills, MD, National Health Publishing, 1990.

such as incontinence, falls and syncope, infections, depression, delirium, malnutrition, and pressure sores, require specific diagnostic treatment strategies. Because of limited access to biotechnology, frequent dependence on nonphysicians for evaluation of medical problems, and cost constraints, the NH approach to these problems often differs from that found in the hospital or office setting. For example, whereas it might be feasible to care for a febrile resident with pneumonia in a NH where parenteral antibiotics are part of routine therapy and laboratory and radiologic services are easily accessible, the same patient might well be transferred to an acute care facility if such services are not readily available. Likewise, whereas evaluation of incontinence might entail extensive invasive tests and therapeutic trials in a functional 85-year-old who resides in the community, a similar strategy might be inappropriate for an 85-year-old NH resident who is severely demented and bedbound.

Although the interplay between acute and chronic disease adds a dimension of complexity that requires all the ingenuity of the physician and health care team, the opportunity to maintain health and prevent disease in the NH should not be forgotten. Mandated visitation schedules

TABLE 9–3	**ROLE OF THE ATTENDING PHYSICIAN IN THE NURSING HOME**

1. Comprehensively assess each resident and coordinate all aspects of medical care. Implement specific treatments and services to enhance or maintain physical and psychosocial function.
2. Participate in the development of individual care plans and review and revise such plans periodically in conjunction with the health care team.
3. Review progress of each resident relating to individualized therapy (i.e., speech, occupational therapy, physical therapy) and, in concert with appropriate therapists, approve continued use.
4. Evaluate the need for rehabilitative services. Order appropriate measures and assistive devices to reduce the risk of accidents.
5. Evaluate the need for physical or chemical restraints, minimizing their use whenever possible.
6. Periodically review all medications and monitor for both continued need and adverse drug reactions. Respond appropriately to periodic review and recommendations of the consultant pharmacist.
7. Physically attend to each resident in a timely fashion consistent with established state and federal guidelines. Document progress and changes in care plans.
8. Respond in a timely fashion to medical emergencies.
9. Facilitate information transfer when possible and appropriate between acute and long-term care facilities.
10. Inform residents of their health status and, whenever possible, optimize each resident's ability for self-determination; determine each resident's decision-making capacity while assisting in establishing advance directives.

in the NH allow the physician ample opportunity to perform a complete and thorough geriatric assessment. Whereas review of medications, nutritional status, need for restraints and urinary catheters, and changes in physical or psychological status should be sought at each encounter, an annual review of immunizations, tuberculin skin test reactivity, and screening tests related to cancer detection is recommended. Screening in the NH must, of course, be individualized in accordance with its potential impact on the quality of life and the existence of cost-effective treatment interventions that are acceptable to the resident. Periodic review of Advance Directives should also be sought. Surprisingly, despite a dismal success rate for cardiopulmonary resuscitation in nursing homes, a majority of NH residents prefer to maintain the option of resuscitation. In one recent study, only one in eight residents with decision-making capability had had a previous discussion of preferences with their health care providers.[37]

Ensuring high-quality care in the NH setting remains a challenge. Numerous reports continue to document the presence of inappropriate care practices. For example, in a study of Maryland nursing homes involving almost 4000 residents in a 1-year period, only 11% of cases involving four common infections received even a minimally appropriate evaluation.[38] In addition to individual physician traits, the characteristics of the medical staff (i.e., open versus closed) may predict the quality or intensity of the services delivered.[39] The reader is referred to a number of texts devoted exclusively to NH care that discuss in detail many of the pertinent clinical and administrative issues alluded to here (see Additional Readings).

ROLE OF THE FAMILY

Contrary to popular belief, families do not abandon their loved ones following institutionalization. Indeed, only a minority of NH residents are truly "familyless" in a functional sense. Each family's function obviously varies from patient to patient but may involve simple companionship, assistance with ADL, and advocacy of resident rights. Forging an effective alliance with the family so that they become an important part of the "total institution" will go a long way toward ensuring an optimal quality of life for each resident.

SUMMARY

The continued growth of nursing homes and the increasing complexity of care required will present an ever-increasing challenge to the health care system during the next several decades. Needless to say, physicians, nurses, and other professionals require special skills and sensitivities to ensure delivery of optimum care in an environment that is likely to become even more highly regulated. It is hoped that the opportunity to affect significantly the quality of life of millions of elderly people in need will provide the lure to attract and retain dedicated health care professionals to the NH.

References

1. Doty P, Liu K, Wiener J: An overview of long-term care. Health Care Finance Rev 1985;6(3):69.
2. Johnson CL, Grant LA: The Nursing Home in American Society. Baltimore, Johns Hopkins Press, 1985.
3. Institute of Medicine, Committee on Nursing Home

Regulation: Improving the Quality of Care in Nursing Homes. Washington, D.C., National Academy Press, 1986.

4. Elon RD: Medical practice in nursing facilities: Assessing the impact of OBRA. *In* Katz PR, Kane RL, Mezey M (eds): Quality of Care in Geriatric Settings. New York, Springer, 1995.

5. Zimmerman DR, Karon SL, Arling G, et al: Development and testing of nursing home quality indicators. Health Care Finance Rev 1995;16:107–127.

6. Kapp MB: Limiting medical interventions for nursing home residents: The role of administrative law. *In* Katz PR, Kane RL, Mezey M (eds): Advances in Long-Term Care, Vol. I. New York, Springer, 1991.

7. Strahan GW: An overview of nursing homes and their current residents: Data from the 1995 National Nursing Home Survey. Advance data from Vital and Health Statistics, No. 280. Hyattsville, MD, National Center for Health Statistics, 1997.

8. Schneider EL, Guralnik JM: The aging of America: Impact on health care costs. JAMA 1990;263:2335–2340.

9. Cohen MA, Tell EJ, Wallack S: The lifetime risks of costs of nursing home use among the elderly. Med Care 1986;24:1161–1172.

10. Mulrow CD, Chiodo LK, Gerety MB, et al. Function and comorbidity in south Texas nursing home residents: Variations by ethnic group. J Am Geriatr Soc 1996;44:279–284.

11. Feather J: Resource Utilization Groups (RUGs): An Introduction for Health Care Professionals. Information on Aging Series. Buffalo, Network in Aging of Western New York, 1986.

12. Meiners MR, Thorbum P, Roddy PC, Jones BJ: Nursing Home Admissions: The Results of an Incentive Reimbursement Experiment. A NCHSR Report. Washington, D.C., U.S. Dept. Health and Human Services, 1985.

13. Fitzgerald JF, Moore PS, Dittus RS: The care of elderly patients with hip fracture: Changes since implementation of the Prospective Payment System. N Engl J Med 1988;319:1392–1397.

14. Tresch DD, Duthie EH, Newton M, Bodin B: Coping with diagnosis related groups: The changing role of the nursing home. Arch Intern Med 1988;148:1393–1396.

15. Sager MA, Easterling DV, Kindig DA, Anderson OW: Changes in the location of death after passage of Medicare's prospective payment system. N Engl J Med 1989;320:433–439.

16. Sager MA, Easterling DV, Leventhal EA: An evaluation of increased mortality rates in Wisconsin nursing homes. J Am Geriatr Soc 1988;36:739–746.

17. Holtzman J, Lurie N. Causes of increasing mortality in a nursing home population. J Am Geriatr Soc 1996;44:258–264.

18. Zimmer JG, Eggert GM, Treat A, Brodows B: Nursing homes as acute care providers: A pilot study of incentives to reduce hospitalizations. J Am Geriatr Soc 1988;36:124–129.

19. Spillman BC, Kemper P: Lifetime patterns of payment for nursing home care. Med Care 1995;33:280–296.

20. Waldo DR, Lazenby HC: Demographic characteristics and health care use and expenditures by the aged in the United States: 1977–1984. Health Care Finance Rev 1984;6:1.

21. Murtaugh CM, Kemper P, Spillman BC: Risky business: Long term care insurance underwriting. Inquiry 1995;32:271–284.

22. Boaz RF, Muelleur CF: Predicting the risk of permanent nursing home residents: The role of community help as indicated by family helpers and prior living arrangements. Health Services Research 1994;29:391–414.

23. Jette AM, Tennstedt S, Crawford S: How does formal and informal community care affect nursing home use? J Gerontol 1995;50:S4–S12.

24. Wallace SP: The no-care zone: Availability, accessibility and acceptability in community-based long-term care. Gerontologist 1990;30(2):254–261.

25. Weissert WG, Hedrick SC: Lessons learned from research on effects of community-based long term care. J Am Geriatr Soc 1994;42:348–353.

26. Liu K, McBride T, Coughlin T: Risk of entering nursing homes for long vs. short stays. Med Care 1994;32:315–327.

27. Spence DA, Wiener JM: Nursing home length patterns: Results from the 1985 National Nursing Home Survey. Gerontologist 1990;30(1):16–20.

28. Lewis MA, Kane RL, Cretin S, Clark V: The immediate and subsequent outcomes of nursing home care. Am J Public Health 1985;75:758–762.

29. Katz PR, Seidel G: Nursing home autopsies: Survey of physician attitudes and practice patterns. Arch Pathol Lab Med 1990;114:145–147.

30. Freiman MP, Murtaugh CM: Public Health Reports 1995;110:546–554.

31. U.S. Department of Health and Human Services: Vital and Health Statistics. Chart Book on Health Data on Older Americans, United States, 1992 (Series 3, No. 29). Washington, D.C., U.S. Department of Health and Human Services, 1993.

32. Kayser-Jones JS, Wiener CL, Barbaccia JC: Factors contributing to the hospitalization of nursing home residents. Gerontologist 1989;29(4):592.

33. Tresch DD, Simpson WW, Burton JR: Relationship of long term care and acute care facilities. The problem of patient transfer and continuity of care. J Am Geriatr Soc 1985;33:819–826.

34. Mezey M, Knapp M: Nurse staffing nursing facilities: Implications for achieving quality of care. *In* Katz PR, Kane RL, Mezey M (eds): Advances in Long Term Care, Vol. II. New York, Springer, 1993.

35. Katz PR, Karuza J, Kolassa J, Hutson A: Medical practice with nursing home residents: Results from the national physician professional activities census. J Am Geriatr Soc 1997;45:911–917.

36. Katz PR, Karuza J, Counsell SR: Academics and the nursing home. Clin Geriatr Med 1995;11(3):503–516.

37. O'Brien LA, Grisso JA, Maislion G, et al: Nursing home residents' preferences for life sustaining treatments. JAMA 1995;274:1775–1779.

38. Warren JW, Palumbo FB, Fitterman L, et al: Incidence and characteristics of antibiotic use in aged NH patients. J Am Geriatr Soc 1991;39:963–972.

39. Karuza J, Katz PR: Physicians staffing pattern correlates of nursing home care: An initial inquiry and consideration of policy implications. J Am Geriatr Soc 1994;42:1–7.

Additional Reading

Psychiatric Care in the Nursing Home. Reichman W, Katz PR (eds). New York: Oxford University Press, 1996.
Medical Direction in Long Term Care. Levenson SA (ed). Durham, NC: Carolina Academic Press, 1993.
Medical Care in the Nursing Home. Ouslander JG, Osterweil D, Morlew J (eds). New York: McGraw Hill, 2nd ed, 1997.
Principles and Practice of Nursing Home Care. Katz PR, Calkins E (eds). New York: Springer, 1989.

10 Home Care

George Taler, M.D.
Timothy J. Keay, M.D., M.A.-Th.

Home care is the fastest growing sector of health services delivery in the United States.[1] Medicare expenditures for home health care increased from $2.12 billion in 1988 to approximately $16 billion in 1995. Estimated national expenditures were $33 billion, or nearly one third of the total cost of long-term care services. The 1992 National Home and Hospice Care Survey conducted by the National Center for Health Statistics found that over 1 million patients receive in-home services on any given day.

Growth of home care services is stimulated by many factors and is expected to continue during the next several decades. Most patients (75%) who receive in-home services are over the age of 65; their average age is 70 years. For every resident in a nursing facility, there are three to four patients with conditions of equal medical complexity and debility residing in the community with the assistance of family, friends, and the intermittent services of home health care agencies. The swelling ranks of the elderly population, especially the oldest cohorts, will place increasing demands on supportive services.[2] Changes in the hospital environment prompted by the prospective payment system and pressures from managed care organizations to reduce admissions and lengths of stay will dictate that most convalescence, rehabilitation, and terminal care be provided in post-acute care settings. But as restrictive policies imposed by state governments continue to limit the licensure of more post-acute care and long-term care beds, it is expected that an increasing proportion of these services will be delivered in the patient's home.

Contrary to popular belief, a survey of primary care physicians shows that the majority make house calls, although they limit this practice to episodic visits to a few selected patients.[3] However, a myriad of forces within the health care arena will probably lead to significant changes in the way home care is viewed by the medical community. Efforts to reduce the costs of care to the chronically ill are leading practitioners to explore increasingly more complex care in the home. Advances in technology resulting in minia-turization and automation of high-tech supportive equipment, such as ventilators, feeding pumps, dialysis machines, and medication delivery devices, coupled with a loosening of restrictions on location of service, have allowed patients with severe disabilities to remain in the community. Societal trends toward self-reliance, the financial implications of nursing home placement, and the increasing acceptance of long-term care insurance policies that include provisions for home care are stimulating the desire to gain access to these services.

BENEFITS OF HOME CARE

There are many advantages for both patient and physician in using home care. Patients who are appropriately included in home care benefit from the convenience of the physician's visits. In addition, a house call obviates the costs of specialty transport and unwelcome public exposure. Furthermore, in-home supports improve overall health and both functional and cognitive status.[4]

Functional assessment is best accomplished in the environment in which the patient lives. Caregiver issues are more clearly recognizable, including the burdens of providing support, financial concerns, depression, and possibly abuse. The added costs and inconvenience of diagnostic testing and consultation promote a step-wise, algorithmic strategy that is generally more appropriate in geriatric practice. Finally, negotiating with patients on their own "turf" reinforces the importance of patient autonomy and ethical decision making and reaffirms the balance in the doctor-patient relationship.

House calls benefit the physician by adding an important dimension to the knowledge of the patient's circumstances, by sharpening primary care skills, and by developing a greater appreciation for the costs and invasiveness of medical interventions in other settings. Ramsdell and colleagues[5] found that an average of two new problems per patient were discovered among those who first underwent an interdisciplinary comprehensive geriatric assessment in the office and were subsequently evaluated at home. Twenty-three percent of these new problems involved potential mortality or significant morbidity and were distributed equally among medical, psychiatric, and safety concerns.

Another advantage is that the office practice is more predictable and more efficient when patients appropriate for house calls are seen at home. Physically impaired and behaviorally disruptive patients require additional office staff time to assist with dressing and mobility; it takes far more of the physician's time to review a complex medical care plan (especially if the patient is not accompanied by the primary caregiver), to perform the examination, and to adjust the treatment regimen; diagnostic testing is more difficult; and problems frequently arise with continence. Following the visit, a stretcher-bound patient who occupies an examination room waiting for ambulance transport can seriously impede office flow. Also, a sizable home care practice can enhance the volume and efficiency of the group's hospital practice. Homebound patients experience 0.5 hospital admission per patient per year, the highest rate among ambulatory patients and even higher than those in nursing homes.[6] Once the acute illness has stabilized, familiarity with the range of in-home services and a willingness to visit the patient at home for follow-up care facilitates discharge planning. Also, home care may reduce hospitalizations among certain populations. Respiratory, cardiac, endocrine, and mental illnesses that result in repeat hospital admissions may all respond to intensive in-home monitoring and support.

DEVELOPING AN OFFICE-BASED HOUSE CALL PROGRAM

It is to the advantage of every primary care physician to develop the knowledge and skills that will enable him or her to manage patients at home. However, it is also necessary to develop a well-conceived and deliberate plan to run an efficient house call program.

Choosing Appropriate Patients for House Calls

The best candidates for house calls are chronically or terminally ill patients who have impaired mobility or disruptive behaviors (Table 10–1). Patients with dementia, terminal illness, or severe psychiatric disorders may decompensate in a public waiting room, causing discomfort for all involved. Terminally ill patients often find it a hardship to come to the office and are more effectively seen at home to address their physical

TABLE 10–1	**PATIENTS APPROPRIATE FOR HOME CARE**

Require special transport
Are behaviorally disruptive
Have complex medical and psychiatric problems
Are terminally ill
Have failed to respond to the medical regimen
Caregiver burn-out is evident
Elder abuse is suspected
Are chronic "no-shows" at the office

and emotional needs. Bereavement issues may require more time than is convenient in the office and may have more meaning for the family when they are addressed at home. Other patients who could be considered for house calls are those with functional and caregiving problems that need to be addressed at each visit. Also to be considered are those patients to whom the physician is committed but who are chronic "no-shows" and thereby disrupt office scheduling.

For some patients, house calls are indicated for only one or two visits. For example, when an illness has resulted in a significant change in function, a home visit following hospital discharge will highlight the appliances and services needed for support during convalescence and rehabilitation. Patients who fail to respond to what should be adequate therapy or whose response is inconsistent may benefit from a diagnostic home visit. In these perplexing situations, a house call will often elucidate nutritional problems or indiscretions, verify the purchase of prescribed medications, or reveal the presence of medications from other sources that interfere with the expected response. Situations in which there is suspected caregiver burnout or elder abuse are usually better assessed by a diagnostic house call.

Establishing an Office Organizational Structure

Two components are necessary to establish a successful house call program based in a private office setting. First is organizing the information flow, and second is establishing a house call team from community resources. The house call team is composed of the physicians who make house calls, the house call coordinator, representatives from the home care agency, and other health care professionals with whom the program has an informal working arrangement. The objective is to manage this aspect of the service spectrum with maximum efficiency and minimum disruption of the ambulatory practice.

HOUSE CALL COORDINATOR

A house call coordinator is the pivotal individual around whom the home care practice is organized. All calls are channeled through the coordinator, including those from patients and their families, home care agency staff, pharmacists, and vendors. Providing a central focus through which all information flows facilitates communication, saves everyone a great deal of time on the telephone, and assists in documentation. Emergency triage is managed through simple algorithms. The coordinator may offer the patients and their caregivers emotional support, encouragement, and practical advice from a lay perspective. Home care nurses can leave messages and updates, reassured that there will be a written note documenting their report and that true emergencies will be conveyed promptly. Telephone consultations between team members and the physician can be coordinated, ensuring that the parties will be available at the designated time and that the chart information for an efficient interchange will be accessible. The coordinator also organizes the correspondence, charting, and scheduling arrangements for diagnostic testing, delivery of medications and supplies, special clinic appointments, and consultations.

HOME CARE NURSING

The practice should align itself with a limited number of home care agencies—preferably just one. The choices are based on several factors, which include the service area involved, affiliation with the major hospital or hospitals where the physicians have privileges or nurse liaison services that facilitate discharge planning and communication with the agency, adequate size to provide timely services, and a solid reputation. For larger house call practices, the agency should be willing to assign the patients to a small pool of nurses, social workers, and therapists who may also participate in team meetings. This gives the physicians sufficient experience to learn the capabilities of the agency staff, and the agency can become more comfortable with the style of the physicians and their office routines. Likewise, the physicians and practice administrators can influence the policies and procedures of the agency to better coordinate their services.

Subacute problems that arise between visits can be managed effectively by initiating a nursing visit and in-home laboratory or radiographic tests, according to the history. The nurse can usually examine the patient within 24 hours and can provide an assessment. The information gathered through these sources provides a rea-

sonably accurate basis for diagnosis and therapy. Subsequent nursing visits can be scheduled as often as twice daily for a short time. However, house calls are generally not appropriate for a patient with an acute and serious illness. An emergency department is better suited to evaluate efficiently a patient with unstable vital signs, acute delirium, or significant trauma. One exception is the patient with an imminently terminal disease who has elected to forego hospitalization. Because the medical care plan in such cases requires careful consideration and negotiation with the family, an intercurrent house call often results in more humane care for the dying.

OTHER TEAM MEMBERS

The physician should recruit the other members of the house call team and encourage them to attend regularly scheduled meetings. A community pharmacist can work in consultation with the physician to review drug profiles, monitor regimens through a drug-drug interaction program, and alert the team to the availability of new medications and formulations. By delivering medications and disposable supplies to the home, the pharmacist is more likely to increase the number of referrals to the business; by assuming responsibility for oversight of patient compliance as part of the team, account retention is ensured. Pharmacists who have earned a Pharm D degree can assume the management of selected regimens—for example, anticoagulation, pain control for hospice patients, and adjustment of insulin dosage for new-onset diabetics. Affiliation with the house call program can increase referrals from the practice as a whole. Similarly, a durable medical equipment vendor benefits by new referrals and by the built-in forum for marketing new products at team meetings. Regular meetings with the physicians and their staff greatly facilitates completion of the often complex and arcane certificate of medical necessity forms required for the vendor's billing procedures.

HOUSE CALL TEAM MEETINGS

The house call team meetings are important for communication, interdisciplinary consultation, and timely completion of required documentation. A regular agenda facilitates the flow of information. While one physician reports on recent patient encounters, the others review paperwork associated with their house call patients and listen for information that may be pertinent for cross-covering. The nurse reports on the patients who require skilled services; the home care liaison supervisor conveys information from the physical therapists, occupational therapists, or other nurses who have seen patients under the practice's care. The pharmacist reports on compliance issues and reviews any intercurrent changes in the medical regimen. Should new orders for nursing, medications, equipment, or other services be issued during the presentations, these can be written and signed immediately. Weekly meetings generally last an hour for programs that cover 100 patients.

Financial Considerations

Financial viability is essential to the success of the program. The first issue involves determining the size of the home care practice to ensure an appropriate number of calls to warrant the time commitment. The second pertains to ensuring appropriate remuneration for the services rendered.

TIME MANAGEMENT AND DETERMINING PRACTICE SIZE

Specific half-day sessions should be set aside for house calls, preferably at the same time of the week and during daylight hours. Coordination of the office schedule with staff and other practitioners minimizes overhead expenses. House calls made during normal working hours ensure ready telephone access to other providers and support personnel as well as safety. Recent surveys of physicians who are active in house call practice have found that the typical house call takes approximately 20 to 30 minutes in the home. Travel time should be minimized by defining a geographic radius divided into quadrants, each visited monthly, or by clustering patients along specified routes. The physician should have a copy of the calendar and plan the return visit at the conclusion of each house call. This allows the flexibility to see the patient as often as appropriate for his or her condition, coordinate the visit with other house calls in the neighborhood, fit the visit into the family's schedule, and prevent physician overscheduling.

Five to seven patients can be seen in their homes in a half-day session; 10 to 12 patients can be seen when multiple visits can be scheduled in a few locations. Therefore, the size of the practice is determined by either the number of available half-day sessions or the number of patients available to the practice. Generally, a half day per week is sufficient to manage 60 to 80 patients who are seen quarterly for routine visits and as needed when their condition is less stable.

ENSURING APPROPRIATE REMUNERATION

The current procedural terminology (CPT) descriptions for house call services are listed in Table 10–2. Because homebound patients are most similar to those in nursing homes (i.e., they have multiple concurrently active diagnoses), the higher code numbers are most often applicable. Documentation is the key to verifying the requested remuneration. Records of telephone contacts with patients, family, and home care staff, as well as team meetings are advisable. Progress notes should include historical data, physical examination findings, pertinent diagnostic test results, a therapeutic reassessment reflective of all active diagnoses, an evaluation of the patient's functioning, caregiver issues, and evidence of a medical care plan for the ensuing period. There are no Medicare restrictions on the number of visits as long as there is sufficient justification in the progress notes.

As of 1995, Medicare has agreed to pay on a monthly basis for care plan oversight (CPO) at a rate comparable to that allowed for a high-level, established-patient home visit. Criteria defining eligibility for remuneration under the CPO code are different than those used for any other evaluation and management service; early experience suggests that approximately one quarter of the home care case load may be eligible. The patient must be under the active care of the physician as demonstrated by a face-to-face encounter within the 6 months prior to the initiation of CPO billing and must be under the care of a Medicare-certified home care agency for a Medicare-covered service (for example, home infusion therapy is excluded under Medicare, and so is excluded under CPO as well). A minimum of 30 minutes per calendar month of documented time devoted exclusively to the coordination, monitoring, and adjustment of the medical care plan is needed.

Billable time includes only interactions with other health professionals through meetings, telephone calls, or review of correspondence and medical records beyond that needed for routine care. Services usually provided as part of followup care after office or home visits do not contribute to CPO time. Therefore, telephone calls with the patient or family, contacts with other office staff, and routine matters, such as prescription renewals or signing home care agency orders, may not be counted. CPO may not be billed for care covered under a global fee arrangement, such as for follow-up of a surgical procedure or services provided by the medical director or an employee of a Medicare hospice. Finally, certain

TABLE 10–2 **CPT CODES FOR HOME VISITS***

Home visit for the evaluation and management of a **New Patient**, which requires these three key components:

Home Visit Code	99341	99342	99343
History	Problem focused	Expanded problem focused	Detailed
Examination	Problem focused	Expanded problem focused	Detailed
Decision Making	Low complexity	Moderate complexity	High complexity
Nature of Problem(s)	Low severity	Moderate severity	High severity

Home visit for the evaluation and management of an **Established Patient**, which requires these three key components:

Home Visit Code	99351	99352	99353
History	Problem focused	Expanded problem focused	Detailed
Examination	Problem focused	Expanded problem focused	Detailed
Decision Making	Low complexity	Moderate complexity	High complexity
Nature of Problem(s)	Low severity	Moderate severity	High severity

Counseling and/or coordination of care with other providers or agencies are provided consistent with the nature of the problem(s) and the patient's and/or family's needs.

Care Plan Oversight (CPO): 99375

Physician supervision of patients under care of home health agencies, hospice, or nursing facility patients (patient not present) requiring complex or multidisciplinary care modalities involving regular physician development and/or revision of care plans, review of subsequent reports of patient status, review of related laboratory and other studies, communication (including telephone calls) with other health care professionals involved in patient's care, integration of new information into the medical treatment plan and/or adjustment of medical therapy, within a 30-day period 30–60 minutes.

From American Medical Association: Physicians' Current Procedural Terminology Manual. Chicago, American Medical Association, 1996.
    CPT codes, descriptions, and numeric modifiers only are copyright 1995 American Medical Association. All rights reserved.
    *Extensive revisions to the CPT codes for home visits and care plan oversight are expected in early 1998. Please refer to the updated CPT manual for billing purposes or call the American Medical Association for CPT information at 1-800-634-6922.

professional relationships may exclude physicians from billing under the CPO code. Physicians who hold a 5% or greater ownership share in the home care agency providing services or receive more than $25,000 in compensation from the agency are not eligible to bill for CPO provided through that agency. Because CPO is a new code with a novel set of criteria, the Medicare intermediaries are likely to scrutinize carefully the documentation supporting the charges, underscoring the importance of maintaining comprehensive medical records.

A medical director contract with a home care agency is a different way to enhance practice revenue. Such contracts require approximately 4 to 8 hours a week for chart reviews for quality assurance purposes, in-service training for the agency staff, liaison with other physicians, and policy review and development. Criteria must be met to ensure compliance with certain "self-referral" statutes enacted in many states. It is prudent not to own stock in the home care agency or any other entity that is financially

aligned with it. No more than 25% of the home care agency's revenues may be derived from affiliation with the practice, and the services rendered must not be either those that would normally be given without compensation or those that are reimbursable through patient care. Under no circumstances can the physician accept remuneration for referrals.

Conducting a Home Visit

The house call presents an array of professional challenges for which the physician must be prepared, mostly through self-study. Few residency training programs incorporate adequate home care experiences, and there are few role models in the academic world from whom to learn. Physicians have a natural sense of trepidation in venturing outside the familiar surroundings of the hospital or ambulatory setting without the immediate support of the nursing staff, availability of diagnostic facilities, and easy accessibility of colleagues and consultants. Practicing in the

---

TABLE 10–3 **THE "ADVANCE PACKET"**

Letter of introduction to the house call program:	Questionnaires and forms:
1. The names and telephone numbers of the personnel in the office with whom the patient can expect to interact.	1. Past medical, family, and social histories.
2. House call visit policies for regular, subacute, and acute care visits.	2. Review of systems and preventive medicine review.
3. Affiliations with hospitals, home care agencies, and other vendors.	3. List of prescription and over-the-counter medications taken both regularly and as needed.
4. Telephone availability.	4. Medical allergies.
5. Charges for services.	5. Nutritional review.
	6. Functional assessment.
	7. Advance directive form.

---

patient's home tests one's bedside clinical skills in obtaining a history, performing a physical examination, and developing a diagnostic differential on which to base therapy. Seeing the patient in the home also uncovers situations that require knowledge that is usually in the province of other health professions, such as family counselling, financial planning, home safety, assessment for the use of rehabilitative equipment, and linkage with community resources. As advances in miniaturization and technology allow life-support equipment to be used in the home, practitioners will be called on to deal with devices previously encountered only in the hospital. Mastering patient management in this setting opens the door to some of the most personally rewarding experiences in all of primary care.

For patients new to the practice who will be managed under the house call program, the physician should give and get as much information before the visit as practicable. An "advance packet" of information about the services available through the program and selected questionnaires and requests for copies of recent medical records, including hospitalizations, will streamline the first visit (Table 10–3). An Advance Directive form will encourage the patient and family to express their values and opens a discussion about the nature and extent of care desired and expected.

The appointment should be scheduled to allow adequate time (usually at least 1 hour is needed) and with assurances that responsible family members will be present. Clear directions to the home and any special travel information are essential. Observation begins with the neighborhood, its cleanliness, access to convenience stores, pharmacy, and so on, and the condition of the other houses in relation to the patient's home. Disparities between the patient's house and those surrounding it offer clues to the level of functioning of the patient, his financial status, and the likely availability of friendly neighbors for assistance. After reviewing the "advance packet" materials, the priorities on the initial visit are to obtain a working history based on the chief complaints and current problems, to perform a targeted physical examination, to assess mental function and the ability to perform activities of

---

TABLE 10–4 **HOUSE CALL BAG: EQUIPMENT**

Blood pressure cuffs with interchangeable bulb
  and gauge:
  Regular
  Obese
  Pediatric
Gloves with lubricant and hemoccult slides
Otoscope/ophthalmoscope kit
Glucometer
Peak flow meter
Digital thermometer
Tape measure
Hammer and tuning fork
Bandage scissors
Toenail clippers
Portable bathroom scale
Optional:
  Sterile scissors, forceps, and disposable scalpel
  Sterile 4 × 4 gauze and tape
  Hand-held electrocardiogram device

TABLE 10–5 **HOUSE CALL BAG: STATIONERY**

Prescription blanks
Appointment cards
Progress note paper, history forms, drug flow
  sheets, etc.
Advance directive forms
Release of information forms
Informed consent forms for tetanus, Pneumovax,
  and influenza vaccinations, and debridement or
  other procedures
Assessment forms such as mini-mental state
  examination, elder abuse checklist, and home
  safety assessment checklist
Information and referral phone numbers

TABLE 10-6 **THE PHYSICIAN'S ROLE IN CAREGIVER SUPPORT**
---

1. The patient and caregiver must be perceived as a single unit. The dependencies of the patient must be matched by the capabilities of the caregiver and the willingness of the caregiver to provide assistance and support.
2. A comprehensive home-based approach to care can provide the full range of treatment and service resources necessary to support the patient-caregiver unit. Formal supports through public and private agencies may complement those skills and abilities that the caregiver cannot provide.
3. Caregivers and patients must be frequently assessed and re-assessed in order to identify behavioral, functional, and physiologic problems that may threaten the patient-caregiver unit.
4. Training of the caregiver in order to meet the needs of the patient assures the caregiver's competence and the safety and well-being of the patient. Most families are highly motivated and can be successfully trained in a wide variety of therapeutic, diagnostic, and behavioral management skills. Educating the family to the specific signs and symptoms of illness as pertains to their loved one, greatly facilitates clinical management and avoids untoward developments.
5. Behavioral problems must be managed expeditiously. When brought to the attention of the physician, aberrant behaviors have led to a high level of concern in the caregiver. Often, these behaviors are the first manifestations of an acute delirium requiring prompt diagnostic and therapeutic intervention. If not based on a clinical change, specific recommendations involving either behavioral management or psycho-pharmacologic therapies must be provided. Recognition of the caregiver's frustration is an important element in preventing abuse or premature institutionalization.
6. Validate the caregiving role by affirming the work of caregiving and acknowledging the stress and burden. A home visit provides as much emotional support to the caregiver as it provides a means for continuing medical management.
7. The primary care physician is the case manager and provides appropriate connections with health, social service agencies, and specialty referrals to assist in clinical management. Caregivers often feel a sense of isolation and are very dependent on their relationship with the primary care physician.

From American Medical Association, Council on Scientific Affairs: Physicians and family caregivers: A model for partnership. JAMA 269:1282–1284, 1992. Copyright 1992, American Medical Association.

daily living and instrumental activities of daily living, to review home safety, and to evaluate the capabilities and emotional well-being of the caregiver. Documentation should include a problem list, a medication list, and decisions concerning the advance directives. This information helps to develop the management goals (e.g., to provide maintenance care or terminal care) and to determine the need for further laboratory tests and consultations. A scheduled follow-up appointment completes the visit.

On subsequent visits, a review should encompass the ongoing problems (check the problem and medication lists and monitoring parameters), any intercurrent problems, the functional status, and health maintenance (e.g., vaccinations). Some time should be set aside with the caregiver to answer questions, clarify monitoring parameters, and provide emotional support.

The tasks entailed in the house call are more readily performed if the proper instruments and forms have been brought to the home (Tables 10–4 and 10–5). It is better not to carry any medications, needles, or syringes except as needed for vaccinations. Bring all "sharps" back to the office for proper disposal.

SPECIAL CONSIDERATIONS

Care in the home presents many issues that are outside the usual practice of medicine in the hospital, office, or nursing home. Special issues beyond the scope of this chapter include detailed consideration of the ideal site of medical care for particular patients, safety in the home, family dynamics (especially the role of caregiver [Table 10–6]), detection and treatment of elder abuse, functional supports and knowledge of available durable medical equipment, and the use of high-tech options in the home setting. The knowledge gained from house call experiences broadens the scope of concerns that are included in the primary care considerations of patients with multiple impairments and generally lead to the most appropriate care in the least restrictive environment.

SUMMARY

Home care is a useful option for medical management of a particular group of functionally impaired people. The population for whom this type of care is most appropriate is burgeoning, as is the home care industry. These patients are often very ill with progressive debilitating diseases that frequently lead to death, yet they receive great benefit from care given in their homes. Physicians who are contemplating incorporating a house call component into their practice need to acquire the knowledge and skills that aid in providing effective care in the home and work within an organized, interprofessional supportive system that maximizes team efficiency.

References

1. Kavesh WN: Home care: Process, outcome, cost. Ann Rev Gerontol Geriatr 1986;6:135–195.
2. Pawlson LG: Health care implications of an aging population. *In* Hazzard WR, Andres R, Bierman EL, Blass JP (eds): Principles of Geriatric Medicine and Gerontology. New York, McGraw-Hill, 1990, pp. 157–166.
3. Keenan JM, Boling PE, Schwartzberg JG, et al: A national survey of the home visiting practice and attitudes of family physicians and internists. Arch Intern Med 1992;152:2025–2032.
4. Council on Scientific Affairs: Home care in the 1990s. JAMA 1990;263:1241–1244.
5. Ramsdell JW, Swart JA, Jackson JE, Renvall M: The yield of a home visit in the assessment of geriatric patients. J Am Geriatr Soc 1989;37:17–24.
6. Master RJ, Feltin M, Jainchill J, Mark R, Kavesh WN, Rabkin MT, Turner B, Bachrach S, Lennox S: A continuum of care in the inner city: Assessment of its benefits for Boston's elderly and high-risk populations. N Engl J Med 1980;302:1434–1440.

Additional Reading

American Medical Association: Guidelines for the Medical Management of the Home Care Patient. Chicago, Department of Geriatric Health, American Medical Association, 1992.

11 Office Practice

Eric G. Tangalos, M.D., C.M.D.

The office practice of geriatric medicine offers primary care physicians as well as subspecialists a greater opportunity to provide preventive services to patients. It also allows physicians to evaluate issues that confront the elderly in everyday life at a more measured pace. An office-based functional assessment of an older patient may include evaluation of daily activities, cognition, continence, special senses, mobility, and specific psychosocial issues. This is the time and the place to discuss immunizations, advance directives, the game of golf, and grandchildren. This is also the setting in which a practice must run most efficiently because reimbursement in such situations is weakest for those who still provide primary care in the fee-for-service environment. A few selected items in this context are discussed in this chapter. In the following pages the author's experiences at the Mayo Clinic are offered not necessarily as gold standards but rather as examples of approaches that have proved to be of some benefit.

Studies have shown that formalized comprehensive geriatric assessment can result in improved survival, reduced hospital and nursing home stays, lower medical costs, and improved functional status for individuals undergoing such assessments. The modern office and the web of services available to today's practitioners allows all of the individual elements of geriatric assessment to come forward on behalf of patient care. Simple measures that are part of most office practices do make a difference.

Office-based geriatric assessment can help in determining patient placement, assistance needed for daily activities, medication selection, and prognosis. A shift from disease-oriented to function-oriented care entails a knowledge of social, cognitive, and mobility factors that are all elements of geriatric care. Older persons can benefit from this broadened definition of health and from preventive services. The clinician who can help patients achieve small improvements in functional, psychological, or cognitive abilities may provide significant benefits to the patient's quality of life.[1] Although the elderly can be categorized by age cohorts, there is no consensus about which age groups are considered the "young old" or the "old old."[2] Categorization by functional ability, number of co-morbid conditions, and presence of infirmity has also been recommended. Those with the poorest health status are considered frail or "at risk" elderly.[3]

HEALTH RECOMMENDATIONS FOR DISEASE PREVENTION

Most studies evaluating preventive services use reduction of disease-specific mortality as an outcome. In the elderly there are clearly additional and more relevant health outcomes to be considered. Health in old age can be said to consist of three related factors: (1) the absence of disease, (2) the maintenance of optimal function, and (3) the presence of an adequate support system.[4] However, while older adults tend to have a greater burden of disease than younger persons, individuals may still be considered "healthy." Therefore, the major goals of preventive care in the elderly are a delay or reduction in morbidity and prevention of disease to maximize the quality of life, satisfaction with life, and productivity.

The primary physician must also navigate a variety of practice environments. For the best care of the patient all these different worlds come into play as part of a continuum. An understanding of the patient's environment is as important as an assessment of his or her physical well-being in evaluating a patient's ability to be healthy. The physician's ability to maintain good health in an elderly patient goes beyond knowing what drugs are appropriate therapy. Understanding their environment, how they perceive it, and how they move around in it are hallmarks of geriatric care. Environmental modification can be a shared responsibility with other disciplines such as occupational therapy. Protecting brittle bones from injury should be a consideration at all times. Handrails on stairways and in the bathroom may prevent falls. Removing throw rugs and using night lights may also prevent accidents.

Sensory deprivation is another important determinant in the health and well-being of elderly patients. Bright colors and adequate lighting can help counter the loss of depth perception that comes with age. Hearing aids may transform a dull withdrawn individual back into a person in touch with his family and environment. Poor vision and cloudy mental images may both regain clarity with cataract surgery. For the patient with poor position sense, poor balance, or peripheral neuropathy, a cane provides not only support but the reassurance of additional sensory input.

Demented patients present a particular challenge because the pharmacologic agents capable of treating these disorders are still limited. Care of the individual is enhanced at any stage of disease if the environment is stable and certain needs are met. Caregivers should not disrupt familiar routines, and habits should be maintained. For example, brushing teeth in the safety of one's own bathroom requires almost no cognition or memory function, yet the same task during a visit to a son or daughter may unmask severe intellectual deficits. Encouraging these patients to keep lists and keep paper and pen close to the telephone are helpful strategies. For patients with more limited function, habits should be vigorously maintained, and overlearned behaviors should be reinforced.

Environmental modifications and adequate sensory input are only some of the truly preventive measures available to the practitioner and patient. Exercise to preserve mobility and improve cardiovascular tone should be encouraged. Weight loss should be accomplished by dieting, and efforts should continue to get patients to stop smoking and maintain good control of their blood pressure. Influenza vaccination should be offered yearly. Tuberculosis surveillance is extremely important in today's environment, and testing should be maintained, especially on nursing home admission. Chapter 13 gives further details about disease prevention.

PREOPERATIVE ASSESSMENT OF OLDER ADULTS

The physician is responsible for assisting elderly patients who face surgery. Clearly, older patients can do quite well with elective operations and even have excellent survival curves for emergent procedures. Morbidity and mortality related to emergency situations are generally related to the severity of the incident and the burden of disease patients take with them into the operating room. Surgical rates are 55% higher in persons over the age of 65, and older persons are disproportionately represented in surgical admissions. Older patients account for 75% of all postoperative deaths, and there is a nearly linear increase with each passing decade of life.[5]

Age remains the most important risk factor for the elderly in surgery of any type. The general trend is to accept age as an independent variable in assessing risk. A useful tool for assessing preoperative general status is Dripp's American Society of Anesthesiology (ASA) physical status scale.[6] Class I comprises healthy persons less than 80 years of age. Class II includes otherwise healthy patients 80 years of age or older or those who have mild systemic disease. Class III patients have a severe systemic disease that is not incapacitating. Class IV patients have an incapacitating systemic disease that is a constant threat to life. Class V patients are moribund and are not expected to survive 24 hours with or without the operation. Activity of daily living (ADL) scales, nutritional status, and cognitive function all help to predict surgical complications. Next to age, dementia is the most important predictor of poor outcome; surgical mortality is increased by 52% compared to nondemented general surgery patients in one series.[7] It is important for mental status to be assessed preoperatively to anticipate surgical risk and possible postoperative complications such as delirium.

Table 11–1 outlines an approach to assessing a patient's risk for cardiac complications with noncardiac surgery. This system, reported by Detsky and colleagues, lets the clinician score patients according to clinical variables. The risk of postoperative cardiac complications can then be estimated from the patient's score as noted in the table.

Yet another popular approach to the issue of preoperative cardiac risk assessment has been to use imaging techniques (dipyridamole-thallium scans or dobutamine stress echocardiography). These techniques can detect occult coronary disease and define known cardiovascular disease. Fleisher and Eagle have argued that the primary benefit of these studies has been to identify patients who should undergo preoperative coronary revascularization.[8] These authors believe that these studies are best used in patients who are at moderate risk of cardiac perioperative morbidity (i.e., one or two risk factors only: Q waves on electrocardiogram, angina, diabetes mellitus, age over 70 years, and treated ventricular ectopic activity). For this group of patients, these imaging techniques seem best suited to further stratifying a patient's risk of postoperative complications.

Many surgical procedures are intended to be used in the elderly and carry relatively low risk. These include cataract surgery, prostatectomy, and hip surgery (both elective joint replacement and emergent surgery for fracture). Risky surgery involves procedures on the biliary tract and all

TABLE 11–1 **THE MODIFIED MULTIFACTORIAL INDEX FOR PREOPERATIVE ASSESSMENT OF CARDIAC PATIENTS**

	Points
Coronary artery disease	
Myocardial infarction less than 6 months ago	10
Myocardial infarction more than 6 months ago	5
Canadian Cardiovascular Society angina:	
Class III (walk 1 to 2 level blocks or 1 flight of stairs)	10
Class IV (with any activity)	20
Unstable angina within 6 months	10
Alveolar pulmonary edema	
Within 1 week	10
Ever	5
Valvular disease (suspect critical aortic stenosis)	20
Arrhythmias	
Rhythm other than sinus or sinus plus atrial premature beats on last preoperative electrocardiogram	5
More than five premature ventricular contractions at any time prior to surgery	5
Poor general medical status (Po_2 <60 mmHg, Pco_2 >50 mmHg, potassium level <3.0 mEq/liter, bicarbonate <20 mEq/liter, blood urea nitrogen >50 mg/dL, creatinine >3 mg/dL, abnormal serum glutamic-oxaloacetic transaminase, signs of chronic liver disease, bedridden from noncardiac causes)	5
Age over 70	5
Emergency operation	10

Likelihood ratio for complications for score 0–15 is 0.43; for score 16–30 is 3.38; and for score >30, is 10.60.

Modified from Detsky AS, Abrams HB, McLaughlin JR, et al: Predicting cardiac complications in patients undergoing non-cardiac surgery. J Gen Intern Med 1986;1:211–219.

trauma surgery. The elderly have become major consumers of cardiovascular surgery, and age should not be a determinant in either approving or denying an appropriate procedure. Severe left ventricular dysfunction remains the greatest predictor of mortality, followed by such complicating factors as renal insufficiency, chronic obstructive pulmonary disease, other vascular disease, and low body weight.[9] Social support and home care also play extremely important roles in helping the patient return to function.

Other areas of preoperative management include antibiotic prophylaxis (see Chapter 44 for details) and anticoagulation. Numerous regimens have been advocated to reduce the perioperative risk of deep vein thrombosis or pulmonary embolism. Generally, for procedures with a high risk of thromboembolic complications (e.g., hip fracture or knee-hip replacement), more aggressive measures such as full-dose warfarin therapy or low-molecular-weight heparin are advocated. For lower risk procedures (e.g., abdominal procedures), more modest regimens such as fixed-dose subcutaneous heparin have been employed.

Preanesthetic Medical Evaluation

It is advisable to evaluate the general physical status of all patients scheduled for general anesthesia, regional anesthesia, or intravenous sedation. At the Mayo Clinic, for example, only patients with no complicated medical problems are eligible for such a preanesthetic medical evaluation (PAME). Patients with significant cardiovascular disease, bleeding diathesis, significant pulmonary disease, uncontrolled diabetes mellitus, uncontrolled hypertension, renal disease, hepatitis or jaundice, or substance abuse go on for complete medical evaluation before surgical clearance is approved.

All patients have an examination in which height, weight, vital signs, medications, allergies, review of systems, and physical examination results are recorded, with emphasis on cardiopulmonary status. Table 11–2 lists the minimum laboratory tests required before an anesthetic is administered to a healthy patient. Other tests may be indicated by the patient's medical history, medications, and examination results.

- A complete blood count (CBC) is indicated in all patients who are typed and screened or cross-matched for blood transfusions.
- Measurement of a potassium concentration is indicated in patients who are taking diuretics or are undergoing bowel preparation.

TABLE 11–2 **PREANESTHETIC LABORATORY TESTS**

Age	Tests Required
Under 40	None
40–59	ECG
	Creatinine/Glucose
Over 60	CBC, ECG, CXR
	Creatinine, glucose

Abbreviations: ECG, electrocardiogram; CBC, complete blood count; CXR, chest radiograph.

- A chest radiograph is indicated for patients who have a history of cardiac or pulmonary disease or recent respiratory symptoms.
- A history of cigarette smoking in patients over the age of 40 who are scheduled for upper abdominal or thoracic surgery is an indication for spirometry.

The electrocardiogram (ECG) is the principal test used for early detection of coronary atherosclerotic disease. However, there are important limitations in the sensitivity and specificity of electrocardiography when it is used as a screening test. A normal resting ECG does not rule out coronary disease.[10] Conversely, an abnormal ECG does not reliably predict the presence of coronary artery disease.[11] Some practitioners advocate obtaining a baseline ECG to assist in interpreting subsequent ECGs, but recent studies indicate that in actual practice, most baseline tracings uncommonly provide information that affects treatment decisions.[12]

THE STRUCTURED OFFICE VISIT

Two relatively new tools are used at the Mayo Clinic to assist physicians with history-taking and documentation. Current visit information (CVI) is required for each major access visit or "new" problem. It includes information provided by the patient except for the chief complaint, which is taken directly from the patient during the face-to-face interview. The patient-family history (PFH) form is required of patients every 3 years but is reviewed, updated, and signed each time the patient returns for a major access visit or "new" problem. Medications are updated on the CVI form along with advance directives, a systems review, ADL status, and the authorization to release medical information. The past medical history including hospitalizations, family history, social history, and other risk factor information is recorded on the PFH form.

Standardized forms were developed to save precious office time, avoid missed information, and establish a pattern of care that would be easy to understand by outside review agencies and third-party payers. Patients and families are asked to complete these forms before arriving at the office. They are mailed out in advance with the appointment reminders. At best, they each take 20 minutes to complete; very old patients are often best assisted by other family members. Once this information is placed in the permanent record it is available to all Mayo physicians to use in both the outpatient and hospital settings. Work is also underway to record this information electronically so that it can be instantly incorporated into summary letters and carried forward into subsequent examinations.

Information from the physical examination is also recorded on a structured form. This can be either handwritten or recorded through dictation, kept electronically, and printed when needed. Again, a standard check-off form is used to prevent missing information. By convention, underlined parts of the examination are recorded as normal, circled organ systems require explanation, and areas of the body not notated are considered not examined. This system works well to document for third-party payers that the examination proceeded in a logical fashion. The recorded information matches the clinical findings, diagnoses, test ordering, and billing records. In the future, the electronic record will prohibit ordering tests that are not backed up by the appropriate clinical diagnosis and plan of care.

All examination rooms are set up in the same way. No matter what floor or what building the room is in, throughout the Mayo campus there are really no surprises. By convention, speculums and gloves can always be found in the same place. The same holds true for sheets, gowns, and even tongue depressors. The standard examination table was changed a few years ago to accommodate the aging population. The earlier version had a step that was a full 12-inch lift: a great quick screen for motor dysfunction from thyroid disease but quite a struggle for a frail 80-year-old. This step is now only 5 inches high, and with fixed stirrups almost anyone who can come to the office can lift up high enough to get onto the table. As an additional compromise for the elderly body, the examination table now breaks at midbody rather than just at the head. With so many arthritic spines and poor hearts and lungs it was very difficult to get patients to lie flat safely. Now a pneumatic cylinder assists with the appropriate positioning to get the best examination possible without compromising the patient's comfort.

OFFICE TIDBITS

Fax Machines

Office automation in the form of fax machines reached the author's practice in late 1988. In an attempt to streamline the transfer of information and orders from the office back to the nursing home, nurse practitioner assessments and physician orders were initially routed back and forth to the nursing home. Although the facilities were skeptical at first, the time and cost savings have proved to be significant and have made the fax machine an indispensable tool.[13, 14] Building on this practice, dedicated facsimile access and auto dial functions have been provided to all local pharmacies. Prescription refills are handled through templates that have been mutually agreed to by pharmacists and physicians.

Managing Anticoagulation

Standardized protocols provide a great opportunity for the use of nonphysicians in the office to deliver care. One of the best examples of this may be the regulation of anticoagulation therapy. For example, at the Mayo Clinic international normalized ratio (INR) values are currently followed, allowing registered nurses (RNs) to adjust therapy in patients whose condition demands either a range of 2.0 to 3.0 or 2.5 to 3.5 by following defined adjustment protocols.[15] The following recommendations are also posted for use by the RN.[16]

MECHANICAL HEART VALVES

1. Target INR 2.5 to 3.5 for all mechanical heart valves.
2. Aspirin 100 mg/day with warfarin INR 3.0 to 4.5.
3. Dipyridamole 400 mg/day may offer added benefit.
4. If full-dose warfarin is contraindicated, use warfarin INR 2.0 to 3.0 + aspirin 660 mg + dipyridamole 150 mg/day.

TISSUE HEART VALVES

1. Mitral valves: INR 2.0 to 3.0 for 3 months.
2. Aortic valves: when in normal sinus rhythm, anticoagulation is optional.
3. Atrial fibrillation with tissue valve: INR 2.0 to 3.0 long-term.
4. Left atrial thrombus at surgery: INR 2.0 to 3.0 long-term.
5. History of thromboembolism with tissue valve: INR 2.0 to 3.0 for 3 to 12 months.
6. Tissue valves in normal sinus rhythm: aspirin 325 mg/day optional.

When to stop and start warfarin (Coumadin) in the presence of elective surgery remains something of an art form in the hands of the surgeon. As a general rule, the author stops anticoagulant therapy 7 to 10 days prior to surgery and resumes it on the day of hospital dismissal. Patients are not given a loading dose when they restart the drug but resume their regular preoperative regi-

men. The drug can be expected to reach therapeutic levels 7 to 10 days after treatment resumes.

Information Kiosks

For patients and families who must spend some time in a waiting room (what else can you call it but a waiting room?), a series of videotapes on given disease conditions can be effective educational-entertainment vehicles. Access to understandable medical information is critical for patients in view of the fact that, no matter what is said to a patient when a diagnosis is established, very little is comprehended during that first office visit. In addition to videos, informational brochures on disease-specific conditions and medication use including cross-reactivity can be very helpful. A list of family and support services available in the community specifically for the elderly can be invaluable. Additional resources exist at the senior citizens' center and through Mayo's patient education library.

Transportation

The availability of transportation service varies greatly with locale. Nursing homes and retirement centers may provide their own services for patients. Facilities that lack these services may have access to the full complement of wheelchair cabs and specialized van services for the handicapped. Some cities subsidize door-to-door service for people who are too impaired to use public transportation. Given the frequency of inclement weather throughout the country, the process of moving people from one indoor environment to another indoor environment often becomes a major challenge. Skyways and subways can only do so much. The Baldwin Building for community medicine at the Mayo Clinic, for example, has an easy access drive-up area that is protected from wind and snow. An outer series of sliding doors can accommodate wheelchairs and stretchers. Patients then face two inner doors and can choose from either the energy-saving revolving door or another set of sliding doors large enough to allow assisted entry. Skilled help is readily available regardless of weather conditions.

Patient Correspondence

If at all possible, a central office should remind patients of appointments through the mail or by phone. The PFH and CVI previously discussed are sent to patients before annual examinations and major access visits. In that the author's clinic is a primary care practice, very few letters have to be sent to referring physicians. However, there is significant correspondence with home health agencies, nursing homes, and equipment suppliers. Until recently, special forms that made use of carboned duplicates for handwritten notes were used to communicate with other providers of care to patients. Recently the Mayo Clinic's electronic record has been more fully implemented, and all physicians now use full dictation. Duplicates of transcribed notes are either mailed or faxed to the appropriate parties. Although the immediacy of a handwritten progress note that is identical to the clinical record has been sacrificed, significant gains in legibility have been made.

Physicians at Mayo follow a dictation template in preparing their remarks for the electronic medical record. Transcriptionists are responsible for this specific task. A complete discussion of the development of an electronic record and the different data elements that go into making such a record is unfortunately beyond the scope of this chapter.

THE ORGANIZED OFFICE

One might think that tremendous uniformity of action would result from 31 salaried physicians working collaboratively in a practice of primary care established 50 years ago to provide community care in the nation's first group practice of medicine. Think again! True growth comes from experimentation, and within the four sections of the Division of Community Internal Medicine at the Mayo Clinic, different activities abound. All sections participate in the implementation of guidelines including uncomplicated urinary tract infection (UTI), smoking cessation, preventive services, and immunizations. However, the use of nurses and clinical assistants for office and telephone help in the different sections varies tremendously.

Emerging patterns of practice include one-on-one accountability with an "assistant." Given the limited time physicians now have to spend with patients, more cost-effective use of additional personnel is required. In addition, the myriad of rules and responsibilities, guidelines to be followed, and documentation required for billing procedures further moves the physician away from the patient. All nonphysician activities should be done by somebody else, leaving the evaluation and management responsibilities that require physician time to the physician. Straightforward problems such as uncomplicated UTIs, sore throats, viral upper respiratory infections (URIs), and sinusitis are now handled by RN

staff using standardized algorithms (although not in the geriatric population).

In modern practice the volume of telephone calls has gone up dramatically, first because patients are too busy to come in, and second because health plans and incentive systems encourage patients to stay away. The Mayo Careline (a contract service) provides 24-hour nurse advice and appropriate triage guidance. This helps to ensure that patients receive the appropriate level of service for their particular problem. Telephone triage is handled divisionally by nurses stationed on clinical floors who work with only some protocols and even fewer algorithms.

Disease management services remain a developing concept. Although the health care team is in favor of providing better information to patients, the "fax on demand" at Mayo is used only in continuing medical education. Consideration has been given to providing multilingual instructions to patients using "smart" fax machines (computers), but this process has yet to begin. Mayo's Web sites offer patients information about specific disease entities and provide enough information to make appointments. Questions may be answered in the public forum, much as is done with the Mayo Health Letter, but individualized responses may constitute the practice of medicine across state lines. Patients requesting appointment information are for the most part given a phone number to call when they are ready to come.

MEDICATION REVIEW

Compliance remains a major difficulty in the management of medications in the elderly. Elderly Americans spend approximately $3 billion per year on prescription medications, little of which is reimbursed by third-party payers. There is a direct correlation between advancing age and the number of drugs prescribed. At least 90% of Americans over age 65 take at least one prescription medication daily, and a majority take two or more.[17] Cardiovascular drugs, antihypertensive agents, analgesics, anti-inflammatory drugs, sedatives, and gastrointestinal preparations are the most commonly used medications in the elderly.[18] The more medications an individual takes, the more frequent the dosing, the more complicated the instructions, and the more expensive the drugs, the less likely it is that the patient will take the pills as prescribed. A well-informed patient and meticulous control over medication use are the keys to success. Reminders to patients to bring all their drugs (including over-the-counter medications) in for review at each office visit is critical (Fig. 11–1).

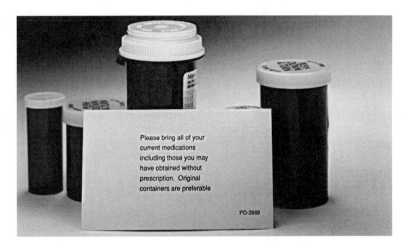

Figure 11–1 Mail reminder to patients to bring medications to office visit.

Please bring all of your current medications including those you may have obtained without prescription. Original containers are preferable

PD-2868

The medications are reviewed against hospital discharge summaries, home care orders, and the patient's own schedule. Every attempt should be made to put all prescriptions under one physician's name (again for ease of review) and rigorously scrutinize each program to make sure it is as simple to understand and as easy to follow as possible. Patients should be encouraged to use only one pharmacy for their business, which makes an occasional call to double-check a prescription much easier for all parties. When possible, patients should know the names of each of their drugs and should have a good understanding of why they are being used.

Breaking pills in half and using a dosing schedule of more than three times a day should be discouraged. By convention, in the author's practice warfarin (Coumadin) is dispensed only in 2.5-mg tablets, making the "currency of exchange" less complicated for anticoagulation protocols and less likely to create error among all caregivers. Examples of pill boxes that can be

purchased are also made available to patients both in the office and through the hospital pharmacy. Boxes should have lids that are easy to open and be able to handle a week's worth of medication, usually seven columns and four rows. Most important, the cover must be transparent so that one can see in a matter of seconds what is inside (Fig. 11–2). Medication organizers should not be a game of hide and seek. The newer electronic dispensers may catch on, but for now they are complex, expensive, and intimidating.

ADVANCE DIRECTIVES

Hospitals, nursing homes, and physicians have been required since the passage of the Omnibus Budget Reconciliation Act (OBRA) 1990 and the Patient Self-Determination Act to provide information about advance directives to all patients. If possible, it is preferable to organize the patient record to accommodate advance directives with

Figure 11–2 Medication organizer.

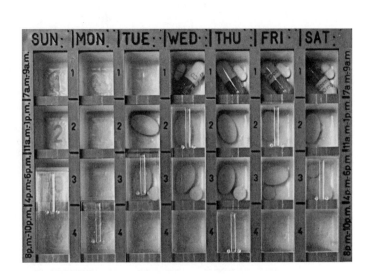

both a notifier to physicians that one exists and a repository to contain the actual documents. The information contained in the record may include a living will, an autopsy directive, an anatomic bequest, and information about a durable power of attorney. The availability of living will templates as well as information about counseling, such as that obtained through local senior citizens' centers, can be quite helpful.

Advance directives include living wills and the durable power of attorney (DPoA) for health care matters. Living wills are explicit value-based declarations used by patients to refuse or accept various life-sustaining medical interventions in the event of terminal illness. Alternatively, the durable power of attorney is designed to allow someone to speak for the patient when the patient with certain medical conditions cannot make his or her wishes known. Despite enthusiasm for written advance directives, few adults have completed them.[19] A randomized controlled trial from Kaiser Permanente found that mailing an educational pamphlet and form about the durable power of attorney to patients over 65 years of age significantly increased the number who completed the durable power of attorney form.[20] The living will is an easy first start, but in some states it is less useful than the DPoA because of restrictions on implementation.

SOCIAL SERVICES

Social workers in the office setting are a luxury few can afford. Even in the hospital this resource seems to be extremely difficult to find. At times, resources available through the county or local ombudsman can augment services that are accessible through the office or hospital system. Minnesota's legislation on vulnerable adults for example is quite strong and provides county support to at least investigate potential abuse. The ombudsman system can handle patients in the community, but its greatest impact is on nursing home patients. Home health agencies have a vested interest in generating business, as do nursing homes, and often the best service and most accurate financial advice comes from these businesses. Area Agencies on Aging, through provisions specified in the Older Americans Act (1964), provide free legal services to those in need. The "circuit rider," often a paralegal, can usually be found holding court at the local senior citizens' center.

SUMMARY

Functional assessment of older persons can best be carried out in an office practice set up to handle a more complex population of patients.

Activities of daily living, mobility, cognition, special senses, and psychosocial issues are only a few of the problems facing clinician and patient alike. Several tools are available to increase the effectiveness of the clinical examination (see Chapters 1 and 2). The goals of these evaluative measures are to identify impairments, prevent disabilities, and remove barriers to independence. These goals are accomplished through efforts to improve function, modify medical and social boundaries, and increase assistance given to the patient when needed. Identification of risk factors for geriatric syndromes may promote restoration of compensatory ability and prevent the onset of functional dependence. The primary care physician's ability to attend to these functional goals may improve a patient's quality of life and can assist in directing the management of associated chronic medical disorders.

Other chapters in this text highlight areas that should be emphasized in office geriatric practices. These include the appropriate history and physical examination (Chapter 1), functional assessment (Chapters 1 and 2), cognition assessment (Chapters 1, 26, and 27), driving (Chapter 7), prevention assessment (Chapter 13), nutritional assessment (Chapter 15), gait and fall assessment (Chapters 1 and 19), and sensory assessment (Chapters 41 and 42).

References

1. Rubin CD, Sizemor MT, et al: A randomized, controlled trial of outpatient geriatric evaluation and management in a large public hospital. J Am Geriatr Soc 1993;41:1023–1028.
2. Stults BM: Preventive health care for the elderly. West J Med 1984;141:832–845.
3. Pace WD: Geriatric assessment in the office setting. Geriatrics 1989;44:29–35.
4. Kennie DC, Warshaw G: Health maintenance and screening in the elderly. In Reichel W (ed): Clinical Aspects of Aging, 3rd ed. Baltimore, Williams & Wilkins, 1989, pp. 13–25.
5. Thomas DR, Ritchie CS: Preoperative assessment of older adults. J Am Geriatr Soc 1995;43:811–821.
6. Dripps RD, Lamont A, Eckenhoff JE: The role of anesthesia in surgical mortality. JAMA 1961;778:261–266.
7. Bernstein GM, Offenbartl SK: Adverse surgical outcomes among patients with cognitive impairments. Am Surg 1991;57:682–690.
8. Fleisher LA, Eagle KA: Screening for cardiac disease in patients having noncardiac surgery. Ann Intern Med 1996;124:767–772.
9. Higgins TI, Estafanous FG, Loop FD, et al: Stratification for morbidity and mortality outcome by preoperative risk factors in coronary bypass patients: A clinical severity score. JAMA 1992;267:2344–2348.
10. Detrano R, Froelicher V: A logical approach to screening for coronary artery disease. Ann Intern Med 1987;106:846–852.
11. Kannel WB, Anderson K, McGee DL, et al:

Nonspecific electrocardiographic abnormality as a predictor of coronary heart disease: The Framingham study. Am Heart J 1987;113:370–376.

12. Sivaram CA, Ahmed N, Lestina JR: Electrocardiogram in the ambulatory clinic in older patients with cardiac disease: An assessment of the contribution to management. J Am Geriatr Soc 1996;44:452–455.

13. Tangalos EG, Freeman PI, Garness SL: Nursing homes and fax machines. JAMA 1990;264(6):693–694.

14. Tangalos EG, Freeman PI: Nursing homes and fax machines (in reply). JAMA 1990;264(23):2296.

15. Hirsh J, Poller L: The international normalized ratio. A guide to understanding and correcting its problems (review). Arch Intern Med 1994;154(3):282–288.

16. Stein PD, Alpert JS, Coplan J, et al: Antithrombotic therapy in patients with mechanical and biotic prosthetic heart valves. ACCP guidelines. Chest 1992;102(Suppl 4):445S–455S.

17. Moellar JF, Mathiowetz NA: Prescribed medications: A summary of use and expenditures by Medicare beneficiaries. National Center of Health Services Research and Health Care Technology Assessment. DHHS Publication No. (8HS)89-3448. National Medical Expenditure Survey Research Findings, Vol. 3 (Sept.). Rockville, MD, Department of Health and Human Services, 1989.

18. Hale WE, May FE, Marks RG, Stewart RB: Drug use in an ambulatory elderly population: A five-year update. Drug Intell Clin Pharm 1987;21:530–535.

19. Steiber SR: Right to die: Public balks at deciding for others. Hospitals 1987;61(5):72.

20. Rubin SM, Strull WM, Fialkow MF, Weiss SJ, Lo B: Increasing the completion of the durable power of attorney for health care: A randomized controlled trial. JAMA 1994;271(3):209–212.

12 Palliative Care

Diane E. Meier, M.D.

R. Sean Morrison, M.D.

Judith C. Ahronheim, M.D.

The dramatic advances in medical care that have taken place during the past century have had the untoward side effect of changing the definition of death from the natural culmination of life into an unwanted outcome of disease and a failure of medical intervention. A century ago the majority of Americans died in their homes, but of the 2 million deaths that now occur annually in the United States, more than 80% occur within a health care institution (65% in hospitals and 15% in nursing homes). The causes of death have also changed during the past 100 years. Whereas in 1900 five of the ten leading causes of death in the geriatric population were infectious diseases, in 1995 only pneumonia and influenza remained in the top ten. Our enhanced ability to manage successfully and significantly extend life for patients with chronic disease (diabetes, congestive heart failure, coronary artery disease, renal failure) and to cure previously fatal diseases (e.g., cancer, bacterial infections, tuberculosis) has blurred the boundary between curable diseases and those that inexorably result in death. It is not an understatement to suggest that many patients and health care providers regard the prolongation of life and the cure of disease as the fundamental and exclusive goals of modern medicine. The inability of our medical culture to regard the quest for a peaceful death as a legitimate medical enterprise has rendered a profound disservice to millions of dying persons in this country and has led to a demonstrable inability to meet the needs of such persons and their families. Caring for dying patients is not easy. It requires an ability to address and balance the needs of patients and families, to communicate about intimate and existential issues, to use one's expertise in pain and symptom management, and to coordinate and function within an interdisciplinary team.

CONFRONTING DEATH

Discussions about end-of-life care should ideally begin well before patients and physicians are confronted with a life-threatening event. A routine office visit presents an opportune time to inquire about whether an advance directive has been completed and to explore patients' attitudes, values, and beliefs about their life and their medical care. All too often, however, advance care planning does not occur, and physicians face the challenge of exploring these issues after the patient has lost decision-making capacity with family members who may not know the patient's wishes about care.

Breaking Bad News

Informing a patient that he or she has a fatal disease, even when advance care planning has been undertaken, is one of the most stressful tasks a physician faces. Yet the manner in which such news is delivered and the plan of care that is developed ultimately have a significant impact on the quality of life remaining for a patient. Although there are many forms of "bad news" and an equal number of clinical situations in which such news is delivered, the following framework provides some useful general guidelines for how to share such news with patients.[1, 2]

Establishing the proper physical context before initiating the patient encounter is critical. Ideally, bad news should be delivered in person in a private area in which there will be no interruptions. One should sit down, make eye contact with the patient, and then begin the discussion by exploring the patient's knowledge of the illness. Grasping the patient's comprehension of the disease and his or her understanding of its impact on the future provides the physician with a useful starting point for the remainder of the conversation. Patients with a thorough understanding of the complexities of their disease require a different approach than uninformed or less sophisticated patients. The next step is to ascertain how much information the patient wants to know. For example, "Would you like me to give you the full details of the situation or is there someone else with whom you would rather I discuss it?" Although the majority of patients desire to be fully informed about their condition and the options facing them, some may not, or they may prefer family members to be so informed and to make decisions for them. Recent research suggests that this may be particularly true for patients of certain ethnic groups in the United States.[3]

Once it has been established how much information the patient wants, it is time to share the information with the patient—a process that has been referred to as aligning and educating.[1] The discussion should begin at the patient's level of understanding and should make use of common words and phrases. Throughout the conversation, the physician should listen to the patient's concerns, frequently reinforce and clarify information, assess the patient's comprehension of what has been said, and, very importantly, avoid the temptation to present too much information all at once. Finally, the clinician should respond to the patient's feelings and organize an immediate therapeutic plan that includes specific references to the patient's concerns and incorporates the patient's agenda.

The question about whether to inform a patient of a diagnosis of Alzheimer's disease has received little attention in the literature and remains controversial. Arguments against such truth-telling cite the uncertainty of the diagnosis in the early stages of the disease, the fact that patients are often brought to medical attention by concerned family members who may ask that the diagnosis not be shared, and the fact that patients with dementia may not have the capacity to fully comprehend the nature of the diagnosis or to take appropriate action based on the information. Authors favoring full disclosure cite the principle of patient autonomy and the need for patients to be aware of their diagnosis to plan appropriately for their future medical care and indeed, for their remaining life.[4] The few empirical studies that have examined this question are limited by small sample sizes but have found that a majority of patients want to be told of a diagnosis of dementia.[5]

Eliciting Patient Preferences

Once a terminal diagnosis has been made and the information has been shared, the discussion should shift to an attempt to elicit patient preferences and goals of care. On a global level, one wants to determine whether the patient prefers to direct treatment toward achieving maximum life prolongation or whether optimization of comfort is more important given the limited life expectancy. Outlining a realistic evaluation of the available treatment options (e.g., probability and extent of response to treatment, duration and quality of extended life, anticipated side effects), identifying patients' short- and long-term goals and needs, discovering their expectations about therapy, and evaluating their coping strategies are critical components of this discussion. The goal of this conversation is to lead the patient to an understanding of the benefits and burdens of the available treatment options and to develop an individualized plan of care that is acceptable to them and is in keeping with their values and goals. This is also an appropriate time to elicit from patients their preferences about specific life-sustaining treatments such as cardiopulmonary resuscitation, artificial nutrition and hydration, and mechanical intubation. It is also appropriate to review with them the potential indications for such therapies and to offer a realistic appraisal of the outcome in their situation. A review and revision, if necessary, of a previously completed advance directive or the execution of a new directive are natural prologues to such a discussion.

PALLIATIVE CARE

As defined by the World Health Organization, palliative care is the active total care of a patient whose disease does not respond to curative treatment. Control of pain, of other symptoms, and of psychological, social, and spiritual problems is paramount. The goal of palliative care is the achievement of the best quality of life that is possible for the patient and the family.[6] Whereas the model disease for palliative care has traditionally been cancer, palliation is also appropriate for patients with other chronic illnesses such as congestive heart failure, chronic obstructive pulmonary disease, renal failure, and degenerative neurologic conditions such as Alzheimer's disease, amyotrophic lateral sclerosis, and Parkinson's disease. Although many speak of switching from life prolongation to palliation, or from cure to care, it is rare for such a defining moment to be clearly evident in the course of most chronic illnesses. Rather, it is more reasonable to begin a dialogue with the patient at the time of diagnosis, emphasizing that the initial focus of care will be directed toward life prolongation, if indeed this is appropriate and desired by the patient. A continual reassessment of the benefits and burdens of treatment is necessary as the disease advances so that as the ratio of benefits to burdens shifts, there will be an accompanying increase in the proportion of palliative interventions.

Hospice Care

Patients for whom the sole focus of care is palliation can and should be offered the option of hospice care. Hospice provides interdisciplinary team care (physicians; nurses; social workers; home health aides; clergy and spiritual advisors; speech, language, occupational, and physical therapists; and volunteers) to dying patients, primarily in the home, although some hospices serve patients in long-term care facilities and residences. Since 1982, hospice care has been available under the Medicare program for all part A beneficiaries who have a life expectancy of 6 months or less and are willing to forego standard Medicare-reimbursed services in favor of palliative care. Services covered under this program include physician and nursing care, medical equipment and supplies, outpatient medications for symptom management and pain relief, short-term inpatient care, up to 4 hours per day of a home health aid, and physical and occupational therapy. Hospice is also covered by the Civilian Health and Medical Program for Uniformed Services (CHAMPUS), many third-party insurers and managed care organizations, and Medicaid in 36 states.

Despite the existence of the Medicare benefit, a substantial number of dying patients are unable to utilize hospice services. Patients living in rural areas and inner cities often have very limited access to hospice services because of a scarcity of programs in these areas. Patients without family or significant others or patients with working family members may also be unable to avail themselves of hospice. The hospice benefit typically provides for only 4 hours of custodial home health aide services, thus requiring the family to provide the remaining 20 hours—a time commitment or financial obligation that is impossible for many families to meet. Although inpatient hospice care might be considered an alternative, the financial limitations of the hospice benefit (inpatient costs must be paid out of the hospice per-diem rate) preclude this option except in situations of brief intercurrent illnesses or terminal care in the last few days of life. Lack of knowledge also contributes to the underuse of hospice palliative care services. Despite the fact that hospice has existed in this country for more than 20 years, many physicians and patients are still not aware of the availability of hospice or fail to consider hospice as an option early enough in the course of the disease. Indeed, a substantial number of hospice referrals are made after the patient has become moribund and is not able to benefit from the interdisciplinary services that hospice provides. Finally, the difficulty of determining a 6-month prognosis in dying patients, particularly those with chronic illnesses (e.g., chronic obstructive pulmonary disease, congestive heart failure) or slowly progressive neurologic disorders such as Alzheimer's disease often inhibits referral to hospice for palliative care.

Prognostication

The ability to predict the course of disease accurately becomes increasingly important in terminally ill patients. Patients and families desire a reasonable estimate of life expectancy to plan for their remaining time and to get their affairs in order. Physicians must be able to prognosticate accurately to time the referral to hospice appropriately. Despite the importance of this topic, relatively little attention has been paid to prognostication in the professional literature, and there exist very few instruments that can be used to estimate life expectancy accurately for individual patients. Life expectancy for patients with dementia, motor neuron disease, acquired immune deficiency syndrome (AIDS), and advanced cardiac or pulmonary disease is highly variable, making prognostication even more difficult. Most studies that report *objective* prognostic data do so for very select patient populations and often do not take into account such variables as comorbid conditions or health-related quality of life. A task force from the National Hospice Organization recently reviewed the available data on prognostication and has published guidelines to aid physicians in determining when hospice referral is appropriate for patients with noncancer diagnoses.[7] Until future research further defines this issue, the following guidelines have been suggested as a reasonable approach for clinicians faced with estimating life expectancy for an individual patient: (1) Identify objective measures of prognosis if available; (2) assess the validity and reliability of the measures; (3) assess the relevance and utility of the measures; and (4) evaluate how the patient's unique clinical or social attributes modify the prognosis.[8]

SYMPTOM MANAGEMENT

Pain Assessment

Relief of pain and other physical symptoms is one of the central goals of palliative care. A review of multiple surveys in cancer patients demonstrates that more than half of patients have pain that is unrelieved.[9] The recent SUPPORT (Study to Understand Prognoses and Preferences for Outcomes and Risks of Treatment) study[10] found that 50% of conscious seriously ill,

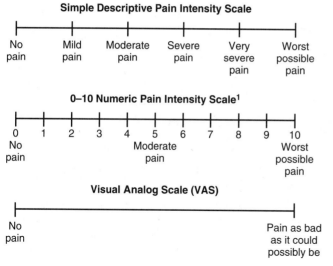

Figure 12–1 Pain intensity scales. (From Jacox A, Carr D, Payne R, et al: Management of Cancer Pain. Clinical Practice Guideline No. 9. AHCPR Publication No. 94-0592. Rockville, MD, U.S. Department of Health and Human Services, Public Health Service, Agency for Health Care Policy and Research, 1994.)

hospitalized patients suffered moderate to severe pain at least half the time during their last 3 days of life. In studies of institutionalized elderly, the prevalence of pain ranges from 45% to 80%[11] and is associated with musculoskeletal and degenerative joint disorders, neuropathies, ischemic vascular disease, and cancer. Significant functional consequences follow from untreated pain in this population, including depression, social withdrawal, immobility, sleep disturbance, cognitive impairment, and malnutrition, among others.[11] These data demonstrate the problem of underrecognition of pain in our medical culture and emphasize the need for enhanced identification of pain and suffering through formal assessment procedures.

Pain is a subjective sensation that is influenced by many physical, emotional, and social factors and requires comprehensive assessment of these domains to permit proper treatment. Formal pain assessment procedures permit rational choices of diagnostic and therapeutic interventions, ensure that pain and other distressing symptoms are actually recognized if they are present, and convey the message to the patient that the presence of pain is important and of interest to the health care professional.

Pain assessment is particularly complex in elderly patients, who typically underreport their symptoms and usually present with several medical comorbid conditions in addition to the main disease process; in addition, the prevalence of cognitive impairment is significantly higher in this group than in the general population. Published instruments that measure pain intensity have not been well validated in elderly populations. Brevity, use of a visual-analog or numerical scale, and ease of administration are critical to

the usefulness of these instruments in the practice setting. Commonly used and validated tools include the Edmonton Symptom Assessment Scale,[12] the Wisconsin Brief Pain Inventory,[13] and the Memorial Pain Assessment Card (Fig. 12–1).[14] Patients with visual, hearing, or motor impairments may be unable to complete the instrument without help, and no valid tools for assessment of pain in the moderately or severely cognitively impaired are currently available. In all patient populations it is critical to take seriously the patient's expression of distress, particularly if it represents a change from baseline status. Grimacing or avoidance behaviors during movement or during a physical examination are obvious signs of pain or discomfort and should prompt a search for the source of the symptom, and appropriate therapy. A change in functional capacity is another marker for the presence of physical distress when patients are unable to self report. Agitation and screaming commonly attributed to the underlying dementia in cognitively impaired patients and managed with neuroleptics may be due to untreated physical pain, a possibility that should be assessed by thorough physical examination and appropriate diagnostic studies.

Pain Management

Because pain research has focused almost exclusively on young and middle-aged patients, the applications of currently available data in older adults are limited. The difficulty of balancing therapeutic benefits in terms of symptom relief with the burden of drug side effects is particularly challenging in this age group, mandating aggressive and preventive approaches to predictable side effects such as constipation and implementation of a knowledgeable and rapid response to less common side effects such as hallucinations. The essential principles of pain management, based on recommendations of the United States Agency for Health Care Policy and Research, are listed in Table 12–1.[14] All clinicians should be familiar with the World Health Organization (WHO) three-step analgesic ladder, which is a validated, simple, and effective method of ensuring pain relief.[15] Step 1, for mild to moderate pain, recommends the use of a nonopioid analgesic with or without an adjuvant agent and followed in patients with worsening or unresponsive pain, by the addition of a so-called weak opioid such as codeine or oxycodone (step 2). Pain that is moderate to severe at baseline or that does not respond adequately to a step 2 regimen, should be treated with larger doses of a weak opioid or a more highly potent opioid such as morphine, hydromorphone, levorphanol, or fentanyl (step 3). An adjuvant analgesic agent

may be added at any step on the ladder (see later under Adjuvant Analgesics for a discussion of adjuvant agents). Frequent upward dose titration may be necessary as the disease progresses.

There is no ceiling or maximum permitted dose for opioid agonists (although codeine doses above 65 mg are associated with dose-limiting side effects), and some patients require large doses for control of severe pain. Development of unmanageable side effects from one agent may be addressed by lowering the dose and increasing dose frequency (if adequate analgesia is present) or by switching to a different agent and taking advantage of incomplete cross-tolerance. The new agent should be started at approximately half the equianalgesic dose of the initial drug (Table 12–2). Appropriate initial dose reductions should be employed for elderly patients, particularly those with renal or hepatic disease or congestive heart failure. In some elderly patients the risks of renal injury or hepatotoxicity associated with acetaminophen and the risks of renal injury,

---

TABLE 12–1 **ESSENTIAL PAIN MANAGEMENT GUIDELINES***

1. Individualize the regimen to the patient.
2. Use the simplest dosing schedule and least invasive treatment modalities first. Begin analgesics at half the usual recommended adult starting dose and titrate slowly, watching for side effects as the drug accumulates.
3. Use acetaminophen or a nonsteroidal anti-inflammatory agent (NSAID) for mild to moderate pain unless there is a contraindication. Long-term use of NSAIDs is associated with a high risk of gastropathy and bleeding in the elderly. First-line use of a "weak opioid" may be safer in this population.
4. Add an opioid for persisting or worsening pain, beginning with codeine or oxycodone.
5. Change to higher potency opioids (morphine, hydromorphone, or levorphanol) for persistent or worsening pain that is unresponsive to appropriate doses of codeine or oxycodone.
6. Chronic or persistent pain should be treated with an around-the-clock regimen with additional "rescue" or prn doses to maintain a steady drug level and avoid pain recurrence.
7. Meperidine should not be used in treatment of pain because of the accumulation of toxic metabolites that may cause confusion, especially in the elderly. Mixed agonist-antagonist opioids (such as pentazocine) may cause agitation and will precipitate opioid withdrawal in patients taking opioid agonists.
8. Tolerance and physical dependency are expected consequences of opioid therapy and are not the same thing as psychological addiction.
9. The oral route is preferred when possible, but rectal and transdermal opioids are available to permit avoidance of parenteral administration of opioid analgesics. Intramuscular administration should not be used because it is painful and leads to unreliable absorption and serum levels.
10. Patients with pain unresponsive to maximal systemic opioids should be considered for intraspinal analgesia.
11. Constipation is a nearly universal side effect of opioids and should be treated preventively, with close monitoring for development of fecal impaction. Fecal impaction may present with diarrhea, urinary retention, or delirium, especially in the elderly.
12. Placebos should not be used in the management of pain.
13. The medication and other treatment regimens should be written out for the patient and family.
14. Clear communication about the pain management regimen should occur prior to any transfers between care settings.

*Adapted from Jacox A, Carr D, Payne R, et al: Management of cancer pain. Clinical Practice Guideline No. 9. AHCPR Publication No. 94-0592. Rockville, MD, U.S. Department of Health and Human Services, Public Health Service, Agency for Health Care Policy and Research, 1994.

TABLE 12-2 **DOSE EQUIVALENTS FOR OPIOID ANALGESICS IN OPIOID-NAIVE ADULTS >50 kg BODY WEIGHT**[a]

| Drug | Approximate Equianalgesic Dose | | Usual Starting Dose for Moderate to Severe Pain | |
	Oral	Parenteral	Oral	Parenteral
Opioid Agonist[b]				
Morphine[c]	30 mg q 3–4 h (repeat around-the-clock dosing) 60 mg q 3–4 h (single dose or intermittent dosing)	10 mg q 3–4 h	30 mg q 3–4 h	10 mg q 3–4 h
Morphine, controlled-release[c,d] (MS Contin, Oramorph)	90–120 mg q 12 h	N/A	90–120 mg q 12 h	N/A
Hydromorphone[c] (Dilaudid)	7.5 mg q 3–4 h	1.5 mg q 3–4 h	6 mg q 3–4 h	1.5 mg q 3–4 h
Levorphanol (Levo-Dromoran)	4 mg q 6–8 h	2 mg q 6–8 h	4 mg q 6–8 h	2 mg q 6–8 h
Meperidine (Demerol)	300 mg q 2–3 h	100 mg q 3 h	N/R	100 mg q 3 h
Methadone (Dolophine, other)	20 mg q 6–8 h	10 mg q 6–8 h	20 mg q 6–8 h	10 mg q 6–8 h
Oxymorphone[c] (Numorphan)	N/A	1 mg q 3–4 h	N/A	1 mg q 3–4 h
Combination Opioid/NSAID Preparations[e]				
Codeine[f] (with aspirin or acetaminophen)	180–200 mg q 3–4 h	130 mg q 3–4 h	60 mg q 3–4 h	60 mg q 2 h (IM/SC)
Hydrocodone (in Lorcet, Lortab, Vicodin, others)	30 mg q 3–4 h	N/A	10 mg q 3–4 h	N/A
Oxycodone (Roxicodone, also in Percocet, Percodan, Tylox, others)	30 mg q 3–4 h	N/A	10 mg q 3–4 h	N/A

[a]Caution: Recommended doses do not apply for adult patient with body weight <50 kg.

[b]Caution: Recommended doses do not apply to patients with renal or hepatic insufficiency or other conditions affecting drug metabolism and kinetics. Smaller starting doses should be used in elderly, opioid naive patients.

[c]Caution: For morphine, hydromorphone, and oxymorphone, rectal administration is an alternative route for patients unable to take oral medications. Equianalgesic doses may differ from oral and parenteral routes because of pharmacokinetic differences.

[d]Transdermal fentanyl (Duragesic) is an alternative. Transdermal fentanyl dosage is not calculated as equianalgesic to a single dose of morphine. Doses above 25 mcg/h should not be used in opioid-naive patients.

[e]Caution: Doses of aspirin and acetaminophen in combination opioid/NSAID preparations must also be adjusted to the patient's weight.

[f]Caution: Codeine doses above 65 mg are not appropriate because of diminishing incremental analgesia with increasing doses but continually increasing nausea, constipation, and other side effects.

NOTE: Published tables vary in suggested doses that are equianalgesic to morphine. Clinical response is the criterion that must be applied for each patient; titration to clinical response is necessary. Because there is not complete cross-tolerance among these drugs, it is usually necessary to use a lower than equianalgesic dose when changing drugs and to retitrate.

Abbreviations: q, every; N/A, not available; N/R, not recommended; IM, intramuscular; SC, subcutaneous.

From Jacox A, Carr D, Payne R, et al. Management of cancer pain. Clinical Practice Guideline No. 9. AHCPR Publication No. 94-0592. Rockville, MD, U.S. Department of Health and Human Services, Public Health Service, Agency for Health Care Policy and Research, 1994.

gastrointestinal toxicity, or bleeding associated with nonsteroidal anti-inflammatory agents may support the initial use of step 2 weak opioids (codeine or oxycodone alone) rather than the nonopioid step 1 agents.[11]

MANAGEMENT OF OPIOID SIDE EFFECTS

Because of the high prevalence of constipation, cognitive impairment, and polypharmacy in the elderly, skilled preventive efforts and management of the side effects of opioids are critical to the successful use of analgesics in this population. The most common side effects of opioids are constipation and sedation, but confusion, nausea, dry mouth, urinary retention, hallucinations, dysphoria, euphoria, altered cognition, and the syndrome of inappropriate secretion of antidiuretic hormone are also seen. Because of their high risk of toxicity, several opioids should not be used or should be used only with great caution in elderly patients. These include meperidine (accumulation of toxic metabolites); propoxyphene (no more effective than nonopioids as an analgesic but has all the side effects and toxicities of an opioid); pentazocine (associated with agitation in elderly patients); and long-acting opioids such as methadone and transdermal fentanyl (which may accumulate to dangerous levels in elderly persons with impaired drug metabolism).

Gastrointestinal and Urologic Side Effects. Constipation is a nearly universal side effect of opioid analgesics that can lead to serious and sometimes life-threatening complications if not identified and treated appropriately. Unlike the tolerance that develops to other side effects of opioids, constipation does not diminish over time and requires preventive and combined use of stool softeners, rectal suppositories, "irritant" laxatives (e.g., bisacodyl or senna), and hyperosmotic agents (milk of magnesia, lactulose). Fecal impaction may present with a change in mental status, diarrhea, or urinary retention and should always be ruled out when there is any change in clinical status in a patient receiving opioid agents.

Nausea and vomiting may occur as a drug side effect, as a consequence of intestinal obstruction due to fecal impaction, or as a result of another underlying disease process. Antiemetic agents (ondansetron, cisapride, metoclopramide, haloperidol, prochlorperazine, scopolamine, or hydroxyzine) given at regular dosage intervals are usually effective in treating opioid-induced nausea. The side effects of phenothiazine derivatives, antihistamines, and scopolamine as antiemetics include anticholinergic effects, hallucinations,

and extrapyramidal disorders, and these side effects pose relative contraindications to the use of these agents in the elderly. Ondansetron and cisapride have fewer antidopaminergic effects but are costly. Dry mouth may be treated with oral lubricants (lemon glycerin swabs), ice chips, artificial saliva, and frequent sips of fluid.

Urinary retention may result from the anticholinergic effect of the opioid, drug interactions with other anticholinergic agents, fecal impaction, prostatic hypertrophy, or progression of tumor. It is common in patients who are receiving spinal opioid analgesics. If a change in opioid type or route of administration is ineffective, intermittent urethral catheterization or an indwelling catheter may be necessary to allow continued administration of the drug.

Central Nervous System Side Effects. Sedation is a common early side effect of opioids, but patients can be reassured that tolerance to this symptom usually develops over several days. Because of the risk of confusion, falls, and other central nervous system effects of multiple drug-drug interactions in older patients, close supervision at home is necessary early in the course of therapy for opioid-naive patients. Persistent sedation should be managed by ruling out other causes of delirium (including interaction with other sedating medications), reducing the dosage and increasing the frequency of administration of the lower dose, switching to a different opioid, or adding psychostimulants (e.g., methylphenidate, 2.5 to 5 mg morning and early afternoon) if the previous measures fail. Hallucinations and confusion should also be managed by ruling out other causes of delirium, reducing the opioid dose, increasing the dosage frequency, switching to an alternative opioid, or, if these measures fail, adding a low dose of a major tranquilizer such as haloperidol or resperidol.

Respiratory depression may occur in opioid-naive patients until tolerance develops to this side effect or, rarely, when a pain stimulus suddenly ceases and sedative effects predominate. A build-up of agents with a long half-life in the elderly (methadone, sustained-release morphine sulfate, transdermal fentanyl, levorphanol), especially in patients with comorbid cardiac, renal, or liver disease, typically results in progressive sedation that will lead to respiratory depression if it is not identified and corrected early. Withholding the next one or two doses and reducing the 24-hour dosage total by about 25% will usually correct the oversedation before it is necessary to resort to opioid antagonists. If opioid antagonists (naloxone) are needed to prevent respiratory arrest, they must be slowly titrated to avoid the recurrence of severe pain and opioid withdrawal symptoms.[14] When adequate pain control cannot be achieved without risking respiratory depression, careful review of the goals of therapy is mandated. If the patient is near death and is suffering greatly, the benefits of pain relief and a peaceful death usually outweigh the risk of a slightly hastened death.

ADJUVANT ANALGESICS

Adjuvant agents are used to supplement analgesia when opioids are insufficient, to manage concurrent symptoms (such as anxiety or depression contributing to pain) or side effects (such as sedation), and to treat symptoms that are relatively unresponsive to opioid agents (such as neuropathic pain syndromes). Tricyclic antidepressants are widely used for the treatment of neuropathic pain and as supplements to opioid analgesia through their direct analgesic effects, potentiation of opiates, and mood elevation. Amitriptyline is the best studied agent for these indications, but its strong anticholinergic profile with the associated side effects of constipation, urinary retention, orthostatic hypotension, risk of falls, dry mouth, and sedation make it a difficult drug to use safely in the elderly, especially in combination with opioids.

Although there are fewer data to support their use as adjuvant analgesics, nortriptyline and desipramine have fewer associated side effects and should be tried first. Maximum benefits of therapy may not be seen for 4 to 6 weeks after initiation of a tricyclic antidepressant agent. Other commonly used adjuvant agents include corticosteroids (for appetite stimulation and treatment of brain edema, cord compression, and plexopathies), anticonvulsants for neuropathic pain (e.g., gabapentin, carbamazepine, phenytoin), systemic administration of local anesthetic (e.g., oral mexiletene or tocainide, or intravenous lidocaine), neuroleptics (e.g., methotrimeprazine [a phenothiazine with analgesic properties], haloperidol, or resperidol) for delirium, restlessness, and agitation, and psychostimulants (methylphenidate) for treatment of sedation, lack of energy, and depressed mood.

NONPHARMACOLOGIC PAIN MANAGEMENT APPROACHES

Physical therapy, occupational therapy, massage, music, psychotherapy, support groups, biofeedback, hypnosis, meditation, and relaxation techniques may significantly reduce pain and enhance the quality of life in selected patients.

Management of Other Symptoms

GASTROINTESTINAL SYMPTOMS

Anorexia. Loss of appetite is a nearly universal accompaniment of terminal illness and may not require intervention if the patient is near death and does not express a desire to eat. Earlier in the course of a serious illness, improved appetite and nutrition may contribute to higher energy levels, well-being, and functional capacity. Elderly patients should be encouraged to eat whatever is most appealing without regard to fat, sugar, and salt restrictions if possible. Appetite stimulants including corticosteroids and megestrol acetate may help in some patients, but their potential for side effects and toxicity is substantial.

Nausea and Vomiting. Common causes of nausea and vomiting (ulcers, gastritis, obstipation, drug side effects) should be sought and treated if present. Antiemetic agents are usually effective in ameliorating nausea, but the extrapyramidal and anticholinergic side effects of metoclopramide and phenothiazine derivatives often limit the use of these drugs in the elderly. Cisapride or ondansetron, although expensive, are likely to be better tolerated.

Constipation. Constipation has been discussed earlier in the section on Management of Opioid Side Effects.

Diarrhea. Often due to fecal impaction or antibiotic-associated colitis, diarrhea is a particularly distressing and exhausting symptom in the terminally ill. Once these common causes have been ruled out, kaolin-pectin or psyllium may be used effectively to reduce diarrhea. Loperamide or tincture of opium may be used if these measures fail.

Mouth Care. Dry mouth and lips are a common consequence of diminished oral intake and anticholinergic medications. Lip lubricants, lemon glycerin swabs, and artificial saliva are helpful.

URINARY SYMPTOMS

The differential diagnosis of urinary incontinence in the terminally ill includes functional incontinence, overflow incontinence due to fecal impaction or other source of obstruction, vaginal atrophy, infection, and spinal cord or neurologic disease. If the postvoid residual urine volume exceeds 200 cc after impaction is ruled out, an indwelling urethral catheter may be necessary for patient comfort and easing the burden of personal care tasks for the caregivers. In the absence of obstruction, detrusor instability may be treated with the bladder smooth muscle relaxant and anticholinergic agent oxybutynin or a low dose of a tricyclic antidepressant agent, observing carefully for the development of urinary retention and other anticholinergic side effects.

PSYCHIATRIC SYMPTOMS

Depression. Depression is discussed in detail in Chapter 28 but several aspects of depression in the terminally ill deserve review. Because of the underlying physical illness, the standard DSM IV criteria for vegetative symptoms (sleep disturbances and appetite and weight changes) are not useful. The clinician should watch for evidence of withdrawn or depressed mood, loss of interest, and suicidal ideation. Studies have shown that coexisting and untreated major depression is present in a majority of terminally ill patients with a serious desire to die. Depression may be underdiagnosed in this population because of the clinician's belief that depression is "appropriate" in the context of a terminal illness. In fact, only 25% of terminally ill persons have evidence of depression,[16] which is often unrecognized and untreated. Expression by the patient of a desire to hasten death should be openly discussed in an effort to discover the possible alternative meanings of the request to the patient and to respond as directly as possible to the identified sources of the patient's suffering. Escalation of efforts to control distressing pain and other symptoms, a trial of antidepressant therapy, and a psychiatric consultation are appropriate initial responses. The patient should be reassured that she can discontinue life-sustaining interventions (such as chemotherapy, antibiotics, corticosteroids, and artificial nutrition and hydration) when their burdens outweigh their benefits to the patient and that any otherwise uncontrollable suffering can be managed with terminal sedation. A continued dialogue with the patient about the wish to die often reveals a change of mind as time goes on.

Standard antidepressant agents are effective for treatment of depression in the terminally ill but may have a delayed (2- to 6-week) onset of action. Psychostimulants (methylphenidate) are well tolerated and effective alternatives that have a rapid onset and a beneficial effect on energy, mood, appetite, and mental alertness. Methylphenidate (starting with 2.5-mg doses) or dextroamphetamine should be given in the early morning and early afternoon to avoid night-time sleep disturbances, and they can be used while therapy with a standard antidepressant is being initiated.

Delirium. Delirium, agitation, and confusion are extremely distressing to patients and families alike and are common among terminally ill elderly patients. Initial efforts to identify reversible medical causes (especially drug side effects and fecal impaction or urinary retention in patients receiving opioids) should precede pharmacologic intervention. Major tranquilizers (haloperidol, resperidol) in low doses are effective for treatment of agitated delirium. Benzodiazepines may be useful in treating patients with agitated delirium who respond inadequately to a neuroleptic agent, but they should not be used as first-line agents.

Anxiety. Anxiety secondary to pain or dyspnea can be managed by treating the underlying symptoms, but persistent anxiety is often a manifestation of depression. Antidepressants and benzodiazepines with a short half-life are appropriate initial steps in management.

Dementia. End-of-life care in patients with dementia requires recognition of the terminal nature of the disease and a shift from life-prolonging therapies to palliative interventions. Factors associated with a poor prognosis in dementia include dependency in all activities of daily living, urinary and fecal incontinence, nonverbal and nonambulatory state, aversive feeding behavior or malnutrition, and recent medical comorbid conditions (such as pneumonia, sepsis, and pressure sores). Avoidance of burdensome and risky interventions that are of minimal benefit in the end stages of a dementing illness (e.g., tube feeding, restraints, urethral catheters, needle sticks, and intravenous lines) are major components of palliative care in this population. Treatment of agitation requires assessment for painful stimuli before major tranquilizers are initiated.

DYSPNEA

Dyspnea refers to the subjective symptom of breathlessness. Dyspnea is mediated variously through chemoreceptors in the respiratory tract and central nervous system, stretch receptors in the chest wall skeletal muscles that participate in respiration, and the pulmonary vasculature. The quality and intensity of dyspnea depend on the individual patient and are related to ill-defined psychological factors that determine specific reactions to physical stimuli. For these reasons, the extent of dyspnea experienced by the patient may be vastly different from "objective" signs, such as respiratory rate or auscultatory abnormalities, and measurements, such as hypoxia or hypercarbia. The pathophysiology of dyspnea is complex and has been reviewed in detail elsewhere.[17]

Dyspnea in people with a terminal illness can be due to multiple causes, including pulmonary edema, ascites, bronchospasm, respiratory infection, pleural effusion, acidosis, anemia, and other problems. An effort should be made to determine the underlying cause, and therapy should be directed toward reversing treatable contributing factors. Invasive or noninvasive testing is often inconsistent with the goals of care for the patient, but careful clinical diagnosis is generally revealing, and the standard medical treatments, such as diuretics for pulmonary edema or bronchodilators for wheezing, may provide significant relief. In patients with malignant pleural effusion, thoracentesis may be helpful, but these effusions often recur quickly. Recurrence can be prevented with chemical pleurodesis, but, unlike simple needle thoracentesis, pleurodesis can be very painful. Thus it is essential to provide adequate analgesia during and after this procedure. Nonrespiratory causes of dyspnea such as anemia and, less often, acidosis may also respond to specific therapies.

Oxygen is an important supplement to any active treatment for dyspnea. Although the concentration of oxygen must be carefully adjusted for patients who retain carbon dioxide, the symptomatic benefits generally outweigh the potential hazards even in these circumstances. In certain situations, oxygen may reduce dyspnea even if the oxygen saturation is 90% or more. Although specific requirements, such as an oxygen saturation of less than 90%, are required by most U.S. insurance plans to pay for the apparatus used at home, the hospice benefit covers home oxygen use independent of such stipulations.

A cool breeze on the face, through an open window or a fan, may reduce dyspnea. Under experimental conditions, cool air breathed through the nose reduces the ventilatory response to carbon dioxide, which in turn may improve dyspnea by reducing ventilatory effort. This temperature-sensitive or touch-sensitive response may be mediated by reduction in brain temperature or through cold or other receptors in trigeminal nerve afferent fibers.

Systemic opioids are effective in managing dyspnea caused by a variety of factors and need not be reserved for the last days of life. The initial doses for patients with dyspnea are subject to the geriatric prescribing principles outlined in Chapter 5. Opioids act by reducing central respiratory center responsiveness to carbon dioxide tension in a dose-dependent manner. This results in decreased respiratory drive and an increase in partial pressure of carbon dioxide, which sometimes limits this approach to management of dyspnea. However, the decreased perception of dyspnea may also be centrally mediated directly, or it may due to decreased sensitivity of carbon dioxide receptors at the level of the lungs, independent of reduced respiratory drive or rate.[18] Likewise, the mood-altering effects of opioids may contribute indirectly to a reduced sensation of dyspnea.

Nebulized inhaled morphine may sometimes be useful as an alternative or adjunctive treatment. The theoretical basis for this result is that the opioid receptors in the afferent sensory nerves of the respiratory tract are involved in reflex responses that can be inhibited by opioid antagonists that act only at these peripheral sites. There are anecdotal reports of dyspneic patients with end-stage chronic obstructive pulmonary disease, heart failure, cancer, and pulmonary fibrosis who have obtained significant relief of dyspnea with nebulized morphine,[19] although controlled trials in diverse groups, including normals, have not shown consistent benefit. Only 10% of nebulized morphine is systemically absorbed, and medicinal use as described in published reports appears to be well tolerated. The recommended starting dose is 5 mg of morphine in 2 mL of saline at approximately 4-hour intervals, with dose increases titrated to the patient's symptoms. The potential dose range is wide, and high doses may be required in patients who are undergoing chronic systemic opioid treatment.

Nebulized morphine should not be relied on to the exclusion of systemic opioids, particularly in patients with severe shortness of breath. The dose of systemic or nebulized opioids should be titrated according to the patient's report, not "objective" guidelines such as respiratory rate or breathing pattern.[18] A dose as low as 2 to 5 mg of parenteral morphine sulfate is often effective.

Anxiety heightens dyspnea, and relief of anxiety is very important in management. Oxygen may help to relieve anxiety and may also relieve dyspnea directly. Sedatives, including neuroleptics, benzodiazepines, and barbiturates, can be given. Frequent reassurance and companionship are very important.

Morphine and virtually all sedatives depress respiration, and this can become clinically significant. However, there may be no alternative in patients with intractable dyspnea. This dilemma is particularly profound in ventilator-dependent patients who have decided to discontinue ventilator support knowing this will result in death. Patients undergoing such terminal weaning may experience intense dyspnea if ventilator withdrawal is abrupt and if sedation is not given. Suffering is heightened if the patient is conscious and has a feeling of suffocation until the moment of death. The natural coma of carbon dioxide narcosis can sometimes be induced quickly by adjusting the respirator settings. If not, adequate sedation must be given before respirator support is withdrawn. Most, although not all, alert ventilator-dependent patients have been receiving morphine or other sedating medications and will require more than a small dose of sedative for this withdrawal process; the dose should be strictly titrated according to the patient's needs. Although doctors and nurses may be concerned that this sedation is hastening the patient's death, it is impossible to know whether the actual moment of death was determined by the medication or the disease.[20] The ethical principle of double effect that governs this clinical situation permits use of treatments intended to relieve terminal suffering even though an unintended side effect may be a slight hastening of death. When a patient is near death and will suffer without the sedation, the benefits of the treatment outweigh its risks.

USE OF LIFE-SUSTAINING TREATMENTS IN THE TERMINALLY ILL

An important component of palliative care is the avoidance of treatments and diagnostic tests that are painful or intrusive yet fail to contribute to the overall goal of preventing suffering. However, blanket policies, such as "no antibiotics," should be avoided, and each situation should be evaluated on its own merits. Each test or treatment should be considered negotiable. For example, a patient who wishes to avoid resuscitation may still wish to receive antibiotics; one who wishes to avoid amputation may still wish to receive intravenous hydration. A patient who cannot direct care still has the right to make these choices through an authorized surrogate decision maker.

Artificial Nutrition and Hydration in Terminal Care

Artificial nutrition and hydration (ANH) is among the most controversial life-sustaining treatments in patients with incurable illness. Much of the controversy may stem from misconceptions about the medical aspects of this treatment as well as the notion that withholding ANH is "wrong" according to religious or personally held beliefs. However, foregoing ANH at the end of life is fully consistent with the principles of palliative care.[21, 22]

Total parenteral nutrition (TPN) has been used to treat the "anorexia cachexia" syndrome

of AIDS and cancer. This is a complex metabolic abnormality associated with wasting and weakness but not due primarily to inadequate caloric intake. Extensive study of parenteral and enteral calorie replacement in these patients has failed to show that it improves the quality of life. Enteral tube feeding is commonly employed in patients with end-stage dementia or other advanced neurologic impairment who have feeding disorders, but there is no evidence that tube feeding in most of these situations is palliative. Tube feeding has a number of side effects, including pain and discomfort, tube trauma with bleeding, dislodgement leading to reinsertion of the tube or the imposition of restraints, and aspiration. Since the advent of percutaneous endoscopic gastrostomy, gastrostomy tubes have increasingly replaced nasogastric tubes for long-term feeding. However, gastrostomy and jejunostomy tubes may produce serious side effects such as peritonitis or abdominal wall cellulitis, and unusual though devastating problems such as bowel perforation and obstruction and death. These tubes may require revision or replacement, which sometimes leads to hospitalization. Finally, gastrostomy and jejunostomy tubes are often inserted for the explicit purpose of preventing aspiration pneumonia, but there is no evidence that any form of enteral tube feeding reduces the risk of pneumonia in debilitated patients.[21]

Enteral tube feeding is unlikely to be palliative in patients with incurable neurologic impairments or terminal illness. Theoretically, a patient with an obstructing gastroesophageal, head, or neck tumor who is alert and otherwise well enough to experience hunger might be more comfortable with complete or partial gastrostomy or jejunostomy tube feeding. Likewise, a patient with neurologic disease who visibly and consistently chokes on food despite careful spoon feeding with food of appropriate consistency might be more comfortable with tube feeding; however, such a patient must be distinguished from one who develops pneumonia from subclinical aspiration or one whose cough during feeding may be protective. In patients who visibly choke, tube feeding should prevent discomfort, apnea, and hypoxia. There is no evidence that omitting tube feeding in patients with terminal illness leads to discomfort. Even in situations such as those just cited, in which tube feeding might be temporarily palliative, the patient or his authorized surrogate has the option of forgoing tube feeding and gaining relief of symptoms by other means, such as sedation.

Doctors, nurses, and family members sometimes believe that hydration should be provided even in patients who refuse enteral tube feeding, but this practice is illogical in a patient who wishes to forgo life-sustaining treatment. Although providing hydration may sometimes comfort the caregiver, the palliative effect of hydration in patients with terminal illness is limited. Weakness and confusion are common symptoms at the end of life, and although dehydration could be a factor, such symptoms are generally multifactorial in origin and are unlikely to be reversed for any length of time with rehydration. Furthermore, an intravenous line can be intrusive and painful, especially in very ill patients with limited venous access. Hypodermoclysis, or subcutaneous infusion, is sometimes used when venous access fails, but the palliative effect is no greater. Sips of water as tolerated, ice chips, and gentle mouth care are likely to be more palliative than parenteral fluids.[22]

The medical aspects of artificial nutrition and hydration and the misconceptions surrounding their use have recently been reviewed in detail.[21]

Antibiotic Use in Terminal Illness

The treatment of infections in patients with terminal illness is complex. When antibiotics reduce symptoms caused by an infection (such as dysuria, fever, cough, or cellulitis), they are potentially palliative. However, treatment of a life-threatening infection may not be consistent with the goals of a patient who wishes to avoid treatment that is expected to prolong the process of dying. The dilemma is illustrated by the example of pneumonia, which may produce distressing symptoms that could be relieved by antibiotics, but when cured, the patient is restored to the ravages of the underlying terminal illness. In many patients, especially those with severe dementia, a serious infection may lead rapidly to coma, in which case antibiotics would not only fail to contribute to symptom relief but would reverse the natural palliation of coma. In alert patients, symptomatic treatment such as antitussives, antipyretics, or sedation is appropriate if this is consistent with the patient's goals.

BEREAVEMENT

The experience of loss and separation begins well before the actual death of the patient, and the health professional can contribute a great deal toward initiating an effective bereavement process. The opportunity to provide direct care to the dying person is an important means of expressing love and connection. Overzealous delivery of professional services can take this role away from loved ones, who may begin to worry about their own "lack of expertise." Family members may need to be explicitly encouraged to say good-bye, to try to think of the things they want to be sure to have said and to try to say them. This process should occur even if the patient is unresponsive or is unable to speak; she or he may hear and understand the tone of the words or the meaning of a touch or embrace. Families should be given information about what the actual death may be like and what various signs and symptoms mean (e.g., the "death rattle"). The actual time immediately after death is a shock no matter how surely the event is anticipated, and families need privacy and quiet together without undue staff intrusion. Respectful treatment of the body with attention paid to cultural norms and rituals, and allowing family members to participate in washing and dressing the body may all contribute to initiation of a healthy grieving process.

The main tasks of mourning—to accept the reality of the loss, to experience the pain of grief, to adjust to life without the dead loved one, and to reinvest emotional energy in living—occur in highly individual modes without a set pattern.[23] Efforts to avoid the grieving process may be associated with depression, somatization, and social withdrawal, and professional facilitation of the process of mourning in such cases may be crucial to the later well-being of the family. Spouse, friends, and older relatives of an elderly person who has recently died may feel a strong sense of abandonment and isolation as fewer and fewer of their peers remain. A clinician's acknowledgment of this reality, a willingness to begin the process of remembering the deceased by describing memories and listening to those of others, validating the family's role in the caregiving process, and establishing clear expectations about the mourner's future relationship with the doctors and nurses are all helpful approaches. Risk factors for a complicated bereavement process include a difficult or painful death, a sudden death, a suicide, or a death that occurred when the patient was alone. Other major losses, medical illness in the mourner, prior psychiatric history, especially of depression, and an absent or unsupportive family are other indicators of risk and should prompt an offer of professional support.[23]

References

1. Buckman R: How to break bad news: A guide for health care professionals. Baltimore, Johns Hopkins University Press, 1992.
2. Quill TE, Townsend P: Bad news: Delivery, dialogue, and dilemmas. Arch Intern Med 1991;151:463–468.
3. Blackhall LJ, Murphy ST, Frank G, Michel V, Azen S: Ethnicity and attitudes toward patient autonomy. JAMA 1995;274:820–825.

4. Drickamer MA, Lachs MS: Should patients with Alzheimer's disease be told their diagnosis? N Engl J Med 1992;326:947–951.

5. Halroyd S, Snustad DG, Chalifoux SL: Attitudes of older adults on being told the diagnosis of Alzheimer's disease. J Am Geriatr Soc 1996;44:400–403.

6. World Health Organization: Cancer pain relief and palliative care. Geneva, WHO, 1990.

7. National Hospice Organization: Medical guidelines for determining prognosis in selected non-cancer diseases. Arlington, VA, National Hospice Organization, 1995.

8. Christakis NA, Sachs GA: The role of prognosis in clinical decision making. J Gen Intern Med 1996;11:422–425.

9. Bonica J, Loeser J, Chapman C, Fordyce W: The Management of Pain. Philadelphia, Lea & Febiger, 1990, pp. 563–580.

10. Principal Investigators for the SUPPORT Project: A controlled trial to improve care for seriously ill hospitalized patients: The study to understand prognoses and preferences for outcomes and risks of treatments (SUPPORT). JAMA 1995;274:1591–1598.

11. Ferrell B: Pain evaluation and management in the nursing home. Ann Intern Med 1995;123:681–687.

12. Bruera E, Kuehn N, Miller MJ, Selmser P, Macmillan K: The Edmonton Symptom Assessment System (ESAS): A simple method for the assessment of palliative care patients. Palliative Care 1991;7:6–9.

13. Daut R, Cleeland C, Flanery R: The development of the Wisconsin Brief Pain Questionnaire to assess pain in cancer and other diseases. Pain 1983;17:197–210.

14. Jacox A, Carr D, Payne R, et al: Management of cancer pain. Clinical Practice Guideline No. 9. AHCPR Publication No. 94-0592. Rockville, MD, U.S. Department of Health and Human Services, Public Health Service, Agency for Health Care Policy and Research, 1994.

15. Jacox A, Carr DB, Payne R: New clinical practice guidelines for the management of pain in patients with cancer. N Engl J Med 1994;330:651–655.

16. Massie M, Holland J: Depression and the cancer patient. J Clin Psychiatry 1990;51:12–17.

17. Manning H, Schwartzstein R: Pathophysiology of dyspnea. N Engl J Med 1995;333:1547–1553.

18. Bruera E, MacEachern T, Ripamonti C, Hanson J: Subcutaneous morphine for dyspnea in cancer patients. Ann Intern Med 1993;119:906–907.

19. Farncombe M, Chater S: Clinical application of nebulized opioids for treatment of dyspnoea in patients with malignant disease. Support Care Cancer 1994;2:184–187.

20. Wilson W, Smedira N, Fink C, et al: Ordering and administration of sedatives and analgesics during the withholding and withdrawal of life support from critically ill patients. JAMA 1992;267:949–953.

21. Ahronheim J: Artificial nutrition and hydration in the terminally ill patient. Clin Geriatr Med 1996;12:379–391.

22. McCann RM, Hall WJ, Groth Juncker A: Comfort care for terminally ill patients. The appropriate use of nutrition and hydration. JAMA 1994;272:1263–1266.

23. Saunders C, Sykes N: The Management of Terminal Disease, 3rd ed. London, Edward Arnold, 1993.

Prevention/ Rehabilitation in Geriatric Practice

13 Preventive Health Maintenance

Mark Joseph Magenheim, M.D., M.P.H.

Attention to clinical preventive services has increased in the past decade, as managed care, managed demand, and health maintenance programs have expanded. As managed *care* (control of access to providers) has been supplemented (or even replaced) by managed *demand* (control of access to services), implications for the geriatric population are becoming problematic in that needed services may not remain readily available. In this more restrictive environment, preventive health services have a higher priority. For the elderly, the focus of clinical prevention is primarily on maintaining functional *ability* rather than on identifying new *disabilities*, although both activities are important. Health assessment of the elderly includes review and follow-up of health issues *primarily* from the perspective of the patient as well as from that of health professionals and payers. Successful health assessment of elderly patients depends on keen observation, sound applied logic, and full use of the "sixth sense."

Screening is central to preventive health assessment of the elderly. As a point of reference, screening is defined generally as "the presumptive identification of unrecognized disease or defect by the application of tests, examinations, or other procedures which can be applied rapidly to sort out apparently well persons who probably have a disease from those who probably do not. A screening test is not intended to be diagnostic. Persons with positive or suspicious findings must be referred to their physicians for diagnosis and necessary treatment."[1]

Two forms of health screening are commonly recognized: (1) *epidemiologic community surveys*, which are used to identify or describe a population that *has not* sought medical assistance and (2) *case-finding* among those who *have* sought medical assistance. Within the category of case-finding, interventions are either provided incidentally to individuals who have not sought screening directly (as when office staff check the blood pressure of every adult at each office visit), or, alternatively, they are provided to populations who have sought screening assistance for self-identified purposes to maintain or improve personal health (as when individuals check their own blood pressure at home or at shopping malls or in drugstores). One difference between these two forms of case-finding is that the first type is offered in a health care setting by a health services *provider*, whereas the second type is initiated in a non–health care setting by the health services *consumer*.

Screening strategies, benefits, costs, and outcomes vary according to the objectives, test features, and points of view of the screening program and its participants. This chapter focuses on provider-initiated screening in the context of preventive health assessment for case-finding of functional impairments or conditions. The aim of this form of professionally based *prescriptive screening* is early detection of important conditions or diseases for which efficacious and efficient interventions exist to prevent or postpone disability and premature death.[2] For the elderly, the goal of prescriptive screening is to improve the quality of life by enhancing functional capacity and reducing disability.

Early efforts at preventive health assessment and screening of the elderly were conducted in the form of epidemiologic community surveys rather than as office-based case-finding. In general, these findings did not show enough benefit to justify mass community screenings. Even when such services were conducted by mobile units or in the homes of the elderly by physician-extenders with back-up laboratory services, the results were not cost-effective.[3-14] Results of Lowther's pioneering studies showed that "the end result of all our early diagnostic activities has thus been an improvement in 23% of the whole group and ... it is unlikely that many general practitioners will be able to accept this further burden in the near future."[4]

Currie and his associates in Scotland reported that "the results of the [Glasgow] survey were perhaps incommensurate with the effort expended since most of the unreported morbidity was trivial, . . . and community health screening of the elderly may be very time-consuming and expensive in time and money."[5] Results of other studies of office-based and special population case-finding among the elderly have been weak owing to limitations of study design and lack of efficacy. Freedman and colleagues report that the low incidence of serious illness (2.8%) among 682 elderly patients screened in Newcastle "revealed that the vast majority of positive symptoms and physical signs were either already known to the patient's general practitioner or were of no real significance to the health and well-being of the patient . . . including previously undiagnosed mental and emotional illness."[13]

One of the most rigorous evaluations of preventive health maintenance screening was the randomized controlled trial done by Tulloch and Moore in 1979.[14] In 295 elderly patients assessed over 2 years, results "in both screened and unscreened groups showed that patients were well adapted in most cases to their problems so that the quality of life of these old people was relatively unimpaired."[14] No significant impact on socioeconomic, functional, and medical disorders affecting health was made, risk rating in the two groups differed only marginally, and screening and surveillance had little impact on health status or vulnerability to stress as represented by risk rating. McKeown's landmark review corroborated the conclusions of many of these rigorous pioneering studies from the United Kingdom.[15]

In North America, studies by Breslow and Somers, Somers and associates, Frame and Carlson, Frame and Kowulich, the Canadian Task Force on the Periodic Health Examination, and the U.S. Preventive Services Task Force of the U.S. Department of Health and Human Services have shown that rigorous, comprehensive health maintenance guides are useful when they emphasize age-related risk assessment targeted to specific groups and conditions.[16–21] Although health maintenance recommendations for many conditions are still under development,[22–26] a number of preventive health assessment protocols have now been adequately validated to warrant routine use in clinical practice.[27–36] As with all screening recommendations, specific protocols for screening the elderly need to be based on general principles and evidence-based, scientifically grounded methodologic criteria.

METHODOLOGIC CRITERIA FOR SCREENING

Screening standards were set forth in 1961, and general principles were adopted by the World Health Assembly in 1971.[37–39] Practical methodologic criteria and guidelines developed during the past 25 years now include the following:

Burden of Disease or Disability

1. Is the condition an important health problem for the individual and for the community? (What is the prevalence and the types and magnitude of suffering among those affected?)

Etiology and Clinical Course

2. What is the natural history of the condition from the latent stage to overt disease or disability? (Is there an early asymptomatic stage?)
3. Will early detection alter the course of the condition?
4. Is effective treatment for the condition available if it is identified before or at an early symptomatic stage?

Efficacy of Screening

5. Is there a suitable screening test to detect the condition at the latent or early symptomatic stage?
6. Is the screening test likely to do more good than harm?
7. Is the test valid for the condition being assessed?
8. What is the effect of the condition's prevalence in the population on the predictive value (yield) of the screening test?

Effectiveness of Preventive Assessment

9. Is the screening test acceptable to patients, to health professionals, and to payers of the preventive health assessment?
10. What is the labeling effect of a positive test result?
11. What is the level of compliance with screening protocols among patients, professionals, and payers? (That is, do patients and clinicians adhere to recommended screening procedures? Do insurers pay for such services? Do prevention incentives exist, and do they work?)

Community Effectiveness

12. Are diagnostic facilities available, accessible, and affordable for those with positive results on screening tests?
13. Is treatment available, accessible, and affordable?
14. What is the level of compliance with treatment among patients, health professionals, and payers of treatment services?
15. Is there suitable coverage? (That is, do those in need receive effective services and treatments after screening?)
16. What is the impact of effective diagnosis and treatment on the burden of suffering, in magnitude, type, or other costs?

Efficiency (Economic Evaluation)

17. Is screening cost effective when compared with other means of diagnosis and treatment? (What is the relative benefit of preventing, arresting, or curing the problem early?)
18. Is screening for condition A cost effective compared with screening for condition B in terms of screening efficacy and effectiveness?
19. Is diagnosis and treatment of condition A cost effective compared with diagnosis and treatment of condition B in terms of community effectiveness and the population's burden of suffering?
20. What are results of cost-utility analyses of screening and treatment alternatives? (That is, do screening and early detection lead to an improvement in end results as measured by quality-adjusted life-years, or is it merely "staging-migration"?)

Consistent use of these criteria helps to promote rational evaluation of screening and preventive assessment protocols and fosters effective clinical policies and practices. Although the "spectrum of evidence" is still incomplete, it is nonetheless important to conduct a critical review of any proposed health screening technique, procedure, or method intended for the elderly to develop and implement appropriate periodic assessments and to avoid inefficacious, ineffective, and potentially harmful interventions. The recommendations for preventive assessment of the elderly in this chapter focus on burden of suffering, natural history (etiology and clinical course), efficacy, and effectiveness. Issues of community effectiveness and economic analysis, although relevant, are beyond the scope of this chapter. In the following section, the condition of essential hypertension among the elderly is used as an example to show how these guidelines and methodologic criteria can be applied to determine appropriate specific preventive recommendations for this common problem.

APPLICATION OF PREVENTIVE ASSESSMENT RECOMMENDATIONS

Essential hypertension is a common geriatric problem that can be used as an example for applying rules of evidence to preventive assessment guidelines.

Step One: Burden of Disease or Disability

Approximately 5% to 35% of North American adults have an elevated diastolic and/or systolic blood pressure depending on age, sex, and race. (The wide range of prevalence is itself a useful measure of the difficulty of determining the true burden of disability.) The peak prevalence of diastolic hypertension (more than 95 mmHg) is 16% in males and 19% in females at 55 to 64 years, and the peak of isolated systolic hypertension (more than 160 mmHg) occurs in about 28% of males and 33% of females aged 75 to 79. Results are inconsistent for those over age 80.

Determining the true prevalence of hypertension among those over 65 years old is difficult because of frequent misreporting and misclassification in this group, and the burden of suffering among elderly hypertensives is problematic because of the usually asymptomatic nature of the condition and the adverse side effects of treatment. However, target organ damage occurring as a consequence of untreated hypertension poses a huge burden to society, to individual patients and their families, and to the health care system. Disability and premature death from congestive heart failure, myocardial infarction, coronary heart disease, cerebrovascular accidents, and atheromatous brain infarction due to untreated hypertension remain major health problems.

Step Two: Etiology and Clinical Course

Information about the etiology of essential hypertension is limited, but data on the clinical course of the condition are substantial. Among those aged 65 to 74, data consistently show significantly higher rates of congestive heart failure and death from cardiovascular disease in diastolic hypertensive women compared to age-matched nonhypertensive women. Risks associated with isolated systolic hypertension in those 65 to 79 years and for those over age 80 are now quite well documented.[40]

Efficacy studies of compliant patients under 65 years old with treated hypertension have shown an 83% reduction in mortality and 92% reduction in morbidity among those with severe diastolic hypertension (more than 115 mmHg before treatment), a 67% reduction in events among those with moderate diastolic hypertension (105 to 114 mmHg), and a 17% reduction in mortality in those with mild hypertension (90 to 104 mmHg). Optimal control can be achieved after 5 years for two thirds of young adults needing hypertensive therapy, but control among the elderly is inconsistent.

The results of the VA Cooperative Study and the Hypertension Detection and Follow-up Program (HDFP) for elderly patients unequivocally demonstrated benefits of therapy for those aged 60 to 74 with moderate (105 to 114 mmHg) or severe (over 115 mmHg) diastolic hypertension. Efficacy of treatment was not demonstrated for those over age 60 with mildly elevated diastolic (less than 104 mmHg) or isolated systolic hypertension. Reliable results have been reported from the Systolic Hypertension in the Elderly Program (SHEP) study,[41] but consistent findings for those aged 75 and over have been limited in most studies to date.

Newer methods of antihypertensive treatment and questions about the efficacy of stepped care have further complicated management of this problem among the elderly. Negative side effects include postural hypotension, urinary incontinence, confusion, sedation, abrupt changes in blood pressure, hypokalemia, depression, fatigue, weakness, and anorexia. The case for treatment thus needs to be established clearly before subjecting an elderly patient to the rigors of daily antihypertensive therapy.

Although there is a high burden of suffering among untreated hypertensives with a diastolic pressure of more than 105 mmHg, the evidence for intervening in elderly patients with *mild* diastolic hypertension or isolated systolic hypertension is not as firm. These forms of high blood pressure are the most common among those aged 65 or over, and treatment recommendations for this group have recently been better validated. Although they are based on good evidence from well-designed studies, preventive assessment and health maintenance guidelines for mild hypertension in the elderly are not yet conclusive.[41]

Step Three: Efficacy of Preventive Assessment

The foremost technical aspect of screening, which determines efficacy, is the establishment of test validity. Validity here refers to the ability of the test to identify individuals with the condition correctly (sensitivity) and to identify individuals without the condition correctly (specificity). The extent to which screening test results conform to those derived from an acknowledged gold standard of diagnostic accuracy provides a measure of sensitivity, specificity, and overall test validity. Table 13–1 shows these concepts of determining validity algebraically.

As shown in Table 13–1, it is possible to place each screened individual into cells labeled (a), (b), (c), or (d) and to compute the respective percentages in each cell. In this hypothetical example, the hypertension screening program is being conducted in a community of 1000 adults where population screening has not previously been available. We assume that measuring devices are reliable and that the blood pressure readings taken are diagnostically accurate and are not affected by observer bias. Given the suitability of the screening test and good information on the benefits of early detection and treatment,

---

TABLE 13–1 **RESULTS OF SCREENING TEST ILLUSTRATING SENSITIVITY AND SPECIFICITY**

Results of Screening Test	"True" Condition or Disease State		Total Number Screened
	Condition or Disease (+)	*No Condition or Disease (−)*	*Total Number Screened*
Positive (+)	True positive (TP) a	False positive (FP) b	Total positive a + b
Negative (−)	False negative (FN) c	True negative (TN) d	Total negative c + d
	TP + FN[a] a + c	TN + FP[b] b + d	Total screened a + b + c + d

[a]Sensitivity $= \dfrac{TP}{TP + FN} = \left(\dfrac{a}{a + c}\right) \times 100.$

[b]Specificity $= \dfrac{TN}{TN + FP} = \left(\dfrac{d}{b + d}\right) \times 100.$

we now wish to determine the validity of the screening test.

In the perfect screening test (i.e., one with 100% sensitivity, 100% specificity, and no false-positive or false-negative results), all diseased subjects would be in cell (a) and all nondiseased subjects would be in cell (d). In actual practice, however, this is neither attainable methodologically nor desirable. (To achieve "perfection," the tests would have to be exceedingly costly and inefficient, and the potential benefits derived from early screening of asymptomatic persons would be lost.)

Instead of perfection, the goal of preventive assessment in the form of screening for case-finding is to achieve the highest levels of both sensitivity and specificity consistent with other screening criteria deemed essential for the given condition. To achieve this balance, the approach taken in case-finding is to "trade off" the sensitivity and the specificity of a test. Operationally, this is done by setting a level in advance that must be met for a test outcome to be deemed "positive." This "criterion of positivity"[42] is determined clinically and statistically as that point on the spectrum of measurement (from "definite health" to "definite disease") that affords optimal sensitivity and specificity for the condition in question—at the lowest cost, pain, inconvenience, and risk. The criterion of positivity is affected by value preferences for "health," "acceptable risk," cost-benefit ratios for different points on the full spectrum of measurement, and the prevalence of the condition of interest. As

shown later, different cut-off points can lead to substantial variations in the screening results obtained.

Using validated standards, our example (Table 13–2) uses a fifth-phase Korotkoff level of 105 mmHg as the cut-off point for diastolic hypertension. Patients labeled hypertensive (those who have a diastolic reading of 105 mmHg or greater on screening) would be referred for definitive diagnosis and treatment (the so-called gold standard). From the results of our screening program (shown in Table 13–2), we conclude that the screening test for hypertension appears to be very good at correctly identifying individuals with diastolic hypertension (sensitivity = 95.0%) and without diastolic hypertension (specificity = 95.0%). At this cut-off level of 105 mmHg in an unselected population, this test shows good predictive value for positive test results (88.0%) and very good predictive value for negative test results (98.0%). This means that the post-test likelihood of correctly identifying an individual as hypertensive or as nonhypertensive based on this screening test alone is quite good. We also conclude that the prevalence of diastolic hypertension (more than 105 mmHg) among these 1000 persons is 280/1000 or 28%, which is within the expected range based on the results of other surveys. Thus, we conclude that this screening test appears to be valid.

Let us now apply the same screening test to a population of 1000 persons over age 65 who live in a retirement community in the Sun Belt. In Table 13–2 we determined that our hypertension

TABLE 13–2 **EXAMPLE FOR CALCULATING SCREENING TEST SENSITIVITY AND SPECIFICITY FOR DIASTOLIC HYPERTENSION (≥105 mmHg)**

Result of Blood Pressure Screening Test	True Disease State		Total Number Screened
	Disease (+) Hypertensive	*Disease (−) Not Hypertensive*	
Positive test (≥105 mmHg)	a 266	b 36	a + b 302
Negative test (<105 mmHg)	c 14	d 684	c + d 698
	a + c 280	b + d 720	a + b + c + d 1000

Percentage sensitivity $= \dfrac{a}{a + c} = \dfrac{266}{280} \times 100 = 95.0\%$

Percentage specificity $= \dfrac{d}{b + d} = \dfrac{684}{720} \times 100 = 95.0\%$

Post-test likelihood of a positive test (positive predictive value) $= \dfrac{a}{a + b} = \dfrac{266}{302} \times 100 = 88.0\%$

Post-test likelihood of a negative test (negative predictive value) $= \dfrac{d}{c + d} = \dfrac{684}{698} \times 100 = 98.0\%$

Prevalence of diastolic hypertension $= \dfrac{a + c}{\text{Total}} = \dfrac{280}{1000} \times 100 = 28.0\%$

screening program had a sensitivity of 95% and a specificity of 95% and that the prevalence was 28% in this general population. Although the test *characteristics* do not change in different populations (test sensitivity and specificity remain unchanged), what happens to test *validity* if the prevalence changes?

First, we begin with previous information that the prevalence of *undetected* diastolic hypertension among those over age 65 in this Sun Belt population may be only 8% because most people in this population already know their blood pressures and are in fact under medical care. Combining this figure with the known sensitivity of 95% and specificity of 95% gives the results shown in Table 13–3.

Working backward, we start with a total population of 1000 and an expected prevalence of 8% in the population of interest. The resulting N of a + c (prevalence) equals 80 (8% of 1000). The total population (a + b + c + d) of 1000 less the expected prevalence a + c (80) equals 920 nondiseased (which equals b + d). Using the known percentages for sensitivity (95%) and specificity (95%), we then calculate values for all the remaining cells. From Table 13–2, we know that the sensitivity and specificity remain unchanged, and thus the percentages of false-negatives and false-positives will also remain the same. However, when we compare the predictive values of the same screening test in these two settings (but with prevalences of 28% and 8%, respectively), the results are quite different.

The predictive value of a screening test refers to the likelihood that the subject with a positive test result actually has the disease of interest (positive predictive value) or that a subject with a negative test result does not have the disease of interest (negative predictive value). The calculation of predictive value is derived by computing the ratio of true outcomes to all outcomes for both negative and positive test results, based on Bayes' probability theorem.[43] Expressed mathematically, the predictive value of a positive test result is TP/TP + FP (or a/a + b, where TP = true positive and FP = false positive), and the predictive value of a negative test result is TN/TN + FN (or d/c + d, where TN = true negative and FN = false negative). From Table 13–2, the positive predictive value is 266/302 × 100 or 88.0%, and the negative predictive value is 684/698 × 100 or 98.0%. As shown in Table 13–3, the positive predictive value is 76/122 × 100 or 62.3%, and the negative predictive value is 874/878 × 100 or 99.5%.

Comparison of these values shows us that a difference in prevalence can have a major impact on the predictive value of a screening test. In the first example (see Table 13–2), the predictive value of a positive test result was more than 88%. Thus, 88 persons of every 100 with a positive test result would be true positives, and 12 would *not* be true positives. In the second example shown Table 13–3, the predictive value of a positive test result was less than 63%. Here, only 62 elderly persons of each 100 with a positive test

TABLE 13–3 **CALCULATION OF EXPECTED DIASTOLIC HYPERTENSION SCREENING OUTCOMES (PREVALENCE OF 8 PERCENT, TEST SENSITIVITY OF 95 PERCENT, AND SPECIFICITY OF 95 PERCENT)**

Result of Blood Pressure Screening Test	True Disease State		Total Number Screened
	Disease (+) Hypertensive	*Disease (−) Not Hypertensive*	
Positive test (≥105 mmHg)	a 76	b 46	a + b 122
Negative test (<105 mmHg)	c 4	d 874	c + d 878
	a + c 80	b + d 920	a + b + c + d 1000

Given sensitivity: $95\% = \dfrac{a}{a + c} = \dfrac{a}{80}$

then: $a = 0.95 \times 80 = 76$

Given specificity: $95\% = \dfrac{d}{b + d} = \dfrac{d}{920}$

then: $d = 0.95 \times 920 = 874$

Positive predictive value $= \dfrac{a}{a + b} = \dfrac{76}{122} = 62.3\%$

Negative predictive value $= \dfrac{d}{c + d} = \dfrac{874}{878} = 99.5\%$

result would be true positives, and 38 screened persons with a positive result would in fact *not* be hypertensive.

The problem of limited predictive value is even greater when prevalence is very low (below 3%, for instance). As Vecchio has shown, the predictive value of a single diagnostic test in unselected populations is markedly affected by the prevalence of the condition and by the pretest "likelihood of positivity."[44] Thus, even when test sensitivity and test specificity are high, there may still be an unacceptably large number of false-positive results when prevalence is low. This relationship is displayed in Figure 13–1, and it has been confirmed for many disorders, including diabetes mellitus and lung, breast, and cervical cancer. In addition to these limitations, many biases can affect preventive assessment efforts, such as unmasking (signal detection) bias, diagnostic suspicion bias, lead time (starting time) bias, volunteer bias, exposure-suspicion bias, diagnostic access bias, mimicry bias, previous opinion bias, and Neyman (prevalence-incidence) bias. Biases produce screening results that differ systematically from "the truth," and the extent to which bias is controlled increases overall validity of screening and case-finding.

Step Four: Effectiveness of Preventive Assessment

Blood pressure screening is well accepted by patients, providers, and the health care system. However, labeling of individuals as hypertensive

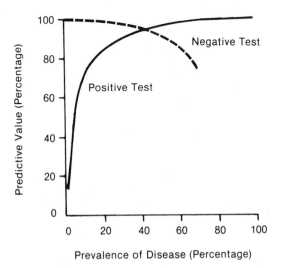

Figure 13–1 Relationship between prevalence of disease and predictive value, with sensitivity held constant at 95% and specificity held constant at 95%. (Adapted from Vecchio TJ: Predictive value of a single diagnostic test in unselected populations. N Engl J Med 274:1171, 1966.)

often leads to new problems such as lowered self-esteem, higher work absenteeism, lower productivity, and "sick role" behavior. These phenomena have occurred among untreated hypertensives and among mislabeled normotensives. Such problems can thus be attributed to the labeling process itself and are not necessarily due to the disease process of hypertension (which is asymptomatic in most patients) or to the side effects of treatment. Diagnostic labeling is especially important in assessing the elderly.

Compliance also affects clinical outcomes. Compliance for keeping appointments following screening for blood pressure ranges from 50% to 83% and is affected by the demographics of the patient, features of the screening test, clinical setting, condition of interest, perceived therapeutic regimen, patient-therapist interaction, and sociobehavioral aspects of the patient and the therapist. Even the most rigorous and valid screening test (one with high sensitivity and high specificity as well as a high predictive value) may lack adequate effectiveness if it is unacceptable to patients or practitioners or if compliance is too low.

Step Five: Community Effectiveness

This process is concerned with the availability, accessibility, and validity of definitive diagnostic services and with the efficacy and effectiveness of therapies for individuals with positive results on screening or preventive assessment tests. For hypertension, interobserver and intraobserver variations in measuring blood pressure limit the accuracy of this diagnosis, and this is further complicated by controversy about what constitutes hypertension that warrants treatment among persons over the age of 65 years.

Although the efficacy of treatment is well established for some forms of hypertension in some populations, diagnostic inaccuracy, clinical disagreement, and lack of compliance by patients and providers markedly reduce the effective coverage and impact of appropriate services and treatment of hypertension among the elderly.[45]

Step Six: Efficiency (Economic Evaluation)

The final (and usually the most difficult) step in analyzing the evidence on preventive assessment is an evaluation of its cost-effectiveness. For hypertension, cost-effectiveness was analyzed early by Weinstein and Stason.[46] Their *cost* estimates of hypertension screening and care per year of increased quality-adjusted life expectancy (impact) were lowest when services were provided in the form of office-based case-finding rather than as community-wide screening.

Logan and colleagues published a pioneering cost-effectiveness analysis of nurse practitioner care of hypertensives at work sites with physician office care. They found that nurse care was more effective and less costly.[47] Cost-benefit and cost-utility analysis of treating hypertension has not yet been well analyzed, nor has the cost-effectiveness of treating hypertension been compared with that of treating other disorders.

Economic analysis of hypertension screening or care among the elderly is further complicated by the finding that different high blood pressure cut-off levels markedly affect the results of cost-effectiveness analysis. It has been demonstrated that procedures that are cost effective for screening hypertension at age 30 are not cost effective when they are used for screening at age 60. As Weinstein pointed out, "These analyses underline the principle that even though screening (for hypertension) is relatively inexpensive, the large attrition between detection and ultimate blood pressure control severely compromises its cost-effectiveness. . . . [P]rograms to screen for hypertension are indicated on cost-effectiveness grounds only if adequate resources are available to ensure that detection is translated into effective long-term blood pressure control."[46]

GOALS OF PREVENTIVE ASSESSMENT OF THE ELDERLY

In the context of the foregoing general screening principles and methodologic criteria, what goals are reasonable for prescriptive preventive geriatrics? The United Kingdom has advocated screening the elderly "to preserve physical health, to maintain mental health, and to preserve social standing and circumstances,"[3] and to discover minor disabilities that can limit coping ability and enjoyment of life. Other screening goals have included establishing comprehensive baselines, devising forms and systems to promote periodic health assessments as integral elements of office practice, fostering teamwork, and developing information about elderly problems.

Others support screening to detect early problems among those with locomotor difficulties, those recently discharged from the hospital, those bereaved or living alone, those with financial troubles, and those over age 80 regardless of health status.[14] The World Health Organization advises geriatric screening "to keep the elderly in good health and happiness in their own houses for as long as this is possible," and Breslow and Somers define health monitoring for those 60 to 74 years old to prolong optimum physical, men-

tal, and social activity and to minimize handicaps from chronic conditions. For those over age 75, health goals are to prolong effective activity, to live independently, to minimize inactivity and discomfort, to avoid institutionalization, and, when illness is terminal, to ensure minimal distress and maximum emotional support to dying patients and their families.[16]

The Report of the U.S. Preventive Services Task Force in its 1996 Guide to Clinical Preventive Services devotes over 900 pages and thousands of references to support appropriate recommendations that meet the methodologic criteria outlined in this review.[21] Based on these and other rigorously conducted studies, mainly in the United States and Canada, specific recommendations can be made at this time for appropriate periodic health assessment of the elderly; these are summarized in the following sections.

SPECIFIC RECOMMENDATIONS

These guidelines are based on the general principles described earlier. Preventive assessment of the young elderly (those aged 65 to 74 years) focuses mainly on health problems that can be eliminated or controlled, and assessment of those over age 75 emphasizes reducing problems that impair function but for which cure or optimal control is less likely. Further, tests and procedures should be limited to those that meet standards of sufficient validity and that are acceptable and likely to make a difference to the person's overall health status. Although some scientific evidence that allows fully informed decision-making about office-based elderly screening and follow-up is available for some conditions found in the elderly, other evidence is often lacking at the level of the individual patient. Thus, definitive recommendations for preventive assessment of the elderly for a number of conditions and problems remain incomplete.

In categories for which information is incomplete, guidelines are based on the best available data using the methodology of the U.S. Clinical Preventive Health Services Task Force and others.[20, 21, 27, 29, 31, 33, 48–53] When a recommendation is either absent or equivocal, individual clinical judgment based on general screening principles, guidelines, and methodologic criteria is suggested.

Tables 13–4 and 13–5 and Figure 13–2 display periodic health assessment and health maintenance recommendations for the elderly based on the foregoing general principles, criteria, and quality of the evidence. Table 13–4 lists conditions for which direct intervention and follow-up are warranted (many such interventions can be

TABLE 13–4 **RECOMMENDED HEALTH ASSESSMENT AND HEALTH MAINTENANCE ACTIVITIES FOR ELDERLY PATIENTS**

Condition	Recommended Intervention	Follow-up Action
Accidents	Careful history in the office once between ages 65 and 70 years, then every 2 years to age 75, and then annually in home visits	With positive history, monitor very closely; conduct comprehensive history and physical examination as appropriate
Alcohol abuse or dependency	Careful history/review in the office once between ages 65 and 70 years and once between 70 and 75 years and then regularly during home assessments	Nutrition review and assessment of social support and personal status to link with community resources as needed
Breast cancer	Annual office examination and teaching/reinforcement of self-breast examination regularly at home	Refer for mammography if clinically indicated or if previously equivocal between ages 50 and 59 years
Colorectal cancer	Flexible sigmoidoscopic examination in the office every 3 to 5 years to age 80; annual stool examination for occult blood to age 80	Depending on clinical findings, monitor and assess closely; refer as indicated
Depression	Careful history at least once between ages 65 and 70 and 70 and 75 and then annually during home assessments; monitor closely after loss; anticipate risk of self-harm and/or suicide	Home assessment and review when findings indicate closer attention warranted; brief therapy with drugs and possibly counseling is useful in some cases
Drug hazards	Comprehensive review of all drugs prescribed and taken from all sources at every visit from age 65 years, plus annual home assessments from age 75 years; periodic tests of renal function are useful	Monitor drug actions, interactions, and adverse reactions on regular basis and seek to reduce type, number, and dosages to bare minimum
Falls	Detailed history at least once between ages 65 and 70 years, then every 2 years to 75 years, and then annually	Monitor closely with history of one fall; investigate when history is positive for two
Foot care	Assess once by history and inspection between ages 65 and 70 years, then every 2 years to age 75, and then annually during course of regular home assessments	Regular assessments during visits for blood pressure and weight checks in the office; refer for chiropody or orthopedics as indicated
Hearing impairment	Discretionary assessment in office once between ages 65 and 70 years and 70 and 75 years, and then every 2 years or more often if high-risk or previous history of loss	Office audiometry and/or referral for tests or aids/enhancements; office procedures such as syringing of canals frequently sufficient
Hypertension	Blood pressure check yearly in office and discretionary during visits for other reasons, annually during regular home assessments after age 75	Monitor according to step-care protocols and consider carefully before instituting drug therapy in this group
Immunization status	History of previous immunizations and documentation in office chart; for high-risk patients, immunize for influenza annually to age 75, and then annually for all over 75; discretionary for international travelers, BCG test,[a] and diphtheria immunizations	Tetanus booster every 10 years; polio (Salk) vaccine discretionary every 10 years; influenza annual vaccine for some to age 75, and for all over 75 years; pneumonia vaccine once only
Impaired mobility	Careful history in the office once between ages 65 and 70 years, and then each year in home assessments and in office for other reasons	Careful review of all medications, social situations, nutritional status, musculoskeletal system; investigate and treat as appropriate
Loss and bereavement	Comprehensive history and inspection during course of office visits for other reasons to age 75 and then annually at home also; short-term drug therapy or counseling can help	Special attention to hidden "signals" during office visits; monitor closely after death of spouse or pets or change in status, e.g., income or residence

Table continued on following page

TABLE 13–4 **RECOMMENDED HEALTH ASSESSMENT AND HEALTH MAINTENANCE ACTIVITIES FOR ELDERLY PATIENTS** *(Continued)*

Condition	Recommended Intervention	Follow-up Action
Obesity	Weight check during physical examination once from ages 65 to 70 and with every blood pressure check in office; annually at home during assessments after 75 years	Diet counseling can help in some patients; food purchase/preparation assistance; exercise and peer support useful for some patients
Periodontal disease and dental caries; oral cancer	History and inspection of oral cavity discretionary to age 75 years and then each year in home assessments in reference to dentures/oral cancer or for dental care needs	Investigate if suspicious lesions seen; refer for proper assessment of dentures; link patient to community resources in reference to nutrition if indicated or for dental restoration
Progressive incapacity with advanced age	Annual office visits for review of functional status, abilities, and impairments; home assessments at least once yearly for all patients over age 75 years	Depending on level of abilities and extent of support system, refer to community resources when appropriate
Skin cancer	Assess every 2 years from ages 65 to 74, then each year from age 75	Refer to dermatologist for more specific evaluation and/or biopsy for pathologic assessment
Stature/height	Check height during examination in office once between ages 65 and 70 years with weight check, and then every 3 to 5 years in the office; reassess annually at home at each assessment in patients over 75 years	Monitor weight for height and document shortening of stature and development of any obesity, kyphosis, knee and/or hip flexion, and spinal osteoporosis with or without neurologic deficits; investigate/refer/treat with diet, analgesics, other medications, braces and supports, walkers, and/or rehabilitation as appropriate
Urinary incontinence	Establish trusting rapport with patients over time; obtain careful history in office at least once between ages 65 and 70 and 70 and 75 and then follow closely each year at home assessments; anticipate problem in high-risk patients or circumstances	Investigate reversible causes such as urinary tract infection, stress, detrusor instability; organize support in community to maintain person at home as long as possible with treatment or referral as needed
Victimization and abuse	Careful history in office at any time when suspicion index is high or when clinical evidence suggests physical, psychologic, or material abuse, nutritional deprivation, or intentional over-medication (chemical straight-jacketing); regular review during annual home assessments in patients after 75 years in all settings; use of home safety and medication check lists is often helpful in monitoring	Thorough documentation to identify and distinguish areas of intentional and unintentional neglect, misinformation, ignorance, or direct or indirect abuse; development of personal advocacy role to counsel caregivers; referral to self-help and support groups, information and education resources, and community liaison
Visual impairments	Obtain history of visual function and refractive corrections during visits for other reasons up to age 70 years and then follow more closely, with annual review during assessments at home after age 75 years. For diabetic patients, do fundoscopic exam with dilation in office every year	Office examinations and/or referral as indicated; glaucoma tonometry may be warranted; monitor all previously diagnosed patients; marshal community resources, e.g., special visual aids. Refer all diabetics to ophthalmologist annually

[a]BCG = Bacille Calmette-Guerin: Immunization for *Mycobacterium tuberculosis* administered to select populations at special risk.

TABLE 13–5 **CONDITIONS REQUIRING FURTHER RESEARCH TO DETERMINE APPROPRIATENESS OF SCREENING AND CASE-FINDING IN ASYMPTOMATIC ELDERLY**

A. Conditions for Which Periodic Assessment May Be Warranted in the Asymptomatic Elderly[a]

Condition	Suggested Approach
Anemia, iron-deficiency type; malnutrition	Periodic hemogram (every 2 to 5 years) with follow-up and treatment prn
Glaucoma, chronic open-angle type	Ocular tonometry or tonography every 3 to 5 years with referral prn *may* be useful despite low sensitivity, low specificity, and diagnostic inaccuracy
Gynecologic neoplasia 　Cervical 　Endometrial 　Ovarian	Pap smears are *not* warranted after age 70 when previously negative; pelvic examination every 2 years potentially useful for uterine or ovarian enlargement; jet washings and biopsy only for high-risk women with postmenopausal bleeding
Hyperglycemia	Fasting serum glucose (or 2-hour postcibal) or Hgb A1c at 2- to 5-year intervals
Prostatic carcinoma	Rectal palpation annually at time of assessment for colorectal carcinoma; urinary cytology, serum acid phosphatase levels and PSA may be warranted
Renal impairment	For monitoring—creatinine clearance useful (if obtainable); chemical urinalysis, blood urea nitrogen, and serum creatinine (every 2 to 5 years) at time of hemogram and serum glucose determinations
Tuberculosis	Intradermal purified protein derivative-Tween (5 T.U.) tuberculin sensitivity testing every 5 years in two-step procedure (7 to 10 days apart, although 10% to 20% of elderly will have anergy); sputum staining. Culture; chest x-ray as appropriate; treat prn

B. Conditions That Do Not Presently Warrant Periodic Assessment in the Asymptomatic Elderly[b]

Condition

Confusion/dementia
Hyperlipidemia
Hypothyroidism
Lung cancer
Osteoporosis

[a]However, data are equivocal or insufficient for definitive recommendations at this time.
[b]Based on established scientific principles and screening criteria.

efficiently and effectively conducted by supervised nonphysician health personnel). Home follow-up (often in conjunction with community resources), where available, is often necessary and appropriate in many instances. With elderly patients, the medical practitioner's role includes a large element of coordination of services to maintain health and to preserve independent functioning.

Table 13–5 contains a list of conditions that require further research to determine whether preventive assessment among the elderly is warranted (either as screening or as case-finding) and if so, in what form, how often, for how long, and to what end. Problems listed in Part A do warrant periodic assessment at this time, but problems shown in Part B do not presently warrant either screening or case-finding based on the methodologic criteria and quality of the evidence now available.

Figure 13–2 is a health maintenance flow sheet for elderly patients. This recommended schedule of preventive interventions is based on current knowledge and principles consistent with methodologic criteria for preventive assessment in general. Modifications of Figure 13–2 and of Tables 13–4 and 13–5 are anticipated as more information becomes available through advances in clinical prevention research in the areas of periodic health assessment and health maintenance of the elderly.

Listed below are principles and guidelines for preventive assessment of the elderly.

1. Use of nonphysician health personnel is central to sound preventive assessment and health surveillance of the elderly.
2. Preventive assessment of the elderly is acceptable and preferable when it is conducted in health facilities or the home rather than in the community at large.

Name of Patient: _____

Birthdate: _____

Sex: Male ___ Female ___

Date (day/month/year)

MARK AN "X" OVER EACH BOX WHEN ASSESSMENT IS DONE

Age at this Assessment

RECOMMENDED INTERVENTION

O = Office ● = Home

Intervention	65	66	67	68	69	70	71	72	73	74	75	76	77	78	79	80	81	82	83	84	85	86	87	88	89	90
Comprehensive Functional Assessment in the Office	O		O		O		O		O		O	O	O	O	O	O	O	O	O	O	O	O	O	O	O	O
Full Medication Review	O	O	O	O	O	O	O	O	O	O	O	O	O	O	O	O	O	O	O	O	O	O	O	O	O	O
Blood Pressure Check	O	O	O	O	O	O	O	O	O	O	●	●	O	●	O	●	●	●	●	●	●	●	●	●	●	●
Weight Check	O	O	O	O	O	O	O	O	O	O	●	●	O	●	O	●	●	●	●	●	●	●	●	●	●	●
Influenza Immunization	O	O	O	O	O	O	O	O	O	O	●	●	O	●	O	●	●	●	●	●	●	●	●	●	●	●
Breast Examination	O	O	O	O	O	O	O	O	O	O	●	●	O	●	O											
Stools for Occult Blood	O	O	O	O	O	O	O	O	O	O	O	O	O	O	O											
Skin Assessment	O		O		O		O		O		O	O	O	O	O	O										
Prostatic Examination (*)	O	O	O	O	O	O	O	O	O	O																
Pelvic Examination (*)	O		O		O		O		O		O															
Pneumonia Immunization	O										O										O					
Tetanus (Td) Booster	O										O										O					
Poliomyelitis Booster	O										O										O					
Comprehensive Phys. Exam.	O										O															
Home Assessment	●										●	●	●	●	●	●	●	●	●	●	●	●	●	●	●	●
Accident Prevention	O						O		O		O	●	●	●	●	O	●	●	●	●	O	●	●	●	●	●
Alcohol Dependency Review	O						O		O		O	●	●	●	●	O	●	●	●	●	O	●	●	●	●	●
Depression Review	O						O		O		O	●	●	●	●	O	●	●	●	●	O	●	●	●	●	●
Falls and Gait Review	O						O		O		O	●	●	●	●	O	●	●	●	●	O	●	●	●	●	●
Foot Care/Podiatry Check	O						O		O		O	●	●	●	●	O	●	●	●	●	O	●	●	●	●	●
Loss/Bereavement Review	O						O				O	●	●	●	●	O	●	●	●	●	O	●	●	●	●	●
Psychosocial Review	O						O				O	●	●	●	●	O	●	●	●	●	O	●	●	●	●	●
Urinary Continence Review	O						O				O	●	●	●	●	O	●	●	●	●	O	●	●	●	●	●
Victimization/Abuse Check	O						O				O	●	●	●	●	O	●	●	●	●	O	●	●	●	●	●
Vision Assessment	O						O				O	●	●	●	●	O	●	●	●	●	O	●	●	●	●	●
Mental Status Examination	O						O				O	●		●		O	●	●	●	●	O	●	●	●	●	●
Hearing Assessment	O						O				O	●		●	O		●		O		●		●	O	●	●
Periodontal/Oral Check	O						O				O	●		●	O		●		O		●		●	O	●	●
Hemogram Check (*)	O						O				O			O												
Fasting Serum Glucose (*)	O						O				O			O												
BUN/Serum Creatinine (*)	O						O				O			O												
Chemical Urinalysis (*)	O						O				O			O												
Tuberculin Sensitivity (*)	O						O				O					O										
Measurement of Height (*)	O						O				O					O										
Glaucoma Assessment (*)	O						O				O					O										
Flexible Sigmoidoscopy (*)	O						O				O					O										

O = Office ● = Home Address _____ Telephone _____

(*) Research is needed to determine the validity and appropriate frequency of this intervention; use individual discretion for patients in advanced years. ©

Figure 13–2 Health maintenance flow sheet for older adults (65 to 90 years of age).

3. Regular episodic "health maintenance" activities intended to preserve function and prevent or reduce impairment are more appropriate than exhaustive, expensive, and often ineffective searches for new diseases or diagnoses, especially in persons over age 80.

4. Systematic checklists and office flow sheets are expeditious methods for monitoring screening results and the health status of elderly patients.

5. Technologic advances enhance elderly preventive assessment, but use of procedures or methods that have not been validated should be limited until they have been evaluated.

6. The periodic health examination has a relatively low sensitivity for the detection of major disorders that have lethal outcomes, and extensive health surveillance programs for the elderly are not currently justifiable on methodologic grounds.

7. The frail elderly in the community are especially susceptible to the "inverse care law." That is, those in greatest need and for whom preventive assessment and surveillance have the highest potential benefit are most likely to be missed or to default. Active case-finding and close follow-up of elderly with particularly high risk (the lonely, the recently bereaved, and the poor) are especially important health intervention priorities.

8. Lifetime health monitoring is a useful process in the spectrum of risk-based preventive assessment. Extension of this approach among the elderly is particularly worthwhile when it is conducted in accordance with guidelines of the U.S. Preventive Services Task Force, the American Academy of Family Physicians, the American College of Physicians, and the Canadian Task Force on the Periodic Examination.[20, 21, 48, 49, 53]

9. Research aimed at further defining and delineating the efficacy of specific preventive assessment interventions based on sound clinical and epidemiologic principles continues to be needed because of the urgency of the "geriatric imperative" in the United States.

10. The ultimate dictum of *primum non nocere* ("first, do no harm") is highly germane in preventive assessment of the elderly. Holland's insight in 1974 remains true today: "In the middle-aged and elderly, simple tests for vision and hearing and tests to identify people in need of chiropody or walking aids may be far more effective than more complex biochemical and laboratory-oriented procedures in improving the 'quality of life.' "[50]

Although more scientifically based recommendations either for or against specific preventive assessments in the elderly are becoming validated,[25–29] the quality of much evidence at this time remains inadequate to justify high-level intervention.[22–24] However, "therapeutic nihilism" is also a risk in that appropriate interventions might *not* be undertaken based solely on one's age rather than on the full range of factors relevant to the individual patient and his or her wishes.[54]

SUMMARY

The challenge, then, is to find the right balance between the value of screening the elderly through periodic health assessments to identify and correct or minimize treatable problems on the one hand, and, on the other hand, to avoid the very real problem that clinically or biochemically inapparent (and most often insignificant) "abnormalities" may lead to overzealous investigation and overtreatment of the elderly at high cost, inconvenience, and risk.[55, 56] Conversely, reflex ageism that denies otherwise appropriate interventions based on age discrimination alone also warrants cautious monitoring.[57] In the end, sound clinical judgment is always necessary. Especially for those caring for the elderly in times of critical change in health care structure, finance, and accessibility, it is also irreplaceable.

References

1. Commission on Chronic Illness: Chronic Illness in the United States, Vol. 1. Prevention of Chronic Illness. Cambridge, Harvard University Press, 1957, p. 45.
2. Sackett DL: Screening in family practice: Prevention, levels of evidence, and the pitfalls of common sense. J Fam Pract 1987;24:233–234.
3. Whitby LG: Screening for disease: Definitions and criteria. Lancet 1974;2:819–822.
4. Lowther CP, Macleod RDM, Williamson J: Evaluation of early diagnostic services for the elderly. Br Med J 1970;3:275–277.
5. Currie G, MacNeil RM, Walker JG, et al: Medical and social screening of patients aged 70–72 by an urban general practice health team. Br Med J 1974;2:108–111.
6. Milne JS, Maule M, Williamson J: Method of sampling in a study of older people with a comparison of respondents and non-respondents. Br J Prev Soc Med 1971;25:37–41.
7. Powell C, Crombie A. The Kilsyth questionnaire: A

method of screening elderly people at home. Age Ageing 1974;3:23–28.

8. Burns C: Geriatric care in general practice. A medico-social survey of 391 patients undertaken by health visitors. J R Coll Gen Pract 1969;18:287–296.

9. Tomlinson JM: Setting up a geriatric survey in general practice. Update 1976;8:277–281.

10. Taylor GF, Eddy TP, Scott DL: A survey of 216 elderly men and women in general practice. J R Coll Gen Pract 1971;21:267–275.

11. Steel K, Williams F, Fairbank M, Knox K: Laboratory screening in the evaluation and placement of geriatric patients. J Am Geriatr Soc 1974;22:538–543.

12. Brocklehurst JC, Carty MH, Leeming JT, Robinson J: Medical screening of old people accepted for residential care. Lancet 1978;2:141–142.

13. Freedman GR, Charlewood JE, Dodds PA: Screening the aged in general practice. J R Coll Gen Pract 1978;28:421–425.

14. Tulloch AJ, Moore V: A randomized controlled trial of geriatric screening and surveillance in general practice. J R Coll Gen Pract 1979;29:733–740.

15. McKeown T (ed): Screening in Medical Care: Reviewing the Evidence; A Collection of Essays. Neufield Hospitals Providence Trust. London, Oxford University Press, 1968.

16. Breslow L, Somers AR: The lifetime health-monitoring program: A practical approach to preventive medicine. N Engl J Med 1977;296:601–605.

17. Somers AR, Bruch TL, Frame PS, et al: Lifetime health monitoring: A whole life-plan for well patient care. Patient Care 1979;13:83–86, 120–126, 160–164, 201–205.

18. Frame PS, Carlson SJ: A critical review of periodic health screening using specific screening criteria. J Fam Pract 1975;2:29–36, 123–129, 189–194, 283–289.

19. Frame PS, Kowulich BA: Stool occult blood screening for colorectal cancer. J Fam Pract 1982;15:1071–1075.

20. Canadian Task Force on the Periodic Health Examination: Canadian guide to clinical preventive health care. Ottawa, Canada Communication Group, 1994.

21. U.S. Preventive Services Task Force: Guide to Clinical Preventive Services, 2nd ed. Alexandria, VA, International Medical Publishing, 1996.

22. Stewart KJ: What are we really accomplishing with screening for disease? Fam Pract Mgmt 1996;3:29–31.

23. Fetters MD, Fischer G, Reed BD: Effectiveness of vaginal Papanicolaou smear screening after total hysterectomy for benign disease. JAMA 1996;275(12):940–947.

24. Leininger L: Overperformance of preventive care procedures in primary care practice. J Gen Intern Med 1994;9:88–90.

25. Catalona WJ, Smith DX, Ratliff TL, Basler JW: Detection of organ-confined prostate cancer is increased through prostate-specific antigen-based screening. JAMA 1993;270:948–954.

26. Voelker R: Population-based medicine merges with clinical care: Epidemiologic techniques. JAMA 1994;271:1301–1302.

27. Kellie SE, Griffith H: Emerging trends in assessing performance and managing in health care: Expectations for implementing preventive services. Am J Prev Med 1995; 11:388–392.

28. Wagner EH: Managing medical practice: The potential of HMOs. *In* Gelijns AC (ed): IOM Workshop Proceedings. The Changing Health Care Economy: Impact on Physicians, Patients, and Innovators. Washington, DC, National Academy Press, 1992, p. 51–61.

29. Thompson RS, Taplin SH, McAfee TA, Mandelson MT, Smith AE: Primary and secondary prevention services in clinical practice: Twenty years' experience in development, implementation, and evaluation. JAMA 1995;273(14):1130–1135.

30. Kottke TE, Brekke ML, Solberg LI: Making "time" for preventive services. Mayo Clin Proc 1993;68:785–791.

31. Walsh JME, McPhee SH: A systems model of clinical preventive care: An analysis of factors influencing patient and physician. Health Educ Q 1992;19:157–175.

32. Lomas J, Haynes RB. A taxonomy and critical review of tested strategies for the application of clinical practice recommendations: From 'official' to 'individual' clinical policy. Am J Prev Med 1988;4:77–94.

33. Handley MR, Stuart ME: An evidence-based approach to evaluating and improving clinical practice: Implementing practice guidelines. HMO Pract 1994;2:75–83.

34. Taplin SH, Thompson RS, Schnitzer F, Anderman C, Immanuel V: Revisions in the risk-based breast cancer screening program at Group Health Cooperative. Cancer 1990;66(4):812–818.

35. Pearson DC, Thompson RS: Evaluation of Group Health Cooperative of Puget Sound's Senior Influenza Immunization Program. Public Health Rep 1994;109:571–578.

36. Stuart ME, Handley MA, Thompson RS, Conger M, Timlin D: Clinical practice and new technology: Prostate-specific antigen (PSA). HMO Pract 1992;6:5–11.

37. Thorner RM, Remein QR: Principles and Procedures in the Evaluation of Screening for Disease. Monograph No. 67, Publication No. 846. Washington, DC, U.S. Public Health Service, Division of Chronic Disease, 1961.

38. Wilson JMG, Jungner G: Principles and Practice of Screening for Disease. Public Health Papers No. 3. Geneva, World Health Organization, 1968.

39. Wilson JMG, Hilleboe HE: Mass Health Examinations as a Public Health Tool. Technical Report Series No. A24. Public Health Papers No. 45. Geneva, World Health Organization 1971.

40. The Systolic Hypertension in the Elderly Program (SHEP) Cooperative Research Group: Rationale and design of a randomized clinical trial on prevention of stroke in isolated systolic hypertension. J Clin Epidemiol 1988;41:1197–1208.

41. The Systolic Hypertension in the Elderly Program (SHEP) Cooperative Research Group. Prevention of stroke by antihypertensive drug treatment in older persons with isolated systolic hypertension. JAMA 1991;265(24):3255–3264.

42. Cole P, Morrison A: Basic issues in population screening for cancer. J Natl Cancer Inst 1980;64:1263–1272.

43. Last J (ed): A Dictionary of Epidemiology, 3rd ed. New York, Oxford University Press, 1995, p. 14.

44. Vecchio TJ: Predictive value of a single diagnostic test in unselected populations. N Engl J Med 1966;274:1171–1173.

45. Mulrow CD, Cornell JA, Herrara CR, et al: Hypertension in the elderly: Implications and generalizability of randomized trials. JAMA 1994;272:1932–1938.

46. Weinstein MC, Stason WB: Economic considerations in the management of mild hypertension. Ann NY Acad Sci 1978;304:424–440.

47. Logan AG, Milne BJ, Achber C, et al: Worksite treatment of hypertension by specially trained nurses—a controlled trial. Lancet 1979;2:1175–1178.

48. American Academy of Family Physicians. Age Charts

for Periodic Health Examination. Kansas City, American Academy of Family Physicians, 1993.

49. Eddy DM (ed): Common Screening Tests. Philadelphia, American College of Physicians, 1991.
50. Holland WW: Taking stock: Screening for disease. Lancet 1974;2:1494–1497.
51. United Kingdom, National Health Service: Health Service Guidelines—NHS Management Executive, Sheffield, England, National Screening Programme; 1993.
52. American College of Obstetricians and Gynecologists: Recommendations on Frequency of Pap Test Screening. Washington, DC, American College of Obstetricians and Gynecologists, 1995.

53. Sox HC Jr, Woolf SH: Evidence-based practice guidelines from the U.S. Preventive Services Task Force (editorial). JAMA 1993;269:2678.
54. Avron J: Benefits and cost analysis in geriatric care: Turning age discrimination into health policy. N Engl J Med 1984;310:1294–1295.
55. Levkoff SE, Cleary PD, Wetle T, Besdine RW: Illness behavior in the aged: Implications for clinicians. J Am Geriatr Soc 1988;36:622–629.
56. Sackett DL, Holland WW: Controversy in the detection of disease. Lancet 1975;2:357–359.
57. Halpern J: Can practice guidelines safeguard patient values? J Law Med Ethics 1995;23:75–81.

14 Exercise

Julie Chandler, Ph.D.

Stephanie Studenski, M.D., M.P.H.

Regular exercise offers an attractive approach to preventing decline and restoring function in older adults. While the effects of exercise are known and formal guidelines exist for younger adults,[1] less is known about exercise later in life, especially in people with multiple illnesses or existing functional limitations. Programs for such special populations have been the subject of intense study in recent years. Can exercise be used to improve health status in the frail person with limited mobility, muscle weakness, poor balance, and poor endurance? The evidence, though incomplete, is encouraging. Some limitations in frail elders may be the result of deconditioning due to inactivity, which is often a final common pathway entered from a classic geriatric vicious cycle of illness and complications.[2, 3] Some impairments due to disuse and deconditioning (such as strength, balance, and endurance) can be modified with exercise, just as they are in younger, healthier adults.[4, 5] Whether a reversal of impairments such as weakness translates into improved function and mobility is less clear, but the initial findings hold promise. The purpose of this chapter is to review exercise programs intended to increase strength, aerobic conditioning, and balance in older adults and to make recommendations for clinical practice.

The conceptual basis for exercise intervention in frail older adults rests on a model of disability that describes disability as the result of a mix of organ system–based impairments. Muscle weakness, limited joint mobility, poor aerobic capacity, and poor balance are all potentially reversible impairments that have been associated with mobility problems (walking, climbing stairs, rising from a chair), [6–9] routine activities (showering, housekeeping, shopping),[10, 11] and falls.[12–14] In a deconditioned older person, walking, showering, or rising from a chair can represent up to 80% of maximum oxygen uptake (VO_2 max).[5] Poor joint mobility has been associated with difficulty in using public transportation.[7] The accumulation of multiple impairments may be an especially stressful burden for a frail elderly person; multiple deficits in strength, range of motion, central processing, and sensation predict poor endurance and poor performance in tasks such as walking, reaching, and climbing stairs, better than any single impairment or disease.[15] These observations from cross-sectional data have led to the hypothesis that treatment of reversible physiologic deficits may lead to improved function.

STRENGTH TRAINING PROGRAMS IN THE ELDERLY

High-Intensity Strengthening

Numerous studies have convincingly shown that gains in strength are achievable with high-intensity strength training even in nursing home residents in their nineties[16–24] (Tables 14–1 and 14–2). Programs consist of progressive resistive training in which the participant lifts 70% to 90% of a one-repetition maximum (the amount of weight that can be lifted fully through the range of motion one time only) three times per week for at least 8 to 10 weeks. The load is increased weekly to maintain the intensity of the stimulus. Usually two to three sets of 10 are repeated per muscle group per exercise session. Strength gains of up to 200% have been reported using these exercise programs.

The impact of high-intensity resistance training on physical performance has been more variable than its impact on strength. Significant increases in habitual gait speed, maximum gait speed, tandem gait speed and stair-climbing power have been reported in some studies[16, 17, 22] but not others.[21] The magnitude of benefit in physical performance may be directly related to the initial performance level of patients. More impaired participants who have initial habitual gait speeds of 0.7 meter per second or less tend to gain more after resistance training[17] than those with initial gait speeds of over 1 meter per second.[21] On the other hand, healthier individuals with initial gait speeds of over 1 meter per second may show increased *maximum* (fastest) gait velocity after strength training.[22] These findings suggest that improvement in habitual gait speed

TABLE 14–1 **STRENGTHENING INTERVENTIONS IN HEALTHY ELDERLY**[a]

Author	Population Studied	No. Patients	Design	Intervention	Outcomes Impairments	Outcomes Physical Performance	Outcomes Disability	Limitations
Frontera et al, 1988[19]	Older men 60–72 yr	12	Before/after	Dynamic strength training	• Knee strength ↑ significant (107%–226%) ($p <$ .0001) (1 repetition max) • Isokinetic strength ↑ 10%–18% ($p <$ .05)	N/T	N/T	Small sample
Grimby et al, 1992[50]	Men 78–84 yr	9	Before/after	Isometric concentric and eccentric strength training 2–3 ×/wk × 25 sessions	10% ↑ in concentric strength	N/T	N/T	Limited sample size, no control group, limited outcome measures
Charette et al, 1991[20]	Women 69 ± 1 yr	27	RCT	Resistance strength training of lower extremity 3 ×/wk × 12 wk	28%–115% Δ in strength ($p <$ .05) in exercise group	N/T	N/T	
Judge et al, 1994[21]	Men + women ≥75 yr	28 resistance, 27 control, 55 other	RCT	Resistance training vs. control vs. other	Significant ↑ in strength in resistance group only ($p ≥$ .005)	• Significant ↑ in gait velocity in resistance group and control group • No significant Δ in chair rise time	N/T	
Era, 1988[51]	Healthy men 74–84 yr	42	RCT	Strengthening (isometric, dynamic) vs. flexibility vs. control 2 ×/wk × 1 hr × 8 wk	Significant Δ in knee strength in both exercise groups; no Δ in static sway	N/T	N/T	

Study	Subjects	N	Design	Intervention	Outcome	Function		Limitations
Brown et al, 1990[24]	Community-dwelling men 60–70 yr	14	Before/after	Dynamic resistance training 3 ×/wk × 12 wk	Isokinetic strength ↑ by 17%–18%; no Δ in isometric strength; evidence of hypertrophy	N/T	N/T	Small sample, no control group
Hunter et al, 1997[22]	Healthy women 60–70 yr	14	Before/after	Strength training—total body	Significant ↑ in strength (31%–52%)	• Significant ↑ in maximal gait velocity (18%) • NIEMG of biceps ↓ 36% during carrying activities • NIEMG of rectus femoris ↓ 40% during chair rise task	N/T	No control group
Frontera et al, 1990[18]	Healthy men 60–70 yr	12	Before/after	High-intensity resistance training of knee flexors and extensors at 80% of 1 repetition max 3 ×/ wk × 12 wk	• 10% ↑ in 1 repetition max • 10% ↑ in isokinetic strength of 60% • 23% ↑ in total work • ↑ in VO₂ max (p = .03)	N/T	N/T	No control; no integrated measure of performance
Ades et al, 1996[23]	Healthy men + women 65–79 yr	24	RCT	Progressive resistive training strength 3 ×/wk × 12 wk	• Significant ↑ in exhaustive submax walking endurance (time) • Significant ↑ in arm and leg strength (29%–65%) of a 1 rep max)	N/T	N/T	No integrated measures of performance

Abbreviations: ↑, ↓, increase, decrease; Δ, change; RCT, randomized controlled trial; N/T, not tested; NIEMG, needle insertion electromyogram.

[a]See also Table 14–8 for definitions pertaining to this table.

TABLE 14–2 **STRENGTHENING INTERVENTIONS IN IMPAIRED ELDERS**[a]

Author	Population Studied	No. Patients	Design	Intervention	Impairments	Physical Performance	Disability	Limitations
						Outcomes		
Fiatarone et al, 1994[17]	Nursing home men and women	100	RCT	High-intensity strength training vs. strength/nutrition vs. nutrition vs. placebo 3 ×/wk × 10 wk	113 ± 8% ↑ in strength in exercise group (1 repetition max) vs. 3 ± 9% in control (p < .001)	• Gait velocity ↑ by 11.8% ± 3.8% in exercise (p = .02) • Stair climbing power ↑ by 28.4% vs. 3.6% ± 6.7% in control (p = .01)	Level of spontaneous activity ↑ in strength training groups only (p = .03)	
Fiatarone et al, 1990[16]	Nursing home nonagenarians (6 women, 4 men) 90 ± 1 yr	10	Before/after	High-intensity strength training 3 ×/wk × 8 wk	174% ± 31% gain in quadriceps strength (one repetition max)	Tandem gait speed ↑ by 48%	N/T	
Fisher et al, 1991[25]	Elderly men with OA of knee 67.6 ± 6.1 yr	15	Before/after	Isometric and isotonic strengthening 3 ×/wk × 1 hr × 16 wk	Muscle strength ↑ 23%–47% Muscle endurance ↑ 25%–40%	Gait speed ↑ significant (12%)	Functional status index scores improved: • dependency ↓ 10% • difficulty ↓ 25% • pain ↓ 40%	
Fisher et al, 1991[26]	Nursing home residents (10 women, 4 men) 60–90 yr	14	Before/after	Isometric and isotonic strengthening of knee extensors 3 ×/wk × 6 wk	Significant ↑ in muscle endurance (p < .05) Significant ↑ in strength (p < .05)	N/T	Nursing reports of ↑ in spontaneous activity and ↓ in dependency	No control group; ? statistical significance

Abbreviations: RCT, randomized controlled trial; OA, osteoarthritis; ↑, ↓, increase, decrease.
[a]See also Table 14–8 for definitions pertaining to this table.

is likely to occur with strength training especially in more impaired individuals, while in healthier elders strength training affects mostly the elements of physiologic reserve such as maximum gait speed.

Low-Intensity Strengthening

Lower-intensity resistance training has also been used successfully to increase strength, although the magnitude of strength gain is not as marked.[25] In older persons with osteoarthritis, resistance training that includes both isotonic (lifting a weight through the range of motion) and isometric (static) contractions (three to five repetitions each) at an intensity of 50% of a maximum effort, three times a week for 16 weeks, has been shown to increase strength (35%), muscle endurance (35%), and speed of limb movement (50%).[25] With use of a similar program in nursing home residents, strength improved by 15%, endurance by 35%, and speed of limb movement by 35%.[26] Another study showed only modest gains (5% to 10%) in strength in deconditioned nursing home patients after a three day per week, 12-week program of resistance training at 40% to 60% of a one-repetition maximum.[27] A supervised in-home progressive resistive exercise program using graded elastic bands in frail older men and women showed gains of 10% to 15% in lower extremity strength after 10 to 12 weeks of three times per week exercise.[28] In healthier community-dwelling older women, a 25-week program of light resistance exercise increased shoulder strength by about 20% and lower extremity strength modestly (10%).[29]

In patients who have conditions that make it difficult to exercise, lower-intensity training is an acceptable alternative method for achieving modest increases in strength. Can lower-intensity strength training achieve the same effects on gait and function as high-intensity strengthening? The few studies that have looked specifically at measures of performance after low-intensity strength training have shown mixed results. Osteoarthritis patients showed improvement in the functional status index with decreases in dependency, difficulty, and pain.[25] Nursing home residents showed some evidence of increased spontaneous activity in one study and improvement in mobility in another.[26] An in-home supervised exercise program that increased lower extremity strength in frail elderly men and women showed no improvement in measures of gait or mobility.[28] Because there are many other determinants of mobility performance besides strength, such as the presence of co-morbid conditions, depression, and cognition, it is unclear who is likely to benefit from low-intensity exercise and how much strength gain is required to enhance performance. Integrated treatment approaches that incorporate low-intensity strength exercise with interventions for other impairments may be more successful in improving function than strength training alone.

AEROBIC EXERCISE TRAINING IN THE ELDERLY

High-Intensity Endurance Training

Aerobic exercise programs in healthy older adults improve aerobic capacity as measured by maximum oxygen uptake (VO_2 max) and resting heart rate (Tables 14–3 and 14–4). Aerobic activities are those that require continuous exercise of large muscle groups to raise the heart rate above the resting level for a sustained period of time. Examples of aerobic activity are walking, biking, running, and swimming. Guidelines for aerobic exercise prescription for healthy adults recommend an intensity of 60% to 75% of maximum heart rate (as measured by an exercise stress test), three days per week for at least 6 weeks.[1] Appropriate adaptations for impaired older persons with mobility limitations have not been clearly established.

In healthy men and women over the age of 64, supervised high-intensity aerobic training at 70% of maximum heart rate for 30 minutes, three times per week for 16 weeks, results in increased VO_2 max and a significantly decreased incidence of new cardiac conditions.[30] In healthy men and women in their 70s, Hagberg and colleagues showed that high-intensity aerobic exercise (35 to 45 minutes at 75% to 85% of maximum heart rate, three times per week for 6 months) results in significantly greater gains in VO_2 max than high-intensity strength training.[31]

Low-Intensity Exercise Training

Like high-intensity aerobic exercise, low-intensity aerobic exercise (30% to 45% of maximum heart rate for 25 minutes, three times per week) can significantly increase VO_2 max in healthy men and women over the age of 60.[32, 33] The magnitude of effect on VO_2 max is related to both the intensity and the duration of exercise. The higher the intensity and the longer the duration of exercise, the greater the effect on aerobic capacity. These findings, though made in healthy older adults, have important implications for more impaired persons who cannot tolerate high-intensity exercise. Studies of aerobic conditioning pro-

TABLE 14–3 **AEROBIC EXERCISE IN HEALTHY ELDERS**[a]

Author	Population Studied	No. Patients	Design	Intervention	Outcomes Impairments	Physical Performance	Disability	Limitations
Posner et al, 1990[30]	Elderly men and women ≥ 65 yr	184	RCT	70% of VO_2 max. 30 min 3 ×/wk × 16 wk (supervised)	Significant ↑ in VO_2 max	N/T	↓ in incidence of new cardiac conditions compared with that of those who did not exercise	
Hagberg et al, 1989[31]	Older men and women 70–79 yr	—	Random assignment to exercise group	35–45 min 3 ×/wk × 26 wk at 75%–85% max HR vs. 30 min 3 ×/wk on Nautilus	Aerobic group ↑ in VO_2 max 22% vs. 5% ↑ in strength group; aerobic group ↑ in strength by 5%; Nautilus group ↑ 9%	N/T	N/T	
Seals et al, 1984[33]	Community-dwelling men and women 63 ± 2 yr	11	Before/after	6 mo low-intensity training followed by 6 mo of higher intensity	Significant ↑ in VO_2 max with low-intensity training (p < .05); greater ↑ in VO_2 max with higher intensity (p < .01); overall ↑ of 30% in VO_2 max	N/T	N/T	
Badenhop et al, 1983[32]	Community-dwelling men and women ≥ 60 yr	32	RCT (low intensity [n = 14] vs. high intensity [n = 14]) vs. control	Cycle ergometry: LI: 30%–45% max HR HI: 60%–75% max HR 25 min 3 ×/wk × 9 wk	Significant ↑ in VO_2 max in both exercise groups; significant ↓ in resting HR in both groups	N/T	N/T	

Abbreviations: RCT, randomized controlled trial; ↑, ↓, increase, decrease; N/T, not tested; HR, heart rate; HI, high-intensity; LI, low-intensity.
[a]See also Table 14–8 for further definitions pertaining to this table.

TABLE 14-4 AEROBIC CONDITIONING IN IMPAIRED ELDERS[a]

Author	Population Studied	No. Patients	Design	Intervention	Outcomes			Limitations
					Impairments	Performance	Disability	
Naso et al 1990[34]	Nursing home patients without dementia and/or significant cardiac disease	15	RCT	Intervention 3 ×/wk upper and lower extremity conditioning; low intensity × 1 yr	Small but significant ↑ in aerobic capacity (with arm ergometry)	N/T	N/T	

Abbreviations: RCT, randomized controlled trial; N/T, not tested.
[a]See also Table 14-8 for further definitions pertaining to this table.

TABLE 14-5 BALANCE INTERVENTIONS IN HEALTHY ELDERS[a]

Author	Population Studied	No. Patients	Design	Intervention	Outcomes			Limitations
					Impairments	Physical Performance	Disability	
Province et al, 1995[43] Wolf et al, 1996[39]	Community-dwelling men and women 76 yr ± 5 yr	72	RCT	Static balance vs. dynamic balance (Tai Chi) vs. wellness discussion 1-2 ×/wk × 15 wk	N/T	N/T	Incidence ratio for falling: IR = .87 – static balance (.62, 1.23) IR = .63 – Tai Chi (.64, .89) p = .01	
Judge et al, 1994[21] Wolfson et al, 1996[38]	Community-dwelling men and women ≥ 75 yr	110	RCT	Balance platform training 3 ×/wk; 45-min sessions × 3 mo	No Δ in strength	No Δ in gait velocity or chair rise time		

Abbreviations: RCT, randomized controlled trial; N/T, not tested; Δ, change; IR, incidence ratio.
[a]See also Table 14-8 for further definitions pertaining to this table.

grams in frail populations suggest that low-intensity training three days per week can lead to small but significant training effects.[34] Concurrent illnesses that prevent continuous training are common in this population and may dampen the potential effect of such a program on cardiovascular outcomes. Sidney and Shephard advocate frequent repetition of a low-intensity (30% to 40% of maximum heart rate) program in the very deconditioned older person to achieve the desired increase in aerobic capacity and avoid undue stress.[35] In addition to physiologic benefits, aerobic exercise has a positive impact on depression and other markers of psychological well-being in elderly men and women.[36, 37]

BALANCE TRAINING IN THE ELDERLY

Specific balance training programs have been advocated as a means of improving postural reactions and reducing falls in older persons. The impact of static and dynamic balance training on measures of gait and balance in healthy and impaired older persons has been reported in a few studies[21, 38, 39] (Table 14–5).

Static balance training involving balance recovery activities on the balance platform has been compared with dynamic balance training involving a set of slow, smooth, and rhythmical movements found in the ancient Chinese martial art form of Tai Chi.[39] Persons who participated in the 15-week (one to two times per week) Tai Chi program had a lower incidence of falling than persons in the static balance training group. Tai Chi also was effective in lowering the fear of falling among participants. Training in neither group significantly affected strength, joint range of motion, or cardiovascular endurance.

In healthy women over the age of 75, balance training included three 45-minute sessions of training on a computerized balance platform and floor-based exercises such as standing on one leg, standing on foam, tandem walking forward and backward, walking on a narrow beam, and sitting on a rubber ball.[21, 38] This balance intervention significantly improved performance on all balance measures tested including loss of balance on the sensory organization test, single leg stance time, and functional base of support, but it was not associated with an increase in walking velocity or with improvement in chair rise time. Interestingly, balance training was actually associated with a decrease in gait speed.

These recent results suggest that an integrated dynamic movement approach to balance training may be an effective approach to reducing falls in active community-dwelling elderly men and women. The success of balance interventions in more impaired populations such as nursing home residents has not been reported.

COMBINED EXERCISE PROGRAMS

The principle of specificity of exercise dictates that the physiologic effects of training will be limited to the physiologic systems stressed most by the exercise intervention. Aerobic conditioning programs have marked effects on VO_2 max but little or no effect on muscle strength.[31, 40] In healthy persons, high-intensity strength training significantly increases muscle strength but has little effect on aerobic capacity,[18, 31] although recent studies suggest that in sedentary older persons, strength training alone may lead to a modest improvement in walking endurance.[23] Balance interventions have little effect on either strength or endurance.[38, 39] Because of limited cross-training ability, a single mode of exercise is not likely to maximize the rehabilitation potential of the deconditioned older person with multiple impairments. In healthy older men and women, studies that have combined aerobic and strengthening interventions have demonstrated their anticipated beneficial effects on physiologic outcomes of strength and aerobic capacity and possibly on some markers of static balance[38, 41] (Table 14–6). For the most part, combined exercise programs in healthy elderly persons have not shown gains in gait or other markers of mobility. Because high-functioning elderly people may perform at or near a perfect score at baseline on many common mobility tests, there may be no room in which to detect improvement—a ceiling effect.

A low-intensity program of progressive resistive plus aerobic conditioning exercise delivered to male nursing home residents three times per week for 12 weeks produced modest physiologic changes in strength and aerobic capacity and significant changes in the Tinetti mobility score and gait velocity[27] (Tables 14–7 and 14–8). An individualized physical therapy program stressing low-intensity progressive resistive exercise, range of motion, balance, and mobility training delivered to very frail nursing home residents failed to improve measures of strength, balance, and joint range of motion but did have a modest effect on physical mobility.[42]

DISCUSSION

Exercise interventions in older adults in general produce positive physiologic effects in persons of all ages and levels of impairment. Musculoskeletal and cardiovascular systems respond to both resistance and aerobic training as measured by

TABLE 14–6 **COMBINED EXERCISE PROGRAMS IN HEALTHY ELDERS**[a]

Author	Population Studied	No. Patients	Design	Intervention	Outcomes			Limitations
					Impairments	Physical Performance	Disability	
Judge et al, 1993[41]	Community-dwelling women 62–75 yr	21	RCT	Lower extremity resistance training, brisk walking, and balance (Tai Chi) vs. flexibility alone 3 ×/wk × 6 mo	Balance: single-stance center of force displacement ↓ 18% in strength/balance group (p = .02), but not in flexibility group	N/T	N/T	Small healthy sample
Rikli and Edwards, 1991[44]	Community-dwelling women 57–85 yr	31 exercise 17 control	Exercise vs. control	Aerobic training and calisthenics 3 ×/wk × 3 yr	• Choice reaction time ↓ in exercise subjects (p < .0001) • Single leg stand time ↑ (p < .015) • Flexibility ↑ (p = .0004) • Grip strength ↑ (p = .006)	N/T	N/T	Not RCT; volunteer bias may account for higher scores in exercise subjects
Agre et al, 1988[29]	Community-dwelling women 63–88 yr	47	Exercise vs. control	Aerobic exercise and resistance training and flexibility training 3 ×/wk × 1 hr × 25 wk	Significant difference in shoulder rotation and knee flexion strength between exercise and control groups	N/T	N/T	Exercise/control group not randomly assigned

Table continued on following page

TABLE 14–6 **COMBINED EXERCISE PROGRAMS IN HEALTHY ELDERS**[a] *Continued*

Author	Population Studied	No. Patients	Design	Intervention	Outcomes				Limitations
					Impairments	*Physical Performance*	*Disability*		
Morey et al, 1991[40]	Community-dwelling male veterans ≥ 65 yr	25	Before/after	Aerobic training, strengthening, and flexibility 3 ×/wk × 90 min × 2 yr	• Met level ↑ 20% • Submax HR ↓ by 7% • RHR ↓ by 8% • No Δ in strength • Grip strength ↑ by 11%	N/T	N/T		No control group for comparison
Judge et al, 1994[21]	Community-dwelling men & women ≥ 75 yr	28 exercise 27 control	RCT	Balance training and strength training	No Δ in strength	No Δ in gait speed or chair rise			
MacRae et al, 1994[45]	Women in senior centers ≥ 60 yr	80	RCT	Low-intensity balance, strength, and flexibility 1 hr 3 ×/wk × 1 yr	• Control group ↓ in strength (p < .002) • Intervention group did not Δ	No significant difference in gait characteristics or one-legged stand in either group	No significant difference in falls incidence		Limited measures of performance; healthy sample of women; low power for detecting falls
Hornbrook et al, 1994[46]	Community-dwelling men and women ≥ 65 yr	1611 intervention 1571 control	RCT	Education on falls risk factors, home exercise including strength, balance, and endurance	N/T	N/T	Risk of falling: OR: 0.85 (p < 0.05)		Exercise program not closely monitored

Abbreviations: RCT, randomized controlled trial; N/T, not tested; HR, heart rate; RHR, resting heart rate; ↑, ↓, increase, decrease; Δ, change; OR, odds ratio.
[a]See also Table 14–8 for further definitions pertaining to this table.

TABLE 14-7 **COMBINED EXERCISE PROGRAMS IN IMPAIRED ELDERS**[a]

Author	Population Studied	No. Patients	Design	Intervention	Outcomes			Limitations
					Impairments	Physical Performance	Disability	
Crilly et al, 1989[47]	Women in residential care facilities	50	RCT	Coordination, flexibility, and strength	No significant Δ in postural sway	N/T	N/T	Limited outcomes measured
Tinetti et al, 1994[48]	Community-dwelling men and women ≥ 70 yr at risk for falls	301	RCT	Individualized intervention to reduce risk factors for falls, including exercise intervention for some people	N/T	N/T	Significant ↓ in falls rate RR 0.69 (0.52, 0.90)	Exercise stimulus not measurable
Sauvage et al, 1992[27]	Deconditioned male nursing home residents 73.4 ± 4 yr	14	RCT	Progressive resistive exercise plus aerobic conditioning (70% max HR) 3 ×/wk × 12 wk	• No significant Δ in VO$_2$ max • Marginal Δ in strength	• Significant ↑ in Tinetti mobility score • No change in stride or step length • Gait velocity ↑ (p = .013)	N/T	Limited sample size
Thompson et al, 1988[49]	Community-dwelling men and women with noncardiac health problems	22	RCT	Aerobic conditioning, strength, ROM, and coordination 3 ×/wk × 1 hr for 16 wk	No significant Δ in leg strength or aerobic capacity	No significant Δ in timed obstacle course or one-legged stance	No significant Δ in self-evaluation of life function	Small sample; low power
Mulrow et al, 1994[42]	Male and female nursing home residents > 60 yr dependent in ≥ 2 ADL	194	RCT	Individualized physical therapy 3 ×/wk × 4 mo (active, passive ROM, progressive, resistive exercise, balance and mobility training)	N/T	Significant improvement (15.5%) in physical subscale of physical disability index	No significant Δ in SIP or ADL scale	N/T

Abbreviations: RCT, randomized controlled trial; N/T, not tested; ↑, increase; ↓, decrease; HR, heart rate; RR, relative risk; ROM, range of motion; ADL, activities of daily living; SIP, sickness impact profile.

[a]See also Table 14-8 for further definitions pertaining to this table.

141

TABLE 14–8 **DEFINITIONS PERTAINING TO TABLES 14–1 TO 14–7**

Isometric strength training	Muscle contracts forcefully, but neither shortens nor lengthens; no joint movement takes place
Isotonic strength training	Set resistance, such as an ankle weight, is applied throughout the specified range of motion, resulting in shortening and/or lengthening contractions of muscle
Concentric strength training	Resistance is applied as muscle shortens
Eccentric strength training	Resistance is applied as muscle lengthens
Dynamic strength training	Resistance is applied as muscle shortens or lengthens, resulting in movement of the limb; isotonic or isokinetic
Static balance	Ability to keep center of gravity over base of support during upright stance when no trunk or limb movement is taking place
Dynamic balance	Ability to keep upright during movement of center of gravity over base of support
↑, ↓	Increase, decrease
N/T	Not tested
Δ	Change
RCT	Randomized controlled trial
HI	High intensity
LI	Low intensity
IR	Incidence ratio
HR	Heart rate
RHR	Resting heart rate
OR	Odds ratio
ROM	Range of motion
SIP	Sickness impact profile
ADL	Activities of daily living
NIEMG	Needle insertion electromyogram
VO_2 max	Maximum oxygen uptake
RR	Relative risk
Met level	Level of work

impairment level outcomes such as strength and maximum oxygen uptake. The magnitude of the physiologic effect may be dampened in frailer individuals in response to lower exercise stimuli. Nevertheless, there is promising evidence that even low-intensity aerobic and strengthening programs result in physiologic gains in moderately frail individuals. In the most impaired elders, exercise may not lead to substantial gains but may help to forestall further declines in physiologic reserve.[42]

The extent to which exercise programs enhance performance and reduce disability is less clear. High-intensity interventions are most likely to improve physiologic reserve in relatively healthy elders. Low-intensity interventions may or may not produce enough effect to truly influence function. Interpretations of these programs are confounded by the limitations of our current measures of function, which may have ceiling effects or be insensitive to change.

The impact of specific balance training on function is unclear at this time. Variability in the measures used to assess balance as well as variability in the exercise programs delivered makes it difficult to evaluate the impact of balance training alone. Programs such as Tai Chi are promising as an effective means of reducing the risk of falls in community-dwelling elderly. Their impact on frailer individuals and on other aspects of performance has not been reported.

Studies of exercise interventions of all types have largely targeted healthy community-dwelling elderly because exercise programs are often delivered in group settings and require sufficient function to travel and perhaps walk some distance to an exercise site. Group exercise has many benefits in addition to the training effects; it may have a positive influence on psychological and social factors. However, frailer community-dwelling individuals may have difficulty in accessing group exercise sessions and have not been extensively studied. Low-intensity home exercise programs may be an alternative means of providing an exercise stimulus to the more frail community-dwelling elders.

CHOICE OF EXERCISE PROGRAM

The data currently available suggest that high-intensity strength (80% of a one-repetition maximum) and aerobic training (60% to 75% of maximum heart rate) programs given three times per week for at least 6 weeks can lead to substantial gains in physiologic function. Low-intensity strength (light resistance, body weight) and endurance training (30% to 45% of VO_2 max) programs carried out over longer periods of time (at least 9 weeks) can also lead to significant gains in physiologic function.

The intensity, duration, and content of exercise prescription for the geriatric patient should be based on individual need. The higher functioning older adult can tolerate high-intensity training in one or more systems (strength, endurance, balance). Such an older adult might be prescribed a program of aerobic activity such as walking, swimming, or bicycling at least three times a week and a strength training program using weights two to three times a week. More impaired individuals are likely to demonstrate deficits in more than one system and thus would probably benefit from a low-intensity program of longer duration of combined strength, aerobic, and balance training. The program may have to be supervised if the patient is unstable during movement. Otherwise, the choice of group or individual exercise can be left to personal preference. Since the risk of musculoskeletal injury is increased with poor weight-lifting technique, older adults should be encouraged to learn good form under supervision as they begin weight training. For all persons, exercise should be carried out at a level that is challenging but sustainable. For example, during aerobic exercise, the patient should have the breath to talk and keep up a conversation. During strength training, the individual should be able to complete a set of lifts in good form. All exercise programs should include warm-up and cool-down periods and flexibility exercises to avoid cardiovascular and musculoskeletal injury. Cardiac stress testing prior to a high-intensity exercise program is indicated for individuals with multiple cardiac risk factors, and thus probably for many older adults. There is no clear evidence of the need to undergo stress testing prior to a more moderate program.

Geriatric rehabilitation is based on the assumption that an improvement in modifiable impairments provides the resources to compensate for fixed deficits. Even individuals with several reversible impairments may have the potential for functional gain if the aggregate burden is reduced. Exercise training is a potential avenue for reducing the burden of impairments to pave the road toward improved function.

References

1. American College of Sports Medicine: The recommended quantity and quality of exercise for developing and maintaining cardiorespiratory and muscular fitness in healthy adults. Med Sci Sports Exerc 1990;22:265–274.
2. Bortz WM: Disuse and aging. JAMA 1982;248:1203–1208.
3. Mor V, Murphy J, Masterson-Allen S, Willey C, et al: Risk of functional decline among well elders. J Clin Epidemiol 1989;42:895–904.
4. Fiatarone M, Evans W: The etiology and reversibility of muscle dysfunction in the aged. J Gerontol 1993;48:77–83.
5. Bruce RA: Exercise, functional aerobic capacity and aging. *In* Andres R, Beirman EC, Hazzard WR (eds): Principles of Geriatric Medicine. New York, McGraw-Hill, 1985, pp. 87–103.
6. Bassey EJ, Fiatarone M, O'Neill E, et al: Leg extensor power and functional performance in very old men and women. Clin Sci 1992;832:321–327.
7. Bergstrom G, Aniansson A, Grimby G, Lundgren-Lindquist B, Svanborg A: Functional consequences of joint impairment at age 79. Scand J Rehab Med 1985;17:183–190.
8. Bassey EJ, Bendall MJ, Pearson M: Muscle strength in the triceps surae and objectively measured customary walking activity in men and women over 65 years of age. Clin Sci 1988;74:85–89.
9. Buchner DM, de Lateur BJ: The importance of skeletal muscle strength to physical function in older adults. Ann Behavioral Med 1991;13:91–98.
10. Gersten JW, Agre C, Anderson K, Cenkovich P: Relation of muscle strength and range of motion to activities of daily living. Arch Phys Med Rehabil 1970;3:137–142.
11. Jette AM, Branch LG: Impairment and disability in the aged. J Chron Dis 1985;38:59–65.
12. Studenski SA, Duncan PW, Chandler JM: Postural responses and effector factors in persons with unexplained falls: Results and methodologic issues. J Am Geriatr Soc 1991;39:229–234.
13. Gehlsen GM, Whaley DM: Falls in the elderly: Part II. Balance, strength and flexibility. Arch Phys Med Rehabil 1990;71:739–741.
14. Whipple RH, Wolfson LI, Amerman P: The relationship of knee and ankle weakness to falls in nursing home residents. J Am Geriatr Soc 1987;35:13–20.
15. Duncan PW, Chandler JM, Studenski SA, et al: How do physiological components of balance affect mobility in elderly men? Arch Phys Med Rehabil 1993;75:1343–1349.
16. Fiatarone M, Marks E, Ryan N, et al: High intensity strength training in nonagenarians. JAMA 1990;263:3029–3034.
17. Fiatarone M, O'Neill E, Doyle R, Clements K, Solares G, Nelson M, Roberts S, Kehayias J, Lipsitz L, Evans W: Exercise training and nutritional supplementation for physical frailty in very elderly people. N Engl J Med 1994;330:1769–1775.
18. Frontera W, Meredith C, O'Reilly KP, Evans WJ: Strength training and determinants of VO_2 max in older men. J Appl Physiol 1990;68:329–333.
19. Frontera W, Meredith C, O'Reilly KP, et al: Strength conditioning in older men: Skeletal muscle hypertrophy and improved function. J Appl Physiol 1988;64:1038–1044.
20. Charette SL, McEvoy L, Dyka G, et al: Muscle hypertrophy response to resistance training in older women. J Appl Physiol 1991;70:1912–1916.
21. Judge J, Whipple R, Wolfson L: Effects of resistive and balance exercises on isokinetic strength in older persons. J Am Geriatr Soc 1994;42:937–946.

22. Hunter G, Treuth M, Weinsier R, Kekes-Szabo T, Kell S, Roth D, Nicholson C: The effects of strength conditioning on older women's ability to perform daily tasks. J Am Geriatr Soc 1975;43:756–760.

23. Ades PA, Ballor DL, Shikaga TA, Utton JL, Nair KS: Weight training improves walking endurance in healthy elderly persons. Ann Intern Med 1996;124:568–572.

24. Brown A, McCartney N, Sale D: Positive adaptations to weight-lifting training in the elderly. J Appl Physiol 1990;69:1725–1733.

25. Fisher N, Pendergast DR, Gresham GE, Calkins E: Muscle rehabilitation: Its effect on muscular and functional performance of patients with knee osteoarthritis. Arch Phys Med Rehabil 1991;72:367–374.

26. Fisher NM, Pendergast DR, Calkins EC: Muscle rehabilitation in impaired elderly nursing home residents. Arch Phys Med Rehabil 1991;72:181–185.

27. Sauvage L, Myklebust B, Crow-Pan J, Novak S, Millington P, Hoffman M, Hartz A, Rudman D: A clinical trial of strengthening and aerobic exercise to improve gait and balance in elderly male nursing home residents. Am J Phys Med Rehabil 1992;71:333–342.

28. Studenski SA, Chandler JM, Duncan PW: A home based strength training program for frail elders. Gerontologist 1993;34:21.

29. Agre J, Pierce L, Raab D, McAdams M, Smith E: Light resistance and stretching exercise in elderly women: Effect upon strength. Arch Phys Med Rehabil 1988;69:273–276.

30. Posner J, Gorman K, Gitlin L, Sands L, Kleban M, Windsor L, Shaw C: Effects of exercise training in the elderly on the occurrence and time to onset of cardiovascular diagnoses. J Am Geriatr Soc 1990;38:205–210.

31. Hagberg JM, Graves JE, Limacher M, Woods DR, Leggett SH, Cononie C, Gruber JJ, Pollock ML: Cardiovascular responses of 70–79 yr old men and women to exercise training. J Appl Physiol 1989;66(6):2589–2594.

32. Badenhop DT, Cleary PA, Schaal SF, Fox EL, Bartels RL: Physiological adjustments to higher-or-lower intensity exercise in elders. Med Sci Sports Exerc 1983;15(6):496–502.

33. Seals DR, Hagberg JM, Hurley BF, Ehsani AA, Holloszy JO: Endurance training in older men and women. I. Cardiovascular responses to exercise. J Appl Physiol 1984;57(4):1024–1029.

34. Naso F, Carner E, Blankfort-Doyle W, Coughey K: Endurance training in the elderly nursing home patient. Arch Phys Med Rehabil 1990;71(3):241–243.

35. Sidney KH, Shephard RJ: Frequency and intensity of exercise training for elderly subjects. Med Sci Sports 1978;10(2):125–131.

36. Blumenthal JA, Emery CF, Madden DJ, et al: Long-term effects of exercise on psychological functioning in older men and women. J Gerontol 1991;46(6):P352–P361.

37. McMurdo ME, Burnett L: Randomized control trial of exercise in the elderly. Gerontology 1993;38(5):292–298.

38. Wolfson L, Whipple R, Derby C, et al: Balance and strength training in older adults. Intervention gains and Tai Chi maintenance. J Am Geriatr Soc 1996;44(5):498–506.

39. Wolf SL, Barnhart HX, Kutner NG, et al and the Atlantic FICSIT Group: Reducing frailty and falls in older persons: An investigation of Tai Chi and computerized balance training. J Am Geriatr Soc 1996;44(5):489–497.

40. Morey M, Cowper P, Feussner J, DiPasquale R, Crowley G, Sullivan R, Jr: Two year trends in physical performance following supervised exercise among community-dwelling older veterans. J Am Geriatr Soc 1991;39:549–554.

41. Judge J, Lindsey C, Underwood M, Winsemius D: Balance improvements in older women: Effects of exercise training. Phys Ther 1993;73:254–265.

42. Mulrow C, Gerety M, Kanten D, Cornell J, DeNino L, Chiodo L, Aguilar C, O'Neil M, Rosenberg I, Solis R: A randomized trial of physical rehabilitation for very frail nursing home residents. JAMA 1994;271:519–524.

43. Province M, Hadley E, Hornbrook M, Lipsitz L, Miller P, et al: The effects of exercise on falls in elderly patients: A preplanned meta-analysis of the FICSIT trials. JAMA 1995;273:1341–1347.

44. Rikli RG, Edwards D: Effects of a three year exercise program on motor function and cognitive processing speed in older women. Res Q Exerc Sports 1994;62:61–67.

45. MacRae P, Feltner M, Reinsch S: A 1-year exercise program for older women: Effects on falls, injuries, and physical performance. J Aging Phys Act 1994;2:127–142.

46. Hornbrook M, Stevens V, Wingfield D, et al: Preventing falls among community-dwelling older persons: Results from a randomized trial. Gerontologist 1994;34:16–23.

47. Crilly RG, Willems DA, Trenholm K, et al: Effect of exercise on postural sway in the elderly. Gerontology 1989;(35):137–143.

48. Tinetti M, Baker D, McAvay G, Claus E, Garrett P, Gottschalk M, Koch M, Trainer K, Horwitz R: A multifactorial intervention to reduce the risk of falling among elderly people living in the community. N Engl J Med 1994;33:821–827.

49. Thompson RF, Crist DM, Marsh M, Rosenthal M: Effects of physical exercise for elderly patients with physical impairments. J Am Geriatr Soc 1988;36:130–135.

50. Grimby G, Aniansson A, Hedberg M, et al: Training can improve muscle strength and endurance in 78–84 year old men. J Appl Physiol 1992;23:2517–2523.

51. Era P: Posture control in the elderly. Int J Tech Aging 1988;1:166–179.

15 Nutrition

Adil Abbasi, M.D.

Nutritional problems frequently complicate the course of medical illness. Nutritional problems in hospitalized and institutionalized patients have been linked to increased morbidity, mortality, and medical care expenditures. Prevention, early diagnosis, and treatment of such problems are therefore prudent to increase the chances of favorable clinical outcomes. This chapter reviews the principles of clinical nutrition, pertinent age-related pathophysiologic changes, nutritional assessment, nutritional requirements, and nutritional problems of older people.

PRINCIPLES OF CLINICAL NUTRITION

Food provides essential and nonessential nutrients for the metabolic needs as well as the growth and maintenance of our body systems. An essential nutrient is defined as one that cannot be produced in the body from ingested food and therefore must be supplied by the diet. Identification of essential nutrients became feasible when investigators in the field of nutrition and metabolism developed purified diets. An animal or a human being under study was fed a mixture consisting of known purified nutrients. Failure of growth or other indications of illness were identified when they accompanied a diet deficient in one or more essential nutrients. Useful indicators that reflect the withdrawal of an essential nutrient in healthy older adults are nitrogen balance and body weight.

The essential nutrients that have been identified in this fashion can be divided into macronutrients and micronutrients based on the daily amount of the essential nutrient required in humans. For macronutrients this amount is more than 100 mg/day, and for micronutrients it is less than 100 mg/day. Nutrients can also be divided into organic products (proteins, essential fatty acids, vitamins) and inorganic factors (water, minerals, trace elements).

For each essential nutrient there are three dosage thresholds: minimal daily requirement (MDR), recommended daily allowance (RDA), and maximum daily tolerance. The MDR is determined in a group of healthy subjects of specified age, sex, and physiologic status and represents the mean value, in the subjects tested, of the lowest amount of the nutrient that will prevent clinical or chemical manifestations of a deficiency illness. The RDA, the amount estimated to prevent deficiency in at least 97% of the population, takes into account the interindividual variation in MDR and is usually 30% to 100% higher than the MDR. The maximum daily tolerance reflects the fact that every dietary component, essential or nonessential, will cause illness if sufficient excess is taken for a sufficient time period. RDAs that specifically address the needs of the geriatric age group, 65 years and older, do not exist. According to current recommendations, the RDAs are the same for all subgroups 51 years and older.

AGE-RELATED PATHOPHYSIOLOGIC CHANGES AND THEIR INFLUENCE ON NUTRITIONAL STATUS OF OLDER PEOPLE

Normal aging is associated with profound developmental changes in cells, tissues, and organs as well as changes in physiologic processes. It is important to remember that older people are the most hetergeneous group of our population, and therefore wide interindividual variations in age-related physiologic changes are seen. Some of the pathophysiologic changes that influence the nutritional status of older people are discussed in the following sections.

Changes in Height, Weight, and Body Composition

For a variety of reasons, including decline in bone mineral density, older people tend to lose height with age. The mean height loss over the life span for women and men is 4.9 cm and 2.9 cm, respectively. Body weight also changes with age. It increases in both men and women until the late sixties and tends to decline thereafter. Total body fat as a proportion of total body composition increases with age and doubles between the ages of 25 and 75. This increase in total body fat is associated with a corresponding decline in lean body mass. Age-associated changes in height, weight, and body composition are important in nutritional planning and assessment of older people. Some age-associated changes in body composition and the significant interindividual variations in these changes make it difficult to interpret some of the anthropometric measurements commonly used in older people. A balanced diet and an exercise program may retard the proportional decrease in lean body mass and increase in total body fat associated with aging.

Oral Cavity

Oral health is often related to dietary habits and nutritional status. Some of the oral health problems that affect the elderly include dental caries, periodontal disease, and changes in salivary gland function resulting in xerostomia, mucositis, and tooth loss. According to some reports, up to 40% of the older population is edentulous. Some recent surveys have shown that the prevalence of edentulous adults is decreasing. This decline in prevalance of edentulous adults is most likely due to the better dental care available to the population in general. Lack of teeth leads to difficulty in chewing food, which makes it difficult to eat a regular diet and thereby increases the likelihood of undernutrition. Prosthetic replacement of teeth reduces taste sensation and does not fully restore the ability to masticate. Older people do not chew as efficiently as younger people and tend to swallow larger pieces of food. Owing to subtle neuromotor changes in the swallowing mechanism, the oral phase of swallowing takes 50% to 100% longer. Some recently published studies have shown an association between loss of teeth, oral problems, and undernutrition in older people. Some other oral health problems common in the elderly that may increase the risk of undernutrition include mouth dryness (xerostomia), dental caries, temporomandibular joint dysfunction, periodontal disease, and ill-fitting dentures.

Gastrointestinal System

The gastric mucosa changes with age, leading to an increase in nonparietal cells. This may result in a decline in gastric acid output, which may influence the absorption of certain essential nutrients, including vitamin B_{12}, folic acid, and iron. The intestine's ability to absorb food particles generally does not change significantly, but declines in the metabolism and absorption of carbohydrates (especially lactose), calcium, and iron may occur.

Taste and Smell Sensation

Several changes take place with age in the senses of taste and smell. Taste sensitivity may decline with age, but the evidence is inconclusive and varies significantly among individuals. Age-associated declines in the number of lingual papillae and salivary flow may be associated with diminished taste sensation. The sense of smell declines rapidly after the fifth decade, and by the eighth decade smell detection is almost 50% poorer than it was at its peak, but there is wide individual variation. Age-associated changes in taste and smell sensation make the discrimination and enjoyment of food difficult and therefore may contribute to undernutrition.

NUTRITIONAL REQUIREMENTS OF OLDER PEOPLE

For optimum management of nutritional problems, a knowledge of the nutritional requirements of older people and the impact of disease on these requirements is essential. Caloric balance indicates energy intake that maintains steady body weight. Caloric insufficiency or caloric undernutrition is reflected by weight loss, and excess caloric intake may cause weight gain. Conditions that can modify nutritional requirements include infection, surgery, trauma, medications, alcohol abuse, and malabsorption.

Caloric Requirements

Caloric requirements decline by approximately 22% from age 30 to age 80. One third of this decline is believed to be due to a decrease in metabolic rate secondary to a decline in lean body mass with age. The remaining two thirds of this decline are due to a decline in energy expenditure secondary to a decrease in physical activity. Furthermore, some investigators have reported that caloric intake also declines in older people. According to one report, 17% of subjects 60 years and older consumed less than 1000 calories/day. The decline in caloric requirements and caloric intake in older people puts them at high risk for undernutrition of various essential nutrients.

A useful approximation of the actual caloric needs of patients in the clinical setting can be obtained from the following chart:

- No stress, minimal activity   25 kcal/kg/day
- Mild stress (e.g., upper respiratory tract infection, grade I to II pressure ulcer)
                                                    30 kcal/kg/day
- Moderate stress (e.g., grade III pressure

ulcer, urinary tract infection, pneumonia)
35 kcal/kg/day
- Severe stress (e.g., sepsis, grade IV pressure ulcer)
40 kcal/kg/day

Protein Requirements

The current recommendations for protein intake in older people is 0.8 g/kg body weight. A balanced diet of a healthy older adult should contain 12% to 14% of the total caloric intake from various protein sources. During periods of stress, such as during infection or trauma, the protein intake should be increased to 1.0 to 1.5 g/kg body weight.

Vitamin and Mineral Requirements

Recommended dietary allowances (RDAs) for various vitamins and minerals are shown in Table 15–1. In a recent review by Russell and Suter, the authors concluded that, based on the current body of knowledge, the 1989 RDAs are too low for the elderly population for riboflavin, vitamin B_6, vitamin D, and vitamin B_{12}.[1] The authors also concluded that present RDAs for older people appear to be appropriate for thiamine, vitamin C, and folic acid but are probably too high for vitamin A. In general, healthy older people eating a balanced diet do not need a multivitamin and mineral supplement. However, such supplements may be valuable in a subgroup of older people who are at higher risk for developing deficiencies of calories, proteins, and micronutrients. Older people who are at high risk for developing nutritional deficiencies include eating-dependent nursing home residents and house-bound elderly. Some studies have shown that underweight, hypoalbuminemia, anemia, and an incidence of pressure sores are higher in eating-dependent nursing home residents.

A number of studies have shown that up to three fourths of older people have intakes of vitamin D that are less than two thirds of the RDA. Older people are at higher risk for vitamin D deficiency because of insufficient dietary vitamin D intake, impaired renal synthesis of 1,25-dihydroxyvitamin D, and inadequate sunlight exposure. High-risk groups of older people for low vitamin D level include nursing home residents living in the northern climates, residents taking chronic anticonvulsant therapy, and house-bound patients. Similarly, a large proportion of older Americans fail to meet the currently recommended guidelines for optimal calcium intake. A National Institutes of Health (NIH) consensus statement for calcium and vitamin D intake suggests that the current RDAs for calcium and

TABLE 15–1   RECOMMENDED DIETARY ALLOWANCES FOR THE ELDERLY[a]

Nutrient	Recommended Daily Allowance (RDA)	
	Women	*Men*
Protein (g/kg)	0.8	0.8
Vitamins		
A (μg)	800	1000
D (μg)	5.0	5.0
E (mg)	8.0	10
K (μg)	65	80
C (mg)	60	60
Thiamin (mg)	1.0	1.2
Riboflavin (mg)	1.2	1.4
Niacin (mg)	13	15
B_6 (mg)	1.6	2.0
Folate (μg)	180	200
B_{12} (μg)	2.0	2.0
Biotin (μg)[b]	30–100	30–100
Pantothenic acid (mg)[b]	4–7	4–7
Minerals		
Calcium (mg)	800	800
Phosphorus (mg)	800	800
Magnesium (mg)	280	350
Iron (mg)	10	10
Zinc (mg)	12	15
Iodine (μg)	150	150
Selenium (μg)	55	70
Trace elements		
Copper (mg)[b]	1.5–3.0	1.5–3.0
Manganese (mg)[b]	2.0–5.0	2.0–5.0
Fluoride (mg)[b]	1.5–4.0	1.5–4.0
Chromium (μg)[b]	50–200	50–200
Molybdenum (μg)[b]	75–250	75–250

[a]Adapted from Food and Nutrition Board, National Academy of Sciences, National Research Council: Recommended Dietary Allowances. Washington, DC, National Academy of Sciences, revised 1989.
[b]Estimated safe daily intakes.

vitamin D are suboptimal and therefore should be revised.[2] Table 15–2 summarizes the optimum daily calcium requirements as recommended by the NIH consensus statement. Since vitamin D metabolites enhance calcium absorption and vitamin D deficiency has been shown to be associated with an increased risk of fractures, the NIH consensus statement recommends a higher daily intake of vitamin D than the current RDA. It recommends a vitamin D intake of 200 to 400 IU or 5 to 10 mg cholecalciferol/day.

Fluid or Water Intake

Older people are at increased risk for dehydration due to age-associated declines in thirst sen-

TABLE 15–2 **OPTIMUM DAILY CALCIUM REQUIREMENTS**

	Age (yr)	Milligrams
Men	25–65	1000
	>65	1500
Women	>50	
	On estrogen	1000
	Not on estrogen	1500
	>65	1500

National Institutes of Health: NIH Consensus Statement: Optimum Calcium Intake. Washington, DC, National Institutes of Health, 1994, pp. 1–31.

sation, inadequate fluid intake, and excessive fluid loss. Subgroups of older people at highest risk for dehydration include nursing home residents, patients with dementia, patients with chronic debilitating illness, and patients taking multiple medications. Recommended fluid intake (water) is 30 mL/kg body weight/day.

NUTRITIONAL ASSESSMENT

Nutritional assessment involves gathering data such as dietary history, clinical observations during physical examination, anthropometric and biochemical measurements, and possible drug-nutrient interactions. The assessment starts with a dietary history followed by physical examination and biochemical measurements.

Dietary History and Physical Examination

The dietary history begins with a history of recent unintentional weight gain or weight loss, recent surgery, or trauma; a history of any chronic illness such as diabetes, hypertension,

renal failure, hepatic failure, heart failure, malignancy, or peptic ulcer disease; a history of any recent illness such as recurrent nausea, vomiting or diarrhea, drug or alcohol abuse; use of multiple medications; and a detailed social history. The patient's recent dietary intake is estimated as accurately as possible from either a diet history or, if possible, an actual calorie count based on meals eaten, preferably spanning a period of the previous 5 to 7 days and including a weekend.

A careful physical examination including a search for signs of nutritional deficiencies is important in performing a nutritional assessment. Evidence of body fat and muscle wasting is characteristic of marasmic malnutrition. Loss of skin turgor, loss of hair color and softness, pitting edema, and enlargement of the liver and parotid glands are more characteristic of a kwashiorkor type of malnutrition. Some of the characteristics of kwashiorkor and marasmic malnutrition as listed in the American Medical Association's International Classification of Diseases (ICD-9-CM) are outlined in Table 15–3. Signs and symptoms of various nutrient deficiencies are outlined in Table 15–4. Findings characteristic of trace element deficiencies should also be recognized. Examples include the association of zinc deficiency with diarrhea, dermatitis, hair loss, poor wound healing, and alteration in the senses of taste and smell; chromium deficiency with weight loss, glucose intolerance, and diabetic neuropathy; copper deficiency with anemia and leukopenia; and iron and iodine deficiency with anemia and goiters, respectively.

Anthropometric Measurements

Anthropometric measurements include measurements of height, weight, body mass index, and skin and muscle folds.

TABLE 15–3 **ICD-9-CM CODES FOR CLASSIFICATION OF MALNUTRITION**

ICD-9-CM Code	Diagnostic Category	Selected Diagnostic Criteria
260	Kwashiorkor	1. Body weight >90% of ideal 2. Transferrin <200 mg/dL, or albumin <3.5 g/dL 3. Decreased oral intake for more than 2 weeks 4. Anorexia, nausea, vomiting for more than 2 weeks
261	Marasmus	1. Body weight <90% of ideal or <90% of usual 2. Transferrin >200 mg/dL or albumin >3.5 g/dL 3. Weight loss >10% in 6 months 4. Decreased oral intake for more than 2 weeks 5. Anorexia, nausea, vomiting, diarrhea for more than 2 weeks

From International Classification of Diseases, Clinical Modifications, 9th revision: Dover, DE, American Medical Association, 1996.

TABLE 15–4 **SYMPTOMS AND SIGNS OF NUTRIENT DEFICIENCY IN ELDERLY PERSONS**

Nutrient	Clinical Presentation
Vitamins	
A	Dryness of skin, xerophthalmia, Bitot's spots, increase in dark adaptation time
D	Osteomalacia
E	Anemia
K	Bleeding diathesis
C	Petechiae, ecchymoses, perifollicular hemorrhage, bleeding gums (scurvy)
Thiamine (B_1)	Muscle weakness and pain, hyporeflexia, hypoesthesia, cardiomegaly, encephalopathy (beriberi)
Riboflavin (B_2)	Angular stomatitis, cheilosis, magenta tongue
Niacin	Raw tongue, tongue fissuring, dermatitis, diarrhea, dementia (pellagra)
Pyridoxine (B_6)	Glossitis, peripheral neuropathy, anemia
Folacin	Pallor, glossitis, anemia, stomatitis
B_{12}	Paresthesias, ataxia, memory loss
Minerals	
Calcium	Osteoporosis, osteomalacia
Phosphorus	Weakness, osteomalacia
Magnesium	Weakness, tremor, tetany seizures
Iron	Weakness, angular stomatitis, koilonychia, anemia
Zinc	Rash and scaling of skin, hypogonadism, delayed wound healing, hypogeusia
Iodine	Goiter
Copper	Anemia
Chromium	Glucose intolerance
Selenium	Cardiomyopathy, cancer

BODY WEIGHT

Weight loss is considered the strongest predictor of morbidity and mortality in hospitalized and institutionalized patients. Expressing body weight as a percentage of the ideal weight is one method of assessing optimum body weight. Metropolitan Insurance Company height and weight tables are the most commonly used reference source for estimating ideal body weight. The most current Metropolitan table was derived from the 1983 Build Study on Americans and was based on subjects aged 25 to 59 years old who carried life insurance. However, these tables do not include subjects over 65 years of age. Master and colleagues reported data on the weights and heights of white Americans aged 65 to 94 years.[3] According to this report, body weight continues to increase into the late sixties and then gradually declines in the later decades of life. This is the best available information on height and weight for people 65 years and older (Tables 15–5 and 15–6).

Use of the patient's own best weight for a reference standard is preferable for nutritional assessment because it allows a more accurate determination of recent or chronic weight loss than a weight as a percentage of the ideal. This weight is also called the percentage of usual body weight (UBW). The best source of this information is the patient's previous medical record. The percentage of UBW can be determined by the following formula:

$$\text{Percent UBW} = \frac{\text{actual weight}}{\text{UBW}} \times 100$$

Hamwi's method is quick and is probably the most commonly used method of estimating ideal body weight, but it tends to underestimate ideal body weight, especially for people older than 60 years of age. Hamwi's formula for estimating ideal body weight is as follows:

Men: ideal body weight = 106 lb + 6 lb for every inch over 5 feet

Women: ideal body weight = 100 lb + 5 lb for every inch over 5 feet.

BODY MASS INDEX

Body mass index (BMI) is a ratio of body weight (kg) to the square of body height (m²). BMIs of 23 or less and 30 or more have been shown to be associated with increased mortality in the 60-year and older age group. In other words, the association of BMI and mortality is a U-shaped curve in people 60 years and older. Furthermore, the BMI associated with minimal mortality increases with advancing age. Therefore, a BMI that may be considered excessive in a 20-year-old person may be normal for a person who is

TABLE 15–5 **AVERAGE WEIGHT IN POUNDS FOR MEN AGED 65 TO 94 YEARS**

Height (inches)	Age (yr)					
	65–69	**70–74**	**75–79**	**80–84**	**85–89**	**90–94**
61	142	139	137	—	—	—
62	144	141	139	135	—	—
63	146	143	141	136	133	—
64	149	146	143	138	135	—
65	151	149	145	141	139	130
66	154	152	148	144	142	133
67	156	155	151	147	145	136
68	159	158	154	150	148	140
69	163	162	158	154	152	144
70	167	165	162	159	156	149
71	172	169	166	164	160	154
72	177	173	171	170	165	—
73	182	178	175	—	—	—

Adapted from Master AM, et al.: Tables of average weight and height of Americans aged 65 to 94 years. JAMA 1960;172(7): 658–662.

60 years old. The formula for calculating BMI is as follows:

$$BMI = \frac{\text{body weight (kg)}}{\text{height}^2 \ (\text{m}^2)}$$

SKIN FOLD AND MUSCLE MASS MEASUREMENTS

The mid-arm circumference can be used to estimate the body's skeletal muscle mass, whereas the triceps skin fold and subscapular skin fold thickness can be used to estimate the subcutaneous fat reserves. These measurements are less reliable in people 60 years and older due to age-related declines in lean body mass and increases in body fat. Chumlea and colleagues reported anthropometric measurements in 119 white men and 150 white women aged 60 to 104 years living in Ohio.[4] These are the best available standards for skin fold and muscle mass measurements in older people to date.

ALTERNATE METHODS FOR MEASURING HEIGHT AND WEIGHT IN PATIENTS WITH DISABILITIES AND DEFORMITIES

In patients who have lost a body part, estimation of desirable body weight is more difficult. Total

TABLE 15–6 **AVERAGE WEIGHT IN POUNDS FOR WOMEN AGED 65 TO 94 YEARS**

Height (inches)	Age (yr)					
	65–69	**70–74**	**75–79**	**80–84**	**85–89**	**90–94**
58	133	125	123	—	—	—
59	134	127	124	116	110	—
60	135	129	126	118	113	—
61	137	131	128	121	116	—
62	139	134	131	124	120	118
63	141	137	134	128	124	119
64	144	140	137	132	128	120
65	147	144	140	136	133	124
66	151	147	143	140	138	129
67	155	151	146	144	142	—
68	159	155	—	—	—	—
69	164	160	—	—	—	—

Adapted from Master AM, et al.: Tables of average weight and height of Americans aged 65 to 94 years. JAMA 1960;172(7): 658–662.

arm length measurement, arm span measurement, and knee height measurements are alternative methods of measuring height in nonambulatory patients and patients with disabilities and deformities. The following list of percentages of total body weight contributed by individual body parts, described by Grant and Dehoog,[5] can be used to estimate desirable weight in these patients.

Lower leg with foot	7.1%
Entire leg	18.6%
Trunk without limbs	42.7%

Biochemical Indicators of Nutritional Status

Several biochemical indicators can be used to assess nutritional status. Kwashiorkor-type malnutrition is associated with depletion of the visceral protein mass. Affected patients may not have any evidence of weight loss and may even be overweight. It is therefore sometimes difficult clinically to diagnose this type of malnutrition on the basis of the physical findings alone. Because visceral protein mass cannot be measured directly, the serum concentration of proteins synthesized by the liver is used as an indirect method of determining visceral protein mass. Serum transport proteins that have been found useful for this purpose include albumin, transferrin, thyroxine-binding prealbumin, and insulin-like growth factor-1 (IGF-1).

ALBUMIN

Several investigators have shown that hypoalbuminemia (serum albumin levels of less than 3.5 g/dL) is associated with increased morbidity and mortality in hospitalized and institutionalized patients. It is easily measured and quite accurately reflects the visceral protein status in the absence of acute changes in hydration or stress. The total albumin pool varies from 3 to 4 g/kg for women and 4 to 5 g/kg for men. The half-life of albumin has been estimated to be 18 to 21 days. Protein undernutrition has been shown to be associated with a decrease in albumin synthesis by the liver. Because of its large body pool and long half-life, the serum concentration of albumin changes slowly with malnutrition, thereby limiting its clinical usefulness in hospitalized or institutionalized patients with acute malnutrition. Furthermore, several investigators have reported that because albumin is a negative acute-phase reactant, its concentration in the serum may decline during an acute illness. It is therefore not considered a reliable marker of nutritional status. However, this does not diminish the association of hypoalbuminemia with increased morbidity and mortality in hospital and institutional settings.

THYROXINE-BINDING PREALBUMIN

Prealbumin plays a major role in the transport of thyroxine and serves as a carrier molecule for retinol-binding protein. It has a short half-life of 2 to 3 days, and its serum concentration changes rapidly with changes in protein nutrition status. It has also been shown that the prealbumin concentration increases with improvements in nutritional status. Therefore, it can be used not only as a marker of malnutrition but also as a method of monitoring response to therapy in patients with malnutrition. Prealbumin levels of between 10 and 15 mg/dL, 5 and 10 mg/dL, and less than 5 mg/dL are labeled mild, moderate, and severe visceral protein depletion, respectively.

TRANSFERRIN

Transferrin is a beta globulin that transports iron in the plasma. Its serum concentration appears to be less significantly altered by the state of hydration than that of albumin owing to its smaller body pool mass. Several conditions other than malnutrition can alter its serum concentration. The serum concentration of transferrin falls markedly with liver disease and in conditions that lead to protein loss. Its serum half-life ranges from 8 to 10 days. Because of the shorter half-life and the smaller body pool, the serum concentration of transferrin is considered a better marker of protein malnutrition than the serum albumin level. Serum concentrations of transferrin of 150 to 200 mg/100 mL, 100 to 149 mg/100 mL, and less than 100 mg/100 mL are considered reflective of mild, moderate, and severe visceral protein depletion, respectively.

INSULIN-LIKE GROWTH FACTOR-1

Insulin-like growth factor-1 (IGF-1) is a peptide synthesized primarily in the liver (although smaller concentrations are secreted by a number of other tissues in the body) that mediates the growth-promoting effects of growth hormone. It has been shown that the serum concentrations of IGF-1 decline with malnutrition, falling as rapidly as less than 5 days after starvation, and they recover just as quickly with refeeding. Studies have shown that a rapid decline in IGF-1 level is associated with both protein and calorie undernutrition. It has also been shown that the

IGF-1 level declines with aging. Therefore, its usefulness as a marker of nutritional status in older people remains to be defined.

Subjective Global Assessment

The traditional methods of nutritional assessment rely heavily on objective anthropometric and laboratory test results. Some investigators have proposed basing the nutritional assessment on the findings of the history and physical examination, a method called subjective global assessment (SGA). SGA can be used to identify hospitalized patients at risk for malnutrition. The five guidelines obtained from the history and physical examination for SGA include (1) weight loss, (2) dietary intake, (3) gastrointestinal symptoms that may influence nutritional status, (4) functional capacity, and (5) physical signs. SGA is a subjective screening tool and has various categories that can be interpreted as follows:

- *Class A* indicates less than a 5% weight loss or more than a 5% weight loss but recent evidence of weight gain and improved appetite (well-nourished).
- *Class B* indicates a 5% to 10% weight loss without recent weight gain, poor dietary intake, and mild (1+) loss of subcutaneous fat (moderately malnourished).
- *Class C* indicates weight loss of more than 10% with severe loss of subcutaneous fat and muscle wasting, often with edema (severely malnourished).

The effectiveness and usefulness of SGA in a clinical setting have yet to be established.

Nutrition Screening Initiative

The nutrition screening initiative was developed by the American Academy of Family Physicians, the American Dietetic Association, and the National Council on the Aging Inc. to screen older Americans who are at increased nutritional risk.[6] Older people may have an increased nutritional risk due to a variety of factors, including a decline in caloric intake after age 60 and increased prevalence of functional disability, undesirable psychological or social environment, one or more medical problems, and use of multiple medications. Since a compromised nutritional status has been shown to be associated with increased morbidity and mortality, early recognition and treatment of increased nutritional risk in older people is recommended.

The nutrition screening initiative is a tiered approach to screening. The first level of screening is a checklist completed by the older people or caregiver; this is followed by a two-level approach accomplished in a professional setting. The nutrition screening initiative is designed to facilitate early recognition and treatment of nutritional deficiencies in older Americans.

Drug-Nutrient Interactions

Drug-induced nutritional deficiencies result from drug-induced malabsorption, renal loss of a nutrient, or inhibition of biosynthesis of a nutrient. These deficiencies are more common in patients with poor oral intake, compromised nutritional status, or prolonged or chronic illness. Older adults are at increased risk for drug-induced deficiencies because they consume proportionately larger numbers of prescription medications and because malnutrition is common, particularly in institutionalized older people, in whom, coincidentally, polypharmacy is also more common.

Several drugs (e.g., digoxin) can cause anorexia, thereby leading to lower caloric intake. A variety of drugs (e.g., antihistamines, antipsychotics, tricyclic antidepressants) can cause dryness of mouth because of their anticholinergic side effects and therefore can impair oral intake. Diuretics can cause deficiencies of various electrolytes, including sodium, potassium, and magnesium, as well as dehydration. Concurrent use of a laxative and a diuretic can cause the electrolyte deficiency and dehydration to become worse. Several drugs can adversely influence calcium and vitamin D metabolism, including phenytoin, phenobarbital, and isoniazid. In addition, drugs such as anticonvulsants, corticosteroids, heparin, thyroxine, and loop diuretics can negatively influence bone mineral density. A careful review of all medications taken should be part of the nutritional assessment of an older person.

NUTRITIONAL PROBLEMS
Protein-Calorie Undernutrition

Surveys of community-dwelling healthy elderly people have shown that up to one third of subjects have a caloric intake below the RDA and that mineral and vitamin intake is below the RDA in up to 50% of subjects. In these surveys, the blood levels of various vitamins and minerals were subnormal in up to 30% of subjects. Despite low intake and subnormal nutritional indicators, body weight, adipose mass, and muscle mass were rarely depleted, and protein intake was generally adequate. The interpretation of these findings is that the diminishing energy expenditures of the elderly lead to a lower energy requirement and therefore to a reduced food intake. But unless the nutrient density of the diet is simultaneously increased, subclinical mineral and vitamin deficiencies are likely to occur.

Several surveys have shown that the nutritional status of institutionalized elderly is less favorable than that of those living independently in the community.[7] In institutionalized elderly low caloric and protein intake is common, and up to 50% of residents are underweight or hypoalbuminemic or show evidence of significant depletion of muscle mass and adipose mass. Blood levels of both water-soluble and fat-soluble vitamins are frequently low.

Protein-calorie undernutrition is associated with increased morbidity, mortality, and medical expenditures in both hospitalized and institutionalized elderly. Several reports have shown that weight loss, body weight below 90% of ideal, cholesterol level of less than 160 mg/dL, and albumin concentration of less than 4 g/dL are associated with increased morbidity and mortality. Therefore, knowledge of the potentially reversible causes of protein-calorie undernutrition as well as its early recognition and optimum treatment are important.

Patients with a significant weight loss—i.e., more than 5% in 1 month, more than 7.5% in 3 months, or more than 10% in 6 months—or with a body weight of less than 90% of ideal or a serum albumin level of less than 3.5 g/dL are at increased risk for developing protein-calorie undernutrition. Several reports have shown that subjects who require feeding assistance are at increased risk for undernutrition of various vitamins and minerals as well as calories and proteins. Poverty, isolation, and depression are some of the other common risk factors for protein-calorie undernutrition in old people. Table 15–7 can be used to identify subjects at increased risk for undernutrition.

In the institutionalized setting, where protein-

calorie undernutrition is most common, an interdisciplinary team approach is the ideal way of managing this problem. The physician should help in recognizing the problem early and treating it optimally. The dietitian and nurses play vital roles in estimating caloric intake, satisfying caloric needs, and monitoring the response to therapy by taking frequent body weights. Periodic blood tests for some of the readily available biochemical markers can help in monitoring progress as well.

The role of various pharmacologic agents in the management of protein-calorie undernutrition in older people has not yet been proved. No pharmacologic agents have been approved by the Food and Drug Administration (FDA) for use in the treatment of protein-calorie undernutrition in older people. Some studies have shown that use of anabolic hormones such as growth hormone has a beneficial effect, but larger trials are needed to prove the efficacy of hormonal intervention in the management of protein-calorie undernutrition. Megestrol acetate, which has been shown to be helpful in some patients with acquired immunodeficiency syndrome (AIDS) and malignancy, has not been shown to be effective in older people with protein-calorie undernutrition.

Vitamin B₁₂ and Folic Acid Deficiency

It is well known that the prevalence of low serum vitamin B_{12} is higher in older people.[8] Since the majority of older people with low serum B_{12} levels do not develop megaloblastic anemia, the significance of low serum vitamin B_{12} levels is questionable. Many studies have shown that a low serum B_{12} level is not very specific in diagnosing a tissue deficiency of vitamin B_{12}. It has been reported that up to 50% of subjects with low serum B_{12} levels do not have tissue deficiency of vitamin B_{12}. A number of studies have shown that elevation of serum and urinary methylmalonic acid and total serum homocysteine levels are more specific and sensitive markers of tissue vitamin B_{12} deficiency. Using these markers and serum vitamin B_{12} level, it has been shown that the prevalence of vitamin B_{12} deficiency in older people varies from 5% to 15%.

The exact cause and mechanism of vitamin B_{12} deficiency in older people cannot be clearly explained at this time. Pernicious anemia, a disease of late middle age, is uncommon in older people. The majority of older people with vitamin B_{12} deficiency do not show positive results on the Schilling test or have anti-intrinsic factor antibodies. It is believed that vitamin B_{12} defi-

---

TABLE 15–7 **RISK FACTORS FOR NUTRITIONAL PROBLEMS IN THE ELDERLY**

Alcoholism
Debilitating illness
Dementia
Depression
Inadequate eating assistance
Inappropriate use of restricted diet
Infectious illness
Isolation
Multiple medical problems
Polypharmacy
Poor oral and dental status
Poverty

ciency in older people is, at least in part, due to a defect in extraction and absorption of protein-bound vitamin B_{12} in food. Other risk factors for vitamin B_{12} deficiency in older people include a high prevalence of atrophic gastritis (40%) and frequent use of antacids and H_2 blockers. It is well known that vitamin B_{12} deficiency can cause memory impairment and dementia and gait and balance disorders, all of which occur in the absence of specific hematologic or neurologic signs. It is therefore recommended that a serum vitamin B_{12} level be determined in older people (65 years and older), and if it is found to be less than 350 pg/mL, a serum or urinary methylmalonic acid with or without a serum homocysteine level should be obtained. If the methylmalonic acid and homocysteine levels are elevated, vitamin B_{12} deficiency is confirmed.

In patients with severe vitamin B_{12} deficiency and associated clinical symptoms a daily dose of 1000 μg of vitamin B_{12} should be given intramuscularly for 7 days. This is followed by weekly injections for 6 weeks and monthly injections thereafter. In patients with milder forms of this deficiency, 100 to 1000 μg of vitamin B_{12} per month can be administered intramuscularly. The role of high-dose oral vitamin B_{12} supplements (1000 μg or 1 mg/day) in patients with mild vitamin B_{12} deficiency needs more clinical investigation.

Low serum folic acid levels[8] have been found in 10% to 20% of older people. This problem is believed to be due to poor oral intake as well as poor absorption due to gastric atrophy. Folic acid is an essential cofactor in amino acid and nucleic acid metabolism. Folic acid depletion therefore must be recognized and treated. The vitamin B_{12} level should be determined before folic acid supplements are initiated because repletion doses of folic acid in the presence of vitamin B_{12} deficiency can precipitate neurologic damage due to vitamin B_{12} deficiency.

Obesity

Obesity can be defined as a body weight greater than 130% of ideal, or a body mass index greater than 28 kg/m². According to some surveys, up to 26% of white men and 37% of white women over the age of 65 are overweight. With advancing age, the waist-to-hip ratio increases (upper body obesity as opposed to lower body obesity). This increase has been associated with an increased risk for diabetes, hypertension, and coronary artery disease. Furthermore, in older people obesity is associated with a decline in functional status and an increased incidence of pressure sores and sleep apnea syndrome.

TABLE 15–8 **HYPERVITAMINOSIS**

Vitamin A	Gastrointestinal symptoms, liver dysfunction, headache, desquamation, xerosis
Vitamin C	False-positive fecal occult test, renal stones, decreased Vitamin B_{12} absorption, rebound scurvy
Vitamin D	Hypercalcemia, hyperphosphatemia, confusion, lethargy, ectopic calcification
Vitamin E	Potentiates the effect of coumadin by inhibiting vitamin K
Vitamin B_6	Ataxia, loss of vibration and position sense, perioral numbness

A combination of diet, exercise, and behavior modification should be the mainstay of therapy for obesity. Weight loss can be achieved through decreased caloric intake and increased energy expenditure, or both. A balanced, low-calorie diet should be designed with the goal of achieving 1 to 2 pounds of weight loss per week. An exercise program designed to increase energy expenditure will not only help the patient lose weight, it will help to maintain that weight once a desirable weight has been achieved.

Hypervitaminosis

It has been shown that up to 10% of healthy older people consume 10 times the RDA of certain vitamins. Excess consumption of vitamins A, C, D, E, K, B_6, and niacin can result in toxicity syndromes (Table 15–8). Several reports have shown that vitamin E is a protective antioxidant and membrane stabilizer. An association between higher vitamin E concentration or vitamin E intake and lower prevalences of cataracts, cancer, and reduced high-density lipoproteins has been reported. However, the data are considered inconclusive, and the current recommendations for vitamin E intake therefore remain unchanged.

TUBE FEEDING FOR ENTERAL NUTRITION

Advances in medical technology during the past two decades have made tube feeding a more acceptable and readily available procedure for enteral nutrition.[9] Tube feeding for enteral nutrition may be used for a short time or as a permanent method of nutritional support. Tube feeding is indicated in patients with a functional gastrointestinal tract who

• Cannot swallow because of a disease

process, for example, head and neck malignancy, untreated esophageal cancer, or major trauma.

- Have had protein-calorie undernutrition and continued suboptimal nutritional intake for more than 1 to 2 weeks despite all efforts to improve oral intake.

Recently, it has been shown that without intraluminal nutrients, intestinal integrity may deteriorate, allowing translocation of bacteria in the gastrointestinal tract to invade local intestinal defense barriers, which may result in systemic invasion of the body by the gastrointestinal bacteria. Therefore, it is recommended that prolonged starvation (more than 7 days for most healthy and well-nourished people) should be avoided and the gastrointestinal tract should be used as soon as is safely possible, not only for growth and maintenance of the body but also to protect the local defense barriers of the gastrointestinal tract.

Methods of Tube Feeding

NASOENTERIC TUBES

Nasogastric, nasoduodenal, and nasojejunal tubes are referred to as nasoenteric tubes. Nasoenteric tubes are used when a patient needs enteral nutritional support for less than 30 days. Nasoduodenal and nasojejunal tubes may be indicated in patients who are at high risk for aspiration. Tubes placed past the ligament of Treitz have been shown to be associated with a decreased risk of aspiration. Nasogastric tubes can be placed at the bedside with the head of the bed elevated to 45 degrees or more. Nasoduodenal and nasojejunal tubes generally are smaller in size than nasogastric tubes, and therefore clogging of the tubes with nutrients and medications is more common. Metoclopramide, cisapride, or erythromycin given prior to placement of a nasoduodenal or nasojejunal tube may be beneficial in helping to position these tubes beyond the ligament of Treitz. In general, it is easier to insert an unweighted tube. Usually, depending on the expertise of the clinician, nasoduodenal and nasojejunal tubes can be placed at the bedside. In selected patients, nasoduodenal and nasojejunal tubes can be placed under endoscopic or fluoroscopic guidance.

GASTROSTOMY TUBES

Gastrostomy tube placement is indicated in patients who require tube feeding for more than 30 days. In general, gastrostomy tubes are inserted through a percutaneous gastrostomy under endoscopic or fluoroscopic guidance. Gastrostomy tubes have been shown to be safe, effective, and more acceptable for long-term nutritional support than nasogastric tubes.

JEJUNOSTOMY TUBES

Jejunostomy tubes are indicated in patients who need tube feeding for more than 30 days and are at high risk of gastric retention or aspiration due to gastroparesis, reflux esophagitis, or gastrectomy; occasionally they are indicated in patients with gastric or pancreatic cancer. Jejunostomy tubes have been shown to be associated with a decreased risk of aspiration. Data about the efficacy of feeding through a jejunostomy tube as a long-term feeding option are lacking. It has been assumed, without adequate support in the literature, that elemental diets should be fed through a jejunostomy tube.

Techniques of Tube Feeding

Tube feeding may be delivered by bolus, gravity, or pump-controlled techniques. Bolus feeding is the administration of formula using a 50-mL syringe. Depending on the patient's caloric needs, 400 to 500 mL may be delivered over a period of 10 to 15 minutes every 4 to 6 hours. It is a convenient method that can easily be taught to family members or the patient himself for use at home. Bolus feedings, however, are more likely to generate higher residuals. The tube must be flushed with at least 30 to 50 mL of plain water at the end of each feeding.

Gravity feedings can be delivered through intermittent or continuous drip. The rate of delivery is not precise and may result in high residuals. Intermittent gravity feedings are generally the preferred modality. New closed enteral feeding systems allow the delivery of a specified measured amount of formula. An alternative method is to pour the cans of tube feeding formula into the delivery system. At the end of intermittent feeding, the system should be flushed with plain water.

Tube feeding using a pump-controlled technique is the preferred route for intrajejunal feedings. Feedings can be delivered by either intermittent or continuous technique. Since the delivery is accurately controlled, high residual volumes and the risk of aspiration are less likely than with bolus and gravity feeding techniques.

Continuous intragastric feedings are associated with fewer episodes of diarrhea and aspiration than intermittent feedings. Continuous feedings in infants with diarrhea are associated with fewer fecal losses, more positive nitrogen balance, and weight gain compared with intermittent feedings. Also, continuous feedings have been associated with less energy expenditure, primarily due to diet-induced thermogenesis and more effective prophylaxis against stress ulcers.

Some earlier reports recommended withholding tube feeding for at least 2 hours if the residual volume is high. A recently published report does not agree with the earlier recommendations. The authors of this recent study conclude that tube feeding should not be delayed following a single high residual volume (more than 200 mL obtained from a nasogastric tube and more than 100 mL from a gastrostomy tube) because often the next measured residual value is within an acceptable range.[10] The higher the infusion rate, the higher the expected residual volume. Positioning of the patient (in the supine versus the right lateral decubitus position) seems to have no impact on residual volume. Tubes smaller than 10 French have been shown to be unreliable for determining residual volume.

Most institutions have a specific enteral feeding protocol following placement of a new tube.

Complications of Tube Feeding

METABOLIC COMPLICATIONS

Fluid and electrolyte problems are common in patients receiving tube feedings. Hyponatremia, hyperglycemia, hypokalemia, hypophosphatemia, and hypomagnesemia are among the most common metabolic complications. Most institutions have standard guidelines for monitoring body weight, fluid intake and output, and serum glucose and electrolytes for patients on tube feedings.

NONMETABOLIC COMPLICATIONS

Diarrhea

Diarrhea is the most commonly reported complication of tube feeding. The incidence varies from study to study, depending on the definition of diarrhea, from 2.3% to as high as 68%. Some reports have suggested that the severity of illness is the most important factor predicting diarrhea. Besides medications, several pathophysiologic factors, including infection and changes in absorption, blood supply, influence of cytokines, and motility, may predispose tube-fed patients with multiple medical problems to diarrhea.

Medications are a common cause of diarrhea in tube-fed patients. Elixirs of acetaminophen, cimetidine, and theophylline (among others) contain large amounts of sorbitol, which may cause diarrhea. Antacids, laxatives, and drugs containing magnesium may also cause diarrhea. Antibiotics may cause diarrhea owing to the overgrowth of *Clostridium difficile* or other bacteria and *Candida.*

The composition of the formula is a less likely cause of diarrhea. In one study, normal volunteers tolerated full-strength isotonic polymeric small bowel tube feedings at rates as high as 340 mL/hour without incurring significant diarrhea.[11] The use of fiber-containing formulas to control diarrhea related to tube feeding is controversial. Several studies have shown that no significant difference occurs in the incidence of diarrhea in patients receiving enteral formula with fiber compared with those receiving enteral formula without fiber.[9]

Data on low serum albumin levels (less than 2.6 g/dL) in relation to diarrhea are controversial. Hypoalbuminemia (serum albumin less than 3.5 g/dL) is a well-established marker of morbidity and mortality and may identify patients with advanced disease and critical illness who are more prone to diarrhea induced by tube feeding.

Aspiration

Aspiration is a serious complication associated with tube feeding. Patients with an altered gag reflex, a swallowing disorder, or an altered level of consciousness are at higher risk for aspiration. Either aspiration of oropharyngeal secretions or gastric aspiration of the tube-feeding formula may occur. The risk of gastric aspiration can be minimized by elevating the head of the bed 30 to 45 degrees during tube feeding and for up to 1 hour afterward. Intermittent and continuous feeding rather than bolus feeding have been associated with a reduced risk of aspiration. Tubes placed in the small intestine beyond the ligament of Treitz (e.g., jejunostomy tubes) may lower the risk of gastric aspiration and should be considered in patients with recurrent gastric aspiration (tube feeding aspiration), not oropharyngeal aspiration.

Administering Medications Through Feeding Tubes

Feeding tubes are commonly used to administer medications. Certain guidelines must be followed to avoid complications that may result from administration of medications in this manner. Clogging of the tube may result when medications are administered through a tube smaller than 10 French. Flushing the tube with 20 to 30 mL of plain water following administration of medication may minimize the risk of clogging.

Drug absorption and drug metabolism may be altered during tube feedings. Slow-release medications and enteric-coated medications should not be crushed because crushing these medications may increase the rate of absorption and expose them to degradation in the stomach. Absorption of phenytoin may be reduced in some patients when it is given with continuous tube feedings. This change in rate of absorption of phenytoin may or may not influence its bioavailability. Therefore, blood levels of phenytoin should be monitored and the dose adjusted if necessary in patients who require continuous tube feedings and phenytoin. Similarly, the dose of phenytoin may have to be adjusted when a patient is switched from continuous to intermittent tube feedings or oral feedings.

The vitamin K in tube feeding formulas may interfere with the effect of warfarin. Prothrombin time should be monitored when tube feedings are initiated, discontinued, or interrupted.

References

1. Russell RM, Suter PM: Vitamin requirements of elderly people: An update. Am J Clin Nutr 1993;58:4–14.
2. National Institutes of Health: NIH Consensus Statement: Optimum calcium intake. National Institutes of Health. Washington, D.C., 1994, pp. 1–31.
3. Master AM, Lasser RP, Beckman G: Tables of average weight and height of Americans aged 65 to 94 years. JAMA 1960;172:658–662.
4. Chumlea WC, Steinbaugh ML, Roche AF, Mukherjee D, Gopalaswamy N: Nutritional anthropometric assessment in elderly persons 65 to 90 years of age. J Nutr Elderly 1985;4:39–51.
5. Grant A, Dehoog S: Anthropometrics. *In* Grant A, Dehoog S (eds): Nutritional Assessment and Support, 3rd ed. Seattle, self-published by Grant and Dehoog, 1985, p. 12.
6. Nutrition Screening Initiative: Nutrition Screening Manual for Professionals Caring for Older Americans. Washington, DC, Nutrition Screening Initiative, 1991.
7. Abbasi A, Rudman D: Undernutrition in nursing homes: Prevalence, consequences, causes, and prevention. Nutr Rev 1994;52(4):113–122.
8. Stabler SP: Screening the older population for cobalamin (vitamin B_{12}) deficiency. J Am Geriatr Soc 1995;43:1290–1297.
9. American Gastroenterological Association: Technical review on tube feeding for enteral nutrition. Gastroenterology 1995;(108)4:1282–1301.
10. McClave SA, Snider HL, Lowen CC, McLaughlin AJ, et al: Use of residual volume as a marker for enteral feeding intolerance: Prospective blinded comparison with physical examination and radiographic findings. JPEN 1992;16:99–105.
11. Kandil HE, Opper FH, Switzer BR, Heiser WD: Marked resistance of tube-feeding induced diarrhea: The role of magnesium. Am J Clin Nutr 1993;57:73–80.

16 Rehabilitation

Helen M. Hoenig, M.D.

Rehabilitation is a restorative process that aims to maximize a patient's functional abilities through the treatment of impairments, disabilities, and handicapping circumstances. This process can occur through many different interventions, and it can be carried out by a variety of people and in a wide variety of settings. This chapter provides a conceptual framework for the use of rehabilitation and for development of a rehabilitation plan that is suitable for geriatric patients. In particular, this conceptual framework helps to provide an understanding of the determinants of functional dependence and independence in the geriatric population and of the role of specific rehabilitative interventions. The most commonly used interventions will be described and their use outlined for the conditions seen most frequently in the geriatric population.

Approximately one in every seven Americans has a disabling condition that interferes with his or her life activities. Annual disability-related costs total more than $170 billion.[1] Disabilities are disproportionately represented among the elderly and lower socioeconomic populations.[1] Rehabilitation is the primary means of treating disability; its goals are independence in daily living skills and independent functioning in the community.

The success of rehabilitative treatment depends largely on patient participation. Therefore, an agreement between the patient and the provider on the goals of treatment is particularly important. Patients and health care providers sometimes disagree with each other about treatment because they have different beliefs about the origin of disease and how it should be treated and about what constitutes wellness. All of us, patients and providers alike, subconsciously or consciously have a conceptual model of the causes of health and ill health. This model determines the person's approach to coping with illness and influences the goals of health care. The pertinence to rehabilitation lies in the effect of the model on the strategies chosen to cope with chronic illness and during the recovery period after acute illness. People with chronic arthritic pain may be reluctant to engage in regular exercise because they believe that the best treatment for pain is rest. After a heart attack some patients may be fearful about resuming vocational or avocational activities. Similarly, some patients may be reluctant to forgo personal assistance with self-care to achieve greater independence if they come from a family milieu in which a primary means of expressing love is caretaking during illness, especially if assistance with self-care is their only source of caring touch. By the same token, the physician's underlying conceptual model of the illness in question drives the interventions he or she may select to treat the illness. As with other medical diseases, the sophistication of our understanding of the disablement process, i.e., our conceptual model of disability, determines both the diagnostic and therapeutic approaches to the treatment of disability. It is important, therefore, to understand our own models of disease and illness and how they may conflict with those of our patients. The next section will focus on conceptual models of disability.

THE DISABLEMENT PROCESS

We will begin by reviewing two traditional models of health and illness. The first is the biomedical model, and the other is the quality-of-life model. The biomedical model is the model most familiar to physicians and to many health care providers. The focus of this model is on the "etiologic agents and processes that affect biologic, physiologic, and clinical outcomes. It focuses on understanding causation and is derived from biology, biochemistry, and physiology."[2] This model is the basis for many of the advances in medicine that have occurred during the last 100 years and is most useful for unicausal processes. The quality-of-life model, on the other hand, focuses on "function and well-being. It is most useful for understanding complex behaviors and is derived from the fields of social science, psychology, and economics."[2] Because functional disability is a complex behavior caused by biologic, physiologic, psychological, economic, and social factors, effective treatment requires a combination of the two models.

Several attempts have been made to meld these two conceptual models.[1-4] For example, function or behavior can be considered as the product of biologic factors, environmental factors, and psychological factors[3] (Fig. 16–1). Losses in any of these three areas can cause a decrement in function. For example, someone who has been able to live independently in the community after a stroke through the use of paid personal assistance may no longer be able to maintain himself in the community if he suffers a loss of income. Similarly, someone with paraplegia who has been able to manage wheelchair mobility and transfers independently may no longer be able to function this way if she develops degenerative arthritic disease of the shoulders.

The World Health Organization (WHO) adopted a conceptual framework for disability in 1980.[4] The WHO model has been criticized, primarily because of measurement and semantic issues in regard to disability and handicap. In 1991 the Institute of Medicine published a revision of the WHO model that takes into account some of these concerns.[1] However, the WHO model remains the most widely accepted one and will be used throughout this chapter.

In the WHO model, disease is defined as "an intrinsic pathology or disorder that gives rise to changes in the structure or function of the body. Pathologic changes may or may not be evident clinically."[4] Disease, if sufficiently severe, may result in an impairment. Impairment is defined as a "loss or abnormality of structure or function at the organ system level. At this stage, an affected individual becomes aware of the pathology or, in behavioral terms, becomes aware that he or she is unhealthy."[4] So, for example, a person who has had untreated hypertension for a long time may have a stroke. If an impairment is

severe enough or if other facilitating factors are present, the impairment may become manifest as a disability. Disability is a "restriction or lack of ability to perform an activity in a normal manner or a disturbance in the performance of daily tasks. Disabilities are the functional consequences of impairments."[4] Thus, a stroke may or may not be severe enough to interfere with walking.

Finally, depending on societal circumstances, a disability may become manifest as a handicap. Specifically, a handicap is a "disadvantage due to impairment or disability that limits or prevents fulfillment of a role that is normal (depending on age, sex, and social and cultural factors) for the affected individual. The nature and severity of a handicap are determined in large part by the interaction of the person with his or her social and environmental surroundings and the adjustments made by society to it."[4] Thus, for example, if the workplace and home environment are wheelchair accessible, vocational pursuits and independent function in the community may continue despite inability to walk after a stroke.

Disability can be unicausal or multicausal in origin. Multicausal disability is more common in the geriatric population. A number of factors can affect the disablement process (Fig. 16–2). These factors can be thought of as external to the individual (extrinsic factors) and internal to the individual (intrinsic factors).[5] In general, intrinsic factors include such things as comorbid disease, disease severity, and comorbid impairments such as poor cognition. They include the patient's education, culture, and motivation. Extrinsic factors include medical treatment, preventive health care, rehabilitative treatment (e.g., physical therapy), the physical environment, social supports, finances, and so on. Disability and impairment

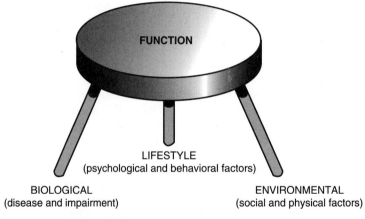

Figure 16–1 Conceptual model of disablement process.

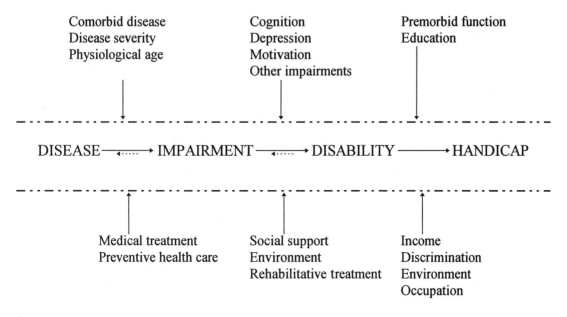

INTRINSIC FACTORS

Comorbid disease	Cognition	Premorbid function
Disease severity	Depression	Education
Physiological age	Motivation	
	Other impairments	

DISEASE ⟵⟶ IMPAIRMENT ⟵⟶ DISABILITY ⟶ HANDICAP

Medical treatment	Social support	Income
Preventive health care	Environment	Discrimination
	Rehabilitative treatment	Environment
		Occupation

EXTRINSIC FACTORS

Figure 16–2 Conceptual model of disablement process and the role of specific factors in that process.

can themselves cause additional diseases and impairments. For example, a patient who is bedbound because of a stroke may develop pressure sores. It is through a thorough understanding of these factors and their relationship to disability that we can reduce disability and handicap.

Since disability in the geriatric population is often multicausal, effective treatment usually requires consideration of the many underlying causes at work. One of the clearest examples of multiple causation is seen in the ability to ambulate after an amputation. Ambulation with a prosthesis significantly increases the work of walking; the higher the amputation, the greater the energy requirement. Typically, patients slow their gait speed to compensate for the increased work required. However, in the presence of significant heart or lung disease, a patient may not be able to meet the energy requirement for independent ambulation. Optimizing cardiac and lung function is a priority in these patients. In some patients with severe cardiopulmonary disease, particularly those with high-level or multiple amputations, independent ambulation may not be a realistic goal. Rehabilitation resources would then be better directed toward obtaining a wheelchair, teaching the patient safe transfer techniques, and ensuring that the patient's environment is wheelchair accessible. Thus, the reha-

bilitation plan must consider all intrinsic and extrinsic factors that contribute to the disablement process. Figure 16–3 is an example of a rehabilitation plan for a specific patient that shows the typical complex interacting factors that often affect function in older patients.

Identification of the intrinsic causes of disability requires the diagnostic input of the physician about the underlying disease states; it is assisted by diagnostic input from rehabilitation therapists about coexisting impairments that may be contributing to the disablement process. Identification of the intrinsic causes of disability in a given patient (i.e., the diagnostic work-up) is aided by an understanding of the prevalence and impact of diseases and impairments seen generally in older people. Some diseases carry a greater likelihood of causing disability—that is, they have a high disabling impact. These include diseases such as hip fracture and stroke. Among older persons, a stroke doubles the odds of developing disability, and arthritis increases the likelihood of developing disability by 50%.[6] More than 60% of persons suffering a hip fracture will incur a reduction in functional ability.[7] On the other hand, hip fracture is a relatively rare occurrence compared with arthritis, so the overall impact of hip fracture on disability in the population as a whole is smaller than that of arthritis. Diseases

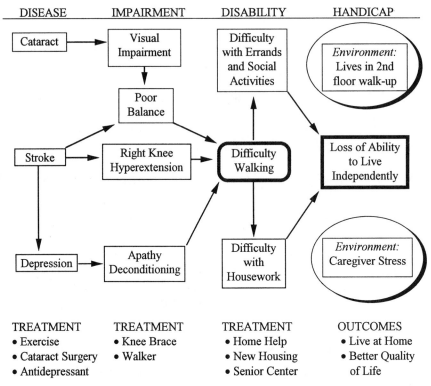

Figure 16–3 Clinical assessment and management map of the results of a disability assessment. Each column heading indicates the type of information listed below it. For example, column one lists three diseases responsible for significant impairment in a person (cataract, stroke, and depression). Different types of management are needed for diseases, impairments, disabilities, and handicaps.

In the Disability column, walking is the key disability from which the patient's other problems stem. If the patient's mobility can be improved, many of the other problems can be improved.

In the Handicap column, the key issue is the patient's ability to live independently (role functioning). Because of social and environmental circumstances, the patient's difficulty with walking threatens to force him to move into a nursing home. However, nursing home placement may not be necessary if treatment of the patient's disease, impairment, and disability is undertaken, along with other environmental modifications (e.g., moving to the first floor). Improvement in the remaining environmental stressor (e.g., spouse's caregiver stress) can be expected as the patient becomes more mobile. (From Rubenstein LV: Using quality of life test for patient diagnosis or screening, or to evaluate treatment. *In* Spilker B [ed]: Quality of Life and Pharmacoeconomics in Clinical Trials. Philadelphia, Lippincott-Raven, 1996, pp. 363–374.)

that cause significant disability and also are highly prevalent in the older population include arthritis, cardiopulmonary disease, and eye disease.[8]

One can also characterize the effect of intrinsic impairments on the likelihood of developing functional disability. Specifically, in the geriatric population, lower extremity impairments such as difficulty in rising from a chair (which requires both strength and balance), limitations in upper extremity strength, visual or hearing impairments, and affective disorders all have been found to predict functional disability. Persons with none of these impairments have a 7% likelihood of developing functional dependence, whereas persons with three of these limitations have a 60% chance of developing functional dependence.[9] Obesity and cognitive impairments are also significant risk factors, but the magnitude of their risk has not been well characterized.

Extrinsic factors can also affect the likelihood of disability in a given individual. Extrinsic factors include psychosocial factors that modify the likelihood or extent of disability and handicap as well as many of our traditional medical and rehabilitative interventions. Extrinsic factors can affect the disablement process at the disease level, the impairment level, the disability level, and the handicap level, and this is a useful way of thinking about treatment of disability.

At the disease level, preventive health care, like regular exercise, appears to prevent development of disability. For example, one recent study found that members of a running club developed disability more slowly than community controls. There were no differences in the two groups in the development of osteoarthritic changes, and the study adjusted for age, obesity, baseline function, and comorbid disease.[10] Again at the disease level, medical and surgical care can affect function. For example, in patients with visual deficits due to cataracts, surgery was shown to improve performance of activities of daily living and timed manual performance.[11] Similarly, use of anti-inflammatory medications can improve function by reducing pain and inflammation in patients with rheumatoid arthritis.

At the impairment level is the process that is classically thought of as rehabilitation. Rehabilitative interventions at this level are often directed toward improving strength and range of motion. For example, in one study, a resistive exercise program (which treats muscle weakness caused by deconditioning) significantly improved stair climbing and gait speed, and increased general physical activity in the very elderly.[12] Impairment-related rehabilitation may also include specific equipment items such as hearing aids.

Classic rehabilitative techniques are also often used at the disability level. These techniques include interventions such as assistive devices and adaptive equipment that make functional tasks easier. Hart and colleagues showed that provision of assistive devices significantly reduced difficulty with activities of daily living and the time required for their performance.[13]

Finally, handicap level interventions include techniques such as patient and family education, for example, to alter beliefs about the sick role in patients with chronic illness. Such education may be needed so that people will return to an active lifestyle even if they still have physical symptoms of disease rather than staying in bed as if they were sick. Other handicap level interventions include reducing architectural barriers, increasing financial resources, and vocational retraining.

REHABILITATION ASSESSMENT (APPROACH, SPECIFIC TESTS, AND EXAMINATIONS)

Clinical assessment for rehabilitation[14] begins by characterizing the disability or disabilities and then proceeds with the differential diagnosis accordingly. To characterize the disability one needs to determine (1) the severity of the disability (e.g., how far the patient can walk, the frequency of the falls, and how much help is required for bathing); (2) any compensatory techniques or adaptations the patient has made (e.g., use of a cane or a shower seat); and (3) any symptoms associated with the complaint (e.g., pain, shortness of breath, weakness, etc.). Pain and affective disorders commonly contribute to disability and should be specifically investigated. Complaints about pain should be evaluated for

the location, quality, radiation, and timing of the pain. It is also important to question the patient about disabilities he or she may not have mentioned. For example, someone who presents with a chief complaint of falls is also likely to have difficulty in rising from the toilet and getting into and out of the tub.

Once the disability or disabilities have been characterized, the assessment should proceed to identification of the relevant causes, i.e., the differential diagnosis. In approaching a differential diagnosis of disability, it is best to start with the impairment level before specific disease diagnoses are considered—otherwise, the differential is overwhelmingly long. For example, more than 50 different diseases can cause difficulty with walking; however, there are only nine basic impairments that can primarily affect walking. Similarly, difficulty with self-feeding in a nursing home patient may be due to cognitive impairment, hand and arm weakness, impaired vision, swallowing difficulties, or abdominal pain. The differential diagnosis varies substantially according to which body system the clinician believes is the most likely culprit; however, the assessment is much more straightforward once the relevant body system has been identified. Thus, if the diagnostician can narrow down the causal factors at the impairment level, the workup and treatment will be more manageable, in that most of the standard differential diagnoses taught in medical school relate specific impairments to possible underlying diseases.

Thus, the clinical assessment in patients with a new-onset disability should be directed first at defining the relevant impairments. As previously discussed, the likely culprits are lower and upper extremity impairments (e.g., weakness, contractures, incoordination), sensory deficits (e.g., reduced proprioception, visual deficits), obesity, impaired cognition, and affective disorders. Thus, the clinical examination should focus on these areas. Special attention should also be directed toward any specific complaints the patient may have mentioned (e.g., shortness of breath with exertion would prompt the diagnostician to perform a thorough cardiopulmonary examination).

If data from the history point to particular impairments, the physical examination targets those areas. Otherwise, the physical examination can begin in the traditional fashion with the head and neck. Examination of the head and neck should include a thorough assessment of vision, including visual acuity, visual fields, and nystagmus. Hearing can be examined with the whisper test. The oral examination should include inspection of the tongue for asymmetry and appreciation of any speech abnormalities (e.g., hypophonia is common in parkinsonism, and a scanning speech pattern should alert the diagnostician to possible cerebellar dysfunction). The clinician should also test for dysphagia by asking the patient to drink some water and observing for any cough or drooling (which would alert the clinician to the possibility of amyotrophic lateral sclerosis or other neurologic disease). Key tactile senses are light touch and position sense. A Romberg test provides a gross assessment of position sense.

The back and neck should be inspected for scoliosis, kyphosis, or other loss of range of motion (spinal stenosis is a fairly common cause of functional impairment in older patients). Functional range of motion for the upper extremity is tested by asking the patient to (1) clasp the hands behind the head; this tests external rotation and abduction of the shoulder as well as elbow flexion; (2) clasp the hands behind the back, which tests internal rotation of the shoulder. Limitations in upper extremity range of motion are likely to affect dressing, bathing, and housework.

Functional range of motion for the lower extremity is tested by asking the patient to (1) place the ankle on the opposite knee, which tests external rotation of the hip, hip flexion, and knee flexion. While the patient is in this position, examine the ankle to determine whether the patient has at least 90 degrees of dorsiflexion. (2) With the patient supine on the examination table, flex the knee of one leg to the chest. The patient should be able to keep the other leg flat on the examining table. This maneuver tests both hip and knee extension in the extended leg, and hip and knee flexion in the flexed leg. At this time the knee of the extended leg can be examined to confirm the presence of 180 degrees of hip and knee extension and to detect any varus or valgus deformity of the knee or any medial or collateral ligmentous laxity. With the foot of the flexed leg firmly on the examination table, the flexed knee can be examined for laxity of the anterior or posterior cruciate ligament. Hip, knee, and ankle range of motion are particularly pertinent to walking and mobility in the community because even a loss of 5 degrees of hip or knee extension can markedly increase the work of walking and may preclude functional ambulation. Loss of ankle range of motion to less than 90 degrees of dorsiflexion (e.g., during prolonged hospitalization) can adversely affect balance and can interfere with ambulation. Similarly, loss of hip and knee flexion makes rising from a chair much more difficult.

Strength in both the upper and lower extremities should be tested. Functional arm strength can be checked by asking the patient to put a heavy book on a shelf; functional pinch strength is assessed by asking the patient to grasp a piece of paper and then resist its removal. Useful screening tests for lower extremity strength include ability to stand on one foot (assistance with balance may be needed), the number of times a patient can stand from a sitting position (normal is five times without using the arms to assist), and the number of times the patient can rise on tiptoe (normal is five to ten times). If any abnormalities are found in either upper or lower extremity screening tests, manual muscle testing should be performed.

Coordination can be easily assessed by asking the patient to perform rapid alternating movement (e.g., toe taps) and/or the finger-nose-finger maneuver (which simultaneously checks functional vision, arm strength, and coordination). Static and dynamic sitting and standing balance are examined by asking the patient to assume independent seated and standing positions and then challenging him or her with a gentle push (be sure to be able to assist the patient to resume balance should it be necessary). A useful test of standing balance is the functional reach test (in which the patient reaches as far forward as he or she safely can while remaining in a standing position; see Duncan and colleagues[15] for details). Finally, the examination should include an assessment of the patient's gait (e.g., using the Tinetti gait and balance test or the Get Up and Go test).[16, 17] Last but not least, cognition and affect should be examined. Useful screening tests for these include the mini-mental state examination and the geriatric depression scale, although many others exist.[15]

At the end of the history and directed physical examination, the diagnostician should have a clear impression of the likely contributory impairments. If the case remains unclear, referral is indicated.[18] Assuming that the causal impairments have been identified, the diagnostic workup is then directed toward determining which underlying diseases are responsible according to standard medical procedure (e.g., the differential diagnosis for monoarticular arthritis includes trauma, infection, gout, and so on, and the clinician would proceed with arthrocentesis). After the disablement process has been characterized according to causative diseases and impairments and any contributory intrinsic or extrinsic factors, an appropriate treatment plan can be developed.

REHABILITATION TREATMENT

The rehabilitation treatment plan is developed after the disablement process has been characterized, a process that includes identification of intrinsic and extrinsic factors. Interventions can then be specifically directed at the identified causal factors and can also be considered systematically according to the point in the disablement process where they may be effective—i.e., one should systematically review whether any useful interventions are possibly at the disease level, at the impairment level, and so on. By using the conceptual model of disability, the clinician can develop a rehabilitation plan that is specifically designed for the needs of the individual patient. Figure 16–3 is an example of the causal pathway of disability and appropriate related treatment interventions in a specific patient. In developing the treatment plan, consideration should be paid to both the suitability of a rehabilitative intervention and its timing in relation to other interventions (Table 16–1). Owing to the multicausal nature of geriatric disabilities, successful treatment often requires a multidisciplinary approach using the expertise of many professionals. The role and training of the individuals in the multidisciplinary rehabilitation team, and where and how their services can be obtained, are reviewed in the next two sections.

REHABILITATION PROVIDERS

Who provides rehabilitation interventions?[19] A number of different professionals can provide important rehabilitative interventions and may have to be included in the health care team for an individual patient. As outlined in the following paragraphs and as shown in Figure 16–4, these providers can be thought of in terms of their impact at different levels of the disablement process. There is a great deal of overlap and variability in the roles played by rehabilitation providers; the descriptions that follow are therefore generalities and may differ significantly among specific providers and facilities.

Treatment provided by physicians largely acts at the disease or impairment level. For example, an internist may give a patient a cortisone injection to reduce inflammation caused by trochanteric bursitis. When the inflammation in the bursa is decreased, the patient experiences a reduction in impairment (reduced pain), a reduction in disability (improved gait), and a possible improvement in ability to maintain social roles through participation in leisure activities, (such as playing golf or hiking). Similarly, a surgeon may place an artificial knee in a patient with severe osteoarthritis. Physicians may also act as leaders of the rehabilitation team, particularly physiatrists, neurologists, orthopedists, and geriatricians. Physician referral is often required for

TABLE 16–1 **GUIDELINES FOR GERIATRIC REHABILITATION**

Cognitive impairment (ability to learn and follow directions, behavior and attention span)—treat if
    Goal is specific and well defined
    Requires no carryover from one day to the next
    Uses what the patient already knows (e.g., overlearned habits)
Prolonged disability (present for many years)—treat if
    Goal is reachable and realistic
    Goal is agreed on by patient, family, and treatment team
Motivation limited (either by patient or caregiver)—treat if
    Goal is well defined and can be reached in well-defined steps
    Treatment team or family can help motivate the patient
Previous rehabilitation—treat if
    Prior rehabilitation was for a different problem
    Adequacy of prior treatment unknown or questionable
Terminal illness—treat if
    Treatment is palliative (e.g., pain relief, reduced caregiver burden)
Comorbid illness—treat if
    Cardiovascular system is stable
    Fractures are stabilized
    Modify treatment in the presence of open wounds or severe osteoporosis
Social circumstances (absent caregiver, environment or finances inadequate)—treat if
    Goals are specific

From Hoenig H, Mayer-Oakes SA, Siebens H, Fink A, Brummel-Smith K, Rubenstein LV: Geriatric rehabilitation: What do physicians know about it and how should they use it? J Am Geriatr Soc 1994;42:341–347.

the patient to gain access to rehabilitation providers, i.e., the physician acts as gate keeper. Thus, it is incumbent on the geriatric physician to be familiar with the role and function of specific rehabilitation providers. The actual rehabilitation services are traditionally delivered by physical, occupational, and speech and language therapists. Other personnel routinely involved with rehabilitation care include nursing personnel, social workers, and dietitians. In addition, some programs have kinesiotherapists, recreational therapists, vocational rehabilitation therapists, psychologists, psychiatrists, and prosthetists who may also contribute to the overall rehabilitation effort.

Physical therapy (PT) affects primarily the im-

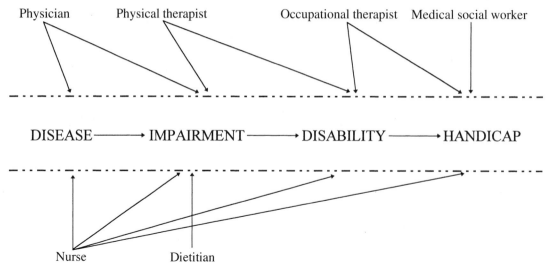

Figure 16–4 The role of different health care providers in the disablement process. For reasons of space and clarity, not all rehabilitation providers are depicted. Please see text for details.

pairment and disability levels. Physical therapists work most specifically with the musculoskeletal and neurologic systems. They provide the following kinds of services: (1) evaluation of joint range of motion and muscle strength; (2) exercise training to increase range of motion, strength, endurance, and coordination; (3) evaluation of mobility (gait or wheelchair) and need for mobility aids and training in their use; (4) treatment with physical modalities, including heat, cold, ultrasound, massage, electrical stimulation, iontophoresis, and so on; and (5) home safety evaluation, sometimes in conjunction with occupational therapy.

Occupational therapy (OT) is largely directed at the disability and handicap levels, although OT hand therapy specialists also provide impairment level interventions. Occupational therapists (OTs) evaluate and train patients in self-care activities and activities of daily living. They recommend and train patients in the use of assistive devices and adaptive equipment for self-care. OTs also work with the cognitive aspects of independent living skills such as the handling of money, safety in the kitchen, and other issues requiring proper judgment. Compensatory techniques to adjust for sensory-perceptual or motor deficits are taught by OTs. They may address prevocational and leisure time issues with patients and their families. OTs and physical therapists (PTs) work together to maintain the patient's range of motion and strength, especially in the upper extremities. OTs may also work in conjunction with speech therapists and nutritionists to help treat difficulties with self-feeding and dysphagia.

Speech therapists work mainly with patients with impairments and disabilities and secondarily with handicapping circumstances. They help patients with all aspects of communication, and they participate in the evaluation and management of patients with swallowing disorders. Because communication involves many components, the speech pathologists intervene at several levels, including evaluation of cognitive skill and aphasia in patients with cortical dysfunction. Management of patients with laryngectomy and other head and neck surgical procedures is also within the scope of the speech pathologist, as is evaluation of swallowing on radiographs, by endoscope, and at the bedside.

Nursing personnel have roles and functions that span the entire spectrum from disease to handicap. Some nurses have specialized training in rehabilitation. Nurses function in an important way in facilitating the patient's independent performance of activities of daily living during daily care. They are an important source of information and education for caregivers and as such may act to reduce both disability and handicap. Nurses help patients manage self-medication, independent bowel and bladder activity, and prevention of secondary complications such as pressure ulcers, as well as provide medication, nutrition, and wound care.

Social workers direct their efforts primarily toward reducing handicapping circumstances. They perform tasks of evaluation, disposition counseling, and liaison with the community. They evaluate the patient's social, physical, and financial home environment. They engage family, community, government, and other resources to assist patients in returning to an appropriate setting for their new level of function. Social workers also provide individual and family counseling. They make home visits and interact with entitlement providers such as Medicare on behalf of the patient.

Dietitians have the greatest impact at the impairment level by preventing or reducing nutritional deficiencies, which can retard recovery from a disability (e.g., reduction of muscle mass due to protein malnutrition reduces strength and exacerbates disability). Dietitians assess the patient's nutritional status and suggest alterations in the patient's diet to maximize nutrition. In conjunction with speech pathologists and occupational therapists, they may treat eating disorders, for example, by altering the consistency of the diet for patients with dysphagia.

Recreational therapists influence the patient at the level of handicap—that is, the ability to maintain social roles and carry on leisure activities. They facilitate the use of organized leisure activities and usually work with patients in group settings, emphasizing social interactions. Personal leisure activities such as hobbies and avocations are used by the recreational therapist to improve self-reliance and self-care. Such activities may help the patient adjust to a new disability. Recreational therapy can be helpful in achieving the goal of community reintegration.

Vocational counselors influence the level of handicap by helping patients return to the work environment. Patients may be able to return to their previous employment with adaptations, or they may be assessed for alternative employment. Vocational counselors usually see patients near the end of their inpatient rehabilitation stay or after discharge. Even in the geriatric setting, vocational counseling may be an important component of the rehabilitation process.

Psychologists are included on the rehabilitation team if testing is needed to assess the patient's psychological or cognitive abilities or if there is a need for counseling. Psychiatrists may be consulted for assessment and pharmacologic treatment of patients with disorders such as depression or dementia, which can interfere with the rehabilitation process. Both psychologists and psychiatrists may be involved in providing counseling and psychotherapy to assist the patient in making adjustments to changes resulting from the new disability.

Prosthetists fabricate and fit braces and other orthotic devices, particularly those for the feet, lower limbs, and back. When an individually fitted orthotic device or splint is needed for the upper extremity, it is usually fabricated by the occupational therapist.

In different settings, other professionals may also participate in the rehabilitation process. In Department of Veterans Affairs hospitals, kinesiotherapists (also known as corrective therapists) work alongside physical and occupational therapists. Kinesiotherapists emphasize long-term maintenance of fitness and conditioning. Music therapists and horticulture therapists can also provide useful services in the treatment of disabled elderly patients and can have beneficial effects on the quality of life of these patients.

SITES AND REIMBURSEMENT FOR REHABILITATION

Rehabilitation is usually reimbursed by one of three major sources. The site in which rehabilitation is offered may be affected by the available reimbursement. Most geriatric rehabilitation services have generally been reimbursed through Medicare; other sources include private insurance (which usually reimburses in a manner similar to that of Medicare), Medicaid, and the Department of Veterans Affairs.[19] Changes in Medicare are expected as prospective payment for rehabilitation and ambulatory care is enacted, and this change may affect the use of rehabilitation services. Health maintenance organizations often use nursing homes for rehabilitation rather than rehabilitation hospitals for their covered patients.

The major sites in which rehabilitation services are currently offered include acute care hospitals, rehabilitation hospitals, skilled nursing care facilities, outpatient settings, and at home. There is some evidence that the site where rehabilitation services are provided can affect treatment outcomes for patients with strokes; however, such evidence is still limited. The following list is a summary of the kinds of rehabilitation services typically available in different settings and the goals typical of rehabilitation treatment in each setting.[20]

1. Acute care hospital. Generally, patients can receive only short-term therapy in this setting because of constraints on the length of stay. The intensity of therapy may vary widely according to staff availability and hospital policy. Typical goals of therapy in acute care hospitals may include diagnostic and prognostic evaluation (e.g., gait assessment, assessment of the patient's functional abilities and home situation for discharge planning), patient and family education, and short-term therapeutic interventions to facilitate early discharge or improve recovery.

2. Inpatient rehabilitation hospital. Inpatient rehabilitation may be provided by freestanding hospitals or by distinct units of acute care hospitals. These hospitals are staffed by a full range of rehabilitation professionals, and an interdisciplinary team provides a comprehensive rehabilitation program for each patient. Hospital inpatient rehabilitation is generally more intense than rehabilitation offered in other settings and requires greater mental and physical effort from the patient.
3. Skilled nursing facilities. Rehabilitation programs in nursing facilities vary widely in the spectrum of services provided. Hospital-based nursing facilities are located in or adjacent to acute care hospitals. They provide rehabilitation services designed primarily for patients who have the potential to improve enough during 2 or 3 weeks of treatment to become candidates for inpatient, home, or outpatient rehabilitation. Programs in community-based nursing homes also vary. Some are nearly as comprehensive as inpatient rehabilitation hospital programs, whereas others are very limited in scope.
4. Outpatient rehabilitation programs. These programs are offered by both hospital outpatient departments and by freestanding outpatient facilities. They can provide either a comprehensive rehabilitation program (i.e., multidisciplinary rehabilitation treatment) or individual rehabilitation services (i.e., services offered by a single provider type, for example, physical therapy). An advantage of outpatient programs is that they enable the patient to live at home while retaining access to an interdisciplinary program and to rehabilitation equipment. The patient also has opportunities to make social contacts and obtain peer support. Although they are frequently more intense, day hospital programs are otherwise similar to outpatient programs. The patient spends several hours, 3 to 5 days per week, in a typical day hospital program. Availability of transportation is a prerequisite for both outpatient and day hospital programs.
5. Home rehabilitation programs. These programs usually provide physical therapy, occupational therapy, and nursing services. Some of these programs also offer speech therapy and social work services. Programs are expanding their capabilities, and some now provide comprehensive services, including home visits by physicians and intense rehabilitation services. An advantage of home rehabilitation programs is that new skills are learned in the same environment where they will be applied. An additional advantage is that many patients function better in a familiar environment.

REHABILITATION FOR SPECIFIC DISEASES

The following section offers an overview of rehabilitation interventions for specific syndromes and conditions. These suggestions should be modified according to individual patient needs.

Stroke

Rehabilitation is commonly used after an acute stroke. Depending on the specific impairments caused by the stroke, rehabilitative interventions may include physical therapy, occupational therapy, and speech therapy. For moderate to severe strokes, all members of the rehabilitation team may be involved. Rehabilitation after a stroke can be provided in any of the rehabilitation settings mentioned earlier. The choice of rehabilitation setting depends on the following factors: (1) the patient's medical stability; (2) the patient's physical endurance; (3) the degree of functional impairment; and (4) the kinds and amount of support available in the home. The Agency for Health Care Policy and Research (AHCPR) recently issued clinical practice guidelines for post-stroke rehabilitation, and they provide an excellent review of pertinent evaluation tools, scientific data supporting specific rehabilitation interventions for stroke, and recommendations for their use.[20] Figure 16–5 depicts the treatment algorithm used by the AHCPR. Further information on cerebrovascular disease in older persons is found in Chapter 32.

Arthritic and Soft Tissue Musculoskeletal Disorders

Rehabilitation is often used in patients with musculoskeletal disorders. The most beneficial rehabilitation intervention varies with the underlying pathophysiology of the disorder and its location. Recent data indicate that walking and resistive knee-strengthening exercises are beneficial for patients with osteoarthritis of the knee.[21] Exercise interventions may also be beneficial for arthritic disease of the shoulder. On the other hand, degenerative joint disease of the hip is

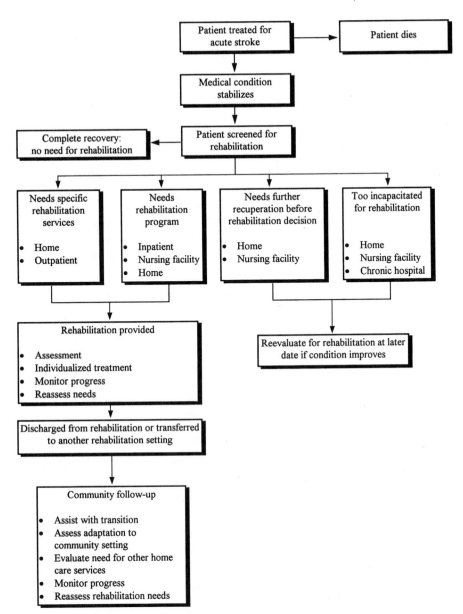

Figure 16–5 Clinical flow diagram for stroke rehabilitation. (From Gresham GE, Duncan PW, Stason WB, et al: Post-stroke rehabilitation: Assessment, referral, and patient management. Clinical Practice Guideline. Quick Reference Guide for Clinicians No. 16. AHCPR Publication No. 95-0663. Rockville, MD, U.S. Department of Health and Human Services, Public Health Service, Agency for Health Care Policy and Research, 1995.)

better treated by reducing the weight borne across the joint through the use of a mobility aid (e.g., a cane) or by altering the activity (e.g., by using a raised toilet seat or shower seat). Chronic but not acute low back pain appears to respond to comprehensive exercise and rehabilitation interventions; however, there is little evidence of benefit from transcutaneous electrical nerve stimulation (TENS).[22, 23] Little is known about the efficacy of other modalities, although use of heat and cold can provide significant symptomatic relief.[24] Corticosteroid injections can be ben-

eficial in patients with inflammatory bursitis or tendonitis; however, the activities that led to the bursitis or tendonitis should be examined simultaneously and appropriate interventions made (e.g., use of a lift on the shoe if a leg length difference caused trochanteric bursitis, or range of motion exercise if tightness of the iliotibial band is present). Orthotics can be beneficial for arthritic problems of the feet, and input from an expert in podiatry can be most helpful. Splinting can provide significant relief from carpal tunnel syndrome and tenosynovitis of the thumb; similarly, padding may be beneficial in patients with ulnar nerve entrapment. Further information on musculoskeletal diseases in the elderly is found in Chapter 39.

Amputation

Amputation of the lower extremity in older persons usually results from vascular insufficiency due either to diabetes mellitus or peripheral vascular disease. The level of the amputation is the major factor affecting the likely functional outcome. Preservation of the knee markedly increases the likelihood of functional ambulation. A below-knee amputee uses 40% to 60% more energy walking on level ground than does a non-amputee, and an above-knee amputee uses 90% to 120% more energy.[25] Other factors affecting the patient's probable functional outcome include diabetic retinopathy or neuropathy. Cardiac disease and cerebrovascular disease are also more common in older amputees and may interfere with functional outcomes. Preoperative consultation with a physiatrist, physical therapist, or prosthetist can be most beneficial.

Postoperative care is dictated in part by the patient's functional goals. If functional ambulation is likely, great care must be taken with the stump to ensure that the stump will support use of a prosthesis. Careful attention must be paid to prevention of contractures. Use of a rigid removable dressing may permit earlier weight bearing, preventing development of deconditioning. If possible, the patient should be fitted with a prosthesis as soon as wound healing permits; a temporary prosthesis is sometimes used while the stump is maturing. The prosthesis should be selected in consultation with a physical therapist and a prosthetist. Pain can be a problem after amputation and may have multiple causes including neuromas, bone spurs, biomechanical pain, or phantom pain. Phantom pain differs from phantom sensations, which are quite common but not painful. Treatment of pain after amputation can be challenging and differs according to the cause; expert consultation is recommended. Cutson and Bongiorni recently reviewed rehabilitation of the elderly lower limb amputee.[25]

Cardiac Rehabilitation

The goal of cardiac rehabilitation is to maximize patient outcome after a myocardial infarction. This goal can be achieved through patient education and graded exercises. Cardiac rehabilitation has been found to reduce mortality significantly at 1 year.[26] It is not clear how much of this benefit is due to the educational component and how much is due to the exercise component. Cardiac rehabilitation may be most beneficial, particularly for reducing disability, among patients with underlying anxiety or depression. AHCPR has recently published clinical guidelines for the use of cardiac rehabilitation.[28] Reimbursement for cardiac rehabilitation can be problematic.

Hip Fracture Rehabilitation

Rehabilitation is commonly used after an acute hip fracture. The goals are to restore functional ambulation and independent self-care. Early mobilization after the hip fracture has been repaired is desirable; otherwise, deconditioning and other bedrest-related complications can be a major cause of morbidity and mortality.[27] Many older patients are unable to comply with "touch-down weight-bearing" or "non–weight-bearing" ambulation, particularly if they have cognitive deficits. These patients often do well with "weight-bearing as tolerated" or "partial weight-bearing" if adequate fracture stability has been achieved. Consultation with the orthopedic surgeon about the surgical technique that is most likely to permit early mobilization may be helpful. Most hip fracture rehabilitative treatment consists of physical therapy. The occupational therapist may help in assessing the patient's need for adaptive equipment or methods used to achieve independent bathing and dressing. Rehabilitation typically begins in the acute care hospital. Rehabilitation may be continued after discharge from the acute care hospital by means of home health aides or subacute rehabilitation care in a nursing home.

Pulmonary Rehabilitation

Pulmonary rehabilitation is usually directed toward patients with chronic obstructive pulmonary disease (COPD). Typical components are patient education, including instruction in physical and respiratory care, psychosocial support, and supervised exercise training. Comparison of an educational program alone with a 2-month comprehensive rehabilitation program that included the aforementioned components showed significantly better exercise tolerance, fewer symptoms of breathlessness and fatigue, and trends toward better survival and shorter hospital stay in the comprehensive program.[29] An extensive review of exercise training (respiratory and endurance) for patients with COPD can be found in an article by Reid and Samrai.[30] Reimbursement for pulmonary rehabilitation can be problematic.

SUMMARY

This chapter has provided a comprehensive review of the concepts and principles underlying the use of rehabilitation services for older persons. Disablement is a complicated process, and its treatment is equally complicated. Rehabilitative interventions are noninvasive, have few complications, and have broad clinical acceptability, all of which make them appealing for use in treating disability among older persons. Although we still have much to learn about the optimal use of rehabilitation, the principles outlined in this chapter will help clinicians to select and apply the rehabilitation interventions most likely to be of benefit to their patients.

ACKNOWLEDGMENT   This work was supported in part by the National Institutes of Health, National Institute on Aging, Geriatric Research and Training Centers, National Grant No. 1 P30 AG09463, and the Claude D. Pepper Older Americans Independence Center, Grant No. 5 P60 AG11268.

References

1. Pope AM, Tarlov AR (eds): Disability in America. Washington, DC, National Academy Press, 1991; pp. 1–15.
2. Wilson IB, Cleary PD: Linking clinical variables with health-related quality of life. A conceptual model of patient outcomes. JAMA 1995; 273:59–65.
3. Trieschmann RB: Aging With a Disability. New York, Demos Publications, 1987.
4. World Health Organization: International Classification of Impairments, Disabilities, and Handicaps: A Manual of Classifications Relating to the Consequences of Disease. Geneva, World Health Organization, 1990.
5. Verbrugge L: Physical and social disability in adults. Primary care research: Theory and methods. AHCPR Conference Proceedings. Rockville, MD, U.S. Department of Health and Human Services, Public Health Service, Agency for Health Care Policy and Research, 1991.
6. Boult C, Kane RL, Louis, TA, Boult L, McCaffrey D: Chronic conditions that lead to functional limitations in the elderly. Gerontol 1994;49(1):M28–36.
7. Marottoli RA, Berkman LF, Cooney LM: Decline in physical function following hip fracture. J Am Geriatr Soc 1992;40(9):861–866.
8. Verbrugge IM, Patrick DL: Seven chronic conditions: Their impact on U.S. adults' activity levels and use of medical services. Am J Publ Health 1995;85:173–182.
9. Tinetti ME, Inouye SK, Gill TM, Doucette JT: Shared risk factors for falls, incontinence, and functional dependence. JAMA 1995;273(17):1348–1353.
10. Fries JF, Singh G, Morfeld D, Hubert HB, Lane NE, Brown BW Jr: Running and the development of disability with age. Ann Intern Med 1994;121(7):502–509.
11. Applegate WB, Miller ST, Elam JT, Freeman JM, Wood TO, Gettlefinger TC: Impact of cataract surgery with lens implantation on vision and physical function in elderly patients. JAMA 1987;257(8):1064–1066.
12. Fiatarone MA, O'Neill EF, Ryan ND, Clements KM, Solares GR, Nelson ME, Roberts SB, Kehayias JJ, Lipsitz LA, Evans WJ: Exercise training and nutritional supplementation for physical frailty in very elderly people. N Engl J Med 1994;330(25):1769–1775.
13. Hart D, Bowling A, Ellis M, Silman A: Locomotor disability in very elderly people: Value of a programme for screening and provision of aids for daily living. Br Med J 1990; 301(6745):216–220.
14. Rubenstein LV, Trueblood PR, Rubenstein LA, Hoenig H: A brief evaluation for patients with difficulty walking. Intensive Course in Geriatric Medicine. Los Angeles, UCLA Multicampus Division of Geriatrics, 1994.
15. Duncan PW, Weiner DK, Chandler J, Studenski S: Functional reach: A new clinical measure of balance. J Gerontol 1990;45(6):M192–197.
16. Lachs MS, Feinstein AR, Cooney LM Jr, Drickamer MA, Marottoli RA, Pannill FC, Tinetti ME: A simple procedure for general screening for functional disability in elderly patients. Ann Intern Med 1990;112(9):699–706.
17. Tinetti ME: Performance-oriented assessment of mobility problems in elderly patients. J Am Geriatr Soc 1986; 34(2):119–126.
18. Hoenig H, Mayer-Oakes SA, Siebens H, Fink A, Brummel-Smith K, Rubenstein LV: Geriatric rehabilitation: What do physicians know about it and how should they use it? J Am Geriatr Soc 1994;42(3):341–347.
19. Gorman PH, Hollander L: Geriatric rehabilitation in MEGA: Multidisciplinary Education in Geriatrics and Aging, a computer-assisted educational program for health practitioners. Baltimore, University of Maryland, Geriatric Gerontology Education and Research, 1992.
20. Gresham GE, Duncan PW, Stason WB, et al: Post stroke rehabilitation: Assessment, referral, and patient management. Clinical Practice Guideline. Quick Reference Guide for Clinicians, No. 16. AHCPR Publication No. 95-0663. Rockville, MD, U.S. Department of Health and Human Services, Public Health Service, Agency for Health Care Policy and Research, 1995.
21. Kover PA, Allegrante JP, MacKenzie CR, Peterson MG, Gutin B, Charlson ME: Supervised fitness walking in patients with osteoarthritis of the knee. A randomized, controlled trial. Ann Intern Med 1992;116(7):529–534.
22. Difabio RP: Efficacy of comprehensive rehabilitation programs and back school for patients with low back pain—A meta analysis. Physical Therapy 1995;75(10):865–878.
23. Deyo RA, Walsh NE, Martin DC, Schoenfeld LS, Ramamurthy S: A controlled trial of transcutaneous electrical nerve stimulation (TENS) and exercise for chronic low back pain. N Engl J Med 1990;322(23):1627–1634.
24. Puett DW, Griffin MR: Published trials of nonmedicinal and noninvasive therapies for hip and knee osteoarthritis. Ann Intern Med 1994;121(2):133–140.
25. Cutson TM, Bongiorni DR: Rehabilitation of the elderly lower limb amputee: A brief review. J Am Geriatr Soc 1996;44:1388–1393.
26. O'Connor GT, Buring JE, Yusuf S, Goldhaber SZ, Olmstead EM, Paffenbarger RS Jr, Hennekens CH: An overview of randomized trials of rehabilitation with exercise after myocardial infarction. Circulation 1989;80(2):234–244.
27. Hoenig H, Rubenstein LV, Sloane RS, Horner R, Kahn K: What is the role of timing in the surgical and rehabilitative care of community-dwelling older persons

after acute hip fracture? Arch Intern Med 1997;157:513–520.

28. Nenger NK, Froelicher ES, Smith LK, et al: Cardiac Rehabilitation. Clinical Practice Guideline. Quick Reference Guide for Clinicians, No. 7. AHCPR Publication No. 96-0672. Rockville, MD, U.S. Department of Health and Human Services, Public Health Service, Agency for Health Care Policy and Research, 1995.

29. Ries AL, Kaplan RM, Limberg TM, Prewitt LM: Effects of pulmonary rehabilitation on physiologic and psychosocial outcomes in patients with chronic obstructive pulmonary disease. Ann Intern Med 1995;122:823–832.

30. Reid WD, Samrai B: Respiratory muscle training for patients with chronic obstructive pulmonary disease. Physical Therapy 1995;75(11):996–1005.

31. Rubenstein LV: Using quality of life test for patient diagnosis or screening, or to evaluate treatment. *In* Spilker B (ed): Quality of Life and Pharmacoeconomics in Clinical Trials. Philadelphia, Lippincott-Raven, 1996, pp. 363–374.

17 Assistive Devices

John Burdett Redford, M.D.

Assistive technology and environmental adaptations for the disabled are seen widely on TV, in newspapers and magazines, and on the streets with curb cuts, ramps, parking spaces, and so forth. Assistive devices and other appliances that provide more independence to the elderly and disabled are commercially available in department stores, drug stores, specialized medical equipment stores, and catalogs as well as health care facilities. It is estimated that there are nearly 2000 sources of equipment worldwide offering approximately 20,000 to 30,000 products for sale. Not all assistive technology is promoted commercially; in many communities there are assistive technology exhibit areas, usually office space staffed by specialists who provide advice and sometimes services and who demonstrate various kinds of adaptive equipment. Physicians and other health care professionals can refer patients to community adaptive equipment centers for selection and comparison of different products. These displays of assistive devices are often adjacent to offices of voluntary health agencies, and such agencies should be helpful in identifying where they are located in the community.

A national long-term care survey of those over age 65 in 1989 found that about 7 million people were totally disabled. In this population 65% were using assistive equipment.[1] According to a recent study the mean number of assistive devices owned by disabled elderly people was 9.[2] Primary care providers are the most commonly reported source of information on disability services, but many physicians have limited knowledge of assistive technology. The greatest concern of most elderly people, even those with minimal impairment, is how to maintain independence at home and stay out of institutions; they often require assistive technology in the home to do this. All physicians in clinical practice should be aware that for disabled elderly persons assistive devices or environmental adaptations may mean the difference between totally or partially independent living and the complete reliance on others to assist in performing daily personal care. The purpose of this chapter is to help steer the medical practitioner through the maze of options in assistive technology by categorizing devices and providing guidelines on their prescription or use. Various kinds of orthoses and prostheses are not reviewed here; rather, the emphasis is on the equipment needs of the disabled elderly individual.

SOURCES FOR REFERRAL AND SUPPLY

The attentive primary care physician should be prepared to give advice on assistive devices or home adaptations or refer patients with disability to rehabilitation specialists or a rehabilitation facility, when proper selection and training with assistive devices require specialized knowledge. Occupational therapists are the most readily available source of information and evaluation because they are specially trained in activity analysis and disability. Occupational therapists can also train individuals in adaptive techniques when specialized equipment may not be necessary. Nevertheless, for many simpler or inexpensive items, such as feeding adaptations or clothing modifications, the physician can refer patients to special stores featuring assistive devices or provide catalogs without involving the expense of engaging special expertise. Several catalogs are listed under Resources at the end of this chapter.

Therapeutic adaptation is the design or modification of the physical environment to assist the performance of self-care, employment, and play or leisure activities. Therapeutic adaptation includes selecting, obtaining, and modifying equipment as well as instructing the patient and family in its proper use and care. An assistive technology device is an essential aspect of therapeutic adaptation. Such a device is defined as any item, piece of equipment, or product system, whether acquired commercially off-the-shelf, modified, or customized, that is used to increase, maintain, or improve functional capability of individuals with disabilities.[3] Devices range from simple objects for daily use (e.g., spoons with built-up handles, elastic shoelaces, doorknobs with rubber levers) to complex electronic devices such as voice-activated environmental control systems.

Most small or disposable pieces of equipment are not funded by third-party payers, generally because they are considered a "convenience" rather than a "medical necessity." Large items such as wheelchairs and special beds, which are defined as durable medical equipment, frequently are funded but require prescription by a specialist physician knowledgeable in rehabilitation of the disabled. Whatever the kind of equipment ordered it must be properly evaluated and explained to patients; the many choices can be confusing, and over-reliance on commercial promotion may prove expensive.

PRESCRIPTION

Prescription for an elderly patient who needs special assistive devices may require a full rehabilitation assessment to integrate the device effectively into the patient's total rehabilitation program. Figure 17–1 proposes a decision-making process for prescribing assistive technology.

Physicians should be aware of the costs of the assistive technology they prescribe and be able to justify the need for the equipment to insurance companies. They should also help patients identify potential funding sources or refer patients to social workers for such help. Efforts to obtain money for assistive technology must consider initial costs, expenses for maintenance, need for patient instruction, and the economic benefit the technology may provide. Funding by an insurance company often requires certification for medical necessity with written evidence by the physician. Usually completing standard forms is sufficient, but if complex assistive technology is required, dialogue with insurance companies may be needed to prove medical necessity. Advice on how to certify for medical necessity is found in *Guidelines for the Use of Assistive Technology,* published by the American Medical Association (see Resources).

REFERRAL TO SPECIALISTS

Referral to a physiatrist or other medical rehabilitation specialists concerning rehabilitation and assistive technology is recommended for patients with severe strokes or other disabling neurologic disorders; spinal cord injuries; brain injuries; neuromuscular disorders; or advanced, disabling arthritis. Medical advice about assistive technology is also needed with disorders requiring home ventilators, with major amputations, and with severe disorders of communication, vision, and hearing. Consider consultation with a physiatrist when there are unresolved questions about diagnosis and prognosis or when programs and treatment require customized and expensive equipment. If additional consultation is suggested by rehabilitation therapists, referral to a physiatrist is also desirable for additional advice concerning treatment or prognosis.

Occupational therapists generally provide and

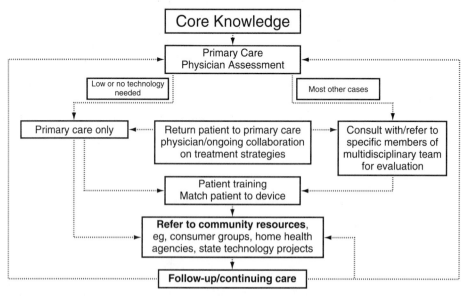

Figure 17–1   Primary care physicians are usually the first to see a person with functional limitations to determine if, when, and by whom assessment will be done. Their longitudinal care responsibilities include acting as a skilled observer of progress, monitoring maintenance of skills, and advising the team of new or changed health care status and loss or change of support systems. (Source: Guidelines for the Use of Assistive Technology: Evaluation Referral Prescription. Chicago, American Medical Association, Copyright 1994.)

recommend self-help aids and orthotic devices. Examples of patients who should be referred to an occupational therapist include those needing assistance in activities of daily living (ADL), splints or orthotic fabrication (primarily for the upper limb), adaptive equipment for work, or assessment of a home environment.

Physical therapists provide help with mobility aids for walking, including assistance and prescription of wheelchairs. Examples of patients needing referral to a physical therapist include those with specific balance or gait disturbances, seating or positioning problems in a wheelchair, or significant range-of-motion or muscular strength impairment.

Speech–language pathologists are experts in the treatment of communication or swallowing disorders. Examples of patients needing referral to speech–language pathologists include those with dysphagia or verbal or written language deficits. When the physician is uncertain of the patient's cognitive ability with language, a referral to a speech–language pathologist may be of assistance.

SELECTION, EVALUATION, AND TRAINING

Some points are worth considering before prescribing any equipment, especially for very old patients. First the practitioner should pay careful attention to the patient's functional disability and proposed living arrangements. If the patient can function reasonably well without the aid or rejects the idea of using an aid to help reduce the impairment, the equipment may never be used. Furthermore, if much training is needed to use the device, it is likely the equipment will be discarded unless training is readily available. Often sufficient time for training is needed before a definite decision can be made.

Another point to consider is cost. Simple aids are better than complex ones often because they are more affordable. In addition, the less conspicuous the aid, the more acceptable it will be. Unfortunately, the walking cane, one of the most effective and cheapest aids, is the most conspicuous. It is often discarded by elderly people who worry over their appearance and freely admit that they are too proud to use a cane. In a lament over this situation, a well-known orthopedic surgeon wrote a memorable editorial, "Don't Throw Away the Cane."[4]

The most decisive basis for evaluation of adaptive equipment is whether it gratifies the need of the user from his or her point of view. Batavia and Hammer[5] have identified four key evaluation and selection criteria for long-term users of assistive devices:

1. Effectiveness—the extent to which the function of the device improves one's living situation, functional capability, or independence
2. Affordability—the extent to which the purchase, maintenance, or repair of the device causes financial difficulty
3. Operability—the extent to which the device is easy to operate and responds adequately to demands
4. Dependability—the extent to which the device operates with repeatable and predictable levels of accuracy under conditions of reasonable use

Decisions made in choosing assistive technology should consider these factors, and written descriptions of equipment should address all or most of them.

PUBLICATIONS

Of the many publications providing information about assistive technology, the *Assistive Technology Sourcebook* by Enders and Hall seems the most complete (see Resources, at the end of this chapter, for more information on this and the following publications). This directory, which has 576 pages, provides the names and addresses of vendors and rehabilitation equipment sources and also includes lists of books and other literature that give further sources of practical information. Another older but excellent guide with outstanding illustrations is edited by Hale. This book ends with eight pages and almost 400 references to resources for the disabled, including extensive literature, national and international organizations, and sources of special supplies. A recent 58-page publication by the American Medical Association, already mentioned above, that gives guidelines for the use of assistive technology is an outstanding summary of information, resources, and services for the disabled. I, along with Basmajian and Trautman, recently edited a book on clinical practice in rehabilitation technology. For sources of information on all aspects of rehabilitation, including evaluation, prescription, and training in the use of assistive technology applied to physical disability, we recommend the textbooks edited by Trombly and DeLisa.

CLASSIFICATION

Most assistive aids fall into one of the following major categories: mobility, eating, dressing, hygiene, communication, and recreation. This classification is used for the headings in this section.

Mobility Aids

Most patients with lower limb disorders benefit from a cane, crutches, or a walker for ambulation. Usually, the more disabled the individual, the more complex the walking device required. In nearly all clinical situations the cane should be held in the side opposite the affected lower limb. A cane can transmit up to 25% of body weight away from the lower limb; crutches or walkers can improve balance more effectively and reduce weight-bearing on both limbs by 50%. Canes and crutches should always be inspected to be sure the rubber tips are effective and safe. Details of different designs of walking aids and methods of gait training are widely available.[6, 7] The most useful aid for most elderly hemiplegic persons is the four-legged or quad cane and the pyramid-shaped folding cane/walker, which combines features of a walker and the quad cane. The latter is more versatile and safer because some patients may tend to trip on quad canes (Fig. 17–2).

An important aspect of mobility is the ability to transfer in and out of beds and chairs. A patient who is able to walk may not be able to get up without help. Simple aids such as bed rails, an overhead trapeze, a rope ladder, or a braided bed pull attached to the foot of the bed may be all that is needed for improved bed mobility (Fig. 17–3). For the elderly patient with arthritic knees, or other disorders that make it difficult to rise from low chairs, recessed wooden blocks may be placed under the feet of furniture

to elevate them several inches. Chairs are also available with either a spring- or motor-driven rising seat. Some elderly patients have found that these chairs aid them in getting up and are well worth the additional cost. To make dressing simple and safe, the elderly person's bedroom should have chairs with arm supports for stability and firm seats that are not lower than the height of the knees.

WHEELCHAIRS

A wheelchair to suit the individual's lifestyle is often the key element in maintaining independence. Physicians should realize that a wheelchair is more than "a chair with wheels." For the patient unable to walk, his or her whole life and interaction with the environment will revolve around the wheelchair. It is an independence-giving, energy-saving substitute, essential for disabled people to participate in the world around them. Wheelchairs come in a wide variety of models and sizes, few of which can be reviewed here. Any patient with special problems who requires a permanent wheelchair should be referred to rehabilitation programs for advice. When a patient is simply advised to go to the nearest wheelchair dealer for an opinion, a needlessly expensive solution may be offered. However, hospital equipment dealers can be very helpful by listing the various features available—depending on the patient's requests and personal requirements—and discussing these with the prescribing physician.

For the elderly person who needs a wheelchair mainly as an accessory aid to mobility, the basic rear-wheel drive or standard wheelchair with a seat that allows at least 2 inches of clearance on either side should be adequate. This chair may be selected with a standard adult, 18-inch-wide seat or a narrow adult, 16-inch-wide seat, depending on the build of the patient. The chair should be as narrow as possible because every inch saved is important in entering doorways. The standard wheelchair has 8-inch casters in front, a straight back (about 100 degrees in relation to the seat), brakes, and fixed or removable footrests. The arms should be padded (Fig. 17–4). In some wheelchairs, the arms are stepped down in front (desk arms), allowing the chair to slide under a desk or a table. The arms can also be removed or swung away to permit sideways transfer to a bed, toilet, or commode, with or without the help of a transfer board.

Powered wheelchairs, using a standard type of frame as just described, have limited application and generally are prescribed only for those unable to operate a manual chair. They are usually

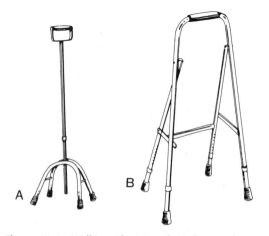

Figure 17–2 Walking aids. *A,* Four-legged, or quad, cane. *B,* Hemiwalker or walk cane. (From Varghese G: Crutches, canes, and walkers. *In* Redford JB [ed]: Orthotics Etcetera, 3rd ed. Baltimore, Williams & Wilkins, 1986.)

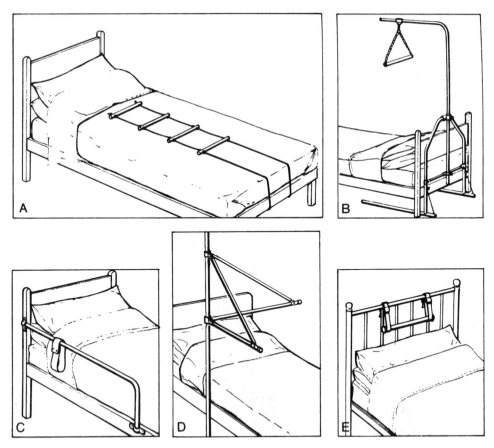

Figure 17–3 Bed aids. *A*, Rope ladder. *B*, Free-standing trapeze. *C*, Handrail with leather loop. *D*, Swivel bar assembly with upright that attaches to floor and ceiling. *E*, Bed bar. (From Hale G [ed]: The Source Book for the Disabled. Philadelphia, WB Saunders, 1979.)

useful only indoors; unless the user has a specially equipped van, they are of little use outside the home. However, in recent years, a vast array of three- or four-wheel powered vehicles, sometimes called "powered scooters," have become available. Most of these scooters are narrower than standard wheelchairs and so are more useful in entering narrow doorways, but, as most are longer than standard wheelchairs, there may be serious problems in turning them indoors. Most scooters are also more unstable than standard wheelchairs and harder to mount. These vehicles are generally usable only by persons with relatively good upper limb function and upper trunk control who are without postural problems or spinal deformities. Many can be easily disassembled into parts and carried in a standard automobile, but the parts can be very heavy for older persons to lift. Because many elderly persons requiring a wheelchair lack the energy to push manual chairs any distance, a scooter will provide them with much better outdoor mobility than a

manual wheelchair. Although many third-party payers have regarded these vehicles as a "luxury item," the scooters have provided invaluable mobility to many disabled persons with multiple medical problems. A great variety of seating and assembly options are available in scooters. Potential users should be advised to shop around among the various models, choose the one most suitable for their functional needs, and rent it for a trial before making a final purchase. However, before any powered wheelchair or scooter is purchased one must consider how it will be transported, because in some instances the user will have to buy a van with a powered lift in order to be able to use the equipment anywhere but around the yard.

Most manual wheelchairs weigh 40 lb or more, but more expensive lightweight chairs are available that weigh 24 lb or even less. Lightweight chairs are most useful if the user or caregiver has to move them frequently in and out of vehicles. Most chairs should be provided with wheel-

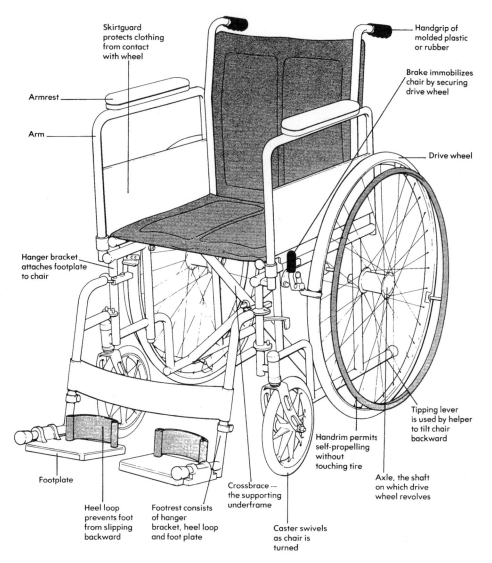

Figure 17–4 Features of a standard wheelchair. (From Hale G [ed]: The Source Book for the Disabled. Philadelphia, WB Saunders, 1979.)

chair cushions. Foam cushions are generally sufficient, but special cushions—filled with air, water, or special gels to minimize pressure over bony points—are absolutely essential for patients with poor sensation or limited sitting tolerance. Many other wheelchair features and accessories are available but need special forms proving medical necessity for prescription. Information on wheelchairs is readily obtained from rehabilitation catalogs, local dealers, or textbooks, including an excellent monograph on wheelchairs published by the Department of Veterans Affairs (see Resources). A new one has just been published by the Rehabilitation Engineering Society of North America (RESNA).[8] I have prepared specific information on various options for wheeled mobility in the elderly.[9]

ENVIRONMENTAL MODIFICATIONS

If a person must be confined to a wheelchair at home, there are a few general considerations regarding home arrangements. Ramps for entrances should be at least 36 inches wide (surfaced with nonskid materials and rising no more than 1 foot in height for every 12 feet of length). Handrails are also very useful on ramps and should be positioned so that the patient can reach both handrails from the chair. The handrails should also be alongside all outside entrances of elderly persons' homes to assist in stair climbing. For wheelchairs, the area at the top of the ramp should be at least 5 feet in depth if the door opens outward. Portable ramps are available but are quite heavy and thus not very practical.

For special situations in which the height of the ground floor is too great, precluding even a two-section ramp and platform, outdoor self-operating elevators can be substituted but are more expensive. Further information on home modifications may be found in the Resources at the end of the chapter.

Doorways should be at least 30 inches and preferably 36 inches wide. Doorknobs and night locks can be fitted with levers for those with poor grasp and limited reach. Indoor stair lifts are available but are very expensive; it is usually cheaper for the family to modify the home to enable the disabled adult to live on the main floor. Floors should be smooth and kept in good repair, and carpets, if used, should have minimal pile. Plastic runners are helpful if the carpet has thick pile. Mossy carpet or loose throw rugs are not only difficult for the wheelchair user but may create mobility problems even for elderly people able to walk unaided.

In a wheelchair, a person's standing height is decreased by one-third and his or her width is doubled. Therefore, to maneuver a turn in a wheelchair a circumference of at least 5 feet is needed. This merits consideration, particularly in the kitchen, bedrooms, and bathrooms. Reach from a wheelchair is very limited and usually done from the side, although forward reach can be aided by removable foot rests. A variety of reachers are available, especially for wheelchair users and others with limited mobility. Length, width of opening, and degree of grasp required should be considered in advising potential users about reachers.

Eating Aids

For persons with poor grasp, impaired coordination, and disorders affecting the shoulder and elbow, many attractive and durable mealtime aids are available from medical supply houses. Poor grasp can be improved readily by enlarging silverware handles either with foam padding, such as pipe insulation, or other materials. A universal cuff that encircles the hand and holds utensils by a sleevelike opening is a useful option. If the patient is one-handed, rocker knives and pizza cutters can replace regular knives. For cooking, microwave ovens or crock pots usually prove simpler to use than the standard oven. Patients with impaired coordination or tremor may be aided by plate guards, scoop dishes, suction cups, or thin Dycem mats made of a versatile sticky plastic material that holds on to furniture (Fig. 17–5). Most occupational therapy departments have kitchens in which therapists can provide excellent advice to families about meal preparation and special equipment such as one-handed kitchen aids and electric devices. An excellent description

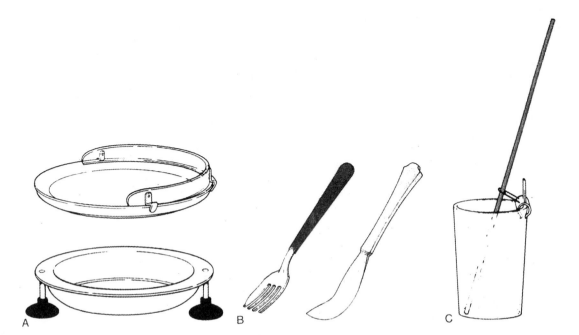

Figure 17–5 Mealtime aids. *A,* Plates with plate guards and suction cups. *B,* Large-handled fork and rocker knife. *C,* Plastic straw with bulldog clip attached to side of glass. (From Hale G [ed]: The Source Book for the Disabled. Philadelphia, WB Saunders, 1979.)

of mealtime aids and food preparation, as well as general advice on housekeeping for handicapped persons, is found in the books edited by Trombly and Hale (see Resources).

Dressing Aids

Clothing for the disabled elderly should be adjustable and expandable, easily put on and taken off, and reinforced against wear by braces and crutches. Above all, it should look attractive. With today's informal fashions of stretchable fabrics, well-chosen garments can enhance physical attributes and conceal flaws. As expressed by a patient who wrote a self-help guide for those with amyotrophic lateral sclerosis, "To feel good, you need to look good."[10]

Easy-to-fasten garments that open in the front provide freedom of movement and eliminate the need to reach upward (e.g., front-fastening brassieres). Such clothing, often using Velcro closures, is now marketed widely and can be bought through many department stores. Enlarging zipper pulls by using a loop or tab makes zipper closure easier. Zipper rings are sold in all fabric stores. Button hooks are also a great aid to those who have inadequate fine grasp to manipulate small buttons. Reachers and a dressing stick tipped with foam allow an elderly person to remain seated while dressing and reduce the risk of falling. Dressing the lower limbs is often difficult for those with poor reach or balance, especially those with stiff hips. A variety of sock donners and reachers are available for such persons. Shoes can be converted to slip-ons with elastic shoelaces, or zippers or Velcro closures can be stitched in by any shoemaker. "No-Bows," used to prevent young children from untying shoes, are sold at shoe stores.

Ideas for aids to dressing and adaptive clothing are readily available in any occupational therapy department. Information is also available in texts on ADL or general rehabilitation, and aids are illustrated in many manuals distributed by voluntary health organizations. Various catalogs provide sources of dressing aids (see Resources). Sears Roebuck now publishes a home health catalog that features clothing as well as many health care aids, and companies have specialized in designing clothing for the disabled and elderly. The Arthritis Foundation's *Guide to Independent Living* provides an extensive list of over 60 of these companies (see Resources).

Hygiene Aids

The bathroom, with its slippery floors and narrow spaces, is the most dangerous place in the home for anyone with impaired balance, joint limitation, or slowness of movement. A call for help may not be heard, especially when water is running or the bathroom door is closed. Thus the bathroom should be made as safe as possible and equipment provided to increase ease in bathing and grooming without mishap.

Grab bars should be placed where needed around tubs, showers, and toilets. Nonskid stripes should be attached to the tub or shower floor, or rubber mats should be placed on such surfaces. Raised toilet seats for persons with weakness or stiffness of the lower limbs are readily available in many medical supply stores (Fig. 17–6). Seats for the bathtub or shower and bath lifters are also widely available. Those with restricted lower limbs who cannot actually sit down in the bottom of a tub can benefit from a hand-held shower. Washing aids include wash mitts, soap-on-a-rope, brushes with suction backs, and long-handled sponges. If the individual cannot walk into the bathroom (for anyone permanently in a wheelchair, bathroom entrances are usually too narrow), a bedside commode may have to be substituted for the bathroom toilet. It should be a sturdy structure with side arms and arranged to permit the feet to touch the floor. Of course, the bathroom doorway can be widened, but this may be very costly. As an alternative, a wheelchair narrower fits almost any folding wheelchair; its crank squeezes the seat to narrow it by 3 to 5 inches.

To compensate for limited grasp, handles of combs, brushes, and fingernail files can be enlarged with foam padding or other material, as previously described for eating utensils. Electric toothbrushes and razors are much easier to use than manual ones for individuals with hand coordination problems.

A discussion of equipment for bowel and bladder incontinence is beyond the scope of this chapter. However, patients with such problems should be aware that there are many types of collecting devices for bladder care and bowel care that make it possible for them to lead a normal life. In most large medical centers, nurses who specialize in colostomy care are a good source of information on such products.

Communication Aids

Many elderly people with motor or sensory impairment have very limited ability to communicate. As a result, their isolation increases, their safety is endangered, and they are cut off from normal sources of intellectual and emotional stimulation, which may even lead to cognitive deterioration.

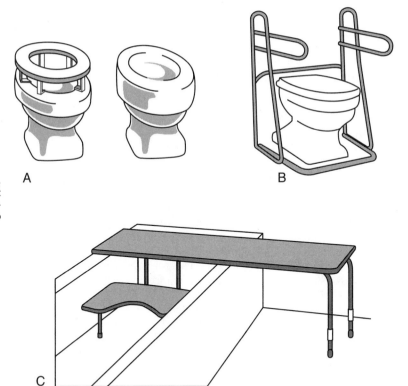

Figure 17–6 Bathroom aids. *A,* Kinds of removable elevating toilet seats. *B,* Grab bars that fit any toilet seat. *C,* Bath bench and tub seat.

Reading materials have been widely adapted for the handicapped, with large-print books and special magnifiers, and magnifying television screen systems are also available. Many large teaching institutions have aid programs for those with low vision that are helpful in providing information in this regard. Reading machines like the Optacon and the Reading Edge (Xerox Imaging Systems, Inc) are available for the severely visually impaired. Research is promising to lower the costs and increase portability of such devices.

If the person's main problem is inability to hold reading matter in a comfortable position, help is readily obtained by a variety of aids. The simplest reading aids are angled book stands that can be placed on tables or on the floor like a music stand, or even racks suspended over beds with the reading material upside down. People with difficulty turning pages can use rubber thimbles or rubber-tipped pencils to grip the pages. Although they cost several hundred dollars, electric page turners are available for the severely handicapped. Prismatic glasses make it possible to see objects at right angles and may aid in reading if a person must lie flat. They can reduce eye strain and neck pain, particularly when neck motion is limited. For those unable to use magnification, even to read or watch television, but who still wish to "keep up with the world," there are now many "talking books."

Many of these are on cassette tapes in local bookstores. Services are also available through the local or national Federation for the Blind or the National Council of the Blind. The Library of Congress, Division of Blind and Physically Handicapped, will, on request, send information on reading aids and the availability of "talking books."

Aids can be used to help those lacking good hand grip or coordination in their writing. Handles of writing instruments can be enlarged with many special types of grips; for example, the handle of a pen can be enlarged by sticking it through a plastic practice golf ball. Occupational therapy departments feature a wide variety of special writing aids, many of which are widely available commercially. Notepads are usually easier to use than loose sheets; clipboards often help to stabilize the paper if one hand is weak, as in hemiplegia; and various types of reading stands can double as writing stands for those who are too seriously disabled to write at a table or desk.

Many elderly people cannot write easily; for them, the electric typewriter—and lately the computer—have been a great benefit, especially if the person lacks strength and coordination to use the controls on a manual typewriter. An electric typewriter or computer keyboard can be operated by a hand-held stick or even a stick attached to a mouthpiece. For those who find both writing and typing a problem, a cassette tape recorder is a useful substitute. When selecting such a recorder, one should consider how difficult it is to operate and select one with simple controls.

ELECTRONIC DEVICES

Without a doubt, the computer has changed almost every aspect of daily life—written and verbal communication, transportation and other scheduling, and employment practices, to name only a few. For the disabled, it has provided almost unbelievable advances to control the environment: switching on lights, television, or radio; changing position in bed; opening doors; and even preparing food can be done with a touch of a finger or even the blink of an eye. Thus, many severely disabled persons are in almost complete charge of their environment.

Electric typewriters have been very helpful in providing writing capabilities for disabled persons in the past, but they are being succeeded almost everywhere by computer keyboards, screens, and printers. Although most computer keyboards use the standard Q W E R T Y typewriter layout, they can be modified to provide almost any combination of symbols required by a person. For the person with a tremor or poor limb coordination, keyboards can usually be expanded to make striking the keys easier. For the nonverbal person, head nods or even eye movements can give signals to the computer to generate verbal commands to relatives or attendants.

A great many programs have been advocated to improve cognitive function by computer technology, including many systems adapted primarily for the cognitively impaired, head-injured person. Research involving computer-aided visual communication systems for global aphasic patients is currently being tested clinically. The value of computers as learning aids remains to be scientifically established, but they have proved extremely popular in many rehabilitation centers. What they offer the cognitively impaired elderly person remains to be seen. However, miniature computers have been widely advocated as memory aids; a person who has failing short-term memory can easily be reminded by a touch of a button what tasks or activities are to be done and in what sequence. These computers can easily be carried in a purse or a pocketbook and are relatively inexpensive.

There is little doubt that the telephone is the most vital tool of communication, especially for elderly people who live alone. Advances in telephone design have made it much easier for the disabled to send or receive calls. Obviously, the telephone should be positioned for the most efficient, comfortable use, especially if reach is limited. For dialing the telephone, simple dialing aids such as a pencil or a dialing tool can solve coordination problems, but most persons will use the touch-tone type of telephone. Giant pushbutton telephone adapters are currently available for easy operation by the disabled. New phone systems have one-touch dialing, completely eliminating the need to dial. If a person has limited arm strength, having a telephone mounted on a gooseneck arm or using handsets can eliminate the need to hold it for any length of time. The conventional telephone can be replaced entirely by a dial, microphone, and speaker set in a special boxed unit. A call to the telephone company is the easiest way for handicapped persons to be advised of the options available.

There are many other types of communication aids, such as sophisticated electronic devices that can provide vocal responses for those without speech. When a serious communication problem develops, the physician is well advised to consult a speech–hearing pathologist whose primary purpose is to develop speech and communication skills in patients. The local chapter of the American Speech and Hearing Association can suggest where to turn for consultation.

Recreation Aids

The easiest and perhaps the only way an elderly disabled person may become part of the community, make new friends, or escape from an institutional setting is through participation in recreational activities. Physicians should therefore encourage disabled elderly people to participate not only in group exercises or outdoor sports but also in any recreational activity that interests them. Disabled elderly people can find many indoor sports and games that have been adapted for various disabilities. For example, special card holders and battery-powered card shufflers are now available. Special tools for indoor gardening and shop work have been developed for specific handicaps. The section on leisure and recreation by Hale is an excellent guide (see Resources); this book also lists various organizations promoting leisure activities for the handicapped.

Table 17–1 is a summary of most of the adaptive equipment solutions described in this chapter.

SUMMARY OF RESOURCES

The aim of this chapter has been to provide medical practitioners and other health profes-

TABLE 17–1   **SUMMARY OF COMMON FUNCTIONAL PROBLEMS AND THEIR ADAPTIVE EQUIPMENT SOLUTIONS**

Condition	Equipment	Special Notes
Mobility Aids—Ambulation		
Minimal balance problem or unilateral lower limb pain or mild weakness	Regular cane with safety tip and various types of grips; long walking stick or staff	Train person to use on unaffected side. Use waist belt for safety at first, depending on individual.
Balance problem or paralysis with support required (e.g., hemiplegia)	Pyramidal cane, quad cane (4-footed), hemiwalker (one-handed walker)	Unstable on grass, sand, or uneven surfaces.
Bilateral lower limb problems with pain or balance loss. No or minimal weight bearing on one side	Standard crutches, forearm crutches (Lofstrand)	Need instruction in crutch use and stair climbing. Waist belt for safety, depending on individual.
Painful wrist or hand (e.g., arthritis of wrist, neuropathy)	Special handgrips or cane or crutch with forearm platform	Platform adds extra weight to the walking aid.
Moderate to severe loss of stability	Walker or weighted walker if very unstable or bad tremor of upper limbs	All cases need instruction in use. Should fold if needed to be transported.
Unable to lift walker during ambulation	Add wheels to front uprights of walker or use 3- or 4-wheeled walker	More wheels increase instability but walkers with 3 or 4 wheels move faster.
Difficulty in climbing stairs and risks of safety on stairs from poor vision or balance	Well-placed and supported hand rails, fully extended; steps with nonskid surfaces and tread markings; stair-climbing walker	
Mobility Aids—Transfer		
Difficulty turning and arising from bed to chair, commode, and so forth	Bed rails; overhead trapeze, manual or electric controls on bed; transfer board—various types	Need instruction in use.
Limited ability to transfer	Transfer board, various types	Need instruction in use.
Total inability to transfer from bed to chair, commode, and so forth	Pneumatic or electric patient lifters	Occupy considerable space. Caregiver needs training in use.
Difficulty arising from chairs (e.g., parkinsonism, lower limb arthritis, weak hip and knee extensors)	Raise legs of furniture, mechanical lifts, or electric seat-lift chairs	Portable seat lifts are heavy. Electric seat-lift chairs are very expensive and limited to use in one area.
Eating Aids		
One-handed: cannot cut food, problems pushing food onto fork or spoon, problems holding plates steady	Rocker knife, pizza cutter; plate guard scooper dish, partitioned plate; Dycem place mats or suction cup on plates	Need occupational therapy advice and trial for best selection.
Limited grasp	Finger loops or built-in handles to utensils for eating; Universal cuff with Velcro closure and a pocket for utensil	Need occupational therapy advice and trial for best selection.
Severe tremor or incoordination	Weighted utensils; use of special cups or straws for drinking	Need occupational therapy advice and trial for best selection.
Dressing Aids		
Difficulty with mobility or weakness in upper extremity; trouble closing fasteners	Reacher, dressing hook or stick, button hook, zipper, Velcro closure	Seek occupational therapy advice.
Difficulty with lower extremity dressing (e.g., pants, shoes, socks)	Reachers, dressing loops on pants with Velcro closures, sock donner, long shoe-horns, Velcro shoe closures, elastic shoelaces	Seek occupational therapy advice.

Table continued on following page

TABLE 17–1 **SUMMARY OF COMMON FUNCTIONAL PROBLEMS AND THEIR ADAPTIVE EQUIPMENT SOLUTIONS** *Continued*

Condition	Equipment	Special Notes
Hygiene Aids		
Inability to use regular toilet	Bedside commode, raised toilet seat, grab bars around toilet; individually designed hygiene aids for cleanup	Selection depends on space in bathroom and ability to enter its narrow doorway.
Inability to use regular bathtub or shower	Bathtub bench with hand-held shower, grab bars on tub or shower; shower chair; inflatable bathtub for use in bed	Survey of home by occupational therapist or other trained person helpful in deciding best arrangement.
Poor grasp or hand coordination for bathing, toilet	Wash mitts, soap-on-a-rope, long-handled sponges, suction-cup soap holders	Seek occupational therapy advice.
Problems with grooming hair, face, teeth	Long-handled or built-up combs or brushes, electric toothbrush, electric razor with custom handle; custom-made makeup kit	Seek occupational therapy advice.
Communication Aids		
Impaired vision for reading	Special magnifiers; large-print book or magnifying television screens	All cases need full ophthalmologic assessment.
Difficulty in using phone	Pushbutton dialing or one-touch dial, speaker phones; various portable phones with special hand sets	Speech and hearing therapy and/ or occupational therapy advice.
Writing or typing difficulty	Individual writing aids, typing sticks with various attachments for gripping	Speech and hearing therapy and/ or occupational therapy advice.
Inability to dial phone or call for help due to severe paralysis or immobility	Voice-activated tape recorders; electronic speaking devices; simple buzzers or other signaling devices operated by switches needing minimal pressure	Speech and hearing therapy and/ or occupational therapy advice.

Developed in collaboration with Eugene Steinberg, M.D., Medical Director, Hospital Based Home Care Program, Buffalo VA Medical Center, Buffalo, NY.

sionals with a short guide to resources in assistive technology for the elderly disabled. A complete list of resources would be impossible to summarize in any meaningful fashion, but the *Assistive Technology Sourcebook* by Enders and Hall (see Resources) can largely serve this purpose. For a shorter summary of sources of information, we recommend the American Medical Association's *Guidelines to Assistive Technology,* prepared by Schwartzberg and Kakavas. The National Rehabilitation Information Center (NARIC) is a source of information funded by the National Institute on Disability and Rehabilitation Research (NIDRR) and, on request, will send fax sheets providing information on almost any form of adaptive equipment (see Resources). Another good source of such information for patients is the *Buyers' Guide,* available from Accent on Living.

There are now a number of on-line databases on electronic networks to assist disabled people and others in obtaining information. ABLEDATA has a database of over 21,000 products and services pertaining to children and adults with disabilities. REHABDATA has a database of over 46,000 documents pertaining to assistive technology and rehabilitation. These data are collected by NARIC from anyone who submits the information to its office and are available to anyone who calls or writes to the National Rehabilitation Information Center (see Resources). For information on more databases, the Rehabilitation Engineering Society of North America (RESNA) produces a book entitled "On-line Access to Disability-Related Information." These data bases provide information, lists of vendors and consultants, sources of fabrication of customized equipment, repair sites, and names of organizations and facilities serving the disabled nationwide. For some data bases you may consult information brokers who are trained to search the data base and provide interface between computer hardware and a person needing information. If a person requires a specific rehabilitation product, local information brokers will provide this information free of charge. Their names can be obtained from the state vocational rehabilitation division or by contacting the National Rehabilitation Information Center.

Under the Technology-Related Assistance for Individuals with Disabilities Act of 1988 (commonly known as the "Tech Act") all states were granted funds to set up regional assistive technology resource projects.[3] The Tech Act as amended in 1994 directs each project to effect "systems change" within its state, namely, to identify barriers that people encounter when trying to obtain assistive technology, such as lack of information, inadequate funding resources, limited expertise among service providers, and gaps in services from public and private agencies. The project should reduce or eliminate those barriers. Many of these projects use electronic mail and are on the World Wide Web, which includes such information as resource lists, where to go locally for assistive technology products and services, and advice regarding funding sources and strategies (Website for Hyper ABLEDATA is http://trace.wisc.edu/tcel/abledata/index.Rtml).

Links are available to local, national, and international resources. Information about any new assistive devices developed by these state projects is sent to NARIC, so this national resource is kept abreast of any new information about rehabilitation technology. Most of these projects are associated with the state's division of rehabilitation services. To find out if there is a center near you, call the rehabilitation office and ask about your state's technology act project for special assistive technology for disabled patients.

The Yellow Pages of the telephone directory may be consulted for volunteer organizations or social service agencies that assist people with various diseases. If a person has a specific chronic disabling disease, a call to the local branch of the national organization should provide information about assistive devices. Voluntary health organizations such as the Muscular Dystrophy Association or the Multiple Sclerosis Society may have equipment pools or "loan closets" near their offices, and this equipment can be made available to needy patients for no charge or sometimes for a small fee. The American Cancer Society is particularly noteworthy in this regard. Information about equipment for handicapped individuals is also available in some large department stores. Local medical supply dealers generally carry an extensive selection of rehabilitation equipment. Their salespersons are usually well informed about living aids or equipment and the options available for different disabling conditions. Many suppliers now employ specialists in

assistive technology who can be very helpful to customers. Finally, exhibitions are held annually in large cities to show disabled people, vendors, and other rehabilitation personnel the latest equipment and devices to aid the disabled.

RESOURCES

Catalogs

Abbey Medical Catalog Sales
American Hospital Supply Corporation
13782 Crenshaw Blvd.
Gardena, CA 90249

Alimed Inc. Catalog
297 High St.
Dedham, MA 02026

Sammons Preston Catalog
P.O. Box 5071
Bolingbrook, IL 60440

Publications

Schwartzberg JG, Kakavas VK: Guidelines for the Use of Assistive Technology: Education, Referral, Prescription. Chicago: American Medical Association, 1994

Enders A, Hall M (eds): Assistive Technology Sourcebook. Washington, DC, RESNA Press, 1990

Hale G (ed): The Source Book for the Disabled. Philadelphia, WB Saunders, 1979

Redford JB, Basmajian JV, Trautman P (eds): Orthotics, Clinical Practice and Rehabilitation Technology. New York, Churchill Livingstone, 1995

Trombly CA (ed): Occupational Therapy for Physical Dysfunction. Baltimore, Williams & Wilkins, 1983

DeLisa JA (ed): Rehabilitation Medicine: Principles and Practice. Philadelphia, JB Lippincott, 1993

Letts RM: Principles of Seating the Disabled. Boca Raton, FL, CRC Press, 1991

Department of Veterans Affairs: Choosing a wheelchair system. J Rehabil Res Dev Clin Suppl 2, 1986

Council of American Building Officials/American and National Standard Institute Inc.: Accessible and Usable Buildings and Facilities. Falls Church, VA, Council of American Building Officials, 1992

Sources of Information

Arthritis Foundation: Guide to Independent Living for People with Arthritis
The Arthritis Foundation

1314 Spring St. N.W.
Atlanta, GA 30309

National Rehabilitation Information Center
(NARIC)
8455 Colesville Rd. Ste 935
Silver Spring, MD 20916
(800) 346-2742

Accent on Living Buyers Guide 1995
P.O. Box 700
Bloomington, IL 61702
(309) 378-2961

References

1. Manton KG, Corder L, Stallard E: Changes in the use of personal assistance and special equipment from 1982 to 1989: Results from the 1982 and 1989 National Long Term Care Survey. Gerontologist 1993;33:168–176.
2. Mann WC, Tomita M, Packard S, et al: The need for information on assistive devices by older persons. Assistive Technology 1994;6:134–139.
3. Technology-Related Assistance for Individuals with Disabilities Act of 1988, Public Law 100-407 (Technology Act).
4. Blount WP: Don't throw away the cane. J Bone Joint Surg [Am] 1956;38:695.
5. Batavia DI, Hammer CS: Toward the development of consumer-based action for the evaluation of assistive devices. J Rehabil Res Dev 1990;27:419–424.
6. Bohannon R, Mahoney J, Portnow J: Self-help aids for minor disabilities. Patient Care 1994;28:141–148.
7. Varghese G: Crutches, canes, and walkers. *In* Redford JB (ed): Orthotics Etcetera, 3rd ed. Baltimore, Williams & Wilkins, 1986, pp. 453–463.
8. Thacker J, Sprigle S, Morris B: Understanding the Technology when Selecting Wheelchairs. Washington, DC, RESNA Press, 1993.
9. Redford JB: Seating and wheeled mobility in the disabled elderly population. Arch Phys Med Rehabil 1993;74:877–885.
10. Hamilton MR: Why Didn't Somebody Tell Me about These Things? Sherman Oaks, CA, Amyotrophic Lateral Sclerosis Society of America, 1984.

Syndromes in Geriatric Practice

18 Urinary Incontinence

Gabriel H. Brandeis, M.D.

Neil M. Resnick, M.D.

Urinary incontinence is the involuntary loss of urine that leads to a hygienic or social problem.[1] The scope of incontinence is enormous because it afflicts at least 10 million adult Americans. The elderly are especially vulnerable; approximately 15% to 30% of community-dwelling elders, one third of those in acute care settings, and 50% of nursing home residents suffer from urinary incontinence.[2, 3]

Its consequences are far-reaching and must be considered in medical, psychosocial, and economic terms. Medically, urinary incontinence is associated with pressure ulcers, skin irritation, and falls, and occasionally with subsequent fracture.[4] The psychological and social impact can be devastating. Urinary incontinence can lead to anxiety, depression, dependency, embarrassment, and isolation. Activities outside the home, social interactions, and sexual relationships may be severely curtailed, placing stress not only on the individual but also on the caregiver, spouse, family, friends, and health care provider. Furthermore, the presence of incontinence is often a major factor in considering institutionalization.[5]

The monetary costs of managing urinary incontinence in the United States are substantial. In 1994 dollars, the direct costs are conservatively estimated at $16.4 billion per year, divided between $11.2 billion for community-dwelling residents and $5.2 billion for nursing home residents. The financial impact of urinary incontinence is considerable and is 60% greater than it was just 4 years ago.[3, 6]

Although incontinence in the elderly is common, morbid, and costly, it remains a neglected problem, both for those afflicted and for those who care for them. More than 50% of the incontinent elderly do not seek help. Reasons include embarrassment, belief that it is part of aging, an assumption that nothing can be done to correct it, and fear that surgery may be the only option.[5] The reality is that incontinence is not an inevitable consequence of aging. Instead, it is a symptom for which a cause can be determined and for which treatment can be prescribed and may even lead to cure.[3, 4] Because many elderly patients will not discuss this problem, it is incumbent on the clinician to ask specifically if there are any voiding difficulties or involuntary loss of urine.

This chapter briefly reviews the basics of anatomy and physiology of the lower urinary tract, the influence of aging, and the causes of urinary incontinence. Building on this base, detailed information is then provided about diagnosis, therapeutic options, and appropriate consultation, with the overall goal of keeping the individual as independent as possible.

ANATOMY AND PHYSIOLOGY OF THE LOWER URINARY TRACT

Normal Anatomy and Physiology

The anatomy and neurophysiology of normal micturition are complex, and disagreement exists about the finer points.[7, 8] In this chapter, the essentials are reviewed to establish a working knowledge, which then can be applied to gain an understanding of voiding dysfunction and its treatment.

The lower urinary tract consists of three parts—a muscular storage and contractile organ called the detrusor, the essentially smooth muscle sphincter located in the proximal urethra (internal sphincter), and the more distal periurethral striated muscle (external sphincter). The detrusor is smooth muscle that accommodates increasing volume at low intravesical pressure. In men the internal sphincter has no distinct landmarks, and blends with the trigone proximally and the membranous urethra distally. In women it is also ill defined and extends throughout most of the urethra. The external sphincter is well defined, particularly in men, with striated muscle arranged in an annular fashion in the urogenital diaphragm. This sphincter helps to maintain storage of urine and can voluntarily interrupt micturition. Continence is maintained by the compressive properties of the urethra, whose smooth and striated muscle components allow coaption of the submucosal tissue to prevent urinary leakage.

Both the autonomic (sympathetic and parasympathetic) and the somatic (voluntary) nervous systems coordinate micturition. The parasympathetic efferent (cholinergic) nerve fibers emanate from the gray matter of spinal cord segments S2 to S4 and are conveyed by the pelvic nerve to the bladder. The afferent fibers carry pain, temperature, and distention perception from the bladder. Physiologically, cholinergic stimulation increases the force and frequency of bladder contractions[9] (Fig. 18–1).

The sympathetic (adrenergic) nervous system's effect on the lower urinary tract is modulated by the presacral or hypogastric nerve, which emanates from spinal segments T10 to L2 and inner-

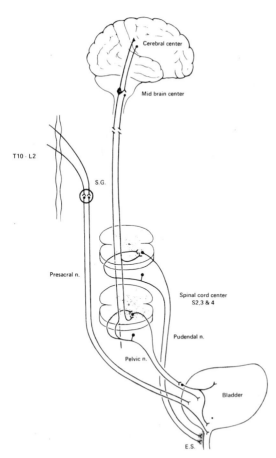

Figure 18–1   Cerebral spinal pathways of micturition. Input from various parts of the brain synapse in the midbrain at the pontine-mesencephalic micturition center. These nerves then synapse in the spinal cord segments S2–S4 and innervate the lower urinary tract. Somatic control from T10–L2 reaches the lower urinary tract via the presacral nerve. (S.G., spinal ganglia; E.S., external sphincter)

vates both the bladder and the urethra. Although beta-adrenergic receptors are predominant in the bladder body or fundus and their stimulation relaxes the detrusor, their numbers in humans are few. On the other hand, the bladder base or trigone, as well as the proximal urethra, is rich in alpha-adrenergic receptors, and their stimulation leads to contraction of the internal sphincter[9] (see Fig. 18–1).

The somatic nerves emanate from spinal cord segments S2 to S4, are carried in the pudendal nerve, and innervate the urogenital diaphragm and external sphincter. Control over micturition resides at higher central nervous system sites. The pontine micturition center coordinates detrusor contraction with sphincter relaxation. Higher central nervous system sites, including the cerebellum, basal ganglia, and frontal lobe, seem to function in an inhibitory mode.[9]

In summary, the normal bladder fills passively with little change in intravesical pressure, and the sphincters remain closed. Filling is facilitated by central nervous system inhibition of parasympathetic activity. Concurrently, reflex increases in alpha-adrenergic and somatic tone maintain sphincter closure. For voiding to occur, a parasympathetic-mediated bladder contraction must coincide with coordinated sphincter relaxation.

Changes with Aging

Detailed studies of aging changes associated with the lower urinary tract are still scarce. Nevertheless, available data indicate that bladder capacity, contractility, and the ability to postpone voiding decrease with age in both men and women, and urethral closure pressure and length decrease in women. In both sexes, the prevalence of involuntary bladder contractions, bacteriuria, and postvoiding residual volume all increase. Although the bladder should empty completely, a 50- to 100-mL postvoid residual can be still considered normal. Prostatic size increases with age in men. In both sexes, fluid excretion patterns change, so that the elderly may excrete most of their ingested fluid during the night, leading to nocturia. Consequently, up to two episodes of nocturia may be considered normal and do not necessarily indicate the presence of a specific disease.[10] When electron microscopy is used to examine bladder biopsy specimens in the elderly, a unique "dense band pattern" of sacrolemmal bands with depleted caveolae is seen.[11] This aging change may be the reason for the decrease in bladder contractility. In addition, the bladder smooth muscle cells can form scattered protrusion junctions, named a "dysjunction pattern."[11]

These changes may be the cause of increased uninhibited contractions in the elderly.

Although urinary incontinence is not a result of aging, each of these factors predisposes a person to incontinence because the overall reserve capacity of an individual is reduced. It must be emphasized that incontinence in the elderly is usually multifactorial, and factors from outside the lower urinary tract often contribute to it. For example, functional status (ability to transfer and dress independently) and medical conditions (Parkinson's disease, dementia, stroke, and diabetes) have been independently associated with the presence of incontinence.[12] These factors, especially when coupled with the additional stress of an acute illness, can cause incontinence.

Incontinence can thus be divided into broad categories—transient, in which alleviation of the stressor can improve or eliminate incontinence, and established, in which no readily identifiable stressor is found.

TYPES OF URINARY INCONTINENCE

Transient Incontinence

Transient incontinence is often acute in onset and is the result of non–lower urinary tract illness; reversal of the illness frequently resolves the incontinence. A mnemonic to aid in remembering transient causes is Resnick's DIAPPERS (*d*elirium, *i*nfection, *a*trophic urethritis or vaginitis, *p*harmaceutical, *p*sychologic, *e*xcessive urinary output, *r*educed mobility, and *s*tool impaction).[2] The primary care provider who is caring for the elderly should become adept at diagnosing and treating these transient causes.

Delirium or acute confusion can result from hospitalization, an acute illness (e.g., pneumonia or myocardial infarction), or medication. The delirium interferes with a person's ability to care for his or her needs, including toileting. As the delirium clears, the incontinence should improve. *Symptomatic infection* of the urinary tract can precipitate incontinence, but asymptomatic bacteriuria cannot. Treatment should restore continence. *Atrophic urethritis or vaginitis*, due to decreasing estrogen effects with age, is common in elderly women. It is identifiable on examination by vaginal mucosal dryness, friability, and telangiectasia; estrogen replacement therapy is effective for this condition. However, estrogen replacement must be considered in relation to the other body systems this hormone affects.

Pharmaceuticals, both prescription and over-the-counter, should always be considered as a possible contributor to incontinence in the elderly. Table 18–1 lists the categories of medications that may contribute to incontinence, their site of action, and their potential effect on continence. Often the offending medication is not readily apparent, and, whenever possible, discontinuing or changing a suspected drug or dosing schedule should be attempted.

Psychological causes of incontinence, although

TABLE 18–1 **MEDICATIONS IMPLICATED IN ALTERING CONTINENCE IN THE ELDERLY**

Class of Medication	Site of Action	Mechanism	Potential Consequences
Adrenergic agent			
Alpha-agonist	Prostatic urethra	Increase urethral closing pressure	Urinary retention
Alpha-antagonist	Urethra in women	Decrease urethral closing pressure	Stress leakage
Anticholinergic agent	Detrusor	Decrease bladder contractility; some also lead to confusion, rigidity, immobility	Urinary retention, overflow incontinence
Neuroleptic			
Tricyclic antidepressant			
Antiparkinsonian			
Antispasmodic			
Antiarrhythmic			
Opiate			
Calcium-channel blocker	Detrusor	Decrease bladder contraction	Urinary retention
Diuretic	Renal	Increase bladder volume	Urgency, incontinence
Sedative/hypnotic			
Benzodiazepine	CNS	Delirium, sedation, immobility	Urgency, incontinence
Alcohol	CNS, renal	Delirium, sedation, diuresis	Frequency, urgency, incontinence

Abbreviation: CNS, central nervous system.

rare, include depression, in which the individual no longer cares about remaining dry, or attention-getting or manipulative behavior. *Excessive urine output* can be caused by large fluid consumption, diuretic therapy, alcohol, or mobilization of fluid resulting from pedal edema or congestive heart failure. In addition, metabolic conditions leading to hypercalcemia or hyperglycemia can lead to polyuria, which may overwhelm the bladder.

Restricted mobility, common in the elderly, lengthens the time required to reach the bathroom. The causes of decreased mobility are often multifactorial and include arthritis, fear of falling, visual impairment, cardiac disease, and physical or chemical restraints. *Stool* or fecal impaction is a common problem, especially in bedbound elderly (in either acute or chronic settings). The mechanism by which fecal impaction results in loss of continence has not been fully elucidated, but it may involve opioid receptor stimulation.[13] Clearing the impaction restores continence.

If the preceding factors have been investigated and continence is not restored, attention must be directed to the established causes.

Established Causes

Functional incontinence has traditionally been defined as incontinence that exists when the lower urinary tract function is presumed to be intact and outside influences contribute to the incontinence. For example, impaired mobility or severe dementia in an elderly person may hinder the person's ability to reach the bathroom in time, resulting in urinary leakage. However, the lower urinary tract is rarely completely intact, and the functional impairment may just overwhelm the individual's ability to compensate. Therefore, this type of incontinence should be thought of as a functional impairment that contributes to rather than causes incontinence.[2]

Although established or persistent forms of incontinence have been classified in different ways (e.g., urge incontinence or detrusor overactivity), the basic pathophysiology remains the same. The abnormality resides in either the bladder or the urethral outlet, or both. The bladder may contract prematurely (detrusor overactivity) or too weakly (detrusor underactivity). Urethral outlet resistance may be inappropriately increased (obstruction) or inappropriately decreased (incompetent). The underlying cause of each type of incontinence may be neurogenic or non-neurogenic. Combinations of each type may also exist in the elderly. An understanding of the four types allows the physician to focus the history and physical examination to establish the diagnoses and prescribe initial treatment.

Detrusor overactivity, which is usually the mechanism underlying urge incontinence, is the most common cause of established geriatric incontinence. It occurs when inhibition of bladder contractions is impaired and the bladder contracts precipitantly, leading to urinary leakage. The patient feels a sudden, strong desire to void, which is associated with involuntary loss of urine. Usually a moderate to large amount of urine is lost, but a small amount does not preclude this diagnosis. Detrusor overactivity may also be associated with nocturia and frequent, periodic incontinent episodes. If the person has a neurologic lesion, detrusor overactivity is termed *detrusor hyperreflexia;* if no neurologic lesion is detected, it is termed *detrusor instability.* Detrusor overactivity is an intrinsic bladder phenomenon. At the cellular level, bladder smooth muscle cells form abnormal "protrusion junctions," which are hypothesized to allow electrical conduction between cells, resulting in involuntary detrusor contractions.[14] Local bladder pathology such as a urinary tract infection, carcinoma, or stones may also cause the bladder to contract involuntarily. Abnormalities of the urethral outlet (obstruction or incompetence) are considered secondary causes because correction of the urethral abnormality leads to reversal of the detrusor overactivity in most younger adults; similar data are not yet available for older patients. Detrusor overactivity can also be divided into two subsets based on detrusor contractility. The first type is detrusor overactivity with normal contractility (i.e., the bladder is able to empty most of its contents), and the second is detrusor hyperactivity with impaired contractility (DHIC), in which the bladder cannot empty and usually more than 100 mL of urine remains after an involuntary contraction.[15]

Detrusor underactivity occurs when the bladder's contractile capacity is so reduced that overflow incontinence ensues. It differs from detrusor overactivity in that in the latter condition, the bladder contracts without the patient's awareness, whereas the underactive detrusor contracts (if at all) only when the patient tries to void. Detrusor underactivity is uncommon in the geriatric population. It may be neurogenic in origin due to nerve damage from diabetes mellitus, alcohol, tabes dorsalis, or vertebral disease, or it may be secondary to long-standing obstruction. At the cellular level, degeneration of both smooth muscle and nerves is seen.[11]

Outlet incompetence, or stress incontinence, is common in women. The patient notes involuntary loss of urine during physical activity or coughing, for example. Usually the leakage is small in amount and is rare in the supine position. It is usually due to weakening of the supporting structures of the pelvic floor or, less commonly, to damage or incompetence of the urethral sphincter itself. Although uncommon in men, stress incontinence can occur after transurethral surgery or radiation therapy that damages the anatomic sphincter.

Urethral obstruction is a common cause of incontinence in elderly men.[4] It may lead to urinary retention and bladder distention with overflow incontinence, postvoid dribbling, or urge incontinence due to associated detrusor overactivity. Non-neurologic causes include prostatic hyperplasia, medications (e.g., an alpha-adrenergic agonist), tumors, and strictures. Spinal cord lesions are neurologic causes. An important but uncommon type of outlet obstruction is detrusor-sphincter dyssynergia, in which the sphincter contracts inappropriately or remains closed instead of relaxing normally and opening when the bladder contracts.

Mixed incontinence is present when a combination of the preceding types exists. Most often it is a combination of detrusor overactivity and outlet incompetence.

CLINICAL ASSESSMENT

Once the preceding causes are understood, the clinical evaluation can be tailored to gather the appropriate information to establish a diagnosis. Clinical assessment of patients with urinary incontinence requires a complete history, physical examination, and laboratory tests. The goals of the evaluation include (1) identification and treatment of the transient causes of incontinence, (2) detection of any serious underlying condition (e.g., brain or spinal cord lesions, bladder stones, bladder or prostate carcinoma, hydronephrosis, or poor bladder compliance), and (3) determination of the lower urinary tract cause of established incontinence to the extent that it affects therapy.[16] Additional laboratory tests, specialized studies, or urodynamics and consultation may be needed in selected cases. Since the information needed is comprehensive, the evaluation may require several visits.

The *history* of the incontinence should be obtained from the patient or caregivers. It should include information about onset, precipitating factors, frequency, volume, dysuria, straining, feeling of incomplete emptying, daily pattern of voiding, medications, surgery, and previous attempts to treat the incontinence. The severity of the problem should be ascertained because evaluation and treatment options may be altered

according to the degree of interference with the patient's daily life. The history should also include any related illnesses such as stroke, spinal cord injury, immobility, or diabetes. Information on functional status and how the person copes with the problem (e.g., use of sanitary napkins or knowledge of every bathroom in town) can be revealing.

The voiding diary is an essential component of the history. It need not be complex and may be completed by the patient or caregiver. It should be kept for a minimum of 48 hours and should have four columns: (1) *time* of each void or leakage noted; (2) measured *volume* of urine volitionally voided; (3) *estimate* of the volume of each incontinent episode (mild, moderate, severe); and (4) *comments* such as the number of pads used or any activities that provoked the leak.[17]

Information from the history and voiding diary and determination of the presence of precipitancy or stress leakage usually allow the physician to establish the probable diagnosis and devise a treatment plan. For example, if the history reveals that a woman leaks only when coughing and laughing, is dry at night, and voids 200 mL in the morning on awakening, a diagnosis of stress incontinence should be entertained. If the voiding diary reveals nocturia in a person with pedal edema or congestive heart failure (and the majority of fluid is excreted during the night), a diuretic taken in the afternoon or early evening may decrease night-time fluid shifts and resultant voids.

The *physical examination* should focus on the neurologic aspects of the problem, including the patient's mental status and the status of sacral nerve segments S2 to S4 (bulbocavernosus and anal wink reflexes and resting and volitional anal sphincter tone and control). The presence of either the anal wink or bulbocavernosus reflex establishes the integrity of the motor innervation of the external urethral sphincter and the anal sphincter because both are innervated by the same sacral roots. The anal wink reflex is assessed by pricking or scratching the skin of the perianal area and noting whether an immediate contraction ("winking") of the external anal sphincter occurs. The bulbocavernosus reflex is elicited during the rectal examination either by pinching the glans penis or by gently stroking the clitoris and feeling contraction of the external anal sphincter.

In addition, the physical examination should concentrate on such medical aspects as congestive heart failure or pedal edema, functional abilities such as mobility and dexterity, a rectal examination for fecal impaction, and a pelvic examination to detect atrophic vaginitis. The size of the prostate on rectal examination correlates poorly with outlet obstruction, and the presence or absence of a cystocele correlates poorly with the cause of leakage.[17] If indicated, a clinical stress test should be performed. The patient should be as upright as possible and should have a full bladder and a relaxed pelvic musculature; he or she should then be asked to cough vigorously. If immediate leakage is seen, the test is positive for stress incontinence. The test should reproduce the patient's clinical symptoms. A negative test, when performed properly, is specific for ruling out stress incontinence. The void should be observed for straining, strength, and interruption of stream, and a postvoid residual (PVR) should be obtained by catheterization or bladder ultrasound. If the residual volume is greater than 100 mL, bladder weakness or retention should be considered.

Basic *laboratory tests* recommended for each patient include a urinalysis and serum creatinine or blood urea nitrogen. If indicated, other tests such as a urine culture, serum glucose, and cytology may be obtained.

Although the next step in the assessment is somewhat controversial, a stepped noninvasive approach seems to be most appropriate. First, overflow incontinence should be considered if the PVR exceeds 450 mL. Depending on the patient's overall condition, referral for further testing may be appropriate; alternatively, it may make more sense merely to place an indwelling catheter to reduce the high residual urine and reduce the risk of infection and hydronephrosis. Fortunately, overflow is rare, especially in women, in whom urethral obstruction is uncommon. Therefore, in women, differentiation between stress incontinence and detrusor overactivity must be made. In men, stress incontinence is uncommon in the absence of previous urethral surgery. Thus, the differential diagnosis in men is usually between urethral obstruction and detrusor overactivity. If the PVR exceeds 200 mL, hydronephrosis must be excluded. Regardless of the result, referral for surgery should be considered if clinically appropriate. For the others, empirical treatment for detrusor overactivity with close monitoring of the PVR can be prescribed. The same process can be employed for nursing home residents, as outlined in the resident assessment protocol (RAP) for urinary incontinence associated with the Minimum Data Set (MDS).[18]

Consultation for *specialized tests* or *urodynamics* may be needed if treatment without definitive diagnosis would be deleterious to the patient, for example, an elderly man with symptoms of urgency, frequency, leakage of a moderate amount of urine, and a PVR of 100 mL. While this description is consistent with outlet obstruction, it is also consistent with detrusor overactivity. If the man undergoes prostatectomy, for example, to relieve the presumed obstruction and the diagnosis is incorrect, the incontinence may become worse. Conversely, if an incorrect diagnosis of detrusor overactivity is made and anticholinergic treatment (discussed later) is prescribed, urinary retention may result. In cases like this, consideration should be given to urodynamic evaluation. Urodynamics include a cystometrogram (to evaluate bladder function during filling, not voiding), which is optimally performed with simultaneous measurement of abdominal pressure; uroflowmetry (to evaluate urine flow); urethral profilometry (to evaluate urethral function); and radiographic monitoring. Complex invasive urodynamic investigation is feasible and safe in the elderly in the hands of an experienced laboratory.[15] Bedside cystometry has been described but requires caution to avoid misdiagnosis.[19] Since bedside cystometry depends on large changes in bladder pressure, it will miss subtle pressure changes as seen in detrusor hyperactivity with impaired contractility. Furthermore, it may detect uninhibited contractions that may not be related to the cause of the incontinence.[2]

TREATMENT

The treatment program must be individually tailored to the patient and the pathophysiology. For example, pelvic floor muscle exercises (Kegel exercises) may be tried for a cognitively intact woman with stress incontinence, but they are inappropriate for women with considerable dementia. A stepwise approach to therapy is discussed in the following sections and is outlined in Table 18–2.

Transient Incontinence

Treatment of the underlying condition cures the incontinence. Some patients, such as those with delirium, must be supported while the underlying illness resolves, and management may include scheduled toileting and use of disposable or absorbent undergarments and condom catheters for men.

Detrusor Overactivity

Several treatment options exist for a diagnosis of detrusor overactivity. Behavioral measures, such as bladder training or prompted voiding,[20, 21] should be tried initially. For the cognitively intact

TABLE 18–2 **STEPPED APPROACH TO TREATMENT OF URINARY INCONTINENCE**

Condition	Clinical Type of Incontinence[a]	Treatment
Detrusor overactivity with normal contractility	Urge	1. Bladder retraining ± biofeedback or prompted voiding techniques 2. ± Bladder relaxant medication, if needed and not contraindicated 3. Indwelling catheterization alone often leads to bladder "spasm" and leakage around the catheter 4. If needed, induce urinary retention pharmacologically and add intermittent or indwelling catheterization[b]
Detrusor hyperactivity with impaired contractility	Urge[c]	1. If bladder empties adequately with straining, use behavioral methods ± bladder relaxant medication (see text) 2. If PVR > 150 mL, use augmented voiding techniques[d] or intermittent catheterization (± bladder relaxant medication). If neither is feasible, use undergarment or indwelling catheter[b]
Stress incontinence	Stress	1. Conservative methods (weight loss if obese; treatment of cough or atrophic vaginitis; physical maneuvers [cross legs, tighten pelvic muscles]; rarely, pessary) 2. If leakage threshold ≥150 mL, adjust fluid excretion and voiding intervals 3. Pelvic muscle exercises ± biofeedback and weighted intravaginal cones 4. Imipramine (or doxepin) or alpha-agonist ± estrogen if not contraindicated 5. Surgery, periurethral bulking injections, artificial sphincter
Urethral obstruction	Urge or overflow[e]	1. Conservative methods (fluid excretion adjustment, bladder retraining or prompted voiding) if hydronephrosis, elevated PVR, recurrent symptomatic UTI, and gross hematuria have been excluded 2. Bladder relaxants if DO coexists, PVR is small, and surgery is not desired or feasible 3. Alpha-adrenergic antagonists, finasteride, antiandrogens, and/or LHRH analogs as appropriate and the patient either prefers them or is not a surgical candidate 4. Surgery (incision, prostatectomy)
Underactive detrusor	Overflow	1. If duration is unknown, use decompression for several weeks and perform a voiding trial 2. If patient cannot void, PVR remains large, or retention is chronic, try augmented voiding methods[d] ± alpha-adrenergic antagonist, but only if some voiding is possible; bethanechol is rarely useful unless bladder weakness is due to an anticholinergic agent that cannot be discontinued 3. If these measures fail, or if voiding is not impossible, try intermittent or indwelling catheterization[b]

Adapted from: Resnick NM: Voiding dysfunction and urinary incontinence. *In* Beck JC (ed): Geriatric Review Syllabus. New York, American Geriatrics Society, 1991, pp. 141–154; and Resnick NM: Urinary incontinence. Lancet 1995;346:94–99.

Treatment should be initiated only after adequate toilet access has been ensured, contributing conditions have been treated (e.g., atrophic vaginitis, heart failure), fluid management has been achieved, and unnecessary or exacerbating medications have been discontinued. For additional details, see text.

[a] Urge, leakage in absence of stress maneuvers and urinary retention, usually preceded by abrupt onset of need to void; stress, leakage that coincides instantaneously with stress maneuvers, in absence of urinary retention; overflow, frequent leakage of small amounts associated with urinary retention.

[b] Prophylaxis can be used for recurrent symptomatic UTI, but only if catheter is not indwelling.

[c] But may also mimic stress or overflow incontinence.

[d] Augmented voiding techniques include Credé and Valsalva maneuvers (see text for details). They should be performed only after commencement of voiding.

[e] Also can cause postvoid "dribbling" alone, which is treated conservatively (e.g., by sitting to void and allowing more time, "double voiding," and gently "milking" the urethra after voiding).

Abbreviations: PVR, postvoid residual; UTI, urinary tract infection; DO, detrusor overactivity; LHRH, luteinizing hormone–releasing hormone.

person, *bladder retraining* with or without biofeedback can be attempted. To begin this technique, the person voids at a time interval that is smaller than the incontinent interval shown in the voiding diary. If leakage occurs every 3 hours, the person should void every 2 hours while awake and should resist the desire to void in between. (There is no need to schedule voids at night.) Once incontinence improves, the interval between scheduled voids is progressively increased by half an hour until an interval of 3 to 4 hours is reached. This should allow adequate dry time between voids for most activities.[20] For the demented patient in a nursing home, *prompted voiding* can be tried. With this technique, residents are asked on a regular schedule (usually every 2 hours) whether they need to void. They are toileted if they respond affirmatively, and positive reinforcement is provided. Using this method, 40% of residents demonstrated improvement.[21] Residents who respond within 3 days of initiation of the program are most likely to benefit; for those who do not, prompted voiding should be discontinued.[22]

Anticholinergic or smooth muscle relaxants may be added to reduce the involuntary contractions of the overactive detrusor and increase the volume needed to elicit the involuntary contraction. These medications have systemic anticholinergic side effects (xerostomia, confusion, constipation, urinary retention), especially if outflow obstruction or impaired contractility coexists. Propantheline (15 to 30 mg tid to qid taken on an empty stomach) is a commonly used anticholinergic agent, but its toxic-therapeutic ratio may be less favorable in older individuals. Oxybutynin (2.5 to 5 mg qd to qid) and dicyclomine (10 to 30 mg tid to qid) have both anticholinergic and smooth muscle relaxant properties. Tricyclic antidepressants, particularly imipramine and doxepin (25 to 50 mg tid), have also been employed, although their exact mechanism of action is unknown.[23] Along with anticholinergic side effects, imipramine can cause orthostatic hypotension and confusion. Calcium-channel blockers have also been tried.[23] Frequently, the choice of medication in the elderly is influenced by other factors. For instance, if an incontinent patient needs treatment for angina or hypertension, a calcium-channel blocker could be used. For patients whose incontinence cannot be controlled by these methods, an indwelling catheter may be considered. However, this option entails a serious analysis of the risk-benefit ratio.

Detrusor Hyperactivity with Impaired Contractility

Using detrusor hyperactivity with impaired contractility as an example, an important treatment principle must be noted. Medications, especially those with anticholinergic or bladder relaxant properties, can lead to urinary retention. Although retention can occur in any case, the practitioner must be especially vigilant in patients with detrusor hyperactivity with impaired contractility because contractility in such patients is compromised prior to initiation of therapy. Thus, if the bladder empties adequately (with augmented voiding—straining or Credé maneuver, in which the hand applies pressure over the lower abdomen), and the PVR is low, behavioral methods with or without bladder relaxant therapy should be used. If the PVR is more than 150 mL and concomitant stress incontinence is absent, bladder training should be attempted first. It can be augmented with intermittent straight catheterization with or without judicious use of bladder relaxants. If stress incontinence is present, bladder training should be tried initially, with bladder relaxant medications added if needed. If the PVR increases in this situation, the Credé maneuver will decrease it, thereby reducing the leakage due to stress incontinence.[24] If these techniques are not feasible, pads, undergarments, or an indwelling catheter can be used.

Stress Incontinence

Outlet incompetence is manifested by stress incontinence, which can be treated nonsurgically or surgically. Nonsurgical therapy includes weight loss if the patient is obese, behavioral techniques such as pelvic muscle (Kegel) exercises, use of vaginal cones, and biofeedback to enhance urine storage.[25-27] In addition, if stress leakage occurs when bladder volume is above a certain amount, as evidenced by the voiding diary or clinical examination, this leakage can be minimized by adjusting the fluid intake and voiding frequency. Although these techniques have minimal adverse effects, a great deal of motivation and effort on the part of the patient is needed. Drug therapy can be tried using estrogen alone (especially in patients with atrophic urethritis or vaginitis) or an alpha-agonist such as sustained-release phenylpropanolamine (25 to 100 mg bid) or pseudoephedrine (15 to 30 mg bid to tid). Estrogen (0.3 to 0.625 mg qd or as a vaginal cream, one application qod) has been shown to be effective for urgency, frequency, nocturia, and dysuria; elderly women seem to prefer the oral formulation. The use of estrogen must be considered in light of its risk-benefit profile in elderly women.[3, 28] Side effects of alpha-agonists include tachycardia, hypertension, anxiety, and insomnia.

Periurethral bulking agents, which are injected into the urethra to increase the ability of the sphincter to coapt, are now available and may be appropriate in selected cases. Urethral plugs are now being developed; they require a high degree of manual dexterity to insert. Surgical techniques are successful in managing stress incontinence and have a 70% to 90% 1-year success rate, although success rates decline thereafter.[3] Several procedures exist and should be considered regardless of the patient's age.

Urethral Obstruction

Obstruction of the urethra can present as urge, postvoid dribbling, or overflow incontinence. Because of prostatic enlargement, strictures, or carcinoma, it is more common in men, but up to 5% of incontinence in women is caused by obstruction[10] resulting from a large cystocele, stricture, or meatal stenosis. Conservative therapy, including bladder retraining and prompted voiding, can be used if hydronephrosis, high PVR, recurrent urinary tract infection, and hematuria are not present. Surgical correction is feasible, even in the infirm, to prevent urinary retention, which predisposes an individual to urosepsis, hydronephrosis, and renal failure. If surgical therapy is not an option, alpha-adrenergic blockers such as prazosin, terazosin, or doxazosin (in a dosage titrated according to symptoms and blood pressure) decrease tone in the prostatic capsule and urethra and are often efficacious, especially if prostatism is the cause of the obstruction.[29] Finasteride can be tried, but its benefits are less impressive, occur less often, and take many months to achieve. As a last resort, intermittent catheterization or an indwelling catheter can be used.

Detrusor Underactivity

The patient with detrusor underactivity generally has a large PVR and overflow leakage. The goal is to reduce the urine in the bladder to decrease incontinence and to prevent hydronephrosis and urosepsis. First, a trial of indwelling or intermittent catheterization should be undertaken to decompress the bladder, allowing it to recover its contractile ability. Since intermittent catheterization is often not feasible in the elderly, an indwelling catheter should be placed and should remain for a minimum of 2 weeks. It should then be removed to see if voiding recurs. If not, the catheter can be reinserted for 4 weeks and a voiding trial attempted again. The Credé and Valsalva (straining) maneuvers can also be tried in an attempt to induce or augment bladder contractions. An alpha-adrenergic antagonist can be tried but only if the patient can initiate void-

ing. Bethanechol, a cholinergic agonist, can be tried (10 to 50 mg qid) but is rarely effective. If these maneuvers do not restore voiding, long-term intermittent catheterization or an indwelling catheter is needed.

Mixed Incontinence

Many women show evidence of two kinds of incontinence—urge incontinence and stress incontinence. To determine the predominant cause, urodynamic testing may be necessary. If this is unavailable, empirical treatment based on clinical acumen can be started. Often, treatment that addresses the predominant type of incontinence substantially improves the patient's condition. However, the patient has to be monitored closely in case the selected treatment worsens the incontinence or leads to deleterious side effects.

Functional Incontinence

In patients with normal lower urinary tract function, adjunctive measures are needed.

ADJUNCTIVE THERAPY

If an indwelling urethral catheter is used to prevent skin breakdown, for example, bacteriuria is inevitable and can lead to significant illness and death. If possible, indwelling catheters are best avoided. Self-intermittent catheterization is difficult for the elderly, and catheterization by the caregiver may not be frequent enough to achieve the goal of dryness. Men can use a condom catheter, but it may cause skin irritation or bacteriuria or may be continually dislodged. Female external collection devices exist but are not perfected.[30]

Absorbent pads, garments, and environmental manipulation are extremely helpful in the management of incontinence if it proves refractory to other measures. However, they should not be prescribed as definitive therapy in lieu of a complete investigation, when feasible. During evaluation and after the diagnosis has been confirmed, these products are often excellent adjunctive measures. Because they are unaware of or bewildered by the over-the-counter products available, many elderly women resort to sanitary napkins, facial tissue, or towels to cope with their incontinence. For instance, a disposable pad in a specially designed pant may be useful for small amounts of leakage, while a disposable diaper may be useful for larger amounts.[31] Many products exist, and details about them can be obtained from Help for Incontinent People* or the Simon Foundation.† Changes in the environment, including elevated toilet seats, grab bars, commodes, or hand-held urinals, may allow better access for an elderly person.

SUMMARY

Urinary incontinence in the elderly is prevalent, costly, and ignored. Although it is not part of normal aging, age-related changes predispose the elderly to incontinence, which leads to stigmatization, loss of independence, and medical illness. The majority of afflicted individuals have had no evaluation. Fortunately, most cases of incontinence can be cured or improved, and every person should be evaluated, first for transient causes and then, if the incontinence persists, for established causes. Insight and information allow the health care provider to alleviate most of the unpleasantness associated with incontinence, if not the incontinence itself.

References

1. Abrams P, Blaivas JG, Stanton SL, Anderson JT: The standardization of terminology of lower urinary tract function. Neurourol Urodynam 1988; 7:403–428.
2. Resnick NM: Urinary incontinence. Lancet 1995; 346:94–100.
3. Fantl JA, Newman DK, Colling J, et al: Urinary incontinence in adults: Acute and chronic management. Clinical Practice Guideline, No. 2, 1996 update. AHCPR Publication No. 96-0682 Rockville, MD; U.S. Department of Health and Human Services, Public Health Service, Agency for Health Care Policy and Research, 1996.
4. Resnick NM, Yalla SV: Management of urinary incontinence in the elderly. N Engl J Med 1985; 313:800–805.
5. Wyman JF, Hawkins SW, Fantl JA: Psychosocial input of urinary incontinence in the community dwelling population. J Am Geriatr Soc 1990;38:282–288.
6. Hu TW: Impact of urinary incontinence on health care costs. J Am Geriatr Soc 1990;38:292–295.
7. Elbadawi A: Neuromuscular mechanics of micturition. In Yalla SV, McGuire EF, et al (eds): Neurourology and Urodynamics: Principles and Practice. New York, Macmillan, 1988, pp. 3–35.
8. Wein AJ: Clinical neuropharmacology of the lower urinary tract. In Yalla SV, McGuire EF, et al (eds): Neurourology and Urodynamics: Principles and Practice. New York, Macmillan, 1988, pp. 377–398.
9. Mattiason A: Bladder and urethral physiology and pathophysiology. In Krane RJ, Siroky MB, Fitzpatrick JM, (eds): Clinical Urology. Philadelphia, JB Lippincott, 1994, pp. 536–557.
10. Resnick NM: Voiding dysfunction in the elderly. In Yalla SV, McGuire EF, et al (eds): Neurourology and Urodynamics: Principles and Practice. New York, Macmillan, 1988, pp. 303–330.
11. Elbadawi A, Yalla SV, Resnick NM: Structural basis of geriatric voiding dysfunction II: Aging detrusor: normal vs. impaired contractility. J Urol 1993;150:1657–1667.
12. Resnick NM, Baumann MM, Scott M, et al: Risk factors for incontinence in the nursing home: A multivariate study. Neurourol Urodynam 1988; 7:274–276.
13. Hellstrom PM, Sjoquist A: Involvement of opioid and nicotinic receptors in rectal and anal reflex inhibition of urinary bladder motility in cats. Acta Physiol Scan 1988; 133:559–562.
14. Elbadawi A, Yalla SV, Resnick NM: Structural basis of geriatric voiding dysfunction III: Detrusor overactivity. J Urol 1993;150:1668–1680.
15. Resnick NM, Yalla SV: Detrusor hyperactivity with impaired contractile function. JAMA 1987; 257:3076–3081.
16. Resnick NM: Noninvasive diagnosis of the patient with complex incontinence. Gerontology 1990;36 (Suppl 2):8–18.
17. Resnick NM: Voiding dysfunction and urinary incontinence. In Cassel CK, Riesenberg DE, et al (eds): Geriatric Medicine. New York, Springer, 1990, pp. 510–518.
18. Resnick NM, Baumann MM: Long-Term Care Facility Resident Assessment Instrument (RAI) User's Manual (version 2.0). Washington, DC, Health Care Financing Administration, 1995, pp. 3-105–3-110; C-27–C-35.
19. Resnick NM, Brandeis GH, Baumann MM, DuBeau CD, Yalla SV: Misdiagnosis of urinary incontinence in nursing home women: Prevalence and a proposed solution. Neurourol Urodynam 1996;15:599–618.
20. Fantl JA, Wyman JF, Hawkins SW, Hadley EC: Bladder training in the management of lower urinary tract dysfunction in women. J Am Geriatr Soc 1990; 38:329–332.
21. Schnelle JF: Treatment of urinary incontinence in nursing home patients by prompted voiding. J Am Geriatr Soc 1990;38:356–360.
22. Ouslander JG, Schnelle JF, Uman G, Fingold S, Nigam JG, et al: Predictors of successful prompted voiding among incontinent nursing home residents. JAMA 1995;273:1366–1370.
23. Wein AJ: Pharmacologic treatment of incontinence. Urol Clin North Am 1995;22:557–579.
24. Resnick NM, Yalla SV, Laurino D: The pathophysiology of urinary incontinence among institutionalized elderly persons. N Engl J Med 1989;320:1–7.
25. Wells TJ: Pelvic (floor) muscle exercise. J Am Geriatr Soc 1990;38:333–337.
26. Burgio KC, Engel BT: Biofeedback-assisted behavioral training for elderly men and women. J Am Geriatr Soc 1990;38:338–340.
27. Burns PA, Pranikoff K, Nochajski TH, Hadley EC, Levy KJ, Ory MG: A comparison of effectiveness of biofeedback and pelvic muscle exercise treatment of stress incontinence in older community-dwelling women. J Gerontol 1993;48:M167–M174.
28. Cardozo L: Role of estrogens in the treatment of female urinary incontinence. J Am Geriatr Soc 1990; 38:326–328.
29. Oesterling JE: Benign prostatic hyperplasia: Medical and minimally invasive treatment options. N Engl J Med 1995;332:99–109.
30. Warren JW: Urine collection devices for use in adults with urinary incontinence. J Am Geriatr Soc 1990;38: 364–367.
31. Brink CA: Pads, undergarments, and management strategies. J Am Geriatr Soc 1990;38:368–373.

---

*Help for Incontinent People (HIP), PO Box 544, Union, SC 29379; telephone (803) 579-7900.

†Simon Foundation, 3621 Thayer Road, Evanston, IL 60201; telephone (800) 23-SIMON.

19 Instability and Falls

Stephanie Studenski, M.D., M.P.H.
Lynda Wolter, M.D.

Instability and falls can be markers of generally poor health or declining function.[1] Falls may have serious physical and psychological consequences, including injury, hospitalization, impaired mobility, restricted activity, functional decline, nursing home placement, and fear of falling again. A person who is unsteady but does not actually fall may still restrict his or her activity, resulting in reduced mobility, less independent function, and social isolation. Thus, instability without actual falls is still a serious problem. The ultimate goals of care for these patients are to improve function and prevent injury through a systematic evaluation of the causes of instability. Because many cases of instability and falls in older people are due to multiple interacting problems, management approaches should be multifactorial. Three key strategies are to identify reversible causes, treat modifiable impairments, and adapt to fixed disabilities.

BACKGROUND

Epidemiology

One third of community-dwelling elders and half of nursing home residents fall each year. Falls are the leading cause of accidental death in older persons. One percent of those who fall fracture a hip, 5% sustain another fracture, 5% incur a serious soft tissue injury,[2] and 2% are hospitalized.[3] Hip fracture is a leading cause of morbidity and mortality; 200,000 hip fractures occur each year. A fifth of the victims die within 6 months, and another fifth are admitted to nursing homes. Hip fracture results in a 10% to 15% decrease in life expectancy, and costs are higher than $1 billion per year.[4, 5]

The risk of an injury with falling depends on both susceptibility and exposure. Exposure to high-intensity forces at impact is potentially higher in more active persons. A less active person's risk of injury depends more on susceptibility, that is, the presence of fragile bones or ineffective protective responses.[4] Falls and injuries in frail elders tend to occur within the home during routine activities. Vigorous elders may be more likely to fall and injure themselves while away from home, during dynamic activities, or while negotiating stairs or other environmental hazards.[6] Although the consequences of falls and injuries have been described extensively, the impact of instability and fear of falling in older persons who have not fallen is unknown.[7]

Postural Control Theory

Balance is the ability to remain upright in motion. From a biomechanical perspective, balance is achieved by continuously controlling the displacement of the body's center of mass over a moving base of support. The mass is usually a tall narrow column in the upright human, and the base of support, represented as the two-dimensional contact area between the body and the support surface, is often the area between the two feet. This biomechanical task adapts to constantly changing conditions. For example, the base of support changes in size from a rectangle enclosing both feet while standing to the area under one foot while walking. The center of mass can project directly over the base of support to produce a stable body, called "static equilibrium." To move from one place to another, the mass projection must move outside the base of support, and the body must quickly relocate the base under the moving mass. Such conditions are not stable on a second-to-second basis; thus walking is sometimes called "controlled falling," and movement really represents a dynamic equilibrium.[8]

The postural control system organizes this biomechanical task. The system uses multiple sensory inputs to continuously determine the body's position and trajectory in space, a central nervous system to integrate the sensory information and organize rapid responses, and effector systems such as muscles and joints to carry out the instructions of the central nervous system. The three sensory systems are vision, somatosensation, and vestibular function. The central nervous system uses automatic postural responses to provide rapid reactions. Automatic responses are sometimes called long loop reflexes because they have characteristics that are intermediate between monosynaptic stretch reflexes and typical voluntary responses. Stretch reflexes are extremely stereotyped (the same thing happens every time) and very rapid; they occur in about 50 msec. Voluntary responses are infinitely modifiable and occur in a minimum of 150 to 200 msec. Postural responses lie between the two; they have stereotypical elements and occur in about 100 msec. Classically, stereotypical features include responses about the ankle to small perturbations, responses about the hip to moderate displacements, and stepping responses to more demanding movements of the body mass.

Innumerable changes due to aging and disease can influence the elements of the postural control system, resulting in difficulty in managing the biomechanical task. The postural control system, like many complex physiologic systems, has redundancies and back-up adaptive mechanisms. Thus, the blind person can get about successfully. Failures of postural control can occur when the demands of the biomechanical task overwhelm the system, when a critical element of the system fails, or when the adaptive back-up systems are gradually depleted through multiple accumulating deficits. The clinician can build on a foundation of knowledge about postural control theory, biomechanical mechanisms, and aging effects to construct an organized approach to problems of instability. Excellent reviews of the key issues have recently been published.[8, 9]

A Structured Approach to Fall Risk Factors

Reported risk factors associated with falls vary from study to study and incorporate a broad range of unique perspectives such as demographic, medical, and functional issues. For example, age, female gender, medications, weakness, impaired cognition, low vision, foot problems, acute illness, chronic neuromuscular conditions, environmental factors, trouble rising from a chair, risky behaviors, housebound status, and a history of previous falls or stumbles have all been identified as risk factors for falls.[4, 6, 10–12] The clinician can organize this information into meaningful constructs to foster recall and support clinical evaluation.

Whatever the construct, it is clear that fall risk is cumulative; risk increases as the number of factors increases.[12] An approach that encompasses the range of risk factors and can be used to develop a clinical plan includes (1) functional abilities, (2) environmental context, (3) acute toxic and metabolic stressors, and (4) threats to

TABLE 19–1	**FALLS AND INSTABILITY: EVALUATION AND MANAGEMENT**
Screening	Falls
	Instability
	Fear of falling
Assessment (FEAT)	**F**unctional assessment
	Vigorous, transitional, frail
	Environmental context
	Person-setting interaction
	Environments avoided
	Acute toxic or metabolic factors
	Only if falling is of new onset or a recent change
	Threats to postural control
	Sensory, central, effector
Management	Reverse: Toxic or metabolic factors
	Rare single treatable diagnosis
	Adapt:
	"Friendly" environment, human help, assistive devices
	Modify:
	Vision: optometric factors
	Vestibular function: medication, rehabilitation
	Central nervous system: medication, rehabilitation
	Effector: rehabilitation, exercise

postural control. These four groups produce the mnemonic FEAT (Table 19–1).

Functional abilities are the individual's capacity for specific movements or tasks. Mobility tasks have a natural order; it is easier to sit than to stand and easier to walk than to climb stairs or toe a line. This natural order allows clinicians to assign individuals to general levels of capacity. Tinetti has called these levels vigorous, transitional, and frail.[6] To be useful in a clinical setting, these terms must be defined. Although there are many possible definitions, one brief, efficient, and tested system is presented here.[13] Frail persons meet the criteria for disordered walking; they either use an assistive device or take steps that are shorter than twice the length of the foot. Vigorous persons can walk heel to toe or descend steps step over step. Transitional people function midway between the other two. Frail people have the highest risk for falls and are more likely to have falls indoors. Vigorous people are least likely to fall, and if they do, the circumstances are likely to be more demanding, and the impact force of the fall is likely to be higher. Frail people with limited functional abilities are at risk for the consequences of instability even if they do not fall; they may be characterized by fear of falling, social isolation, and increased dependence.

Environmental context assesses the interaction between an organism and the environment. Environmental factors are sometimes called extrinsic factors, whereas factors that are within an individual are called intrinsic factors. Some falls may be attributable to a purely intrinsic trait such as syncope and others may result from purely extrinsic, environmental factors such as being knocked over by a truck. Most falls in older persons are the result of interactions between the person's current balance capacity and the environmental conditions of the moment. Environmental risk can be based on the degree of threat required to produce a fall. One individual falls only when the environment is quite challenging, for example, on an icy sidewalk at night. Another falls under a minimal challenge, as when getting out of bed. Considering the environmental context as a spectrum, the clinician can identify the degree of environmental challenge that produces falls in a particular patient. This perspective can help to clarify the potential capacity of the individual and the approach to environmental modification and can help in detecting change over time as the ability of the individual to tolerate environmental challenge increases or decreases. In addition, any mismatch between the person's apparent functional capacities and the environmental context of a fall should be explored. A vigorous person who is falling under low stress conditions may have a greater likelihood of transient events like arrhythmias, transient ischemic attacks, or alcohol intoxication.

Acute toxic and metabolic stressors are generally not found in people who have a long-standing problem with falls. However, in general practice and in emergency rooms, the individual who becomes "weak and dizzy" and then falls may be more likely to have an acute illness, such as infection, dehydration, blood loss, electrolyte imbalance, or hypoxemia. Evaluation of a patient for these common problems makes the most sense when a falling syndrome is new or when there has been a recent change in functional abilities or environmental context.

Identifying threats to postural control is a particularly useful clinical approach to identifying risk factors. This approach is well suited to geriatric concepts of accumulating deficits and multiple contributing factors. The sensory, central processing, and effector components of postural control encompass many known risk factors. Deficits in vision (acuity, depth perception, visual fields, dark adaptation), proprioception, and vestibular function are possible. Vestibular deficits can occur in the semicircular canals, where they affect sensations of acceleration, or in the utricle and saccule, where they affect the gravitational

sensation that determines the vertical upright position. Peripheral sensory deficits lead to difficulty in determining the position of the foot and ankle, thereby limiting detection of irregularities in the terrain and reducing the ability to detect sway.[14] Multiple sensory deficits are especially likely to produce a disequilibrium syndrome. Central processing, which coordinates movements smoothly and efficiently, may be impaired. Neurologic conditions such as Parkinson's disease, cerebrovascular disease, cerebellar syndromes, normal pressure hydrocephalus, and spinal cord lesions can impair the organization and speed of postural responses.[9] Dementias may impair judgment and attention, may lead to deconditioning, and are sometimes associated with degeneration of movement-planning areas of the brain.[15] Medications can affect the central nervous system by causing sedation, delayed response time, orthostasis, or extrapyramidal side effects. Decreased cerebral perfusion due to arrhythmias or valvular lesions is very rarely implicated as a cause of chronic falls. Effectors such as muscle strength, joint flexibility, and endurance may be impaired by aging, disease, and disuse and can be additional contributors to a poorly functioning postural control system. Often overlooked are foot problems, such as bunions, hammertoes, elongated nails, and improper footwear.

CLINICAL APPROACH TO INSTABILITY AND FALLS

The older adult with instability or falls may not actively bring these problems to the physician's attention. All health care providers should consider screening their older patients briefly and periodically for both falls and instability. One systematic approach to the evaluation and management of these problems is presented in Table 19–1. Start by inquiring about falls. Find out if the falling syndrome is new, has changed recently (within weeks to months), or is of long standing. In the absence of falls, ask about fear of falling or restrictions of activity due to lack of confidence.[7] Again, inquire whether this is a relatively new problem or a long-standing one. Acquire a general feeling for the functional level of the individual. This can often be done while watching the older adult enter the examination room or move from a chair to the examination table (Table 19–2). Is the individual able to walk without an assistive device, take footsteps of reasonable size (about twice the length of the foot), and rise from a chair without using the arms? If not, the individual is somewhat frail. Can the older adult tandem walk at least four heel-to-toe steps in a row? This is one sign of excellent vigorous balance. In your

TABLE 19–2 **ASSESSMENT OF PHYSICAL FUNCTION**

Basic level
1. Step length at least twice foot length
2. Walks without assistive device
3. Rises from chair without using arms

High level
1. Tandem walks at least four to five steps
2. Descends stairs step-over-step

Categories
1. Frail: Fails basic level
2. Transitional: Passes basic level, fails high level
3. Vigorous: Passes high level

mind, assign the person to one of the three categories: vigorous, transitional, or frail.

Inquire about the environmental context. For patients who have fallen, identify the setting and activity at the time of the fall. In the absence of falls, inquire about the kinds of environments the individual avoids or enters only with support from another person or device.[7] Match the functional capacity with the environmental context. Falls in a person with vigorous function and minimal environmental challenge indicate the presence of transient medical events or perhaps psychologic issues. Similarly, a vigorous individual who restricts activity and avoids environments unnecessarily may benefit from reassurance.

If falls and instability are of recent onset, a physical examination for more acute findings of dehydration or cardiopulmonary or neuromuscular abnormalities should be carried out. Brief screening tests for toxic and metabolic stressors such as electrolyte imbalance or hypoxia should be considered (see later section on diagnostic testing).

The history and physical examination are used to explore threats to postural control. The sensory, central processing, and effector elements are reviewed systematically, and the three sensory systems—vision, somatosensation, and vestibular function—are examined. For vision, one should inquire about the use of eye wear and problems with dark adaptation. Is the patient monocular due to a dense cataract or unilateral blindness? People who have only one functioning eye have reduced stereopsis and more problems with depth perception. The visual fields, including the inferior as well as the lateral fields, should be examined. Peripheral vision loss occurs in patients with glaucoma and stroke as well as in apparently healthy older adults.[16]

Acute vestibular disorders present classically with vertigo, which is defined as a hallucination of motion, often perceived as spinning of the

person or the room. The two most common causes are benign positional vertigo and Meniere's disease. People with chronic, especially bilateral vestibular disorders often lack sensations of vertigo. These individuals are more likely to have movement intolerance, especially when there are strong visual cues of motion. For example, people with chronic vestibular disorders may feel dizzy when they push a grocery cart down an aisle because their vision tells them they are moving but their chronic vestibular deficit does not provide the brain with sensations of acceleration.

Physical examination for vestibular disease is difficult. Traditional tests for nystagmus are frequently negative in people with definite vestibular disease. A Hallpike maneuver, in which the patient is brought from a supine position, with the head rotated sideways and down, to a sitting position can stimulate otolith activity and help in the diagnosis of benign positional vertigo. Chronic vestibular disorders are very difficult to diagnose in the clinic. Tests for body position and acceleration with the eyes closed are sometimes helpful. For example, the patient can be asked to march in place with the eyes closed. A normal person remains in one place, whereas someone with vestibular hypofunction rotates or moves off base.[17] Many high-tech approaches to the diagnosis of vestibular diseases have been developed during the last decade. It is unclear whether they are helpful in older adults with multiple deficits. Some of these approaches were developed for younger persons with very specific isolated vestibular conditions, and they may be confounded in older adults who have multiple interacting disorders.

Older adults who have problems with somatosensation may not necessarily complain of numb feet. They may note a disquieting sense of being unsure of themselves when they are standing and walking, a form of dizziness that is clearly not felt in the head. This sensation, sometimes called disequilibrium syndrome, has been described as a feeling that resembles trying to walk in a rowboat. It occurs when losses of somatosensation are present, often in combination with other sensory deficits. Thus, disequilibrium is often a multiple sensory disorder syndrome. Peripheral sensory deficits may be present on traditional testing for toe position and sharp-dull discrimination but are often normal in people who have a clear-cut disequilibrium syndrome. More frequently, these individuals have several physical findings. A positive result on Romberg's test (increased sway when the eyes are closed) is a sign that stability is dependent on vision. It is not specific for peripheral sensory disorders but can be very sensitive, especially if the patient is asked to put his or her feet as close together as possible (providing the smallest base of support). Another test that is strongly associated with disequilibrium is extensive loss of the vibratory sense. Although many healthy elders cannot feel vibration at the most distal bony prominences, such as the base of the great toe, those with disequilibrium cannot feel vibration at the ankle and often not even at the knee.

Central postural responses can be tested directly in the clinical setting by performing a righting test. The examiner stands behind the patient and tugs at the pelvis. The normal response is to promptly bring one foot backward under the body and sometimes to bring both arms forward. Abnormal reactions include a complete lack of response, sometimes called the "timber reaction," and multiple small ineffective steps. Lack of a righting response suggests a central nervous system condition that affects the basic postural organization. It is often a poor prognostic sign for recovery of balance function. Conversely, an intact righting response implies an excellent basis for recovery of function if other contributors to the problem are identified and treated.

Further neurologic examination is needed to detect specific conditions associated with poor postural responses. Parkinson's disease is much more common in older adults than previously thought.[18] It is frequently associated with a primary loss of righting reactions and can present differently in older people than in younger adults. Older adults are less likely to have tremor and are more likely to have balance problems, gait problems, and cognitive problems. Cogwheeling rigidity is often the best clue to the diagnosis. This sign is sometimes subtle but can be made more prominent by having the patient actively move the contralateral extremity during testing. For example, the patient can tap one hand against the knee while the examiner moves the other elbow through the range of motion, feeling for the characteristic cogwheeling sign.

Righting responses may also be lost at some point in the course of many dementias, including Alzheimer's disease, white matter disease, multi-infarct syndromes, and normal pressure hydrocephalus.[8]

Spinal cord syndromes such as cervical and lumbar stenosis can cause sensory and motor deficits that affect the components of balance. These problems are not necessarily associated with pain and can be diagnosed by detecting sensory deficits, localizing weakness and reflex changes. It is important not to make the diagnosis by radiologic scans alone because many structural abnormalities occur without accompanying neurologic deficits.

Drugs can affect central responses in four major ways—causing delayed reaction time, sedation, decreased cerebral perfusion, or extrapyramidal effects.[19] It can be difficult to remember a laundry list of medications that could possibly affect balance but is easier to remember and review the four mechanisms. Consider all prescription and over-the-counter formulations of drugs that are known to affect the central responses directly as well as those that have such consequences indirectly as unintentional side effects. For example, benzodiazepines, especially those with long half-lives, clearly increase the risk of falls, even if the individual does not knowingly feel sedated. Antihistamines can also cause sedation and may be present in over-the-counter formulations available for colds and sinus disorders. Decreased cerebral perfusion may be the result of orthostasis and may be due to antihypertensive agents. Other drugs can affect blood pressure as an unintentional side effect. For example, antianginal agents such as nitrates and levodopa for Parkinson's disease can cause orthostasis. Drugs can also cause extrapyramidal consequences, most commonly recognized as a side effect of major tranquilizers, but such effects can also occur with other drugs such as metoclopramide.

Cardiovascular causes of falls are largely mediated by decreased cerebral perfusion. It is always worth checking for orthostasis, although mild degrees of this condition, such as systolic changes of 20 mmHg, are common and are often clinically unimportant. Of greater interest is either a large drop of 30 mmHg or more or a drop to a systolic blood pressure of under 100 mmHg. The detection of arrhythmias or valvular lesions has generally not proved to be helpful in the management of falls. These abnormalities are often simply common comorbidities that are not contributing to the problem and require treatment that has a substantial morbidity of its own. The threshold for pursuing evidence of decreased cerebral perfusion may be lowered if frank syncope is present, if there is a clear mismatch between functional capacity and environmental threat, and perhaps if the syndrome is of recent onset.

Diagnostic Testing

Because falls have a heterogeneous origin, both diagnostic tests and management plans must be individually tailored based on the clinical information obtained; a nonspecific cookbook approach should be avoided. One study found, during a complete post-fall assessment, that most diagnoses (95%) are determined from the history and physical examination alone.[20] A chemistry profile, complete blood count, oxygen saturation, drug levels, electrocardiogram, and chest radiograph are most likely to be helpful when falls have begun recently or when there has been a recent change. A Holter monitor is rarely useful. If focal neurologic findings are noted, an imaging study or electromyogram (EMG) may be needed. Specialized vestibular or visual testing may be productive in selective cases, but costly, low-yield tests should not be obtained indiscriminately. The goal is to confirm the diagnostic impressions and quantify the degree of functional impairment. At times, a home evaluation to assess the environmental hazards and directly observe the patient's performance of activities of daily living and instrumental activities of daily living can be revealing (Table 19–3).

MANAGEMENT APPROACH

Individualized Multidisciplinary Modifications

Given the multifactorial causes of falls, management strategies must be multifaceted and comprehensive yet individualized. The goal is to maximize function and independence while minimizing injury. A multidisciplinary approach engages various personnel to address the disability and help to lower the cumulative burden of deficits as well as the risk of falling. This may involve treating reversible disease, modifying impairments, and adapting to fixed disabilities. For example, an optometrist, physical therapist, social worker, and physician may all make significant contributions to reducing the risk of falls in a visually impaired, frail individual with limited mobility who is taking multiple medications.

If reversible conditions such as metabolic disturbances are found, they can be treated. Rarely, treatment of some patients with normal pressure hydrocephalus, subdural hematoma, or arrhythmia results in a complete cure. More likely, the clinician will find himself working on multiple modifiable impairments. Among the sensory deficits, those of vision and vestibular function are most likely to respond to treatment. Visual field deficits may be helped by corrective lenses that include prisms.[16] Vestibular disorders may respond to medications such as meclizine and are often improved by training or desensitization programs provided by therapists.[17] Central disorders are often not curable but may be somewhat responsive to treatment. Medication for Parkinson's disease may result in improved ease of movement but unfortunately does not change the postural control deficit itself. Sometimes an individual who is starting treatment for Parkinson's disease may actually fall more often. Although he or she can walk faster, the sense of balance is still defective, a situation that can lead to more opportunities for mishaps and injuries.

Many medications are potential contributors to instability. Because impairments may accumulate over time, it is even possible for a drug to begin to cause problems only after many years as other adaptive mechanisms become compromised. A systematic approach to reducing medications can identify which agents are required for cure, for symptomatic relief, or for prevention of long-term complications. In each area, the agent can be deemed essential, useful, or less likely to be necessary. If a drug is thought to contribute to instability, it may be eliminated if deemed unnecessary or replaced with an alternative agent if considered important. Real controversies sometimes occur about the best decision if treatment for a dangerous condition such as heart disease results in dysfunctional consequences such as dizziness and instability.

Primary direct intervention on balance function may reduce falls and improve balance.[21, 22] Exercise can be adapted to the functional abilities of the person. Some techniques have been

---

TABLE 19–3 **ENVIRONMENTAL MODIFICATIONS AND HOME SAFETY CHECKLIST**

Flooring

Secure rugs (nonskid backing) and carpets (tack down, no tears)
Remove clutter and obstacles from stairs, hallways
Keep cords out of traffic areas
Use nonskid wax

Access

Store frequently used items within reach
Repair unstable railings and other handholds
Provide handrails the full length of the stairway

Lighting

Ensure adequate lighting, especially on stairways
Check for lights or light switches near doorways, bed
Provide night lights for bathroom, stairway, etc.

Bathroom

Install grab bars for tub, toilet
Place rubber mat or decals in tub or shower

Outdoors

Be sure sidewalks and driveway are free of cracks and breaks
Examine lawn and garden for holes, rocks, loose boards, etc.
Keep walkways free of leaves, snow, etc.

developed that are based on high-tech computer programs or body consciousness approaches such as tai chi. Water exercise may be helpful[23] in that elderly people can practice balance maneuvers without the fear of falling; the water will cushion them if they lose their balance.

The effector system is clearly responsive to treatment. Strength, flexibility, and endurance remain highly modifiable, even in many frail elders.[24] There is no clear consensus about the best way to exercise. Some programs use formal weight-training equipment, and some use low-tech strategies such as Theraband and body weight for resistance.

Some degree of instability may persist after efforts to reverse disease and modify impairments have been pursued. Many approaches can be used to help the patient adapt to fixed disabilities. Mobility and self-care assistive devices can extend the person's functional abilities. An emergency call system may also be beneficial and can improve safety while allowing independence. The patient's home or living environment can be made more "friendly" by improving lighting, visual contrast, and available handholds.[25] New flooring materials may help to reduce the impact of a fall.[26] In places where very frail older adults congregate, like nursing homes, staffing patterns can be adapted to increase supervision of those known to be likely to fall. Here the answer, in part, may be to offer periodic supervised physical activity and to anticipate needs such as toileting. Restriction of activity should be a last resort.

The Frailty and Injuries: Cooperative Studies of Intervention Techniques (FICSIT) trials included eight multisite clinical trials that investigated interactions among biomedical, behavioral, and environmental factors contributing to functional loss and disability in the elderly.[26] Exercise was emphasized, and a range of interventions and populations was tested. The overall results of the FICSIT trials revealed a modest but significant decrease in the incidence of falls, particularly for those interventions that specifically addressed balance. Because of low statistical power to detect a treatment effect in reducing injurious falls, which occurred rarely, no significant change was noted in incidence of injurious falls.[3] Tinetti and colleagues reported a reduction in the falls incidence ratio to 0.69 using a multidimensional intervention that addressed and modified medications, behavior, education, and exercise.[27]

Falls in Nursing Homes

Residents who fall in nursing homes present some unique challenges and issues. Persons in nursing homes are more likely to take many medications, have more disability, and suffer from poor cognition and impaired judgment. Some residents are unable to clearly express their needs. Use of passive injury protection is one attractive approach. Hip protectors used in a nursing home population reduced risk, but patient compliance was a notable problem.[28] A trial of thorough post-fall assessment found no change in the incidence of falls but a significant decrease in hospitalization due to falls. The falls may have triggered an earlier and more thorough evaluation of the patients' overall medical condition.[20] Physical restraints have never been shown to decrease the incidence of falls. Currently, the challenge in nursing homes is to reduce all forms of restraint while maintaining patient safety. Key elements include attempts to (1) screen for and treat reversible contributors to instability, (2) use supervised exercise to reduce physical restlessness, and (3) anticipate the needs that precipitate unsupervised activity, such as a desire for toileting, food, drink, symptom relief, or diversion.

SUMMARY

Instability, fear of falling, and falls themselves are common contributors to restricted activity and reduced health in older adults. It is important to screen for instability and fear of falling in addition to actual fall events. Assessment includes functional evaluation, an environmental history, screening for acute toxic or metabolic conditions when the situation is new or changing, and a systematic review of threats to postural control. Management includes identification of reversible causes, modification of impairments, and adaptation to fixed disabilities. Multiple contributing factors are often present that require an individualized, multidimensional approach to evaluation and management. The ultimate goals are to improve function, maximize independence, and reduce risk of injury.

References

1. Tinetti M, Inouye SK, Gill TM, Doucette JT: Shared risk factors for falls, incontinence and functional dependence: Unifying the approach to geriatric syndromes. JAMA 1995;273:1348–1353.
2. Kennedy TE, Coppard LC: The prevention of falls in later life. Dan Med Bull 1987;34(Suppl):1–24.
3. Province MA, Hadley EC, Hornbrook MC, et al: The effects of exercise on falls in elderly patients. A preplanned meta-analysis of the FICSIT trials. JAMA 1995;273:1341–1347.
4. Tinetti ME, Doucette J, Claus E, Marottoli R: Risk factors for serious injury during falls by older persons in the community. J Am Geriatr Soc 1995;43:1214–1221.
5. Kiel DP: The evaluation of falls in the emergency department. Clin Geriatr Med 1993;9:591–598.

6. Speechley M, Tinetti M: Falls and injuries in frail and vigorous community elderly persons. J Am Geriatr Soc 1991;39:46–52.

7. Powell LE Myers AM: The activities-specific balance confidence scale. J Gerontol 1995;50A:M28–M34.

8. Maki B, McIlroy W: Postural control in the older adult. Clin Geriatr Med 1996;12:635–658.

9. Alexander N: Postural control in older adults. J Am Geriatr Soc 1994;42:93–108.

10. Cummings SR, Nevitt MC: A hypothesis: The causes of hip fractures. J Gerontol 1989;4:M107–M111.

11. Teno J, Kiel DP, Mor V: Multiple stumbles: A risk factor for falls in community dwelling elderly. A prospective study. J Am Geriatr Soc 1990;38:1321–1325.

12. Tinetti ME, Speechley M: Prevention of falls among the elderly. N Engl J Med 1989;320:1055–1059.

13. Studenski S, Duncan PW, Chandler J, et al: Predicting falls: The role of mobility and nonphysical factors. J Am Geriatr Soc 1994;42:297–302.

14. Richardson JK, Hurvitz EA: Peripheral neuropathy: A true risk factor for falls. J Gerontol 1995;50A:M211–M215.

15. Morris JC, Rubin EH, Morris EJ, Mandel SA: Senile dementia of the Alzheimer's type: An important risk factor for serious falls. J Gerontol 1987;42:412–417.

16. Maino J: Visual deficits and mobility: Evaluation and management. Clin Geriatr Med 1996;12:803–823.

17. Herdman SJ: Assessment and treatment of balance disorders in the vestibular deficient patient. *In* Duncan P (ed): Balance. Alexandria, VA, American Physical Therapy Association Publications, 1990, pp. 87–94.

18. Bennett DA, Beckett LA, Murray AM, et al: Prevalence of parkinsonian signs and associated mortality in a community population of older people. N Engl J Med 1996;334:71–76.

19. Campbell AJ: Drug treatment as a cause of falls in old age. A review of the offending agents. Drugs Aging 1991;1:289–302.

20. Rubenstein LZ, Robbins AS, Josephson KR, Schulman BL, Osterweil D: The value of assessing falls in an elderly population. A randomized clinical trial. Ann Intern Med 1990;113:308–316.

21. Wolf SL, Barnhart HX, Kutner NG, et al: Reducing frailty and falls in older persons: An investigation of tai chi and computerized balance training. J Am Geriatr Soc 1996;44:489–497.

22. Wolfson L, Whipple R, Derby C, et al: Balance and strength training in older adults: Intervention gains and tai chi maintenance. J Am Geriatr Soc 1996;44:498–506.

23. Simmons V, Hansen PD: Effectiveness of water exercise on postural mobility in the well elderly: An experimental study on balance enhancement. J Gerontol 1996;51A:M233–M238.

24. Chandler J, Hadley E: Exercise to improve physiologic and functional performance in older adults. Clin Geriatr Med 1996;12:761–784.

25. Connell BR: Role of the environment in falls prevention. Clin Geriatr Med 1996;12:859–880.

26. Ory MG, Schectman KB, Miller JP, et al: Frailty and injuries in later life: The FICSIT trials. J Am Geriatr Soc 1993;41:283–296.

27. Tinetti M, Baker D, McAvay G, et al: A multifactorial intervention to reduce the risk of falling among elderly people living in the community. N Engl J Med 1994;331:821–827.

28. Wallace RB, Ross JE, Huston JC, Kundel C, Woodworth G: Iowa FICSIT trial: The feasibility of elderly wearing a hip joint protective garment to reduce hip fractures. J Am Geriatr Soc 1993;41:338–340.

20 Orthostatic Hypotension, Dizziness, and Syncope

Scott L. Mader, M.D.

Hypotension, whether it occurs after administration of medications, standing, or meals, is an important and often reversible disorder in older persons. It can cause dizziness and syncope, which are common clinical problems in older patients. The purpose of this chapter is to (1) review the age- and disease-related changes in physiology that can predispose a patient to hypotension and cerebral hypoperfusion, and (2) to formulate a process of evaluation and treatment for the patient with orthostatic hypotension, dizziness, or syncope.

AGING AS A RISK FACTOR

Some known age-associated changes in physiology would be expected to favor development of hypotension after cardiovascular stressors in elderly persons.[1] There are changes in arterial compliance and venous system tortuosity with age. Cardiac hypertrophy may impair diastolic filling. Renal sodium conservation is impaired, and neurohypophyseal release of vasopressin is blunted after standing. Renin, angiotensin, and aldosterone levels are lower in elderly subjects and also have a blunted response to upright posture. Atrial natriuretic peptide (ANP) levels increase with age, and the hypotensive response to ANP infusion increases with age.[2] The change in heart rate after hypotensive maneuvers and the maximum heart rate during exercise or isoproterenol infusion are decreased.

Other age-related changes decrease the likelihood of hypotension. The vasoconstrictor response of blood vessels to alpha-adrenergic agonists probably does not change with normal aging. In contrast, beta-adrenergic vasodilation is impaired despite an intact response to nonreceptor-mediated vasodilators such as nitroglycerine. Plasma norepinephrine levels increase with age under both basal and stress conditions such as standing, isometric exercise, and cold stimulation. These changes suggest that vasoconstriction would be enhanced in elderly persons after standing.

Clinical data suggest that the balance of these age-related changes is toward an increase in the risk of hypotension. Diuretic-induced volume depletion or vasodilation with nitrates causes greater orthostatic blood pressure declines in elderly than in younger subjects. Postprandial blood pressure declines occur in healthy elderly subjects but not in younger controls.[3] For any decrease in blood pressure, elderly persons are also more likely to become symptomatic because of the high likelihood of cerebral vascular disease and the shift in cerebral autoregulation that occurs with hypertension, another common disorder.

ORTHOSTATIC HYPOTENSION

Orthostatic or postural hypotension (OH) is a common clinical problem in elderly persons seen in a medical practice. It is associated with dizziness, pre-syncope, syncope, falls, cerebral vascular accidents, and myocardial infarction. OH is a side effect of many common medications used by older persons and often results from multiple causes. It is usually reversible, and appropriate treatment will likely improve function and independence.

Epidemiology

The prevalence of OH depends on the patient group studied and the definition used. Most studies use a fall in systolic blood pressure of at least 20 mmHg after standing. Elderly subjects with no medical problems or medications have a low prevalence (6%) of OH.[4] In inpatient, outpatient, and nursing home surveys, 11% to 33% of subjects have significant falls in blood pressure after standing. A study of more than 5000 subjects aged 65 and older found an overall prevalence of OH of 16% to 18%.[5] OH was significantly associated with difficulty in walking, falls, a history of myocardial infarction, and a history of transient ischemic attacks. Therefore, OH can be anticipated in patient populations in which the appropriate risk factors (see next section) are present. Conversely, this finding should not be expected in otherwise healthy elderly persons.

Postprandial hypotension is also an important cause of hypotension in elderly patients.[3] In a study of 113 nursing home residents, 96% experienced a reduction in systolic blood pressure after eating. Thirty-six percent had a reduction in systolic blood pressure of 20 mmHg or more, 11% had a measured systolic blood pressure of less than 100 mmHg, and two subjects developed symptoms (angina, transient ischemic attack).

Differential Diagnosis

There are many causes of OH.[6] Table 20–1 shows some common and uncommon diagnostic categories found in older persons. Many medications associated with OH are commonly used by elderly persons.[7] These drugs can cause OH by many mechanisms including volume decrease, vasodilation, impairment of autonomic reflexes, and central nervous system depression. They include alcohol, antihypertensive, antiadrenergic, antiparkinsonian, antianginal, antiarrhythmic, anticholinergic, antidepressant, diuretic, narcotic, neuroleptic, and sedative agents.

Old age alone is not a sufficient explanation for OH, and when elderly patients are found to have OH, it is not unusual to find multiple contributing factors. For example, an elderly person hospitalized for pneumonia may have several coexisting conditions: diuretic therapy, previous stroke, malnutrition, hypokalemia, anemia, and deconditioning, all of which contribute to the problem.

Idiopathic orthostatic hypotension (IOH) and multiple system atrophy (MSA, Shy-Drager syndrome) are uncommon causes of OH in elderly persons. These disorders should be considered in patients who have supine hypertension and an

TABLE 20–1	**DIFFERENTIAL DIAGNOSIS OF ORTHOSTATIC HYPOTENSION**

I. Common

    Anemia, blood loss
    Bed rest, deconditioning
    Dehydration, malnutrition
    Hypokalemia
    Medications

II. Neurologic

    Central: cerebrovascular accidents, Parkinson's disease, tumors
    Peripheral: peripheral neuropathy (amyloid, diabetes, uremic, viral), sympathectomy

III. Cardiovascular

    Cardiac: aortic stenosis, hypertrophic cardiomyopathy, mitral valve prolapse
    Vascular: large varicose veins

IV. Endocrine or Renal

    Adrenal insufficiency
    Diabetes insipidus
    Hypoaldosteronism
    Pheochromocytoma
    Renal concentrating defect

V. Less Common

    Baroreceptor destruction (neck radiation, surgery)
    Idiopathic orthostatic hypotension (IOH)
    Multiple system atrophy (MSA or Shy-Drager syndrome)
    Tumor-associated (carcinoid, bradykinin)

impressive orthostatic blood pressure drop in the absence of other conditions or medications associated with OH.

Evaluation

All elderly patients should have their postural blood pressure determined as part of the routine assessment and whenever potentially hypotensive medications are started. Patients who complain of dizziness, syncope, falls, transient ischemic attacks, or other cerebral symptoms should always be evaluated for postural hypotension even in the absence of a clear-cut postural component.

The history should focus on previous medical and surgical problems, medications, alcohol use, and dietary intake of salt, water, and calories. An autonomic, neurologic, cardiovascular, and endocrine review of systems should be performed. The autonomic review of systems is often confusing in older persons because of the large number of positive responses in this population (presence of constipation, urinary difficulties, sexual dysfunction, night blindness). However, a negative review of systems is helpful in ruling out significant autonomic dysfunction.

The physical examination should begin with the blood pressure determination. A greater difference in blood pressure is seen if supine to standing rather than sitting to standing readings are compared. After 5 minutes of supine rest, the blood pressure should be taken until it is stable. After the person stands, the blood pressure is measured 1 minute later. For screening purposes, a 1-minute reading is usually sufficient. However, depending on the history, blood pressure taken at 3 minutes, 5 minutes, after walking or climbing stairs, and after prolonged standing may be useful.[8] OH is diagnosed if there is a 20-mmHg decrease or more in systolic pressure, or a 10-mmHg decrease or more in diastolic pressure. A single OH determination can be misleading because serial determinations in patients can be variable. If symptoms compatible with cerebral hypoperfusion occur without a significant change in blood pressure, the patient may have "orthostatic cerebral hypoperfusion." This occurs particularly in patients with carotid stenosis. Volume should be assessed by examination of the jugular venous pressure. The carotid arteries should be examined for the presence of bruits. The heart should be auscultated while the patient is supine as well as upright because the murmurs of idiopathic hypertrophic cardiomyopathy or mitral valve prolapse may be more prominent in the standing position. A careful neurologic examination is necessary to assess for depression, cognitive impairment, previous stroke, Parkinson's disease, and peripheral neuropathy.

Routine laboratory assessment need not be extensive. In patients without specific indications, a complete blood count (CBC), electrolytes, blood urea nitrogen (BUN), creatinine, glucose, albumin, calcium, phosphorus, urinalysis with specific gravity, and an electrocardiogram should be performed. More extensive testing should be limited to patients in whom suggestive abnormalities appear on the history, physical examination, or laboratory screening. Commonly ordered additional tests include echocardiography, cosyntropin stimulation test, and urine electrolytes. Autonomic function testing, adrenergic drug infusions, and supine or standing plasma catecholamine measurements can be useful if the diagnosis is unclear and the patient fails to respond to conservative therapy.

Treatment

In a few patients a specific cause of OH is found, and this should be addressed. However, most older persons are found to have multiple causative factors, some of which are correctable and some of which are fixed deficits.[6, 9]

The initial steps are to (1) evaluate the patient's medications, (2) increase fluid, salt, and nutritional intake, (3) increase activity level, and (4) provide patient education. Medications can be reduced, changed, or stopped completely. Patients with hypertension and OH can be treated with beta-blockers or vasodilator agents (calcium channel blockers, angiotensin-converting enzyme inhibitors, or angiotensin receptor blockers). Diuretics, central sympatholytic agents (alpha-methyldopa) and peripheral alpha-adrenergic blockers are more likely to cause or exacerbate OH. Treatment of hypertension is reported to improve postprandial hypotension.[3] For patients with depression, the newer serotonin-reuptake inhibitors are preferred and have even been used to treat OH.[10] In some instances, it may be difficult to stop the offending medications. In these cases, treatment strategies including the use of salt tablets, elevation of the head of the bed, and fludrocortisone administration (see following discussion) may be instituted prior to or while continuing the offending medication.

Another useful measure is to increase salt intake. Many older persons follow a low-salt diet even in the absence of a history of hypertension. Salting food with one packet of salt (approximately 1 gm) at each meal can improve blood pressure tolerance and food intake in these patients. Exercise and reconditioning are extremely important. Patients who spend most of the time in bed will continue to have OH despite other treatment measures. Isometric exercise of the arms, legs, and abdominal muscles before standing decrease blood pooling and can improve blood pressure tolerance.

Education is important so that patients and families will understand the cause and management of the symptoms. Patients should be instructed to rise slowly from the supine to a sitting posture, and then to wait a few minutes before standing up. They should stand only when there is a support available to prevent falling. Isometric tensing of the legs, arms, and abdominal muscles decreases venous pooling and helps maintain blood pressure during position changes or prolonged standing. A urinal or bedside commode should be provided so that patients do not have to get up quickly or without assistance. Finally, they should be instructed to take extra salt and fluid during times of volume stress such as during extreme heat, febrile illness, and episodes of gastroenteritis.

For patients who do not respond to these simple measures, additional treatments may be tried. A head-up tilt at night is effective and is often easier with older patients who may not be sharing a bed with another person.[11] This is best accomplished with books or 2- by 6-inch blocks placed under the legs at the head of the bed. The bed can be raised in small increments to tolerance. Salt tablets can be prescribed for patients with poor oral intake in 1-gm tablets. One gram of NaCl equals 17 mEq of Na, and treatment can start at 1 to 2 gm twice a day and can be increased if necessary and tolerated. Fludrocortisone acetate (Florinef) is an effective treatment that acts by promoting salt retention and sensitizing the blood vessels to catecholamines. It can be started at 0.1 mg qhs and increased on a weekly basis up to 0.5 mg twice a day. The most common side effect is hypokalemia (which can exacerbate OH) and mild dependent edema. Precipitation of new congestive heart failure is a theoretical but uncommon occurrence. Adequate salt intake must be part of this regimen. Support hose are a widely recommended therapy for OH, but they are difficult to put on and are only really effective when fitted thigh or waist-high stockings are used.

DIZZINESS

The complaint of dizziness is frequent among elderly persons. It is the third most common reason why patients 65 and older visit family physicians and the fifth most common reason why this age group visits general internists. It is the most common presenting complaint of persons 75 and older.[12] It is implicated in up to 25% of falls and restricts activity in up to one third of subjects. An understanding of the differential diagnosis, work-up, and management of this symptom is important in providing optimal care to elderly patients.

Epidemiology

When patients say they are dizzy, they are generally referring to one or more of the following symptoms:

- Vertigo
- Pre-syncope
- Imbalance, or
- Nonspecific lightheadedness

The prevalence of dizziness ranges from 5% for persons aged 65 to 69 to 20% for those 85 or older in one study.[13] Another group found that the lifetime prevalence of dizziness severe enough to see a physician or take a medication was 30%.[14] They found four clinical characteristics that were significantly related to dizziness:

multiple neurosensory deficits, the presence of cardiovascular risk factors, depressive symptoms, and the perception of being nervous. The general symptom of dizziness was not associated with an increased risk of death or institutionalization after 1 year of follow-up.

Two studies have reported on the final diagnosis in elderly patients who were evaluated for dizziness. Sloane and Baloh reported on 116 patients over age 70 who were referred for dizziness to a neuro-otology clinic.[15] They found that the clinical history provided the key diagnostic data in 70% of the cases. After evaluation, they made the following diagnoses: 46% had peripheral vestibular disorders, 19% had cerebrovascular disorders, 7% had other central disorders (cerebellar atrophy, acoustic neuroma [previously diagnosed], drug toxicity), and 15% had other disorders (anxiety or depression, multiple sensory deficits, vasovagal attack, cardiac arrhythmia, postcataract surgery). No cause was determined in 14%. Half of the patients with peripheral vestibular disorders were thought to have benign positional vertigo (described in detail later in this section). A Canadian dizziness program reported on 1194 patients 70 years or older at the time of their first visit.[16] These patients represented 12% of the patients referred to the program. The most common diagnoses were suspected or confirmed positional vertigo (40%), unknown (27%), nonvestibular or non-neurologic medications, cardiovascular disease, diabetes, or psychogenic causes (9%), and cerebrovascular disease (6%).

These studies provide important information about patients referred to specialty clinics for the evaluation of dizziness. However, in a nonreferred population, the distribution of diagnoses may be somewhat different. In a primary care geriatric practice, dizziness may be more commonly caused by multiple sensory deficits, cervical spondylosis, and orthostatic hypotension than these referral studies suggest.

Evaluation

Because dizziness is a symptom that cannot be measured objectively, the history is essential.[17, 18] After the patient's initial description, the following questions should be asked.

1. How many kinds of dizziness does the patient have? It is not uncommon to hear a very contradictory history only to find that the patient has more than one kind of symptom.
2. What does the patient mean when he says he is dizzy? Dizziness is usually categorized into one of four groups:

- Vertigo (sense of rotation or being pushed)
- Pre-syncope or impending faint
- Imbalance (sensation localized to the body, relieved by sitting or lying down)
- Ill-defined lightheadedness (cerebral sensation of being woozy, floating, swimming, visual abnormalities)

Forty percent of patients have characteristics in more than one category. If the history remains unclear, the patient should be asked to keep a log of symptoms and activities that can be reviewed at a follow-up visit.

3. What is the symptom pattern (acute, recurrent, positional, or continuous)? Are all of the episodes the same?
4. Are there any associated symptoms (hearing loss, tinnitus, nausea, sweating)?
5. What medications (including alcohol) does the patient take or has taken recently (aspirin-like agents, anticonvulsants,

antidepressants, aminoglycoside antibiotics, vasodilators, antihypertensives)?
6. What diseases does the patient have? Has he or she been sick recently?
7. What is the general level of activity, and how has this been affected?

In patients with vertigo, the differential diagnosis varies by symptom pattern (acute, recurrent, positional; see Table 20–2).[18] In addition, one must determine whether the vertigo is related to peripheral neurologic dysfunction (e.g., a labyrinth disorder) or central neurologic dysfunction (e.g., brain stem, cerebellum). Vertigo of peripheral origin is generally worst at onset, is markedly aggravated by position, and often is associated with tinnitus or hearing changes. The onset of vertigo in relation to recent events helps in suggesting a diagnosis. Symptoms that appear after a viral illness suggest vestibular neuronitis. Symptoms appearing after other systemic illnesses suggest acute toxic labyrinthitis. Symptoms occurring after head trauma, whiplash, or loud noise suggest a traumatic etiology. Symp-

TABLE 20–2 **DIFFERENTIAL DIAGNOSIS OF DIZZINESS**

I. Vertigo

Acute	*Recurrent*	*Positional*
Infectious	Hypothyroidism	Benign positional vertigo
Seizure	Meniere's disease	Central causes
Toxic (illness or drug)	Migraine	Cervical
Trauma	Multiple sclerosis	Postinfectious
Tumor	Seizure	Post-trauma
Vascular event	Syphilis	
	Transient ischemic attack	

II. Pre-Syncope

See Tables 20–1 and 20–3
Hyperventilation

III. Imbalance

Cervical spine disease
Medication toxicity
Multiple sensory impairments
Muscle weakness
Neurologic disease
  Cerebellar degeneration
  Myelopathy
  Parkinson's disease
  Peripheral neuropathy
  Stroke
Unstable joints

IV. Ill-Defined Lightheadedness

Carbon monoxide intoxication
Hyperventilation
Medications
Psychiatric disorders
Stroke
Visual disorders

toms not associated with these precipitants suggest a peripheral vascular event. Vertigo associated with the Valsalva maneuver or sneeze suggests the infrequent possibility of a fistulous tract in the labyrinth. Episodic vertigo that is associated with hearing loss suggests Meniere's disease.

Vertigo of central origin almost always has other neurologic findings referable to the brain stem or cerebellum, such as visual changes (diplopia or blindness), cerebellar signs, and other indications of brain stem involvement. This type of vertigo is more likely to be continuous, is only variably affected by position, and may not be maximal at onset. Primary brain tumors or metastatic brain tumors are uncommon causes of vertigo. Even acoustic neuroma does not typically present as vertigo. Hearing loss, tinnitus, and frequently neurologic abnormalities occur first. Multiple sclerosis can occur in elderly persons but is unusual. Seizures rarely present with dizziness or vertigo as the sole manifestation.

A special category of vertigo is positional vertigo.[18, 19] It usually indicates a benign disorder and is almost always caused by a peripheral vestibular disturbance, although in rare cases it can be associated with a central lesion. The main historical features of benign positional vertigo (BPV) are (1) the symptoms occur *only* with a change in position, and (2) after a change in position, the symptoms last less than 1 minute. These features distinguish BPV from other conditions causing vertigo in which the sensation of rotation is generally continuous but is exacerbated by movement. BPV is an episodic condition that lasts weeks to months, but it recurs frequently. Patients may complain of mild postural instability between attacks. It is often precipitated by lying down, rolling over in bed, or sudden head movements that the patient often learns to avoid. In about half the cases, a prior ischemic, infectious, or traumatic insult can be identified; in the remainder, no cause can be identified. BPV can be distinguished from central positional vertigo with the Hallpike maneuver (described later).

If the problem is not vertigo, the next line of questioning is to determine whether the problem is one of an impending faint. This category includes patients with OH, hyperventilation, and cardiac disorders (see later section on syncope). Hyperventilation is usually associated with lightheadedness and circumoral and digital paresthesias.

If the patient describes imbalance, questions should focus on vision (glaucoma or refractive error), hearing, arthritis of the neck or extremities, alcohol use, and symptoms of peripheral neuropathy. The effect of support while walking (holding the elbow or carrying a cane) is important because a marked improvement in stability with only minimal support is characteristic of multiple sensory deficit. The possibility of Parkinson's disease should be considered. Dilated cerebral ventricles or a midline cerebellar tumor can also produce these symptoms without other specific neurologic findings.

The final category is ill-defined lightheadedness. Generally, this symptom usually does not suggest a serious underlying disorder. This symptom may be secondary to medication, hyperventilation, or a previous stroke. In the winter months in conjunction with headache, carbon monoxide poisoning should be considered. Affective or anxiety disorders can also be associated with complaints of chronic lightheadedness.

The *physical examination* is tailored to the history as described previously. Time spent taking a careful history can save time on the physical examination. Some of the following tests may be useful in evaluating the dizziness whose cause is unclear from the history:

1. Blood pressure taken in the supine position and after standing for 1 minute
2. Head turning (side to side and up and down)
3. Hyperventilation
4. Valsalva maneuver
5. Carotid sinus stimulation (see later section on syncope)
6. Ear inspection and hearing test
7. Neurologic examination including:

   - Evidence of previous stroke or parkinsonian features
   - Sensory examination including joint position and vibration sense
   - Cerebellar testing (past pointing suggests vestibular lesion; intention tremor and abnormal alternating movements suggest cerebellar dysfunction)
   - Romberg's test
   - Gait assessment

8. Hallpike's maneuver

The Hallpike maneuver can be useful for assessment of some patients with true vertigo. Under ideal conditions, the patient should wear Frenzel's glasses. These have 20-diopter lenses with accompanying illumination so that the patient is unable to fixate visually and the eyes are under magnification. Peripheral vertigo is easily suppressed if the patient is allowed to focus on an object. The test begins with the patient in a sitting position on the examination table. The examiner quickly lays the patient down with the head hanging over the back of the table at approximately a 30-degree angle and the face turned 45 degrees to the right. The patient is observed for nystagmus and queried about vertigo or reproduction of the symptoms. The head is held there for 1 minute. The patient is then returned to the sitting position and again observed for 1 minute. The test is then repeated with the head held at 45 degrees to the other side. If vertigo is reproduced, the test should be repeated two or three times on the side that caused the most pronounced symptoms to see if the nystagmus and symptoms fade.

If BPV is present, after being positioned in the supine head-turned position, there will be a short *latency period of 5 to 15 seconds*, and then the patient will complain of severe vertigo, and J-shaped, rotatory nystagmus may be observed. This will *fade in less than a minute*. Back in the sitting position, transient vertigo and nystagmus may be observed again. When tested on the other side, only 20% of patients have recurrent symptoms and findings. *The vertigo will fade with repeated testing.* During remissions or mild episodes of BPV, the Hallpike maneuver may be negative, and the diagnosis must be made on the history alone. When no nystagmus is elicited, BPV is still a more likely diagnosis than dizziness due to a central cause. A central lesion should be suspected if vertigo is dissociated from the nystagmus and if the nystagmus begins immediately on positioning, is primarily horizontal or vertical, lasts longer than 1 minute, or does not fade with repeated testing.

Laboratory testing depends on the working diagnosis and the site of presentation. In the emergency room, routine glucose determination (for hypoglycemia) and cardiac rhythm monitoring are useful in patients over age 45 who present with dizziness. In patients with acute vertigo, a CT scan to rule out a cerebrovascular event should be considered.

In less acute settings, testing of patients with vertigo should include glucose determinations (to exclude hyperglycemia), thyroid function tests, and serologic tests for syphilis to identify potentially reversible causes. When the diagnosis remains unclear, consultation with a subspecialist from either the ear, nose, and throat (ENT) department or neurology department should be considered. They may perform dynamic tests of vestibular function such as electronystagmography and caloric testing. If there is evidence of a central lesion, a computed tomographic (CT) scan directed through the petrous pyramids or a magnetic resonance imaging (MRI) scan may be considered, although many asymptomatic elderly patients have abnormal findings on MRI.[20] These imaging techniques are not usually necessary and are best ordered after consultation with a subspecialist.

Those with pre-syncope should be evaluated in the same way as patients with syncope. Patients with a balance problem should undergo testing as dictated by the history and physical findings. In those with lightheadedness, drug level testing should be performed if appropriate. These patients do not require other diagnostic evaluation unless abnormalities on the above evaluation are identified.

Treatment

Therapy for vertigo is discussed initially; then recommendations for nonvertiginous dizziness are reviewed. If an elderly patient without a previous history of vertigo develops an acute episode of moderate or severe vertigo, hospital admission for observation and symptom control may be appropriate. It can be very difficult at times to rule out a brain stem or cerebellar infarction. Treatment of symptoms associated with acute vertigo usually includes medications with anticholinergic and antiemetic properties. A good initial choice is promethazine (Phenergan), which has both characteristics. It can be given orally, rectally, or intramuscularly in a dose of 12.5 to 50 mg. If the patient is excessively anxious, a benzodiazepine may also be a useful adjunctive therapy. For patients with mild or moderate bouts of vertigo, promethazine can be used if nausea is present, and meclizine (Antivert) if nausea is not present. One should start with a low dose of either agent (12.5 mg) at bedtime, gradually titrating the dose to the level tolerated. In general, medication should be used for only short periods of time. Chronic therapy is rarely indicated. A set of exercises has been developed to shorten the duration and impact of benign positional vertigo, but these should be reserved for the robust and interested patient.[21]

For those with pre-syncope, the specific etiology should be addressed (e.g., orthostatic hypotension, hyperventilation). For patients with balance problems or a multisensory deficit, a referral to physical therapy for gait evaluation, strengthening, and a gait-assist device is important, as is audiologic assessment and ophthalmologic screening. Appropriate treatment of patients with ill-defined lightheadedness begins by discontinuing any offending medications and also includes ophthalmologic assessment. Psychiatric evaluation is appropriate if other features suggest a psychiatric disorder. Physical therapy and exercise programs may be useful. Reassurance and regular follow-up are important.

SYNCOPE

Syncope is a common and potentially serious problem in elderly persons. It accounts for approximately 3% of emergency room visits and 1% of medical admissions to a general hospital.[22] The causes of syncope in elderly patients are different from those in younger individuals. A syncopal episode can lead to injury, fear, and functional limitation. Proper evaluation and management are essential to maintain maximum patient independence.

The term syncope is used to denote a transient loss of consciousness and postural tone that resolves spontaneously without resuscitative intervention and without residual symptoms. This disorder should be differentiated from other states of altered consciousness such as cardiac arrest, coma, and seizure.

Epidemiology

Syncope is common in patients of all ages. Thirty-seven percent of younger individuals have had a syncopal episode.[22] A study of elderly nursing home residents showed a 23% prevalence over 10 years, a 1-year incidence of 6%, and a recurrence rate of 30%.[23]

In studies by Kapoor and colleagues, which evaluated 210 patients 60 years and older presenting to emergency rooms, clinics, and inpatient services, the causes of syncope were evenly split between cardiac, noncardiac, and unknown.[24] Almost half the cardiovascular causes were ventricular tachycardia, and the next largest category was sick sinus syndrome (17%). Orthostatic hypotension and situational events (cough, defecation) constituted 60% of the noncardiac causes. Vasovagal syncope was an unusual cause of syncope in the elderly group. Forty percent of the patients had sustained trauma. Cardiovascular causes were much more common in elderly persons than in younger subjects. Lipsitz and associates reported on 97 institutionalized elderly with syncope.[25] They found that the causes were evenly split between specific diseases, situational stressors, and unknown causes. The most common specific causative conditions were myocardial infarction, aortic stenosis, and volume depletion. The most common situational stressors were hypotension induced by drugs, eating, defecation, and postural changes. Recurrence rates were approximately 30% for all etiologic classes (cardiovascular, noncardiovascular, and unknown) of syncope. Recurrence only

rarely (5%) provided new information that allowed a specific diagnosis to be made in a patient who had been previously evaluated.[22]

The prognosis for younger patients with syncope depends on its cause. The highest 2-year mortality occured in patients with syncope due to cardiac causes (32%); lower rates apply to noncardiac (5%) and unknown causes (2%). In elderly patients, the 2-year mortality rates were 38%, 22%, and 20% for cardiovascular, noncardiovascular, and unknown causes, respectively.[24]

Evaluation

Initial evaluation for syncope begins with a careful history.[26] If an observer was present at the time of the episode, he or she should be questioned. Patients should be allowed to describe the event in their own words and encouraged to suggest a possible diagnosis. Then the following information should be obtained. Table 20–3 shows the differential diagnosis to keep in mind when beginning the evaluation.

1. How many times has this occurred? Recurrent episodes are common. Has near syncope as well as syncope occurred?
2. What has been the patient's general health in the last few days? Has he been eating and taking fluids and medications in the usual manner? This question may uncover illnesses (e.g., diarrhea) that in combination with a usual medical regimen may result in hypotension.
3. How did the episode begin? What activities was the patient engaged in? Were there any associated symptoms? Shaving (carotid sinus), recent meal

---

TABLE 20–3 **DIFFERENTIAL DIAGNOSIS OF SYNCOPE**

I. Reflex
   Carotid sinus, cough, defecation, micturition, swallowing, vasovagal
II. Hypotensive
   Medication, multiple diseases and impairments, orthostatic, postprandial, volume depletion
III. Cardiac
   Arrhythmias, atrial myxoma, aortic dissection, cardiomyopathy (dilated or hypertrophic), myocardial infarction, pulmonary hypertension or embolism, valvular disease
IV. Central nervous system
   Psychiatric, seizure, subclavian steal syndrome, transient ischemic attack, tumor
V. Abnormal blood composition
   Anemia, hyperventilation, hypoglycemia, hypoxia

(postprandial hypotension), standing (orthostatic hypotension), difficult urination or defecation (bradycardia or hypotension), climbing stairs (hypoxia, aortic stenosis), chest pain (angina or myocardial infarction), and palpitations (arrhythmia) are some of the possible responses to this question.

4. What occurred during the episode? Was incontinence present or tonic-clonic movements, suggesting a seizure?
5. How did the episode end? Slow onset and slow recovery suggest hyperventilation or hypoglycemia. Sudden onset but slow recovery (more than 15 minutes) suggest a seizure disorder, transient ischemic attack, or head trauma. Sudden onset and sudden resolution suggest hypotension, outflow obstruction, or arrhythmia. Did any injury occur?

The history should then focus on a careful review of medications, alcohol use, and eye drops. The past medical history should focus on cardiovascular risk factors.

The physical examination should include blood pressure measurements in both arms to rule out subclavian steal syndrome or aortic dissection, and an orthostatic blood pressure measurement should be done as well (see previous discussion). Blood pressure should also be measured after walking or climbing stairs if the history is suggestive, as described in the previous section.

A careful cardiopulmonary examination should be done to check for volume status, aortic stenosis, hypertrophic cardiomyopathy, pulmonary embolism, or pulmonary hypertension. Stool guaiac and neurologic examinations should be performed.

Laboratory tests should include a complete blood count, blood chemistries, urinalysis (specific gravity), and an electrocardiogram (ECG). On electrocardiography, frequent ectopic beats, bradycardia, abnormal PR interval, long QT interval, conduction delay, or bundle branch block may suggest a rhythm disturbance as a cause. However, even in patients with bifascicular or trifascicular block, syncope is more commonly due to another cause than to complete heart block.

With this data base, the diagnosis will be apparent in a third of patients, and the work-up or treatment can proceed accordingly. If the diagnosis is still unclear, carotid sinus massage can be performed to test for carotid sinus hypersensitivity. This maneuver should not be performed in patients who have carotid bruits or digitalis toxicity. In these instances, Holter monitoring should be considered. There are rare reports of asystole,

complete heart block, and stroke occurring in elderly patients after carotid sinus massage, and some authors recommend having intravenous access, atropine, and resuscitation equipment available. Carotid sinus massage can be performed as follows. With an electrocardiogram running, a baseline blood pressure is taken. The carotid bifurcation is *gently* massaged for 5 seconds, the ECG observed, and the blood pressure is rechecked. The test is then repeated on the opposite side. Criteria for abnormal response include symptoms, sinus pause of 3 seconds or longer, or systolic blood pressure decline of more than 50 mmHg or systolic pressure of less than 90 mmHg. Some investigators also perform this test with the patient upright, but this increases the false-positive rate.[27]

For patients with suspected defecation or micturition syncope, or digitalis toxicity, the Valsalva maneuver can be performed. The patient forces air against a closed glottis for 15 seconds under ECG monitoring while the physician looks for excessive bradycardia.

If these evaluations are negative and a cardiac cause is still suspected, Holter monitoring and echocardiography are useful because of the high prevalence of rhythm disturbances, valvular disorders, and myocardial disease in this population. In one study, Holter monitoring in 17% of elderly subjects led to diagnoses that were not identified on initial assessment.[24] Prolonged ambulatory Holter monitoring, transtelephonic event monitoring, treadmill testing, ambulatory blood pressure monitoring, cardiac catheterization, signal-averaged ECG, electrophysiologic studies, and tilt-table testing may ultimately be useful but should be performed in conjunction with a cardiologist. Tilt-table testing in conjunction with isoproterenol infusion does not appear to be as useful in the evaluation of elderly patients with syncope as it is in younger patients.[28]

Head CT scans and electroencephalography are very low yield studies in patients who do not have clinical evidence of a cerebrovascular event or seizure.

Treatment

The goal of treatment is to prevent recurrence or death. If a specific cause is defined, appropriate treatment options can be discussed. If no specific disorder is identified, careful consideration should be given to the possibility of multiple causes. Empirical therapy with pacemakers, digoxin, antiarrhythmics, or antiseizure medications does not appear to reduce subsequent syncopal events.[29] The following interventions may be useful:

1. Medications should be reviewed. Medications whose therapeutic benefit is unclear or that have a hypotensive effect should be tapered or discontinued.
2. For patients with postprandial hypotension, smaller and more frequent meals with less carbohydrate and more protein should be considered along with a liberalized salt intake.[3] A caffeinated beverage before the meal may also be helpful.
3. Extreme neck rotation and tight shirt collars should be avoided.
4. A regular exercise program should be initiated with supervision.
5. Urination and showering should be performed while sitting.
6. Prolonged, quiet standing should be avoided. If any symptoms develop, the patient should assume a supine or sitting position.
7. Hypotensive stressors should be avoided (hot tubs, sauna).
8. After a prolonged time in a supine or sitting position, isometric exercises of the upper and lower extremities should be performed, and the patient should be cautioned to stand slowly with support assistance.

Patients should be monitored carefully, and further episodes should be reported immediately. Patients should be instructed not to drive until their evaluation is completed. It is important to remember that the cause remains unknown in approximately one third of patients after evaluation. Caregivers or spouses should be trained to take a pulse so that they can check the rate and strength of the pulse wave during subsequent episodes if witnessed.

References

1. Mader SL: Aging and postural hypotension. An update. J Am Geriatr Soc 1989;37:129–137.
2. Hausdorff JM, Clark BA, Shannon RP, Elahi D, Wei JW: Hypotensive response to atrial natriuretic peptide administration is enhanced with age. J Gerontol 1995;50(3):M169–M172.
3. Jansen RWMM, Lipsitz LA: Postprandial hypotension: Epidemiology, pathophysiology, and clinical management. Ann Int Med 1995;122:286–295.
4. Mader SL, Josephson KR, Rubenstein LZ: Low prevalence of postural hypotension among community-dwelling elderly. JAMA 1987;258:1511–1514.
5. Rutan GH, Hermanson B, Bild DE, Kittner SJ, LaBaw F, Tell GS: Orthostatic hypotension in older adults. The Cardiovascular Health Study. Hypertension 1992;19:508–519.
6. Robertson D, Robertson RM: Causes of chronic orthostatic hypotension. Arch Intern Med 1994;154:1620–1624.
7. Mets TF: Drug-induced orthostatic hypotension in older patients. Drugs Aging 1995;6(3):219–228.
8. Streeten DHP, Anderson GH: Delayed orthostatic intolerance. Arch Intern Med 1992;152:1066–1072.
9. Ahmad RAS, Watson RDS: Treatment of postural hypotension. A review. Drugs 1990;39:74–85.
10. Grubb BP, Samoil D, Kosinski D, Wolfe D, Lorton M, Madu E: Fluoxetine hydrochloride for the treatment of severe refractory orthostatic hypotension. Am J Med 1994;97:366–368.
11. Ten Harkle ADJ, van Lieshout JJ, Wieling W: Treatment of orthostatic hypotension with sleeping in the head-up tilt position, alone and in combination with fludrocortisone. J Intern Med 1992;232:139–145.
12. Weindruch R, Korper SP, Hadley E: The prevalence of dysequilibrium and related disorders in older persons. Ear Nose Throat J 1989;68:925–929.
13. Hale WE, Perkins LL, May FE, Marks RG, Stewart RB: Symptom prevalence in the elderly J Am Geriatr Soc 1986;34:333–340.
14. Sloane P, Blazer D, George LK: Dizziness in a community elderly population. J Am Geriatr Soc 1989;37:101–108.
15. Sloane PD, Baloh RW: Persistent dizziness in geriatric patients. J Am Geriatr Soc 1989;37:1031–1038.
16. Katsarkas A: Dizziness in aging: A retrospective study of 1194 cases. Otolaryngol Head Neck Surg 1994;110:296–301.
17. Ruckenstein MJ: A practical approach to dizziness. Postgrad Med 1995;97(3):70–81.
18. Leigh RJ, Zee DS: The Neurology of Eye Movements. Philadelphia, F.A. Davis, 1991, pp. 411–419.
19. Baloh RW, Honrubia V, Jacobson K: Benign positional vertigo: Clinical and oculographic features in 240 cases. Neurology 1987;37:371–378.
20. Day JJ, Freer CE, Dixon AK, Coni N, Hall LD, Sims C, Gehlhaar EW: Magnetic resonance imaging of the brain and brain stem in elderly patients with dizziness. Age Aging 1990;19:144–150.
21. Brandt T, Daroff RB: Physical therapy for benign paroxysmal positional vertigo. Arch Otolaryngol 1980;106:484–485.
22. Kapoor WN: Evaluation and outcome of patients with syncope. Medicine 1990;69:160–175.
23. Lipsitz LA, Wei JY, Rowe JW: Syncope in an elderly, institutionalized population: Prevalence, incidence, and associated risk. Q J Med 1985;55:45–54.
24. Kapoor W, Snustad D, Peterson J, Wieland HS, Cha R, Karpf M: Syncope in the elderly. Am J Med 1986;80:419–428.
25. Lipsitz LA, Pluchino FC, Wei JY, Rowe JW: Syncope in institutionalized elderly: Impact of multiple pathological conditions and situational stress. J Chronic Dis 1986;39:619–630.
26. Bonema JD, Maddens ME: Syncope in elderly patients. Why their risk is higher. Postgrad Med 1992;91:129–144.
27. MacIntosh S, Da Costa K, Kenny RA: Outcome of an integrated approach to the investigation of dizziness, falls, and syncope in elderly patients referred to a "syncope" clinic. Age Ageing 1993;22:53–88.
28. Sheldon R: Effects of aging on responses to isoproterenol tilt-table testing in patients with syncope. Am J Cardiol 1994;74:459–463.
29. Aronow WS, Mercando AD, Epstein S: Prevalence of arrhythmias detected by 24-hour ambulatory electrocardiography and value of antiarrhythmic therapy in elderly patients with unexplained syncope. Am J Cardiol 1992;70:408–410.

21 Osteoporosis

Luis R. Navas, M.D.

Kenneth W. Lyles, M.D.

Osteoporosis is a systemic skeletal disease characterized by a reduction in the amount of bone mass, microarchitectural impairment of bone tissue, and a subsequent increase in fractures. This disease is present in epidemic proportions in the United States, affecting between 20 and 25 million people. Because osteoporosis is characterized by a long latency period and a lack of symptoms, many patients' first encounter with the disease is a skeletal fracture with minimal trauma. The resulting physical deformities can lead to functional impairments that may have a significant impact on quality of life, mobility, and mortality. The primary care physician should have a high level of suspicion for this disease because it is much easier to prevent bone loss than it is to manage the sequelae of skeletal fractures.

EPIDEMIOLOGY AND COST OF OSTEOPOROSIS

Life expectancy at birth has improved in the United States and is projected to increase to 82 years for women and 74.2 years for men by the year 2020. Furthermore, the older population (over age 65) is projected to reach 52 million people by the year 2020. Because osteoporotic fractures occur more commonly in people over 65 years old, the burden of this disease is expected to increase during the next few decades.[1] It was estimated in 1990 that approximately 1.7 million hip fractures occurred throughout the world, and about 50% of these fractures occurred in North America, Europe, and Oceana.[2] There are more than 1.5 million osteoporotic fractures annually in the United States, and these fractures are expected to increase in the next 50 years.[3] The annual cost of care for osteoporosis in the United States is now approximately $10 to $20 billion, but within 50 years this cost may exceed $240 billion.[4] In the United States 265,000 hip fractures occur each year, most of them in patients over the age of 70 years.[3] There is a perception that money is being wasted on individuals who have a short life expectancy, but in fact, the cost of hip fracture treatment per quality-adjusted life year compares favorably with that for renal transplant or coronary artery bypass.[5] By the age of 90, 32% of women (one in three) and 17% of men (one in six) will have suffered a hip fracture.[3, 6]

Vertebral fractures are more common than hip fractures, and frequently patients may not seek medical attention for these. The lifetime risk of vertebral fractures for a woman aged 50 is estimated at 32%, whereas her lifetime risk of hip fracture is 15.6%.[7] Although early work suggested that vertebral fractures were not clinically significant, several more recent studies have shown that vertebral compression fractures in older patients have a major impact on their physical, functional, and psychosocial status.[8, 9] Osteoporotic fractures at any site are associated with an approximate doubling of the risk of physical limitations and an even higher risk of functional limitations.[2, 9] Combining information about bone mass and prevalent (existing) fractures is a powerful means of predicting the occurrence of new vertebral fractures. A reduced initial bone mass of 2 standard deviations (SD) at a given age is associated with a fourfold to sixfold increase in the risk of new vertebral fracture. A single fracture at the baseline examination increases the risk for a new vertebral fracture fivefold. The presence of two or more fractures at baseline increases the risk twelvefold.[10, 11]

Mortality in patients with osteoporosis is increased. Older women with low bone density have a significant increased risk of a nonfracture-related death within 3 years. For each standard deviation decrease in bone mineral density in the proximal radius there is a 1.19-fold increase in nontraumatic mortality.[12] Also, it is well known that there is an increased risk of death after a hip fracture. The death rate within 1 year of hip fracture ranges from 12% to 24% and increases with age.[2, 13, 14] The coexisting chronic diseases and frailty that are present in some older patients sustaining a hip fracture may be the cause of the increased mortality.[2, 13] Because of the excess morbidity and mortality suffered by patients with osteoporosis and the services needed by impaired patients after sustaining a skeletal fracture, early diagnosis and appropriate treatment are crucial to try to prevent the disease or slow its pathologic progression.

SKELETAL FUNCTION AND REMODELING

The skeleton has three distinct functions. First, it serves as a lightweight frame to which the muscles and tendons are attached, thus allowing movement and change of position. Second, it provides protection for important organs like the brain, spinal cord, heart, lungs, and bone marrow. Finally, the skeleton provides a reservoir of minerals and buffers (i.e., calcium, phosphorus, magnesium, sodium, and carbonate). When an excess amount of acid occurs in the diet of a patient with chronic acidosis, skeletal phosphate and carbonate can serve as buffers. Likewise, when dietary calcium is not sufficient, calcium will be resorbed from the skeleton. Because the metabolic function of the bone precedes its structural function, in states of calcium deficiency or chronic acidosis bone growth or remodeling (formation and resorption) is impaired.

The skeleton is formed of two type of bones: cancellous or trabecular bone and cortical bone. Cancellous bone is a series of trabeculae (plates) that form the meshwork in the vertebral body and at the end of the long bones. It represents 20% to 25% of the skeleton. The cortical bone is the compact bone that forms the outer shell of the bones. It provides most of the support for the body and represents 75% to 80% of the skeleton. Long bones such as the femur are at least 90% cortical bone. Trabecular bone is more sensitive to changes in bone remodeling than cortical bone because it has a greater surface-to-volume ratio.

The bones grow in two ways: longitudinal growth, which ceases with the closure of the epiphyses in the early twenties, and bone mass growth. The bone mass reaches a peak at about the age of 30 years. After a period of stabilization, when the rates of bone formation and bone resorption are in equilibrium, bone loss begins in both sexes. Over her lifetime a female loses approximately 35% of her cortical bone mass and 40% to 50% of her trabecular bone mass. Two rates of bone loss have been identified.[3, 15-18] First, slow loss, or "normal bone loss," is a slow and gradual loss of both trabecular and cortical bone that affects males and females equally. Second, the so-called fast bone loss is a transient and more rapid phase of bone loss. This rapid phase of bone loss occurs in approximately 35% of early postmenopausal women and in some men who develop hypogonadism. At this time it

cannot be predicted who will undergo such rapid bone loss. Local production of selected cytokines may mediate this effect. In women identified as "fast losers" at menopause, about 50% of bone mass has been lost within 12 years of menopause.[16, 17] The loss of bone that occurs during the menopause is a transient phase that usually lasts 5 to 8 years.

All areas of the skeleton undergo a complex remodeling process. In areas of increased skeletal loading, the remodeling process increases the bone mass, a phenomenon referred as Wolf's law.[3] The bone remodeling process is carried out by cellular units called the bone morphologic units in which osteoclasts, osteoblasts, and osteocytes are the cellular elements. The osteoclast, a multinuclear cell derived from granulocyte-macrophage colony-forming units, resorbs bone, forming a resorption cavity. Osteoblasts, derived from fibroblast colony-forming units in the bone marrow, fill the resorption cavity, depositing a protein collagen matrix called osteoid. Osteoblasts then mineralize the osteoid tissue over a period of 2 months. Twenty percent of osteoblasts become surrounded by calcified matrix and become osteocytes. The process of remodeling takes 100 to 150 days to complete, and about 5% of the bone mass is undergoing remodeling at any one time.

Recently, it has been proposed that interleukin-1 beta (IL-1β) and other cytokines such as tumor necrosis factor alpha and beta (TNFα and β) produced by osteoclasts in the bone morphologic unit stimulate the production of osteoclast precursor cells. The production of interleukin-6 (IL-6) and anexin II by osteoclasts also stimulates and promotes adhesion of circulating osteoclast precursor cells to the endothelium of the capillary supplying the bone morphologic unit.[19]

The process of bone formation and resorption in a young adult results in conservation of bone mass. Imbalance of these processes may result in bone loss when more bone resorption occurs than bone formation. Two histologic forms of bone loss have been described. High-turnover osteoporosis occurs when bone resorption is increased. The activity of both osteoclasts and osteoblasts is increased, but the osteoblasts fail to keep pace with the accelerated resorption, and the net result is a reduction in bone mass. As a result of the high turnover, the resorption cavities or lacunae in the bones become deeper. The second type of bone loss is the low-turnover type, which is more common in older patients. In this type, the function of the osteoclasts is normal, but the osteoblasts fail to refill the resorption cavities completely, causing a reduction in bone mass.

HORMONAL CONTROL AND EFFECTS ON THE SKELETON AND MINERALS

The three major hormones involved in the regulation of mineral metabolism (calcium and phosphate) in the skeleton are parathyroid hormone (PTH), calcitonin, and 1,25-dihydroxycholecalciferol (the active form of vitamin D).[20] PTH is secreted by the parathyroid glands and regulates the serum ionized calcium level by directly increasing bone resorption and increasing reabsorption of calcium in the distal tubules of the kidneys. It also increases phosphate excretion in urine. PTH increases the conversion of 25-hydroxycholecalciferol to 1,25-dihydroxycholecalciferol in the renal tubule. Serum levels of PTH are increased with aging, probably in response to decreased gastrointestinal absorption of calcium and a reduction in the glomerular filtration rate.

Vitamin D is involved in the absorption of calcium and phosphate in the gastrointestinal system. Vitamin D_3, or cholecalciferol, is produced in the skin from 7-dehydrocholesterol by the action of ultraviolet rays in sunlight. In the liver, the cholecalciferol is hydroxylated to 25-hydroxycholecalciferol or calcidiol. Calcidiol is converted in the proximal tubules of the kidney into the active metabolite 1,25-dihydroxycholecalciferol, or calcitriol. Calcitriol supplies adequate calcium and phosphate for mineralization by increasing calcium and phosphorus absorption by the intestine. In bone, calcitriol improves mineralization and probably stimulates osteoblastic activity. With aging, absorption of calcium and phosphate in the gastrointestinal tract is decreased, especially after age 70, and the serum level of calcitriol is decreased about 50%. The production of vitamin D in the skin is also reduced with age, particularly in institutionalized elderly patients. Several studies have shown evidence of a primary impairment in the renal production of calcitriol in elderly patients with osteoporosis.

Calcitonin is secreted by the C cells or parafollicular cells in the thyroid gland and acts to reduce the serum calcium concentration by inhibiting bone resorption. The relationship of calcitonin in mineral metabolism is not clear, and its role in osteoporosis is also unclear. Calcium metabolism and bones are affected by various other hormones. Long-term use of or excessive endogenous production of glucocorticoids causes bone loss by altering bone remodeling. Glucocorticoids increase bone resorption by osteoclasts and decrease bone formation by osteoblasts.[21] Also, they reduce gastrointestinal calcium-phosphorus absorption by exerting a direct action on the intestine, and they increase renal calcium-phosphorus excretion. The decreased absorption of calcium by the gut is reported to cause an increase in PTH secretion, causing a secondary hyperparathyroidism.[22]

Thyroid hormone is necessary for normal bone growth and turnover, but excess thyroid hormone may produce hypercalcemia (due to a direct stimulation of osteoclasts) and may lead to bone loss (osteoporosis) and hypercalciuria.

Insulin increases bone formation, and the Rotterdam study[23] demonstrated that women with non–insulin-dependent diabetes mellitus have increased bone density and a lower frequency of nonvertebral fractures. This "protective effect" of insulin in diabetics may be explained by the period of hyperinsulinemia due to insulin resistance before the onset of the diabetes or by the strong binding effect of insulin on sex hormone binding globulin, which may lead to higher levels of free serum estradiol and testosterone during the hyperinsulinemia stage.

Growth hormone is required for growth of the skeleton. Somatomedins and insulin-like growth factor-1 (IGF-1) stimulate protein synthesis in bones. The sex steroids are also required for optimal bone mass and will be discussed subsequently.

FACTORS ASSOCIATED WITH BONE MASS

Bone mass is the net result of the amount of bone formed minus the amount of bone lost. Genetics, race, sex, diet and nutrition, exercise, and the use of tobacco and alcohol are important factors in determining bone mass and bone turnover. In twin studies it has been shown that 60% to 80% of peak bone density is genetically determined.[24, 25] A positive family history of osteoporosis is a risk factor for osteoporosis. In blacks, osteoporosis is rare; whites, Eskimos, and Asians have a higher incidence of osteoporosis. Two factors may explain why blacks may have a low incidence of this disease. First, they have a greater initial bone mass, and second, they have slower bone remodeling rates. Females in general have a lower bone mass than males, and this may explain why women suffer more osteoporosis than men. White, Asian, and Eskimo women have a greater risk of developing osteoporosis than black or Hispanic women.

Nutrition may also play an important role in the development of osteoporosis. An acid-ash diet* may have a negative effect on bone mass.

---

*An acid-ash diet consists largely of meat, fish, eggs, and cereals with little fruit, vegetables, cheese, or milk; when catabolized, it leaves an acid load to be excreted in the urine.[26]

This diet generates a residue of approximately 100 mEq of acid daily. With a chronic acid load, the bones provide buffers (calcium and phosphorus) through increasing bone resorption. This chronic acid diet causes an excessive loss of calcium, which is manifested by hypercalciuria, and may play a role in the development of osteoporosis.[27] There is some suggestion that the incidence of osteoporosis is lower in vegetarians, but appropriate long-term studies are required to verify this hypothesis.[27]

Diets high in phosphorus were formerly thought to have an adverse effect on bone mass. However, diets that contain the average daily phosphate intake of most Americans (800 to 2000 mg) are not harmful to the skeleton.[3]

In the United States, osteoporotic postmenopausal women have been shown to be in negative calcium balance, and most of these women fail to replace these calcium losses. Dietary calcium deficiency has been associated with lactose intolerance and low dietary calcium intake. A consideration that may contribute to the calcium deficiency seen in elderly patients is that they may lack the ability to absorb most of the calcium they ingest. Multiple studies have shown that calcium supplements produce a sustained reduction in the rate of loss of bone mass in postmenopausal women and may reduce the incidence of fractures. So the consensus is that calcium supplements are warranted in older women.[3, 28–31]

Polymorphism of the vitamin D receptor gene allele (genotypes BB, Bb, and bb) has been suggested as a cause of a significant portion of the total genetic effect on peak bone, bone turnover, and rate of bone growth and bone loss.[32] At this time, this effect is controversial, and studies are ongoing to resolve this dilemma. However, it has been found that elderly people with the BB and Bb genotypes were less responsive to calcium supplements for maintenance of bone density.[33] The bb genotype is more common in the Japanese population, whereas the BB and Bb genotypes are more common among Caucasians.[25] In the future, such polymorphisms could be an invaluable aid in selecting the optimal therapy for the prevention and treatment of osteoporosis.

Prolonged immobility is a cause of bone loss. Patients undergoing complete bedrest who experience prolonged absence of weight bearing can lose up to 1% of their bone mass per week. Resuming weight-bearing activity gradually restores the bone mass to normal. Exercise or physical activity such as walking is associated with an increase in bone mass. Obesity appears to protect against bone loss by increasing skeletal loading or by increasing the levels of estrogen.

Intake of a moderate amount of alcohol can have a positive effect on bone mass.[34] However, the bone loss and fractures seen in some people who consume large amounts of alcohol is multifactorial. Alcohol in large amounts may have a direct toxic effect on osteoblasts and produces a low-turnover osteoporosis. It may also reduce the dietary protein intake, lower the calcium intake, and cause low testosterone levels, which can contribute to the development of osteoporosis.[3, 35] Heavy alcohol drinking can impair gait and predispose patients to falls, placing them at higher risk for fractures.

Cigarette smoking is a risk factor for bone loss and may have a secondary effect on ovarian function. Currently it is believed that smoking accelerates estrogen metabolism in the liver. Patients who smoke should be advised not to do so.

A number of conditions, diseases, and drugs have effects on the skeleton (Table 21–1). Conditions and diseases associated with osteoporosis are gastrectomy, castration, thyrotoxicosis (hyperthyroidism), hyperparathyroidism, rheumatoid arthritis, Cushing's syndrome, and possibly diabetes mellitus. Chronic use of glucocorticoids, heparin, and anticonvulsants (e.g., phenytoin) can cause bone loss. Consumption of caffeine can cause mild renal calcium losses. Thiazide diuretics may have a protective role by causing renal calcium conservation.

Osteoporosis can result from multiple factors; however, clinical risk factors may help the clinician predict the bone mass of a patient. Increasing age (over 65 years), low body index, a history of maternal fracture, and smoking are associated clinically with low bone mass. On the other hand, a history of estrogen use, non–insulin-dependent diabetes, thiazide use, increased weight, greater muscle strength, later age at menopause, and greater height are associated with higher bone mass.[36, 37]

CLASSIFICATION OF OSTEOPOROSIS

The World Health Organization (WHO) defines low bone mass or low bone mass density as values that are from 1 to 2.5 SD below the normal mean values for young normal adults in the third or fourth decade of life; values below 2.5 SD are defined as osteoporosis.[15]

Osteoporosis has a variety of presentations. In general, it has been classified as primary or not associated with other diseases, and secondary or associated with inherited disorders or acquired pathologies. Primary osteoporosis can be divided into several types (see Table 21–1). Primary osteoporosis in most patients is classified as involutional osteoporosis, which has two subcategories.

TABLE 21–1 **CLASSIFICATION OF OSTEOPOROSIS**

Primary Osteoporosis
Idiopathic osteoporosis (juvenile and adult)
Involutional osteoporosis
    Type I osteoporosis, postmenopausal
    Type II osteoporosis, age-associated
Secondary Osteoporosis
Inherited
    Ehlers-Danlos syndrome
    Fibrogenesis imperfecta ossium
    Glycogen storage disease
    Homocystinuria due to cystathionine
        synthetase deficiency
    Marfan's syndrome
    Osteogenesis imperfecta
    Wilson's disease
Acquired
    Chronic inflammatory diseases: rheumatoid
        arthritis
    Drugs
        Alcoholism
        Anticonvulsants
        Cisplatin
        Cyclosporine
        Diuretics (except thiazides)
        Glucocorticoids
        Heparin
        Methotrexate
        Thyroid hormone excess
Endocrine and metabolic factors
    Acromegaly
    Adult hyperphosphatemia
    Calcium deficiency
    Cushing's syndrome
    Diabetes mellitus type I
    Hyperparathyroidism
    Hyperthyroidism (thyrotoxicosis)
    Hypogonadism
    Scurvy

Secondary Osteoporosis *(Continued)*
Gastrointestinal
    Chronic liver disease (primary biliary
        cirrhosis, hemochromatosis, Wilson's
        disease)
    Gastrectomy
    Inflammatory bowel disease
    Malnutrition (anorexia nervosa)
    Sprue (gluten-induced enteropathy)
Hemato-oncologic
    Beta-thalassemia
    Leukemia
    Lymphoma
    Metastasis
    Multiple myeloma
    Sickle cell disease
    Systemic mastocytosis
Renal
    Chronic renal failure
    Idiopathic hypercalciuria
    Renal tubular acidosis
Others
    Immobilization
    Post-organ transplantation
    Pregnancy (transitional)

Type I or postmenopausal osteoporosis is found usually in women 15 to 20 years after the menopause. The incidence in women is six to eight times higher than that in men. It has been postulated that the cause of this osteoporosis is accelerated bone resorption. The increased bone turnover results in a secondary decrease in PTH secretion as well as a secondary reduction in the renal production of calcitriol. Patients present with trabecular bone loss with vertebral fractures or distal forearm fractures.

Type II, age-associated, or senile osteoporosis occurs in men or women over the age of 70; it has a female-to-male ratio of 2:1 or 3:1. The mechanisms of this bone mass loss are thought to be increased PTH secretion resulting from decreased gastrointestinal calcium absorption and decreased osteoblast function. Patients usu-

ally present with fractures of the hip or vertebrae, sites that contain cortical and trabecular bone, although fractures of the pelvis, ribs, and tibia can also occur. A great number of these fractures are the result of falls or trauma, which occur frequently in elderly patients.

There are other diseases and medications that are associated with reduced bone formation or accelerated bone loss. These secondary causes of osteoporosis are listed in Table 21–1. The use of some medications can affect the bones. Long-term use of glucocorticoids is a cause of osteoporosis. Two thirds of patients who receive doses of more than 10 mg of prednisone per day are at risk for bone loss and subsequent fractures. Dilantin used over the long term can cause low-turnover osteoporosis. Heparin therapy has also been associated with bone loss resulting from increased amounts of bone resorption. The use of thyroid hormone with significant long-term suppression of thyroid-stimulating hormone (TSH) levels is associated with low bone mass; however, an increase in skeletal fractures has not been demonstrated yet. Another cause of bone loss and subsequent fractures may be either a primary malignancy of the skeleton such as multiple myeloma or a metastatic cancer such as lung or breast carcinoma.

CLINICAL PRESENTATION

Although osteoporosis is a generalized disorder of the skeleton, it is generally a silent disease. There are few if any clinical manifestations until a fracture occurs. Vertebral compression fractures can occur with minimal trauma, such as bending, coughing, sitting down hard, or falling. In general, these fractures affect the lower thoracic and upper lumbar vertebrae. The usual symptom of a compression fracture is severe pain that the patient can localize to the area of the fracture. It may radiate to the abdomen or into the flanks, and occasionally an ileus can develop. Back movement, bending, coughing, straining to have a bowel movement, and sitting or standing for long periods of time may worsen the pain. The pain from a vertebral compression fracture generally lasts 4 to 8 weeks and then gradually subsides. The patient lies on the back or side in a fetal position. To move from a supine to a sitting or standing position, the patient must push up from a lateral position. By careful examination, it is possible to determine by percussion the spinous process affected because tenderness is elicited. Vertebral compression fractures can be associated with lost height. Occasionally in the presence of two or more vertebral compression fractures, the patient complains of intermittent back pain.

After the acute pain of the fracture subsides, recurrent back pain may be present, described by patients as back tiredness. This may represent new fractures or muscle spasm. The natural progression of the clinical problems can be variable. Frequently, there are several years between fracture episodes, and after the first fracture the patient may have several symptom-free years. The patient may develop a deformity of the back with an increase in the curve of the thoracic spine (kyphosis), commonly known as dowager's hump. Flattening of the natural lumbar lordosis also occurs. More fractures of the thoracic and lumbar spine lead to relaxation of the abdominal muscles and angulation of the ribs, resulting in abdominal protrusion; such patients complain of early satiety. Ultimately, the ribs can come to rest on the iliac crests. In the severe forms of the disease the loss of the anterior lumbar curve leads to a hip tilt, hamstring contractures, permanent hip joint flexion, stiff ankles, and pronated feet, resulting in a unsteady gait.

Other fractures can occur in patients with osteoporosis. The clinical picture of the distal forearm or Colles' fracture is that the patient falls and, in an attempt to lessen the impact of the fall, extends the wrist. After the fracture has been reduced and heals, the patient may have a decreased range of motion of the wrist. Hip fracture is the most devastating osteoporotic fracture of the elderly. Falls play a significant role in causing hip fractures. Risk factors that influence the mechanics of falling are the orientation of the fall (especially lateral falls), the amount of soft tissue padding over the hip, and the amount of bone mass. Fortunately, most falls do not result in injury, and only about 5% of falls lead to fractures.

Following a hip fracture community-dwelling elderly subjects experience a substantial decline in physical function. A prospective cohort study of community-living elderly who had a hip fracture showed that 86% of them could dress themselves independently at baseline, but only 49% could do so 6 months after the hip fracture. In the same study, 75% of the subjects could walk across the room independently, but only 15% could do so 6 months after the event.[6] Premorbid physical and mental function prior to the fracture can predict this decline.

DIAGNOSTIC APPROACH AND DIFFERENTIAL DIAGNOSIS

Because a diverse group of diseases can result in bone loss, the etiology of bone loss must be defined if at all possible before therapy is instituted. A history and physical examination are needed when osteoporosis is suspected. The history should include a family history of bone disease. A history of nephrolithiasis and a history of sexual development (in women this may include menarche, number of children, menopause, and hormone replacement therapy; in men it includes potency and libido) should be obtained. A pharmacologic history should focus on prior and current use of glucocorticoids, anticonvulsants, anticoagulants, and thyroid medications. Both tobacco use and alcohol consumption should be quantified. The review of systems should focus on symptoms of malignancy, Cushing's disease, hyperthyroidism, and hyperparathyroidism. A history of skeletal fractures, bone pain, and height loss is also important. An attempt should be made to understand how the fracture or fractures impair the patient's function. A history of back tiredness and back pain triggered by activities that involve bending, such as cooking, removing clothes from the washer and dryer, vacuuming, or pushing a lawn mower, can be a symptom of a vertebral compression fracture. The physical examination should include information about weight, height, size of thyroid gland, spine configuration, and range of motion of the spine in flexion, extension, and side bending. The gait should be noted as well as the ability to handle transfers and climbing and descending stairs. For patients who have had a prior hip fracture, leg length discrepancy should be assessed. With the patient in a supine position, both legs are measured, and the distance from the anterior iliac crest to the medial malleolus in each is compared.

All patients with osteoporosis should be evaluated at least once for treatable conditions; this evaluation should include a complete blood count, urinalysis, calcium, phosphorus, and alkaline phosphatase levels, liver function tests (SGOT, SGPT, bilirubin), thyroid panel (TSH, free T_4), serum creatinine, and blood urea nitrogen (BUN). Further evaluation may be necessary in the presence of abnormal results—e.g., an elevated serum calcium level may be the result of an asymptomatic hyperparathyroidism. If gastrointestinal malabsorption or malnutrition is suspected, a 25-hydroxyvitamin D level should be measured. Bone mass density measurements are useful in the management of patients with osteoporosis. If the bone mass measurement is low, aggressive therapy may be indicated; if the measurement is within normal limits, prophylactic therapy and exercise can be prescribed. Further details about bone density measurements are discussed in the next section, on management and therapy.

Other diseases should be considered in the differential diagnosis of a patient with osteoporosis, including Paget's disease, osteomalacia, and malignancies of various types. Paget's disease of bone is a common disorder that affects 1% to 3% of people over the age of 60 years. The diagnosis is usually made on finding either an elevated serum alkaline phosphatase level or increased excretion of urine hydroxyproline. If Paget's disease presents in the lytic phase it may be confused with osteoporosis, but a bone scan and radiographs can be used to make this diagnosis. Osteomalacia is a disorder in which the newly formed osteoid tissue fails to mineralize normally. Clinically, the disease may present with fractures, bone pain, and osteopenia on radiographs. The diagnosis of osteomalacia is complex, but the most common causes are vitamin D deficiency

and phosphate depletion from antacids or renal phosphate wasting. Neoplasms of several types may cause osteopenia: leukemias, multiple myeloma, lymphoma, and carcinomatosis can result in bone loss, particularly in the vertebral column. Multiple myeloma is frequently present in the elderly and is evident by compression fractures, hypercalcemia, and renal failure.

MANAGEMENT AND THERAPY OF OSTEOPOROSIS

Conventional radiographs can provide some information about the skeleton. At least 30% to 60% of bone mineral must be lost before osteopenia can be seen on radiographs. Radiographs are not useful as a measurement of bone mass. However, radiographs can give useful facts about the skeleton. In osteopenic vertebrae there is a loss of horizontal trabeculae, and the vertical trabeculae appear more prominent. The vertebral end-plate surfaces are accentuated. Biconcave depressions on the superior and inferior surfaces can result from expansion of the intervertebral disks into the vertebral body, giving a codfishlike appearance on radiographs. Osteoporosis does not cause erosion of the vertebral cortex; if this is present, neoplasm should be ruled out. When a compression fracture is seen on radiographs, the apex of the wedge fracture in the lumbar and thoracic vertebrae is usually anterior. Posterior wedging of a fracture suggests another disease process, such as Paget's disease, osteomyelitis, or metastasic malignancy.

New methods have been developed to quantitate the amount of bone mass. These methods include single- and dual-energy photoabsorptiometry, dual-energy x-ray absorptiometry, quantitative computed tomography and neutron activation analysis, and quantitative ultrasound. Each method provides different information, and quality control in the measurement is essential. At present the most widely used method is dual-energy x-ray absorptiometry (DEXA), which measures the bone mass of the proximal femur, lumbar vertebral spine, and radius. These measurements of bone mass are useful clinically.

The Scientific Advisory Board of the National Osteoporosis Foundation[38] has suggested five indications for measurements of bone mass: (1) in estrogen-deficient women, to diagnose significantly low bone mass to make decisions about therapy; (2) in patients with vertebral abnormalities or roentgenographic osteopenia, to diagnose spinal osteoporosis to make decisions about further diagnostic evaluation and therapy; (3) in patients receiving long-term glucocorticoid therapy, to diagnose low bone mass to adjust therapy;

(4) in patients with asymptomatic primary hyperparathyroidism, to diagnose low bone mass to identify those at risk of severe skeletal disease who may be candidates for surgical intervention; and (5) in patients receiving therapy for osteoporosis, to determine the efficacy of the therapy. Bone mass measurements are not recommended for screening. They are valuable when they will determine the institution or withholding of therapy such as estrogen, bisphosphonates, or calcitonin.

Bone biopsy and histomorphometric studies are not commonly used but are useful techniques for determining the effects of experimental interventions on bone resorption and formation indices.

Therapy for a patient with an acute vertebral fracture consists of strong analgesics; narcotics and muscle relaxants may be necessary. Bed rest may be needed until the pain and coexisting muscle spasm subside but should be limited to prevent deconditioning. In some cases a back brace may be helpful in providing support and can aid in relieving the muscle spasm. During the period of bed rest the patient can be given literature about the disease and how to manage it. After the acute episode of pain has subsided, many patients are left with chronic lumbosacral pain that is due to muscle spasm. At this point, the patient should be referred to a physical therapist for instruction and practice in an exercise program. He or she is taught how to lift objects and how to function so that the chances of future fractures are reduced. Because osteoporosis is a chronic disease, therapy should be directed toward preventing further bone loss and teaching the patient strategies for management of the disease.

In patients with established osteoporosis, currently the Food and Drug Administration (FDA) has approved three drugs for its treatment: estrogen, alendronate, and calcitonin. These drugs act by decreasing bone resorption so that the rate of bone loss is decreased. Estrogen is believed to act in part by decreasing the production of local cytokines (IL-6), which increase osteoclastic bone resorption. Estrogen replacement therapy can be given as oral conjugated estrogens or estradiol, or by transdermal patch. For women with an intact uterus progesterone in low doses (2.5 or 5 mg of medroxyprogesterone acetate) daily or cyclic progesterone (5 to 10 mg for 10 to 12 days of the cycle) must be administered to prevent the development of endometrial hyperplasia or endometrial carcinoma. A daily dose of 0.625 mg of conjugated estrogens or 2 mg of estradiol generally is adequate to treat or prevent bone loss. Furthermore, this dose of estrogen reduces both vertebral and hip fractures by 50% if it is given for 10 years.

The problem with estrogen replacement therapy is patient compliance. Less than 30% of patients placed on replacement therapy are still taking it after 1 year.[39, 40] Many factors enter into the decision to start estrogen therapy, but even in a woman who begins therapy 20 years after menopause positive benefits have been shown. Estrogen decreases the incidence of vasomotor symptoms (hot flashes), vaginitis, urethritis, dyspareunia, urinary tract infections, and possibly depression. More than 30 epidemiologic studies indicate that postmenopausal estrogen use is associated with a 44% reduction in the risk of coronary heart disease.

The risks of estrogen therapy are an increase in endometrial hyperplasia and endometrial carcinoma and a possible increase in the risk of breast cancer. Patients receiving estrogens have more abnormal vaginal bleeding, which can lead to endometrial biopsy or dilation and curettage. The relation between estrogen therapy and breast cancer is far from clear. A number of earlier studies found no link between hormone replace therapy (HRT) and the risk of breast cancer.[41–44] A more recent study showed an increased risk of breast cancer after 5 or more years of estrogen therapy.[45, 46] At the present time, the Women's Health Initiative is under way to help determine the risk of breast cancer in postmenopausal women on HRT. Until that study is completed, patients should be informed about the current knowledge of the risks and benefits of HRT and allowed to choose for themselves whether or not to use therapy. In general, patients with hypertension should be monitored to make sure that HRT does not alter blood pressure control. The practitioner should also bear in mind that estrogens increase the incidence of gallstones.

Alendronate (Fosamax), an aminobisphosphonate, was approved by the FDA for the treatment of postmenopausal osteoporosis in 1995. Alendronate reduces bone resorption by decreasing osteoclast activity, causing a premature apoptosis (programmed cellular death) of osteoclasts.[19] This drug increases bone mass in the spine and hip in 96% of patients who receive it. It is also associated with a 48% reduction in the rate of vertebral compression fractures.[47] The major side effect of this drug is esophageal irritation, but more than 95% of people who received this drug in clinical trials had little difficulty with this side effect. Alendronate is poorly absorbed by the gastrointestinal tract, so the patient must take the medication while fasting and wait a minimum of 30 minutes before eating or drinking anything but water. Patients should not be recumbent after taking alendronate. For the treatment of osteoporosis 10 mg of alendronate daily is recommended. Adequate calcium intake of 800 to 1000 mg daily must also be ensured.

Calcitonin has also been approved for the treatment of postmenopausal osteoporosis. It prevents bone loss by inhibiting osteoclastic resorption. Because it can also prevent vertebral bone loss in postmenopausal women, it should be considered as an alternative in women who cannot take or refuse to take estrogen. Previously, only injectable calcitonin (Calcimar) was available, but the FDA approved the use of nasal salmon calcitonin (Miacalcin) in 1995. Nasal calcitonin used in doses of 200 units/day plus calcium supplements increased bone density in the lumbar spine. Calcitonin in the injectable or nasal form has some analgesic effect and can be used to treat the pain caused by vertebral compression fractures.

In addition to the therapies just described, calcium intake should be monitored. Postmenopausal women should have a daily intake of calcium of 1200 to 1500 mg/day. Treatment of elderly patients with vitamin D is effective in maintaining bone mass and may reduce the frequency of hip fractures.[48, 49] Vitamin D has a direct effect on bones. It stimulates the formation of osteoblasts, inhibits osteoclast progenitors, increases inherent bone strength, stimulates the formation of compact bone, and corrects the secondary hyperparathyroidism common in the elderly. Supplementation with 400 to 800 IU daily is sufficient.

Other agents can stimulate bone formation or increase existing bone mass and may reduce the chance of further fractures. Several drugs have been shown to have such properties, including thiazide diuretics, sodium fluoride, and human synthetic 1-34 parathyroid hormone fragments. These agents, particularly the latter two, must still be considered experimental therapies for osteoporosis. The thiazides in some studies have been associated with a decreased incidence of bone loss and osteoporotic fractures. Thiazides probably act by conserving renal calcium, thus reducing bone resorption. Trials are under way to determine if these agents reduce bone loss and prevent fractures.

Fluoride increases the number, activity, and lifespan of osteoblasts. In doses of 40 to 80 mg/day it can increase trabecular bone volume, but it has no effect on cortical bone. When given alone, fluoride causes the formation of abnormal bone, but this effect can be minimized by giving 800 to 1000 mg/day of calcium. Fluoride increases trabecular bone in about half of the pa-

tients, causes a minimal increase in another 25%, and has no effect in the remainder.[50] The bone formed as a result of stimulation by fluoride is less strong than normal bone. There have been divergent results in studies of the incidence of osteoporotic fractures in patients treated with fluoride.[50, 51] A study using a slow-release form of sodium fluoride and calcium citrate administered for 4 years to postmenopausal women showed an increase in bone mass in the spine and hip.[51] This drug also inhibited new vertebral compression fractures. Slow-release sodium fluoride is currently being considered by the FDA for approval as a therapy for postmenopausal osteoporosis. Fluoride has significant side effects: nausea and gastric irritation occur in most patients. About 10% of patients may develop lower extremity pain, which may result from stress fractures or tendonitis.

Exogenous testosterone has also been considered for the treatment of osteoporosis in women. There is one randomized study of the benefit of testosterone on bone density in women with osteoporosis.[52] After 3 years it showed no change in bone density in those receiving estrogen alone, but a 2.5% increase in bone density was evident in those receiving combined therapy with estrogen and testosterone. Further studies are necessary to confirm whether the combination of testosterone and estrogen has a clinical role.

Osteoporosis is less common in men than in women, probably because men have a greater bone mass and do not experience an equivalent of menopause. Among men with osteoporosis, secondary causes are present in 26% to 72% of patients. The most common causes of secondary osteoporosis in men are exposure to high-dose glucocorticoids, hypogonadism, long-term heavy alcohol consumption, smoking, and hyperthyroidism. Also, age-related declines in testosterone, adrenal androgens, and insulin-like growth factor-1 may contribute to a reduction in bone formation and bone loss.[53, 54]

Evaluation of men with osteoporosis should rule out secondary causes. Currently, we lack studies that identify effective therapies in men with osteoporosis; however, studies are under way to test the effects of calcium, vitamin D, testosterone, bisphosphonates, and calcitonin. Testosterone in men is an appropriate treatment in the presence of diagnosed hypogonadism and no history of prostate cancer. Testosterone is available as an intramuscular injection of a long-acting testosterone ester (testosterone cypionate or testosterone enanthate), and there are also two transdermal preparations of testosterone (Testoderm and Androderm). As replacement therapy, the suggested dosage for the injectable preparation is 50 to 400 mg every 2 to 4 weeks. Transdermal delivery through the scrotal skin (Testoderm) has the advantage of requiring only one patch per day but must be worn on the scrotum. Nonscrotal delivery (Androderm) may produce normal plasma concentrations of testosterone and its metabolites when two patches are applied to nonscrotal skin at bedtime. The most common adverse effects of the patch are skin irritation and contact dermatitis, which can lead some patients to stop using it.

A number of new drugs for the treatment and prevention of osteoporosis are under study. Some of them are bisphosphonates (i.e., risedronate and tiludronate), recombinant human parathyroid hormone (ALX1-11), estrogen agonist-antagonist (i.e., droloxifene), selective estrogen receptor modulator (raloxifene), and vitamin D_2 analog, which is intended to improve intestinal absorption of calcium.

PREVENTION OF OSTEOPOROSIS

Prevention is the only intervention that is cost-effective for osteoporosis. The 1994 National Institutes of Health (NIH) Consensus Conference[29] recommended increasing the calcium content of the diet to 1200 to 1500 mg/day for young adults and 1500 mg/day for older patients unless the patient has a history of hypercalcemia or hypercalciuria,. Calcium may be more bioavailable in dairy products than in green vegetables. Calcium therapy should be given to all patients with osteoporosis in three or four doses totaling 1000 to 1500 mg/day of elemental calcium. Once this treatment has been initiated, serum calcium levels should be monitored annually. Recent data have shown also that high calcium intakes are associated with a significantly decreased risk of fractures of the wrist and hip.[28, 55] Excessive calcium intake (more than 2000 mg/day) is to be avoided because it can cause hypercalcemia or the milk-alkali syndrome. Elderly subjects may experience difficulties with flatulence and constipation if calcium intakes exceed 1500 mg./day.

Physical exercise is another form of therapy for all patients, but the amount should be dictated by common sense. Prevention of falls and other trauma may be as beneficial as therapy aimed at preventing further bone loss. Cigarette smoking and heavy alcohol consumption should cease.

Use of estrogen appears to be the most effective therapy in preventing postmenopausal bone loss. Epidemiologic studies suggest that estrogen use can decrease fracture frequency in women. Estrogen should be initiated as soon as possible after the menopause or oophorectomy. It is un-

known how long estrogens should be continued, but at least 10 years is advised; some authorities suggest administering them for life. In women who are currently postmenopausal the only FDA-approved therapy for the prevention of bone loss is estrogen; however, studies are under way to determine whether alendronate and calcitonin can be used to prevent postmenopausal osteoporosis. Hypogonadal young adults should be evaluated, and if the hypogonadism cannot be reversed, sex hormone replacement therapy should be initiated.

References

1. Shneider E, Guralnik J: The aging of America. JAMA 1990;263:2335–2340.
2. Barret-Connor E: The economic and human cost of osteoporotic fractures. Am J Med 1995;98(Suppl 2A):3–8.
3. Lyles K: Osteopenia: Osteoporosis and osteomalacia. Ambulatory Geriatric Care. St. Louis, Mosby-Year Book, in press, 1997.
4. Lindsay R: The burden of osteoporosis: Cost. Am J Med 1995;98(Suppl 2A):9–11.
5. Parker MJ, Myles JW, Anand JK, Drewett R: Cost-benefit analysis of hip fracture treatment. J Bone Joint Surg 1992;74b:261–264.
6. Marottoli RA, Berkman LF, Cooney LM: Decline in physical function following hip fracture. J Am Geriatr Soc 1992;40:861–866.
7. Cummings SR, Black DM, Ruben SM: Lifetime risks of hip, Colles' or vertebral fracture and coronary heart disease among white postmenopausal women. Arch Intern Med 1989;149:2445–2448.
8. Lyles KW, Gold DT, Shipp KM, et al: Association of osteoporotic vertebral compression fractures with impaired functional status. Am J Med 1993;94:595–601.
9. Greendale GA, Barrett-Connor E, Ingles S, Haile R: Late physical and functional effects of osteoporotic fracture in women: The Rancho Bernardo study. J Am Geriatr Soc 1995;43:955–961.
10. Ross PD, Davis JW, Epstein RS, Wasnich RD: Pre-existing fractures and bone mass predict vertebral fracture incidence in women. Ann Intern Med 1991;114:919–923.
11. Silman AJ: The patient with fracture: The risk of subsequent fractures. Am J Med 1995;98(Suppl 2A):12–16.
12. Browner WS, Seeley DG, Vogt TM, Cummings ST: Non-trauma mortality in elderly women with low mineral density. Lancet 1991;338:355–358.
13. Lu-Yao GL, Baron JA, Barrett JA, Fisher ES: Treatment and survival among elderly Americans with hip fractures: A population-based study. Am J Public Health 1994;84:1287–1291.
14. Ray WA, Griffin MR, Baugh DK: Mortality following hip fracture before and after implementation of the prospective payment system. Arch Intern Med 1990;150:2109–2114.
15. Riis BJ: The role of bone loss. Am J Med 1995;98 (Suppl 2A):29–32.
16. Christiansen C: What should be done at the time of menopause? Am J Med 1995;98(Suppl 2A):56–59.
17. Christiansen C, Riis BJ, Rodbro P: Prediction of rapid bone loss in postmenopausal women. Lancet 1987;Vol. I.

18. Hansen MA, Overgaard K, Riis BJ, Chistiansen C: Role of peak bone in postmenopausal osteoporosis: 12-year study. Br Med J 1991;303:961–964.
19. Parfitt AM, Mundy GR, Roodman GD, Hughes DE, Boyce BF: A new model for the regulation of bone resorption, with particular reference to the effects of bisphosphonates. J Bone Miner Res 1996;11:150–159.
20. Ganong WF (ed): Review of Medical Physiology. Norwalk, CT: Appleton & Lange, 1993.
21. Mitchell DR, Lyles KW: Glucocorticoid-induced osteoporosis: Mechanisms for bone loss; evaluation of strategies for prevention. J Gerontol 1990;45:153–158.
22. Prince RL, Dick I, Devine A, et al: The effects of menopause and age on calcitropic hormones: A cross-sectional study of 655 healthy women aged 35 to 90. J Bone Miner Res 1995;10:835–842.
23. Van Daele PL, Stolk RP, Burger H, et al: Bone density in non-insulin dependent diabetes mellitus. The Rotterdam Study. Ann Intern Med 1995;122:409–414.
24. Peacock M: Vitamin D receptor gene alleles and osteoporosis: A contrasting view (editorial). J. Bone Miner Res 1995;10:1294–1297.
25. Eisman JA: Vitamin D receptor gene alleles and osteoporosis: An affirmative view. (editorial). J. Bone Miner Res 1995;10:1289–1293.
26. Stedman's Medical Dictionary, 25th ed. Baltimore, Williams & Wilkins, 1989.
27. Barzel US: The skeleton as an ion exchange system: Implications for the role of acid-base imbalance in the genesis of osteoporosis. J Bone Miner Res 1995;10:1431–1436.
28. Reid IR, Ames RW, Evans MC, et al: Long-term effects of calcium supplementation on bone loss and fractures in postmenopausal women: A randomized controlled trial. Am J Med 1995;98:331–335.
29. NIH Consensus Development Panel on Optimal Calcium Intake. JAMA 1994;272:1942–1948.
30. Cummings SR, Nervitt MC, Browner WS, et al: Risk factors for hip fractures in white women. N Engl J Med 1995;332:767–773.
31. Prince R, Devine A, Dick I, et al: The effects of calcium supplementation (milk powder or tablets) and exercise on bone density in postmenopausal women. J Bone Miner Res 1995;10:1068–1075.
32. Garnero P, Borel O, Sornay-Rendu E, Delmas PD: Vitamin D receptor gene polymorphisms do not predict bone turnover and bone mass in healthy premenopausal women. J Bone Miner Res 1995;10:1283–1288.
33. Ferrari S, Rissoli R, Chevalley D, Slosman D, Eisman JA, Bonjour J-P: Vitamin D receptor gene polymorphisms and change in lumbar spine bone mineral density. Lancet 1995;345:423–424.
34. Felson DT, Zhang Y, Hannan MT, Kannel WB, Kiel DP: Alcohol intake and bone mineral density in elderly men and women. The Framingham Study. Am J Epidemiol 1995;142:485–492.
35. Keck E, Bremer G, Franck H: Alcohol-induced osteopenia. Radiologe 1986;26:587–591.
36. Bauer DC, Browner WS, Cauley JA, et al: Factors associated with appendicular bone mass in older women. Ann Intern Med 1993;118:657–665.
37. Earnshaw SA, Hosking DJ. Clinical usefulness of risk

factors for osteoporosis. Ann Rheum Dis 1996;55:338–339.
38. Jonston CC, Melton LJ, Lindsay R, Eddy D: Clinical indications for bone mass measurements. A report from the Scientific Advisory Board of the National Osteoporosis Foundation. J Bone Miner Res 1989;4 (Suppl 2):1–28.
39. Nachtigall LE: Enhancing patient compliance with hormone replacement therapy at menopause. Obstet Gynecol 1990;75:77s–80s.
40. Genant HK, Baylink DJ, Gallagher JC: Estrogens in the prevention of osteoporosis in postmenopausal women. Am J Obstet Gynecol 1989;161:1842–1846.
41. Belchetz PE. Hormonal treatment of postmenopausal women. N Engl J Med 1994;330:1062–1071.
42. Henrich JE: The postmenopausal estrogen/breast cancer controversy. JAMA 1992;268:1900–1902.
43. Grady D, Rubin SM, Petitti DB, et al: Hormone therapy to prevent disease and prolong life in postmenopausal women. Ann Intern Med 1992;117:1016–1037.
44. Stanford JL, Weiss NS, Voigt LF, et al: Combined estrogen and progestin hormone replacement therapy in relation to risk of breast cancer in middle-age women. JAMA 1995;274:137–142.
45. Colditz GA, Hankinson SE, Hunter DJ, et al: The use of estrogens and progestins and the risk of breast cancer in postmenopausal women. N Engl J Med 1995;332:1589–1593.
46. Colditz GA, Stampfer MJ, Willett WC, et al: Prospective study of estrogen replacement therapy and risk of breast cancer in postmenopausal women. JAMA 1990;264:2648–2653.
47. Liberman U, Weiss S, Broll J, et al: Effect of oral alendronate on bone mineral density and the incidence of fractures in postmenopausal osteoporosis. N Engl J Med 1995;333:1437–1443.
48. Ooms ME, Roos JC, Bezemer PD, et al: Prevention of bone loss by vitamin D supplementation in elderly women: A randomized double-blind trial. J Clin Endocrinol Metab 1995;80:1052–1058
49. Chapuy MC, Arlot ME, Delmas PD, Meunier PJ: Effect of calcium and cholecalciferol treatment for three years on hip fractures in elderly women. Br Med J 1994;308:1081–1082.
50. Riggs BI, Hodgson SF, O'Fallon WM, et al: Effect of fluoride treatment on the fracture rate in postmenopausal women with osteoporosis. N Engl J Med 1990;322:802–808.
51. Pak Ch, Sakhaee K, Adams-Huet B, et al: Treatment of postmenopausal osteoporosis with slow-release sodium fluoride. Ann Intern Med 1995;123:401–408.
52. Barlow Dh, Abdalla HI, Roberts AD, et al: Long-term hormone implant therapy: Hormonal and clinical effects. Obstet Gynecol 1986;67;321–325.
53. Kelepouris N, Harper KD, Gannon F, Kaplan FS, Haddad JG: Severe osteoporosis in men. Ann Intern Med 1995;123:452–460.
54. Seeman E: The dilemma of osteoporosis in men. Am J Med 1995;98(Suppl 2A):76–88.
55. Abelow BJ, Holford TR, Insogna KL: Cross-cultural association between dietary animal protein and hip fracture: A hypothesis. Calcif Tissue Int 1992;50:14–18.

22 Pressure Ulcers

Patricia S. Goode, M.D., M.S.N., E.T.
Richard M. Allman, M.D.

Pressure ulcers are an all too common problem among the elderly, in that more than 50% of persons with pressure ulcers are over age 70.[1] Almost two thirds of pressure ulcers first develop in acute care hospitals. Sixty to seventy percent of these ulcers occur within the first 2 weeks of hospitalization.[1] As many as 20% to 33% of patients admitted to nursing homes have a pressure ulcer that is stage 2 or more severe.[2-4] The true costs of pressure ulcer care are difficult to ascertain. Data indicate that patients with pressure ulcers have increased hospital costs, increased lengths of stay, and increased mortality.[5-7]

DEFINITIONS

Pressure ulcers can be defined as localized areas of tissue injury that develop when soft tissue is compressed between a bony prominence and an external surface for a prolonged period of time.[8] These lesions may present clinically as nonblanchable erythema, blisters, ulcerations, or lesions covered with necrotic eschar. Since pressure is the primary pathophysiologic factor in the development of these lesions, *pressure ulcer* is the preferred term. Previous terminology includes decubitus ulcer and bedsore, which imply that the lesions occur only when lying down; in fact, some of the most severe pressure-induced cutaneous injuries result from prolonged sitting.

Clinical staging or grading of pressure ulcers helps in guiding clinical management decisions. The National Pressure Ulcer Advisory Panel (NPUAP) has suggested adopting a uniform staging system (Table 22–1). There has been considerable controversy about stage 1 pressure ulcers (nonblanchable erythema, darkening or induration of intact skin), but development of a stage 1 ulcer is associated with the subsequent occurrence of a stage 2 or greater ulcer in nearly 60% of cases.[5] Pressure-induced blisters typically occur on the heels and are most often stage 3 if they are unroofed, but this is not recommended because the blister provides a natural "dressing." Most wounds covered with eschar have full-thickness tissue necrosis and are stage 3 or 4, although these wounds cannot be accurately staged until the eschar is removed.

PATHOGENESIS

Pressure is the primary etiologic factor in the development of pressure ulcers. Development of prolonged pressure sufficient to result in ischemic tissue damage is related to the degree of immobility. In a classic study, Exton-Smith and Sherwin[9] used a mattress sensor to monitor spontaneous nocturnal movements in patients at an extended care facility. No patient with 51 or more spontaneous nocturnal movements developed a pressure ulcer, but 90% of patients with 20 or fewer movements did.

Muscle and subcutaneous tissue are more susceptible to pressure-induced injury than are epidermal and dermal tissues. Contact pressures of 60 to 70 mmHg for 1 to 2 hours can cause muscle damage.[10] Pressures under bony prominences such as the sacrum and greater trochanter can be as high as 100 to 150 mmHg on a standard hospital mattress, and pressures under the ischial tuberosities of a seated person can reach 300 mmHg.[11] These pressures are sufficient to decrease the transcutaneous oxygen tension to

---

TABLE 22–1 **PRESSURE ULCER CLASSIFICATION**

Stage 1	Nonblanchable erythema, darkening, or induration of intact skin. Indicates underlying tissue injury.
Stage 2	Partial thickness skin loss involving the epidermis, dermis, or both.
Stage 3	Full thickness skin loss involving subcutaneous tissue which may extend to, but not through, the underlying fascia.
Stage 4	Deeper full thickness lesions extending into muscle, bone, or supporting structures.

Adapted from National Pressure Ulcer Advisory Panel: Pressure ulcer prevalence, cost and risk assessment: Consensus development statement. Decubitus 1989; 2(2): 24–28.

nearly zero.[11] Age-related changes in the skin including thinning of the epidermis, increased skin permeability, flattening of the dermal-epidermal junction, loss of dermal vessels, and loss of elastic fibers may increase the older person's susceptibility to pressure ulcers.

Other factors such as shear, friction, and moisture can also lead to skin breakdown. Shear is generated when tangential forces are applied to the skin surface, causing the dermis and epidermis to shift laterally with respect to the deeper layers, angulating the blood vessels and reducing the amount of pressure needed to cause vessel occlusion. Shear occurs commonly in the tissues over the sacrum when an individual sits up in a chair or a bed and then slides toward the edge of the chair or the foot of the bed. The sacral skin is held in place by friction, and the underlying blood vessels are stretched and angulated, increasing their susceptibility to pressure-induced necrosis. Friction can lead to blister formation and superficial skin erosions. Moisture causes maceration, and incontinence has been found to be a risk factor in several studies. However, two studies[5, 7] have examined fecal and urinary incontinence separately and have found that only fecal incontinence is independently associated with development of pressure ulcers.

RISK FACTORS

Periodic use of a risk assessment tool has been found to decrease the incidence of pressure ulcers.[12] The Norton Scale, the first such instrument, and the Braden Scale have been evaluated most often with respect to reliability and validity. Patients should be assessed on admission to acute care hospitals, rehabilitation centers, nursing homes, home care programs, and other health care facilities, and then should be reassessed at periodic intervals.[13]

Awareness of risk factors helps to target preventive interventions to those patients who are most likely to benefit. Risk factors for pressure ulcer development include bedbound or chairbound status, immobility (i.e., inability to reposition oneself), incontinence, inadequate dietary intake, impaired nutritional status, and altered level of consciousness.[13] Risk factors have been shown to vary by setting; hence risk factors for acutely ill patients in hospitals may be quite different from those for chronically ill patients in nursing homes. Prospective studies are needed to more clearly define the pertinent risk factors in each setting.

PREVENTION

After risk of pressure ulcers has been identified in an individual either by the presence of multi-

---

TABLE 22–2 **PRESSURE ULCER PREVENTION**

1. Use a risk assessment tool to identify patients at risk for pressure ulcers. Modify risk factors (immobility, moisture or incontinence, nutritional deficiencies) as possible. Reassess patients regularly.
2. Use a repositioning schedule to reposition immobile patients—at least every 2 hours for bedbound patients and every hour for chairbound patients. Avoid positioning directly on the trochanter. Use pillows and other devices to lift heels completely off bed and to keep bony prominences from direct contact. Minimize elevation of head of bed.
3. Use a pressure-reducing seating surface (*not* the donut-type) for chairbound patients and a pressure-reducing mattress or mattress overlay for at-risk patients in bed.
4. Provide skin care: Inspect skin daily, cleanse regularly with a mild cleanser, use moisturizers for dry skin, and avoid massage over bony prominences.
5. For incontinent patients, cleanse skin at time of soiling and use topical moisture barrier ointment. Use underpads or briefs with a quick drying surface against the skin.
6. Maintain adequate dietary intake of protein, calories, and fluids. Give daily multivitamin, multimineral supplement to at-risk patients.
7. Optimize activity level, mobility, and range of motion. Institute a rehabilitation program.
8. Educate patients, family, and caregivers and health care providers about etiology, risk factors, risk assessment tools, skin assessment, selection and use of support surfaces, skin care, positioning, and documentation.

Data from Panel for the Prediction and Prevention of Pressure Ulcers in Adults: Pressure Ulcers in Adults: Prediction and Prevention. Clinical Practice Guideline No. 3. AHCPR Publication No. 92-0047. Rockville, MD, U.S. Department of Health and Human Services, Public Health Service, Agency for Health Care Policy and Research, 1992.

---

ple risk factors or by the use of a risk assessment tool, preventive measures should be initiated. Table 22–2 summarizes the methods used to prevent pressure ulcers. Prevention programs may include adequate nutrition, proper management of co-morbid conditions including incontinence, and rehabilitation to improve mobility and functional status. Educational programs for caregivers, including physicians, nurses, nursing assistants, and family members, are also important. Multidisciplinary teams have been able to reduce the incidence of pressure ulcers by more than 50% in acute care hospitals.[11, 14]

Positioning

The traditional recommendation for preventing pressure ulcers is to reposition at-risk patients every 2 hours. Actually, considerable differences exist among individuals in their tolerance of various pressure-time intervals. The frequency of repositioning required depends on the degree of mobility of the patient and the support surface used. At-risk individuals should be monitored carefully for evidence of nonblanchable erythema and skin discoloration or induration (stage 1 pressure ulcer), which indicate the need for more frequent repositioning or the use of more effective pressure-reducing devices. Generous use of soft pillows between the legs, behind the back, and supporting the arms is helpful to maintain proper position.

A right or left 30-degree oblique position, in which the patient's back is at a 30-degree angle to the support surface, avoids direct pressure on the bony prominences that accounts for 80% of pressure ulcers: the sacrum, ischial tuberosities, trochanters, lateral malleoli, and heels.[11] In contrast, lying with the back at a 90-degree angle to the support surface exposes the greater trochanter and the lateral malleoli to pressure. This side-lying position should be avoided in patients who are unable to reposition themselves. The supine position puts pressure on the sacrum and heels, while sitting exposes the tissues over the ischial tuberosities to pressure. Keeping the head of the bed elevated less than 30 degrees decreases shearing forces, so immobile patients whose heads are elevated more than 30 degrees for bathing or eating should be returned to an elevation of less than 30 degrees within 1 to 2 hours unless this is medically contraindicated.

Pressure Reduction

A number of pressure-reducing devices are marketed to prevent and treat pressure ulcers. Synthetic sheepskins and 2-inch convoluted ("egg crate") foam mattress overlays are very popular and are relatively inexpensive. Although they can increase the patient's comfort, they cannot decrease pressure sufficiently to prevent pressure ulcers. Information such as indention load deflection (ILD—the amount of force required to compress the foam a given percentage of its original height), density (the weight of a cubic foot of foam), and the support factor (the 65% ILD divided by the 25% ILD) can be useful in selecting appropriate foam products.[15] Foam mattress overlays that are specifically designed to prevent pressure ulcers (e.g., BioGard, Derma-Foam, Geo-matt, IRIS) are preferable, since they

reduce pressure under bony prominences to levels that are believed to reduce risk. Foam mattress overlays have a one time cost of $30 to $50. As an alternative, the standard hospital mattress may be replaced with a mattress that has pressure-reducing capability at a cost of less than $200 to $750 (e.g., BioCore, DeCube, PressureGuard). This may be a cost-effective solution for high-risk settings such as intensive care units, general medical floors, and orthopedic wards.

Static air mattress overlays (e.g., K-Soft, Sof-Care) have interconnecting air cells that transfer air among cells as a person changes position on them, equalizing pressure. They are inflated to an appropriate pressure (i.e., when the sacrum is not palpable to the examiner's hand placed beneath the inflated air cells of the mattress overlay). Cost is $25 to $50. Some static overlays have a rental fee of about $25 a day (e.g., ROHO). Dynamic systems, or alternating air mattresses (e.g., AcuCair, BioTherapy, Clini-Care, First Step) have air cells that are alternately inflated and deflated by a bedside pump. Water- or gel-filled mattresses and overlays (e.g., Lotus, TenderGEL) are difficult to move and have not been popular in acute care hospitals but may be appropriate in long-term care settings or in the home. One randomized controlled trial demonstrated a greater than 50% decrease in incidence of pressure ulcers with the use of alternating air mattresses or water mattresses compared with the use of conventional hospital mattresses in an acute care hospital.[14]

Devices such as heel protectors, which are designed to decrease pressure over a localized area, can be useful to reduce pressure over high-risk bony prominences. Patients who are in chairs or wheelchairs for longer than 1 or 2 hours at a time should use an appropriate pressure-reducing chair cushion (e.g., Jay, ROHO, Waffle cushion). These chair cushions have properties similar to those of mattress overlays and can be selected using similar criteria. "Donut" cushions should not be used for pressure relief because they may cause ischemia in the tissues positioned in the center of the donut.[13]

Skin Care

Proper skin care is an important part of a pressure ulcer prevention program. The skin should be inspected daily and cleansed at regular intervals and after each episode of soiling with a mild cleanser (e.g., Dove soap). Since dry skin is a risk factor for pressure ulcers,[5, 16] topical moisturizers (e.g., Bard Skin Care Cream, Nivea Moisturizing Lotion, Vaseline Constant Care) should be used to help increase the resistance of the skin to mechanical trauma. More studies are needed to demonstrate whether moisturizers can actually decrease the incidence of pressure ulcers. Maceration also decreases the resistance of the skin to mechanical trauma. Skin should be protected from incontinence and excessive perspiration by the use of a topical moisture barrier (e.g., A & D Ointment, Peri-Care Moisture Barrier Ointment, Restore Barrier Creme). Underpads or briefs that have a quick-drying surface placed against the skin are also helpful in keeping moisture away from skin. Massage over bony prominences has traditionally been recommended as part of a pressure ulcer prevention program. However, there is evidence that massage actually increases the incidence of pressure ulcers by causing deep tissue trauma,[17] and it should therefore be avoided.[13]

Pressure Ulcers in Terminal Conditions

Despite the use of appropriate preventive care, some pressure ulcers may still occur. The skin is the largest organ of the body, and pressure ulcers may be one part of the syndrome of multiple organ failure that accompanies many terminal conditions. Inability to prevent pressure ulcers in terminally ill patients should be considered when the presence of pressure ulcers is used as an indicator of the quality of care.

TREATMENT

Treatment of All Stages

Treatment of pressure ulcers is summarized in Table 22–3.[18]

ASSESSMENT

A carefully recorded assessment of pressure ulcers at the initiation of therapy is mandatory to provide a baseline against which to judge improvement or deterioration. A complete description includes the number of pressure ulcers and, for each ulcer, the location, stage, size (length, width, depth), description of tunneling or undermining, necrotic tissue, odor or exudate if present, and the condition of the surrounding skin (maceration, abrasions, discoloration, induration, if present). Although stage 2 pressure ulcers usually heal in days to weeks, ulcers in stages 3 and 4 may require months to heal completely. Improvement can by judged by a decrease in size (taking undermining into account), a decrease in odor and drainage, a decrease in the amount of necrotic tissue, improved appear-

TABLE 22–3 **PRESSURE ULCER TREATMENT**

1. Assess ulcer(s) initially and then reassess weekly: size (length, width, depth), description of tunneling, undermining, necrotic tissue, odor, exudate, and cellulitis, if present; and condition of surrounding skin.
2. Relieve pressure: use a repositioning schedule and pressure-reducing support surface.
3. Assess and manage nutritional status: intake goal of 30 to 35 calories/kg/day, 1.25 to 1.50 g protein/kg/day, and daily high-potency multivitamin, multimineral supplement.
4. Use autolytic, enzymatic, mechanical, or sharp debridement to remove necrotic tissue. Dry eschar on heels should be left in place unless evidence of infection is present.
5. Cleanse ulcer at each dressing change with saline or other nontoxic cleanser with technique that minimizes mechanical trauma to wound.
6. Select ulcer dressings that keep ulcer bed continuously moist and surrounding skin dry.
7. Bacteremia, sepsis, or cellulitis require systemic antibiotic therapy. Local infection (colonization) does not require systemic antibiotics and is more appropriately treated with topical antibiotics (*not* topical antiseptics).
8. For nonhealing ulcers, consider adjunctive therapy such as electrical stimulation.
9. Provide adequate pain relief.

Data from Bergstrom N, Bennett MA, Carlson CE, et al: Treatment of pressure ulcers. Clinical Practice Guideline No. 15. AHCPR Publication No. 95-0652. Rockville, Md. U.S. Department of Health and Human Services, Public Health Service, Agency for Health Care Policy and Research, 1994.

ance of granulation tissue, and improved appearance of the surrounding skin. Serial photographs may be useful for monitoring. Tools are also available to guide wound assessment and quantify healing.[19]

The staging system recommended by the NPUAP is useful in guiding initial clinical management but is not intended nor appropriate for monitoring healing. The original tissue layers are not regenerated in a full-thickness wound. Just as a third-degree burn does not become a second-degree and then a first-degree burn as it heals, a pressure ulcer does not progress through reverse staging.

NUTRITION

Optimizing nutritional status cannot be emphasized strongly enough and is all too often neglected. The Agency for Health Care Policy and Research (AHCPR) guideline[18] suggests as markers of clinically significant malnutrition: a serum albumin level of less than 3.5 g/dL, a total lymphocyte count of less than 1800/mm³, and weight loss of more than 15% or a weight of less than 80% of ideal. Tube feeding or parenteral nutrition should be considered for patients with insufficient oral intake, the goal being 30 to 35 calories/kg/day and 1.25 to 1.50 g protein/kg/day. Protein intake has been shown to be one of the most important predictors of improvement in pressure ulcers. A high-potency vitamin and mineral supplement (e.g., Centrum, Theragram M, Unicap M) should be given daily to all geriatric patients with pressure ulcers owing to the high prevalence of subclinical vitamin and mineral deficiencies in this group. Inadequate data are available to support the routine use of additional vitamin and mineral supplements. Megadose vitamin and mineral therapy may even be harmful to patients because of the toxicity of high levels of the supplement itself (vitamin A) or because of side effects (anorexia with oral zinc supplements).

Stage 1 Pressure Ulcers

The appearance of nonblanchable erythema, other discoloration, or induration over a bony prominence signals underlying tissue injury and mandates an evaluation of the preventive measures currently in use. The use and adequacy of pressure-reducing devices, the frequency and techniques of repositioning, and the adequacy of the patient's nutritional status should be assessed and any necessary changes made. Topical application of various pressure ulcer treatment products is unnecessary for stage 1 ulcers, since the epidermis is intact. The goal of intervention at this stage is to halt progression of tissue injury before epithelial breakdown occurs, and this is best done by relieving pressure.

Stage 2 Pressure Ulcers

With appropriate intervention, stage 2 pressure ulcers usually heal in weeks without scarring. Patients with pressure ulcers of any stage are at high risk for additional skin breakdown, so attention to all preventive measures described previously is particularly important. Usually stage 2 pressure ulcers are quite shallow, have minimal necrotic tissue, and are not infected. However, they can be quite painful. Local wound care for stage 2 pressure ulcers should maintain a moist, physiologic environment that facilitates granulation and epithelialization and does not disturb

healing tissue. Occlusive, vapor-permeable dressings (e.g., Bioclusive, OpSite, Tegaderm) and hydrocolloid dressings (Comfeel, Dermiflex, DuoDERM, Intrasite, Tegasorb) permit accumulation of serous fluid on top of the wound, providing a physiologic environment; they also reduce pain and in controlled trials improve healing of shallow pressure ulcers (stage 2 and shallow stage 3). These dressings should be changed every 2 to 7 days, depending on the wound. More frequent dressing changes increase expense, damage the surrounding skin, and are usually unnecessary.

Stage 3 and 4 Pressure Ulcers

Stage 3 and 4 pressure ulcers generally take months to heal and result in scarring. Ulcers may enlarge initially as necrotic tissue is removed. As for treatment of stage 2 ulcers, general systemic measures such as nutritional support, pressure relief, and management of risk factors are essential.

PRESSURE REDUCTION

Positioning patients on a pressure ulcer should be avoided. It cannot be emphasized enough that without relief of local pressure, the pressure ulcer will not heal, and all other therapeutic measures will be futile. Positioning devices such as soft pillows may be used to raise a pressure ulcer off the support surface. A written repositioning schedule should be used. It is particularly helpful to post the schedule on the wall above the patient's bed. A pressure-reducing surface should be used for all patients at risk for developing additional pressure ulcers. A static support surface may be sufficient for patients who can assume a variety of positions without putting weight on a pressure ulcer. A dynamic support surface is usually necessary for patients who are unable to reposition themselves, for those who completely compress a static support surface (i.e., bottom out), and for those with pressure ulcers on multiple turning surfaces. Some mattress overlays may lift the patient so high that the side rails are not high enough to prevent falls in at-risk patients; caution should be used to select an overlay that is compatible with the bed. A mattress replacement or a specialized bed is another alternative.

SPECIALIZED BEDS

Patients with multiple large truncal stage 3 and 4 ulcers, with less than two intact turning surfaces available for repositioning, or with ulcers that fail to heal on a less expensive support surface when all other components of the care plan are optimal, may require the use of a specialized bed. Air-fluidized beds (e.g., Clinitron, FluidAir) contain microspheres of ceramic glass that are covered by a filter sheet. Warm pressurized air is forced up through the glass beads so that they take on the characteristics of a fluid, and the patient floats on the system. Low air-loss beds (e.g., Flexicair, KinAir, Pneu Care Plus) consist of a traditional hospital bed frame fitted with large fabric cushions that are constantly inflated with air. The standard hospital bed frame allows the head of the bed and the bed itself to be raised or lowered, an advantage compared with the air-fluidized bed. The drying effect of the air-fluidized beds (and some dynamic mattress overlays) may be helpful in treating patients with excessive skin moisture, but because it increases insensible fluid losses, the hydration status of the patient requires extra attention. Air-fluidized beds rent for $55 to $100 per day, and low air-loss beds rent for $30 to $80 per day. Low air-loss mattress overlays are available and rent for $20 to $40 per day.

The effectiveness of low air-loss beds has not been compared with that of air-fluidized beds, but both types of beds decrease the healing time of pressure ulcers compared with foam overlays or traditional hospital mattresses. Many beds, overlays, and mattresses are reported to lower pressure under bony prominences to below capillary filling pressure, traditionally considered to be 32 mmHg. However, most of these measurements are made in healthy young volunteers, not in frail elderly patients or patients with neurologic disorders, who may require considerably less pressure to occlude the capillaries. Any pressure-reducing support surface requires monitoring of the patient's skin to ascertain individual efficacy.

DEBRIDEMENT

Removal of necrotic debris is the first step in reducing the bacterial content of the wound. Bacterial counts of greater than 100,000 (10^5) colonies per gram of tissue in pressure ulcers correlate well with impaired wound healing and wound graft failure. Wounds with eschar or large amounts of necrotic debris are best debrided surgically. Debridement is often performed at the bedside with sterile tissue forceps and scissors or scalpel. If there is bleeding, a dry gauze dressing should be applied for several hours before moist therapy is resumed. Lesser amounts of necrotic debris can be removed with irrigation or whirlpool techniques, wet-to-dry saline gauze dressings, or enzymatic debriding agents such as collagenase. Debridement (wet-to-dry dressings, whirlpool, enzymatic agents, and so on) should be discontinued once the wound base is clean to prevent disruption of healthy granulation tissue.

INFECTION

Several issues involving infection and pressure ulcers should be mentioned. The first is culturing. Essentially all stage 2 or more severe pressure ulcers are colonized with bacteria, and routine cultures of a wound that does not appear infected add nothing to the therapeutic plan. Evidence of cellulitis, osteomyelitis, or sepsis is an indication for culturing. Needle aspiration and ulcer biopsy have been recommended as the most reliable culture methods.[18] However, if the wound is first thoroughly cleansed with a nonantimicrobial solution and then a 1 cm² area of the wound base is swabbed for 5 seconds with sufficient pressure to express fluid from the wound tissue, reliable semiquantitative culture data can be obtained.[20]

Systemic antibiotics are not needed for routine treatment of pressure ulcers but are indicated for patients with cellulitis, sepsis, or osteomyelitis. In addition, since debridement results in transient bacteremia, antibiotics for endocarditis prophylaxis should be administered as indicated. In patients with sepsis or suspected bacteremia, broad-spectrum coverage for aerobic gram-negative rods, gram-positive cocci, and anaerobes is indicated pending culture results. Ampicillin-sulbactam, imipenem, ticarcillin-clavulanate, or a combination of clindamycin and an aminoglycoside is an appropriate choice for initial antibiotic therapy. The mortality of patients with sepsis associated with pressure ulcers is high, so treatment should be aggressive. Prompt, thorough surgical debridement of necrotic tissue is also indicated to remove the source of the bacteremia.

Randomized controlled trials suggest that topical antibiotics such as gentamicin and silver sulfadiazine may help infected pressure ulcers to heal. In contrast, antiseptics such as 1% povidone-iodine, 0.25% acetic acid, 0.5% sodium hypochlorite (Dakin's solution), and 3% hydrogen peroxide all are cytotoxic to fibroblasts in culture, may impair wound healing, and should not be used in patients with pressure ulcers.[18] Topical antibiotics effective against gram-negative, gram-positive, and anaerobic organisms (e.g., silver sulfadiazine, triple antibiotic) may be prescribed for specific purposes such as accomplishing an initial decrease of bacterial wound content or decreasing foul odor, or as a therapeutic trial for ulcers that are not healing despite an optimal multicomponent treatment plan. A fixed treatment period (2 weeks) is recommended to avoid adverse local and systemic effects and selection of antibiotic-resistant bacteria.[18]

The Centers for Disease Control (CDC) recommends use of drainage and secretion precautions (gloves for touching infective material, gowns if soiling is likely, handwashing before next patient contact, contaminated articles discarded or bagged and labeled before being sent for decontamination and reprocessing) in managing patients with an infected pressure ulcer. If an infection is caused by a multiply resistant organism or if the drainage is not adequately contained by the dressing, contact isolation (which is the same as drainage and secretion precautions with the addition of a required private room) is indicated. Many nursing homes will not accept patients who have positive cultures for a resistant organism.

ULCER DRESSINGS

Stage 3 and 4 ulcers should be protected with a dressing that keeps the ulcer bed continuously moist and the surrounding skin free of maceration. Intact skin can be protected with an ointment-based moisture barrier. Deep ulcers that have been adequately debrided should be lightly packed with a material that does not inhibit healing; saline-moistened gauze is the standard. The gauze should be kept continuously moist and should be remoistened before removal if necessary to avoid disrupting the granulation tissue. Wet-to-dry dressings should be used only to debride wounds and should be discontinued when the wound bed is clean. A variety of alternatives to saline-moistened gauze dressings exist, and randomized placebo-controlled studies are needed to compare the efficacy of these various dressings and to provide specific indications for use of the different types. Some dressings are particularly formulated for the management of ulcers with large amounts of drainage (e.g., Bard Absorption Dressing, Debrisan). Calcium alginate dressings (e.g., Sorbsan) and combination products (e.g., IntraSite Gel) show promise in their ability to create a therapeutic microenvironment and also are easily removed without disrupting granulation tissue.

Miscellaneous topical agents (e.g., sugar, honey, vitamins, zinc, magnesium, aluminum, gold, phenytoin, insulin, yeast extract, aloe vera gel) have been promoted from time to time but have not been evaluated sufficiently to warrant a current recommendation.[18] Topically applied growth factors (e.g., recombinant platelet-derived growth factor and basic fibroblast growth factor) have shown promising results, and studies are ongoing. Skin equivalents are also currently undergoing clinical trials. Systemic agents such as vasodilators, hemorrheologics (pentoxifylline), serotonin inhibitors, and fibrinolytic agents cannot be recommended for use in treating pressure ulcers because of lack of data on their efficacy.[18] Of the adjunctive therapies (e.g., hyperbaric oxygen; infrared, ultraviolet, and low-energy laser irradiation; and ultrasound), only electrotherapy (electrical stimulation of the wound) has demonstrated sufficient efficacy in treating pressure ulcers. Electrical stimulation is recommended for stage 2, 3, and 4 ulcers that have proved unresponsive to conventional therapy.[18] In addition to promoting more rapid healing, electrical stimulation may assist in controlling pain.

SURGICAL TREATMENT

Surgical treatment of pressure ulcers includes direct closure, skin grafts, skin flaps, musculocutaneous flaps, and free flaps. Ischiectomy (to remove the underlying bony prominences) can lead to perineal ulcers and urethral fistulas and is no longer recommended.[18] Most of these procedures were developed for young patients with spinal cord injuries, although age alone is certainly not a contraindication for surgical treatment. Surgical consultation should be obtained for older persons for whom surgical intervention would be appropriate after considering the patient's rehabilitative potential and ability to tolerate a surgical procedure including the postoperative immobility required. Postoperative care usually involves the use of an air-fluidized or low air-loss bed for at least 2 weeks. Weight bearing is gradually increased after this time, and close observation of tissue tolerance is needed. Education of patients and caregivers is essential to reduce the high rate (10% to 60%) of recurrence of pressure ulcers following surgical repair.

References

1. Petersen NC, Bittman S: The epidemiology of pressure sores. Scand J Plast Reconstr Surg 1971;5(1):62–66.
2. Allman RM: Epidemiology of pressure ulcers in different populations. Decubitus 1989;2(2):30–33.
3. Berlowitz DR, Wilking SVB: The short term outcome of pressure ulcers. J Am Geriatr Soc 1990;38:748–752.
4. Spector WD, Kapp MC, Tucker RJ, Sternberg J: Factors associated with presence of decubitus ulcers at admission to nursing homes. Gerontologist 1988;28(6):830–834.
5. Allman RM, Goode PS, Patrick MM, Burst N, Bartolucci AA: Pressure ulcer risk factors among hospitalized patients with activity limitation. JAMA 1995;273(11):865–870.

6. Allman RM, Goode PS, Bartolucci AA, Burst N: Pressure ulcers and hospital costs. J Am Geriatr Soc 1993;41(10):SA7.

7. Allman RM, Laprade CA, Noel LB, Walker JM, Moorer CA, Dear MR, Smith CR: Pressure sores among hospitalized patients. Ann Intern Med 1986;105(3):337–342.

8. National Pressure Ulcer Advisory Panel: Pressure ulcer prevalence, cost and risk assessment: Consensus development statement. Decubitus 1989;2(2):24–28.

9. Exton-Smith AN, Sherwin RW: The prevention of pressure sores: Significance of spontaneous movements. Lancet 1961;2(7212):1124–1126.

10. Kosiak M: Etiology and pathology of ischemic ulcers. Arch Phys Med Rehabil 1959;40:62–69.

11. Seiler WO, Stahelin HB: Decubitus ulcers, preventive techniques for the elderly patient. Geriatrics 1985; 40(7):53–60.

12. Andersen KE, Jensen O, Kvorning SA, Bach E: Prevention of pressure sores by identifying patients at risk. Br Med J (Clin Res Ed) 1982;284(6326): 1370–1371.

13. Panel for the Prediction and Prevention of Pressure Ulcers in Adults: Pressure ulcers in adults: Prediction and prevention. Clinical Practice Guideline No. 3. AHCPR Publication No. 92-0047. Rockville, MD, U.S. Department of Health and Human Services, Public

Health Service, Agency for Health Care Policy and Research, 1992.

14. Andersen KE, Jensen O, Kvorning SA, Bach E: Decubitus prophylaxis: A prospective trial on the efficiency of alternating-pressure air-mattresses and water-mattresses. Acta Derm Venereol (Stockh) 1983;63(3):227–230.

15. Mulder GD, Fairchild PA, Jeter KF (eds): The Clinician's Pocket Guide to Chronic Wound Repair, 3rd ed. Long Beach, CA, Wound Healing Institute Publications, 1995, pp. 81–96.

16. Guralnik JM, Harris TB, White LR, Cornoni-Huntley JC: Occurrence and predictors of pressure sores in the National Health and Nutrition Examination Survey follow-up. J Am Geriatr Soc 1988;36(9):807–812.

17. Dyson R: Bed sores—the injuries hospital staff inflict on patients. Nurs Mirror 1978;146(24):30–32.

18. Bergstrom N, Bennett MA, Carlson CE, et al: Treatment of pressure ulcers. Clinical Practice Guideline No. 15. AHCPR Publication No. 95-0652. Rockville, MD, U.S. Department of Health and Human Services, Public Health Service, Agency for Health Care Policy and Research, 1994.

19. Bates-Jensen B: New pressure ulcer status tool. Decubitus 1990;3(3):14–15.

20. Stotts NA: Determination of bacterial burden in wounds. Adv Wound Care 1995;8(4):28–36.

23 Sleep and Aging

Sonia Ancoli-Israel, Ph.D.

Daniel F. Kripke, M.D.

With age, many changes occur in sleep. Older people sleep less deeply, wake up more frequently during the night, and awaken earlier in the morning. In the past it was thought that older people need less sleep because they are less active. However, research has shown that physiologic sleep durations in healthy elderly people are about the same as those in younger healthy adults, whereas time in bed is often longer. This chapter examines the sleep of elderly people—how sleep changes, why it changes, and the consequences of these changes.

PATHOPHYSIOLOGY

Sleep can be divided into two types: rapid eye movement (REM) sleep and non–rapid eye movement (NREM) sleep. NREM sleep is further subdivided into four stages: stages 1, 2, 3, and 4. Stage 1 is the very lightest level of sleep, whereas stage 4 is the deepest. Traditionally, polysomnograms using electroencephalography (EEG), eye movement (electro-oculography [EOG]), and electromyographic (EMG) tension of the chin muscles have been recorded.

During NREM sleep, eye movements are slow or absent, and there is a normal degree of muscle tension (Fig. 23–1). During REM sleep, which is the dream state, eye movements are rapid (thus giving rise to the name), and there is almost no muscle tension (Fig. 23–2). In fact, during REM sleep we are paralyzed except for the eyes and the respiratory system. This is a protective mechanism that keeps us from acting out our dreams. When people wake up from their dreams, they sometimes experience a feeling of paralysis, which usually lasts only a few moments and is normal.

During the night we cycle through the different stages of sleep. As we get older, the pattern of the cycles begins to change (Fig. 23–3).[1] Older people experience less sleep in stages 3 and 4 (i.e., deep sleep), less REM sleep, and more awakenings during the night.[2] Sleep efficiency (defined as the amount of time asleep divided by the amount of time in bed) is reduced. In correspondence with poor nocturnal sleep efficiency, the number of naps taken during the day increases with age.

Multiple sleep latency tests indicate that older people are sleepy during the day (i.e., have a shortened sleep-onset latency).[3] This suggests that it is not the need to sleep that is reduced in the elderly but rather the ability to sleep efficiently. This reduction in ability to sleep is secondary to many factors. Two of the main ones are changes in circadian rhythms and a high prevalence of sleep disorders such as sleep-disordered breathing (sleep apnea) and periodic limb movements in sleep.

CLINICAL ASSESSMENT

Using a carefully planned sequence of history-taking and all-night polygraphic recordings (polysomnograms), it is possible to provide specific etiologic diagnoses and treatment recommendations for the majority of patients with sleep complaints.

Evaluation begins with a complete sleep history. Whenever possible, it is important to interview the bed partner because he or she often notices problems in the patient's sleep of which the patient is unaware. A sleep history includes questions about a typical night's sleep, daytime functioning, and details of drug and alcohol use, as well as the medical history. Key data include the following:

1. Time to bed and lights-out time. (Is it the same every night?) Many people with troubled sleep go to bed long before they turn out the lights.
2. Sleep latency. (How long does it take to fall asleep?)
3. Number and duration of awakenings during the night.
4. Final awakening time.
5. Weekday and weekend schedule. (Are times of waking up irregular?)
6. Estimated time spent actually sleeping at night.

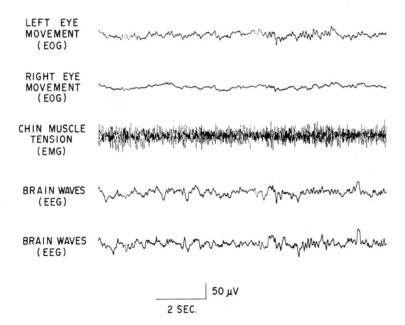

Figure 23–1 Non–rapid eye movement (NREM) sleep. Chin muscle tension is high, and brain waves are slow in frequency and high in amplitude. EOG, electrooculogram; EMG, electromyogram; EEG, electroencephalogram.

These data help to determine the person's sleep pattern. It is often advisable to ask the patient to keep a sleep diary for several weeks prior to the interview to provide a reliable perspective and to help patients learn more about their own sleep patterns.

Other questions attempt to differentiate between specific sleep disorders such as sleep-disordered breathing and periodic limb movements in sleep. Does the patient snore, gasp for breath, stop breathing, or wake up confused (e.g., does he or she show signs of sleep-disordered breathing)? Does the patient kick repetitively or have restless legs (i.e., does he or she show evidence of periodic limb movements in sleep)? It is important to remember that some patients unfortunately will not be aware of any of these symptoms.

Questions about daytime functioning include the following:

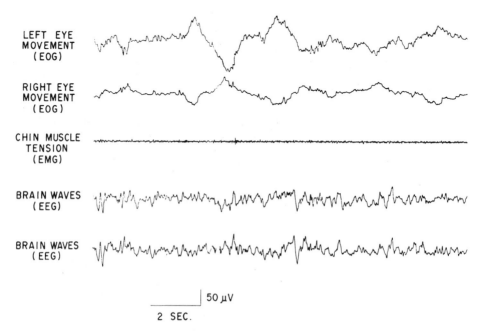

Figure 23–2 Rapid eye movement (REM) sleep. Chin muscle tension is very low, and brain waves are faster in frequency and lower in amplitude than during NREM sleep. EOG, electro-oculogram; EMG, electromyogram; EEG, electroencephalogram.

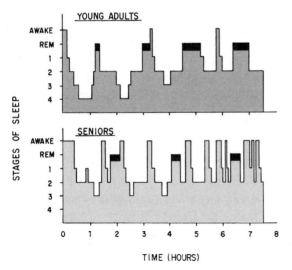

Figure 23–3 Normal sleep cycles. As we get older, it takes us longer to fall asleep and we have less deep sleep, more awakenings, and less REM sleep.

1. How do you feel when you get up in the morning?
2. Do you nap deliberately during the day?
3. Do you find yourself falling asleep while reading, watching television, attending a play or a movie, while talking with friends, or while driving? At what time of day or evening are you sleepy?

These questions try to establish if the patient is falling asleep at inappropriate times, which would suggest disturbed sleep at night.

Drug, alcohol, food (caffeine), and medical histories are all important in determining interactions as well as the causes and effects of the sleep disturbance.

After the history is complete, it is sometimes necessary to refer the patient to a sleep disorders center for evaluation. A full-night recording can then be done. The traditional clinical polysomnogram includes at a minimum EEG, EOG, submental EMG, tibialis EMG, electrocardiography (ECG), two respiration channels, and blood oxygen saturation levels (oximetry). Recordings are made for at least one full night and sometimes for two nights.

Portable recording devices are also available as screening tools.[4] Portable recorders may be connected to the patient in the afternoon or evening, and the patient can be sent home to sleep in his or her own bed. For hospital inpatients, the equipment can be used at the patient's bedside. These systems are more convenient and comfortable for the patient and less expensive than a laboratory polysomnogram but are not appropriate for all situations.[5]

It is only with a full-night recording that one can absolutely rule out sleep apnea. If a polysomnogram cannot be obtained, the clinician must proceed with extreme caution.

DISEASES—DIAGNOSIS AND MANAGEMENT

Circadian Rhythm Changes

With age, the circadian rhythms begin to shift. The average adult begins to become sleepy around 10:00 PM to midnight and wakes up approximately 6 to 8 hours later at 6:00 to 8:00 AM. With age, this circadian rhythm often advances, and thus, older people tend to have an earlier circadian rhythm. People with an advanced sleep phase begin to get sleepy earlier in the evening, for example, around 8:00 to 9:00 PM, but they still awaken about 8 hours later, perhaps between 4:00 and 5:00 AM. Many older people, even though they may feel sleepy, try to stay up until 10:00 or 11:00 PM, yet they still awaken early and thus obtain only 5 or 6 hours of sleep. A combination of poor sleep habits and advanced rhythm may therefore reduce the older person's ability to get a full night's sleep.

The state-of-the-art treatment for advanced sleep phase is exposure to bright light in the evening.[6] The evening light delays the circadian rhythm so that the individual begins to get sleepy later in the evening. A highly effective regimen is 2 hours of bright light (2000 to 2500 lux) from about 7:00 to 9:00 PM. Many people watch television in such dim light in the evening that simply adding additional lighting to the television area may be an effective solution to this problem.

Sleep-Disordered Breathing

Sleep-disordered breathing (SDB), also called sleep apnea, is one of the most serious sleep disorders. SDB is a repetitive process of respiratory cessation during sleep. The SDB syndrome encompasses three types of disorders: (1) obstructive sleep apnea involves the collapse of the pharyngeal airway, with partial or complete blockage of air flow; (2) central sleep apnea results from failure of the respiratory neurons to activate the phrenic and intercostal motor neurons that mediate respiratory movements; (3) mixed sleep apnea is a combination of obstructive and central sleep apnea. Hypopnea is an episode of hypoventilation that may produce anoxia or arousal even when complete sleep apnea (total cessation of air flow) does not occur. SDB is diagnosed when breathing ceases for at least 10 seconds, and at least five episodes of apnea,

TABLE 23–1   **TREATMENT OPTIONS FOR OBSTRUCTIVE SLEEP APNEA**

1. Continuous positive airway pressure (CPAP) or BiPap
2. Uvulopalatopharyngoplasty (UPPP) or other surgeries
3. Tongue-retaining device (TRD) and other oral devices
4. Antidepressants (e.g., trazodone)
5. Weight loss
6. Body position during sleep (avoiding the supine position)

or 15 episodes of apnea plus hypopnea, per hour of sleep. Treatment, however, may not be needed unless the condition is more severe. Most apnea and hypopnea episodes are terminated by transient arousals.

Reviews have suggested that a variety of mechanisms, sometimes working in combination, can cause SDB. These include obesity, micrognathia, jaw or nasal deformities, thyroid, pituitary, or neurologic impairments, and alterations of respiratory reflexes during sleep.[7] Epidemiologic studies, cardiac catheterization studies, and studies done before and after treatment have shown that one of the consequences of SDB is hypertension.[8, 9] Lugaresi and associates[10] have shown that partial obstruction of snoring may also cause nocturnal hypertension. It has also been shown that SDB is associated with increased daytime sleepiness even among elderly subjects who have no sleep complaints. In addition, SDB has been associated with cognitive impairment and dementia.[11] Other consequences of SDB include anoxia, excessive daytime sleepiness, cardiac arrhythmias, cardiorespiratory failure, and ultimately, death during sleep.[12] Treatment options are shown in Table 23–1 for obstructive sleep apnea and Table 23–2 for central sleep apnea.

The prevalence of SDB in the elderly has been shown to be quite high.[13] In a study of randomly selected community-dwelling elderly, Ancoli-Israel, Kripke, and colleagues showed that 24% of those aged 65 years and older had five or more

TABLE 23–2   **TREATMENT OPTIONS FOR CENTRAL SLEEP APNEA**

1. Tricyclic antidepressants
2. Progesterone
3. Acetazolamide
4. Continuous positive airway pressure

apnea episodes per hour of sleep, and 81% had 10 or more episodes of apnea plus hypopnea per hour of sleep.[14] In comparison, in younger adults it has been estimated that 9% of middle-aged men and 4% of middle-aged women have at least 15 episodes of apnea plus hypopnea per hour of sleep.[15] Nevertheless, as with hypertension, this high prevalence does not suggest that this condition is normal with aging. Older adults with SDB should be treated no differently than younger adults with the same symptoms.[16]

Periodic Limb Movements in Sleep

Periodic limb movements in sleep (PLMS), also called nocturnal myoclonus, is characterized by repetitive leg kicks every 20 to 40 seconds during sleep that are followed by brief arousals. The diagnosis is made when there are five or more leg kicks per hour of sleep, each causing an arousal. In this disorder, periodic episodes of leg jerks alternate with normal sleep. Because the patients are repeatedly disturbed, they often complain of both insomnia and excessive daytime sleepiness. Other symptoms of PLMS include leg kicks and restless legs during the day and during relaxation. There is evidence that PLMS is often associated with SDB. Thus, this syndrome may have some pathophysiologic relationship with SDB as well as being an independent syndrome.

Treatment of PLMS is very difficult because the etiology is not known. Three types of medications are generally used, including the sedative-hypnotics (e.g., clonazepam or temazepam),[17] the opiates (e.g., Tylenol with codeine),[18] and levodopa-carbidopa (e.g., Sinemet or Sinemet CR).[19] Each type of treatment has its advantages and disadvantages, and the benefit-to-risk ratio of long-term treatment is unresolved.

The prevalence of PLMS in older populations has been estimated to be 44%.[20] This disorder, therefore, may account for many of the complaints reported by elderly people about difficulty in falling asleep.

Insomnia

Insomnia is defined as difficulty in falling asleep or difficulty in staying asleep. Two factors that can cause the complaint of insomnia in elderly people are medical and psychiatric illness and use of medications. Medical illness, whether it be the pain of cancer or depression, can interfere with sleep. In these situations, it is important to treat the primary medical or psychiatric problem first. Improving the symptoms of the illness should also improve the sleep complaint.

The relationship between medications and

TABLE 23-3 **MEDICATIONS AFFECTING SLEEP**

Medications Known to Cause Insomnia
Alcohol
Beta-blockers
Bronchodilators
Corticosteroids
CNS stimulants (e.g., caffeine, theophylline)
Decongestants (e.g., pseudoephedrine)
Gastrointestinal drugs (e.g., cimetidine)
Cardiovascular drugs
Neurologic drugs
Stimulating antidepressants and fluoxetine
Medications Known to Cause Daytime Sleepiness
Analgesics
Sedating antidepressants
Benzodiazepines

sleep should always be discussed with older patients. Medications that are depressants can cause daytime sleepiness if taken during the day. Medications that are stimulants can cause complaints of insomnia if taken near bedtime. By adjusting the time and dose of the medication, the physician may improve the problem causing the complaint. Examples of medications that can affect sleep are shown in Table 23–3. Note that some drugs, particularly antidepressants such as imipramine, nortriptyline, and desipramine, can cause both insomnia and daytime sleepiness.[21]

As mentioned, treatment of insomnia in the elderly should be geared to treatment of the underlying problem. Sedative-hypnotics should be used only for temporary relief of symptoms and only for short time periods and in conjunction with behavioral techniques. Sedative-hypnotics often increase sleep only modestly. Sedative-hypnotics that have short absorption times are more appropriate for patients complaining of sleep onset difficulties (for example, triazolam or zolpidem). Sedative-hypnotics with longer half-lives are more appropriate for patients complaining of early morning insomnia (for example, temazepam). Sedative-hypnotics are never recommended for long-term use, so they have a limited role in patients with chronic sleep problems.

In summary, sedative-hypnotics should be prescribed only for elderly people with transient insomnia, and no prescription should last longer than about 3 weeks. Older patients with chronic insomnia should use sedative-hypnotics only intermittently, for example, once every two or three nights. Sedative-hypnotics should be prescribed at the lowest possible effective dose and should never be prescribed if SDB is suspected.[22]

Infirm people with arthritis and other chronic illnesses are often inclined to spend extra time in bed, often watching television or reading. Others spend more time in bed (e.g., 10 to 12 hours) because they are concerned that they are not getting enough sleep. A habit of going to sleep promptly after going to bed is desirable, and therefore anything that interferes with this habit may ultimately contribute to insomnia. Spending long hours lying awake in bed is very damaging to sleep patterns. It is often better to read or watch television in a recliner under a favorite quilt, on a couch, or even in another bed, and then going to sleep in one's own bed only when sleep seems imminent. Similarly, the elderly person who awakens in the middle of the night should not remain in bed if he or she feel unable to return to sleep but should get up until he again feels sleepy. Nevertheless, the morning wake-up time should remain the same and should not be extended.

In addition, older insomniacs should be taught good sleep hygiene techniques (Table 23–4). These include exercising regularly, keeping regular hours, avoiding alcohol and caffeine at night, limiting naps, and, as mentioned, not spending excessive time in bed. In addition, because many older insomniacs are sleep advanced, spending more time out of doors to increase overall light exposure will help to stabilize their circadian rhythms.

Behavioral therapies, such as stimulus-control therapy,[23] sleep restriction therapy,[24] and cognitive-behavior therapy,[25] can all be effectively taught to older insomniacs because sleep complaints almost always have behavioral components. Spending less time in bed is one of the most effective treatments for insomnia. It is easy to understand that an elderly person who is advised to restrict time in bed to 6 or 7 hours may become sleepier after a few nights and therefore will fall asleep more rapidly and sleep more soundly. Restricting time in bed is a good treatment because it results in feeling sleepier at bedtime and a greater ability to sleep deeply. What is more surprising to the patient is that restricting time in bed, by correcting bad habits,

TABLE 23-4 **RULES FOR GOOD SLEEP HYGIENE**

1. Exercise
2. Limit naps (less than 30 minutes/day)
3. Take walks to increase light exposure
4. Check medications
5. Avoid caffeine, alcohol, tobacco
6. Limit liquids in the evenings
7. Keep regular hours

may actually result in more physiologic sleep and correspondingly less sleepiness during the day. Often the insomniac who spends 10 to 12 hours in bed can correct the problem by reducing time in bed to 6 to 7 hours, always maintaining a regular wake-up time no matter how little sleep was achieved the night before. Sleep restriction appears to be a safe and lasting treatment.

SLEEP PROBLEMS IN PATIENTS WITH DEMENTIA

Dementia and Institutionalization

Sleep in patients with dementia can be extremely disturbed. These patients have decreased sleep efficiency, and often the circadian rhythms are reversed, with patients sleeping during the day and awake and wandering at night.[11, 26] This extreme disruption of the sleep-wake cycle is the second leading cause of institutionalization, incontinence being the first.[27] Confusion, disorientation, and agitation affect 10% to 30% of institutionalized demented elderly.

In the nursing home, sleep fragmentation is extremely common. Nursing home patients, on average, are never asleep for a full hour and never awake for a full hour. Rather, they are constantly falling asleep and waking up. In one study, nursing home patients were never asleep for more than 40 minutes per hour throughout each hour of the day and night.[28] Many factors contribute to this fragmented sleep. Chronic bed rest is common because the patient is too sick to get out of bed, because of boredom, or because well-meaning staff put the patient to bed too early. Yet the longer one stays in bed, the more fragmented sleep becomes. Sleep-disordered breathing is also extremely common in this population, in which more than 40% of patients meet at least the minimum criteria for diagnosis.[29] Circadian rhythm disturbances are common and are most likely exacerbated by low light exposure. The average amount of bright light exposure in one nursing home was only 11 minutes a day.[30]

Environmental issues also affect the sleep of nursing home patients. Patients in rooms with disruptive roommates tend to have disturbed sleep. Patients who need nursing care during the night will have their sleep disturbed (as will their roommates).

Treating Sleep Problems in the Nursing Home

Treatment of sleep problems in this population should involve a combined approach of behavioral interventions with pharmacologic treatments when necessary. When possible, time in bed should be limited to the night hours only; naps should be restricted to one short nap in the early afternoon, a daily routine should be established with meals served at a table and never in bed, caffeine should be restricted (encourage family members to bring flowers, not chocolate), night-time noise and light should be kept to a minimum, roommates should be matched on the basis of night-time as well as daytime behaviors. Recently, several investigators have begun to examine the use of bright light to treat sleep problems[31, 32] and agitation[33] in the nursing home. Although the full effect of these studies is not yet known, increasing light exposure by taking patients outside more often or increasing the light levels inside may well help many patients.

SUMMARY

When considering sleep problems in the elderly, it is important to remember that the decreased ability to sleep causes sleeplessness, which causes daytime drowsiness and less than optimal functioning. Circadian rhythms naturally advance a few hours with age. Older people may feel sleepy earlier and wake up earlier. Physical activity and natural light exposure can promote better sleep because light exposure may help reset the circadian clock. Sticking to a regular schedule also helps to stabilize the circadian clock. Not sleeping well at night and then napping during the day can cause a disturbed sleep-wake cycle.

Aging by itself does not cause sleep problems. The need for sleep does not decrease with age, although sleep patterns do change. Rather, the ability to sleep decreases with age, due primarily to changes in circadian rhythms and the presence of sleep disorders.

ACKNOWLEDGMENT Supported by NIA AG02711, NIA AG08415, NHLBI HL44915, NIMH MH49671, NIMH MH00117, NIA AG12364, Stein Institute for Research on Aging and the Research Service of the Veterans Affairs Medical Center.

References

1. Webb WB, Roth T, Roehrs TA: Age-related changes in sleep. Clin Geriatr Med 1989;5:275–287.
2. Miles L, Dement WC: Sleep and aging. Sleep 1980;3:119–220.
3. Dement WC, Seidel W, Carskadon MA: Daytime alertness, insomnia and benzodiazepines. Sleep 1982;5:S28–S45.
4. Ferber R, Millman R, Coppola M, Fleetham J, Murray CF, Iber C, McCall V, Nino-Murcia G, Pressman M,

Sanders M, et al: Portable recording in the assessment of obstructive sleep apnea. Sleep 1994;17(4):378–392.

5. Standards of Practice Committee of the American Sleep Disorders Association: Practice parameters for the use of portable recording in the assessment of obstructive sleep apnea. Sleep 1994;17(4):372–377.

6. Campbell SS, Terman M, Lewy AJ, Dijk DJ, Eastman CI, Boulos Z: Light treatment for sleep disorders: Consensus report. V. Age-related disturbances. J Biol Rhythms 1995;10(2):151–154.

7. Shepard JWJ: Cardiorespiratory changes in obstructive sleep apnea. *In* Kryger MH, Roth T, Dement WC (eds): Principles and Practice of Sleep Medicine. Philadelphia, WB Saunders, 1989, pp. 537–551.

8. Fletcher BO: The relationship between systemic hypertension and obstructive sleep apnea: Facts and theory. Am J Med 1995;98(2):118–28.

9. Hla KM, Young TB, Bidwell T, Palta M, Skatrud JB, Dempsey J: Sleep apnea and hypertension: A population-based study. Ann Intern Med 1994;120:382–388.

10. Lugaresi E, Cirignotta F, Montagna P: Snoring: Pathogenic, clinical, and therapeutic aspects. *In* Kryger MH, Roth T, Dement WC (eds): Principles and Practice of Sleep Medicine. Philadelphia, WB Saunders, 1989, pp. 494–500.

11. Bliwise DL: Review: Sleep in normal aging and dementia. Sleep 1993;16:40–81.

12. Ancoli-Israel S, Kripke DF, Klauber MR, Fell R, Stepnowsky C, Estline E, Khazeni N, Chinn A: Morbidity, mortality and sleep disordered breathing in community dwelling elderly. Sleep 1996;19(4):277–282.

13. Ancoli-Israel S: Epidemiology of sleep disorders. Clin Geriatr Med 1989;5:347–362.

14. Ancoli-Israel S, Kripke DF, Klauber MR, Mason WJ, Fell R, Kaplan O: Sleep disordered breathing in community-dwelling elderly. Sleep 1991;14(6):486–495.

15. Young T, Patta M, Dempsey J, Skatrud J, Weber S, Badr S: Occurrence of sleep disordered breathing among middle-aged adults. N Engl J Med 1993;328:1230–1235.

16. Ancoli-Israel S, Coy TV: Are breathing disturbances in elderly equivalent to sleep apnea syndrome? Sleep 1994;17:77–83.

17. Peled R, Lavie P: Double-blind evaluation of clonazepam on periodic leg movements in sleep. J Neurol Neurosurg Psychiatry 1987;50(12):1679–1681.

18. Kavey N, Walters AS, Hening W, Gidro-Frank S: Opioid treatment of periodic movements in sleep in patients without restless legs. Neuropeptides 1988;11(4):181–184.

19. Kaplan PW, Allen RP, Buchholz DW, Walters JK: A double-blind, placebo-controlled study of the treatment of periodic limb movements in sleep using carbidopa/levidopa and propoxyphene. Sleep 1993;16(8):717–723.

20. Ancoli-Israel S, Kripke DF, Klauber MR, Mason WJ, Fell R, Kaplan O: Periodic limb movements in sleep in community-dwelling elderly. Sleep 1991;14(6):496–500.

21. Ancoli-Israel S: All I Want Is a Good Night's Sleep. Chicago: Mosby-Year Book, 1996.

22. Kripke DF, Ancoli-Israel S: Prevalence of sleep apnea with ageing: Implications for hypnotic prescribing. *In* Smirne F, Franceschi M, Ferini-Strambi L (eds): Sleep and Ageing. Milan, Masson, 1991, pp. 233–236.

23. Bootzin RR, Perlis ML: Nonpharmacologic treatments of insomnia. J Clin Psychiatry 1992;53:37–41.

24. Spielman AJ, Saskin P, Thorpy MJ: Treatment of chronic insomnia by restriction of time in bed. Sleep 1987;10:45–56.

25. Morin CM, Kowatch RA, Barry T, Walton E: Cognitive-behavior therapy for late-life insomnia. J Consult Clin Psychol 1993;61(1):137–146.

26. Ancoli-Israel S, Kripke DF: Now I lay me down to sleep: The problem of sleep fragmentation in elderly and demented residents of nursing homes. Bull Clin Neurosci 1989;54:127–132.

27. Pollak CP, Perlick D, Linsner JP, Wenston J, Hsieh F: Sleep problems in the community elderly as predictors of death and nursing home placement. J Commun Health 1990;15(2):123–135.

28. Jacobs D, Ancoli-Israel S, Parker L, Kripke DF: Twenty-four-hour-sleep-wake patterns in a nursing home population. Psychol Aging 1989;4(3):352–356.

29. Ancoli-Israel S, Klauber MR, Kripke DF, Parker L, Cobarrubias M: Sleep apnea in female patients in a nursing home: Increased risk of mortality. Chest 1989;96(5):1054–1058.

30. Ancoli-Israel S, Jones DW, Hanger MA, et al: Sleep in the nursing home. *In* Kuna ST, Surati PM, Remmers JE, (eds): Sleep and Respiration in Aging Adults. New York, Elsevier, 1991, pp. 77–84.

31. Sattin A, Volicer L, Ross V, Herz L, Campbell SS: Bright light treatment of behavioral and sleep disturbances in patients with Alzheimer's disease. Am J Psychiatry 1992;149:1028–1032.

32. Ancoli-Israel S, Kripke DF, Jones DW, Parker L, Hanger MA: 24-hour sleep and light rhythms in nursing home patients. Sleep Res 1991;20A:410.

33. Dovell BB, Ancoli-Israel S, Gevirtz R: The effect of bright light treatment on agitated behavior in institutionalized elderly. Psychiatry Res 1995;57(1):7–12.

24 Hypothermia and Hyperthermia

Calvin H. Hirsch, M.D.

For this relief much thanks, 'tis bitter cold,
And I am sick of heart.

Hamlet I.i

Fear no more the heat o' the sun,
Nor the furious winter's rages . . .

Coriolanus IV.ii

— William Shakespeare

The human organism, like other mammals, is a homeotherm that generates its body temperature principally through metabolism (endothermia) and is capable of maintaining a body temperature that is very close to 37°C (98.6°F) through a wide range of ambient temperatures. Arbitrarily, hypothermia has been defined as a core body temperature (rectal, esophageal, tympanic, or urine) of below 35°C (95°F) and hyperthermia as a core temperature of above 40.6°C (105°F).* As a group, the elderly share with infants a greater vulnerability to the effects of thermal stress and are disproportionately represented among case fatalities due to hypothermia and hyperthermia.

The failure to recognize the contribution of hypothermia and hyperthermia to death and illness has obscured their true incidence. Among susceptible older persons, morbidity from thermoregulatory failure may result from chronic exposure to cold or heat that would not be considered extreme and commonly occurs inside the older person's dwelling. In the United Kingdom, where fuel costs traditionally have been high, it has been estimated that one to five older persons out of 2500 die from illnesses related to hypothermia each year. Between 1979 and 1991, an average of 770 persons died per year in the United States from hypothermia, for an age-adjusted death rate of 0.2 per million. Over half

of these fatalities were in persons aged 65 and older. Neonates and persons over age 65 constituted 64% and 17%, respectively, of the 1815 hospital admissions attributable to hypothermia in New Zealand between 1979 and 1986; nearly all of these patients were admitted from home. Persons over age 65 accounted for 67% of the documented hypothermia-related fatalities in this report. In a survey of British hospitals conducted in the mid 1970s, 3.6% of all patients 65 and older were found to be hypothermic at admission. Average mortality rates from hypothermia increase with age and are nearly 12 times greater in those 75 and over compared to persons aged 15 to 34. Although basal body temperature does not change with healthy aging, surveys conducted in the United Kingdom have revealed a prevalence of 10% to 11.4% of persons with body temperatures at or near hypothermic levels among older persons living at home.

Heat casualty statistics likewise disproportionately represent the elderly. During the summer of 1966 in St. Louis, Missouri, the average temperature exceeded 32°C for nearly 1 month. Of the 246 certified heat-related deaths, 136 (55%) were people 69 years of age and older. That same summer, New York City experienced 200 documented heat-related casualties, among whom the average age was 78. During a heat wave in Memphis, Tennessee, in 1980, the average age of the 483 patients admitted to hospital with a heat-related disorder was 69. Of 28 patients presenting at Parkland Memorial Hospital

---

*Hereafter, only °C will be used. For those readers more comfortable with the Fahrenheit scale, the following conversion may be used: °F = (9/5 × °C) + 32.

244

in Dallas with classic heat stroke in 1978, 89% were over age 64.

HYPOTHERMIA

Pathophysiology

Although socioeconomic conditions, such as poverty, poorly heated or ventilated housing, and undernutrition, may have played a role in these statistics, they demonstrate that older individuals are more likely to present with life-threatening thermoregulatory dysfunction. This increased susceptibility is due to a combination of age-related changes in physiology, a greater prevalence of co-morbid conditions, and a greater likelihood of using medications that affect thermoregulation. The adult human maintains a fine balance between heat gain and heat loss in order to produce a constant optimum temperature that permits intracellular biochemical reactions. Conservation of body heat occurs through the insulating effect of the body's shell (skin, subcutaneous fat, and muscle), basal metabolism, muscular work (including involuntary shivering), and vasoconstriction. About 80% of caloric intake goes into the maintenance of body temperature. When the body's temperature exceeds that of the surrounding air, roughly two thirds of the heat lost occurs by radiation, with variable contributions from conduction and insensible evaporation. Conduction plays a relatively greater role during cold water immersion, since water has 32 times the thermal conductivity of air. Convection (the transfer of heat to currents of passing air or liquid) greatly enhances evaporative and conductive losses.

AGE-ASSOCIATED RISK FACTORS FOR HYPOTHERMIA

In the presence of impaired thermostasis, hypothermia may result from prolonged exposure to an environment that is considered warm yet is cooler than 35°C. Perhaps the most important response of the human organism to cold is behavioral—for example, donning a sweater or moving to a warmer room. An appropriate behavioral response first requires the perception that the environment is too cold. In contrast to young people, healthy older individuals may have difficulty in detecting a 2°C or greater drop in ambient temperature (Table 24–1). In winter, among 72 community-dwelling volunteers in Britain (mean age 77), the average urine temperature was only 36.4°C, yet no subject felt too cold. Seven out of nine subjects with borderline or actual hypothermia claimed they were "comfortable."[1] Peripheral neuropathies, such as those encountered in longstanding or suboptimally controlled diabetes mellitus, may also contribute to diminished thermal sensation.

Second, the individual must be capable of influencing his or her environment. Among the elderly, physical barriers, such as impaired mobility, may impede an appropriate response to being cold. In addition, mobility impairment usually is associated with reduced muscle activity and hence diminished thermogenesis. Cognitive barriers are likewise common; 5% of those over age 65 suffer from dementia and may not know what to do or be able to communicate their discomfort to others. Finally, many older persons on fixed incomes may not be able to afford the cost of heating their homes.

When behavioral responses are insufficient to protect thermostasis, the body must rely on physiologic defenses, which may be impaired by age-associated physiologic changes, chronic illness, and certain medications. The body's first line of defense is its insulation—principally clothing and subcutaneous fat. Normal aging is associated with a loss of subcutaneous fat. When insulation is insufficient to prevent peripheral cooling, local reflex vasoconstriction reduces the surface area of contact of blood with the environment. Using volume plethysmography of the hand, Collins and colleagues[2] observed that in 14% of elderly volunteers (average age 70) vasoconstriction failed to occur upon cooling. In the same volunteers 4 years later, the proportion in whom vasoconstriction failed had increased to one third. Co-morbid conditions and medications that might have influenced vasomotor responses in the subjects unfortunately were not reported. Forty-three percent of those with abnormal vasoconstrictor responses displayed postural hypotension compared with 10% of those with normal vasoconstriction,[3] suggesting that autonomic dysfunction plays a role in increasing susceptibility to hypothermia.

After local vasoconstriction, the body attempts to maintain thermostasis by increasing thermogenesis. The posterior hypothalamus senses cerebral blood temperature and receives input from thermoreceptors via the spinothalamic tract. In response to cooling, the hypothalamus stimulates the sympathetic nervous system to release catecholamines, resulting in further peripheral vasoconstriction and an increase in heart rate, cardiac output, respiratory rate, and blood pressure. Direct stimulation through the extrapyramidal tracts increases muscle tone, which may increase heat production by 50%. When this neuronal stimulation produces rhythmic contraction of the muscles (shivering), heat production may in-

TABLE 24–1 **SUMMARY OF RISK FACTORS FOR THERMOREGULATORY DYSFUNCTION IN THE ELDERLY**

Hypothermia	Hyperthermia
Decreased perception of cold	Decreased perception of heat
Age-related decrease in thermal sensation	Age-related decrease in thermal sensation
Diabetic and other neuropathies	Diabetic and other neuropathies
Ethanol	Ethanol
Benzodiazepines and other sedatives	Benzodiazepines and other sedatives
Maladaptive behavior	Maladaptive behavior
Dementia	Dementia
Immobility	Immobility
Impaired heat retention	Impaired heat loss
Loss of subcutaneous fat	Age-related decrease in vasodilation
Age-related decrease in vasoconstriction	Age-related decrease in cardiac output
Autonomic dysfunction	Peripheral vascular disease
Sympatholytic antihypertensives	Congestive heart failure
Phenothiazines	Cardiovascular deconditioning secondary to
Impaired thermogenesis	immobility, chronic illness
Decreased basal metabolic rate	Obesity
Decreased shivering	Negatively inotropic medications (beta-blockers,
Malnutrition	verapamil)
Hypothyroidism	Decreased sweat response
Drug-induced hypoglycemia	Sweat gland injury (ichthyosis, scleroderma)
Excessive heat loss	Impaired retention of circulating volume
Erythrodermas (psoriasis), burns	Decreased renal concentrating ability
Ethanol	Decreased thirst
Surgery (especially under general anesthesia)	Diuretics
Hypothalamic dysfunction	
Anorexia nervosa	
Parkinson's disease	
Wernicke's encephalopathy	
Medications (ethanol, barbiturates, clozapine,	
caffeine)	
General anesthesia	

crease fivefold in the healthy adult. Although the ability to shiver is retained at least through the ninth decade, the latency of shivering in response to environmental cooling may be longer in older people compared to that in young people, and lower peaks of contraction are attained. It is possible that reconditioning, by restoring muscle mass and the efficiency of muscle work, may reduce or eliminate these age-associated changes in shivering.

Other Conditions Predisposing to Hypothermia

The basal metabolic rate and therefore thermogenesis decrease with aging, related in part to decreasing lean body mass. Metabolic abnormalities, such as hypothyroidism, hypoadrenalism, hypopituitarism, and malnutrition, predispose the body to hypothermia by decreasing thermogenesis. The prevalence of malnutrition among the elderly living in the community approaches 16%

for whites and 18% for blacks but may reach 35% or higher among hospitalized older patients and may exceed 50% among nursing home residents. Protein-calorie malnutrition can easily be overlooked because it may occur without a change in total body weight as a result of replacement of muscle mass by fat. It is diagnosed by finding a serum albumin level of less than 3.5 g/dL in the absence of proteinuria or acute illness. Hypoglycemia, a hazard among alcoholics and the many older patients taking long-acting hypoglycemic medications, may cause hypothermia directly by affecting the hypothalamic thermostat. Hypothermia may also result from diabetic ketoacidosis, presumably due to glucose deprivation of the hypothalamus. Other central nervous system lesions affecting the hypothalamus similarly may induce varying degrees of hypothermia. Wernicke's encephalopathy has been associated with coma, hypotension, and hypothermia. Patients with anorexia nervosa and Parkinson's disease often fail to shiver in the presence of decreasing core temperatures and have defective vasoconstriction, consistent with autonomic dysfunction. Burns and erythrodermas (e.g., severe psoriasis) cause massive radiation of body heat to the environment and impair reflex vasoconstriction to cold. Drugs constitute another important class of contributors to hypothermia. Barbiturates and ethanol interfere with central body temperature regulation, while the latter also induces heat loss through vasodilation. Centrally acting sympatholytic antihypertensive agents, such as clonidine, reserpine, and guanabenz, inhibit reflex vasoconstriction in response to a lowered temperature. Phenothiazines can potentiate hypothermia by inhibiting the shivering response through central mechanisms as well as through alpha-adrenergic blockade. The atypical antipsychotic agent clozapine acts directly on the hypothalamus to induce hypothermia. Even caffeine (as well as other methylxanthines) can predispose to hypothermia, especially when taken in combination with a central or peripherally acting alpha-adrenergic blocking agent.[4]

Unintentional hypothermia occurs in approximately half of patients undergoing surgery and is more likely to occur in patients who are older or who receive general anesthesia. General anesthesia transforms the patient into a poikilotherm whose body temperature varies directly with the temperature of the environment. During mild perioperative hypothermia, catecholamine production increases dramatically; there is a 100% to 500% rise in norepinephrine concentration for each 1° to 2°C reduction in core temperature, resulting in vasoconstriction and frequently in hypertension.[5] Older hypothermic surgical patients generally take longer to return to a temperature of 36°C (often 5 hours or more) unless rewarming procedures are administered. In the immediate postoperative period, Frank and colleagues[6] reported the presence of myocardial ischemia on continuous electrocardiographic monitoring in 36% of hypothermic patients but in only 13% of euthermic patients. Among patients without a preoperative history of coronary artery disease, perioperative hypothermia was associated with a fourfold greater incidence of myocardial ischemia.[6] The shivering that occurs in postoperative older patients produces a 30% to 40% increase in oxygen consumption; narcotic analgesia appears to blunt the shivering response. However, perioperative coronary ischemia is more likely to be related to the catecholamine rise than to the metabolic demands of shivering.[7]

Clinical Assessment

In the elderly, hypothermia often develops insidiously, and subnormal temperatures may be maintained for days or weeks before they finally drop below 35°C. The clinical presentation of hypothermia between 32° and 35°C ("mild hypothermia") mimics that of severe hypothyroidism, with coarse facies, slow, husky speech, impaired mentation, and lethargy. Heterogeneous neurologic symptoms emerge, including confusion, dysarthria, ataxia, focal weakness, sensory loss, depression or loss of the deep tendon reflexes, frontal-release signs, and hallucinations. Hypothermia therefore must be distinguished from other causes of delirium. Pupillary reflexes may be irregular and sluggish, and miosis, mydriasis, or anisocoria may be present. The skin usually is cold to the touch unless external warming has been applied and may appear either pale and corpse-like or show blotchy patches of erythema and purpura. Bullae over pressure-dependent areas have been reported, and the examiner should be alert to signs of frostbite if outside temperatures have been below freezing. A generalized edema may be present owing to the cold-induced shift of intravascular fluid into the interstitium.

Blood pressure, cardiac output, and respiratory rate are characteristically elevated during this phase. Vasoconstriction shunts blood centrally, resulting in increased alveolar and interstitial pulmonary fluid and increased urine output. Hypothermia causes renal tubular glycosuria and a renal concentrating defect, the latter predisposing the individual to hypovolemia. Cold also induces copious bronchial secretions—so-called cold bronchorrhea, which, together with suppression of the cough reflex and increasing lethargy as hypothermia progresses, predisposes the individual to bronchopneumonia. Inspiration of cold air causes an increase in airway resistance owing to increased mucus production, vascular congestion, decreased mucociliary clearance, and bronchial smooth muscle contraction. As the core temperature descends to 32°C, cardiac output along with blood pressure, pulse, and respiratory rate begin to drop. Increasing atrial ectopy occurs, and the electrocardiogram may show inversion of T waves and lengthening of the PR, QT, and QRS intervals. A slowly inscribed terminal force in the QRS (J or Osborn wave [Fig. 24–1]) may appear. Once thought to be pathognomonic for hypothermia, Osborn waves have been reported in patients with massive cerebral injury, hypercalcemia, and interruption of cervical sympathetic pathways.[8] Intestinal motility decreases at a temperature of about 34°C and gradually progresses to ileus. Initially, pancreatic function is undisturbed, but with further cooling, insulin secretion decreases, resulting in hyperglycemia. Hepatic metabolism similarly declines with de-

Upper panel

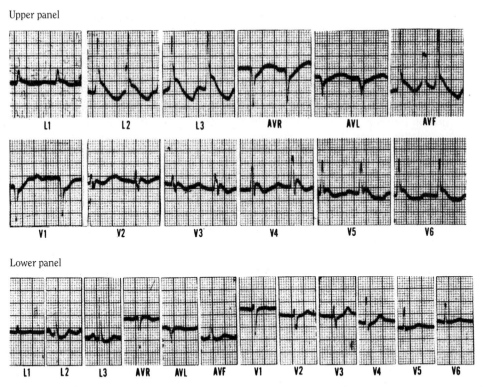

Lower panel

Figure 24–1 Upper panel: Electrocardiogram (ECG) taken during hypothermia showing characteristic terminal J-point elevation of QRS complex (Osborn wave). Lower panel: ECG after normalization of temperature.

creasing core temperature, prolonging the half-life of drugs metabolized by the liver.

Leakage of plasma from the intravascular space and the cold-induced diuresis result in prerenal azotemia and hemoconcentration. The hematocrit increases roughly 2% for each 1 degree drop in core temperature.[9] Hypothermia inhibits platelet function and the enzymes of the clotting cascade, resulting in a coagulopathy that can lead to persistent bleeding or oozing from venipuncture sites and wounds. Hypothermia-related ventilation-perfusion mismatching, increased blood viscosity, and a leftward shift of the oxyhemoglobin curve contribute to hypoxemia. The reduced clearance of lactate produced by shivering muscle and the decreased renal excretion of acid may result in a metabolic acidosis. Serum glucose concentration rises because of decreased insulin secretion. Alcoholics, however, may present with hypoglycemia because of a preexposure depletion of glycogen. Serum potassium levels may be depressed owing to decreased tubular resorption.

At a temperature of between 30° and 31.5°C the last remaining defenses against the cold—shivering and consciousness—cease. At this temperature atrial ectopy gives way to atrial fibrillation with a slow ventricular response. Hy-

poventilation sets in, and respiratory acidosis augments the metabolic acidosis. As core cooling continues, ventricular irritability increases, leading to a high risk of ventricular fibrillation at 28°C and below. Below 28°C the patient may appear dead—cold to the touch, the pulse absent, respirations agonal or undetectable, and the pupils fixed and dilated. Cardiac output drops by 50% at 25°C and by 75% at 22°C, but a parallel reduction in oxidative metabolism spares the vital organs from cell death until extreme hypothermia or prolonged cardiac arrest occurs. At 19° to 20°C the heart stops, and the electroencephalogram becomes flat.

With moderate to severe hypothermia, additional laboratory abnormalities may be found. Signs of pancreatitis are common; pancreatic inflammation and necrosis are seen at autopsy in approximately 50% of patients dying of hypothermia. At or below 20°C leukopenia and thrombocytopenia are commonly observed because of sequestration in the liver and spleen. An elevation in cardiac creatinine phosphokinase (CPK-MB) values to levels suggestive of a myocardial infarction may occur despite the absence of ischemic changes on the electrocardiogram or wall motion abnormalities on the echocardiogram.[10] Although an elevated CPK-MB level may be a benign artifact of cold-induced changes in the membrane permeability of heart muscle, it may also represent subendocardial damage or very small transmural infarctions, which have been detected at necropsy in persons succumbing to hypothermia.[11]

Diagnosis and Management

In hypothermic patients presenting to the emergency department, the lowered body temperature may be a complication of an acute medical condition (for example, overwhelming sepsis or prolonged exposure following a fall and inability to get up). However, hypothermic older patients frequently present with nonspecific symptoms such as shortness of breath, weakness, lightheadedness, confusion, lethargy, or stupor. Overlooking the possible contribution of hypothermia to the patient's symptoms as well as to the physical and laboratory findings could result in inappropriate treatment. Conventional glass and electronic thermometers do not measure temperature below 34°C. Any patient with a temperature of 35°C or below must have his or her core temperature taken with a low-reading thermometer.

In patients with mild hypothermia (core temperatures of over 32°C), passive rewarming with blankets is effective and is probably the safest method of treatment. When active rewarming by externally applied heat is carried out in carefully controlled settings, the outcomes are similar to those achieved with passive rewarming. However, external rewarming generally should be avoided unless the hospital or emergency department has had extensive experience with this technique. The vasodilation that results from external rewarming (e.g., with an electric blanket or currents of warm air) exacerbates the well-described "after-drop" of core temperature that occurs when sequestered cool blood from the surface returns to the core. The vasodilation also increases the risk of hypotension. The complications of external rewarming can be reduced if the application of heat is limited to the trunk.

Unless they are minimally hypothermic, older patients should be admitted to an intensive care unit and placed on telemetry because of the risk of rhythm disturbances and the need for close attention to vital signs, fluid status, and metabolic parameters. Because of the cold-induced diuresis, most hypothermic patients are hypovolemic and require parenteral rehydration, preferably with normal saline warmed to 37° to 40°C. Lactated Ringer's solution should be avoided because of the inability of the hypothermic liver to metabolize lactic acid. As the core temperature returns to normal, third-spaced fluid reenters the vascular space. Thus, fluid resuscitation should proceed cautiously to avoid precipitating congestive heart failure. Monitoring of the central venous pressure may help guide fluid management, but right heart catheterization should be avoided because the catheter tip may induce supraventricular or ventricular arrythmias when it touches irritable mycocardium. Unless the patient has underlying chronic obstructive pulmonary disease, the degree of hypoxemia can be assessed by pulse oximetry. Serum electrolytes, blood urea nitrogen, and serum creatine should be checked and abnormalities corrected. Insulin should not be given unless hyperglycemia is severe (more than 350 to 400 mg/dL) because endogenous insulin secretion increases during rewarming, risking hypoglycemia. The patient should have nothing by mouth until his or her core temperature has risen above 35°C. Unless the patient is able to fully cooperate, bladder (or condom) catheterization is necessary to allow accurate monitoring of urine output. Despite the uncertain clinical significance of the elevated CPK-MB fraction commonly found in hypothermic patients, the high prevalence of coronary artery disease in the elderly, coupled with the documented association of perioperative hypothermia with myocardial ischemia, justifies screening the hypothermic patient for myocardial infarction with serial electrocardiograms and CPK-MB measurements. However, empirical treatment with nitrates and beta-blockers is not justified because it may precipitate or worsen hypotension. Aspirin aggravates the coagulopathy associated with hypothermia.

At a temperature of below 28°C the patient has a depressed level of consciousness. Prophylactic intubation is recommended to prevent aspiration, to control the copious bronchial secretions, and to permit ventilation in the event of cardiac arrest. Intubation should be performed gently and, preferably, after preoxygenation through a mask to minimize the risk of inducing ventricular ectopy. If atrial fibrillation occurs, an agent to slow conduction, such as digoxin or diltiazem, generally is not needed. The atrial fibrillation seen in patients with hypothermia has a slow ventricular response and usually converts spontaneously to normal sinus rhythm following rewarming; such agents may thus induce postrewarming bradycardia or even heart block. A nasogastric tube may be required if ileus is present.

In patients with moderate hypothermia (28° to 32°C), cardiac instability, manifested by ventricular ectopy, warrants active core rewarming. Ventilation with humidified oxygen warmed to 42°C allows the body temperature to rise 1° to 2°C per hour. A popular method of core rewarming is peritoneal lavage with crystalloid dialysate warmed to 40° to 45°C, which achieves rewarming rates of 2° to 4°C per hour. This technique has the advantage of being able to remove dialyzable drugs like barbiturates. Similar rates of rewarming can be achieved with pleural irrigation using large-bore thoracostomy tubes and saline warmed to 40° to 42°C. Recently, hemodialysis has been used successfully for core rewarming; it achieves rewarming rates comparable to those seen with peritoneal dialysis, offers the advantage of more precise correction of acid base and electrolyte disturbances, and eliminates the risk of iatrogenic peritonitis. Because of its ready availability in most hospitals, hemodialysis may replace peritoneal dialysis as a first-line treatment for moderate hypothermia. Gastric, colonic, or bladder irrigation with warmed saline offers relatively little surface area for heat transfer and consequently remains a second-line therapy that can be used when dialysis and pleural irrigation are not available.

At temperatures of below 28°C (severe hypothermia), ventricular fibrillation, the most common cause of death in patients with accidental hypothermia, occurs frequently and is generally refractory to electrical and pharmacologic cardioversion. However, bretylium tosylate has shown some promise at low core temperatures; it is administered as an infusion of 10 mg/kg during ventricular fibrillation.[9] Its efficacy in preventing ventricular fibrillation when given prophylactically is unknown. Extracorporeal rewarming is the most effective method for rapidly raising core temperature and is the treatment of choice in patients with severe hypothermia. Cardiopulmonary bypass can raise core temperature 1° to 2°C every 5 minutes. Femoral vein–femoral artery and atrial-aortic bypass appear to be equally effective, though the the former is less invasive and can be instituted outside the operating room.

A fundamental adage about hypothermia is that the victim is not dead until he or she is warm and dead. The protective effect of hypothermia may permit continued organ survival for many minutes after complete circulatory collapse has occurred. At a core temperature of 25°C, cerebral oxygen requirements are reduced by 70%. Thus, even in the presence of cardiac arrest, cardiopulmonary resuscitation should be continued until the patient has been rewarmed to at least 32°C. The increase in metabolism with rewarming may produce transient hypoxemia that responds to supplemental oxygen. The metabolic acidosis frequently seen in victims of prolonged hypothermia is remarkably well tolerated, and administration of sodium bicarbonate is not generally recommended. In moderate to severe hypothermia, arterial blood gases are useful for monitoring acid base status and oxygenation. Blood gas autoanalyzers warm the blood to 37°C, and the values reported at this temperature should be used for interpretation. For every 1°C drop in temperature, there is a corresponding 0.015 increase in pH and a decrease in the P_{CO_2} due to the direct effect of temperature on the dissociation of hydrogen ions and the partial pressure of dissolved gases. Correcting the blood gas for the patient's temperature consequently may result in an erroneous diagnosis of respiratory alkalosis and an inappropriate reduction in minute ventilation. Maintaining the *uncorrected* pH close to 7.4 appears to result in better myocardial function and electrical stability in both experimental animals and humans.[12] Occult sepsis may complicate hypothermia and has been seen in up to 41% of hypothermic patients presenting to institutions serving a large alcoholic population.[11, 13] Empirical administration of broad spectrum antibiotics therefore appears justified once blood for the appropriate cultures has been drawn. Among victims in whom alcohol abuse is suspected, thiamine should be administered empirically because of the association of Wernicke's encephalopathy with hypothermia.

The published mortality from severe hypothermia ranges from 0% to 80%. Little relationship exists between the core temperature at the time of diagnosis, age, rate of rewarming, and survival. One of the lowest temperatures ever recorded in an elderly patient who fully recovered from accidental hypothermia was 25°C, detected in an 86-year-old man.[14] In patients with hypothermia alone, as among some alcoholics and individuals with mental illness, the prognosis is good, whereas the risk of mortality increases with the severity of underlying disease. Taken as a group, older individuals, with their increased prevalence of predisposing conditions (e.g., hypothyroidism, diabetes mellitus, undernutrition, use of medications), predisposing physiologic changes (e.g., decreased subcutaneous fat, diminished temperature perception, decreased shivering), and the presence of other chronic disease, are more likely to experience and suffer complications from accidental hypothermia.

HYPERTHERMIA

Pathophysiology

AGE-ASSOCIATED RISK FACTORS FOR HYPERTHERMIA

Under conditions of rest and fasting, an average 70-year-old man produces about 65 kcal of heat per hour, about 5 kcal/hour less than an average 40-year-old. While this may be a disadvantage in a cold environment, it may be the one advantage that age confers for protection against hyperthermia. External warming (e.g., the sun) and muscular work add additional heat. An increase in blood temperature is sensed by the anterior hypothalamus, which in turn mediates increased blood flow to the skin and muscle with compensatory vasoconstriction of the splanchnic bed. Cutaneous vasodilation allows heat to be radiated to the environment when ambient temperatures are below 37°C. The increase in peripheral blood flow is accompanied by an increase in heart rate and cardiac output. Impaired cardiovascular performance is therefore an important risk factor for heat-related illness in older individuals (see Table 24–1). Cardiac output declines with age, although the slope of decline is reduced in physically active individuals such as master athletes. Not surprisingly, persons with congestive heart failure are at particular risk for heat-related illness. These individuals cannot acclimatize to the heat and may show signs of worsening congestive heart failure during prolonged exposure to heat. Similarly, common medications among the elderly that reduce cardiovascular function or reduce vascular volume, such as calcium channel antagonists, beta-blockers, and diuretics, increase the risk of heat intolerance. Peripheral vascular disease reduces heat tolerance by interfering with cutaneous vasodilation. Among healthy unacclimatized volunteers with similar proportions of body fat, older subjects (mean age 66) displayed a significantly lower forearm blood flow and a greater esophageal temperature compared to young subjects in response to dry heat exposure.[15] Reduced cardiovascular responsiveness to heat exposure appears to be a concomitant of aging, at least in unacclimatized individuals, and a risk factor for heat intolerance.

When the ambient temperature exceeds 37°C, heat loss from the body depends almost entirely on the evaporation of sweat, which may be enhanced by convective cooling such as that provided by fans. However, as the humidity increases, the ability to lose heat through the evaporation of sweat declines, and fans consequently lose their protective effect. For example, at an ambient temperature of 32.2°C, fans cease to cool when the humidity exceeds 35%. At temperatures of more than 37.8°C, fans may actually contribute to heat stress by increasing the movement of hot air, analogous to the action of a convection oven.

Sweat responses in the elderly have been a subject of controversy. The absolute number of sweat glands per square centimeter of skin does not appear to change with healthy aging, although their function may be altered. Foster and colleagues found a marked reduction in sweating activity in older men compared to younger controls, and an even greater reduction in older women.[16] However, virtually all their older subjects were frail and suffering from a variety of chronic diseases. Among healthy subjects, an age-related decrement in sweat rate can be detected in response to dry but not to moist heat. The sweat rate in the elderly thus appears to be related to the initial hydration of the skin. The threshold core temperature at which sweating occurs also appears to be higher in older persons. Conditions that impair sudomotor activity, such as sweat gland injury from prior heat stroke, ichthyosis, and scleroderma, can predispose to heat intolerance. Medications with anticholinergic effects, such as benztropine, oxybutynin, tricyclic antidepressants, phenothiazines, and antihistamines, directly inhibit sweat production. Benzodiazepines, alcohol, and other sedatives can blunt the patient's awareness of excessive heat and prevent appropriate behavioral responses. Obesity, common in older adults, is associated with an altered sweat gland distribution and results in a decreased surface area to mass ratio and decreased skin blood flow, thus compromising heat loss.

A decrease in the effective arterial volume commonly results from the physiologic response to heat stress. This occurs as a result of loss through sweating, peripheral vasodilation in excess of splanchnic vasoconstriction, and leakage of plasma into myocytes (the latter two occuring during hard muscular work). Although acclimatization reduces the amount of sweat produced for a given amount of work, timely replacement of fluids is a critical behavioral response. After 24 hours of water deprivation, healthy elderly men were less thirsty, drank less water, and failed to dilute their plasma volume to predeprivation osmolality compared to younger subjects.[17] Thirst resulting from heat stress and dehydration is also reduced in the elderly.

As with cold exposure, the most important responses to excessive heat are behavioral, such as removing excess clothing or turning on a fan or air conditioner. However, appropriate behavioral responses depend on the perception of discomfort. Crowe and Moore[18] tested older and younger subjects in a warm chamber with their right hands immersed in a warm water bath that was hot enough to raise core body temperature. The subjects were allowed to obtain a burst of cool air ad libitum. The older subjects availed themselves of the cool air less often than would have been expected, given that their mean tympanic temperature and the mean rate of rise of temperature were significantly higher than these values in the younger subjects. Elderly diabetics and patients with peripheral neuropathies are at substantially increased risk for inability to detect small or gradual increases in ambient temperature. In addition, elderly diabetics may be unable to generate sufficient vasodilation in response to heat stress because of subcutaneous microvascular disease as well as autonomic dysfunction.

Data suggest that acclimatization can reverse or reduce these age-related changes in heat tolerance. Acclimatization involves an increase in circulating blood volume, increased cardiac output for a given level of exercise, an increase in the efficiency of skeletal muscle, a rise in sweat production, an increase in serum aldosterone levels, and increased conservation of sodium in both urine and sweat. Acclimatization thus resembles aerobic conditioning. Tankersley and colleagues[19] compared the responses of seven young men (mean age 29) and 13 older men (mean age 65) to aerobic exercise in a warm environment (30°C, 55% relative humidity). When the young men were compared to the subgroup of older men with comparable levels of physical activity, the older subjects had significantly lower sweat rates and peripheral vasodilation. However, when the younger subjects were compared to seven master athletes who had comparable maximal O_2 uptakes (VO_{2max}—a measure of physical conditioning), the sweat rates and degree of peripheral vasodilation were similar in the two groups. Thus, among healthy, functionally independent older persons, aerobically conditioned individuals can be expected to have greater heat tolerance than their sedentary peers. Conversely, elderly persons who have become cardiovascularly deconditioned due to restricted mobility (e.g., from a stroke or arthritis) are at substantially greater risk for heat intolerance.

Clinical Assessment

Hyperpyrexia supervenes when the body cannot dissipate sufficient heat through radiation, convection, and evaporation. At a core temperature of between 37° and 40°C, the symptoms may appear nonspecific and deceptively flu-like; they include anorexia, nausea, vomiting, diarrhea, lightheadedness, fatigue, headache, myalgias, and muscle cramping. The patient may be confused or display impaired judgment. This type of thermal disorder is termed heat exhaustion or heat prostration, and results from dehydration with varying degrees of salt depletion. Individuals who may have difficulty in gaining access to water, such as patients in nursing homes or those with restricted mobility, are at special risk for heat prostration and characteristically present with hypertonic dehydration. Patients with advanced dementia may not be able to communicate their thirst and may be unable to regulate their environment. Individuals who have lost large quantities of sweat that has been replaced with free water may be eunatremic or hyponatremic. This variant of heat prostration typically occurs in individuals who perform prolonged, intense muscular work in hot environments. The overenthusiastic "weekend gardener" and master athlete are among those prone to this disorder.

Although heat prostration usually responds to simple correction of the fluid-electrolyte imbalance, it can also progress to heat stroke. Heat stroke is defined as a core temperature of over 40.6°C in association with hot, dry skin and functional disturbances of the central nervous system (CNS). At temperatures of over 39° to 40°C, CNS dysfunction occurs, leading to neurogenic hyperventilation, paresthesias, tetany, cerebellar ataxia, agitation, and confusion. As core temperature rises, confusion gives way to lethargy, stupor, and then coma. Sweat gland failure is responsible for the hot, dry skin that is a hallmark of heat stroke.

Heat stroke has two variants: classic and exertional. The latter is the result of large endogenous heat production through intense physical exercise in a hot, usually humid, environment. Clinical and laboratory features of classic and exertional heat stroke are presented in Table 24–2. Hypotension is common in the elderly patient with classic heat stroke (CHS), resulting from dehydration and the inability of cardiac output to maintain a normal blood pressure. Heat stroke induces neurogenic hyperventilation with resulting respiratory alkalosis. However, if hypoperfusion occurs secondary to cardiovascular collapse, lactic acidosis may replace the respiratory alkalosis. Hyperglycemia is observed in up to 60% of patients with CHS, in part due to the stimulation of glycogenolysis and inhibition of insulin secretion by catecholamines, which are elevated during heat stress.[20] Patients with CHS frequently present with diarrhea. Less commonly, cerebellar ataxia may be present and the patient may experience convulsions. Renal tubular damage and hepatocellular necrosis, similar to that seen in shock, also may occur. Disseminated intravascular coagulation, though usually milder than in exertional heat stroke, occurs in about 20% of cases and may cause a diffuse hemorrhagic diathesis. Adult respiratory distress syndrome also has been reported in approximately one fifth of cases.[20] CHS may mimic septic meningitis with the appearance of confusion, nuchal rigidity, and hyperpyrexia. Although the cerebro-

TABLE 24–2 **FEATURES OF CLASSIC AND EXERTIONAL HEAT STROKE**

	Classic	Exertional
Age group	Usually infants or the very old	Usually young, but may include older individuals
Acclimatization	No	No
Baseline health status	Increased prevalence of chronic illness	Usually healthy
Common contributing medications	Diuretics, phenothiazines, haloperidol, anticholinergics	Amphetamines, cocaine
Sweating	Absent	Present or absent
Acid base status	Respiratory alkalosis	Metabolic (lactic) acidosis
Rhabdomyolysis	Mild	May be severe
CPK[a]	Mildly increased	Markedly increased
Acute renal failure	<5% of patients	30% of patients
Hypocalcemia	Unusual	Common
Hypoglycemia	Unusual	Common
DIC[b]	Mild	May be severe
Mortality	Untreated: 70%	Untreated: 30%
	Treated: 17%	Treated: <10%

[a]Creatinine phosphokinase.
[b]Disseminated intravascular coagulation.

spinal fluid may be blood-tinged and show an elevated protein content, pleocytosis is absent.[21] Electrocardiographic changes in CHS are heterogeneous and include nonspecific ST-T wave changes, intraventricular conduction defects, prolonged PR and QT intervals, and supraventricular arrythmias, the most common abnormality being sinus tachycardia. Myocardial ischemia and infarction may complicate CHS, especially in older patients and those with preexisting coronary artery disease. In CHS death usually results from irreversible CNS injury, and necropsy usually reveals signs of neuronal injury and petechial hemorrhages scattered throughout the brain. A small percentage of survivors suffer permanent brain injury, particularly cerebellar injury. In general, however, patients with classic heat stroke suffer less tissue damage than victims of the exertional variant.

OTHER CAUSES OF HYPERTHERMIA

Adverse drug reactions or interactions must be included in the differential diagnosis of hyperthermia. Hyperpyrexia, changes in mental status, and increased muscle rigidity in a patient taking a neuroleptic medication should alert the clinician to the possibility of neuroleptic malignant syndrome (NMS). Although rare (occurring in 0.5% to 1.0% of patients taking neuroleptics), the syndrome has also been reported during withdrawal of dopamine agonists in patients with Parkinson's disease and with the use of metoclo-

pramide. NMS can be effectively treated with bromocriptine or dantrolene. Mortality approaches 20%. Malignant hyperthermia (MH) is a rare, genetically determined syndrome precipitated by certain inhaled anesthetic agents, muscle-blocking agents, and stress. Alterations in the permeability of the sarcoplasmic reticulum to ionized calcium characterize this autosomally dominant trait. The treatment of choice is the muscle relaxant dantrolene. Since mortality approaches 60%, contemplated surgery should be preceded by a careful history to search for any prior adverse reactions to anesthetics in the patient or family members. Although the creatinine phosphokinase level is elevated in approximately 70% of persons at risk for MH, a muscle biopsy is required for definitive diagnosis. Administration of meperidine to an individual taking a monoamine oxidase inhibitor (MAO) may precipitate delirium, hypotension, and hyperthermia. This reaction may occur following a single dose of meperidine. It is thought to be due to accumulated serotonin resulting from the monoamine oxidase blockade. The number of half-lives of the MAO inhibitor that must transpire after the last dose before meperidine can safely be given is unknown. However, the manufacturers recommend that meperidine not be administered within 2 to 3 weeks following discontinuation of the drug.

Diagnosis and Management

The symptoms of heat prostration in the elderly may develop insidiously, may persist for days, and may not all be present simultaneously. In frailer individuals, heat prostration may occur in the absence of thirst. Thus, among patients brought to the physician for one or more of these symptoms, the heat stress causing them may be overlooked, risking the development of life-threatening heat stroke. Assessment of flu-like symptoms in the elderly during periods of hot weather should be accompanied by queries about the patient's living situation. In summer, physicians should educate patients, their families, and caregivers about the symptoms of heat prostration and, for patients living in homes that are poorly ventilated or without air conditioning, encourage them to spend part of the day cooling off in air conditioned public places like shopping malls. When heat prostration is diagnosed, the patient should be placed in a cool room and rehydrated with isotonic or hypotonic saline, depending on the initial sodium and calculated water deficit.

It is important to note that many, if not most, older victims of heat stroke have no prodrome and collapse suddenly. Although heat prostration may progress to heat stroke, it is not a necessary precondition. Heat stroke is a medical emergency, with morbidity and mortality proportional to the delay in recognition and treatment. The presence of sweating should not exclude its diagnosis because the neurologic abnormalities typical of CHS may develop while the patient is still actively sweating. Moreover, generalized sweating may reappear when the victim of CHS is moved to a cool environment. Thus, during hot spells heat stroke should be considered in any patient who presents with a core temperature of over 39°C and mental status changes, even if he or she is sweating.

The cornerstone of therapy is the rapid reduction of core temperature and fluid resuscitation. The patient should be placed in an air conditioned room, if available, and core temperature should be continuously monitored, preferably with a rectal thermistor probe. Acetaminophen and salicylates are ineffective, and the latter paradoxically may increase core temperature. The best method for cooling remains controversial. Chilled intravenuous fluids and gastric, bladder, or colonic lavage with chilled normal saline may produce cooling rates of 0.15°C/minute. Keeping the body wet with cool water applied by wet towels or spray, using a large fan to evaporate the moisture, and placing ice bags in the groin and axillae will cool the patient at a rate of 0.3° to 0.6°C/minute. Rubbing the body with ice bags may expedite cooling, and stimulation of the skin by rubbing reduces reflex vasoconstriction that may delay cooling of the core. Ice water baths

should be avoided because they impair access to the patient, especially during cardiopulmonary resuscitation. Intravenous chlorpromazine (25 to 50 mg) can inhibit reflex shivering but may aggravate hypotension and theoretically can lower the seizure threshold at a time when there is a high risk of convulsions. In the older patient, rehydration should proceed cautiously, and consideration should be given to central venous pressure monitoring or right heart catheterization. Peripheral vasoconstriction during cooling will augment the central circulation, and the victim may have underlying cardiovascular disease or may have sustained myocardial injury as a result of the hyperthermia. Seizures frequently complicate the cooling phase and pose a risk of aspiration as well as an increase in core temperature from the muscular activity. In a comatose patient, prophylactic intubation is therefore recommended. External cooling should be continued until the core temperature reaches 40°C, at which point the body temperature usually continues to fall. However, in patients who are unable to sweat, hyperthermia may recur in 3 to 4 hours. Recovery of the ability to sweat may take several weeks or may be permanently impaired.

Mortality from classic heat stroke approaches 70% in untreated cases but may be reduced to around 17% with treatment. Mortality increases with the duration and severity of the hyperthermia and is higher in those presenting in coma or shock.

CONCLUSION

Hypothermia and hyperthermia disproportionately affect older individuals. Although age-related physiologic changes contribute to thermoregulatory dysfunction in the elderly, the type and severity of underlying chronic diseases, together with the medications used to treat them, confer the greatest risk of morbidity and mortality during periods of thermal stress (see Table 24–1). Physical conditioning has the potential to improve the older person's adaptation to heat, but its ability to slow or reverse age-associated changes in response to cold stress is unknown.

References

1. Fox RH, MacGibbon R, Davies L, Woodward PM: Problem of the old and the cold. Br Med J 1973;1:21–24.
2. Collins KJ, Dore C, Exton-Smith AN, Fox RH, MacDonald IC, Woodward PM: Accidental hypothermia and impaired temperature homeostasis in the elderly. Br Med J 1977;1:353–356.
3. Collins KJ, Exton-Smith AN, James MH, Oliver DJ: Functional changes in autonomic nervous responses with ageing. Age Ageing 1980;9:17–24.

4. Durcan MJ, Morgan PF: Opioid receptor mediation of the hypothermic response to caffeine. Eur J Pharmacol 1992;224:151–156.

5. Frank SM, Higgins MS, Breslow MJ, et al: The catecholamine, cortisol, and hemodynamic responses to mild perioperative hypothermia. A randomized clinical trial. Anesthesiology 1995;82:83–93.

6. Frank SM, Beattie C, Christopherson R, et al: Unintentional hypothermia is associated with postoperative myocardial ischemia. The Perioperative Ischemia Randomized Anesthesia Trial Study Group. Anesthesiology 1993;78:468–476.

7. Frank SM, Fleisher LA, Olson KF, et al: Multivariate determinants of early postoperative oxygen consumption in elderly patients. Effects of shivering, body temperature, and gender. Anesthesiology 1995;82:241–249.

8. Gussak I, Bjerregaard P, Egan TM, Chaitman BR: ECG phenomenon called the J wave. History, pathophysiology, and clinical significance. J Electrocardiol 1995;28:49–58.

9. Danzl DF, Pozos RS: Accidental hypothermia. N Engl J Med 1994;331:1756–1760.

10. Husby P, Andersen KS, Owen-Falkenberg A, Steien E, Solheim J: Accidental hypothermia with cardiac arrest: Complete recovery after prolonged resuscitation and rewarming by extracorporeal circulation [see comments]. Intensive Care Med 1990;16:69–72.

11. Fitzgerald FT, Jessop C: Accidental hypothermia: A report of 22 cases and review of the literature. Adv Intern Med 1982;27:128–50.

12. Swain JA: Hypothermia and blood pH. A review. Arch Intern Med 1988;148:1643–1646.

13. Lewin S, Brettman LR, Holzman RS: Infections in hypothermic patients. Arch Intern Med 1981;141:920–925.

14. Scalise PJ, Mann MC, Votto JJ, McNamee MJ: Severe hypothermia in the elderly. Conn Med 1995;59:515–517.

15. Sagawa S, Shiraki K, Yousef MK, Miki K: Sweating and cardiovascular responses of aged men to heat exposure. J Gerontol 1988;43:M1–M8.

16. Foster KG, Ellis FP, Dore C, Exton-Smith AN, Weiner JS: Sweat responses in the aged. Age Ageing 1976;5:91–101.

17. Phillips PA, Rolls BJ, Ledingham JG, et al: Reduced thirst after water deprivation in healthy elderly men. N Engl J Med 1984;311:753–759.

18. Crowe JP, Moore RE: Proceedings: Physiological and behavioural responses of aged men to passive heating. J Physiol 1974;236:43P–45P.

19. Tankersley CG, Smolander J, Kenney WL, Fortney SM: Sweating and skin blood flow during exercise: Effects of age and maximal oxygen uptake. J Appl Physiol 1991;71:236–242.

20. Al-Harthi SS, Karrar O, Al-Mashhadani SA, Saddique AA: Metabolite and hormonal profiles in heat stroke patients at Mecca pilgrimage. J Intern Med 1990;228:343–346.

21. Knochel JP: Heat stroke and related heat stress disorders. Dis Mon 1989;35:301–377.

25 Failure to Thrive

Roy B. Verdery, Ph.D., M.D.

Failure to thrive in older people is a syndrome consisting of progressive loss of physical functioning, weight, and lean body mass.[1, 2] Failure to thrive defined in this way is a process of gradual loss of function due to various causes, both organic (systemic disease) and nonorganic (functional or psychosocial problems). The condition of being at risk for failure to thrive and the condition of impaired function have both been called "frailty."[3] Frailty is obviously closely related to failure to thrive. Another closely related condition is malnutrition. Malnutrition is generally characterized by a loss of fat mass and visceral protein that occurs when nutritional requirements exceed intake and utilization. Malnutrition can cause failure to thrive and result in frailty. Another related problem is sarcopenia,[4] characterized by low muscle mass. Both malnutrition and failure to thrive can lead to sarcopenia, and sarcopenia is a direct cause of frailty because physical function depends, to some extent, on muscle mass.

HISTORY

Failure to thrive, sarcopenia, frailty, and malnutrition in old age have been recognized for a long time. Readers with a literary interest should read the description of the seventh age of man in Shakespeare's *As You Like It* for a poetic description of this problem. In the geriatric and gerontologic literature, these processes have been referred to collectively as "predeath."[5] They have also been studied from a psychological point of view, in which the possibility that there is a "terminal drop" preceding death has been considered.[6] Although the idea that there is a general decline in cognition immediately preceding death in very old people has been refuted,[7] one interpretation of the data is that cognitive impairment may be a cause of failure to thrive, malnutrition, frailty, and sarcopenia, and that these systemic problems accompanying dementia lead to death.

DEMOGRAPHY

Several recent studies have shown that the prevalence of failure to thrive in people older than 65 years is 10% to 25% in general outpatient populations.[8–10] Prevalence is similar whether failure to thrive is defined as functional loss following hip fracture or weight loss in a general outpatient population. In patients older than 65 admitted to an acute care hospital, up to 50% have experienced weight loss before they entered the hospital. Among this number, hospitalization "cures" 50% to 75%.[10] People with prehospital weight loss whose weight loss continues after hospitalization are at high risk of death. Seventy-five to ninety percent of people with persistent weight loss die within 1 year following hospitalization. There has been no careful look at risk factors for failure to thrive in elderly people. Anecdotal evidence suggests that dementia is a significant risk factor.

PATHOPHYSIOLOGY AND ETIOLOGY

Failure to thrive can be divided into two major categories: (1) failure to thrive caused by organic problems, many of which are diagnosable and treatable, and (2) failure to thrive due to nonorganic problems, which are commonly accompanied by starvation.[11] Most nonorganic causes of failure to thrive can be diagnosed by careful functional, psychological, and social assessment, and many can be cured by direct dietary intervention. There remains a group of patients in whom failure to thrive has no clear cause. Idiopathic failure to thrive is a diagnosis of exclusion and can only be used as a diagnosis after the patient has been carefully evaluated for both organic and nonorganic problems.

Almost all chronic systemic diseases can cause failure to thrive in very old people. A list of organic causes of failure to thrive is given in Table 25–1. Although the manifestations are similar, many different mechanisms cause the functional decline, weight loss, malnutrition, sarcopenia, and frailty in these diseases. Cancer cachexia is due to a combination of hypermetabolism and central anorexia, although functional or mechanical gastrointestinal obstruction commonly plays a role. Chronic infections, such

TABLE 25-1 **ORGANIC CAUSES OF FAILURE TO THRIVE**

Organic Causes	Mediator	Anorexia	Hypermetabolism	Other Factors
Cancer	Multiple	+	±	Gastrointestinal obstruction
Infection				
Infective endocarditis	Cytokines	+		
HIV infection, AIDS	Cytokines	+		Malabsorption
Tuberculosis	Cytokines	+		
Inflammation				
Rheumatoid arthritis	Cytokines	+	+	ADL dependency
Temporal arteritis	Cytokines	+	+	
Endocrinopathy				
Diabetes	Insulin		+	Malabsorption
Thyroid disease	Thyroxine	+	+	Malabsorption
Growth hormone deficiency	Growth hormone			
Estrogen deficiency	Estrogens			
Androgen deficiency	Testosterone			
Organ failure				
Heart failure	Cytokines	+	+	Malabsorption
Respiratory failure	Hypoxemia	+	+	ADL dependency
Cirrhosis	Several toxins	+		
Renal failure	Uremia	+		

+ indicates causes of failure to thrive usually associated with the indicated condition; ± indicates causes of failure to thrive sometimes associated with the indicated condition; blank indicates associations are generally absent or have not been reported.

Abbreviations: HIV, human immunodeficiency virus; AIDS, acquired immune deficiency syndrome; ADL, activities of daily living.

as tuberculosis, infectious endocarditis, and human immunodeficiency virus (HIV) infection, cause anorexia probably through a central action of inflammatory cytokines. In HIV infection, in addition to anorexia, malabsorption caused by drugs or opportunistic organisms is often involved. Nonetheless, the specific cause of acquired immune deficiency syndrome (AIDS) cachexia in an individual patient may not be evident. Chronic inflammatory diseases, epitomized by Crohn's disease and rheumatoid arthritis, cause weight loss due to central anorexia produced by the systemic effects of inflammatory cytokines, and, in Crohn's disease, malabsorption. The common endocrinologic diseases of aging—thyroid disease, diabetes, growth hormone deficiency, and deficiency of androgens and estrogens—generally cause failure to thrive, malnutrition, and sarcopenia by directly stimulating catabolism or inhibiting the anabolic response to nutrients. The mechanism behind failure to thrive caused by organ failure depends on the organ that has failed. Respiratory failure leads to failure to thrive through a combination of hypermetabolism, difficulty in eating due to hypoxemia while chewing, drug-induced anorexia, and catabolism stimulated by chronic steroid use. Cardiac cachexia appears to be cytokine mediated, at least in part.[12] Cachexia due to liver failure is probably due to ineffective use of nutrients. Renal failure probably produces failure to thrive both by directly reducing hormones that stimulate cell proliferation (e.g., erythropoietin) and by the central anorectic effects of uremia.

Depending on the specific drug, medications can cause failure to thrive by producing effects on nearly any system or organ.[13, 14] Drugs can directly inhibit appetite, the ability to eat and swallow, absorption of nutrients, the use of energy, protein, and micronutrients, and the ratio of anabolism to catabolism. Among the easiest causes of failure to thrive to treat are single drugs or polypharmacy. Table 25–2 lists groups of medications associated with weight loss and failure to thrive. Anorexia is the most common reason for failure to thrive due to medications. The second most common problem caused by medications is gastrointestinal dysfunction, which is generally a direct effect of gastric motility. A few medications directly affect metabolic rate.

Nonorganic causes of failure to thrive are generally associated with starvation due to inability to get food, lack of interest in food or anorexia, or inability to eat if food is available and the patient is hungry.

Table 25–3 shows the sequence of functions from the desire to eat through swallowing and demonstrates the complex interaction between

TABLE 25–2 **DRUGS THAT CAN CAUSE FAILURE TO THRIVE**

Class of Drug	Anorexia	Hypermetabolism	Gastrointestinal Dysfunction
Benzodiazepines	+		
Opiates	+		+
Thyroxine	+	+	+
Digoxin	+		
Serotonin reuptake inhibitors	+		
Laxatives			+
Chemotherapy	+		+
Antihistamines	+		
Anticholinergics			+
Corticosteroids		+	
Antibiotics	+		+

+ indicates classes of drugs often associated with indicated problem; blank indicates associations are generally absent or have not been reported.

the psychological, social, and functional aspects of eating. In a geriatric assessment paradigm these integrated components of eating behavior can be discussed, and separate emphases can be placed on physical function, psychological problems, and social considerations that affect food intake.

Functional problems can be subdivided into instrumental activities of daily living (IADLs) and personal activities of daily living (ADLs). Among instrumental activities of daily living that affect failure to thrive are the ability to shop and prepare meals, and among the significant personal activities of daily living are the ability to eat, chew, and swallow. While these problems are not independent of dementia and depression or

isolation and poverty, functional assessment must start with consideration of physical ability. In addition to physical problems that impair independent performance of ADLs and IADLs, progressive neurologic and rheumatologic diseases affect these necessary functions. Thus, cerebrovascular disease (stroke) and Parkinson's disease, as well as other, less common progressive neurologic diseases (e.g., Creutzfeldt-Jakob disease, progressive supranuclear palsy, Pick's disease, and so on), can impair independent performance of ADLs and IADLs and lead to starvation. Similarly, osteoarthritis, rheumatoid arthritis, and other diseases associated with joint or muscle inflammation and destruction can cause loss of function and consequent failure to thrive. Last,

TABLE 25–3 **FUNCTIONAL SEQUENCE FROM APPETITE TO ABSORPTION OF NUTRIENTS**

Sequence of Functions	Category	Therapeutic Modality
Desire (appetite) ↓	Physiologic	Medical treatment
Availability (shopping) ↓	Physical	Physical therapy
Preparation (cooking) ↓	IADL	Occupational therapy
Mobility (eating) ↓	ADL	Occupational therapy
Chewing (dentition) ↓	Dental	Dental treatment
Swallowing ↓	Neuromuscular	Speech therapy
Gastrointestinal motility ↓	Physiologic	Medical treatment
Absorption	Physiologic	Medical treatment

Abbreviations: IADL, instrumental activities of daily living; ADL, personal activities of daily living.

TABLE 25–4 **PROBLEMS AFFECTING FUNCTION THAT CAN CAUSE FAILURE TO THRIVE**

Joint diseases
    Rheumatoid arthritis
    Osteoarthritis
Muscular diseases
    Polymyalgia rheumatica
    Muscular dystrophy
Neurologic diseases affecting muscular function
    Cerebrovascular disease
    Parkinson's disease
    Myasthenia gravis
    Progressive supranuclear palsy
Neurologic diseases affecting cognition
    Alzheimer's disease
    Pick's disease
Dental problems
    Caries
    Gingivitis
    Denture problems

problems affecting chewing and swallowing and dental problems are often overlooked by physicians. Conversely, dentists often report weight gain following treatment of dental problems in elderly people. Table 25–4 is a list of diagnoses that can cause failure to thrive by interfering with function.

Psychological problems leading to failure to thrive are generally those that directly affect the desire for food (Table 25–5). The most common of these is depression. It has been proposed that most idiopathic failure to thrive is due to depression.[15, 16] A problem related to depression is intentional starvation or "chronic suicide."[17] This very vexing problem occurs not infrequently in people who have decided that they have no reason to continue living in their present condi-

TABLE 25–5 **INTERACTIONS AMONG SOCIAL AND PSYCHOLOGICAL PROBLEMS CONTRIBUTING TO FAILURE TO THRIVE**

Psychological Problems	Social Problems		
	Poverty	*Isolation*	*Abuse*
Depression	+	+	+
Grief		+	
Dementia			+
Psychosis	+	+	+
Intention	+	+	+

+ indicates psychological problem often associated with indicated social problem; blank indicates associations are generally absent or have not been reported.

tion. This problem must be very carefully separated from depression because depression is a treatable disease that may have to be addressed despite the patient's wishes. An intentional decision not to eat may be the last autonomous decision a person makes. The moral and ethical dilemmas raised by people who decide to end their lives by not eating are profound.

As mentioned earlier, dementia can cause starvation and failure to thrive through its effect on independent performance of ADLs and IADLs. Anecdotally, it has been suggested that people with Alzheimer's disease experience periodic drops in weight caused by decreases in food intake and increases in activity. The picture of the hyperactive, wandering patient with end-stage Alzheimer's disease who nonetheless eats only four cans of commercial nutritional supplement is common. Such patients should be carefully assessed to be certain that medications, particularly neuroleptics or benzodiazepines, are not making this problem worse. Neuroleptics can cause akathisia characterized by increased agitation and activity and can precipitate failure to thrive. Benzodiazepines can cause anorexia and are known to predispose elderly people to falling.

Social disability also causes failure to thrive. As shown in Table 25–5, social problems are closely related to psychological problems. Older people are commonly isolated. They often have left family and friends in other states when they moved to retirement communities. Many widows and widowers live out the last years of their lives alone. Eating is a social event, and the absence of social contacts can directly lead to decreased food intake. Poverty, too, is a major contributor to failure to thrive in very old and oldest-old people. Most people have used up their retirement savings by the age of 75 to 85, and the amount of money available from public assistance programs may be inadequate to provide rent and medications as well as adequate food. The combination of isolation and poverty can lead to unusual eating behaviors and even the consumption of food that is not intended for people (e.g., cat or dog food).

Neglect and abuse are also causes of failure to thrive in the elderly. As people become more dependent on families and friends and less able to defend themselves because of physical impairment and cognitive deficits, they become more vulnerable to people who take advantage of them. People may take advantage of elderly individuals either by not feeding them as much as they should (that is, neglecting them) or by deliberately starving them for personal gain. Because of their vulnerability, failure to thrive in elderly people due to neglect or abuse is essentially indistinguishable from the effects of neglect and abuse of children and consequent childhood failure to thrive.

There is anecdotal evidence that, in addition to these well-established diagnoses, there are idiopathic or otherwise unknown causes of organic failure to thrive. One can hypothesize that immune dysfunction may cause centrally mediated anorexia and peripheral hypermetabolism even in the absence of an identifiable inflammatory stimulus.

APPROACH TO THE PATIENT WITH FAILURE TO THRIVE

The geriatric assessment paradigm (Table 25–6) is especially effective in evaluating older patients with failure to thrive. The medical portion of the geriatric assessment is specifically useful for addressing organic causes of failure to thrive. Psychological, functional, and social evaluations are especially useful in evaluating people with nonorganic failure to thrive. The group of patients in whom no clear etiology of failure to thrive emerges after a complete geriatric assessment, those with idiopathic failure to thrive, can then be identified for further observation or evaluation.

MEDICAL ASSESSMENT

Table 25–1 offers a list of common medical problems that cause failure to thrive in older people. These can be used to focus the history and physical examination. Family histories of cancer, exposure to tuberculosis and other chronic pathogens, and familial problems causing organ failure, particularly heart and kidney failure, are useful considerations with which to start the evaluation. Personal behaviors that increase risk for HIV infection, cancer, or heart disease, including sexual preference and tobacco or alcohol use, are equally important in the initial evaluation.

A complete physical evaluation, including careful examination of all major systems and organs, is invaluable. Not only should such an examination focus on possible organ failure, it should also focus on signs of systemic disease such as lymph node enlargement, signs of chronic infection such as subacute bacterial endocarditis, and evidence of chronic inflammatory processes such as inflammatory arthritis, temporal arteritis, and polymyalgia rheumatica.

Judicious use of laboratory testing based on the history and physical examination is essential for cost-effective evaluation of an elderly patient with failure to thrive. Although rare diseases can lead to failure to thrive in their end stages, indiscriminate use of laboratory tests to rule these out is not warranted without support from the history and physical examination. The most useful screening tests are a complete blood count with differential and a comprehensive chemistry panel. If the complete blood count with differential is normal, the likelihood of significant metabolic problems or problems associated with either a pleocytosis caused by inflammatory or neoplastic process or cytopenia due to chronic disease, impaired cytopoiesis, or accelerated cell destruction is decreased. The most common abnormality found on a complete blood count is anemia of chronic disease characterized by a mildly decreased red cell count and hematocrit, normal red cell indices, and decreased reticulocyte count in the absence of vitamin B_{12}, folate, and iron deficiency. A comprehensive chemistry panel provides a rapid screen for chronic diseases affecting the kidneys or liver and for undiagnosed diabetes. The only endocrinologic test that has sufficient sensitivity and specificity to be used as a screening test in a person with failure to thrive is a thyroid function test. The simplest of these is the high-sensitivity measurement of thyroid-stimulating hormone (TSH), which can identify either hypothyroidism or hyperthyroidism. A chest radiograph is useful and cost effective because of the high prevalence of lung cancer, chronic pulmonary disease, tuberculosis, and often lung infection in this population. A screening mammogram, if one hasn't been done recently, is probably also cost effective, although for breast cancer to cause failure to thrive it generally must be accompanied by distant metastases, which

---

TABLE 25–6   **GERIATRIC ASSESSMENT PARADIGM**

Medical evaluation
    Medical, family, and social history
    System review
    Physical examination
    Laboratory and radiologic testing
Cognitive and psychological assessment
    Cognition screen
    Depression screen
    Affect evaluation
Functional assessment
    Vision screening
    Auditory screening
    ADL independence screen
    IADL independence screen
Social assessment
    Living situation
    Availability of family
    Proximity of friends
    Utilization of community resources
    Unmet resource needs

usually cause abnormalities on the physical examination or other tests. HIV testing in people with the appropriate risk factors is sometimes warranted. There is probably no reason to screen for other endocrinologic abnormalities such as growth hormone, estrogen, or testosterone levels. Other radiologic or nuclear medicine scans are also not cost effective. It is common for people with failure to thrive to have a combination of problems including anemia of chronic disease, hypoalbuminemia, hypocholesterolemia, and a mildly elevated fasting glucose level. This group of metabolic problems, however, does not help to identify a specific diagnosis since these abnormalities accompany most chronic inflammatory processes and chronic systemic diseases or organ failure.

PSYCHOLOGICAL ASSESSMENT

Among the nonorganic causes of failure to thrive, one of the most important treatable problems is depression. Depression should be evaluated early in the course of evaluation for failure to thrive using either the Diagnostic and Statistical Manual, 4th edition (DSM-IV) criteria[18] or the Geriatric Depression Scale.[19] The Geriatric Depression Scale has been validated in both demented and nondemented patients. In the absence of an organic cause of failure to thrive and the presence of significant depression, a tentative diagnosis of depression should be entertained and treated aggressively. Untreated depression in an older person with failure to thrive can be fatal within a few weeks. Deliberate self-starvation without depression must be considered in the absence of other signs and symptoms of depression.

The second main area that has to be addressed in evaluating people for psychological problems causing failure to thrive is dementia. As mentioned previously, people with Alzheimer's disease may show episodic decreases in weight and declines in physical function. Any of the popular screening methods for dementia should be used to evaluate a person with failure to thrive. A widely used screening tool is the Folstein minimental state examination.[20] Other screens for dementia are also useful, although they may require the collection of additional information if they show that dementia may be present.

FUNCTIONAL ASSESSMENT

Screening for functional causes of failure to thrive can be accomplished simply and effectively. Vision that is adequate for reading is probably adequate to prevent failure to thrive unless it is causing loss of ability to perform an essential function, such as driving the car to buy food. Deafness by itself seldom causes failure to thrive, although it is sometimes accompanied by severe depression, and a deaf person who is depressed may very well have failure to thrive that can be treated simply by improving the ability to communicate.

Among the best screens for functional problems that cause failure to thrive are the Fillenbaum IADL scale[21, 22] and the Katz ADL scale.[22, 23] Dependence in IADLs often accompanies dementia, and a person who is unable to shop or prepare meals because of dementia may very well have failure to thrive because of starvation. Dependence in IADLs is often not easily addressed through the help offered by physical and occupational therapists. In contrast, dependence in ADLs recognized by the Katz ADL scale is often improved by physical and occupational therapy. Difficulty in performing ADLs can cause failure to thrive directly owing to the inability to ingest food even if it is available. Physicians should keep in mind that evaluation by a dentist is often important.

SOCIAL FACTORS AND ASSESSMENT

There are no good screening tests for social problems causing failure to thrive. Evaluation of income and poverty level is often difficult because of the patient's reluctance to discuss finances even with a social worker. In addition, there are important regional and cultural variations in social ability and disability. For example, a person living in a city may have more social support than an isolated person living in a rural setting who must drive to get to a grocery store. One important cause of failure to thrive is the living situation of the patient. That is, does the patient live alone or with a spouse, family, or significant other? Another useful question that might be asked is, "If you were to break your leg and need some assistance for a week or two, how many people do you know who could help you?" Some people know many people who would be able to help out in the event of a medical emergency, and some people know very few. Living alone and isolation are among the most important risk factors for failure to thrive. Caregiver "burnout" or "fatigue" must also be considered.[24] The physician must also consider whether an element of abuse or neglect exists.

ASSESSMENT CONCLUSION

It should be possible to evaluate an older individual efficiently for medical, psychological, functional, and social causes of weight loss and functional decline. From time to time, physicians encounter people who have idiopathic failure to thrive and have no problem that is easily identified. Anecdotal evidence suggests that even prolonged observation or an autopsy of these people is unable to pinpoint the cause of failure to thrive. Whether the diagnosis of such people should be idiopathic failure to thrive based on the negative work-up for other causes or malnutrition or depression because of the similarity in diagnostic criteria is a matter of professional judgment. Failure to thrive is an acceptable diagnosis of exclusion.

TREATMENT OF THE OLDER PERSON WITH FAILURE TO THRIVE

The mainstay of treatment of a patient with failure to thrive is a careful diagnostic work-up and specific treatment of the underlying problem. The organic causes listed in Table 25–1 can all be specifically diagnosed, and most have specific treatments. Depression is treatable with medications, counseling, or, occasionally, electroconvulsive therapy. Functional abnormalities can be addressed by referral to subspecialists or specific therapists. Social problems causing failure to thrive can be addressed specifically as well. In many cases, nonorganic causes of failure to thrive can be handled by admitting a patient to a nursing home or other long-term care situation.

Often, whether failure to thrive has a specific diagnosis or not, a common problem is inadequate food intake. Ideally, this problem is addressed directly by increasing the caloric and protein intake and prescribing a multivitamin with minerals. Among the best things to offer are high calorie food items such as desserts. One of the most calorically dense foods available is high-quality ice cream. This is generally eaten without any difficulty by most patients with failure to thrive. Other desserts, puddings, pies, and so on are also nutritionally dense. Standard nutritional supplements are also effective, although these supplements are often quite expensive and not as palatable as nutritionally dense ordinary foods. A patient with a treatable cause of failure to thrive may need enteral tube feeding. In general, such aggressive treatment should be restricted to people whose underlying problems are clearly reversible. One thing to avoid in treating a person with failure to thrive is unnecessary use of diets with limited salt, sugar, or cholesterol content. Such special diets are often aimed at preventing chronic diseases or the problems resulting from chronic diseases, which are of lower priority than reversing weight loss and functional decline. As mentioned earlier, weight loss that is not treatable commonly leads to death in over 75% of patients within the first year after it is recognized.

ETHICAL CONSIDERATIONS

Failure to thrive in older patients is often recognized only immediately prior to death. No guidelines are available at this time that indicate when treatment of failure to thrive is futile. Nonetheless, advance directives must be carefully considered in diagnosing and treating failure to thrive in the elderly. Many individuals, particularly the very old, do not fear death as much as they fear disability, discomfort, and loss of dignity. Diagnostic and treatment modalities must be carefully considered with the wishes of the patient in mind. Patient autonomy, the right to make decisions about what is done to one's own body, is one of the more salient ethical principles in this regard.

RECORDS AND ECONOMICS

Failure to thrive has its own International Classification of Diseases (ICD-9) code and can be used as a diagnosis of exclusion. Failure to thrive can also be used as a co-diagnosis when a principal diagnosis is known. Indeed, failure to thrive is one of the few geriatric syndromes that has an acceptable diagnostic code.

In the present health care climate, cost-effective diagnosis and cost-effective treatment are important considerations. A physician evaluating a patient with failure to thrive must develop a differential diagnosis list based on the history and physical examination. Screening tests not based on a defendable differential diagnosis list must be limited to those with very low cost and a high positive predictive value. The tests listed previously are the most useful ones, in the opinion of the author. Similarly, cost-effective treatment must be emphasized. To a great extent, this requirement decreases the usefulness of treating, for example, growth hormone deficiency. Although relative growth hormone deficiency is very prevalent in older people, there are no data suggesting that beginning such an expensive treatment in older people with failure to thrive produces reliable benefit. Among the most cost-effective treatments is simple dietary supplementation, particularly increasing the quantity of nutritionally dense normal foods. Of course, specific treatment of known diseases such as infective endocarditis is almost always highly cost effective.

SUMMARY

Failure to thrive is a syndrome and a diagnosis of exclusion that occurs primarily in individuals of advanced age. It is defined by loss of function and weight loss, and, if it is not treatable, it can lead to death in a fairly short period of time. The prevalence of failure to thrive is 10% to 20% in people older than 65, and it is usually due to either organic disease or nonorganic problems: psychological, functional, or social. Failure to thrive due to diagnosable problems is treatable, although the mainstay of much treatment is nutritional supplementation. Idiopathic failure to thrive is commonly recognized and continues to vex specialists in geriatric medicine. As with other chronic diseases affecting survival near the end of life, careful attention must be paid to the risks, costs, and benefits of diagnostic tests and interventional modalities, taking into account the patient's advance directives.

There are many unanswered questions relating to failure to thrive from both an epidemiologic point of view and a biologic point of view. The need for further research in this area is clearly evident.

References

1. Braun JV, Wykle MH, Cowling WR: Failure to thrive in older persons: A concept derived. Gerontologist 1988;28:809–812.
2. Berkman BL, Foster WS, Campion E: Failure to thrive: Paradigm for the frail elder. Gerontologist 1989; 29:654–659.
3. Fried LP: Conference on the physiologic basis of frailty, April 28, 1992, Baltimore, Maryland, USA. Introduction. Aging (Milano) 1992;4:251–252.
4. Holloszy JO: Workshop on sarcopenia: Muscle atrophy in old age. J Gerontol 1995;50A (special issue):1–160.
5. Isaacs B, Gunn T, McKecham A, et al: The concept of pre-death. Lancet 1971;1:1115–1118.
6. Palmore E, Cleveland W: Aging, terminal decline, and terminal drop. J Gerontol 1976;31:76–81.
7. White N, Cunningham WR: Is terminal drop pervasive or specific? J Gerontol 1988;43:P141–P144.
8. Wallace JI, Schwartz RS, LaCroix AZ, Uhlmann RF, Pearlman RA: Involuntary weight loss in older outpatients: Incidence and clinical significance. J Am Geriatr Soc 1995;43:329–337.
9. Fox KM, Hawkes WG, Magaziner J, Zimmerman SI, Hebel JR: Markers of failure to thrive among older hip fracture patients. J Am Geriatr Soc 1996;44:371–376.
10. Verdery RB, Levy K, Roberts N, Howell W: Natural history of failure to thrive, weight loss, and functional disability in elderly people after hospitalization. Age Nutr 1996;7:70–74.
11. Verdery RB: Failure to thrive in old age. J Gerontol 1997;52A (in press).
12. Levine B, Kalman J, Mayer L, Fillit HM, Packer M: Elevated circulating levels of tumor necrosis factor in severe chronic heart failure. N Engl J Med 1990;323:236–241.
13. Williamson J, Chopin JM: Adverse reactions to prescribed drugs in the elderly: A multicentre investigation. Age Ageing 1980;9:73–80.
14. Harrington C, Tompkins C, Curtis M, Grant L: Psychotropic drug use in long-term care facilities: A review of the literature. Gerontologist 1992;32:822–833.
15. Katz IR, Beaston-Wimmer P, Parmelee P, Friedman E, Lawton MP: Failure to thrive in the elderly: Exploration of the concept and delineation of psychiatric components. J Geriatr Psych Neurol 1993;6:161–169.
16. Morley JE, Kraenzle D: Causes of weight loss in a community nursing home. J Am Geriatr Soc 1994;42:583–585.
17. Butler RN: Are your patients getting away with "chronic suicide"? (editorial). Geriatrics 1989;44:15.
18. American Psychiatric Association: Diagnostic and Statistical Manual of Mental Disorders, 4th ed. Washington DC, American Psychiatric Association, 1994.
19. Yesavage JA, Brink TL, Rose TL, Lum O, Huang V, Adey M, Leirer VO: Development and validation of a geriatric depression screening scale: A preliminary report. J Psychiatr Res 1982;17:37–49.
20. Folstein MF, Folstein SE, McHugh PR: "Mini-mental state." J Psychiatr Res 1975;12:189–198.
21. Fillenbaum GG: Screening the elderly. A brief instrumental measure of daily living measure. J Am Geriatr Soc 1985;33:698–706.
22. Applegate WB, Blass JP, Williams TF: Instruments for the functional assessment of older people. N Engl J Med 1990;322:1207–1214.
23. Katz S: Assessing self-maintenance: Activities of daily living, mobility, and instrumental activities of daily living. J Am Geriatr Soc 1983;31:721–727.
24. Vitaliano PP, Young HM, Russo J: Burden: A review of measures used among caregivers of individuals with dementia. Gerontologist 1991;31:67–75.

SECTION

V

Neuropsychiatric Disorders in Geriatric Practice

26 Dementia

William E. Reichman, M.D.

Jeffrey L. Cummings, M.D.

Dementia is a syndrome of acquired persistent dysfunction in several domains of intellectual function including memory, language, visuospatial ability, and cognition (abstraction, mathematics, judgment, and problem solving). Disturbances of mood and alterations in personality and behavior often accompany the intellectual deterioration. Dementia results from a wide variety of conditions including degenerative, vascular, neoplastic, demyelinating, infectious, inflammatory, toxic, metabolic, and psychiatric disorders (Table 26–1). The onset of dementia may be abrupt (trauma or stroke) but is more often gradual. While the majority of dementing illnesses are progressive, in some cases the course of dementia may be modified by appropriate therapeutic interventions. Despite accurate identification of the cause of dementia and provision of symptomatic treatment, affected patients typically suffer marked and progressive impairment in occupational and social functioning. The economic, social, and psychological cost of dementing illnesses on patients and their families is staggering.

Dementia is a growing public health concern. Although specific figures vary, there is a consensus that the incidence and prevalence of dementia increase with advancing age. In many studies it is reported that dementia affects nearly 5% of the population over age 65. Dementia is most frequent in the fastest growing segment of the population, those over age 75.[1] Studies suggest that 3% of the population between the ages of 65 and 74 may have Alzheimer's disease (AD), the most common cause of dementia. This number increases to nearly 19% of the group aged 75 to 84 years, and among persons aged 85 years and above, the figure may approach 50%.[2] It is estimated that nearly 4 million Americans presently suffer from the disorder. The expense of long-term care for afflicted patients over the age of 65 has been estimated at $40 billion annually.[1]

The anticipated expansion of the number of demented patients in the population and its associated cost raise serious questions for those involved in health care planning. Issues to be resolved include choosing the most cost-effective diagnostic tests for routine evaluation of intellectual deterioration, selecting the most effective therapeutic and management strategies, and planning the most humane and fiscally responsible type of long-term care.

This chapter reviews the clinical features of

TABLE 26–1 **CAUSES OF DEMENTIA**

Degenerative disorders
  Cortical
    Alzheimer's disease
    Frontotemporal dementia, Pick's disease
  Subcortical
    Parkinson's disease
    Wilson's disease
    Progressive supranuclear palsy
    Huntington's disease
    Idiopathic basal ganglia calcification (Fahr's disease)
    Multisystem atrophies
    Thalamic dementia
  Lewy body dementia
Vascular dementias
  Multiple large vessel occlusions
  Lacunar state (multiple subcortical infarctions)
  Binswanger's disease (hemispheric white matter ischemia)
  Mixed cortical and subcortical infarctions
Metabolic disorders
  Cardiopulmonary failure
  Hepatic encephalopathy
  Uremic encephalopathy
  Anemia and hematologic conditions
  Endocrine disturbances
  Vitamin deficiency states
  Porphyria
Toxic conditions
  Medication toxicity
  Alcoholic dementia
  Polysubstance abuse
  Heavy metal intoxication
Myelin disorders
Normal pressure hydrocephalus
Neoplastic and paraneoplastic dementias
Traumatic dementias
Infection-related dementias
Inflammatory disorders
Psychiatric disorders

the major syndromes of dementia and discusses the essential components of an evaluation for dementia. Finally, guidelines for management of the more common behavioral problems and mood alterations encountered in patients with dementia are discussed. Special ethical considerations in the medical and surgical care of demented patients are also reviewed.

RELATIVE FREQUENCY OF CAUSES OF DEMENTIA

A classic study of the underlying neuropathology in dementia was reported in 1970 by Blessed and colleagues.[3] The brains of 50 patients who had died in an institution with chronic fatal dementia were examined. Alzheimer's disease was found in 50%, cerebrovascular disease in 17%, and mixed AD and cerebrovascular disease in 25%. Together, neuropathologic changes consistent with AD and cerebrovascular disease were found in more than 90% of all patients with dementia in this population.

Clinical studies analyzing the frequency of different illnesses in living patients with dementia have used a variety of assessment methodologies, patient selection criteria, and diagnostic approaches. In such studies, AD accounts for 39% to 70% of cases, followed, in decreasing order of frequency, by vascular causes of cognitive impairment (13% to 37%) and depression (1% to 18%). A variety of other conditions have been noted in 26% to 48% of cases. Dementing illnesses that are potentially reversible (including vitamin B_{12} and folate deficiency, hypothyroidism, depression) have been found in 3% to 29%. Dementias whose course could be modified by appropriate therapeutic interventions, such as vascular disease or Parkinson's disease, account for 20% to 46% of cases.[4–6]

As a group, these studies suggest that a host of disease states can cause or contribute to the development of dementia. In some of these disorders, timely identification and subsequent treatment may alter the course of intellectual decline. Larson and co-workers[7] demonstrated that in a group of 200 patients over the age of 60 with suspected dementia, more than 30% had more than one medical condition that contributed to the dementia state. After treatment, 28% experienced cognitive improvement of at least one month's duration.

CAUSES OF DEMENTIA
Degenerative Dementias
DEMENTIA OF THE ALZHEIMER TYPE

Alzheimer's disease is the most common cause of dementia in the elderly. The onset of the disease is insidious, generally occurring after the age of 55 and increasing in frequency of occurrence with advancing age. The course is marked by a gradual deterioration of intellectual function, a decline in the ability to accomplish routine activities of daily living, and enduring changes in personality and behavior. Useful guidelines for the clinical diagnosis of Alzheimer's disease have been established by McKhann and co-workers.[8] These criteria require that the patient be between the ages of 40 and 90 years at the time of disease onset, demonstrate progressive loss of memory, and have impairment of at least one additional neuropsychological function. These required deficits must be documented by a standardized mental status examination and neuropsychological assessment. Finally, no additional systemic or brain disorder may be present that could be the cause of the dementia.

The neurobehavioral features of classic dementia of the Alzheimer type include memory impairment, disturbances in language (aphasia), visuospatial deficits, and impaired ability in calculation and abstraction. Disturbances of other cortical functions such as agnosia (impaired recognition) and apraxia (inability to carry out a motor task in the absence of sensory loss, hemiparesis, or difficulty in comprehension) may be observed. The memory impairment characteristic of AD includes deficits in new learning and an inability to recall previously learned material accurately. The language disturbance typical of AD is best characterized as a transcortical sensory aphasia; there is a fluent verbal output accompanied by anomia, impaired comprehension, preserved repetition, and aphasic writing. Although patients may be able to read aloud, their comprehension for written material is impaired.[9] Visuospatial impairment is evidenced by environmental disorientation and an inability to draw figures or copy designs.

Alterations in personality are an early and ubiquitous finding in AD. Patients become increasingly passive, are more coarse in their display of emotions, and are less spontaneous. Some of these symptoms may mimic depression, but more often they occur in the absence of a clearly depressed mood or thoughts of worthlessness, hopelessness, or guilt. Depressed mood may be evident at some time during the course of the illness in 40% to 50% of patients. However, the percentage of patients with AD who meet strict diagnostic criteria for major depression is considerably less (10% to 20%).[10] In up to half of patients with AD, psychosis with delusions of infidelity, theft, harm, or abandonment is encountered.[11] Hallucinations may also occur in patients with AD but are less common than delusions. Hallucinations may be visual and auditory in nature. Other behavioral abnormalities include motor restlessness, agitation, anxiety (inability to separate from the caregiver), catastrophic reactions, aggression, wandering, and insomnia.[12]

Although patients with AD have striking neuropsychological and behavioral disturbances, their primary motor, somatosensory, and visual functions remain intact throughout most of the disease course. In classic AD, extrapyramidal dysfunction (parkinsonism, tremor, and chorea) is absent, and neurologic abnormalities such as rigidity, myoclonus, ataxia, seizures, and dysarthria do not appear until the late stages.

In the middle stage of AD, electroencephalography (EEG) may show theta-range slowing. Neuroimaging studies such as computed tomography (CT) and magnetic resonance imaging (MRI) are normal or show mild cerebral atrophy. In the later stages of the disease, EEG may show delta-range slowing, and neuroimaging procedures disclose cortical atrophy, sulcal enlargement, and ventricular dilatation. Although they are invariably present, these findings are not specific to AD.

The clinical features of AD reflect the relatively selective involvement of the parietal, medial temporal, frontal convex, and basal forebrain regions found at autopsy. The neuropathologic alterations characteristic of AD include neuronal loss, gliosis, an abundance of neuritic plaques, neurofibrillary tangles, amyloid angiopathy, and granulovacuolar degeneration.[13] Neurochemical abnormalities in AD include cholinergic depletion and more variable disturbances of the noradrenergic and serotonergic systems.

Risk factors for AD have been reported to include age, female gender, head trauma, family history of AD, Down's syndrome, low educational level, and the presence of the apolipoprotein-epsilon 4 (APO-E4) allele on chromosome 19. The extent to which AD is an inherited disease has not yet been fully elucidated. However, several important recent advances have identified three separate chromosomal loci associated with familial AD—the presenillin genes 1 (chromosome 14) and 2 (chromosome 1) and the amyloid precursor protein (APP) gene (chromosome 21). These genes appear to be most frequently associated with early-onset (before age 60) familial AD. In the presence of mutations in these genes, AD appears to be inherited in an autosomal dominant fashion. The APO-E4 allele has been reported to be a significant genetic risk factor for AD. This allele is more common in those with either sporadic or late-onset familial AD. The number of APO-E4 alleles correlates with an earlier age of onset as well as an increased risk of development of the disease.

FRONTOTEMPORAL DEMENTIA

Pick's disease and other frontotemporal dementias (FTD) are a heterogeneous group of disorders that share several clinical features with AD such as rate of progression and duration. Many FTD patients are also aphasic and manifest preserved motor integrity. The language disturbance characteristic of Pick's disease initially includes anomia, but there is a more stereotyped and perseverative verbal output than that found in AD. Unlike AD, in the early stages of FTD, memory, calculation, and visuospatial function are relatively well preserved. The most striking feature of this disorder is an extravagant change in the patient's personality including disinhibition, impulsivity, inappropriate jocularity, and intrusiveness. In some patients, the behavioral changes consist of prominent passivity or atypical depressive symptoms; there may be elements of the Kluver-Bucy syndrome (hyperorality, dietary changes, compulsive exploratory behaviors, hypersexuality, agnosia, and placidity).[14] Motor neuron disease has also been associated with FTD and has a more rapidly progressive course than Pick's disease. In FTD, EEG may show diffuse or frontal-temporal slowing. CT or MRI frequently reveals focal frontal-temporal atrophy. These features are compatible with the frontal or temporal lobar atrophy found on postmortem examination of the affected brain. Neuronal degeneration is the characteristic neuropathologic change of FTD. Argyrophilic neuronal inclusions (Pick bodies) with or without balloon cells are also seen in Pick's disease.[15]

Diagnostically, single-photon emission computed tomography (SPECT) may help to distinguish FTD from AD. SPECT demonstrates selective reductions in cerebral perfusion of the anterior hemispheric regions in FTD. In AD, cerebral blood flow is preferentially diminished in the posterior cerebral regions.[16]

SUBCORTICAL DEGENERATIVE DISORDERS

The clinical features of AD and FTD (aphasia, amnesia, apraxia, agnosia) reflect the predominantly cortical involvement in these disorders. Another group of degenerative disorders that cause dementia involves predominantly the subcortical structures (basal ganglia, thalamus, cerebellum, and rostral brain stem). The major disorders in this category include Parkinson's disease, Wilson's disease, progressive supranuclear palsy,

Huntington's disease, Fahr's disease (idiopathic basal ganglia calcification), multisystem atrophies, and thalamic dementia. Approximately 40% of patients with Parkinson's disease have overt dementia and up to 70% have more subtle neuropsychological deficits. The neuropsychological features of subcortical disorders include disturbances in attention and concentration, poor motivation, impaired information-processing speed, and memory disturbances. Patients appear depressed and apathetic, and their psychomotor responses are slow. On memory testing, they have retrieval failures but improve with cues. This memory deficit is often accompanied by disturbances of executive functions including problem solving and strategy formulation.[17] Unlike patients with AD and FTD, patients with subcortical dementia syndromes have prominent movement disorders. Depending on the specific disease state, patients may present with a hypokinetic, rigid parkinsonian state or a hyperkinetic, choreic, dystonic, or ataxic disturbance (Table 26–2).

LEWY BODY DEMENTIA

Lewy body dementia (LBD) is characterized by a pathologic accumulation of Lewy bodies in the brain stem and cortex. The clinical syndrome consists of marked fluctuations in cognition, vi-

---

TABLE 26–2 MAJOR CLINICAL FEATURES OF THE PRINCIPAL DEMENTIA SYNDROMES

Alzheimer's Disease

Gradual onset and progression, aphasia, amnesia, apraxia, agnosia, visuospatial impairment, concreteness, indifference, preserved motor function

Frontotemporal Dementia

Gradual onset and progression, aphasia, apraxia, agnosia, relative retention of memory and visuospatial skills until later stages, personality changes such as Kluver-Bucy syndrome, disinhibition, apathy, atypical depression, preserved motor function

Subcortical Syndromes

Gradual onset and progression, psychomotor retardation, depression, forgetfulness, impaired strategy formulation, extrapyramidal signs and symptoms

Lewy Body Dementia

Gradual onset and progression, aphasia, amnesia, apraxia, agnosia, fluctuating severity, prominent visual or auditory hallucinations, delusions, clouding of consciousness, extrapyramidal signs and symptoms

Vascular Diseases

Abrupt onset, stepwise progression, cortical and subcortical features, fluctuating course, preservation of personality, emotional incontinence, depression, focal neurologic signs and symptoms

Toxic-Metabolic Conditions

Cortical and subcortical features, inattention, fluctuating arousal, peripheral neuropathy, myoclonus, asterixis, tremor

Myelin Disorders

Cortical and subcortical features, focal neurologic signs, mood disorders

Normal Pressure Hydrocephalus

Cortical and subcortical features, psychomotor retardation, apathy, inattention, poor memory, ataxia, gait disturbance, urinary incontinence

Neoplastic Conditions

Cortical and subcortical features, signs of increased intracranial pressure, cranial nerve palsies

Traumatic Conditions

Cortical and subcortical features, memory loss, personality changes, focal neurologic signs

CNS Infections

Cortical and subcortical features, focal neurologic signs, myoclonus, seizures, headache, fever or signs of infection

Inflammatory Conditions

Cortical and subcortical features, systemic evidence of inflammatory process, increased erythrocyte sedimentation rate and other serologic abnormalities

Psychiatric Disorders

Subcortical features, depressed mood, psychomotor retardation, cognitive slowing, poor motivation

sual and auditory hallucinations, clouding of consciousness, and mild spontaneous extrapyramidal symptoms. In some patients severe extrapyramidal signs may first emerge after exposure to standard doses of neuroleptic agents.[18, 19] Unlike delirium, with which it shares some common clinical features, LBD persists and becomes progressively worse. Pathologically, LBD is characterized by numerous neuritic plaques, rare neurofibrillary tangles, and Lewy bodies in cortical and brain stem neurons. Several authors have argued that LBD may be more common than has been historically reported and in fact may be second to AD as a cause of dementia in the elderly.

Vascular Dementias

Dementia resulting from ischemic cerebral injury, or vascular dementia, is second in frequency to AD as a cause of chronic progressive intellectual decline. The percentage of all cases of dementia due to cerebrovascular disease has been quoted as ranging from 12% to 20%.[20] The neuropsychological deficits seen in patients with vascular dementia result from ischemic damage to multiple areas within the cortex and subcortical structures. The clinical features of vascular dementia are determined by the number, site, and volume of infarctions. There is often a temporal relationship between the onset of cognitive loss and the emergence of neurologic signs or symptoms of stroke. Historical features typically include an abrupt onset of deficits, stepwise progression of deficits, and fluctuation in the severity of symptoms. Relative preservation of personality with emotional lability, depression, somatic preoccupation, and nocturnal confusion are often noted. Patients typically show evidence of associated atherosclerosis (electrocardiographic changes, history of myocardial infarction or angina, retinopathy), history of hypertension, and focal neurologic signs and symptoms. Gait ataxia, parkinsonism, and urinary incontinence are not infrequent. A history of stroke or transient ischemic events further supports the diagnosis of multi-infarct or vascular dementia. The Ischemia Scale (IS)[21] is a checklist of the clinical features of multi-infarct dementia including its onset, course, and neurologic and psychiatric findings. A score of 7 or above for a given patient is considered compatible with a vascular origin of the patient's dementia. Despite a sensitivity and specificity of 70% to 80% in separating vascular dementia from Alzheimer's disease,[22] the IS is less well equipped to diagnose reliably the co-morbid occurrence of these two disorders in the same patient. There is evidence that this scale may overdiagnose vascular dementia in patients who are subsequently found to have AD.[23]

Several different clinical presentations of vascular dementia are possible depending on the predominant site of neuroanatomic involvement. Vascular dementia may be a consequence of multiple cortical infarctions, multiple subcortical infarctions (lacunar state), ischemic injury to the deep hemispheric white matter (Binswanger's disease), or a combination of these. Major depression and psychosis frequently occur in dementia due to cerebrovascular disease.[11] In vascular dementia, CT scans may demonstrate multiple areas of lucency compatible with infarction. MRI is particularly sensitive in that it shows increased signal intensity in areas of ischemic injury. EEG may show multifocal slowing.

Dementia resulting from stroke is most often associated with fibrinoid necrosis of arterioles resulting from sustained hypertension. Other causes of vascular dementia include diabetes mellitus, cardiac embolization, and inflammatory vasculitides.

Metabolic and Toxic Dementias

Elderly patients may suffer from several systemic illnesses that predispose them to the development of chronic metabolic encephalopathies. In the majority of cases, metabolic or toxic disturbances of the central nervous system produce transient effects on cognition (delirium). However, when these effects persist for an extended period of time, dementia is diagnosed. These chronic confusional states accompany a wide variety of systemic disorders, including severe anemia, disturbances of the thyroid, parathyroid, and adrenal axes, cardiac and pulmonary insufficiency, renal and hepatic disease, and vitamin deficiencies (particularly deficiencies of vitamins B_{12} and niacin).

Toxic causes of dementia are of particular concern in the elderly because the aged consume disproportionately large amounts of over-the-counter and prescribed medications. The alterations in drug metabolism, distribution, binding, and excretion that accompany normal aging increase the risks of drug toxicity. In addition, with advanced age, the brain may be more sensitive to the effects of drugs even in the absence of excessive dosing or polypharmacy.[24] Agents that are especially likely to cause chronic confusional states include tranquilizers, sedative-hypnotics, and centrally acting antihypertensive agents. Long-term alcoholism and chronic use of other drugs also cause dementia. Likewise, chronic exposure to industrial solvents and heavy metals may cause dementia accompanied by peripheral neuropathy.

Salient clinical features of the metabolic and toxic dementias include fluctuating arousal, inattention, and impaired memory and orientation. Severe disturbances of language and of higher cortical functions such as agnosia or apraxia are notably uncommon. Motor system disturbances such as myoclonus, tremor, and asterixis are frequently present, and EEG demonstrates diffuse slow-wave activity. With resolution of the responsible metabolic derangement or cessation of exposure to the offending toxin, improvement of neuropsychological deficits usually occurs.

Myelin Diseases with Dementia

In the elderly, diseases affecting the white matter are decidedly less common than those affecting the cortical and subcortical gray matter. However, there are several myelinoclastic disorders that may cause dementia in the elderly. Secondary white matter diseases include Binswanger's disease and viral illnesses such as acquired immune deficiency syndrome (AIDS) dementia complex, and progressive multifocal leukoencephalopathy. Multiple sclerosis is the most common demyelinating disorder, although it rarely begins after the fourth decade of life. The course is relapsing and remitting and involves an accumulation of enduring neurologic deficits. Classic symptoms include optic neuritis, myelopathy with spasticity and incontinence, cerebellar dysfunction, and internuclear ophthalmoplegia. Intellectual decline accompanies these features in nearly 50% of afflicted patients.[25] Psychiatric symptoms often noted are depression and mania. Rarer white matter dementing diseases include metachromatic leukodystrophy, adrenoleukodystrophy, cerebrotendinous xanthomatosis, membranous lipodystrophy, adult Schilder's disease, Marchiafava-Bignami's disease, and hereditary adult-onset leukodystrophy.[26]

Normal Pressure Hydrocephalus

Hydrocephalic dementia is characterized clinically by the triad of dementia, ataxia, and urinary incontinence. The dementia is typified by psychomotor slowing, bradyphrenia, inattention, impaired memory, apathy, and concreteness. Symptoms usually evolve over a period of several months to years. In normal pressure hydrocephalus (NPH), cerebrospinal fluid (CSF) obstruction occurs at the level of the arachnoid granulations responsible for absorption into the venous circulation. This state, associated with normal intracranial pressure, results from trauma, subarach-noid hemorrhage, encephalitis, or meningitis. In some cases it may be idiopathic. CT or MRI confirms the presence of increased ventricular size in hydrocephalus. The pattern of CSF flow is studied by radionuclide cisternography and CSF pressure monitoring.[9] Despite its frequent consideration in the differential diagnosis, NPH is a rare cause of dementia. The triad of dementia, incontinence, and ataxia is more often a sign of vascular dementia than of NPH.

Hydrocephalus with increased intracranial pressure is seen in patients with brain tumors (see next section, Neoplastic Dementias) or inflammatory conditions such as ependymitis or arachnoiditis. Symptoms of increased intracranial pressure include headache, papilledema, nausea, emesis, and lethargy. Somnolence or coma may eventually result.

Neoplastic Dementias

Neoplasms that either arise from the brain or metastasize from extracranial tumors may cause dementia through direct compression, hydrocephalus, infiltration of brain tissue, or increased intracranial pressure. Generally, clinical symptoms arising from intracranial tumors are insidious in onset and gradually progressive. Over a period of several weeks to months, patients may experience lethargy, headache, depression, impaired concentration, and memory disturbance. Focal neurologic symptoms may emerge; gait ataxia and incontinence are sometimes noted. While some tumors such as a subfrontal meningioma can cause dementia without other neurologic features, this is the exception rather than the rule.

Meningeal carcinomatosis, another cause of neoplastic dementia, results from neoplastic invasion of the meninges. It is associated with neoplasms of the breast, lung, gastrointestinal tract, and malignant melanoma. Patients experience increased intracranial pressure, cranial nerve palsies, and a chronic confusional state characterized by disturbed attention and concentration.

Occult systemic neoplasms such as oat cell carcinoma of the lung and carcinomas of the ovary or breast have been associated with dementia as a remote effect. Depression and anxiety have also been noted in the clinical presentation. Patients with this type of paraneoplastic syndrome often have clinical evidence of cerebellar dysfunction, or cerebellar atrophy is noted on neuroimaging studies. Seizures, myeloradiculopathy, and myopathy have also been described in patients with this condition.

Traumatic Dementias

Trauma to the brain often results in alterations in personality and enduring intellectual deficits such as aphasia, amnesia, apraxia, and concreteness. The inferior frontal lobes and medial temporal lobes are particularly susceptible to damage in closed head injury. Such trauma may cause hemorrhage, laceration, contusion, and shearing injuries of the neuronal axons. In the elderly, the formation of subdural hematomas is of special concern. Affected patients may develop a chronic confusional state with fluctuating attention and transient, minor focal neurologic signs. Dementia pugilistica has been noted in older or retired boxers following repeated blows to the head. The dementia is accompanied by ataxia and extrapyramidal dysfunction.

Infection-Related Dementias

Several different types of infections of the nervous system can produce dementia. Bacterial infection usually causes an acute encephalopathy (delirium) rather than a chronic confusional state or dementia. General paresis (neurosyphilis) is a chronic spirochetal infection characterized by dementia with prominent frontal lobe signs. Neuroborreliosis (central nervous system Lyme disease) is another cause of dementia that may or may not have been preceded by the classic "target-like" lesion and erythema migrans. Whipple's disease is a poorly understood bacterial infection characterized by meningeal signs, dementia, supranuclear gaze palsy, and systemic symptoms (lymphadenopathy, malaise, diarrhea, fever, arthralgia). Diagnosis depends on a jejunal biopsy demonstrating the characteristic macrophages.

Chronic meningitis resulting from fungal, protozoan, or helminthic infection can cause a chronic confusional state with increased intracranial pressure and cranial nerve abnormalities.

Acute viral infections such as herpes encephalitis can cause a persistent postencephalitic dementia if the injury to the central nervous system (CNS) is severe. Viruses can also cause dementia through a slowly progressive encephalitis. Slow viral dementias include AIDS dementia complex, subacute sclerosing panencephalitis, and progressive multifocal leukoencephalopathy. AIDS dementia complex results from direct infection of the brain by the human immunodeficiency virus (HIV). Clinically, affected patients present with apathy, depression, psychomotor slowing, forgetfulness, and dilapidated cognition.[27] Headache is a common associated feature. Neurologic symptoms such as motor signs and unusual movements may be noted. Opportunistic infections of the CNS (toxoplasmosis, cryptococcosis, and tuberculosis) occur in patients with AIDS and may also cause or exacerbate dementia.

Jakob-Creutzfeldt disease is a potentially transmissible disorder that begins in the fifth to seventh decades. It has been linked to an infectious membranous protein called a prion. The course is rapidly progressive and leads to death within several months. Patients manifest a progressive dementia, myoclonus, and pyramidal and extrapyramidal signs. During the course of the illness, EEG shows periodic spike discharges with background slowing in the majority of patients. Progressive multifocal leukoencephalopathy results from papovavirus CNS infection in immunocompromised patients. The virus produces the greatest impact on the cerebral white matter.

Inflammatory Dementias

Systemic autoimmune disorders such as systemic lupus erythematosus, sarcoidosis, and temporal arteritis may result in dementia through vascular occlusion and direct inflammatory and immunologic effects on the brain parenchyma. Diagnosis depends on an elevated sedimentation rate and confirmatory serologic abnormalities.

Psychiatric Disorders with Dementia

One of the more common causes of intellectual decline in the elderly has been historically called depressive "pseudodementia" but is now referred to as the dementia syndrome of depression (DOD). The syndrome includes forgetfulness, psychomotor retardation, poor motivation, and cognitive slowing. Patients have evidence of depressed mood and may have a personal or family history of depression. Following treatment of the depression, neuropsychological improvement is noted. Dementia has been identified occasionally in patients with other psychiatric disturbances such as acute mania and schizophrenia.[28]

EVALUATION OF DEMENTIA

Comprehensive evaluation of acquired intellectual impairment and associated behavioral and mood disturbances has several purposes: (1) to establish the cause for dementia, (2) to guide appropriate treatment, (3) to identify reversible or treatable concurrent medical illnesses, (4) to determine prognosis, (5) to facilitate education and counseling of family members, (6) to provide genetic advice when appropriate, and (7) to identify pertinent psychosocial stressors and family concerns that directly affect caregiving. To best accomplish these goals, a thorough assessment, consisting of a careful medical and psychiatric history, physical, neurologic, and mental status examinations, laboratory evaluation, and, often, neuroimaging procedures, is mandatory (Table 26–3). The mini-mental state examination[29] provides a brief method of recording and following the changes in mental state of the patient with dementia (Table 26–4).

No battery of laboratory tests is completely

TABLE 26–3 **STANDARD EVALUATION OF DEMENTIA**

History
  History of illness
  Review of systems
  Past medical history
  Medication review
  Family history
  Psychiatric history

Physical Examination
  Neurologic examination
  Mental status examination (with rating of
    dementia severity)

Laboratory Assessment
  Mandatory
    Complete blood count with differential
    Electrolytes, blood urea nitrogen, creatinine,
      blood glucose
    Serum calcium
    Liver function tests
    High-sensitivity thyroid-stimulating hormone
    Serum vitamin B_{12} level
    Syphilis serology
  Selective
    Erythrocyte sedimentation rate
    Human immunodeficiency virus antibody
    Lyme disease antibody titer
    Endocrine studies (serum cortisol,
      parathyroid hormone, etc.)
    Rheumatologic studies (rheumatoid factor,
      antinuclear antibody titer, etc.)
    Arterial blood gas determination

Neuroimaging
  Usually necessary
    Computed tomography or magnetic
      resonance imaging of the head
  Selective
    Single-photon emission computed
      tomography
    Positron-emission tomography

Ancillary Studies
  Lumbar puncture
  Electroencephalogram
  Electrocardiogram
  Neuropsychological evaluation
  Chest radiograph

---

applicable to all demented patients. Individualized investigations are dictated by the particular constellation of signs and symptoms presented. However, in all patients with dementia certain initial studies should be done. Routine tests of greatest diagnostic use include a complete blood count, serum electrolytes (including calcium, serum glucose, creatinine, blood urea nitrogen, bilirubin, and alkaline phosphatase), syphilis serology, vitamin B_{12} level, and thyroid function tests (especially thyroid-stimulating hormone). If pertinent risk factors are identified and the clinical state is compatible with AIDS dementia, antibody testing may be indicated. In the presence of the appropriate clinical history, serologic tests for Lyme disease may be warranted. Lumbar puncture may be appropriate if a demyelinating disorder is suspected, the dementia syndrome is atypical, or evidence of infection or inflammation of the CNS (headache, meningeal signs, fever, seizures) is present.

A neuroimaging study such as MRI or CT scanning of the head is a necessary component of most evaluations for dementia. MRI offers more accurate structural and pathologic assessment but is more time consuming and costly to perform. It cannot be used in patients who have a pacemaker or metallic intracranial objects such as surgical clips. Whichever study is selected, MRI or CT adds to diagnostic precision by detecting stroke, mass lesions, areas of demyelination, hydrocephalus, or atrophy. The routine applicability of newer modalities such as SPECT or position emission tomography (PET) awaits further confirmation. However, SPECT may be useful in helping to distinguish FTD from AD. EEG is helpful diagnostically when infections, Jakob-Creutzfeldt disease, inflammatory disorders, or toxic-metabolic causes of dementia are under consideration. Additionally, EEG is needed for the evaluation of seizure activity. In the evaluation of AD, routine clinical use of serum APO-E4 testing or CSF analysis of tau protein or beta amyloid is discouraged until additional data regarding the sensitivity and specificity of these tests emerge.

The role of cerebral biopsy in the evaluation of dementia is restricted. This procedure rarely leads to the diagnosis of a reversible condition and often results in substantial morbidity.[30] Cerebral biopsy is most often justified in the evaluation of Jakob-Creutzfeldt disease when special precautions may be needed to limit transmission during postmortem study.[31]

MANAGEMENT OF DEMENTIA

The neuropsychological deficits, neuropsychiatric symptoms, and medical illnesses that afflict de-

TABLE 26–4 **MINI-MENTAL STATE EXAMINATION**

Maximum Score	Score	
		Orientation
5	( )	What is the (year) (season) (date) (month) (day of week)?
5	( )	Where are we: (state) (county) (town) (hospital) (floor)?
		Registration
3	( )	Name 3 objects: 1 second to say each. Then ask patient all 3 after you have said them.
		Give 1 point for each correct answer. Then repeat them until the patient learns all 3. Count trials and record.
Trials		
		Attention and Calculation
5	( )	Serial 7's. 1 point for each correct. Stop after 5 answers. Alternatively, spell "world" backwards.
		Recall
3	( )	Ask for 3 objects repeated above. Give 1 point for each correct.
		Language
9	( )	Name a pencil, and watch. (2 points)
	( )	Repeat the following, "No ifs, ands, or buts." (1 point)
	( )	Follow a 3-stage command: "Take a paper in your right hand, fold it in half, and put it on the floor." (3 points)
	( )	Read and obey the following: "Close your eyes." (1 point)
	( )	Write a sentence. (1 point)
————	( )	Copy a design. (1 point)
Total Score		

ASSESS level of consciousness along a continuum   Alert   Drowsy   Stupor   Coma

From Folstein MF, Folstein SE, McHugh PR: Mini-mental state. J Psychiatr Res 1975; 12:189.

mented patients pose significant clinical challenges for physicians and caregivers. Effective treatment and management involve both pharmacologic and nonpharmacologic interventions.

Restoration of Intellectual Function

At the present time, no single pharmacologic agent has shown clear efficacy in reversing or halting the intellectual deterioration accompanying the two most common dementia syndromes, AD and vascular dementia. In patients with AD, however, the cholinesterase inhibitors tacrine and donepezil have produced clinical benefit in approximately 30% to 50% of treated patients. When evident, the clinical response to these drugs is approximately the amount of cognitive decline that would otherwise have been noted after 6 to 12 months of disease progression. Tacrine may produce liver function abnormalities and requires serum studies when the dose is increased; donepezil has no associated liver function abnormalities. Both agents may cause gastrointestinal distress. In vascular de-

mentia, optimal control of hypertension and hyperlipidemia and cessation of smoking help to prevent recurrent stroke; many clinicians advocate the use of one daily enteric-coated aspirin to further diminish the risk.

For the other nondegenerative dementing disorders, improvement in cognitive function following therapy is rarely complete. Replacement of vitamin B_{12}, ventricular shunting for patients with NPH, or correction of hypothyroidism often leads to symptomatic improvement but rarely to complete recovery. Importantly, these interventions can halt disease progression and are thus of considerable benefit.

Several nonpharmacologic techniques can aid caregivers and physicians in helping the demented patient remain as functional as possible throughout the course of the illness. These include (1) maintaining eye contact and speaking to the patient in a simple, distinct, and calm manner, (2) asking only one question at a time and allowing ample time for a response, (3) establishing a regular, structured daily routine while encouraging the patient's active participation, (4) calmly reorienting the patient when necessary, (5) breaking down all tasks into several simple steps, and (6) setting realistic expectations for what the patient can and cannot do.

Management of Neuropsychiatric Symptoms

In contrast to the largely unsuccessful experience in arresting or reversing the intellectual deficits of AD and vascular dementia, many of the psychiatric and behavioral disturbances commonly encountered in these patients are directly amenable to nonpharmacologic and pharmacologic intervention (see also Chapter 25).

Nonpharmacologic interventions for severe anxiety and psychosis include gentle reassurance and distraction. It is rarely helpful to attempt to convince patients that their beliefs are false or that they are hallucinating. Such confrontation by the caregiver or physician can escalate any concomitant agitation.

Occasionally, demented patients may become agitated or aggressive. If the patient is physically violent, caregivers should remove any potentially dangerous objects and ensure their own safety. If distraction or reassurance does not improve the patient's behavior, medication may be the only available option.

For the treatment of psychosis, neuroleptics are the agents of choice. Although there are few double-blind placebo-controlled trials that compare the efficacy of different classes of agents, neuroleptics such as haloperidol, thiothixene, and thioridazine are commonly used with moderate benefit. Unfortunately, in many patients the use of these drugs is complicated by increased confusion and other side effects. Older patients may be particularly susceptible to the tendency of higher potency neuroleptics (haloperidol, thiothixene, fluphenazine) to cause extrapyramidal reactions such as bradykinesia, rigidity, tremor, and restlessness. Use of lower potency agents (thioridazine, chlorpromazine) may result in orthostatic hypotension, sedation, and anticholinergic side effects (dry mouth, constipation, urinary retention, blurred vision, and tachycardia). As a result, and despite the increased risk of extrapyramidal side effects, higher potency agents such as haloperidol and thiothixene in low doses (0.5 to 2 mg po qd) have generally been the drugs of first choice to treat psychoses. Recently, atypical neuroleptic medications such as risperidone have been used to treat such symptoms. This medication causes less extrapyramidal dysfunction but may be associated with hypotension. In patients who are particularly sensitive to the extrapyramidal effects of

neuroleptic medications (e.g., those who have Lewy body dementia), clozapine may be efficacious and better tolerated. However, the risk of agranulocytosis associated with the use of this drug warrants weekly determinations of white blood cell counts.

If neuroleptic-induced extrapyramidal signs appear, lowering the dosage and treating the patient with amantadine 100 mg po bid or tid is often effective. Chronic use of neuroleptics may lead to tardive dyskinesia or one of its variants, such as tardive dystonia or tardive akathisia (restlessness).

In patients with mild anxiety or restlessness, moderately short acting benzodiazepines such as oxazepam 10 to 15 mg po qd or bid, or lorazepam 0.5 to 1 mg po qd or bid may be useful. Buspirone (15 to 45 mg po qd) also may be of benefit.

The pharmacologic management of nonpsychotic agitation or combativeness may include use of neuroleptics, benzodiazepines (for minor agitation or anxiety), or agents such as anticonvulsants, beta-adrenergic blockers, and serotonin-enhancing agents. Although no particular neuroleptic is especially superior in controlling aggression, a more sedating agent such as thioridazine in starting doses of 10 to 25 mg po bid may be preferred. The dose can be increased carefully, watching for the emergence of orthostasis and anticholinergic side effects.

If an aggressive or agitated patient fails to respond to either low- or high-potency neuroleptics or if significant side effects develop that preclude continuation of a chosen agent, alternative classes of psychotropic drugs may be employed. Carbamazepine in doses of 400 to 1200 mg po qd may have some use in treating aggressive, agitated behavior. Valproic acid in a dose range of 250 to 1000 mg po qd has also been proved effective for these symptoms. Monitoring of serum levels of these drugs and complete blood counts and liver function tests are required in these patients. Other agents that may be helpful include serotonin-enhancing drugs such as trazodone 50 to 400 mg po qd or clonazepam 0.5 to 4 mg po qd in divided doses. Buspirone 15 mg po bid or fluoxetine 20 to 40 mg po qd may also serve as alternatives. Finally, some authors have advocated the use of propranolol to control aggressive, violent behavior. The dose ranges vary considerably (60 to 1500 mg po qd in divided doses); in older patients, doses in the lowest ranges are most safely employed. Contraindications include sinus bradycardia, congestive heart failure, and asthma.[32] Cholinergic agents may decrease psychosis or agitation in some patients.

Pharmacologic management of depression and

other mood disturbances in patients with dementia is similar to that employed in the nondemented elderly patient. Initially, physical contributors to the alteration in mood state should be investigated such as co-existing medical illnesses and drug or medication toxicity. Patients' feelings about their loss of intellectual ability, associated social and financial problems, and guilt about increased caregiver burden must be thoroughly explored and addressed. While these factors are being dealt with, pharmacologic treatment can be directed to target symptoms such as dysphoric mood and disturbances of sleep, appetite, and energy. Treatment with antidepressant agents that have few anticholinergic side effects such as bupropion, sertraline, fluoxetine, paroxetine, venlafaxine, trazodone, and nefazodone may afford some relief without producing additional confusion. Pharmacotherapy should be commenced with the lowest possible dose, and upward titration should be performed judiciously.

Patients with dementia frequently have sleep disturbances. They may be restless or wander aimlessly in the night. Initial interventions should be directed toward improving sleep hygiene. Tactics include (1) avoiding caffeinated beverages and medications with stimulant effects in the afternoon or evening, (2) limiting eating or watching television in bed, encouraging only sleeping, (3) discouraging excessive intake of fluids in the evening to prevent nocturia, (4) investigating other medical causes of insomnia such as pain, cardiac or pulmonary disease, or restless legs syndrome, and (5) discouraging daytime naps. When these interventions are not sufficient to restore adequate sleep, pharmacotherapy is indicated. Although no particular hypnotic agent has demonstrated truly superior efficacy in patients with dementia, chloral hydrate 500 to 1000 mg po hs is often of benefit. Trazodone 50 to 150 mg po hs is frequently used for this purpose as well. Short-acting benzodiazepines such as oxazepam (10 to 30 mg po hs) or lorazepam (0.5 to 2 mg po hs) may be helpful if given 1 hour before bedtime. If these agents are used for prolonged periods, however, patients may experience early morning awakening. Long-acting benzodiazepines such as flurazepam and diazepam are best avoided because their metabolites often accumulate, leading to daytime drowsiness or increased confusion. A sedating neuroleptic such as thioridazine (25 to 50 mg po hs) may be beneficial in treating nocturnal agitation.

Caregiver Issues

Ongoing surveillance and treatment of caregiver stress and depression is of paramount importance in the successful management of the demented patient. Identification and participation of other potential caregivers should be encouraged. When feasible, primary caregivers should be encouraged to attend caregiver support groups while lessening their own burden of responsibility through the use of ancillary assistance such as daycare, respite services, or home health aides. Referral of caregivers to organizations such as the Alzheimer's Association is often helpful (1-800-272-3900). Early in the course of dementia, referral should be made for financial and legal counseling. Additionally, caregivers should be educated about the signs and symptoms of potentially complicating medical problems such as urinary tract infection and incontinence. Simple strategies such as beginning a regular toileting schedule, using adult diapers, and monitoring fluid intake can aid in the successful management of urinary incontinence. Over time, information should also be gathered about the family's attitudes toward nursing home admission, and appropriate advice about this issue should be given as needed.

References

1. Foley JM, Cassel CK, Eastman P, et al: Differential diagnosis of dementing diseases. Consensus Development Conference Statement, National Institutes of Health, Bethesda, MD, July 1987.
2. Evans DA, Finkenstein HH, Albert MS, et al: Prevalence of Alzheimer's disease in a community population of older persons: Higher than previously reported. JAMA 1989;268(18):2551–2556.
3. Blessed G, Tomlinson BE, Roth M: The association between quantitative measures of dementia and of senile change in the cerebral grey matter of elderly subjects. Br J Psychiatry 1968;114:797–811.
4. Erkinjuntti T, Wikstrom J, Palo J, Autio L: Dementia among medical inpatients: Evaluation of 2000 consecutive admissions. Arch Intern Med 1986; 146:1923–1926.
5. Van Horn G: Dementia. Am J Med 1987;83:101–110.
6. Thal LJ, Grundman M, Klauber MR: Dementia: characteristics of a referral population and factors associated with progression. Neurology 1988; 38:1083–1090.
7. Larson EB, Reifler BV, Sumi SM: Diagnostic evaluation of 200 elderly outpatients with suspected dementia. J Gerontol 1985;40(5):536–543.
8. McKhann G, Drachman D, Folstein M, et al: Clinical diagnosis of Alzheimer's disease: Report of the NINCDS–ADRDA Work Group under the auspices of Department of Health and Human Services Task Force on Alzheimer's Disease. Neurology 1984;34:939–944.
9. Cummings JL: Dementia syndromes: Neurobehavioral and neuropsychiatric features. J Clin Psychiatry 1987; 48(5 Suppl):3–8.
10. Wragg RE, Jeste DV: Overview of depression and psychosis in Alzheimer's disease. Am J Psychiatry 1989; 146:577–587.
11. Cummings JL, Miller B, Hill MA, Neshkes B: Neuropsychiatric aspects of multi-infarct dementia and

dementia of the Alzheimer type. Arch Neurol 1987; 44:389–393.

12. Reisberg B, Borenstein J, Salob SP, et al: Behavioral symptoms in Alzheimer's disease: Phenomenology and treatment. J Clin Psychiatry 1987;48(5 Suppl):9–15.
13. Brun A, Gustafson L: Distribution of cerebral degeneration in Alzheimer's disease. Arch Psychiatr Nervenkr 1976;223:15–33.
14. Cummings JL, Duchen LW: The Kluver-Bucy syndrome in Pick's disease. Neurology 1981;31:1415–1422.
15. Verity MA, Wechsler AF: Progressive subcortical gliosis of Neumann: a clinicopathologic study of two cases with review. Arch Gerontol Geriatr 1987;6:245–261.
16. Neary D, Snowden JS, Northen B, Goulding P: Dementia of frontal lobe type. J Neurol Neurosurg Psychiatry 1988;51:353–361.
17. Cummings JL: Subcortical dementia. Neuropsychiatry, neuropsychology, and pathophysiology. Br J Psychiatry 1986;149:682–697.
18. McKeith G, Perry H, Fairbairn AF, et al: Operational criteria for senile dementia of Lewy body type (SDLT). Psychiatr Med 1992;22:911–912.
19. Kalra S, Bergeron C, Lang AE: Lewy body disease and dementia. Arch Intern Med 1996;156:487–493.
20. Kase CS: Epidemiology of multi-infarct dementia. Alzheimer Dis Assoc Disord 1991;5(2):71–76.
21. Hachinski VC, Iliff ID, Zilhka E, et al: Cerebral blood flow in dementia. Arch Neurol 1975;32:632.
22. Chui HC, Victoroff JI, Margolin D, et al: Criteria for the diagnosis of ischemic vascular dementia proposed by the State of California Alzheimer's Disease Diagnostic and Treatment Center. Neurology 1992; 42:473–480.
23. Roman GC: The Epidemiology of Vascular Dementia in Cerebral Ischemic Dementias. New York, Springer-Verlag, 1991, pp. 9–15.
24. Mahler ME, Cummings JL, Benson DF: Treatable dementias. West J Med 1987;146:705–712.
25. Filley CM, Heaton RK, Nelson LM, et al: A comparison of dementia in Alzheimer's disease and multiple sclerosis. Arch Neurol 1989;46:157–161.
26. Reichman WE, Cummings JL: Diagnosis of the rare dementia syndromes: An algorithmic approach. J Geriatr Psychiatry Neurol 1990;3:73–84.
27. Navia BA, Jordan BD, Price RW: The AIDS dementia complex: I. Clinical features. Ann Neurol 1986; 19:517–524.
28. Cummings JL: Clinical Neuropsychiatry. New York, Grune & Stratton, 1985, p. 86.
29. Folstein MF, Folstein SE, McHugh PR: Mini-mental state. J Psychiatr Res 1975;12:189–198.
30. Kaufman HK, Catalano LW: Diagnostic brain biopsy: A series of 50 cases and a review. Neurosurgery 1979; 4:129–136.
31. Gajdusek DC, Gibbs CS, Asher DM, et al: Precautions in medical care of, and in handling materials from, patients with transmissible virus dementia (Creutzfeldt-Jakob disease). N Engl J Med 1977;297:1253–1258.
32. Zayas EM, Grossberg GT: Treating the agitated Alzheimer patient. Clin Psychiatry 1996;57(Suppl 7):46.

27 Delirium

Joseph Francis, Jr., M.D., M.P.H.

Acute confusional states are common in older patients. The phenomenon of delirium is particularly challenging for clinicians because its outward manifestations vary greatly. As a result, delirium is hard to recognize. Additionally, many complex medical conditions underlie the problem. This creates management problems that test the skill of even the most expert clinicians. There is no easy, formulaic approach to delirium. However, this chapter attempts to provide a basic framework for understanding delirium and practical guidelines for recognizing and managing it in older persons.

BASIC CONCEPTS

Defining Features

The fourth edition of the American Psychiatric Association's Diagnostic and Statistical Manual (DSM-IV) lists four key features that characterize delirium (Table 27–1).[1] First, patients with delirium have a disturbance of consciousness that involves an altered level of awareness of their environment and impaired ability to focus, sustain, or shift their attention. In older persons,

---

TABLE 27–1 **DIAGNOSTIC CRITERIA FOR DELIRIUM**

A. Disturbance of consciousness with reduced ability to focus, sustain, or shift attention.
B. A change in cognition or the development of a perceptual disturbance that is not better accounted for by a preexisting, established, or evolving dementia.
C. The disturbance develops over a short period of time (usually hours to days) and tends to fluctuate during the course of the day.
D. There is evidence from the history, physical examination, or laboratory findings that the disturbance is caused by a medical condition, substance intoxication, or medication side effect.

Adapted from American Psychiatric Association: Diagnostic and Statistical Manual of Mental Disorders (DSM-IV), 4th ed. Washington, DC, American Psychiatric Association, 1994.

---

this disturbance usually appears as drowsiness, lethargy, or stupor but may present as hypervigilance (e.g., alcohol withdrawal delirium) or as subtle deficits of attention (e.g., inability to follow complex commands or maintain a train of thought owing to distractibility).

The second feature of delirium is the presence of cognitive deficits beyond what one would expect from a preexisting or evolving dementia. Again, a wide range of manifestations is possible, from obvious memory loss, disorientation, and hallucinations at one extreme to milder disturbances of language and perception at the other. In patients with delirium, speech is often rambling and incoherent, comprehension is faulty, and writing ability is severely impaired. Frank delusions or hallucinations are uncommon; more typical are misperceptions and faults in recognition (e.g., the nurse entering the room is mistaken for a hostile intruder).

Third, delirium is acute and fluctuating. It develops over hours to days, an aspect of chronology that is critical in differentiating it from dementia. Additionally, its features are unstable and typically are most severe in the evening and at night. Sometimes this fluctuation can lead clinicians to believe that delirium is resolving when in fact the relative lucidity is only temporary.

The final feature of delirium is the presence of one or more medical causes, such as acute illness or drug toxicity. In older persons the precipitating cause of delirium usually resides outside the central nervous system, and multiple contributing factors can be identified. A challenge for clinicians faced with delirium is that, other than the cognitive change, patients often do not look "sick." This can be true even in patients with life-threatening illness, such as acute myocardial infarction or sepsis. Additionally, there is little correlation between the underlying cause of delirium and its clinical manifestations.

Secondary Features

The DSM-IV definition for delirium omits a number of manifestations that may be seen in some individuals but lack sufficient sensitivity or specificity to confer a diagnosis. Such features include sleep disturbances, agitation, and changes in mood and affect. For example, patients with delirium may have insomnia and other sleep problems, including a frank reversal of the normal diurnal sleep-wake cycle. However, other medical illnesses can produce similar findings. Mood and behavior changes, such as depression or combativeness, can occur in people with delirium but may also be a manifestation of dementia.[2]

In lay speech, the term delirium connotes a hyperactive, flagrantly psychotic state, but this, too, is an uncommon manifestation in older patients. Delirium is typically a "quiet" disturbance, which makes it more easily overlooked.[3]

Finally, reversibility is not a necessary feature of delirium. Although the disturbance in consciousness and cognition is potentially correctable when delirium is promptly recognized and its underlying cause effectively treated, a complete return to baseline mental functioning may take weeks or months and often fails to occur.[4]

Prevalence and Impact

Delirium is common. Between 10% and 15% of older patients admitted to hospitals with acute medical illness have evidence of delirium. An additional 5% to 30% develop delirium later in their hospital stay, often as an iatrogenic complication. Among very frail patients, such as those experiencing hip fracture, the prevalence may exceed 50%. These startling figures indicate that delirium is one of the most common functional consequences of acute illness in geriatric populations.[5]

Delirium has been less studied outside of acute care hospitals. It is assumed (but has not been proved) that delirium is less common in ambulatory and long-term care settings. In one study of older patients presenting to emergency rooms, investigators identified cognitive impairment in 40%, of which one quarter met the criteria for delirium; such patients were more likely to require admission to the hospital.[6]

Delirium is harder to recognize in nursing home patients because it is commonly superimposed on a preexisting dementia. Pilot studies using assessment tools from the Minimum Data Set estimated that 9% of all nursing home residents and 16% of residents in special care units for the demented met criteria for delirium.[7]

Delirium has an enormous impact on the well-being of older persons and should be viewed as a sentinel event identifying a high-risk population needing careful attention. Reported mortality

rates vary widely depending on the population studied and the diagnostic criteria employed, but pooled data from several recent cohort studies demonstrate a 1-month mortality of approximately 15% and a 6-month mortality that exceeds 20%, which is twice the rate for patients of similar age without delirium.[8] Among the survivors of an episode of delirium, functional and cognitive decline often persists for months and can lead to institutionalization.[9] Hospital stays are prolonged, and other complications (aspiration pneumonia, pressure ulcers, falls) occur more frequently in patients with delirium.

Risk Factors

As with other geriatric syndromes, delirium is multifactorial. It is helpful to classify risk factors into two categories: those that increase baseline vulnerability (e.g., advanced age, underlying dementia) and those that precipitate the disturbance (Table 27–2).[10] These risk factors can interact in complex ways. For example, patients with high baseline vulnerability may develop delirium with relatively trivial insults, and combinations of risk factors may confer more than an additive effect.

The most consistent risk factor for delirium in recent studies has been the presence of underlying brain disease, particularly dementia, cerebrovascular disease, and Parkinson's disease. Twenty-five to fifty percent of delirious patients have evidence of preexisting dementia. The presence of dementia increases the risk of delirium by nearly threefold. Other chronic brain lesions,

---

TABLE 27–2   **RISK FACTORS FOR DELIRIUM**

Factors that increase vulnerability:
  Advanced age
  Chronic brain disease
    Dementia
    Stroke
    Parkinson's disease
  Sensory impairment
Factors that may precipitate delirium:
  Polypharmacy (especially psychoactive drugs)
  Iatrogenic complications
    Infection
    Dehydration
    Immobility (including restraint use)
    Malnutrition
    Use of bladder catheters

Data from Francis J: Delirium in older patients. J Am Geriatr Soc 1992;40:829–838 and Inouye SK, Charpentier PA: Precipitating factors for delirium in hospitalized elderly persons: Predictive model and interrelationship with baseline vulnerability. JAMA 1996;275:852–857.

such as infarctions, are frequently found on brain imaging studies of delirious patients. Finally, Parkinson's disease can increase the risk of delirium following surgery or electroconvulsive therapy, although the drugs used to treat this disorder may also play a role.

Many different drugs have been implicated in individual cases of delirium, but only a few are regularly associated with delirium in prospective studies. These include narcotics, sedative-hypnotics, and anticholinergic agents. Some members of a drug class have a particular propensity for causing delirium. For example, long-acting benzodiazepines and meperidine are more strongly associated with delirium in the perioperative setting than other sedatives or narcotics. This reflects their pharmacologic properties; for example, meperidine's metabolite, normeperidine, accumulates in older persons with impaired renal function and has anticholinergic and central nervous system (CNS)-excitatory properties.[11]

PATHOPHYSIOLOGY

Basic Considerations

The pathophysiology of delirium is poorly understood. This should not surprise the clinician who is familiar with delirious patients. The severity of the illness, lack of cooperation, and complicating features (e.g., multiple drugs, underlying dementia) make even the most basic investigations challenging.

Additionally, electrophysiologic studies, positron-emission tomography (PET), and other techniques for studying brain function are hard to employ in patients with so transient and fluctuating a disturbance. Animal models of delirium, which examine maze running, locomotion, electroencephalographic (EEG) changes, and subjective changes in behavior following a stressor known to induce delirium in humans, have been proposed but are still in their infancy. Finally, we lack a good conceptual model, since our knowledge of the normal mechanisms of consciousness and arousal remains fragmentary.

Electrophysiology

Despite these limitations, some important facts are known. Romano and Engel performed seminal work in the 1940s using electroencephalography in acutely ill patients.[12] They established that delirium was a disturbance of global cortical function. EEG changes of delirium (slowing of the dominant posterior alpha rhythm and appearance of abnormal slow-wave activity) correlated with the level of consciousness and other observed behaviors. Additionally, a variety of causes induced similar EEG changes, suggesting a final common neural pathway. The major exception appeared to be that of delirium accompanying alcohol and sedative-drug withdrawal, in which low voltage, fast-wave activity predominated.

EEG measures primarily cortical activity, but recent investigations using evoked potential studies support an important role for subcortical structures (e.g., thalamus, basal ganglia, and pontine reticular formation) in the pathogenesis of delirium. Such findings correlate with clinical reports that patients with structural abnormalities of the basal ganglia have a higher susceptibility to delirium.

Neurotransmitter and Humoral Mechanisms

Drugs that are agonists or antagonists of a number of neurotransmitters can produce delirium-like effects, but the precise role of such neurotransmitter systems is difficult to determine. Additionally, measurements of cerebrospinal fluid (CSF) levels of neuropeptides (e.g., somatostatin), endorphins, serotonin, norepinephrine, and gamma-aminobutyric acid (GABA) reveal multiple alterations in patients with delirium, but it is difficult to exclude the potential confounding effects of underlying illness or dementia in such studies.

Of all the neurotransmitters studied to date, acetylcholine appears to play the most important role in delirium. Anticholinergic drugs produce delirium when given to healthy volunteers and are even more likely to produce acute confusion in frail older persons. This effect can be reversed with cholinesterase inhibitors such as physostigmine. Medical conditions that precipitate delirium such as hypoxia, hypoglycemia, and thiamine deficiency have been shown to decrease acetylcholine synthesis in the CNS. Serum anticholinergic activity, measured with binding assays employing purified preparations of brain muscarinic receptors, correlates with the severity of delirium in postoperative and medical patients. Finally, Alzheimer's disease, itself characterized by a loss of cholinergic neurons, increases the risk of delirium due to anticholinergic medication.

It is very important for clinicians to keep in mind the anticholinergic mechanism because so many agents (including many not traditionally viewed as having "anticholinergic" effects) show muscarinic binding. Some older patients with delirium show elevated serum anticholinergic activity even in the absence of anticholinergic drug use, raising the possibility that endogenous anticholinergic substances may play a role in delirium.[13]

Recent investigations have also uncovered an emerging role of inflammatory mediators. Cytokines such as interleukins have strong CNS effects when they are injected into the ventricles of experimental animals. Endogenous cytokine activity may be responsible for delirium in such situations as sepsis (in which mental changes may actually precede fever) and cardiopulmonary bypass.[14, 15] When cytokines are used therapeutically (e.g., interferons in patients with chronic hepatitis or cancer), cognitive and behavioral effects frequently occur, especially in patients who are more susceptible to delirium due to underlying organic brain disease.

CLINICAL ASSESSMENT

Failure to Recognize Delirium

Prompt recognition of delirium and identification of its underlying causes are essential for proper treatment. Unfortunately, clinicians fail to recognize delirium in up to 70% of cases. Usually this is not because behavioral problems or cognitive impairment are inapparent. Rather, clinicians wrongly attribute acute confusion to the patient's age, to his or her dementia, or to other mental disorders. In one study, for instance, over 40% of patients referred to a consulting liaison psychiatrist for evaluation or treatment of depression were ultimately found to have delirium.[16]

Assessing the Presence of Delirium

DSM-IV criteria form a practical framework for the assessment of delirium. Level of consciousness is often the first observable clue. Clinicians must not "normalize" lethargy or somnolence by assuming that illness, sleep loss, fatigue, or anxiety are causing the changes. When the patient appears to be awake, the ability to focus, sustain, or shift attention can be assessed during attempts to obtain a history. A global assessment of the patient's "accessibility" during conversation or the performance of a mental status examination has been shown to be a sensitive indicator of delirium.[17] Conversation with the patient may also elicit memory deficits, disorientation, or speech that is tangential, disorganized, or incoherent. Beware, however, of superficially appropriate conversation that follows social norms but is poor in content. When in doubt, clinicians should perform formal mental status testing, such as the mini-mental state examination or brief bedside tests of attention (e.g., forward digit span; vigilance A test). It is important to empha-

size that no single test can substitute for an astute observer with knowledge of the criteria for delirium.[18]

A determination that cognitive impairment or perceptual problems are not due to a prior or progressing dementia can be challenging and requires knowledge of the patient's baseline functioning. If a clinician has not previously assessed the cognitive abilities of an older patient who is presenting with confusion, capable informants must be immediately sought to establish a chronology. Formal and informal caregivers also are important sources for establishing fluctuations. Not infrequently, the patient who was combative or confused the night before is found to be completely lucid during morning rounds. Clinicians should not rely on a single assessment of mental state but must actively solicit evidence of behavioral change from all available caregivers, especially those caring for the patient during evenings and nights.

Clinicians must also remember the factors that are *not* required in the definition of delirium. Agitated behaviors are infrequent among older persons with delirium despite the popular connotations of the term. "Quiet" delirium, including withdrawal, subtle misperceptions, or passive compliance, is more likely than dramatic outbursts, which makes the disturbance all too easy to mistake for depression or dementia.

Differential Diagnosis

Many authors place great emphasis on differentiating delirium from dementia and other psychiatric disorders. In practice, careful attention to the key features of acute onset, fluctuating course, altered consciousness, and cognitive decline readily distinguish delirium from depression, psychotic illness, and dementia. When in doubt, the most useful rule-of-thumb is to *assume delirium* and attempt to rule out common medical causes. This is true even for patients with known psychiatric illnesses, since they, too, are susceptible to delirium when acutely ill.

A common and particularly challenging clinical situation is the patient with known dementia who experiences a sudden change in behavior. Not all behavioral changes in demented patients are due to delirium. Patients with dementia resulting from diffuse Lewy body disease may, for instance, manifest fluctuating confusion, hallucinations, and delusions with no identifiable medical cause. Other psychiatric illnesses (e.g., depression) as well as catastrophic reactions to stressful situations (loss of spouse, accident, unfamiliar environment) can cause patients with Alzheimer's-type dementia to deteriorate. Differentiating these possibilities is difficult when the patient is unable to give a coherent history or cooperate with the examination. However, it is well known that dementia increases the older patient's susceptibility to delirium, so a wise course is again to assume the latter and evaluate the patient for common medical or drug precipitants.

Finally, delirium should also be distinguished from "sundowning," a frequently seen but poorly understood phenomenon of behavioral deterioration seen in the evening hours, typically in demented, institutionalized patients.[19] Sundowning should be presumed to be delirium when it is a *new* pattern. However, in patients with established sundowning and no obvious medical illness, impaired sleep regulation, circadian disturbances, or nocturnal factors in the institutional environment (e.g., shift changes, noise, reduced staffing) may contribute to this phenomenon.

EVALUATION AND MANAGEMENT

Bedside Assessment

Patients with delirium are sick, so a search for the underlying causes must not be delayed. Although virtually any medical illness can precipitate delirium in the predisposed individual, certain ones are found so frequently that an initial evaluation should consider them in every delirious patient (Table 27–3).

Review of medications heads the list, since drug toxicity accounts for approximately 30% of all cases of delirium.[20] The most common offending drugs are listed in Table 27–4. Clinicians should be careful not to neglect over-the-counter

TABLE 27–4 DRUGS COMMONLY CAUSING DELIRIUM

Anticholinergic medications
  Antidepressants
  Antipsychotics
  Antihistamines
  Antispasmodics
  Antiemetics
  Antiparkinsonian agents
  Cardiovascular drugs
Sedative-hypnotics
Analgesics
  Narcotics (especially meperidine)
  Nonsteroidal anti-inflammatory agents
Histamine-2 receptor antagonists
Digoxin
Antiepileptic drugs
Corticosteroids

Data from Francis J: Drug-induced delirium. CNS Drugs 1996;5:103–114.

agents, drugs prescribed by other physicians, or drugs belonging to other household members. A simple but high-yield diagnostic procedure is to ask a family member to clean out the medicine cabinet and bring the contents in for review.

Performing a comprehensive history and physical examination is often difficult or impossible in the confused or uncooperative patient. Clinicians should instead perform a focused assessment, concentrating on vital signs, state of hydration, skin condition, potential infectious foci, and neurologic findings. Pitfalls must be kept in mind: the temperature may be under 101°F even in patients with serious infections; auscultatory and radiographic findings of pneumonia may be subtle or absent; abdominal catastrophes may present without peritoneal signs in frail older patients. False-positive findings occur as well—for example, nuchal rigidity may not signify meningitis.

The neurologic examination is often discounted because many items have poor interrater reliability (e.g., plantar and deep-tendon reflex testing) or are difficult in uncooperative patients (e.g., sensory testing). However, a basic assessment emphasizing level of consciousness, unambiguous cranial nerve and motor deficits, and, if possible, visual fields, is useful for identifying individuals with a higher likelihood of intracranial disease. For instance, posterior cortical stroke can present as delirium and has few findings other than hemianopsia.[21]

Ancillary Testing

Just as the potential causes of delirium are legion, so also are the laboratory tests that might

TABLE 27–3 MEDICAL CONDITIONS COMMONLY CAUSING DELIRIUM

Fluid-electrolyte disturbances
  Dehydration
  Hyponatremia, hypernatremia
Infections
  Urinary tract
  Respiratory tract
  Skin and soft tissue (e.g., pressure ulcers)
Drug toxicity
Metabolic disorders
  Hypoglycemia
  Hypercalcemia
  Uremia
  Liver failure
Low perfusion states
  Shock
  Heart failure
Withdrawal from alcohol and sedatives

be considered. Unfortunately, a desire for diagnostic completeness not only increases costs, it can also delay prompt treatment of more obvious disorders. Authorities have therefore stressed the importance of targeted testing. Serum electrolytes, creatinine, glucose, and calcium levels, complete blood count, and urinalysis are reasonable tests for most patients with delirium when a cause is not immediately obvious. Drug levels should be ordered when appropriate, but the results should not lull one into complacency because delirium can occur even in the presence of "therapeutic" levels of such agents as digoxin, lithium, or quinidine. Further testing should be based on the history and clinical examination; a report of slow cognitive decline over several months, for instance, increases the importance of evaluating thyroid function and vitamin B_{12} level.

Although older patients with bacterial meningitis are more likely to present with delirium than with the classic triad of fever, headache, and meningismus, this is still an uncommon disorder. In febrile older patients with delirium, routine evaluation of the CSF is usually not necessary as long as other infectious foci are obvious.[22]

Finally, neuroimaging should be performed immediately if a new focal neurologic finding is present or recent head trauma has occurred. In all other patients, selective use is advised. Computed tomographic (CT) abnormalities of the head are commonly seen in patients with delirium but usually represent chronic conditions that may predispose the patient to delirium but less often represent acute, treatable causes. If the initial clinical evaluation discloses an obvious disturbance and the patient improves with treatment, neuroimaging is probably not warranted.

Treatment

The only specific therapy with the potential to reverse delirium is successful treatment of the medical condition or conditions that have caused the disturbance. Because more than one condition is typically present, several lines of treatment are started simultaneously. However, correction of sepsis, dehydration, or drug toxicity may take days. During that period, the patient with delirium is susceptible to intercurrent illness, iatrogenic complications, and further drug exposures that can maintain the delirious state.

Additionally, the uncooperative and disruptive behaviors that characterize delirium in many older patients can threaten the success of therapies directed at specific medical causes. The patient who refuses to eat or drink because of fear of staff or who pulls out his or her intravenous line, nasogastric tube, or oxygen cannula thwarts the therapeutic process and may cause further injury. Most of the pharmacologic therapies (Table 27–5) described for delirium are means of controlling these disruptive behaviors and are themselves nonspecific. One notable exception is physostigmine, which can reverse the effects of anticholinergic intoxication. Because physostigmine has a short duration of action and side effects of its own, most cases of known anticholinergic toxicity are best treated by stopping the offending agent and providing supportive care.

Maintaining this distinction between specific and nonspecific therapy (or "cure" and "control") is important, since there is no ideal drug for managing the behavioral complications, and nearly all the agents used to treat delirium can themselves cause adverse behavioral effects. Benzodiazepines such as lorazepam, for instance, may be useful as short-acting sedatives but can worsen delirium; they are best reserved for patients with delirium due to sedative drug or alcohol withdrawal. Haloperidol has been favored for the treatment of delirium because of its absence of anticholinergic effects and its low potential for cardiac toxicity (even in critically ill patients),

---

TABLE 27–5 **PHARMACOLOGIC TREATMENT OF DELIRIUM**

Physostigmine
  Usual dose: 1 to 2 mg slow intravenous push
  Duration of action is short (15 to 60 minutes)
  Monitor for cholinergic side effects
    Bradycardia
    Bronchospasm
    Seizures
  Rapid response is diagnostic of anticholinergic
    intoxication
Haloperidol
  Usual dose: 0.5 to 1.0 mg by mouth or parenterally
  Onset of action usually delayed (10 to 30 minutes)
  Minimal sedation or hypotension
  High doses may produce QT prolongation,
    torsades de pointes
  Significant extrapyramidal side effects
    Akathisia
    Rigidity or immobility
    Neuroleptic malignant syndrome
Lorazepam
  Usual dose: 0.5 to 1.0 mg orally or intravenously
  Sedation seen in 1 to 5 minutes after parenteral
    dosing
  Useful for withdrawal states and as adjunct to
    haloperidol
  Can worsen confusion

Data from Francis J: Delirium in older patients. J Am Geriatr Soc 1992;40:829–838.

TABLE 27–6 **ENVIRONMENTAL MEASURES THAT REDUCE AGITATION IN CONFUSED PATIENTS**

Avoid restricting patient movement
   Avoid use of restraints
   Mobilize patient up from bed
Minimize stressful stimuli
   Reduce noise
   Avoid indiscreet staff talk within earshot of patient
Provide meaningful orienting stimuli (not calendars)
   Windows
   Routine activities
Promote good sleep hygiene
   Avoid sedative-hypnotics
   Avoid drugs that impair sleep (caffeine, theophylline)
   Keep patient awake and active during daytime
   Provide adequate daytime light exposure
Optimize sensory function
Communicate reassurance
Provide pleasing stimulation
Make environment seem familiar to patient
   Avoid unnecessary room changes
   Provide items from patient's home

although prolongation of the QT interval and torsades de pointes have been reported after administration of high doses.[23] Haloperidol can produce serious adverse effects such as rigidity, akathisia (which sometimes is mistaken for worsening delirium and can lead to escalating doses of the medication), and life-threatening neuroleptic malignant syndrome.

Environmental Measures

An aspect often neglected in the treatment of delirium is the provision of a safe supportive environment; some suggested modalities for achieving this goal are listed in Table 27–6. Modern hospitals are often characterized by pandemonium, and the needs of frail, confused patients for reassurance, gentle stimulation, and orienting stimuli can be lost in the quest for cost-efficiency. Environmental measures have proved helpful in managing disruptive behaviors among demented institutionalized patients and may be useful for delirious patients as well. Simple measures may be the most effective. For instance, a window with a view to the outside may reduce the risk of delirium by half,[24] and bedside sitters (preferably family members and others familiar to the patient) can obviate the application of restraints.

References

1. American Psychiatric Association: Diagnostic and Statistical Manual of Mental Disorders, 4th ed. Washington, DC, American Psychiatric Association, 1994, p. 129.
2. Liptzin B, Levkoff SE, Gottlieb GL, Johnson JC: Delirium. J Neuropsychiatry Clin Neurosci 1993;5:154–160.
3. Francis J, Martin D, Kapoor WN: A prospective study of delirium in hospitalized elderly. JAMA 1990;263:1097–1101.
4. Murray AM, Levkoff SE, Wetle TT, et al: Acute delirium. and functional decline in the hospitalized elderly patient. J Gerontol 1993;48:M181–M186.
5. Francis J: Delirium in older patients. J Am Geriatr Soc 1992;40:829–838.
6. Naughton BJ, Moran MB, Kadah H, Heman-Ackah Y, Longano J: Delirium and other cognitive impairment in older adults in an emergency department. Ann Emerg Med 1995;25:751–755.
7. Fries BE, Mehr DR, Schneider D, Foley WJ, Burke R: Mental dysfunction and resource use in nursing homes. Med Care 1993;31:898–920.
8. Cole MG, Primeau FJ: Prognosis of delirium in elderly hospital patients. Can Med Assoc J 1993;149:41–46.
9. Francis J, Kapoor WN: Prognosis after hospital discharge of older medical patients with delirium. J Am Getriatr Soc 1992;40:601–606.
10. Inouye SK, Charpentier PA: Precipitating factors for delirium in hospitalized elderly persons: Predictive model and interrelationship with baseline vulnerability. JAMA 1996;275:852–857.
11. Marcantonio ER, Juarez G, Goldman L, et al: The relationship of postoperative delirium with psychoactive medications. JAMA 1994;272:1518–1522.
12. Romano J, Engel GL: Delirium: I. Electroencephalographic data. Arch Neurol Psychiatr 1944;51:356–377.
13. Mach JR, Dysken MW, Kuskowski M, et al: Serum anticholinergic activity in hospitalized older persons with delirium: A preliminary study. J Am Geriatr Soc 1995;43:491–495.
14. Bolton CF, Young GB, Zochodne DW: The neurological complications of sepsis. Ann Neurol 1993;33:94–100.
15. Stefano GB, Bilfinger TV, Fricchione GL: The immune-neuro-link and the macrophage: Postcardiotomy delirium, HIV-associated dementia, and psychiatry. Prog Neurobiol 1994;42:475–488.
16. Farrell KR, Ganzini L: Misdiagnosing delirium as depression in medically ill elderly patients. Arch Intern Med 1995;155:2459–2464.
17. Anthony JC, LeResche LA, von Korff MR, Niaz U, Folstein MF: Screening for delirium on a general medical ward: The tachistoscope and a global accessibility rating. Gen Hosp Psychiatry 1985;7:36–42.
18. Pompei P, Foreman M, Cassel CK, Alessi C, Cox D: Detecting delirium among hospitalized older patients. Arch Intern Med 1995;155:301–307.
19. Bliwise DL: What is sundowning? J Am Geriatr Soc 1994;42:1009–1011.
20. Francis J: Drug-induced delirium. CNS Drugs 1996;5:103–114.
21. Benbadis SR, Sila CA, Cristea RL: Mental status changes and stroke. J Gen Intern Med 1994;9:485–487.
22. Warshaw G, Tanzer F: The effectiveness of lumbar puncture in the evaluation of delirium and fever in the hospitalized elderly. Arch Fam Med 1993;2:293–297.
23. Wilt JL, Minnema AM, Johnson RF, Rosenblum AM: Torsade de pointes associated with the use of intravenous haloperidol. Ann Intern Med 1993;119:391–394.
24. Wilson LM: Intensive care delirium: The effect of outside deprivation in a windowless unit. Arch Intern Med 1972;130:225–226.

28 Depression

Donald P. Hay, M.D.

Kari L. Franson, Pharm.D.

Linda Hay, Ph.D.

George T. Grossberg, M.D.

EPIDEMIOLOGY

At any time in life, depression is a devastating illness. It has been found to be more disabling than the other more commonly recognized physical illnesses of diabetes, hypertension, and arthritis. The estimated prevalence of depressive disorders in the elderly varies widely. Clinicians often attribute this variability to the difficulty of recognizing depression in the geriatric population. Because of this, in a recent article it was stated that "at least 15% to 20% of community elders have a type and degree of depression warranting clinical and public health attention."[1] According to the criteria listed in the fourth edition of the *Diagnostic and Statistical Manual of Mental Disorders,* approximately 5 million of 31 million Americans aged 65 or older suffer from depression. It is reported that 1 million of these suffer from major depressive disorder and that minor depression, dementia syndrome of depression, and depression secondary to a medical illness have higher prevalence rates in the elderly than in the adult population as a whole.

The prevalence of depression also varies according to the setting in which the geriatric patient is seen. It is estimated by a Department of Health and Human Services Consensus Panel that 15% to 20% of nursing home patients have symptoms of depression, whereas only 5% of elderly patients seen in primary care clinics report depression. This figure drops even further in healthy, community-dwelling elders, of whom only 3% report depressive symptomatology.[2] However, the highest rate of depression occurs in the elderly, medically ill, inpatient population, in which rates as high as 40% have been found.[3]

Without regard to actual prevalence, late-life depressive disorders are associated with increased morbidity and mortality and take a significant toll on the individual and society. Unfortunately, for every individual who seeks medical attention for depression, a significant number remain unidentified, undiagnosed, or untreated.

DIAGNOSIS

In considering mood disorders in older adults, the clinician must be aware of major depression, which is the most debilitating and most closely associated with suicide risk, chronic low-grade depression or dysthymia, and mood disorders secondary to an underlying medical condition or a prescribed or over-the-counter (OTC) medication.

Major Depression

According to the fourth edition of the Diagnostic and Statistical Manual of Mental Disorders of the American Psychiatric Association (DSM-IV), the diagnosis of major depression requires the presence of five vegetative signs and symptoms, one of which must be either lowered mood or loss of interest and pleasure present on a continuous basis for at least 2 weeks. Table 28–1 lists the DSM-IV criteria for major depression. Cutting back on activities may be an early warning sign of depression in the elderly. Almost always,

---

TABLE 28–1 **DIAGNOSIS OF MAJOR DEPRESSION**

1. Depressed mood or
2. Decreased interest or pleasure in activities and four of the following:
3. Change in appetite, usually weight loss
4. Insomnia or hypersomnia
5. Psychomotor retardation or agitation
6. Lack of energy
7. Worthlessness; excessive or inappropriate guilt
8. Decreased concentration
9. Recurrent thoughts of death or suicide

Adapted from American Psychiatric Association. Diagnostic and Statistical Manual of Mental Disorders, 4th ed. Washington, DC, American Psychiatric Press, 1994.

appetite is adversely affected resulting in concomitant weight loss; weight gain may occur, albeit rarely, especially in younger persons. Sleep is commonly affected, and the most severe depressions are accompanied by terminal insomnia or early-morning awakening. Lack of energy or easy fatigability is often a presenting feature in the elderly, perhaps accompanied by spending *too much* time in bed. If one encounters feelings of worthlessness or excessive or inappropriate guilt or remorse, caution is advised because these individuals may be moving into a major depression with *psychotic* features (accompanied by delusions or hallucinations). The latter have a close association with suicide.

When problems with concentration and thinking are prominent, the dementia syndrome of depression is diagnosed; this is often mistaken for conditions such as Alzheimer's disease. However, if the cognitive changes are due solely to depression, they should resolve once the depression is ameliorated. It is also important to pay attention to recurrent thoughts of death and to inquire about thoughts or plans for suicide. Obviously, anyone who is deemed an active suicide risk requires prompt intervention and close observation.

Dysthymia

Subsyndromal depression and dysthymia are terms used to describe a less acute occurrence of depression. This condition is present when fewer than five of the nine symptoms required for the diagnosis of major depressive disorder have been present for at least 2 years. Dysthymia is similarly treatable with psychopharmacologic and psychotherapeutic measures. Decisions about when and how to treat dysthymia include consideration of the functional level and degree of impairment of the patient. Antidepressants are relatively benign and in many cases prove helpful.

All psychiatric illnesses, including depression and dysthymia, are affected by and in turn affect medical co-morbidities. The geriatric population experiences more medical illnesses of a more chronic nature than younger populations. The symptoms of medical illnesses and the medications used to treat them can contribute to the initiation or worsening of depression. Depression in turn, especially that of a more chronic nature, can exacerbate medical illnesses by many pathways, including decreased physical activity, interference with sleep patterns, and lack of appetite, which sometimes leads to nutritional compromise. Consideration of the evaluation and treatment of subsyndromal depression requires attention to the current and past medical history as

well as assessment of current medications. Table 28–2 lists some of the medical conditions and medications that may be associated with symptoms of depression in the elderly.

The Depression Evaluation

Table 28–3 highlights the fundamental features of a thorough depression assessment. This assessment is done once before treatment is initiated to rule in or out any underlying medical disorders

TABLE 28–2 PHARMACOLOGIC AND MEDICAL CAUSES OF DEPRESSION

Pharmacologic Causes

Alpha-methyldopa	Digitalis
Barbiturates	Estrogens
Cancer chemotherapeutic agents	Guanethidine
	Levodopa
Chloral hydrate	Morphine
Cimetidine	Propranolol
Clonidine	Reserpine
Codeine	Steroids
Diazepam	

Medical Causes

Adrenal disease	Hypokalemia
Alzheimer's disease	Hyponatremia
Anemia	Hypothyroidism
Cancer of pancreas	Multi-infarct dementia
Cerebral tumor	Parkinson's disease
Congestive heart failure	Postmyocardial infarction
Diabetes	Renal disease
Hepatic disease	Stroke
Huntington's disease	Vitamin B_{12} deficiency
Hyperthyroidism	

Adapted from Manepalli J, Grossberg GT: Recognition and treatment of depression. *In* Szwabo PA, Grossberg GT (eds): Problem Behaviors in Long-Term Care. New York, Springer, 1993, pp. 44–58.

TABLE 28–3 THE DEPRESSION EVALUATION

History
Physical, neurologic, psychiatric examination
Medication and substance exposure review
Laboratory studies:
    Chemistry panel (e.g., electrolytes, calcium, phosphorus, glucose, renal/hepatic function tests)
    Complete blood count
    Triiodothyronine (T_3), thyroxine (T_4), thyroid-stimulating hormone
    Vitamin B_{12}, red blood cell folate
    Urinalysis
    Chest radiograph
    Electrocardiogram
    Tests for human immunodeficiency virus (HIV) or rapid plasma reagin (RPR), if indicated
    Computed tomography neuroscan or magnetic resonance imaging, if indicated

that may be contributing to the symptoms of depression. Obviously, the induction process starts with a thorough history obtained from the patient, family, and other available informants in an attempt to tease out the signs and symptoms of depression. It is well known that older adults rarely complain of or use the term depression. Many may present initially with vague, nonspecific somatic complaints. However, lurking in the background is often a clinically significant depression.

A head-to-toe physical and neurologic examination is vital to identify underlying medical problems. A psychiatric evaluation together with the use of a screening tool such as the geriatric depression scale (GDS)[4] will help to solidify the diagnosis (Table 28–4). A laboratory evaluation is important to detect metabolic, infectious, endocrine, hematologic, nutritional, and other abnor-malities that may present with depressive symptoms or exacerbate depression in older adults. Of equal importance is a thorough review of any and all prescribed or over-the-counter medications the patient may have access to including alcohol, which may trigger symptoms of depression.

PHARMACOTHERAPY OF GERIATRIC DEPRESSION

Treating depression in the elderly population is difficult given the high variability in clinical presentation and treatment response. Seventy percent of patients with an acute major depressive episode respond to the first antidepressant used. This response rate increases to 80% to 85% with the trial of a second agent. However, the definitive response to antidepressants is

---

TABLE 28–4 **GERIATRIC DEPRESSION SCALE**

1. Are you basically satisfied with your life?	Yes/No° ____
2. Have you dropped many of your activities and interests?	Yes°/No ____
3. Do you feel that your life is empty?	Yes°/No ____
4. Do you often get bored?	Yes°/No ____
5. Are you hopeful about the future?	Yes/No° ____
6. Are you bothered by thoughts that you can't get out of your head?	Yes°/No ____
7. Are you in good spirits most of the time?	Yes/No° ____
8. Are you afraid that something bad is going to happen to you?	Yes°/No ____
9. Do you feel happy most of the time?	Yes/No° ____
10. Do you often feel helpless?	Yes°/No ____
11. Do you often get restless and fidgety?	Yes°/No ____
12. Do you prefer to stay at home rather than going out and doing new things?	Yes°/No ____
13. Do you frequently worry about the future?	Yes°/No ____
14. Do you feel that you have more problems with memory than most?	Yes°/No ____
15. Do you think it is wonderful to be alive now?	Yes/No° ____
16. Do you often feel downhearted and blue?	Yes°/No ____
17. Do you feel pretty worthless the way you are now?	Yes°/No ____
18. Do you worry a lot about the past?	Yes°/No ____
19. Do you find life very exciting?	Yes/No° ____
20. Is it hard for you to get started on new projects?	Yes°/No ____
21. Do you feel full of energy?	Yes/No° ____
22. Do you feel that your situation is hopeless?	Yes°/No ____
23. Do you think that most people are better off than you are?	Yes°/No ____
24. Do you frequently get upset over little things?	Yes°/No ____
25. Do you frequently feel like crying?	Yes°/No ____
26. Do you have trouble concentrating?	Yes°/No ____
27. Do you enjoy getting up in the morning?	Yes/No° ____
28. Do you prefer to avoid social gatherings?	Yes°/No ____
29. Is it easy for you to make decisions?	Yes/No° ____
30. Is your mind as clear as it used to be?	Yes/No° ____
	TOTAL ____

Scoring:
 Score 1 for °, 0 for not
 0–10 = normal
 11 or more = probable depression

Adapted from Yesavage JA, Brink TL: Development and validation of a geriatric depression screening scale: A preliminary report. J Psychiatr Res 1983;17(1):37–49.

marred by a high placebo response rate, reported to be as high as 40%, and a delay in response of 4 to 8 weeks. When depression is complicated by psychosis, the response rate to an antidepressant alone is less than a 50%. In clinical practice, however, the response rate in elderly patients is reported to be much lower because of subtherapeutic dosing and shorter duration of treatment. Because depression is recognized as a recurrent disease, with a relapse rate of over 50%, the current literature suggests that, following an acute depressive episode, therapy should be continued for 6 to 12 months.[5] In elderly patients, who often have had two previous episodes of depression, maintenance antidepressant therapy is suggested for 4 to 5 years.[6] A history of two previous episodes plus a family history of depression, or a history of three or more episodes brings a recommendation for lifetime maintenance therapy.

To be able to prescribe an antidepressant properly for an elderly patient, the clinician must have knowledge of (1) the specific features of the diagnosis; (2) concomitant diseases that may either contribute to the depression or complicate the treatment; (3) concomitant medications that may either contribute to the depression or complicate the treatment; (4) previous antidepressant response; (5) the family history of response to antidepressant therapy. Choice of the appropriate antidepressant also requires knowledge of the various theoretical mechanisms of action and profiles of adverse effects. The drugs used to manage depression have high interpatient variability. Clinicians should use extra caution: The toxicities seen in the elderly are not dose dependent; rather, they are concentration dependent. This distinction is critical because the elderly normally require only one third to one half the dosage used for a young adult to acquire a therapeutic effect. This reduced dosage requirement results primarily from alterations in volume of distribution and liver metabolism in the elderly. Clinicians should be aware that, owing to these changes, drug accumulation may occur, and drugs with long half-lives are particularly problematic.

Tricyclic Antidepressants

Tricyclic antidepressants (TCAs) remain the gold standard for therapy. Of these, however, only the secondary amines nortriptyline and desipramine are regularly used in the elderly. This restricted use is due to the relatively nonspecific mechanism of action possessed by the tertiary amines amitriptyline, imipramine, trimipramine, and doxepin (Table 28–5). These agents' polypharma-

TABLE 28–5 TRICYCLIC ANTIDEPRESSANT THERAPY

	Adult Dosage (mg/day)	Mechanism
Tertiary Amines		
Amitriptyline	25–300	5-HT>NE
Doxepin	25–300	5-HT>NE
Imipramine	25–300	5-HT>NE
Secondary Amines		
Desipramine	25–300	NE>5-HT
Nortriptyline	10–150	NE>5-HT
Protriptyline	15–60	NE>5-HT

Abbreviations: 5-HT, 5-hydroxytryptophan, serotonin; NE, norepinephrine.

ceutical actions include inhibition of presynaptic serotonin and norepinephrine reuptake and prohibitively high anticholinergic effects, inhibition of alpha-1-adrenergic action (orthostatic hypotension), inhibition of histamine-1 receptor action (sedation), and prolongation of cardiac repolarization (leading to lengthening of the QT interval).[7] Because of these effects, tricyclic agents are contraindicated in many elderly patients who have cardiac conduction defects.

Caution is required in the geriatric patient with cardiovascular disease, narrow-angle glaucoma, benign prostatic hypertrophy, urinary retention, or a history of seizures. Additionally, clinicians should be aware of the relative supersensitivity of the elderly to anticholinergic effects, which can cause profound confusion. These agents should be given at bedtime to avoid the consequences of the previously noted adverse effects. Caution is also required in patients with suicidal ideation because lethal doses can be achieved with as little as a 2-week supply of tricyclics. Many clinicians report that the availability of therapeutic serum drug concentrations of nortriptyline and desipramine favors their use in the elderly. However, in a review of therapeutic serum drug concentration usage, it was reported that toxicity was seen at the same rate in groups that had therapeutic drug monitoring and those that did not. Based on this report, therapeutic drug monitoring may be appropriate in patients with toxic reactions, nonresponders without adverse effects, and the elderly. Even within the therapeutic range, geriatric patients should be monitored for signs and symptoms of overdose, whether mild (confusion and urinary retention) or severe (arrhythmias, hyperpyrexia, and respiratory depression). The general rule when initiating antidepressant therapy (with tricyclic agents or otherwise) in the elderly is to "start low and go slow" and titrate doses to effect.

TABLE 28-6   **ANTIDEPRESSANT THERAPY WITH SELECTIVE SEROTONIN REUPTAKE INHIBITORS**

	Fluoxetine	**Sertraline**	**Paroxetine**	**Fluvoxamine**
Adult dosage	10–40 mg daily	25–150 mg daily	10–40 mg daily	25–300 mg (if > 100 mg, use split dosing)
t1/2	2–3 days	26 hr	21 hr	15 hr
Metabolite	Norfluoxetine	Desmethylsertraline (1/8 as potent)		
Metab t1/2	7–9 days	2–3 days		
CYP450 inhibition	Parent and metabolite inhibit 2D6	Little 2D6 inhibition Possible 3A4 inhibition	Significant in vitro 2D6 inhibition	1A2 inhibition 3A3,4 inhibition
Side effects	Anxiety, anorexia, insomnia	Headache, diarrhea, sexual dysfunction	Nausea, GI upset, constipation	Nausea, insomnia, sedation
Comments	Shown effective for OCD	Possibly effective for OCD	Higher anticholinergic effects than secondary amines	Approved for OCD; no depression indication

Abbreviations: OCD, obsessive compulsive disorder; 2D6, 3A4, 1A2, and 3A3,4 represent specific isoenzymes of the cytochrome P450 (CYP450) system.

Selective Serotonin Reuptake Inhibitors

The selective serotonin reuptake inhibitors (SSRIs) include fluoxetine, sertraline, paroxetine, and fluvoxamine (Table 28–6). These agents are relatively specific for inhibiting the reuptake of serotonin and subsequently increasing serotonin neurotransmission. Because of this selectivity, the SSRIs lack the myriad adverse effects seen with the tricyclic antidepressants. It is for this reason that both psychiatrists and general practitioners are using SSRIs as first-line therapy for the treatment of depression. The SSRIs are structurally unrelated, well absorbed, highly protein bound, and extensively metabolized, yet they have various routes of metabolism.[8] The 7- to 9-day half-life of the norfluoxetine metabolite may lead to significant accumulation of this metabolite in the elderly (see Table 28–6). Compared to tricyclic antidepressants, SSRIs reportedly cause more gastrointestinal side effects including nausea, vomiting, and stomach upset. These adverse effects are believed to be self-limiting and thus may last only 1 to 3 weeks; such adverse effects may also indicate a too-rapid titration of dose that may be alleviated by lowering the dose. Another helpful approach is to recommend eating some food 20 to 30 minutes before the patient takes the medication. The neurologic side effects of SSRIs can be more persistent. Fluoxetine, for example, can cause significant anxiety and insomnia, an occurrence that necessitates a change to a less stimulating therapy. When initiating therapy with SSRIs it is best to start with a morning dose of the drug because of the stimulating effects, but these agents can be given at bedtime if the patient reports sedation.

Atypical Antidepressants

Other options for the treatment of depressed geriatric patients include atypical antidepressants (sometimes termed second-generation or newer antidepressants) (Table 28–7). These agents' proposed mechanisms of action do not fit into the categories listed earlier. Maprotiline is a rarely used tetracyclic antidepressant with a long half-life that is believed to inhibit presynaptic norepinephrine reuptake. Although seizures are reported to occur three times more frequently than with tricylics, maprotiline is associated with fewer cardiac arrhythmias. Amoxapine inhibits presynaptic reuptake of norepinephrine and serotonin, and its metabolite 8-hydroxyamoxapine blocks dopamine activity. Because of this inhibition, the geriatric patient may be at increased risk of developing parkinsonism, akathisia, or possibly tardive dyskinesia. The proposed use of this agent for psychotic depression is not warranted because when psychotic symptoms resolve, the antipsychotic should be discontinued to decrease the neurologic effects. With overdosage, amoxapine causes fewer cardiac effects but carries a risk of seizures, irreversible neurologic damage, and renal failure.

Bupropion is a popular antidepressant in elderly patients who are unable to tolerate other antidepressants because it has minimal sedative, anticholinergic, and cardiovascular properties. The mechanism of action of bupropion was believed to result from inhibition of dopamine reuptake; however, this inhibition has been found to be weak and may affect the norepinephrine and serotonin systems only slightly. Because of the increased threat of seizures with single doses of more than 150 mg, it is recommended that bupropion be given in divided doses despite a half-life that has been reported to be as long as 15 hours. Doses should be initiated at 75 mg twice daily and increased as tolerated. Because insomnia is common, a bedtime dose should be avoided.

Trazodone and nefazodone, which are classified as serotonergic drugs but not SSRIs, are believed to both inhibit serotonin reuptake and antagonize the serotonin-2 postsynaptic receptor. The postsynaptic receptor inhibition is thought to be responsible for the effectiveness of these agents in the anxious patient. Trazodone inhibits alpha-1-adrenergic receptors, giving rise to clinically significant orthostatic hypotension that peaks 1 to 2 hours after the dose and limits the clinical usefulness of this weak antidepressant in the elderly. The alpha-2-adrenergic effects of trazodone can rarely produce priapism. Both agents produce sedation with next to no anticholinergic effects, cardiac conduction abnormalities, or seizures, and both have been found safer than tricyclic antidepressants in overdose.[7] Nefazodone has a 2- to 4-hour half-life and is metabolized into three active metabolites that have half-lives of less than 24 hours; thus it requires twice daily dosing. Because of the possibility of sedation and dizziness, doses should be started at or below 50 mg twice daily.

Venlafaxine selectively inhibits the reuptake of both serotonin and norepinephrine from the synaptic cleft. Interestingly, venlafaxine has been found useful in patients in whom previous treatment has failed. Thus, many clinicians are using this agent as a safer second-line therapy in elderly patients who have failed to respond to an SSRI. In contrast to most psychoactive agents, venlafaxine is metabolized to an active metabolite that is excreted through the kidneys, thus requiring dosage adjustments in elderly patients with renal impairment. Side effects include nausea, somnolence, insomnia, and confusion. Venlafaxine is less arrhythmogenic than tricyclics but can cause small increases in blood pressure.

Monoamine Oxidase Inhibitors

Monoamine oxidase inhibitors (MAOIs) are believed to exert their therapeutic effect by blocking the synaptic destruction of biogenic amines. Phenelzine and tranylcypromine block the enzyme irreversibly; however, a newer reversible MAOI (meclobemide) is being used outside the United States. The MAOIs have not been well studied in the elderly because of their limiting adverse effects and drug interactions. For this reason, these drugs are often reserved for patients who have not responded to tricyclics or SSRIs. Yet there exists a body of literature indicating that the MAOIs may be effective for "atypical depression." The possibility of hyperpyrexia or a serotonin syndrome precludes combination therapy with other antidepressants. Other drug-drug or drug-food interactions can occur with over-the-counter cold products (which contain sympathetic amines), and foods containing high levels of tyramine such as aged cheeses,

TABLE 28–7 **ATYPICAL ANTIDEPRESSANT THERAPY**

	Maprotiline	Amoxapine	Bupropion	Venlafaxine	Trazodone	Nefazodone
Adult dosage	150–225 mg/day	200–600 mg/day	200–450 mg/day	75–375 mg/day	200–600 mg/day	100–600 mg/day
t1/2	21–25 hr	11–16 hr	14 hr	5 hr	4–7.5 hr	2–4 hr
Side effects	Seizures, anticholinergic effects, sedation, orthostasis	EPS/TD, possible seizures, drowsiness	Nausea, vomiting, insomnia, agitation	Confusion, somnolence, nausea, vomiting, hypertension	Sedation, orthostasis, priapism	Sedation, headache, orthostasis
Comments			Avoid in patients with seizures	Dose adjustment in patients with renal impairment	Orthostasis limits use at high doses	Inhibits CYP 3A3,4; Avoid: terfenadine, cisapride, astemizole

Abbreviations: EPS/TD, extrapyramidal symptoms/tardive dyskinesia; CYP3A3,4, cytochrome P450 isoenzymes 3 and 4.

cured meats, and beer. These interactions result in a hypertensive crisis, and the clinician should be aware of the early warning signs such as stiff neck, occipital headache, nausea, vomiting, sweating, flushing, and palpitations. The MAOIs have significant adverse effects as well. Orthostasis is common and is best prevented by increasing the dosage gradually. Weight gain, sexual dysfunction, and edema may also occur. Overdosage results in palpitations, agitation, frequent headaches, hypertension, or severe orthostasis.

Stimulants

Sympathomimetic agents such as methylphenidate and dextroamphetamine stimulate presynaptic catecholamine release and inhibit reuptake. These agents have been shown to provide quick relief of depressive symptoms in small studies of medically ill, elderly patients. Unfortunately, the long-term efficacy or adverse effects of the stimulants are unknown in this population.

NONPHARMACOLOGIC TREATMENT

The nonpharmacologic treatment of depression in the elderly includes a variety of strategies, each reflecting the unique challenges of treating this population. In addition to the difficulty of distinguishing between depression and dementia, a juxtaposition of the two may occur, complicating treatment. Also, it is important to include the entire treatment team as well as the entire support system in the assessment and treatment process. The treatment team frequently consists of the primary physician, consulting psychiatrist, occupational therapist, social workers, and nurses. Proper assessment, education of the patient, day hospital care, social support services, and individual, group, and milieu psychotherapy should be considered to address the wide range of problems that may face the older individual working through issues of chronic illness or a major depressive disorder.

The choice of treatment for the elderly, as with younger populations, depends on the severity of the symptoms. Intensive psychosocial support is recommended in addition to hospitalization, medication treatment, or electroconvulsive therapy for elderly patients with more severe depressive episodes. For patients who have had a severe acute episode and for those who are more moderately depressed or who have dysthymia, long-term outpatient treatment that includes medication and psychotherapeutic strategies may be necessary.[9]

Assessment and education are important from the standpoint of compliance. Cohort issues arise even before the primary physician or geriatric psychiatrist begin to consider the possibility of a diagnosis of a major depressive disorder. The NIMH Consensus Development Conference of 1991 found, among other treatment issues, that depression in later life occurs in the context of numerous social and physical problems, and attentive and focused clinical assessment is essential.[2] Many elderly individuals do not report depressive symptoms to health care providers because they believe these are to be expected. Depression is also often attributed to organic illness.[10] All health care professionals working with the elderly should be well trained and knowledgeable about the symptoms of depression, and they should also know when to try to elicit the less obvious information from patients. Sources of information that may be vital in the assessment of the elderly include the patient's spouse, siblings, and offspring. Family members may have observed details that may be critical for the clinician.

Education is an essential part of the diagnostic and treatment process. This process includes not only the patient and his or her family but also the primary care physician. Many elderly individuals as well as the general population are not aware of the biologic phenomenon of major depressive disorder. In presenting treatment options, an explanation of the rationale for medication treatment must be made to the patient and the family to ensure compliance. Much has been written about the need to coordinate all treatment of the elderly, including medication strategies and psychotherapy with family members.

There are many reports in the literature about the effects of psychotherapy and pharmacotherapy for elderly patients who have depression in the maintenance treatment phase.[9] Most reports indicate that a combination of medications and psychotherapy is more effective than either psychotherapy or medication alone.

Cognitive behavioral techniques have been found to be effective in providing patients with skills such as enhancing coping abilities, promoting health, and improving quality of life. Education about the effects of negative thoughts on mood and training to identify these themes are very helpful. Behavioral techniques include training in ways to increase experience with pleasant events and decrease the occurrence of unpleasant events.

Group therapy provides an orientation to others as well as the use of individual psychotherapy techniques. Life review therapy is helpful in a group and allows individuals to focus on their life memories in a positive environment.

COMPLIANCE

The effectiveness of any type of treatment for depression in the geriatric patient depends on the compliance of the patient with the treatment recommendations. The diagnosis and treatment of depression in the elderly can best be divided into three components: (1) identification of depression symptoms as such and subsequent diagnosis, (2) treatment, and (3) maintenance therapy. All three are critical, and failure in any one may result in continued suffering that could otherwise be treated easily, allowing the affected individual to lead a normal and healthy life. Because of the increase in longevity, diagnosis and effective treatment of an 80-year-old may normalize the quality of life for this individual for many years!

Compliance in the outpatient arena first requires a recognition and understanding by the patient of both the diagnosis and the treatment recommendations. The stigma of mental illness and a general unawareness of depression as a physical illness as well as multiple medical comorbidities, difficulty with transportation, and a fixed income may all lead to noncompliance. For these reasons, there is a special need at the first meeting with the patient and the family to develop a good "treatment alliance" to facilitate further diagnosis and effective treatment.[11]

Understanding the need for medication and the requirements for safe psychopharmacotherapy is similarly critical for successful treatment of the index episode and continued prophylaxis from recurrence in this frequently relapsing chronic illness. Elderly outpatients may not pay adequate attention to medication directions or may continue to take the drugs according to their own prior preference despite current recommendations.

Compliance in this population may be affected by many factors including forgetfulness, poor vision, and self-neglect secondary to an underlying and untreated depression, psychosis, or dementia. Other factors that may contribute to patient noncompliance include medication side effects, perception of lack of efficacy, and the feeling that improvement has been accomplished and taking the medication is no longer necessary.[12]

Side effects are the number one reason why geriatric patients discontinue medications, and it is therefore critical for the physician to choose the appropriate medication at the correct dose. Starting low and increasing the dosage gradually are the recommended methods for treating this population.

Occasionally the physician may encounter a patient who refuses to abandon older medications and older dosing strategies. In such situations it is always helpful to have the family present with the patient to help with a discussion of diagnosis and treatment recommendations.

ELECTROCONVULSIVE THERAPY

Electroconvulsive therapy (ECT) continues to be the single most effective treatment for major depressive disorder with or without psychotic features and for bipolar disorder, and it may be helpful for treating affective and psychotic disorders in elderly patients with movement disorders such as Parkinson's disease and tardive dyskinesia.[11, 13, 14] It is the treatment of choice for patients with psychotic delusional depression because it is usually not possible to treat these patients rapidly, safely, and adequately without incurring significant and dangerous medication side effects.

ECT is effective, works rapidly, and is extremely safe in this population. Unilateral placement of electrodes at adequate stimulation levels along with the use of pulsed square-wave stimulating equipment has been proved safe and effective without worsening of cognitive status.

Issues of compliance for this treatment are critical. Compliance is affected by fear and apprehension engendered by the myths and misrepresentation of this method as well as the difficulty of requiring continuation or maintenance therapy. Given the high incidence of medical comorbidities, which make the logistics for follow-up treatments more difficult, compliance may be further jeopardized. This situation therefore requires extensive effort by the physician to form an effective treatment alliance so that not only the initial treatment but also the continuation and maintenance therapy can be given as required. In this way the elderly patient can be maintained symptom free, and the frequent recurrences of this often recurrent and chronic physical illness can be prevented.

References

1. Gurland BJ, Cross PS, Katz S: Epidemiological perspectives on opportunities for treatment of depression. Am J Geriat Psychiatry 1996;4(4):S7–S13.
2. U.S. Department of Health and Human Services: Consensus Statement: National Institute of Mental Health Consensus Development Conference: The diagnosis and treatments of depression in late life. Bethesda, MD, U.S. Department of Health and Human Services, 1991, pp. 1–6.
3. Koenig HG, Blazer DG: Minor depression in late life. Am J Geriatr Psychiatry 1996;4(4):S14–S21.
4. Yesavage JA, Brink TL: Development and validation of a geriatric depression screening scale: A preliminary report. J Psychiatr Res 1983;17(1):37–49.

5. American Psychiatric Association: Practice Guideline for Major Depressive Disorder in Adults. Am J Psychiatry 1993;150(4)Suppl:1.
6. Kupfer DJ, Frank E, Perel JM, Cornes C, et al. Five-year outcome for maintenance therapies in recurrent depression. Arch Gen Psychiatry 1992;49:769–773.
7. Preskorn SH: Recent pharmacologic advances in antidepressant therapy for the elderly. Am J Med 1993;94(Suppl 5A):2S–12S.
8. DeVane CL: Pharmacokinetics of the newer antidepressants: Clinical relevance. Am J Med 1994;97(Suppl 6A):13S–23S.
9. Schneider LS, Olin JT: Acute therapy for geriatric depression. Int Psychogeriatrics 1995;7:7–25.
10. Martin LM, Fleming KC, Evans JM: Recognition and management of anxiety and depression in elderly patients. Mayo Clin Proc 1995;70(10):999–1006.
11. Hay DP, Hay L, Renner J, Franson K, Hassan R, Szwabo P: Compliance and the treatment alliance in the elderly patient with serious mental illness. *In* Blackwell B (ed): Treatment Compliance and the Therapeutic Alliance. Amsterdam, Netherlands: OPA Overseas Publishers Association, 1997, pp. 295–308.
12. McMullen P, Ross AJ, Rees JA: Problems experienced with medicines by psychogeriatric patients in the community. Pharm J 1991;247:182–184.
13. American Psychiatric Association Task Force Report on Electroconvulsive Therapy: The Practice of ECT: Recommendations for Treatment, Training and Privileging. Washington, DC, American Psychiatric Press, 1990.
14. Hay DP: Electroconvulsive therapy. *In* Kaplan HI, Saddock B (eds): Comprehensive Textbook of Psychiatry, 6th ed, Vol. 2. Baltimore, Williams & Wilkins, 1995.

Additional Readings

Depression Guideline Panel: Depression in Primary Care. Vol. 2: Treatment of Major Depression. Clinical Practice Guideline, No. 5. AHCPR Publication No. 93-0551. Rockville, MD, U.S. Department of Health and Human Services, Public Health Service, Agency for Health Care Policy and Research, 1993.
Hay DP, Hay L: Comprehensive Review of Geriatric Psychiatry, 2nd ed. Washington, DC, American Psychiatric Press, 1996.

29 Emotional and Behavioral Problems

Timothy Howell, M.D., M.A.

This chapter is about problems in older adults that are vexing: those that cause dysphoria in patients, interfere with their functioning, or cause distress in their caregivers, be they family members, peers, or health care professionals. A broad range of problematic behaviors may be brought to the attention of a physician; they are too numerous to address in a brief chapter. Hence the focus here is on some common syndromes and the development of an approach that can help sort through some of the more complicated, unusual, or even novel situations that may arise.

The morbidities associated with problem behaviors are enormous. Their presence in an older adult can interfere with the delivery of optimum health care, and they are common precipitants for institutionalization. They often constitute a rationale for antipsychotic treatment in long-term care (LTC) facilities. Not only are they a source of subjective distress in elderly patients, thereby compromising their quality of life, they are also a source of objective distress for caregivers in forms of anxiety, depression, and burnout.

TYPES OF PROBLEMATIC BEHAVIORS

Many different kinds of problematic behaviors are encountered in the practice of geriatric medicine. These include dysphoric effects, such as depression, anxiety, irritability, and mania. Agitation or aggression may be verbal or physical and may present as resistance to treatments, clinging to caregivers, or disruptiveness (e.g., distressing repetitive behaviors, sundowning, or wandering). Patients may develop suspiciousness, paranoia, or even such frankly psychotic symptoms as delusions or hallucinations. Somatization can be an especially challenging issue for a busy geriatri-

cian. The assessment and management of disorders concerned primarily with disturbances of affect are covered in the chapter on depression (Chapter 28), and those concerned with disturbances of cognition are covered in the chapters on dementia and delirium (Chapters 26 and 27, respectively).

BIOPSYCHOSOCIAL APPROACH

The biopsychosocial approach is a useful one in dealing with vexing behaviors. The rationale for this approach is that clinical problems frequently are multifactorial in origin and typically call for solutions using multiple modalities. This approach facilitates the analysis of such situations and reminds us not to come to premature closure about what may be disturbing a patient but to tease apart the different strands that comprise the problem to ensure that each constituent is optimally addressed.

In developing a strategy to parse the potential components of a problem behavior using a biopsychosocial approach, one focuses first on the biologic aspects. Here the most common factors that may be causing or exacerbating a problem behavior are medications and concurrent medical problems. A newly prescribed drug may be a culprit, or a long-standing medication to which the patient has become more sensitive suddenly (e.g., due to an acute change such as a stroke) or gradually (e.g., due to physiologic changes associated with aging or the gradual progression of a chronic illness). Likewise, an acute medical problem, or the progression or exacerbation of a chronic one, may contribute to a behavioral problem. The most frequent psychobiologic factors are concurrent psychiatric disorders: cognitive (including dementia and delirium), substance-related or psychotic (including schizophrenia), mood (including depression and mania), anxiety, and somatoform (including hypochondriasis and somatization). And the most common psychosocial factors are the physical environment and interpersonal relations, especially in terms of how these may be affected by an individual's personality style and personal history. It is at this level that one is most likely to encounter unique combinations of factors that can be tricky to sort through, and consequently where collateral sources of information can be very helpful.

PROBLEMS IN DEMENTIA

All of the problems delineated previously can occur in the context of a dementing illness. In dementia of the Alzheimer's type (DAT), they tend to occur later in the course of the disease and have a prevalence of 70% to 90% in the moderate to severe stages. A study by Cummings[1] revealed the following prevalences of noncognitive symptoms in DAT: apathy, 72%; agitation, 60%; anxiety, 48%; irritability, 42%; dysphoria, 38%; and delusions, 22%. Such psychiatric problems originate in the underlying neuropathologic processes of DAT. Disturbances of higher cortical function figure prominently. DAT patients with agnosia fail to recognize familiar people and places, and for some, this may precipitate anxiety and a tendency to get lost. With aphasia, the verbal confusion and inability to understand may provoke frustration, irritability, and catastrophic reactions. The apraxias that undermine patients' ability to perform activities of daily living (ADLs) often do the same.

Agitation or Aggression

The word agitation, so frequently used in discussions of the problematic emotions and behaviors of DAT patients, is a term that has mixed blessings. Most everyone familiar with this patient population knows what it means. But there are frequent differences about what the term refers to, and this is a critical factor in conducting research and interpreting the rapidly growing literature on this subject. Some definitions that have been proposed include: (1) an acute or chronic syndrome of pathologic arousal, usually involving repetitive motor or verbal activities[2]; (2) disruptive vocal or motor behavior that causes discomfort, poses a risk, or interferes with care.[3] In the latter definition, context is important. Thus, wandering in a street would be considered risky, whereas wandering in a safe yard could even be beneficial.

There are many types of agitated behaviors in patients with DAT. Among the distressing repetitious behaviors are repeated screams, shouts, complaints, requests, moans, curses, and criticisms. Aggressive behaviors include, but are not limited to, hitting, spitting, scratching, and kicking. Purposeless activities range from throwing objects to pacing, from disrobing to rummaging through drawers. DAT patients may refuse the help they need, wander, or fidget. Because its causes are potentially so numerous, it is best to view such agitation as a nonspecific symptom or sign, analogous to cough or fever, which may have multiple causes.

Further complicating the process of assessing these kinds of problems is the fact that DAT patients may be unable to report or describe their symptoms. This is reflected in the fact that undiagnosed illness is more common in older adults in the early stages of DAT than in nondemented elderly. Agitation may be the only indicator of an underlying illness. Thus, one needs to be alert for concurrent medical problems, such as cardiovascular disorders, pulmonary disorders, diabetes, or neoplasms. Uncomfortable or painful conditions that may generate agitation in a dementia patient but may be inadvertently overlooked include urinary tract infections (UTIs), constipation, fecal impaction, skin breakdown, headache, sinus congestion, dental problems, dislocated joints, arthritis, or fractures. Delirium is another consideration, especially because dementia patients are more vulnerable to being "tipped over" by such causes of excess morbidity as dehydration, electrolyte disturbances, medications with central nervous system (CNS) side effects, or drug interactions. Age-associated declines in liver or kidney function may also play a role here.

Sensory impairments can compound the deterioration of abilities in dementia patients by further compromising their ability to process, interpret, and understand events in their environment. Hence, poor hearing or vision should be assessed and addressed as feasible. Some dementia patients may not be able to use or tolerate prosthetic devices such as eyeglasses or hearing aids, but these devices warrant an adequate trial before such a conclusion is drawn. It may even work out that such items can be used some of the time, and the benefits derived from even partial successes should not be underappreciated.

Among the noncognitive psychiatric problems in patients with dementing illnesses are a loss of adaptive abilities, including poor impulse control, reduced toleration of frustration, and impaired ability to calm oneself down. These difficulties may stem from involvement of the disease process in the frontal lobes and probably underlie the nearly ubiquitous phenomenon of catastrophic reactions in dementia patients. Catastrophic reactions are intense emotional and behavioral responses (e.g., anxious resistiveness, angry outbursts, tearful refusals) precipitated by common situations (e.g., dressing or bathing) in which the demented individual no longer has the cognitive ability to cope (e.g., due to an inability to appreciate the need to accomplish the task, recognize who is trying to help them, or perform the task). Psychotic symptoms occur more commonly in patients with dementia than in age-matched healthy controls and include paranoia, hallucinations, and delusions. Depression occurs in approximately 20% of patients during the course of DAT. It may become manifest as agitation, pacing, insomnia (including sundowning), crying, or refusal to eat.

Treatment strategies for the emotional and behavioral problems that arise in patients with dementia start with a careful differential diagnosis and continue with systematic efforts to address the medical, psychiatric, and social or environmental components identified as contributing factors. Catastrophic reactions can often be managed by discerning the patterns (e.g., time, place, situation) in which they occur, thus identifying their precipitants (e.g., tasks, environmental factors, persons). One can help patients to cope better by foreshadowing, taking more time, and breaking tasks down into simpler steps.

Pharmacotherapy for agitated behaviors should be employed only when psychosocial interventions are insufficient. Such therapy must be judicious because dementia patients are usually more sensitive to the side effects of psychotropic medications and more prone to delirium. Agents that are sometimes useful include trazodone, antipsychotics, anticonvulsants, antidepressants, anxiolytics, and beta-blockers. All these medications have limited efficacy in this patient population, and no signs or symptoms have yet been found that predict a positive response. Hence, it is important to approach each patient with an individualized treatment plan: identify the target symptoms clearly, then track their response to titration of the medication in terms of their frequency and intensity while monitoring for side effects.

When dementia patients become acutely aggressive, safety can be ensured by removing items that could be used as weapons and calling for assistance from police, crisis intervention workers, or other trained staff. Restraints should be employed only on a brief, emergency basis, because their prolonged use is associated with significant morbidities. Dementia patients who engage in activities (e.g., driving; smoking; using appliances, machinery, or firearms; neglecting health and hygiene) that may endanger themselves or others because they have become unmindful of hazards or unable to follow directions or use safeguards raise difficult ethical issues. The challenge here is to achieve an optimal balance of patient autonomy and quality of life with safety. Close supervision, substitutions (e.g., of microwave ovens or hand tools for standard ovens or power tools), limited drivers' licenses, and the provision of home care services (e.g., chore services, meals-on-wheels, health aides) all represent examples of creative ways in which to design individualized interventions that foster such an optimum balance.

Distressing Repetitive Behaviors

Distressing repetitive behaviors such as yelling, demanding, clinging, and criticizing occur in about half of all outpatients with dementia and are often quite taxing to caregivers. They are usually due to the dementing process itself but may be caused by environmental stressors, pain, or depression. Reasoning with or confronting the patient is generally not helpful and may be counterproductive. Trying to determine if the repetitive behavior has some underlying meaning (e.g., fear of abandonment) can sometimes suggest helpful responses (e.g., periodic reassurance). Distraction, behavior modification, and stress reduction may be efficacious. If pain or depression is suspected but is difficult to confirm because of a patient's inability to communicate, an empirical trial of an analgesic or antidepressant may be warranted.

Sundowning

The term sundowning usually refers to late afternoon or nocturnal increases in confusion in dementia patients, typically associated with agitation, restlessness, or wandering. Given the variable definitions of this problem, it is difficult to establish its prevalence, but overall, it appears that nearly half of outpatients with dementia develop sleep problems. Untreated, the nocturnal type of sundowning can rapidly lead to caregiver exhaustion in the home setting and may thereby precipitate institutionalization. Causes to be considered in patients with sundowning include such medical problems as nocturia, congestive heart failure (CHF) with paroxysmal nocturnal dyspnea (PND), and delirium. Most major psychiatric disorders that occur with dementia can be associated with insomnia and sundowning. Psychosocial stressors such as relocation, bereavement, and placement in an institutional setting (e.g., with fewer social cues about when to sleep) may also be contributory factors. Dementias themselves alter sleep architecture and thus may predispose to sundowning. Finally, patients with premorbid histories of being "night owls" or working in such jobs as night watchman or baker may revert to old sleep-wake patterns. Management of sundowning consists of providing a stable sensory environment (e.g., comfortable temperature, quiet surroundings, and perhaps a nightlight to facilitate orientation in the dark) and addressing specific medical, psychiatric, and psychosocial factors identified, as clinically indicated. It is important to use much caution when prescribing hypnotic-sedative medications because these frequently have only time-limited effectiveness, may exacerbate cognitive impairment, and cause paradoxical or other untoward side effects.

Sexual Problems

Sexual problems arise in more than 10% of patients with dementia and cause considerable distress in their partners. Both hypersexuality and loss of interest in sex may result from the dementia itself, from medications, or from a concurrent affective disorder. If the dementia is mild, counseling may enhance communication about specific issues for a couple. Adjustment of prescribed medications associated with impotence or anorgasmia (e.g., antihypertensives, selective serotonin reuptake inhibitors) or hypersexuality (e.g., dopaminergic antiparkinsonian drugs) may restore normal sexual function. Likewise, treatment of a co-morbid depression or mania may restore a diminished libido or a hyperactive libido, respectively. For dementia patients with delusions of infidelity or delusions that others are their spouses, neuroleptic medications may diminish the intensity (if not cause remission) of the delusions. There are case reports of estrogens for the treatment of male patients with dementia whose problems with sexual aggression have proved severe and refractory to other treatments. Teaching caregivers to reframe sexual requests as calls for attention and closeness may also be helpful. Reassuring the unaffected partners that such behaviors are due to the dementia and are not a reflection on their relationships can go a long way toward reducing the embarrassment and distress that they may feel.

Wandering

Wandering is yet another class of behavioral disturbance that can stem from dementia and may have multiple causes. By exposing patients to environmental hazards or causing them

subjective fright, wandering can pose serious problems in the delivery of care, whether at home or in institutional settings. Its prevalence appears to correlate with the severity of the dementia (about 20% of patients with mild dementia, and about 50% of those with severe dementia). Wandering can arise when a patient with Alzheimer's disease gets lost. It can be precipitated by relocation, environmental stimuli, boredom, psychosis, agitated depression, or hypomania. Wandering may be an unanticipated behavioral side effect of medication (e.g., akathisia due to antipsychotics, or looking for a bathroom after administration of a diuretic). Aimless wandering can be a manifestation of the dementia itself.

Wandering in patients with dementia is managed as clinically indicated according to the cause or causes uncovered and the principles discussed earlier. In addition, posting signs may help to direct dementia patients who can still read or recognize icons. Boredom can be alleviated by providing an exercise program and a schedule of meaningful activity. Involving cognitively impaired patients in useful tasks that call on skills they still retain can also enhance their self-esteem. Alarm systems are available to alert others when Alzheimer's patients wander away from supervised areas. Finally, if the wandering is not otherwise problematic, providing an enclosed environment, such as a garden or indoor courtyard, in which the patient can safely wander can meet the needs of both patients and caregivers.

Dealing with Diagnostic and Prognostic Ambiguities

In working with dementia patients who have emotional and behavioral problems, considerable diagnostic ambiguity may be encountered, especially at first, in trying to sort through the multiple factors that may be contributing to any one individual's set of problems. Enlisting the aid of caregivers by forming ad hoc treatment teams facilitates the gathering and sifting of information that can clarify the particular picture of a given patient. Their working knowledge of the patient and ongoing astute observations can provide major dividends. This approach also helps with prognostic ambiguities because very often it is difficult to determine how much improvement is realistic to expect or aim for. Even when an optimal result has been achieved, something else may happen that requires starting the process all over again (e.g., a fall with a hip fracture, or another stroke). One can work with family members or nursing staff to identify target symptoms, develop interventions, and track the results (e.g., using flow sheets). Then, by making modifications according to the results and instituting other changes that may be necessary in the course of the patient's dementia, all participants can be reassured that all that can be done is being done. Thus, the process of developing an ad hoc team can also address the sense of collective helplessness or guilt that is sometimes engendered by these kinds of problems, in which care providers (including physicians) may feel at a loss about what can be accomplished in the presence of a progressive illness for which there is still no definitive cure.

To illustrate these principles, consider the case of Mr. A, an 84-year-old retired baker with CHF and moderate DAT, who lives with his daughter, Mrs. B. She is a 62-year-old widow who brings him with her to the clinic. She is exhausted by his wandering out of their house in the middle of the night and his habit of resistance when she attempts to redirect him. She feels badly that she is becoming so frustrated with him because she realizes that he can no longer be responsible for his behavior. A review of the situation with her reveals a number of possible causes of the behavior: (1) a diuretic that is given bid; (2) symptoms suggestive of a UTI and perhaps PND; (3) a somewhat depressed affect but no apparent psychosocial stressors. An assessment strategy is developed with the daughter, and she returns in a week with a log that reveals that: (1) her 30-year-old son, who still lives at home, has been noisy at night when he returns from his second-shift job; (2) her father has a predominantly sad mood, as well as a poor appetite, low energy, anhedonia, and undue pessimism. This observation confirms that her father indeed has a depressive disorder superimposed on his dementia. In addition, a careful physical examination shows that the CHF is under good control, whereas a urine culture reveals a bladder infection.

Subsequent medication adjustments include changing the diuretic to a once daily schedule in the morning, a course of antibiotic for the UTI, and a sedating antidepressant to help with sleep as well as mood. Mrs. B begins to participate in an Alzheimer's support group and instructs her son to come in quietly through the back door when he returns from work. On follow-up a few weeks later, Mr. A's UTI and depression have resolved, and he is no longer up during the night, distressed and looking for the bathroom. He is, however, awaking regularly at 5 AM, ready to go to work. Mrs. B is able to redirect him by feeding him an early breakfast, and she is much less tired because she is able to go to bed a little sooner and sleep through the night. Less stressed, she feels better about herself and, with support from others in her group, more confident as a caregiver.

ANXIETY AND AVOIDANT OR REPETITIVE BEHAVIORS

To date, anxiety disorders in the elderly have been less well studied than depression or dementia. This may stem in part from the ubiquity of anxiety, which is almost taken for granted and is underappreciated as a clinical problem. Another challenging factor in the study of anxiety in older adults is that of confounding variables. It is often difficult to gauge the significance of anxiety symptoms in elderly patients in whom those symptoms overlap with those arising from medical problems and their treatments. Further, the current cohort of elderly patients may be generally less comfortable in discussing psychological feelings and hence are more likely to focus on the somatic symptoms of anxiety.

Despite these obstacles to research, a picture is emerging from a number of studies indicating that anxiety disorders are some of the most common psychiatric problems encountered in an older population. The National Institute of Mental Health (NIMH) Epidemiologic Catchment Area (ECA) study found a 1-month prevalence of all anxiety disorders in a community-dwelling population 65 years of age and older to be 5.5% (6.8% in women and 3.6% in men). The most common anxiety disorder found was phobic disorder (4.8%), followed by obsessive-compulsive disorder (OCD, 0.8%) and panic disorder (0.1%).[4] The symptoms of anxiety include psychological feelings of uncomfortable apprehension and such psychomotor signs as tremulousness and muscle tension. The autonomic symptoms of anxiety include shortness of breath, tachycardia, diaphoresis, dry mouth, lightheadedness, gastrointestinal distress, and flushing. Signs of vigilance that are also characteristic of the experience of anxiety include edginess, poor concentration, and an exaggerated startle response.

The differential diagnosis of anxiety includes adjustment disorder with anxiety, generalized anxiety disorder (GAD), phobias, panic disorder, OCD, post-traumatic stress disorder (PTSD), and anxiety disorder due to general medical condition (which used to be referred to as organic anxiety disorder). Adjustment disorders with anxiety occur in response to an identifiable stressor, such as a financial setback. But in older adults less severe stressors, such as a relocation from one room to another in a nursing home or a new illness, even if not severe or disabling, may give rise to an adjustment disorder. Interventions are focused on reducing the burden of the stressor or enhancing the coping skills of the patient. GAD is characterized by apprehension that is persistent (at least 6 months and often years in older adults), frequent, and unwarranted by the circumstances (either excessive or unrealistic). Based on the American Psychiatric Association's *Diagnostic and Statistical Manual of Mental Disorders* (DSM-IV) criteria, the patient with GAD finds the anxiety difficult to control and experiences three or more anxiety symptoms.[5] This disorder can be treated with relaxation therapies and judicious use of anxiolytic medications (keeping in mind the side effects of benzodiazepines to which older patients are more vulnerable, such as sedation, falls, and cognitive impairment).

When an older patient shows avoidant behaviors not founded on realistic concerns, it is important to consider the possibility of phobias or panic disorder. Phobias involve fears that are persistent and excessive or irrational and are triggered immediately by exposure to a specific object or situation. Patients with a phobia retain insight into the fact that their reactive fear is unwarranted but continue to feel it nonetheless, to the point where they avoid the precipitating stimulus or endure it only with much subjective distress. A more specific diagnosis of social phobia can be made when the affected individual experiences an unwarranted fear of scrutiny, humiliation, or embarrassment in social contexts. Panic attacks can occur in older as well as younger adults, but when they occur for the first time in late life, they are more likely to be mistaken for myocardial infarctions, transient ischemic attacks, or other acute medical problems. Panic attacks typically involve discrete periods of unwarranted, usually spontaneous, and very intense fear or discomfort; they reach a peak within 10 minutes and are accompanied by strong autonomic anxiety symptoms as well as a fear of dying, losing control, or "going crazy." The diagnosis of panic disorder is made when patients experience recurrent panic attacks and then develop (1) a persistent concern that they may have additional attacks, (2) worries about the implications or consequences of their attacks, or (3) changes in their behavior (typically avoidant in nature). Because of the intense nature of the attacks, such patients often become fearful of the fear itself and thus avoid (or endure only with a lot of subjective distress) the situations in which they first experienced the attacks and in which escape would be difficult or embarrassing. Phobias can be treated with cognitive-behavioral interventions (e.g., systematic desensitization). Panic disorder may respond to similar interventions, antidepressant medications (the selective serotonin reuptake inhibitors have been found to be beneficial, as are the older tricyclics), or sometimes both.

Both OCD and PTSD involve symptoms that are repetitive in nature, although in different ways. Obsessions consist of recurrent persistent thoughts, impulses, or images that are experienced by patients as intrusive and inappropriate. Among the most common themes of obsessions are contamination, pathologic doubt, bodily concerns, need for symmetry, aggression, and sexual images or impulses. They do not include excessive worries about real-life problems. Some obsessions may generate strong feelings of shame, which can prevent the patient from even reporting the symptoms. Compulsions are actions that are analogous to obsessions. They involve repetitive behaviors that patients feel driven to perform because of obsessions and are typically aimed at preventing, or at least reducing the likelihood of, some dreaded event. In OCD, insight is retained; patients realize that these phenomena are products of their own minds, and they initially experience the obsessions or compulsions as distressing and try to ignore, suppress, or otherwise neutralize them. Late-onset OCD is rare. Patients may present for the first time in late life, however, because of age-related changes or other medical or psychiatric problems. Transient OCD symptoms, for example, may occur in the context of a major depressive episode. Another diagnostic concern with geriatric patients who have OCD of long standing is that they may have had to cope with their obsessions or compulsions for so long (even decades) that they have gotten used to them and no longer view them as irrational. If available, information from collateral sources about the early course of the OCD in such patients can help to clarify the nature of the current symptoms.

PTSD involves exposure to a traumatic event in which the individual is confronted by or threatened with death, injury, or violation of the self, and consequently experiences intense fear, horror, or helplessness. As a consequence, PTSD causes persistently increased levels of arousal, and the patients repeatedly reexperience the event and avoid stimuli that remind them of it. Symptoms of increased arousal include insomnia, outbursts of anger, poor concentration, hypervigilance, and an exaggerated startle response. Avoidance behaviors include efforts to steer clear of thoughts, feelings, conversations, people, places, or activities reminiscent of the traumatic event. Patients with PTSD may also have trouble recalling significant aspects of the trauma and have a restricted range of affect or a foreshortened sense of the future. They may feel estranged from other people or lose interest in and drop out of activities in which they used to participate. Repetitive nightmares, flashbacks when awake, and intrusive, distressing memories or images are all ways in which a patient may persistently reexperience the trauma.

Little research has been published thus far on the efficacy of treatments for OCD or PTSD in geriatric patients. Cognitive and behavioral therapies have been used with some success in younger patients. Pharmacotherapy specific for OCD consists of the selective serotonin reuptake inhibitors, including fluvoxamine, and the tricyclic antidepressant clomipramine. The latter may not be well tolerated by older patients, given its strong sedative, anticholinergic, and hypotensive side effects. Medications for PTSD are more empirical: antidepressants, anxiolytics, and mood stabilizers have all been employed with varying degrees of success.

Finally, anxiety in older patients may be a consequence of a concurrent or underlying but still undiagnosed medical condition or a side effect of some medical treatment. Examples of these include cardiopulmonary disorders associated with discomfort or hypoxia, most endocrine disorders, and chronic pain syndromes. Neurologic disorders with which anxiety may be associated include masses, infections, focal seizures, vertigo, and movement disorders. Steroids, sympathomimetics, antidepressants, and stimulants are examples of medications that can cause anxiety as a side effect. Drug toxicity (e.g., excess digoxin or thyroid supplementation) or withdrawal (e.g., alcohol, sedative-hypnotics) may also be a culprit. Treatment strategies depend on the nature of the problems uncovered: eliminating or minimizing anxiogenic substances, reducing or changing anxiogenic medications, and addressing contributing medical problems.[7]

PARANOIA AND PSYCHOTIC SYMPTOMS

Elderly patients occasionally have difficulties in reality testing, such as paranoia, delusions, or hallucinations. Although the NIMH ECA study[4] revealed that schizophrenia, a specific psychotic disorder, has a relatively low prevalence among community-dwelling elderly (0.2% to 0.9%), other research has found higher levels of psychotic symptomatology in certain clinical settings: (1) persecutory ideation in the community, 4%; (2) paranoid disorder in an outpatient geriatric psychiatry clinic, 17%; (3) delusions in a nursing home, 21%.[8] Some risk factors that may predispose older adults to the development of psychotic symptoms include cognitive impair-

ment and sensory deprivation, especially impaired hearing or vision. Recently widowed older adults may occasionally experience the presence of their deceased spouses in the form of auditory or visual hallucinations. These experiences are typically benign and may even be comforting to the surviving partner; hence they do not usually require treatment.

A number of psychiatric disorders affecting older adults are characterized by or associated with psychotic symptoms. Paranoid delusions have been found to occur in up to 40% of older adults with delirium. Recent research in dementia has shown that up to 40% of patients with Alzheimer's disease or vascular dementia develop psychotic symptoms during the course of their illness. Among the most common delusions is the idea that others are stealing, breaking in, or poisoning food. Hallucinations have been reported to occur in up to one third of patients with Alzheimer's disease. Both major depression and mania can appear for the first time in late life and may be associated with psychotic features. The reader is directed to other chapters of this book for a broader discussion of psychosis in the context of dementia, delirium, and mood disorders. Here we will focus on schizophrenia, delusional disorder, and the organic psychoses (i.e., those due to medical problems or drugs).

Schizophrenia, usually a chronic disorder, is characterized by at least two of the following symptoms: delusions, hallucinations, disorganized speech (derailment or incoherence), catatonic or grossly disorganized behavior, and what have come to be called "negative symptoms" (flattened affect, alogia, avolition). In addition, the diagnostic criteria for schizophrenia include a marked decline from baseline in psychosocial functioning as reflected in work performance, interpersonal relations, or self-care. Most adults in late life with schizophrenia have grown old with their illness; in 90% of these, the onset of the disorder occurred prior to age 46. There is a growing body of research on late-onset schizophrenia (LOS). While the diagnostic criteria are the same as those for the early-onset form, in LOS negative symptoms and disorganized speech appear to be less prominent, whereas persecutory delusions tend to be more common. Risk factors associated with LOS include female sex, sensory deficits, social isolation, eccentric personality, and a family history of schizophrenia. A prototypical case might be that of an elderly woman, hard of hearing and with cataracts but no prior overt psychiatric history, who otherwise manages to live alone successfully. She periodically calls 911, fearful that someone is trying to poison her water supply, but she cannot be reassured, much to the consternation of those trying to help.

Diagnosis of a delusional disorder entails the presence of one or more nonbizarre delusions for at least a month in the absence of schizophrenia, a psychotic mood disorder, or organic psychosis. The delusions are usually quite circumscribed; aside from the delusions and their ramifications, the functioning of patients with delusional disorders is not significantly impaired, nor is their behavior otherwise overtly odd or bizarre. Subtypes of delusional disorder include erotomanic, grandiose, jealous, persecutory, somatic, and mixed types.

Organic psychoses include those caused by an underlying medical condition or drug toxicity. Brain disease (cerebrovascular, degenerative, traumatic, neoplastic, infectious, and immunologic) may contribute to the development of psychotic symptoms in older patients. Hydrocephalus, seizure disorders, and hepatic or renal failure can do likewise. Other potential medical causes include electrolyte disturbances, vitamin deficiencies (thiamine, folate, B_{12}, niacin), and hypoactivity or hyperactivity of the thyroid, parathyroid, or adrenal glands. Among medications with the potential to induce psychosis are anticholinergics, dopaminergics, steroids, stimulants, digoxin, cimetidine, benzodiazepines, anticonvulsants, lidocaine, and procainamide. It is especially important to consider all these factors in those elderly patients with long-standing psychoses such as schizophrenia. If their psychotic symptoms become more disorganized, or if they develop new ones out of character with the usual ones, a separate organic psychosis may be superimposed on the chronic disorder.

The treatment of psychotic symptoms in older adults consists primarily of identifying and addressing any contributing medical problems (including difficulties with medications and other substances that may be implicated) and providing the patient with a safe, reassuring, and supportive environment. For delusions or hallucinations that are distressing to patients or that interfere with their function or care, judicious use of an antipsychotic medication is indicated. Here, the choice among the many available neuroleptics is fraught with difficulties because of their many side effects. Whereas the less potent antipsychotics (e.g., chlorpromazine, thioridazine) are often associated with relatively less risk of extrapyramidal side effects (EPSE), they carry relatively more risk for significant sedation, orthostasis, and anticholinergic symptoms (including blurred vision, dry mouth, constipation, urinary retention, and cognitive impairment). And while the risks for such side effects are relatively lower with the highly potent neuroleptics (e.g., haloperidol, fluphenazine, thiothixene, trifluoperazine), their use raises the risks of EPSE, including parkinsonian symptoms, akathisia, and dystonia. Although there are no data available that support this approach objectively, one strategy is to become familiar with the use of neuroleptics of intermediate potency (e.g., molindone, loxapine, perphenazine), which, at least theoretically, have risks intermediate between those of the less and more potent neuroleptics. All these medications, if used on a long-term basis, carry a significant risk in older patients for the development of the abnormal involuntary movements characteristic of tardive dyskinesia (TD). Hence their use in LTC settings is regulated,[10] and patients taking them require periodic screening for TD.

The newer atypical antipsychotics have begun to be used with geriatric patients with some success, but these too require caution. Clozapine can be helpful in some patients with Parkinson's disease with delusions or hitherto refractory schizophrenia, but it has all the side effects of a less potent antipsychotic and also lowers the threshold for seizures. Risperidone and olanzapine appear to be associated with some reduction in the likelihood of EPSE in some older patients if employed at lower doses.

For patients who, given the nature of their delusions (e.g., as in those with LOS), refuse treatment, one can obtain psychiatric consultation and, in cases of imminent danger, court-ordered evaluation and treatment. When danger is not imminent and the patients refuse to see a psychiatrist (as is not infrequently the case), one can attempt to build a therapeutic alliance over a period of time to the point where sufficient trust is established for them to consider taking medication to relieve distress. This may be accomplished by "agreeing to disagree" about the issues about which they are delusional (e.g., whether someone is breaking into their apartment and leaving salt on the table) and working with them on nonanxiety-provoking medical or social concerns for which they are open to interventions (e.g., management of their hypertension or arranging transportation to the clinic).

SOMATIZATION

Not infrequently, geriatricians encounter older patients with troubling somatic complaints that seem to defy even the most thorough diagnostic and therapeutic efforts. These patients often consume an inordinate amount of time and resources, undergo risky procedures and treatments, and generate anxiety and frustration in their health care providers. Many of them are individuals who "transduce" their subjective psychological distress into bodily sensations of discomfort.[11] Such clinical phenomena, referred to generically as somatization, are probably best understood from a biopsychosocial perspective as occurring in the context of an illness. Just as in physics one can meaningfully study light as both a particle and a wave, so also one can fruitfully view illness as both a disease process and how the patient experiences that disease. Thus, somatization can occur not only in clinical situations in which there appears to be no demonstrable organ system or cellular dysfunction but also when patient complaints or responses to treatment appear to be disproportionate to demonstrable disease processes. In both instances, there are problems to be addressed in the patient's experience of internal or interpersonal difficulties. Very little research data on somatization in older populations are available, but it has been estimated that up to 60% of primary care patients present with somatic complaints that express psychological distress. Somatization can occur in the context of transient emotional distress, mood and anxiety disorders, psychophysiologic disorders, psychotic disorders, malingering, factitious disorders, personality disorders, and somatoform disorders.

Hypochondriasis is a somatoform disorder characterized by the fears or beliefs of the patient that he or she has a serious disease, stemming from a misinterpretation of somatic symptoms. These beliefs persist for many months (or even years) despite appropriate medical assessment and reassurance and cause significant subjective distress or impaired functioning. Such beliefs are not delusional in their intensity, which distinguishes them from a psychotic disorder, nor are they limited strictly to concerns about physical appearance, which would constitute a (rare) body dysmorphic disorder. In undifferentiated somatoform disorder a patient has one or more somatic complaints and subsequent distress or functional impairment that, despite an appropriate work-up, cannot be accounted for by a known medical condition or exceeds what is expectable on the basis of the patient's history and clinical findings. Older patients with these disorders may feel misunderstood and abandoned by impatient physicians, become hostile, or resort to doctor-shopping.

A number of theories have been developed to explain the genesis of such somatoform disorders. These have been nicely reviewed by Kaplan and colleagues.[11] Some neurobiologic theories postulate that abnormal processing of afferent sensory information by the central nervous system amplifies normally imperceptible stimuli, which the patient then experiences and labels as problematic. Others propose that some patients have interhemispheric communication problems such that emotions are expressed through physical complaints rather than verbally. Psychodynamic theories interpret somatization as a way of resolving underlying emotional conflicts (e.g., a desire for comfort and nurturance versus a fear of rejection).

Behavioral theories propose that somatization is learned under the influence of environmental reinforcers. A patient may present with an illness, complaining of chest pain and anxiety, for example. By focusing on the chest pain to the exclusion of the anxiety, the physician and others reinforce the somatic complaint while at the same time downplaying the perceived significance of the emotional complaint. For some patients, who have such experiences repeatedly, their "illness behavior" is thus shaped by the interactions into a somatizing pattern. Sociocultural theories of somatization put forth the notion that in a culture one learns socially acceptable ways of handling emotional issues, including those involved in illnesses. The degree to which the direct expression of feelings is permitted, tolerated, or encouraged varies from one culture to another. Somatization may then become a means of indirect expression of emotions in cultures in which open demonstrations of feeling are less acceptable. In such cultures, taking a patient's somatic complaints literally may give rise to significant misinterpretations.

When working with somatizing patients, it is important to do more than "rule in" or "rule out" an underlying medical or psychiatric disease process; it is important to listen actively to the patient to learn the place of the complaints in the context of the person's body, intrapsychic life, and interpersonal relations and culture. In addition to determining the pattern of somatization according to these criteria, one can watch for low self-esteem, guilt, or difficulties with handling anger or assertiveness. The ways in which the patient interacts with other family members and health care providers and how he or she uses medical services can provide significant clues to the roles the symptoms may be playing in everyday life. An understanding of the patient's personal beliefs about the nature and meaning of the symptoms and illness and how he or she copes with stress can be very revealing. Questions about what a patient thinks has caused the problem, why it began when it did, how it affects him, and what kind of treatment he thinks he should receive can help to clarify his experience of the problem. Likewise, eliciting the patient's hopes and fears about the illness may provide important insights.[11]

For patients whose somatization represents a transient response to an acute stressor, the prognosis is generally good. These patients typically respond well to appropriate reassurances and education about their problems. Chronic somatization, however, calls for a more sophisticated approach. A key component is the cultivation of an empathic doctor-patient relationship, the development of a therapeutic alliance characterized by trust and caring. This is often not easy because treating physicians, when confronted with patients who seem to resist their best efforts to help, may find themselves feeling helpless, hopeless, inadequate, angry, guilty, or fearful. Such feelings may be further compounded by another set of feelings about developing such strong reactions in the first place (e.g., feeling guilty about feeling angry).

The first step in addressing such responses is to recognize that one is having them, and allowing oneself to fully feel them rather than dismissing or trying to ignore them can facilitate this process. The next step is to consider what such strong feelings represent, because very often they can provide a great deal of information about these patients. In ways analogous to how the forehead of a febrile patient makes one's hand feel warm, so the feelings engendered by the complaints of somatizing patients can reveal important clues about their condition. A not uncommon phenomenon in patients who have difficulty in directly communicating their ideas and feelings is that, through their behavior, they end up causing others around them to have the same feelings that they have. Thus, some chronically depressed or angry patients, for example, who find it difficult or impossible to articulate their discontents, may generate resonating feelings of sadness or frustration in those who come in contact with them.

The feelings elicited by working with somatizing patients, then, are not something to feel guilty about but rather should be appreciated for what they are: valuable sources of information that can help to clarify the issues involved and can be tapped by shifting diagnostic modalities. The challenging task is to resist the temptation to either suppress them or react blindly to them, but instead to work them through like other clinically demanding diagnostic tasks, thoughtfully, respectfully, and sensitively.

The insights obtained in this manner can be used to overcome the apparent barriers to delivering care to chronically somatizing patients and to gradually build a therapeutic alliance. Seeing such patients on a regular basis at short intervals

"whether they need to be seen or not" can do much to establish a foundation of dependability and constancy on which to build. By not making the follow-up contingent on the presence of somatic complaints, the doctor-patient relationship is reinforced instead. Care should be taken to schedule the frequency of follow-up according to the individual patient's needs. Too short or too long an interval could lead to the symptoms becoming worse. A solicitous approach that communicates acceptance and respect for the patient as a person can promote enhanced self-esteem. It can also help to derail the all-too-common self-fulfilling prophecies through which such patients anticipate rejections from physicians, behave in such a way that they are rejected, and thereby confirm their original expectations. These dynamics are often well-reflected in such clinical phenomena as doctor-shopping and excessive use of medical resources. A consistent approach, in which the reality of the symptoms is not contested but respectfully assessed with a careful physical examination (no matter how strange the complaint) and judicious laboratory testing, will go a long way toward reassuring these patients that they are being taken seriously. Careful attention to patients' affect and nonverbal communications can facilitate this ongoing process.

Premature interpretations connecting somatic complaints with psychological issues are generally best avoided. Usually these patients have heard such responses before and associate them with prior rejections. Over an extended period of time, during which a sound therapeutic alliance is established, it may be possible to learn to make such connections for some, though probably not all patients, particularly if these interpretations are couched in terms of stress (including the stress of the symptoms themselves). In nearly all cases, attending patiently to the patient's story, beliefs about the illnesses, and expectations of care will enhance the doctor-patient relationship. This in turn can enable the treating physician to discover the patient's strengths as well as weaknesses and then support the best ways of coping. If the patient expresses impatience at the length of time it may take to accomplish some of these things, he or she can be reminded that such enterprises take time, and that if the situation were so easily remediable, it would already have been resolved.

Another critical component in the management of chronic somatization is the setting of appropriate, attainable treatment goals. Here is where a strategy of caring, as opposed to curing, can yield substantive results. Instead of aiming for the total elimination of somatic complaints, one can set as "target goals" such things as a reduction in the number of hospitalizations, diagnostic procedures, emergency room visits, or urgent phone calls to the office, or an increase in the number of social outings. These indirect psychosocial markers, when used on an individual basis of how the patient is doing (as opposed to what he may be saying) can be employed as measures of progress.

References

1. Cummings JL: Neuropsychiatry and the neurobiology of behavior. *In* American Association for Geriatric Psychiatry: Partnerships in Care of the Older Patient. Bethesda, MD, American Association for Geriatric Psychiatry Central Office, 1995.
2. Spar JE, LaRue A: Concise Guide to Geriatric Psychiatry. Washington, DC, American Psychiatric Association, 1990.
3. Rosen J, Mulsant BH, Wright B: Agitation in severely demented patients. Ann Clin Psychiatry 1992;4:207–215.
4. Regier DA, Boyd JH, Burke JD, et al: One-month prevalence of mental disorders in the United States. Arch Gen Psychiatry 1988;45:977–986.
5. American Psychiatry Association: Diagnostic and Statistical Manual of Mental Disorders, 4th ed. Washington, DC, American Psychiatric Association, 1994.
6. Rasmussen SA, Eisen JL: The epidemiology and clinical features of obsessive compulsive disorder. Psychiatr Clin North Am 1992;15:743–758.
7. Howell T: Anxiety Disorders. *In* Reichman WE, Katz PR (eds): Psychiatric Care in the Nursing Home. New York, Oxford University Press, 1996, pp. 94–108.
8. Grossberg GT, Manepalli J: The older patient with psychotic symptoms. Psychiatric Services 1995;46(1):55–59.
9. Reichman WE, Rabins PV: Schizophrenia and other psychotic disorders. *In* Reichman WE, Katz PR (eds): Psychiatric Care in the Nursing Home. New York, Oxford University Press, 1996; pp. 109–117.
10. Omnibus Budget Reconciliation Act of 1987, P.L. 100–203, 101 Stat. 1330.
11. Kaplan C, Lipkin M, Gordon GH: Somatization in primary care. J Gen Intern Med 1988;3:177–190.

Additional Readings

Devanand DP, Levy SR: Neuroleptic treatment of agitation and psychosis in dementia. J Geriatr Psychiatry Neurol 1995; 8(Suppl 1):S18–S27.

Fogel BS, Sadavoy J: Somatoform disorders. *In* Sadavoy J, Lazarus LW, Jarvik LF, et al (eds): Comprehensive Review of Geriatric Psychiatry, II. Washington, DC, American Psychiatric Press, 1996.

Kleinman A: The Illness Narratives. New York, Basic Books, 1988.

Mace NL, Rabins P: The 36-Hour Day. Baltimore, Johns Hopkins University Press, 1991.

Pearlson GD, Petty RG: Late-life-onset psychoses. *In* Coffey CE, Cummings JL (eds): Textbook of Geriatric Neuropsychiatry. Washington, DC, American Psychiatric Press; 1994.

Tariot PN, Schneider LS, Katz IR: Anticonvulsant and other non-neuroleptic treatment of agitation in dementia. J Geriatr Psychiatry Neurol 1995; 8(Suppl 1):S28–S39.

30 Alcohol and Substance Abuse

Wendy Adams, M.D., M.P.H.

THE SCOPE OF THE PROBLEM

The importance of alcohol use and misuse as risk factors for health and social problems among elderly people is becoming increasingly evident. In the 1960s and 1970s, alcoholism was thought by many to be a "self-limiting disease"—that is, people had either died of complications of alcoholism or had stopped drinking by the time they reached old age. In recent years, however, numerous epidemiologic studies have shown the substantial public health impact of alcoholism among older people. It is also evident that heavy drinking often has adverse medical consequences even when a formal diagnosis of alcohol abuse or alcoholism is not warranted. On the other hand, potential health benefits from light and moderate drinking have also been recognized. Recent studies have begun to determine the frequency of both heavy drinking and alcohol use disorders (alcohol abuse and dependence) in this population. Consequences of heavy drinking specific to older people are being explored. Instruments are being developed to improve detection of problem drinking in the older population. Treatment programs tailored to the special needs of older people have been developed in some areas. This chapter reviews the epidemiologic data on the frequency and nature of problem drinking among elderly people, discusses age-related pharmacologic changes that affect the body's handling of alcohol, reviews the clinical presentation and sequelae of alcohol problems in older people, and presents treatment options. The extent and consequences of other substance abuse, which have been studied less extensively than alcohol, are also discussed.

Studies of alcohol use and its adverse consequences have employed varying definitions of the terms "heavy drinking," "problem drinking," "alcoholism," and "alcohol abuse." When reading studies of alcohol problems, it is important to bear in mind that the definition of problem drinking may have a major impact on the results

of the study. For instance, studies that employ a strict definition of alcoholism show lower prevalences than studies that use more relaxed criteria, such as heavy drinking. The term heavy drinking itself may mean one drink per day to some and six drinks per day to others. In the 1980s, standardized criteria for alcohol abuse and alcohol dependence were developed and published in the Diagnostic and Statistical Manual of Mental Disorders, 3rd edition (DSM-III). The fourth edition of this manual (DSM-IV) has now been published and has somewhat revised criteria.[1] Studies that use these standard definitions are much easier to compare with one another. However, it is important to bear in mind that these definitions do not include all persons who suffer harm from their use of alcohol. Regular heavy drinking or binge drinking may cause adverse medical or social consequences even when the DSM-III or -IV criteria are not met.

Alcohol Use and Misuse in the Community

Alcohol has been commonly used throughout recorded history. Long ago, the psalmist gave thanks for "wine to gladden the heart of man."[2] Today, approximately 50% of people aged 65 and older report using alcohol, at least on occasion. There is considerable geographic variation in alcohol consumption, however. In the project known as Established Populations for Epidemiologic Studies in the Elderly (EPESE), for instance, 70% of older people surveyed in East Boston reported drinking alcoholic beverages within a year's time, whereas in rural Iowa only 46% did.[3] The frequency of alcohol use also depends on several other factors, including the age range, the sex ratio, and the general health status of the sample surveyed, as well as the method used to measure alcohol use. In general, samples that include more "older old" people (over 75 years old) show lower alcohol consumption and less alcoholism. In every location, men are more likely than women to drink, to be heavy drinkers, and to be alcoholic. Since people tend to give up alcohol consumption as their health declines, populations with a large proportion of chronically ill or disabled people also usually have less alcohol consumption, though such populations also include a certain number of people whose illness or disability has been caused by heavy alcohol consumption.

Light and moderate drinking are not problematic for the most part and may even have health benefits under some circumstances.[4, 5] Heavy drinking, on the other hand, causes considerable morbidity and mortality. Alcohol use disorders (alcohol abuse or dependence) represent the extreme of drinking that is harmful medically or socially or both. Several population-based studies have examined heavier drinking and alcohol use disorders among elderly people. A summary of several of these is shown in Table 30–1. The most methodologically rigorous population-based study of alcohol problems in elderly people is

part of the Epidemiologic Catchment Area (ECA) study.[6, 7] The prevalence of alcohol abuse and alcoholism by DSM-III criteria in that study ranged from 0% of women in rural North Carolina to 3.7% of men in Baltimore. During a 1-year follow-up period, the ECA study investigators calculated incidence rates (i.e., rates of newly developed cases of alcohol abuse and alcoholism). Though these rates declined with age up to age 60, they began to increase again in both men and women after age 60,[8] and were particularly notable in men aged 75 and older. This increasing incidence in older people is based on a very small number of cases, however, and needs confirmation in additional studies. It is also important to note that the figures from the ECA study represent persons with diagnosable alcohol abuse or alcoholism and do not include all heavy drinkers.

Although alcohol problems continue to have an important impact on the public health of older people, fewer elderly than younger people are heavy drinkers or alcoholics. Probably several factors contribute to this decline. Those who are

---

TABLE 30–1 **HEAVY DRINKING AND ALCOHOL PROBLEMS IN COMMUNITY-BASED STUDIES**

Study	Population	Definition of Problem Drinking		Prevalence		
				Overall	*Men*	*Women*
1. EPESE Cornoni-Huntley[3]	14,461 people aged 65 and older in four geographic locations	≥ 2 drinks per day	East Boston	8.4%	16%	1.6%
			Iowa	5.4%	7.9%	2.4%
			New Haven	6.6%		
			White		12.2%	2.2%
			Nonwhite		9.8%	4.3%
			North Carolina	7.2%		
			White		10.1%	6.0%
			Black		5.9%	2.6%
2. Epidemiologic Catchment Area Study Blazer[6] Myers[7]	805 men and 1305 women aged 65 and older in four separate geographic locations	DSM-III alcohol abuse or dependence	North Carolina			
			Urban		0.9%	0.3%
			Rural		2.0%	0%
			New Haven		3.0%	1.9%
			Baltimore		3.7%	1.7%
			St. Louis		3.0%	1.0%
3. Paganini-Hill[13]	11,888 California retirement community residents aged 60–89	3 or more drinks per day			31%	22%
4. Alexander and Duff[14]	260 retirement community residents, median age 76	2 or more drinks per day		20%		
5. Adams[16]	317 retirement community residents in Wisconsin, median age 83	≥ 1 drink per day		8%		
		CAGE positive		1%		

now elderly have, on average, had lighter drinking habits lifelong (a so-called cohort effect). Also, men have higher mortality rates than women at all ages, so the female-to-male ratio of the population increases with age. Since women of all ages are less likely to use or misuse alcohol, the female predominance of the older population contributes to lower alcohol use overall. As noted earlier, older people often decrease their alcohol intake in response to declining health or functional impairment. In addition, many alcoholics and heavy drinkers do not survive to old age because these people are subject to a high risk of alcohol-related illness and injury.

Despite the lower rate of alcoholism among older people, several studies have described a phenomenon known as late-onset alcoholism.[9, 10] In up to one third of elderly alcoholics undergoing treatment the problem drinking has begun relatively recently. Those who begin to misuse alcohol in old age probably have somewhat different social and medical characteristics from long-term alcoholics who survive into old age.[9–12] Long-term alcoholics often have alienated family members and friends, whereas late-onset problem drinkers may have more intact social resources. For example, in one study of elderly alcoholics in a treatment program, late-onset alcoholics were less likely to be divorced or separated than early-onset alcoholics.[11] This finding has not been consistent in all studies, however, and may vary depending on the group studied. In some cases, late-onset alcohol problems may start as reaction to the losses and stresses associated with aging.

People's living situation and level of socialization probably also affect their drinking habits. As they age, many people move to communities designed specifically for older people, and this change may have an impact on their drinking. Two studies of retirement community samples (see Table 30–1) have shown a very high proportion of heavy drinkers.[13, 14] A third, however, with an older mean age and a larger proportion of women, showed lower rates.[15] In these retirement communities, those with more active social lives were more likely to be heavy drinkers than those who socialized less.

Alcohol Misuse in Medical Settings

Since heavy drinking is known to cause increased morbidity and mortality from illness and injury, it is not surprising to find that the prevalence of alcohol problems is considerably higher in older people in health care settings than in the community. Primary care patients show only a slightly increased prevalence, with 4% to 10% meeting the criteria for current abuse or dependence. Heavy drinking is more common than alcoholism in this setting: In Wisconsin, a recent study of more than 5000 primary care patients over age 60 found that 15% of men and 12% of women drank in excess of recommended limits.[16] Among older emergency room patients, the prevalence of alcohol problems is considerably higher. Two studies using interview methods showed that 14% of elderly emergency room patients were current alcoholics.[17, 18] Another study found that 12.6% of elderly trauma patients in the emergency department had blood alcohol concentrations of more than 100 mg/dL.[19] The prevalence of alcohol problems among hospital inpatients has ranged from 10% to 21%, with consistently higher rates among men than women. Psychiatric settings also show a high frequency of alcohol problems among older adults. In one study of 2309 elderly people referred to a geriatric psychiatry outreach program, 10% were referred for alcohol abuse.[20] In another study, 23% of elderly psychiatric inpatients were found to be alcoholic when interviewed.[21]

Another approach to studying the epidemiology of alcohol problems among elderly inpatients has been to examine hospital discharge diagnoses. This allows the researcher access to a larger number of patients than is feasible in an interview study but almost certainly results in a marked underestimate of the frequency of alcohol abuse and alcoholism. Using this method, two studies have shown a high frequency of alcohol-related hospitalizations among people aged 65 and older.[22, 23] In an analysis of Medicare billing records for the entire United States, the frequency of alcohol-related hospitalizations was slightly higher than the frequency of hospitalizations for myocardial infarction.[23]

Alcohol and drug abuse in nursing homes has been recently reviewed.[24] The prevalence of alcoholism in this setting has ranged from 2.8% to 49%. Studies that make use of patient interviews show a higher frequency than those that depend on chart review for the diagnosis. As in other settings, younger people and men are more likely to be alcoholic. Recently, there has been a trend toward using nursing homes for short-term rehabilitative stays. Because nursing homes serve a larger proportion of acutely ill patients, they are likely to see an increase in the number of alcoholics. The nursing home has the potential to be an excellent setting for the treatment of alcoholism, although few currently offer treatment programs.

The prevalence of alcohol problems among elderly people is higher in those in health care settings than in the general population. This very likely reflects the many kinds of illness and injury known to be associated with alcoholism. Alcohol-related problems seem to be most common in medical settings that provide relatively intense levels of medical care, such as hospitals and emergency departments. Although the prevalence of problem drinking in the general population declines with increasing age, the prevalence of alcohol-related hospitalizations does not. Physicians who care for elderly people must be alert to the possibility that alcohol is contributing to the health problems of these patients.

PHARMACOLOGY

Elderly people have higher blood alcohol levels for the amount of alcohol consumed than do younger people. This is mainly the result of age-related changes in the absorption and distribution of alcohol. Some alcohol is metabolized in the stomach before absorption occurs. This "first pass" effect is caused by the enzyme alcohol dehydrogenase (ADH) in the stomach. With aging, the activity of this enzyme appears to decrease, at least in men, which allows more alcohol to be absorbed.[25] Women may not experience this change, but they have higher blood alcohol levels per amount consumed than men even when younger, in part due to a gender-related difference in gastric ADH activity. Age brings with it an increase in body fat and decreases in lean body mass and total body water. These pharmacologically significant changes in body composition lead to an altered distribution of drugs in the body with increasing age. Drugs that are water soluble, such as alcohol, generally have a smaller volume of distribution because of this phenomenon. The effect, on average, is higher blood levels of alcohol per dose in elderly people than in their younger counterparts.[26]

Hepatic metabolism and renal excretion of alcohol do not appear to be altered in clinically important ways with age. Most alcohol is metabolized in the liver by alcohol dehydrogenase. This hepatic metabolism of alcohol changes little with increasing age. Although most people experience a decline in renal function as they age, less than 5% of alcohol is excreted unchanged, so this effect does not have a major impact on the handling of alcohol. There are few studies of the effects of increasing age on the pharmacodynamic effects of alcohol, but those that have been done show some increasing susceptibility to its psychomotor effects as age increases.[27]

CLINICAL PRESENTATIONS OF PROBLEM DRINKING

How Much Drinking Is Harmful?

Although many studies have focused on alcohol use disorders, it is important for physicians to remember that alcohol consumption can be medically hazardous, even when the drinking behavior does not warrant a formal diagnosis of alcohol abuse or alcoholism. For example, consuming between two and three drinks per day has been shown to increase the risk of hypertension.[28] For women, more than one drink per day may increase the risk of breast cancer; the risk increases with increasing level of alcohol use.[29] The risk of certain other cancers, particularly cancers of the head and neck, increases with consumption of more than two alcoholic drinks per day.[30] In some reports, one to two drinks per day appears to increase the risk of hip fracture,[31-33] though this effect has not been seen in all studies. Because of such complications of moderately heavy drinking, the United States Department of Agriculture, in its *Dietary Guidelines for Americans* (3rd edition), has recommended limiting alcohol consumption to a maximum of two drinks a day for men and one drink a day for women.[34] The United States Preventive Services Task Force suggests that physicians counsel their patients to limit consumption but does not set specific limits on quantity and frequency.[35] Since older people obtain higher blood alcohol levels per drink, lower "safe" limits for consumption may be appropriate. The National Institute of Alcohol Abuse and Alcoholism, in *The Physicians' Guide to Helping Patients with Alcohol Problems*, recommends that older people, male and female, keep consumption to a maximum of one drink per day.[36] When heavy drinking is severe, such well-known medical complications as cirrhosis, gastrointestinal bleeding, pancreatitis, cardiomyopathy, and seizures may develop, and dependence on alcohol is commonly seen. A decline in cognitive and physical function can also result from very heavy alcohol consumption. For some complications of alcohol consumption, the pattern of alcohol use may be more important in determining the risk of illness or injury than the overall quantity consumed. In the National Health and Nutrition Examination Survey follow-up study, for instance, the number of drinks consumed per occasion was an important risk factor for death from injury, whereas frequency of drinking was not.[37] Screening for problem drinking among elderly people clearly should aim to detect those whose alcohol use puts them at risk for medical problems whether or not they meet criteria for alcohol abuse or alcoholism.

The amount of drinking that is safe may be much lower when medications are used concurrently. More than 75% of people aged 65 and older use medications. Of the drugs most commonly used by older people, many have the potential to interact adversely with alcohol. Even light or moderate drinking can be problematic when alcohol is consumed concurrently with certain medications. The reader is referred to a recent review for a more comprehensive discussion of drug-alcohol interactions.[38] Some of the most worrisome include the inhibition of gastric alcohol dehydrogenase by cimetidine, ranitidine, and nizatidine, which results in blood alcohol levels that are 30% to 40% higher than those seen after an equal amount of alcohol alone. Even in the absence of these drugs, elderly people have higher blood alcohol levels than younger people because of the mechanisms discussed earlier. A further increase due to an interaction with one of these drugs may cause an unwitting elderly person to experience unexpectedly severe effects from a small amount of alcohol. Other drugs commonly used by older people also have the potential for adverse interactions with alcohol. Concurrent use of benzodiazepines and other agents that suppress central nervous system functions may impair balance and predispose to falls, cause slower reaction times and lead to an automobile accident, or cause excessive sleepiness. Nonsteroidal anti-inflammatory drugs, when used concurrently with alcohol, cause longer bleeding times and increased gastric inflammation. Warfarin dosing can be extremely difficult when a patient is drinking alcohol. Because of these and other potential drug-alcohol interactions, a discussion of the possible interactions of drugs with alcohol should be a regular part of the education of patients about their medicines.

Symptoms of Alcoholism

Traditionally, hallmark symptoms of alcoholism include tolerance to alcohol, symptoms of withdrawal, loss of control of drinking behavior, and social decline. Specific diagnostic criteria can be found in the fourth edition of the *Diagnostic and Statistical Manual of Mental Disorders* (DSM-IV).[1] These features of alcoholism may present atypically in elderly people, which can make the diagnosis challenging. For instance, *tolerance* is usually described as a requirement for more alcohol to achieve the same effect as that occurring previously with a smaller amount. This phenomenon is largely the result of the increased rate of alcohol metabolism that occurs when liver enzyme activity is induced by regular heavy alcohol use. Because older people have higher blood alcohol levels per drink, however, they may quite honestly require less alcohol to achieve the same effect, even though they have the same liver enzyme induction that causes tolerance in younger people. *Withdrawal* symptoms are similar in older people but are often mistaken for other medical conditions. Elderly people may experience such early symptoms of withdrawal as tremulousness, tachycardia, and tachypnea as well as more severe withdrawal symptoms such as delirium, seizures, and hallucinosis. A common scenario is the older alcoholic person who has been hospitalized for surgery and has not had access to alcohol for a couple of days. When tremulousness, tachypnea, and hypertension develop, alcohol withdrawal is often low on the list of suspected causes. While it is certainly appropriate to keep myocardial infarction, infection, or pulmonary embolus high on the differential diagnosis list in such a situation, alcohol withdrawal must also be considered. *Loss of control* of drinking behavior may be subtle in older people. Since each drink beyond the number intended causes a greater increment in the blood alcohol level than in younger people, older drinkers are less likely to consume extremely large quantities. Finally, *social decline* may present differently in older people. Since they are less likely to be working or driving, older problem drinkers are less likely to be recognized by employers or the police. Social decline may therefore present as decreased interest in activities that were previously pleasurable, poor self-care, malnutrition, or failure to thrive.

Contribution to Medical Illness and "Geriatric Syndromes"

No organ system is indifferent to the effects of alcohol. The impact of alcoholism on medical illness has been extensively reviewed elsewhere,[39] and details are beyond the scope of this chapter. Among elderly people, in whom problematic drinking is less likely to be detected by the social and legal systems that often uncover it in younger people, alcoholism may be particularly likely to present with medical illness. There appears to be somewhat less alcohol-related trauma among older people, however. Common clues to unrecognized alcoholism in medical practice include frequent gastrointestinal disturbances, trouble in controlling hypertension or diabetes, peripheral neuropathy, unexplained seizures, or difficulty in adjusting the dose of warfarin or phenytoin. Liver enzyme induction, expressed by elevated gamma glutamyl transferase (GGT), or elevated mean red blood cell corpuscular volume (MCV) should also raise a suspicion of heavy drinking.

Alcoholism among elderly people has often been described as a hidden problem that masquerades as syndromes that are common in nonalcoholic elderly patients. Indeed, alcoholism may either cause or contribute to most geriatric syndromes. For instance, urinary incontinence is often exacerbated by the rapid bladder filling caused by alcohol's inhibition of antidiuretic hormone. Alcohol's effects on neuromuscular control of bladder function have yet to be clearly elucidated. Gait disturbances may result from alcohol-induced cerebellar degeneration, peripheral neuropathy, or acute intoxication. Heavy drinking increases the risk of depression and suicide. Alcohol interferes with normal sleep and can contribute to insomnia. Dementia, a great scourge of elderly people, usually has a relentlessly progressive course, and alcoholism has proved to be one of the most common causes of truly reversible dementia. Although not all alcohol-related dementia can be reversed, it is clearly incumbent on physicians to make every effort to help affected persons achieve abstinence. It is evident that heavy drinking should be kept in the differential diagnostic list for most geriatric syndromes. Further research is needed, however, to clarify how often alcohol contributes to these syndromes and the extent to which abstinence contributes to an improvement in function.

SCREENING AND DIAGNOSIS

Once cognizant of the need to retain alcohol use disorders in the differential diagnosis for many medical problems, the need for good tools to detect these disorders is apparent. Good history-taking is of the essence. Standardized questionnaires can be used, and several have been developed to screen patients for alcoholism. Unfortunately, most have been based on the behavior of young men and may not be applicable to older people. Some are too lengthy to be practical in clinical situations. Probably the most useful screening tool for use in a busy medical practice is the four-item CAGE questionnaire. The CAGE questionnaire consists of four questions about drinking practices: Have you ever thought you should *C*ut down on drinking? Have people *A*nnoyed you by complaining about your drinking? Have you felt *G*uilty about your drinking? Have you ever taken an *E*yeopener to get going in the morning? The CAGE questionnaire has been tested in older people in the primary care setting and has showed good sensitivity and specificity compared to a formal diagnosis of alcoholism based on DSM-III criteria.[40, 41] These questions can be asked in an interview or embedded in a self-administered screening instrument, such as the ones many physicians use for preliminary medical and social history-taking.

Screening instruments do a good job at detecting those with alcohol use disorders. They are unlikely, however, to detect nondependent heavy drinkers who are at risk of medical complications. In medical practice, detection of these heavy drinkers is also tremendously important if reducing alcohol-related morbidity and mortality is the goal. For instance, people who consume three drinks daily are clearly at risk of hypertension and certain cancers, though few would be diagnosed as alcoholic. It is incumbent on practicing physicians to intervene in this situation by warning patients of the health risks incurred by such drinking. For screening purposes, therefore, questions about the quantity and frequency of alcohol consumption should be asked in addition to the CAGE questions. The National Institute of Alcohol Abuse and Alcoholism recommends asking the following three questions: "On average, how many days per week do you drink alcohol? On a typical day when you drink, how many drinks do you have? What is the maximum number of drinks you have had on any given occasion in the last month?"[36] When discussing the quantity and frequency of drinking, questions that specify the type of alcoholic beverage (e.g., beer, wine, or liquor) may elicit more information than less specific questions. It is also important to clarify the quantity of alcohol meant by the term "a drink" because definitions of that term vary.

When screening questions suggest the presence of an alcohol problem or when the physician is concerned about alcohol use for other reasons, further history-taking is indicated. Asking about symptoms of alcoholism, such as loss of control of drinking behavior, tolerance to alcohol, a history of withdrawal symptoms, or previous treatment for alcoholism, may be enlightening. Information about adverse consequences of drinking should be elicited, such as citations for driving while intoxicated, family disturbances, and alcohol-related illness or injury. Sometimes patients are not forthcoming about sensitive issues such as alcohol misuse until a trusting relationship with the physician has been developed. Nonjudgmental questioning about drinking behavior, along with an explanation of the reason for concern, may have to be repeated at several office visits before valuable information is elicited. Persistent, patient efforts at history-taking are therefore well worthwhile.

Sometimes information from sources other than the patient can be useful. Among older alcoholics, cognitive impairment is particularly common and can make history-taking especially difficult. Talking with family members, close friends, or caregivers is essential when one is evaluating the drinking behavior of a cognitively impaired person. Information from others can also be very helpful when a cognitively intact alcoholic denies problematic drinking. Usually, however, unless cognitive impairment exists, the patient will be a more reliable source than family members. It must also be kept in mind that alcoholism is often a family phenomenon, and alcoholic family members sometimes help the patient avoid detection of problem drinking.

In general, laboratory tests are not good screening tools for alcoholism, though under certain circumstances they can be useful diagnostic adjuncts. A blood alcohol level higher than 100 mg per dL in a patient with no signs of intoxication is a good indication of tolerance to alcohol and usually does indicate alcoholism. When a physician suspects alcohol problems in a patient who denies drinking heavily, the constellation of elevated GGT values, which indicate induction of liver enzymes, and elevated MCV supports the physician's suspicion and may be useful in presenting the patient with the possibility that alcohol is damaging his or her health. However, although GGT and MCV may be elevated more commonly in older than younger alcoholic patients, they are also commonly elevated in nonalcoholic elderly people. Other laboratory values that are often elevated in heavy drinkers include uric acid and blood glucose, which are also commonly elevated in nonalcoholic elderly people. New tests, such as carbohydrate-deficient transferrin and hemoglobin-acetaldehyde adducts, are being developed to screen for alcoholism. These tests may prove useful in the future, but none are yet sensitive or specific enough for use or readily available.

TREATMENT

Treatment by Primary Care Physicians

An exciting development in the treatment of problem drinking in recent years has been recognition of the effectiveness of physician brief intervention. Randomized trials have shown that brief counseling by primary care physicians can result in a significant reduction in alcohol consumption as well as improvements in hypertension control and liver function tests.[42, 43] Essential elements of such intervention include education about current and potential adverse effects of the patient's drinking and specific recommendations for limits on drinking. Many heavy drinkers do not realize that the amount of alcohol they consume is unusual or potentially harmful. Specific information about the risks of the current level of alcohol consumption should be communicated. If adverse consequences of the drinking already exist, these should be pointed out clearly

and the relation between the drinking and the health problem confirmed in no uncertain terms. If there are coexisting psychosocial problems that seem to be contributing to the perceived need for alcohol, recommendations for more effective coping strategies or referrals for more lengthy counseling should be made. If chronic pain is a factor, more effective pain management should be instituted.

It is often important to educate family members and caregivers as well as patients themselves about the consequences of problem drinking. Loved ones may be inclined to allow an older relative "her last pleasure in life" without realizing that drinking at a level that contributes to dementia, incontinence, depression, or gait disturbances is not, in fact, pleasurable. Firm advice to loved ones about the harmful effects of the drinking and the benefits of abstinence can be of immeasurable value.

Treating Alcohol Withdrawal

Treating alcohol withdrawal in elderly people follows the same basic principles as treating withdrawal in younger people. Older people are probably more susceptible to both delirium and medical complications during withdrawal, however, and may require a longer time for detoxification. Because of the potential for complications, it is generally advisable to effect detoxification in the hospital. Various medications have been proposed for treating alcohol withdrawal, but benzodiazepines are still the mainstay because they offer the optimal combination of effectiveness and safety. The long-acting benzodiazepines, such as chlordiazepoxide and diazepam, have extremely long half-lives in older people and may cause prolonged sedation or delirium. Short-acting benzodiazepines, such as lorazepam or oxazepam, are therefore preferable. Thiamine should be administered prophylactically to prevent Wernicke's syndrome. Attention to other nutritional deficiencies, fluid and electrolyte balance, and concurrent medical conditions is essential.

Treatment Programs for Elderly Alcoholics

Many people, especially those with severe alcohol dependence, will benefit from formal alcohol treatment programs. Programs designed especially for older people are probably more appealing to them and appear to increase the likelihood that the patient will complete the treatment.[44] Most communities do not have special treatment programs for older people, however, and outcomes for older people in mixed age programs are as good as those of their younger counterparts. Approximately 50% are abstinent 1 year after treatment. In the absence of special programs, it is important for the referring physician to investigate which existing programs are best able to meet the needs of elderly alcoholics. Medical complications and concurrent medical illnesses are more common and more complex in the older population. A somewhat different pattern of concurrent psychiatric illness is seen, there being more depression and cognitive impairment and fewer personality disorders.[9] A different array of social issues is important to older alcoholics. Some need help in coping with retirement and the consequent changes in life role. For others, help in dealing with grief may be critical. An investigation into which local treatment programs are most effective at meeting these special needs of older people may improve the success of referrals. After formal treatment or in lieu of it, Alcoholics Anonymous and other nonprofessional treatment programs can offer tremendous benefits to many older alcoholics.

For alcoholics with dementia, a different approach, which often includes a change of living situation, is needed. Rarely are these patients able to maintain abstinence unless access to alcohol is restricted. Because cognitive impairment may take several months to improve, a long-term alcohol-free residential setting is ideal. For many patients this will mean nursing home placement because long-term treatment programs are hard to come by in most communities.

Management of Alcoholics Resistant to Treatment

When efforts at brief counseling or formal treatment are not successful, care for the patient is still needed. Just as many people with lung disease continue to smoke and many diabetics do not control their diets, many alcoholics are unable to stop drinking. Although caring for these patients is frustrating for the physician, high-quality care is important and beneficial. Alcoholism is best approached as a chronic illness. For patients with most chronic diseases, cures are not expected. Instead, strategies to manage the disease, effect remissions, and minimize suffering are adopted. Optimal care requires consideration of the person's emotional and social needs as well as medical needs. When the disease is terminal, the person may need help in dealing with concerns about dying, getting affairs in order, and making decisions about what medical interventions are desirable under various circumstances. Many of these principles apply to long-

term management of alcoholism. Several components of good primary care for alcoholics who continue to drink despite treatment efforts can be identified. Continued counseling about the benefits of decreasing alcohol intake is important. It may be beneficial to set intermediate goals for reducing alcohol intake, although abstinence remains the ultimate goal for dependent alcoholics. Feedback about biologic indicators of alcohol-induced harm, such as blood pressure, MCV, or GGT can be helpful. Managing medical complications optimally and addressing psychosocial concerns compassionately are also important. Combined with aggressive nursing and social work interventions, such a program may decrease mortality and improve the quality of life for resistant alcoholic patients.[45]

ABUSE OF OTHER SUBSTANCES

The use of substances other than alcohol may also have adverse medical or social consequences or lead to dependence. Tobacco dependence is the only substance-related disorder that is more common than alcoholism. Morbidity and mortality associated with tobacco-related illness are enormous, and the benefits of smoking cessation among elderly people have been well documented. Physician counseling is very effective in helping people quit smoking and should be employed at every opportunity. Illegal drug use, although problematic in younger populations, is uncommon among elderly people. Harm related to the use of prescription and over-the-counter drugs, on the other hand, is not at all uncommon. Benzodiazepines and opiates are the categories of drugs most likely to cause trouble. Because opiate abuse and dependence in this population have been very little studied, this section will concentrate on the most problematic of psychoactive prescription drugs, the benzodiazepines.

Up to 20% of older people use benzodiazepines.[46] In contrast to alcohol use, which is more common among men and younger people, benzodiazepine use is more common among older people and women. Misuse in the sense of using more of the drug than prescribed is probably uncommon. Surveys suggest that most people for whom these drugs are prescribed either use them as directed or use less than directed. However, tolerance, dependence, and adverse consequences may develop even when these drugs are used as directed.

Tolerance to the anxiolytic effects of benzodiazepines is not usually problematic, but tolerance to the hypnotic effects is common. People who use these drugs for insomnia are therefore likely to require increasing doses to induce sleep and are probably more prone to dependence than people who take them for anxiety. Although high doses and long duration of use increase the risk of dependence, it can occur with relatively low levels of use; as little as 6 to 10 mg per day of diazepam or the equivalent may cause dependence in as short a time as 1 to 2 months. Such low-level dependence is probably relatively asymptomatic unless withdrawal occurs. Withdrawal symptoms may be mild, consisting of anxiety, irritability, and tremulousness, or more severe, comprising hallucinations, delirium, and seizures. Even if withdrawal symptoms do not occur, recurrence of the symptoms for which the drug was originally prescribed is common when the drug is stopped. "Rebound" symptoms, including anxiety and insomnia that are more severe than the original symptoms, may also occur.

Toxicity may also occur with prescribed doses of benzodiazepines. Because the half-lives of some benzodiazepines are extremely long in older people, the drug may gradually accumulate in the body to produce a toxic state. When an excessive amount of the drug is present, benzodiazepines may cause such symptoms as slurred speech, ataxia, and delirium. The use of long-acting benzodiazepines also increases the risk of falls and hip fracture markedly.

Management of benzodiazepine dependence is sometimes difficult. People are often reluctant to give up these drugs. If a long-acting benzodiazepine is being used, initial management should include a change to a shorter-acting drug without active metabolites, such as lorazepam. The shorter-acting drugs are less likely to cause falls and fractures, so this step alone will be beneficial to the patient. The dose can then be gradually tapered. At the same time, one should attempt to institute nonpharmacologic approaches to such problems as insomnia or anxiety for which the drug was prescribed. A search for undiagnosed depression is especially important in managing benzodiazepine-dependent patients because depression is quite common among elderly users of these substances and is optimally treated by antidepressant medication or psychotherapy.

SUMMARY

Alcohol problems occur frequently among elderly patients receiving medical care. They range in severity from moderately heavy drinking to severe alcohol abuse or dependence. Because of the morbidity and mortality associated with such problems, screening patients is highly worthwhile. Counseling interventions by physicians have been shown to be effective, especially for nondependent heavy drinkers. For more severely alcohol-dependent patients, formal treatment programs are often successful. The use of other substances may also have adverse consequences. Benzodiazepine use is particularly common among elderly people and may cause dependence or toxicity even at levels of use sanctioned by physicians. In all patients with substance-related problems, it is essential for the physician to become aware of the substance use, assess the potential or actual harm caused by the substance, and address the issue with the patient. Substance use disorders are often chronic and require ongoing attention from physicians.

References

1. American Psychiatric Association: Diagnostic and Statistical Manual of Mental Disorders, 4th ed. Washington, DC, American Psychiatric Association, 1994.
2. Psalm 104:15.
3. Cornoni-Huntley J, Brock DB, Ostfeld AM, Taylor JO, Wallace RB: Established Populations for Epidemiologic Studies of the Elderly. NIH Publication No. 86-2443 Washington, DC, U.S. Department of Health and Human Services, National Institutes of Health, 1986, pp. 196–199.
4. Klatsky AL: Alcohol and mortality. Ann Intern Med 1992;117:646–654.
5. Rimm EB, Giovannucci EL, Willett WC, Colditz GA, Ascherio A, Rosner B, Stampfer MJ: Prospective study of alcohol consumption and risk of coronary disease in men. Lancet 1991;338:464–468.
6. Blazer D, Crowell BA, George LK: Alcohol abuse and dependence in the rural South. Arch Gen Psychiatry 1987;44:736–740.
7. Myers JK, Weissman MM, Tischler GL, Holzer CE, Leaf PJ, Orvaschel H, Anthony JC, et al: Six month prevalence of psychiatric disorders in three communities. Arch Gen Psychiatry 1984;41:959–967.
8. Eaton WW, Kramer M, Anthony JC, Dryman A, Shapiro S, Locke BZ: The incidence of specific DIS/DSM-III mental disorders: Data from the NIMH Epidemiologic Catchment Area program. Acta Psychiatr Scand 1989;79:163–178.
9. Finlayson RE, Hurt RD, Davis LJ, Morse RM: Alcoholism in elderly persons: A study of the psychiatric and psychosocial features of 216 inpatients. Mayo Clin Proc 1988;63:761–768.
10. Atkinson RM, Tolson RL, Turner JA: Late versus early onset problem drinking in older men. Alcoholism: Clin Exp Res 1990;14:574–579.
11. Hurt RD, Finlayson RE, Morse RM, Davis LJ: Alcoholism in elderly persons: Medical aspects and prognosis of 216 inpatients. Mayo Clin Proc 1988;63:753–760.
12. Schonfeld L, Dupree LW: Antecedents of drinking for early and late-onset elderly alcohol abusers. J Stud Alcohol 1991;52:587–592.
13. Paganini-Hill A, Ross RK, Henderson BE: Prevalence of chronic disease and health practices in a retirement community. J Chron Dis 1986;39:699–707.
14. Alexander F, Duff RW: Social interaction and alcohol use in retirement communities. Gerontologist 1988;28:632–636.
15. Adams WL: Alcohol use in retirement communities. J Am Geriatr Soc 1996;44:1082–1085.

16. Adams WL, Barry KL, Fleming MF: Screening for alcohol problems in older primary care patients. JAMA 1996;276:1964–1967.

17. Adams WL, Magruder-Habib K, Trued S, Broome HL: Alcohol abuse in elderly emergency department patients. J Am Geriatr Soc 1992;40:1236–1240.

18. Tabisz E, Badger M, Meatherall R, Jacyk WR, Fuchs D, Grymonpre R: Identification of chemical abuse in the elderly admitted to emergency. Clin Gerontol 1991;11:27–39.

19. Rivara FP, Jurkovich GJ, Gurney JG, Seguin D, Fligner CL, Ries R, Raisys VA, Copass M: The magnitude of acute and chronic alcohol abuse in trauma patients. Arch Surg 1993;128:907–913.

20. Reifler BV, Kethley A, O'Neill P, Hanley R, Lewis S, Stenchever D: Five-year experience of a community outreach program for the elderly. Am J Psychiatry 1982;139:220–223.

21. Simon A, Epstein LJ, Reynolds L: Alcoholism in the geriatric mentally ill. Geriatrics 1968;23:125–131.

22. Stinson FS, Dufour MC, Bertolucci D: Alcohol-related morbidity in the aging population. Alcohol Health Res World 1989;13:80–87.

23. Adams WL, Yuan Z, Barboriak JJ, Rimm AA: Alcohol-related hospitalizations in elderly people: Prevalence and geographic variation in the United States. JAMA 1993;270:1222–1225.

24. Joseph CL: Alcohol and drug misuse in the nursing home. Int J Addictions 1995;30:1953–1984.

25. Seitz HK, Simanowski UA, Waldherr R, Eckey R, Agarwal DP, Goedde HW, von Wartburg JP: Human gastric alcohol dehydrogenase activity: Effect of age, sex, and alcoholism. Gut 1993;34:1433–1437.

26. Vestal RE, McGuire EA, Tobin JD, et al: Aging and ethanol metabolism. Clin Pharmacol Ther 1976;21:343–354.

27. Vogel-Sprott M, Barrett P: Age, drinking habits and the effects of alcohol. J Stud Alcohol 1984;45:517–521.

28. MacMahon S: Alcohol consumption and hypertension. Hypertension 1987;9:111–121.

29. Longnecker MP: Alcoholic beverage consumption in relation to risk of breast cancer: Meta-analysis and review. Cancer Causes Control 1994;5:73–82.

30. Longnecker MP: Alcohol consumption and risk of cancer in humans: An overview. Alcohol 1995;12:87–96.

31. Felson DT, Kiel DP, Anderson JJ, Kannel WB: Alcohol consumption and hip fractures: The Framingham Study. Am J Epidemiol 1988;128:1102–1110.

32. Hemenway D, Colditz GA, Willett WC, et al: Fractures and lifestyle: Effect of cigarette smoking, alcohol intake, and relative weight on the risk of hip and forearm fractures in middle aged women. Am J Public Health 1988;78:1554–1558.

33. Hernandez-Avila M, Colditz GA, Stampfer MJ, Rosner B, Speizer FE, Willett WC: Caffeine, moderate alcohol intake, and risk of fractures of the hip and forearm in middle-aged women. Am J Clin Nutr 1991;54:157–163.

34. U.S. Department of Agriculture and U.S. Department of Health and Human Services: Nutrition and your health: Dietary guidelines for Americans, Dietary Guidelines for Americans, 3rd ed. Washington, DC, U.S. Departments of Agriculture and Health and Human Services, 1990.

35. U.S. Preventive Services Task Force: Guide to Clinical Preventive Services, 2nd ed. Baltimore, Williams & Wilkins, 1996, pp. 575–578.

36. National Institute of Alcohol Abuse and Alcoholism: The Physician's Guide to Helping Patients with Alcohol Problems. NIH Publication No. 95-3769. Washington, DC, U.S. Department of Health and Human Services, National Institutes of Health, 1995.

37. Anda RF, Williamson DF, Remington PL: Alcohol and fatal injuries among U.S. adults. JAMA 1988;260:2529–2532.

38. Adams WL: Interactions between alcohol and medications. Int J Addictions 1995;30:1679–1699.

39. Lieber CS (ed): Medical and Nutritional Complications of Alcoholism: Mechanisms and Management. New York, Plenum, 1992.

40. Buchsbaum DG, Buchanan RG, Welsh J, Centor RM, Schnoll SH: Screening for drinking disorders in the elderly using the CAGE questionnaire. J Am Geriatr Soc 1992;40:662–665.

41. Jones TV, Lindsey BA, Yount P, Soltys R, Farani-Enayat B: Alcoholism screening questionnaires: Are they valid in elderly medical outpatients? J Gen Intern Med 1993;8:674–678.

42. Wallace P, Cutler S, Haines A: Randomised controlled trial of general practitioner intervention in patients with excessive alcohol consumption. Br Med J 1988;297:663–668.

43. Kristenson H, Ohlin H, Hulten-Nosslin MB, Trell E, Hood B: Identification and intervention of heavy drinking in middle-aged men: Results and follow-up of 24–60 months of long-term study with randomized control. Alcohol Clin Exp Res 1983;7(2):203–208.

44. Kofoed LL, Tolson RL, Atkinson RM, Toth RL, Turner JA: Treatment compliance of older alcoholics: An elder-specific approach is superior to "mainstreaming." J Stud Alcohol 1987;48:47–51.

45. Willenbring ML, Olson DH, Bielinski J: Integrated outpatient treatment for medically ill alcoholic men: Results from a quasi-experimental study. J Stud Alcohol 1995;56:337–343.

46. Mayer-Oakes SA, Kelman G, Beers M, DeJong F, Matthias R, Atchison K, Lubben J, Schweitzer S: Benzodiazepine use in older community-dwelling southern Californians: Prevalence and clinical correlates. Ann Pharmacother 1993;27:416–421.

31 Nervous System Disease

Raymond J. Baddour, M.D.

Leslie Wolfson, M.D.

In the past century, life expectancy has increased from 50 to 75 years. In an aging society, disorders of the nervous system are becoming increasingly important in producing functional incapacity. This has made the recognition, evaluation, and treatment of these conditions of real clinical importance. This chapter begins with a review of some age-related changes in function to make the disease-related changes that follow more meaningful.

THE NEUROLOGY OF AGING: NORMAL VERSUS PATHOLOGIC CHANGE

Awareness of the effects of age on the nervous system is fundamental because it is the basis for determining the presence of disease. Age-related changes are additive to disease in producing functional incapacity. Knowledge of what constitutes normal and abnormal function is critical in deciding when medical evaluation is indicated.

Age-related changes in cognitive and sensorimotor function should not interfere with everyday activities. Elderly patients frequently complain of memory and learning deficits, difficulty in recalling names, and poor short-term recall, although the cognitive decline that occurs in normal aging is modest. Short-term recall is the function that is most impaired and requires otherwise intact older persons to devise adaptive strategies (e.g., making lists). By contrast, dementias produce maladaptive decline, and functional independence is ultimately lost.

Cognitive Function

Verbal intelligence peaks in the third decade and then remains stable until the eighth decade. Language function (e.g., vocabulary and comprehension) is generally well preserved, and deficits noted on routine examination should prompt for-

mal mental status evaluation. Psychomotor skills that are speed based (i.e., finger tapping or mental calculation) peak at age 20 and show a steady decline thereafter. Personality changes are unusual in healthy older persons (less than 10% have them), and therefore the possibility of underlying brain dysfunction should be considered in patients who demonstrate such changes (e.g., depression).[1] Although personality change is unusual as a presenting symptom, 80% of patients with Alzheimer's disease experience such changes during the course of the illness.

Sensory Function

Age-related alterations in vision and hearing commence in the third decade. Visual acuity decreases because of degeneration of photoreceptors, presbyopia results from diminished lens accommodation, and cataracts occur. Also, pupillary size is decreased, pupillary response to light and accommodation is sluggish, and upgaze is restricted. Hearing changes do not become significant until after the age of 65, but presbycusis is found in approximately 40% of people over the age of 75.[2] Patients often complain of an inability to understand speech. This can be attributed to both cochlear degeneration and slowed central processing of auditory information.

Clinical and psychophysiologic measurement studies have demonstrated modest age-related decrements in pain and thermal sensitivity, tactile sensation, two-point discrimination, joint position sense, and stereognosis. By contrast, diminished vibratory perception is encountered in more than half of older persons and is of much greater magnitude. This loss of vibratory sensation is much greater than losses of other large-fiber sensory modalities and thus may be caused by receptor changes, although loss of large myelinated sensory fibers of the peripheral nerves remains a possible explanation.

Motor Function

Visual, vestibular, and tactile-proprioceptive data form the inward portrayal of a person's location, movement, and environment and are therefore central to the motor skills that support balance. Age-related changes in these primary sensory modalites are well documented, although they are not of sufficient magnitude to seriously compromise locomotion. Changes in sensory function are not without consequences because they influence the occurrence of sensory misperception, which may be an important factor in causing falls. Furthermore, decreased sensory input may influence our ability to produce an effective balance response. Interpretation of sensory input and the choice of a motor response, termed sensorimotor processing, is influenced by the number and complexity of choices as well as by increasing age.[3] The time needed to perform complex choice reaction tasks in older persons increases more than that needed for simple tasks. Although they increase with age, afferent and efferent transmission times are not responsible for the bulk of the increases in processing time.[3] Changes in sensorimotor processing time or its effectiveness under adverse or complex conditions (e.g., with limited or inappropriate sensory information or in the presence of a severe hazard) may thus be of practical importance in relation to mobility.

Cross-sectional studies show a decrement in strength from young adulthood to older adulthood of 20% to 40%, which is even greater than the losses in muscle mass observed.[4, 5] Age-related loss of strength is probably unimportant for routine activities but could be a factor in the greater strength demanded when swift responses are necessary to act on environmental hazards.

Most older adults have diminished ankle jerks, but otherwise deep tendon reflexes are only modestly decreased, and plantar responses are typically unaffected by age. Conversely, brisk ankle reflexes with clonus accompanied by extensor plantar responses suggest pyramidal tract dysfunction. The occurrence of reflexes such as palmomental and snout reflexes increases with advancing age, but they are of limited diagnostic use.

Essential tremor, which frequently involves the distal upper extremities and head, is common in older persons. The tremor is maximal when a position is maintained by the involved parts (i.e., postural tremor). When the tremor results in physical disability or social embarrassment, treatment with beta-blockers is warranted.

Balance

Under conditions of quiet standing, sway as a measure of balance is only marginally greater in older adults than in younger persons.[6] By comparison, the extent of one's ability to lean in the anteroposterior plane (i.e., the limit of sway or the functional base of support) decreases by about a third from the third to the eighth decades.[7] Similarly, during this age span, the ability to stand on one leg decreases from more than 30 seconds to slightly less than 15 seconds.[8] Finally, under test conditions with limited sensory input (one modality) or with a vigorous perturbation, older persons lose their balance much more frequently than younger persons, although both groups adapt effectively during repetitive testing.[6] Thus, quiet standing is associated with marginal changes in balance, although activity may push an older person toward the limit of stable stance, thereby activating responses to maintain posture. Under most conditions, the balance of older persons functions effectively and can even improve with repetitive testing. By contrast, the dysfunctional balance associated with impaired mobility is of such magnitude that it can only result from age-related diseases. Furthermore, frequent losses of balance in older persons during testing under challenging conditions (limited sensory input or vigorous perturbation) suggest that these modest age-related decrements may be an element in the increased occurrence of falls in older people.[6] We conclude that age-related balance decrements are analogous to those of other central nervous system (CNS)–dependent functions (e.g., cognition) that do not by themselves lead to significant compromise of function (e.g., immobility).

NEUROLOGIC EVALUATION

In older persons, in addition to a general neurologic assessment one must often evaluate cognition as well as the sensorimotor skills required for mobility. The evaluation of patients with cognitive impairment is described in Chapter 26, as well as in numerous other sources. The key elements of an evaluation suitable for patients with mobility disorders are described in the following paragraphs.

Mental status should be evaluated in these patients because it may be an indication of a degenerative or multifocal disease. For similar reasons, the cranial nerves should be carefully tested. How should a clinician approach the evaluation of sensorimotor function? Strength assessment (i.e., manual motor testing) is particularly difficult in older persons because of the age-related changes noted earlier as well as differences in gender and activity levels. To assist in interpreting manual motor test results examiners should compare muscle groups within the same patient (e.g., left versus right or proximal versus distal). Atrophy of intrinsic hand muscles that is unassociated with weakness or other neurologic dysfunction is also frequently present. Due to these problems, functional testing of the motor system is particularly useful in evaluating the strength of older persons.

Functional motor testing should include the following exercises:

1. Rising from a low chair without using the arms. This exercise tests hip and knee extensor strength and balance.
2. Standing on heels and toes. This maneuver tests dorsi and plantar extension strength and balance.
3. Performing a single, tandem, or semitandem stance. Such a stance tests lower extremity strength and balance (e.g., 10 seconds of single stance are normal for an 80-year-old).
4. Graded forward and backward pushes. Pushes test balance. Subjects should always be pulled toward the examiner.
5. Gait and turns. This exercise tests all facets of sensorimotor function and mobility skills. The examiner should observe for patterned dysfunction (e.g., lurches during walking and multistep turns suggest a balance disorder).

Other components of motor function should be assessed as well (tone, coordination, rapid alternating movements, and the presence of intention, postural, or resting tremor). If cognitive function is intact, sensory testing should not be difficult. Age-related changes in pin, touch, joint position sense, and stereognosis are modest. Lower extremity sensory function is an important component in maintaining mobility and balance. The deep tendon reflexes of older persons become less reactive, and the ankle jerk sometimes cannot be elicited.[9] Brisk reflexes and ankle clonus are unusual in older persons. Their existence should lead the clinician to suspect lesions of the pyramidal neurons or tracts. The presence of extensor plantar responses (Babinski's signs) should be similarly interpreted. The frequency of snout and palmomental reflexes doubles between the fifth and ninth decades.[10] These frontal lobe release signs may be present in otherwise normal older persons, and therefore their significance is uncertain. Evaluation of older patients requires medical assessment as well as neurologic evaluation. The examiner should keep in mind that arthritis can produce a surprising amount of immobility, although pain and joint dysfunction usually make this diagnosis evident.

In the sections that follow a number of neuro-logic disorders with significant impact on older persons are reviewed. For certain conditions, specifically those relating to movement disorders and vascular disease, the reader is referred to Chapters 32 and 33, respectively, for a more detailed discussion.

DISORDERS OF MOBILITY

Ischemic White Matter Disease

It is common for persons in their eighth or ninth decade to experience progressive impairments in gait and balance. Frequently, the pattern of gait and balance dysfunction suggests a bifrontal syndrome. The gait of these patients consists of small steps with the feet adhering to the floor (magnetic gait). Balance is severely impaired. Bradykinesia and rigidity are often present. There may be associated urinary dysfunction as well as slowed cognitive processing, although dementia, if present, is mild. It is likely that this syndrome is caused by the presence of subcortical lesions that compromise the complex frontal processing required for gait and balance. The combination of signs and symptoms can be difficult to distinguish from parkinsonism, and often these patients receive an unsuccessful trial of L-dopa.

The causes of the bifrontal syndrome include ischemic small vessel disease, bilateral frontal disease (e.g., tumor) and normal pressure hydrocephalus. Ischemic small vessel disease involving the subcortical frontal white matter is associated with increased age, hypertension, and the occurrence of silent strokes.[11] The patient develops a progressive bifrontal syndrome that evolves over a period of years. Several studies have demonstrated a relationship between white matter lesions demonstrated on computed tomography (CT) or magnetic resonance imaging (MRI) and impaired gait and balance.[12, 13] A recent clinico-pathologic correlative study determined that these lesions may represent astrocytosis within the white matter that the authors suggest may be activated by localized ischemic changes.[14] Although the pathology described in this study does not clearly indicate a cause for the white matter lesions, localized ischemia fits with clinical and pathologic data and thus is a logical point of departure.

Normal Pressure Hydrocephalus

There are patients with hydrocephalus associated with gait disturbance, dementia, and urinary incontinence who improve after performance of a cerebrospinal fluid (CSF) shunting procedure.

For the past 30 years clinicians have attempted to find a means to predict who will respond to a shunt. Although much clinical experience has accumulated in the intervening years, this question remains only partially answered today.[15]

Normal pressure hydrocephalus (NPH) is not a common disease. The incidence has been estimated at 2.2 per million per year, and the prevalence has been estimated at 5000 to 10,000 patients in the United States.

Studies have shown that the underlying defect in NPH is impaired CSF flow because of obstruction of CSF pathways in the basal cisterns. Acquired communicating hydrocephalus can be produced by subarachnoid hemorrhage, meningitis, cranial trauma, or intracranial surgery, although the cause is unknown in about half the cases. To compensate for the obstruction, alternative absorptive pathways develop, producing a reversal of CSF flow through the ependymal lining of the ventricle into the extracellular space of the white matter, from where it is absorbed through the capillary bed into the venous system. This causes disruption of the periventricular white matter, perhaps by the production of localized ischemia. It is this damage to the periventricular tissue that produces the clinical manifestations of NPH.[16]

Difficulty with gait is often the first and occasionally the only clinical manifestation of NPH. It is also the sign that is most likely to respond to a shunting procedure. Patients have difficulty in initiating gait, walk with small steps, and are unable to lift their feet ("magnetic gait"). These gait abnormalities are associated with postural instability.

Cognitive impairment is usually mild and consists of poor memory, inertia, inattention, decreased speed of processing complex information, and impaired manipulation of acquired knowledge. The mini-mental state examination is not useful for detecting cognitive loss in patients with NPH because the degree of mental impairment is mild and the test is insensitive to subcortical frontal impairment. Both the cognitive impairment and the gait abnormalities resemble those seen in patients with disorders caused by subcortical frontal lobe dysfunction. When intellectual impairment is pronounced, other causes of dementia should be considered. Urinary incontinence is a late sign and has been attributed to damage to the periventricular pathways extending to the bladder control center; the result is an inability to control bladder contractions despite normal sphincteric function.[17]

Computed tomographic (CT) scans in patients with NPH usually show ventricular enlargement that is out of proportion to cortical atrophy. The frontal horns are rounded and the temporal horns are enlarged, but there is no hippocampal atrophy. Atypical features such as mild or moderate cortical atrophy or periventricular abnormalities of white matter suggestive of ischemic lesions are sometimes present but do not preclude the possibility of clinical improvement after a shunt.

Lumbar puncture with removal of 40 to 50 mL of CSF may be followed by a transient or, rarely, prolonged clinical improvement. This procedure has been used as a method of preoperative assessment of the likelihood of operative success. Recent analysis, however, has raised questions about the predictive value of the procedure, although use of the test is still widespread. Continuous external lumbar drainage, in which approximately 150 to 200 mL of CSF are removed daily for 3 to 5 days, has been suggested to predict the outcome of shunt placement more accurately. Other techniques used in investigation, including isotope cisternography, which measures CSF flow dynamics, and single-photon emission computed tomography (SPECT) scanning, which determines the pattern of cerebral blood flow, have been inconsistent in predicting shunt success.

A recent review, which assessed more than 1000 patients with NPH retrospectively, found that 30% of patients who underwent shunting procedures for idiopathic NPH showed significant improvement. When a cause was identified, the success rate increased to 50% to 70%. Approximately 35% of patients with shunts had surgical complications, and approximately 10% of these resulted in death or severe residual morbidity.[18]

Ataxia

A wide-based, unsteady gait characterized by poorly controlled turns and staggering is associated with cerebellar or brain stem dysfunction but sometimes is seen as part of a sensory ataxia (limited proprioceptive and visual input) or in patients with acute vestibular abnormalities (often benign positional vertigo). The history and physical examination often allow one to differentiate among the possibilities. Abnormal neurologic findings suggest brain stem or cerebellar abnormalities, whereas positionally dependent vertigo and nausea associated with gaze-evoked nystagmus and an otherwise normal examination suggest benign positional vertigo. Sensory ataxia can be produced by proprioceptive and visual loss. An MRI is often warranted to look for lesions within the posterior fossa. In older patients, ataxia is often produced by brain stem or cerebellar infarction, multisystem atrophy, or alcoholism.

PAROXYSMAL DISORDERS

Seizure Disorders

After the age of 60, the incidence of seizures increases.[19] The annual incidence of epilepsy in persons aged 65 years and older is 134 per 100,000.[20] The majority of seizures occurring in this population are secondary to strokes, brain tumors, toxic-metabolic disturbances, and Alzheimer's disease. Primary seizure disorders with a late-life onset are rare. Stroke accounts for 30% to 50% of seizures occurring in the elderly population. Tumors and toxic-metabolic causes (e.g., renal failure, alcohol, medication) are each responsible for approximately 10% to 15%. Head trauma may cause another 10%, and 30% are idiopathic.[21, 22]

Initial evaluation of elderly patients with seizures should include a history, and information should be obtained from family members or caregivers whenever possible. A medication history should be elicited as well as information about previous head injuries. Physical examination, serum electrolyte determination, electrocardiography, electroencephalography, head CT scans without and with contrast should also be done. MRI is helpful when CT is negative or inconclusive and the patient's history suggests the possibility of seizures of focal onset. MRI is also effective for identifying abnormalities such as mesial temporal sclerosis and other small cortical scars as well as abnormalities such as hippocampal atrophy. Because MRI provides high-resolution images that are sensitive to differences in tissue constituents, it may also be effective in evaluating patients with underlying brain tumors. Depending on the history and physical findings, other studies that may be considered include lumbar puncture, blood cultures, and toxicology screening tests.

Management of seizures should focus on minimizing the impact of this disorder on the patient's lifestyle while setting guidelines to maximize the patient's safety. Patients should be instructed to avoid driving until they have been free of seizures for 3 to 6 months, avoid swimming alone, and use a shower for bathing.

In patients with toxic or metabolic abnormalities, correction of the abnormality usually suffices for preventing further seizures. In other circumstances, anticonvulsant therapy may be indicated, taking into consideration the fact that drug metabolism changes in older persons, and careful observation of blood levels, is required. The aim

should be to control the seizures with a single drug at the lowest effective dose. Phenytoin (Dilantin), carbamazepine (Tegretol, Epitol), and valproic acid and its derivatives (Depakene, Depakote) are all effective against a wide range of partial and generalized seizures and are generally well tolerated in older patients. Benzodiazepines should be avoided because of their potential for accumulation and toxicity in older patients. Barbiturates should also be avoided because of their sedating potential.[21]

Older patients who develop seizures have an excellent prognosis. In one study, 62% of patients in whom epilepsy began after age 60 remained seizure free for at least 1 year while they received anticonvulsants.[23]

Trigeminal Neuralgia

The pain from trigeminal neuralgia can be among the worst pain that can be experienced. It is lancinating and usually has a duration of seconds. The central and lower portions of the face are commonly affected. These areas are innervated by the maxillary (cranial nerve V_2) and mandibular divisions (V_3) of the trigeminal nerve. The pain can be elicited by stimulation of trigger points. Talking, chewing, shaving, and applying cosmetics, among others actions, can provoke an attack. Early in the course of the disease remissions are common, but later the frequency and severity of the attacks often increase.

Females are affected more than males in a 3:2 ratio. The incidence in the United States is estimated to be 15,000 new cases per year.[24] Onset is most common in the fifth to seventh decades of life.

For many people (particularly older patients) the cause of trigeminal neuralgia is probably demyelination of the retrogasserian ganglionic fibers in the pontine root entry zone.[24] In most patients, this demyelination is initiated by vascular compression (especially compression of the superior cerebellar artery). In a small number of patients (particularly younger patients) other precipitants (e.g., multiple sclerosis or tumor) may damage the nerve, so that neuroimaging may be warranted.

Carbamazepine is an effective treatment for trigeminal neuralgia, producing relief that begins within hours of administration. Side effects are uncommon but can include impaired hematopoietic and liver function, lethargy, and ataxia. There are analogs of carbamazepine that have shown promise in controlling pain and have fewer side effects.[25] Phenytoin has been used successfully, although it is not as effective as other medications. Its effectiveness can be enhanced by using it in combination with carbamazepine and baclofen. Baclofen may be successful in patients who have become resistant to carbamazepine or phenytoin. Its mechanism of action is similar to that of carbamazepine; it depresses excitatory transmission input from the afferent trigeminal fibers and facilitates segmental inhibition of the trigeminal complex.

In some patients drug therapy becomes ineffective, or the side effects become intolerable. For these patients, ablative surgical lesions of the trigeminal nerve should be considered. These procedures provide transient relief accompanied by sensory loss as well as occasional formation of neuroma with anesthesia dolorosa. The best long-term results have been achieved by microvascular decompression of the posterior circulation. This is a major surgical procedure that has a 60% to 80% chance of producing long-term relief and up to a 95% chance of producing a partial remission.[26] The procedure is most appropriate for younger and healthier patients.

Transient Global Amnesia

Transient global amnesia (TGA) is a benign syndrome characterized by sudden onset of memory loss with retention of personal identity. Consciousness and motor skills are unimpaired.[27] The amnesia may last up to 24 hours. In patients over the age of 50 the incidence of transient global amnesia is 23.5 to 32 per 100,000 per year.[28] The prevalence of risk factors for vascular disease, stroke, and dementia are not increased in these patients.[27] Patients are left with an amnestic gap for the event.

Transient memory loss can also occur following seizures, drug intoxication, head trauma, or ischemic events. Epilepsy, migraine, and cerebrovascular accidents have been implicated as causes of TGA, although no cause is generally accepted. Electroencephalograph studies after a TGA episode are usually normal. Epileptic discharges have not been identified.[27] Imaging studies are also commonly normal,[29] although MRIs with signal abnormalities in one or both temporal lobes have been reported.[30, 31] SPECT scans have shown temporary regional hypoperfusion, most commonly localized to the medial temporal lobes.[27] Several reports have noted that the incidence of TGA in patients with migraine is higher than expected, although the exact relationship is unclear.[27]

The prognosis of TGA is good. Other than a permanent memory gap for the attack itself, no neuropsychological sequelae have been noted.[29] There is a 3.6% chance of recurrence.[32]

Vertigo

Dizziness represents a spectrum of symptoms that requires clarification by the examiner during the course of the medical history. For older patients, dizziness may represent (1) lightheadedness, which is a nonspecific symptom, (2) pre-syncope, (3) unsteadiness while walking, which is usually a product of impaired mobility skills, or (4) vertigo, which is an illusion of motion, usually rotational. The diagnostic approaches to and medical implications of the four sensations are quite different. Evaluation of ligtheadedness is rarely productive. A pre-syncope assessment should be directed at entities that produce loss of consciousness. Unsteadiness while walking is often related to impaired sensorimotor function of the lower extremities. Vertigo is produced by brainstem or vestibular dysfunction.

Unlike the situation in younger persons, persistent dizziness in the great majority of older persons has a demonstrable cause.[33] Approximately half have peripheral vestibular abnormalities, and more than 20% have dizziness related to cerebrovascular disease.[33] A key part of the examination is the Nylen-Bárány maneuver, in which a sitting patient is rapidly moved to a prone position with the head hanging downward and is then rotated 45 degrees to one side and then to the other side. In patients with vestibular dysfunction, this maneuver often elicits contralateral rotatory nystagmus from the dependent horizontal canal. Patients with labyrinthitis show a combination of positional vertigo associated with nausea and vomiting, positionally induced rotatory nystagmus, and an absence of associated neurologic signs and symptoms. Approximately half of patients have idiopathic labyrinthitis, and one third have a recent history of head trauma or findings suggestive of viral labyrinthitis.[33] Although vertigo due to vertebrobasilar ischemia can occur in isolation,[34] it is almost always associated with other neurologic findings.

STRUCTURAL DISEASE OF THE BRAIN

Tumors and Chronic Subdural Hematoma

In the past 23 years, the incidence of brain tumor has doubled in patients over age 70 and quintupled in those over 85. It is likely, however, that this increase in the rate of occurrence is related both to an increased incidence of tumors (including malignant glioma) and improvements in diagnosis and attitudinal changes to disease in older persons.[35–37] Other tumors commonly encountered in older persons include metastatic cancer, meningiomas (brain and spine), and neurilemomas, all of which have a higher incidence in persons older than 65 years. Chronic subdural hematomas occur predominantly in the very old and the very young. In recent years neurosurgeons have been increasingly willing to operate on older persons. In one series of operations for removal of a meningioma (elective first-time surgery), older persons had approximately 25% more postoperative complications, although overall, the outcome at 4 months was no different in patients aged 45 to 64 years than in those aged 65 and over.[38] In one series of 103 older patients (median age, 76; range, 70 to 89) with a diagnosis of malignant supratentorial glioma, the overall outcome was worse than the outcome in younger patients; patients who were functionally impaired or over 80 years old were less likely to benefit from radiotherapy.[38] Surgery is more often considered in older patients who are symptomatic or have impending major complications from the tumor. The data indicate that it is these patients who tend to have the poorest outcome. The more medically impaired or frail the patient or the more difficult the surgery, the stronger the indications for surgery must be.

Glioblastomas and metastatic tumors often present with focal or multifocal symptoms occurring over weeks to months, whereas meningiomas and neurilemomas often have a history that extends over a period of years. Glioblastomas and metastatic lesions usually occur within the hemispheres and produce characteristic deficits (e.g., hemiparesis, sensory loss, hemianopsia, aphasia). Metastatic involvement of the extradural spinal canal resulting in rapidly evolving spinal cord compression is common. Meningiomas and neurilemomas are extrinsic to the nervous system but also compress the brain or spinal cord. The myelopathy produced by metastatic lesions, meningiomas, and neurilemomas can usually be distinguished by clinical and imaging criteria.

Subacute subdural hematomas are formed within 2 weeks of an acute bleeding episode by blood breakdown, membrane formation, and accumulation of additional fluid, forming a mass. The symptoms associated with subacute and chronic subdural hematoma evolve over days to weeks. A substantial portion of older persons (30%) have no history of head trauma, and one quarter are taking antithrombotic medications (warfarin [Coumadin], heparin, or platelet antiaggregants).[39] Subdural hematomas may become quite large, compressing the hemispheres over a wide area and producing both diffuse (e.g., headache, delirium) and focal findings. Although subdural hematomas may resolve on their own,

patients who are symptomatic should have surgical treatment. In two recent studies that evaluated the clinical factors associated with mortality, the level of consciousness was most predictive of mortality, but age was still a factor.[39, 40]

SPINAL CORD DISEASES

Cervical Spine

With advancing age, the water content of the nucleus pulposus, the central portion of the disk, decreases, resulting in loss of the disk space, bulging of the annulus, increased movement of the vertebral bodies, and osteophyte formation. In addition, the mobility of the cervical spine, in particular the C5 to C6 interspace, predisposes the patient to degenerative joint changes. As a result, patients develop radiculopathy, myelopathy, or a combination of both. Acute cervical radiculopathy is usually caused by disk herniation. It rarely occurs after the age of 50. When radiculopathy secondary to degenerative spine disease occurs in older people it is usually secondary to spondylitic changes. It presents with neck pain that radiates to one or both arms. Irritation of the C6 root causes paresthesias over the thumb and index finger, whereas a C7 lesion involves the middle three fingers. Associated numbness and weakness may be present. Deep tendon reflexes corresponding to the involved nerve roots may be depressed. A history of prior similar episodes that have resolved is often present in patients with spondylitic radiculopathy. Neck movements may be restricted.

Chronic cervical myelopathy results in a spastic paraparesis. Although they are sometimes present, sensory symptoms and urinary dysfunction are not prominent. A cervical radiculopathy is often present. Examination may reveal signs of spastic paraparesis with diminished reflexes in the upper extremities.

The differential diagnosis of cervical radiculopathy includes primary or metastatic tumors in the cervical region, lesions of the brachial plexus (e.g., Pancoast's tumor), and mononeuropathy (e.g., carpal tunnel syndrome). The differential diagnosis of cervical myelopathy includes cervical tumors, combined system disease, and motor neuron disease. Radiographic evaluation includes spinal radiographs, MRI, and CT myelography.

A trial of analgesics, rest, and use of a soft collar should first be tried in patients with cervical radiculopathy. If this treatment is not beneficial, surgical intervention may be indicated. Surgical decompression is often used for cervical myelopathy, although in patients with high-risk medical conditions and slowly progressive myelopathy, immobilization with a collar may be preferred.[41]

Motor Neuron Disease

Motor neuron disease (MND, amyotrophic lateral sclerosis [ALS]) is produced by degeneration of the anterior horn and cortical motor neurons that results in asymmetrical limb weakness, atrophy, bulbar signs and symptoms, and pyramidal tract dysfunction. The diagnosis can be suspected from the history based on the evolution and distribution of weakness and is supported by the combination of upper and lower motor neuron signs. Patients may also report paresthesias, pain, and muscle cramps.[42] The presence of electromyographic (EMG) evidence of chronic denervation in the absence of neuropathy further supports this diagnosis. Occasionally nerve or muscle biopsy (or both) are required. Progression of the weakness, which is variable, is a feature of the illness. The differential diagnosis of MND includes neoplastic disease of the brain stem and spinal cord, cervical spondylosis, multiple sclerosis, and neuropathy and myopathy. The time course as well as other associated clinical and laboratory features allows the correct diagnosis. In addition to EMG studies, other tests that should be considered include a complete blood count, erythrocyte sedimentation rate, serum chemistries, muscle enzymes (creatine kinase, alanine amino transferase), cryoglobulins, serum protein electrophoresis, urinalysis, chest radiograph, CSF examination, head and spine MRI, and myelography.[43]

Pathologically, the primary feature of MND is the degeneration and loss of the anterior horn and cortical motor neurons. Glial replacement also occurs, resulting in atrophy of the spinal cord and motor cortex as well as gliosis of the lateral columns of the spinal cord.

The etiology of MND remains unknown, although in familial cases abnormalities in the superoxide dismutase gene suggest the possibility of oxidative cell death.[44]

Symptomatic therapy is of great value in augmenting both the quality and duration of life. Treatments to slow the progression of the disease are being developed. Riluzole, a glutamate antagonist, has shown marginal benefit in prolonging survival, and insulin growth factor has also shown some promise.[45]

NEUROMUSCULAR DISEASE

Neuropathy

Peripheral neuropathies may affect predominantly the sensory fibers, motor fibers, or a combination of both. The underlying pathologic process may be demyelination, or it may involve the axon (axonopathy). Electrophysiologic studies are valuable in characterizing the neuropathy and quantifying its extent and severity, although they rarely provide a precise diagnosis. The rate of progression, modality (motor, sensory, mixed, or autonomic), pattern of nerve involvement, past medical history, and laboratory evaluation often allow a correct diagnosis. Following is an overview of three of the neuropathies most often seen in the elderly population.

About 15% of patients with diabetes mellitus have both signs and symptoms of neuropathy. Onset usually occurs after age 50. Several clinical patterns have been identified,[46] although the slowly progressive, distal, symmetrical, predominantly sensory, lower extremity neuropathy is commonly encountered. The axon is the primary site of involvement. In general, patients who are able to maintain strict control of blood glucose levels have fewer neuropathic complications.

Uremic neuropathy presents as a slowly progressive, distal symmetrical, sensorimotor neuropathy whose initial symptoms include numbness or tingling in the legs.[47] Burning dysesthesias in the feet may occur. Motor symptoms begin with distal lower extremity weakness. The condition occurs in at least 60% of patients on dialysis. Electrophysiologic and pathologic studies have shown that the condition is an axonopathy with secondary demyelination. The neuropathy is probably produced by toxins, usually excreted by the kidneys. Renal transplantation may result in resolution of the neuropathy, although recovery may be incomplete. Chronic hemodialysis may halt progression or improve the neuropathy.[48]

Guillain-Barré syndrome (GBS) or acute inflammatory demyelinating polyneuropathy (AIDP) is presumably the result of an aberrant immune response to a preceding infection or other trigger.[49] It has an annual incidence of up to 2 cases per 100,000 population. The condition often begins with paresthesias in the toes and fingers, followed over a period of days by weakness of the lower extremities. Arm, facial, and oropharyngeal weakness may follow. Pain, which is described as aching or sciatica, is common. Neurologic examination reveals symmetrical weakness, absent or diminished deep tendon reflexes, and little loss of sensation despite the presence of paresthesias. In severe cases, respiration, deglutition, and autonomic function may be affected. Progression of weakness reaches a plateau in 1 to 3 weeks. Approximately two thirds of cases occur following an infection, usually a viral upper respiratory tract infection. Complete or near-complete recovery over a period of weeks or months is seen in the majority of patients.

Nerve conduction abnormalities indicating demyelination of the roots and proximal nerves are the most specific and sensitive laboratory findings in GBS. To demonstrate these abnormalities, one must request a specific neurophysiologic test that examines proximal nerve function (i.e., F waves and H reflexes). This test has supplanted the CSF examination, which reveals an elevated protein concentration and few or no cells, as the primary diagnostic tool.

Patients with GBS should be observed in the hospital. Those with very mild cases involving only distal paresthesias and mild limb weakness may not need treatment, but it is advisable to wait approximately 2 weeks before concluding that there will be no progression. Patients with a declining vital capacity or cardiovascular dysautonomia should be observed in an intensive care unit.

Plasma exchange is an effective treatment for GBS, although intravenous immunoglobulin (IVIG) has become the preferred treatment because of its relative safety and equivalent efficacy.[50] Corticosteroids are of no benefit in the treatment of GBS.

Neuromuscular Transmission

Myasthenia gravis is produced by impaired cholinergic transmission due to autoimmune destruction of the nicotinic receptors of the motor end plates. In addition to its high incidence in young women, myasthenia gravis also occurs frequently in older men. The usual symptoms, which may be accentuated by fatigue, include diplopia, ptosis, dysarthria or dysphagia, and weakness. Once suspected, the diagnosis can be confirmed by the occurrence of improvement following an intravenous dose of a short-acting anticholinesterase agent (edrophonium). Elevated cholinergic receptor antibodies and EMG may be useful in supporting the diagnosis. Other autoimmune problems (e.g., thyroiditis, systemic lupus erythematosus) as well as thymoma may be present in these patients. Effective treatment options include anticholinesterases, thymectomy, steroids, and plasmapheresis.

Myopathy

Myopathies result in weakness of the proximal muscles and cause difficulties in arising from a chair or climbing stairs. The medical history may indicate the presence of an endocrinopathy, collagen vascular disease, or cancer. The presence of myopathic findings on EMG confirms the clinical impression. Laboratory evaluation should include creatine kinase determination, erythrocyte sedimentation rate, serum electrolytes, phosphorus and calcium levels, complete blood count, liver enzymes, and thyroid function tests. Muscle biopsy is used to confirm the presence of a specific myopathy for which no other diagnostic test will suffice (e.g., polymyositis or inclusion body myositis).

Idiopathic inflammatory myopathies are the most common histologically proven muscle diseases affecting the elderly. The incidence of dermatomyositis and polymyositis is 2 to 5 per million. The peak incidence of polymyositis occurs in the fifth decade, whereas dermatomyositis peaks in childhood as well as in the fifth decade. Females are more frequently affected than males.

Both conditions typically present with a subacute to chronic progression of proximal weakness. The neck flexors are commonly affected, whereas the facial, respiratory, and extraocular muscles are not. Patients may report myalgias and dysphagia. Patients affected by dermatomyositis have a butterfly facial rash or a rash over the knuckles. They may develop cardiomyopathy, interstitial lung disease, or gastric ulcers. Connective tissue diseases are present in 20% of cases. In 10% to 15% of cases there is an associated malignancy.[51] Diagnosis is based on the clinical features, myopathy on EMG, elevated creatine kinase, and histologic evidence of muscle inflammation and necrosis.

Treatment consists of steroid therapy (prednisone 60 to 100 mg/day), the length of therapy being determined by improvement in strength, a decrease in creatine kinase levels, and the occurrence of side effects. Most patients require low-maintenance doses of prednisone for years. Immunosuppressive agents such as azathioprine are sometimes required in patients who do not respond to corticosteroid therapy or in whom such therapy is contraindicated. IVIG may be useful in patients with dermatomyositis.[52]

Two thirds of patients improve with corticosteroid therapy and have no functional deficits at 3-year follow-up. In patients without cancer, the 5-year mortality ranges from 11% to 25%. Patients with dysphagia or severe weakness have a less favorable outcome.

Inclusion body myositis is another idiopathic inflammatory myopathy that is seen predominantly in the older population; its onset occurs after 50 years of age. Men are affected more frequently than women. Patients present with a slowly progressive, painless weakness that involves both distal and proximal muscles. Dysphagia is a common component. Muscle enzymes may be normal or mildly elevated. EMG is myopathic. Muscle biopsy reveals marked variation in fiber size, endomysial inflammation, grouped atrophy of muscle fibers, and fibers with rimmed vacuoles containing amyloid and abnormal filamentous material. Unlike the idiopathic inflammatory myopathies, inclusion body myositis does not usually respond to immunosuppressive therapy, although a trial of corticosteroids is reasonable. IVIG may be of benefit.[53]

References

1. Rubin EH, Kinscherf DA, Morris JC: Personality and dementia. Bull Clin Neurosci 1989;54:88–94.
2. Rees TS, Ducker LG: Auditory and vestibular dysfunction in aging. *In* Hazzard WR, Andres R, Beirman EL, Blass JP (eds): Principles of Geriatric Medicine and Gerontology. New York, McGraw-Hill, 1990, pp. 432–44.
3. Welford AT: Reaction time, speed of performance and age. Ann NY Acad Sci 1988;515:1–17.
4. Stalberg E, Borges O, Ericsson M, Essen-Gustavsson B, Fawcett PRW, Nordesjo LO, Nordgren B, Uhlin R: The quadriceps femoris muscle in 20–70 year old subjects: Relation between knee extensor torque, electrophysiologic parameters and muscle fiber characteristics. Muscle Nerve 1989;12:382–389.
5. Frontera WR, Hughes VA, Lutz KJ, et al: A cross-sectional study of muscle strength and mass in 45- to 78-year-old men and women. J Appl Physiol 1991;71:644–650.
6. Wolfson L, Whipple R, Derby CA, Amerman P, Murphy T, Tobin JN, Nashner L: A dynamic posturography study of balance in healthy elderly. Neurology 1992;42:2069–2075.
7. King MB, Judge JO, Wolfson L: Functional base of support decreases with age. J Gerontol Med Sci 1994;48:M258–M263.
8. Bohannon RW, Larkin PA, Cook AC, Gear J, Singer J: Decrease in timed balance test scores with aging. Phys Ther 1984;64:1067–1070.
9. Klawans HL, Tufo HM, Ostfeld AM: Neurologic examination in an elderly population. Dis Nerv Syst 1971;32:274–279.
10. Jacobs L, Gossman MD: Three primitive reflexes in normal adults. Neurology 1980;30:184–188.
11. Longstreth WT Jr, Manolio TA, Arnold A, Burke GL, Bryan N, Jungreis CA, Enright PL, O'Leary D, Fried L: Clinical correlates of white matter findings on cranial magnetic resonance imaging of 3301 elderly people. Stroke 1996;27:1274–1282.
12. Baloh RW, Yue Q, Socotch TM, Jacobson KM: White matter lesions and disequilibrium in older people. l. Case-control comparison. Arch Neurol 1995;52:970–974.
13. Masdeu JM, Wolfson L, Lantos G, Tobin J, Grober E, Whipple R, Amerman P: Brain white matter changes in the elderly prone to falling. Arch Neurol 1989;48:417–420.
14. Baloh RW, Vinters HV: White matter lesions and disequilibrium in older people. II. Clinicopathologic correlation. Arch Neurol 1995;52:975–981.
15. Vanneste J: Three decades of normal pressure hydrocephalus: Are we wiser now?. J Neurol Neurosurg Psychiatry 1994;57:1021–1025.
16. Turner D, McGeachie R: Normal pressure hydrocephalus and dementia—Evaluation and treatment. Clin Geriatr Med 1988;4(4):815–830.
17. Ahlberg J, Norlen L, et al: Outcome of shunt operation on urinary incontinence in normal pressure hydrocephalus predicted by lumbar puncture. J Neurol Neurosurg Psychiatry 1988;51:105–108.
18. Vanneste JAL, Augustin P, Davies GA, Blomstrand C: Shunting normal pressure hydrocephalus: Do the benefits outweigh the risks? A multicenter study and literature review. Neurology 1992;42:54–59.
19. Hauser WA, Annegers JF, Kurland LT: Prevalence of epilepsy in Rochester, Minnesota: 1940–1980. Epilepsia 1991;32:429–445.
20. Hauser WA, Annegers JF, Kurland LT: Incidence of epilepsy and unprovoked seizures in Rochester, Minnesota: 1935–1984. Epilepsia 1993;34:453–468.
21. Drury I, Beydoun A: Seizure disorders of aging: Differential diagnosis and patient management. Geriatrics 1993;48:52–58.
22. Scheuer ML, Cohen J: Seizures and epilepsy in the elderly. Neurol Clin 1993;11:787–804.
23. Luhdorf K, Jensen LK, Plesner AM: Epilepsy in the elderly: Prognosis. Acta Neurol Scand 1986;74:409–415.
24. Rosenkopf KL: Current concepts concerning the etiology and treatment of trigeminal neuralgia. Craniomandib Pract 1989;7:312–318.
25. Farago F: Trigeminal neuralgia: Its treatment with two new carbamazepine analogues. Eur Neurol 1987;26(2):73–83.
26. Janetta PJ: Microvascular decompression for trigeminal neuralgia. Surg Rounds 1983;6:24–35.
27. Frederiks JAM: Transient global amnesia. Clin Neurol Neurosurg 1993;95:265–283.
28. Zorzon M, Antonutti L, Mase G, Biasutti E, Vitrani B, Cazzato G: Transient global amnesia and transient ischemic attacks: Natural history, vascular risk factors and associated conditions. Stroke 1995;26:1536–1542.
29. Hodges JR, Warlow CP: The aetiology of transient global amnesia. A case control study of 114 cases with prospective follow up. Brain 1990;113:639–657.
30. Zinelli P, Nasuto S, Miari A: Transient global amnesia: Case reports. Ital J Neurol Sci 1988;9(Suppl 9):19–20.
31. Friend HC: Transient global amnesia (letter). Neurology 1987;37:1889–1890.
32. Hinge HH, Jensen TS: The prognosis of transient global amnesia. *In* Markowitsch HJ (ed): Transient Global Amnesia and Related Disorders. Toronto, Hogrefe & Huber, 1990, pp. 172–180.
33. Baloh RW, Honrubia V, Johnson K: Benign positional vertigo: Clinical and oculographic features in 240 cases. Neurology 1987;37:371–378.
34. Gomez CR, Cruz-Flores S, Malkoff MD, Sauer CM, Burch CM: Isolated vertigo as a manifestation of vertebrobasilar ischemia. Neurology 1996;47:94–97.
35. Boyle P, Maisonneuve P, Saracci R, Muir CS: Is the increased incidence of primary malignant brain tumors in the elderly real? J Natl Canc Inst 1990;82:1594–1596.
36. Bodan B, Wegner DK, Feldman JJ, et al: Increased mortality from brain tumors: A combined outcome of diagnostic technology and change of attitude towards the elderly. Am J Epidemiol 1992;135:1349–1357.
37. Meckling S, Dold O, Forsyth PAJ, Brasher P, Hagen NA: Malignant supratentorial glioma in the elderly: Is radiotherapy useful? Neurology 1996;47:901–905.
38. Maurice Williams RS, Kitchen N: The scope of neurosurgery for elderly people. Age Ageing 1993;22:337–342.
39. Rozzelle CJ, Wofford JL: Predictors of hospital mortality in older patients with subdural hematoma. J Am Geriatr Soc 1995;43:240–244.

40. Krupp WF: Treatment of chronic subdural hematoma with burr-hole craniotomy and closed drainage. Br J Neurosurg 1995;9:619–627.

41. Cartlidge N, Al-Hakim M, Bradley W: Disorders of bones, joints, ligaments, cartilage, and meninges. *In* Bradley W, Waroff R, Finichel G, Marsden C (eds): Neurology in Clinical Practice, 2nd ed. Boston, Butterworth-Heinemann, 1996, pp. 1804–1806.

42. Gubbay SS, Kahana E, Zilber N, Cooper G, Pintov S, Leibowitz Y: Amyotrophic lateral sclerosis: A study of its presentation and prognosis. J Neurol 1985;232:295–300.

43. Williams DB, Windebank AJ: Motor neuron disease (amyotrophic lateral sclerosis). Mayo Clin Proc 1991;66:54–82.

44. Siddique T, Figlewicz DA, Pericak-Vance MA, Haines JL, Rouleau G, Jeffers AJ, Sapp P, Hung WY, Bebout J, McKenna-Yasek D, et al: Linkage of a gene causing familial amyotrophic lateral sclerosis to chromosome 21 and evidence of genetic-locus heterogeneity. N Engl J Med 1991;324:1381–1384.

45. Bensimon G, Lacomblez L, Meininger V, and ALS/ Riluzole Study Group: A controlled trial of riluzole in amyotrophic lateral sclerosis. N Engl J Med 1994;330:585–591.

46. Adams R, Victor M: Diseases of the peripheral nerves. *In* Principles of Neurology, 5th ed. New York, McGraw-Hill, 1993, p. 1136.

47. Asbury AK: Neuropathies with renal failure, hepatic disorders, chronic respiratory insufficiency and critical illness. *In* Dyck PJ, Thomas PK, Griffin JW, Low PA, Paduslo JK (eds): Peripheral Neuropathy, 3rd ed. Philadelphia, WB Saunders, 1993, pp. 1251–1265.

48. Fraser CL, Arieff A: Nervous system complications in uremia. Ann Intern Med 1988;109:143–153.

49. Ropper AH: The Guillain-Barré syndrome. N Engl J Med 1992;326:1130–1136.

50. Van Der Meche FGA, Schmitz PIM, and the Dutch Guillain-Barré Study Group: A randomized trial comparing intravenous immune globulin and plasma exchange in Guillain-Barré syndrome. N Engl J Med 1992;326:1123–1129.

51. Sigurgeirsson B, Lindelof B, Edhag O, Allander E: Risk of cancer in patients with dermatomyositis or polymyositis. N Engl J Med 1992;326:363–367.

52. Dalakas MC, Illa I, Dambrosia JM, et al: A controlled trial of high dose intravenous immune globulin infusions as treatment for dermatomyositis. N Engl J Med 1993;329:1993–2000.

53. Soueidan SA, Dalakas MC: Treatment of inclusion body myositis with high dose intravenous immunoglobulin. Neurology 1993;43:876–879.

32 Cerebrovascular Disease*

Linda Ann Hershey, M.D., Ph.D.

Stroke is the third leading cause of death in the developed world. With heart disease and cancer, it ranks among the most costly of all health care problems. Transient ischemic attacks (TIAs) are important predictors of stroke, myocardial infarction, and death. One third of all patients with TIAs have a stroke within 5 years. Strokes may be either hemorrhagic or ischemic, and hemorrhagic strokes carry a higher mortality (30% to 50%) than ischemic infarction (15% to 20%). Seizures at the onset of a stroke are predictive of subsequent epilepsy. Ischemic vascular dementia develops in 10% to 25% of stroke patients, depending upon age and the number of previous strokes. Just as stroke can be prevented by maintaining blood pressure control, ceasing smoking, and initiating antiplatelet or anticoagulant therapy, vascular dementia can be prevented by controlling stroke risk factors. This chapter reviews the epidemiology, pathophysiology, clinical assessment, and management of cerebrovascular disease in the elderly.

EPIDEMIOLOGY

Transient Ischemic Attack

TIAs are brief episodes of focal loss of brain function that are due to transient hypoperfusion of a portion of the brain supplied by a specific vessel or group of vessels.[1] Most TIAs last less than 24 minutes, but studies usually define them as lasting less than 24 hours. It has been shown by computed tomography (CT) that many TIAs that last longer than 6 to 8 hours are associated with infarction of the brain. Half of all strokes that follow TIAs occur within a year of the last TIA, making TIA an urgent medical condition requiring early evaluation and intervention.[2] Some TIAs are better predictors of myocardial ischemia than of stroke. Retinal TIAs, for example, are more likely to be followed by myocardial infarction than by stroke.

Atherothrombotic Infarction

Stroke is defined as a focal neurologic deficit of vascular origin that is sudden in onset and lasts longer than 24 hours. Hemorrhages account for only 15% of all strokes, while ischemic infarctions account for 80% to 85%. Infarction is divided into three broad categories based on the most common pathologic mechanisms: atherothrombotic, cardioembolic, and lacunar. Atherothrombotic infarcts are associated with plaques of the carotid arteries, the vertebrobasilar arteries, or the aortic arch.

A history of TIAs and the presence of a cervical bruit are more frequently found in persons with atherothrombotic infarction than in those with other types of stroke.[1] In patients who have symptomatic carotid stenosis of 70% or more and no significant cardiac source of emboli, the risk of stroke following a TIA is directly proportional to the percentage of carotid stenosis.[3]

Ischemic stroke patients who have no significant carotid stenosis, no pattern of lacunar infarction, and no cardiac source of emboli may experience stroke because of embolic material that breaks off an atheromatous plaque in the aortic arch.[4] The most common reversible risk factors associated with atheromatous disease of the carotids or the aorta are hypertension and cigarette smoking.

Small Deep Infarction

About 15% of all strokes are due to occlusion of small penetrating vessels in deep structures of the brain, such as the internal capsule, the thalamus, or the brain stem. Over a period of time these small deep infarcts become cystic and filled with fluid, giving rise to the name lacunar because of their resemblance to small lakes.[1] Brain imaging with CT may not identify lacunar infarcts, since they are by definition less than 15 mm in diameter. Magnetic resonance imaging (MRI) is a more sensitive tool than CT for docu-

---

*All material in this chapter is in the public domain, with the exception of any borrowed figures or tables.

menting their presence. The most prevalent reversible risk factor for small deep infarcts is essential hypertension.[5]

Cardioembolic Infarction

Cardiac emboli are responsible for about 15% of all strokes. Patients with atrial fibrillation (AF) are five times more likely to have a stroke (5% per year) than age-matched controls (1% per year). AF patients who have had a previous stroke have an even higher risk of recurrence (12% per year). Not only does the risk of AF increase with age, but the risk of stroke in AF patients is also age related.[6] Other cardiac sources of embolism besides AF include acute anterior wall myocardial infarction, left atrial thrombus, spontaneous echocardiographic contrast, left ventricular thrombus, dilated cardiomyopathy, mitral stenosis, prosthetic heart valves, mitral annulus calcification, subacute bacterial endocarditis, and atrial septal aneurysm.

Hemorrhage

Subarachnoid, intracerebral, and subdural hemorrhages account for another 15% of all strokes. Hemorrhage should be the primary diagnostic consideration in patients who appear in the emergency room with early headache, loss of consciousness, stiff neck, vomiting, agitation, or seizures. Subarachnoid hemorrhage (SAH) is more likely to occur in women than in men, and in blacks than in whites.[7] Intracerebral hemorrhage (ICH) is also more prevalent in blacks except for those over the age of 65 years; in this group whites are at greater risk. Both SAH and ICH are associated with high cost and high mortality (40% to 50%). The most prevalent risk factor associated with SAH is cigarette smoking, whereas for ICH it is hypertension.[8]

Stroke-Related Seizures

Cerebrovascular disease accounts for 30% to 50% of all seizures occurring in the elderly. Early seizures are thought to be more common at the onset of hemorrhagic infarction than at the onset of ischemic infarction. Among the various infarct types, early seizures are more likely to be associated with cardioembolic than with atherothrombotic or lacunar strokes.[9] Late postinfarction seizures may occur months to years following a stroke. Recurrent seizures (epilepsy) develop in about 15% to 20% of all stroke patients.

Ischemic Vascular Dementia

Vascular dementia is a general term used to describe several subtypes of cognitive decline: multi-infarct dementia, lacunar dementia, Binswanger's disease (subcortical arteriosclerotic encephalopathy), and single-infarct dementia. Vascular dementia and mixed dementia (a combination of vascular dementia and Alzheimer's disease) are second only to Alzheimer's disease as the most prevalent causes of cognitive impairment in the elderly. Epidemiologic studies of large populations have supported the findings of smaller autopsy studies: Vascular and mixed dementia account for 20% to 30% of all patients with severe dementia.[10] Hypertension has been shown to be the most important risk factor for both lacunar dementia and Binswanger's disease.[5]

PATHOPHYSIOLOGY

Transient Ischemic Attacks

For many years, TIAs were thought to have a hemodynamic basis rather than an embolic one. Cerebral bypass surgery was originally designed to correct what was thought to be a hemodynamic problem in patients with carotid occlusion or high-grade carotid stenosis. Nevertheless, a large randomized trial showed that this type of surgery produced no significant reduction in the number of subsequent strokes in patients with severe carotid disease.[11]

The embolic hypothesis for TIAs received support on two occasions during the bypass study when surgeons photographed platelet-fibrin material in branches of the middle cerebral artery. Similar platelet-fibrin material had been visualized previously in vessels on the fundi of patients who happened to have been examined during a retinal TIA. Further evidence of a causal link between platelet-fibrin emboli and clinical symptoms is shown by the response of patients with TIAs and small strokes to antiplatelet agents such as aspirin or ticlopidine. Both of these drugs are effective in reducing the frequency and severity of recurrent TIAs and strokes.[12]

Transcranial Doppler (TCD) ultrasonography is a technique that allows investigators to monitor the frequency of emboli arriving in intracerebral vessels of patients with symptomatic carotid stenosis. One group showed that endarterectomy could reduce or eliminate the number of embolic signals recorded by TCD in the middle cerebral artery distal to a high-grade stenotic lesion of the internal carotid artery.[13] This study strengthened the idea that atheromatous plaque could serve as a nidus for platelet-fibrin or cholesterol emboli.

Even though most TIAs are embolic in origin, there are some that are caused by hemodynamic compromise. For example, if there is poor collateral flow through the circle of Willis, a patient with carotid occlusion may experience ischemic symptoms when making rapid postural changes. The phenomenon of unilateral limb-shaking upon standing has been observed in patients with unilateral carotid occlusion. In the extracranial/intracranial (EC/IC) bypass study, there were 74 patients with bilateral carotid occlusion. A few of them experienced focal ischemic events on standing. These symptoms abated after a few months in patients in both the medical and surgical arms of the study. Improvement was probably due to the spontaneous development of collateral circulation.[11]

Noncardioembolic Ischemic Infarction

Patients with stenosis of 70% or more of a symptomatic carotid artery are at high risk (about 25%) for having an ipsilateral infarct within the first 2 years after their TIA or small stroke. This compares to a stroke risk of 2% in asymptomatic patients with carotid stenosis. Among patients with carotid stenosis assigned to the medical treatment arm of the North American Symptomatic Carotid Endarterectomy Trial (NASCET), stroke risk varied not only as a function of the severity of carotid stenosis but also as a function of the number of vascular risk factors present.[3]

Hypertension increases the risk of both ischemic infarction and intracerebral hemorrhage. About 40% of all strokes are associated with systolic pressures of over 140 mmHg.[8] In patients with chronic hypertension, vascular remodeling results in thickening of the media and narrowing of the lumen of small vessels.[5] Normal vessels can dilate to compensate for low perfusion pressures (autoregulation), but as arteriosclerosis progresses, the thickened vessels respond less efficiently to sudden changes in perfusion pressure. As a result, chronically hypertensive individuals who experience acute lowering of systemic blood pressure to normal levels may develop global ischemic symptoms such as dizziness or syncope. Autoregulation is also lost soon after a stroke, which explains why acute lowering of blood pressure in patients with fresh infarcts can cause focal neurologic signs to become worse.

Cautious lowering of blood pressure into the normal range in hypertensive rats can reduce the medial thickness of large cerebral arteries. Similarly, judicious control of blood pressure in patients with chronic hypertension decreases the likelihood of future strokes.[5]

Cigarette smoking is another important reversible risk factor for ischemic stroke. Women who smoke triple their stroke risk, while men who smoke double theirs. Cigarettes augment stroke risk by facilitating atherogenesis and increasing platelet aggregability and hematocrit and fibrinogen levels. Long-term smokers have reduced cerebral perfusion compared to nonsmokers. Just as the risk of stroke can be reversed in hypertensives if blood pressure is controlled over time, so stroke risk can be reversed in light smokers (less than 20 cigarettes/day) who stop smoking.[14] According to a new study, heavy smokers cannot completely reverse their stroke risk by ceasing to smoke, nor can those who switch from cigarettes to cigars or pipes.

Cardioembolic Infarction

Atrial fibrillation associated with rheumatic heart disease and mitral stenosis has long been recognized as a risk factor for stroke. It is now known that chronic AF without valvular heart disease also increases stroke risk.[6] Women in their eighties with nonvalvular AF are at particularly high risk for stroke. In general, women are less likely than men to have AF, but the prevalence of AF becomes nearly equal in men and women by the eighth decade. The risk of stroke in patients with AF rises as a function of age, just as it does with other stroke risk factors such as hypertension, congestive heart failure, previous stroke, or echocardiographic evidence of either left atrial enlargement or left ventricular dysfunction.

Subarachnoid Hemorrhage

Patients with SAH are often younger and less likely to have hypertension than those with ICH.[1] SAH is usually caused by the rupture of a saccular aneurysm or arteriovenous malformation. The risk of aneurysmal rupture usually depends on the size of the aneurysm, with those less than 3 mm in diameter carrying the lowest risk of hemorrhage and those above 10 mm carrying the highest. The clinical severity of the condition at the initial assessment is usually a good index of short-term prognosis.

Ischemic stroke may develop in patients with SAH as a result of vasospasm, particularly when the brain tissue distal to the site of vasospasm remains hypoperfused for longer than 24 hours. In most cases, vasospasm develops within 3 to 5 days of the hemorrhage and resolves over 2 to 4 weeks. The severity of vasospasm usually varies as a function of the size of the clot. Recurrent hemorrhage, a serious consequence of SAH, is associated with a mortality as high as 70%.

Subdural Hemorrhage

Subdural hemorrhage is due to rupture of the bridging veins that extend from the pia mater to the dura mater. Subdural bleeding is more likely to occur in the elderly because the bridging veins become increasingly fragile with age-related atrophy of the brain. Even minor head injuries in the elderly can result in subdural hemorrhage. Patients who are receiving anticoagulation therapy or are alcoholic, thrombocytopenic, or uremic are particularly vulnerable to this complication of a simple fall.

Intracerebral Hemorrhage

ICH represents arterial bleeding directly into the brain parenchyma. The most common locations of hypertensive ICH are the basal ganglia, thalamus, cerebellum, and pons.[1] Anticoagulated patients with ICH are more likely to die than those with spontaneous hemorrhage because hematomas in patients who are being treated with heparin or warfarin are larger. The active bleeding of a spontaneous ICH usually lasts less than an hour, but that of a hypertensive hemorrhage can continue over several hours if the blood pressure is not promptly brought under control. Small deep vessels of hypertensive patients develop both microaneurysms and lipohyalinosis, which are thought to be related to the development of ICH. This fact explains why hypertensive bleeds occur in the same parts of the brain where small deep infarcts are found.

Hemorrhages associated with either cerebral amyloid angiopathy (CAA) or thrombolytic agents are usually cortical, not deep. Patients with these types of hemorrhage often complain of headache, but they rarely lose consciousness. Patients with ICH resulting from CAA are typically over the age of 60 and are usually normotensive. Many of them have recurrent hemorrhages. Autopsy studies have shown that the prevalence of CAA in the general population increases linearly with age, and CAA affects the cerebral vessels in as many as 40% of those in their eighties. Amyloid deposits in the vessel walls are associated with vasculopathy in patients with CAA. Weakening of the vessel wall is thought to lead to hemorrhage.

Stroke-Related Seizures

Infarcts that produce early seizures are usually larger than those not associated with seizures. Cortical strokes are more likely to produce seizures than subcortical ones. Early seizures and stroke recurrence are both predictors of the development of epilepsy.[9] It is not clear what causes an ICH to produce seizures, but seizures associated with SAH are related to the volume of blood in the basal cisterns.

Ischemic Vascular Dementia

The three most important risk factors for vascular dementia are hypertension, advanced age, and recurrent stroke.[10] These are the same risk factors that cause changes in the subcortical white matter in the brains of community-dwelling nondemented elderly individuals.

Pathophysiologically, a critical cascade may account for the relationship between subcortical white matter changes and progressive cognitive decline in elderly hypertensive individuals.[15] Patients with untreated chronic hypertension have been shown to have hypoperfusion in the deep white matter, presumably because of the narrowing of deep penetrating arteries by lipohyalinosis. Nondemented hypertensive patients may be able to compensate for subcortical hypoperfusion by extracting more oxygen from the blood. White matter changes may develop when compensation is no longer possible. This is likely to occur when viscosity rises in association with high hematocrit, hypercholesterolemia, or hyperfibrinogenemia. Ultimately, dementia develops when a critical mass of white matter has undergone demyelinization and other ischemic changes.

CLINICAL ASSESSMENT

Clinical Symptoms of Brain Ischemia

Symptoms of TIAs and infarction vary according to the vessel that has been occluded, either temporarily or permanently (Table 32–1). Symptoms of small deep infarcts differ from those of atherothrombotic infarcts depending upon the location of the lacunae (Table 32–2). If pure motor hemiparesis is associated with nausea or ataxia, the infarct is more likely to be pontine in location

TABLE 32–1 **SYMPTOMS OF BRAIN ISCHEMIA**

Symptom	Corresponding Arterial Territory
Monocular blindness	Internal carotid artery
Unilateral leg weakness	Anterior cerebral artery
Aphasia	Middle cerebral artery
Face and arm weakness (unilateral)	Middle cerebral artery
Homonymous hemianopsia	Posterior cerebral artery
Cortical blindness or diplopia	Basilar artery
Spastic quadriparesis	Basilar artery
Crossed sensory loss, nystagmus, ataxia	Vertebral artery

TABLE 32–2 **SYMPTOMS OF SMALL DEEP INFARCTS**

Symptoms	Corresponding Brain Area
Hemiparesis (no sensory loss)	Internal capsule or pons
Hemianesthesia (no motor loss)	Thalamus
Hemichorea	Caudate, putamen, or subthalamic nucleus
Clumsy hand/dysarthria	Pons
Ataxic hemiparesis	Pons or corona radiata

than capsular. If sensory symptoms march up the arm, a focal seizure is more likely than a TIA. If hemianopsia is associated with headache, nausea, and photophobia, complicated migraine is a better clinical diagnosis than TIA.

Transient vertigo associated with ataxia, diplopia, tinnitus, or nausea is likely to be due to vertebrobasilar insufficiency. Vertigo that develops in a diabetic patient along with tachycardia or tremor may be a symptom of hypoglycemia rather than a TIA. When vertigo is accompanied by bilateral paresthesias and anxiety, it may be a manifestation of hyperventilation or a panic attack.

Emergency Assessment of Brain Ischemia

It is important to order a head CT scan for all patients with symptoms of acute ischemia because tumor, SAH, subdural hematoma, and ICH can all mimic the symptoms of TIA and stroke.[1, 16] Intravenous contrast medium is not needed for the admission head CT scan because the main purpose is to exclude hemorrhage. Only about 50% of acute ischemic infarcts appear on the first CT scan. Infarcts that are already large on the admission CT scan are more likely to bleed if the patient is anticoagulated. Large infarcts carry a poor prognosis in general because they are likely to be associated with edema and increased intracranial pressure.

An electrocardiogram (ECG) is recommended for every new TIA or stroke in order to identify patients who have AF, acute myocardial infarction, or left ventricular hypertrophy.[2, 16] If the admission ECG detects serious cardiac abnormalities, telemetry is usually indicated for at least the first 24 hours. A chest radiograph is also needed on admission to look for cardiomegaly and signs of possible aortic dissection. Blood tests needed in acute TIA and stroke patients include a complete blood count, prothrombin time, partial thromboplastin time, creatinine, glucose, and creatine kinase (CK).

Nonemergent Assessment of Ischemia

If the admission CT scan for a stroke patient is normal, a repeat scan without contrast can be done 4 to 7 days later to document the location and to clarify the pathogenesis of the infarct. This scan will help in selecting the proper therapy. Some small cortical infarcts, for example, may produce a pure motor deficit that mimics a lacunar stroke. After the repeat CT scan has verified a cortical location for the infarct and a carotid source of emboli has been excluded by carotid ultrasound, the clinician is justified in pursuing a cardiac source of emboli (an echocardiogram is recommended at this point).

Carotid ultrasonography should be scheduled within the first week of new ischemic symptoms provided they are in the distribution of the carotid arteries. TCD ultrasound is a noninvasive method of examining the posterior circulation in patients with symptoms of vertebrobasilar insufficiency. If carotid ultrasound suggests high-grade (70% to 99%) stenosis of the symptomatic vessel, cerebral angiography is the next step for patients who are good surgical candidates.[3] This technique is needed to rule out the presence of distal disease of the internal carotid that might be more severe than that in the cervical portion of the artery. Transesophageal echocardiography is justified when no lacunar, cardioembolic, or atherothrombotic sources can be identified.[4]

Subarachnoid Hemorrhage

Sudden onset of severe headache followed by nausea, vomiting, stiff neck, or altered mental state should lead the clinician to suspect SAH. If a noncontrast CT scan shows no evidence of fresh blood in the subarachnoid space, then a lumbar puncture should be done to confirm the diagnosis (10% of SAHs must be diagnosed in this way). If fresh blood is apparent on CT scan, a lumbar puncture is usually contraindicated because changes in hydrostatic pressure could dislodge the clot and facilitate rebleeding. Selective catheter angiography is the next step in localizing the aneurysm or arteriovenous malformation. Nevertheless, 15% to 25% of angiograms performed to detect SAH do not show a source of the hemorrhage. SAH patients with no identifiable aneurysm or arteriovenous malformation on angiography are less likely to experience rebleeding following SAH.

Intracerebral Hemorrhage

Besides hypertension, anticoagulation, alcohol abuse, and amyloid angiopathy, another cause of ICH is brain tumor. Glioblastoma and metastases from lung, melanoma, or kidney are more likely to bleed than other tumor types. A tumor should be suspected if focal symptoms precede the hemorrhage or if bleeding occurs into unusual sites such as the corpus callosum. If the admission CT scan suggests a tumor, contrast CT or MRI should be scheduled the next day to clarify the diagnosis. Treatment for brain tumor differs considerably from that for acute stroke.

Stroke-Related Seizures

In the emergency room, the condition most commonly mistaken for stroke is seizure. The short-term hemiparesis that follows a partial seizure (Todd's paralysis) can be clinically indistinguishable from the weakness associated with a small stroke. On the other hand, 5% of all ischemic stroke patients may develop seizures during the acute stages of an infarct.[9] Only about 20% of EEGs in patients with postinfarction seizures show paroxysmal activity. The presence of early seizures and recurrent strokes is a better predictor of epilepsy in stroke patients than are focal abnormalities on EEG.[9]

Ischemic Vascular Dementia

Multi-infarct dementia is usually distinguished from Alzheimer's dementia by its sudden onset, fluctuating course, focal neurologic signs, and the presence of multiple infarcts as shown by the history or CT.[10] In contrast, the cognitive and gait impairments characteristic of Binswanger's disease may develop subacutely, without cortical infarcts on head CT (which may show only periventricular white matter lucencies and ventricular atrophy). Patients with Binswanger's disease may come to medical attention with a TIA, seizure, repeated falls, pseudobulbar affect, or acute confusional state.

MANAGEMENT

Transient Ischemic Attacks

Recent changes in the practice of medicine have resulted in more frequent management of TIA patients in the outpatient setting. Nevertheless, patients with a high risk of stroke should still be admitted to the hospital, especially those with a probable cardiac source of emboli and those who have had more than two TIAs within the last 2 weeks.[2] Since retinal TIAs carry a lower risk of stroke than hemispheric TIAs, patients with retinal TIAs can usually be evaluated on an outpatient basis.

If cerebral angiography confirms the presence of high-grade stenosis (70% to 99%) of the symptomatic carotid artery, the treatment of choice is endarterectomy and aspirin.[3] In a large randomized trial of aspirin alone versus aspirin combined with endarterectomy, TIA patients treated with both surgery and aspirin were found to have a 9% risk of stroke over 2 years, whereas those treated with aspirin alone had a 26% risk. Patients were not permitted to enter that study if they were over the age of 80 years, were mentally incompetent, had more severe siphon stenosis than proximal carotid stenosis, or had a limited life expectancy owing to cancer or organ failure.

If there is no evidence of either significant carotid stenosis or a cardiac source of emboli, antiplatelet therapy with aspirin or ticlopidine is indicated for stroke prophylaxis.[12] Dipyridamole is usually reserved for patients who cannot tolerate either aspirin or ticlopidine. Most practitioners start therapy for TIA patients with one aspirin per day (325 mg/day), although some patients with recurrent TIAs may benefit from as many as four tablets per day (1300 mg/day). If TIA or stroke patients are intolerant of aspirin or if they continue to have strokes while taking aspirin, ticlopidine is indicated for stroke prophylaxis (250 mg bid). Hematologic monitoring is required during the first 3 months of ticlopidine therapy because about 1% of patients treated with this drug develop severe (rarely fatal) neutropenia during the first 12 weeks of therapy.

There is good evidence from clinical trials that TIA patients with nonvalvular AF should receive anticoagulation with warfarin, especially if they are women over the age of 75 or if they have other thromboembolic risk factors such as left ventricular dysfunction, hypertension, or prior stroke. Aspirin may be preferred, however, for AF patients who are at high risk for falls, have poorly controlled hypertension, or are unlikely to comply with close monitoring of coagulation parameters.

Acute Ischemic Infarction

New data are now appearing in the literature suggesting that thrombolytic agents can improve the functional outcome of survivors of acute ischemic stroke regardless of cause (atherothrombotic, cardioembolic, or lacunar). The most promising agent is tissue plasminogen-activating factor (tPA).[17]

The key to successful use of thrombolytic agents is administration of the drugs within the first 3 hours after the onset of symptoms. Despite the tenfold increase in cerebral hemorrhage, patients receiving tPA were at least 30% more likely to have a good functional outcome at 3 months. Current studies with tPA are examining ways of predicting in advance who might benefit the most and who is at highest risk of hemorrhage.

There is general agreement that most patients with acute ischemic stroke should not be treated with antihypertensive agents unless their calculated mean blood pressure is greater than 130 mmHg.[16] The other exceptions include patients with acute myocardial infarction, acute renal failure, dissection of the thoracic aorta, or hemorrhagic transformation of a cerebral infarction. The best parenteral drugs for treating hypertension in patients with acute stroke are labetalol and nitroprusside.

Early mobilization of stroke patients should aid in preventing pneumonia and other complications. Corticosteroids should be avoided in those with acute ischemic stroke because their use is more detrimental than beneficial (more infections). If there are signs of increased intracranial pressure in a patient with an acute stroke, a trial of hyperventilation is recommended. Surgical intervention is necessary on the rare occasions when hydrocephalus develops or when a large cerebellar infarction is found. Use of heparin in acute stroke cannot be justified by scientific studies, but it is the standard of care in some communities.[16] Prophylactic heparin, on the other hand, is strongly recommended for stroke patients who are immobilized.

Subarachnoid Hemorrhage

The treatment of SAH depends on the patient's neurologic status. Patients who are asymptomatic except for headache or a stiff neck should have early angiography with the goal of performing early surgical clipping of the aneurysm. During close monitoring prior to surgery, these patients need strict bed rest, oral nimodipine, and prophylaxis for deep vein thrombosis. Patients who are drowsy or obtunded may have to be intubated to protect the airway. SAH patients whose condition deteriorates rapidly may be taken to surgery for immediate clot removal and clipping of the aneurysm.

Intracerebral Hemorrhage

If CT of an ICH patient shows no evidence of midline shift and the patient is alert and awake, management on a general medical floor is feasible provided the nurses are given guidelines about the treatment of hypertension, headache, and changes in mental state. If the patient's condition deteriorates, transfer to an intensive care unit is indicated. Families should be made aware of the high mortality rate in patients with ICH. There is general agreement that patients with cerebellar hemorrhages that cause signs of brain stem compression should receive mannitol and surgical decompression.[16]

Ischemic Vascular Dementia

There is good evidence that risk factor management is useful in treating patients with vascular dementia just as it is in those with TIA and small strokes.[10] Occasionally these patients deteriorate if their blood pressure has been reduced excessively, so the goal should be to keep the systolic pressure in the range of 135 to 150 mmHg. Antiplatelet agents have been shown to be beneficial not only for stroke prevention but also for cognitive benefit in patients with vascular dementia. In a double-blind placebo-controlled trial, pentoxifylline produced improvement in cognitive function in patients with vascular dementia who had CT evidence of ischemic changes. The multiple mechanisms of action of this drug probably explain its therapeutic effect. It increases red cell deformability, inhibits platelet aggregation, lowers plasma fibrinogen levels, and decreases the viscosity of whole blood.

SUMMARY

We must communicate to our patients that 40% of all strokes can be prevented with better management of reversible risk factors such as smoking and hypertension. Patients also must learn that stroke is an emergency and that beneficial treatment of acute stroke can only be achieved in those who seek treatment within the first few hours of symptom onset. In addition to thrombolytic agents that dissolve the clots causing acute ischemic stroke, new protective agents are being developed to reduce the size of the infarct. Similar agents are being tested in patients with SAH to prevent infarcts from developing in association with vasospasm. If strokes can be prevented by reducing risk factors, we should see fewer patients with postinfarction epilepsy and vascular dementia. Patient education is the key.

References

1. Whisnant JP, Basford JR, Bernstein EF, et al: Classification of cerebrovascular disease III. Stroke 1990;21:637–676.
2. Brown RD, Evans BA, Weibers DO, Petty GW, Meissner I, Dale AJD: Transient ischemic attack and

minor ischemic stroke. Mayo Clin Proc 1994;69:1027–1039.

3. North American Symptomatic Carotid Endarterectomy Trial Collaborators: Beneficial effect of carotid endarterectomy in symptomatic patients with high-grade carotid stenosis. N Engl J Med 1991;325:445–453.

4. Amarenco P, Cohen A, Tzourio C, et al: Atherosclerotic disease of the aortic arch and the risk of ischemic stroke. N Engl J Med 1994;331:1474–1479.

5. Strandgaard S, Paulson OB: Cerebrovascular consequences of hypertension. Lancet 1994;344:519–521.

6. Wolf PA, Abbott RD, Kannel WB: Atrial fibrillation as an independent risk factor for stroke: The Framingham Study. Stroke 1991;22:983–988.

7. Broderick JP, Brott T, Tomsick T, Huster G, Miller R: The risk of subarachnoid hemorrhage and intracerebral hemorrhage in blacks compared to whites. N Engl J Med 1992;326:733–736.

8. Marmot MG, Poulter NR: Primary prevention of stroke. Lancet 1992;339:344–347.

9. So EL, Annegers JF, Hauser WA, O'Brien PC, Whisnant JP: Population-based study of seizure disorders after cerebral infarction. Neurology 1996;46:350–355.

10. Hershey LA, Olszewski WA: Ischemic vascular dementia. *In* Morris JC (ed): Handbook of Dementing Illnesses. New York, Marcel Dekker, 1994, pp. 335–351.

11. The EC/IC Bypass Study Group: Failure of extracranial-intracranial arterial bypass to reduce the risk of ischemic stroke. N Engl J Med 1985;313:1191–1200.

12. Hass WK, Easton JD, Adams HP, et al: A randomized trial comparing ticlopidine with aspirin for prevention of stroke. N Engl J Med 1989;321:501–507.

13. Siebler M, Sitzer M, Rose G, Bendfeldt D, Steinmetz H: Silent cerebral embolism caused by symptomatic high-grade carotid stenosis. Brain 1993;116:1005–1015.

14. Wannamethee SG, Shaper AG, Whincup PH, Walker M: Smoking cessation and the risk of stroke in middle-aged men. JAMA 1995;274:155–160.

15. Yao H, Sadoshima S, Ibayashi S, et al: Leukoaraiosis and dementia in hypertensive patients. Stroke 1992;23:1673–1677.

16. Adams HP, Brott TG, Crowell RM, et al: Guidelines for the management of patients with acute ischemic stroke. Stroke 1994;25:1901–1914.

17. NINDS Stroke Study Group: Tissue plasminogen activator for acute stroke. N Engl J Med 1995;333:1581–1587.

33 Parkinson's Disease and Parkinsonian Syndromes

David Gordon Lichter, M.B., Ch.B., F.R.A.C.P.

Parkinson's disease (PD) currently affects approximately 1 million people in North America and is particularly common in those over age 60, of whom 1% to 2% are afflicted. Prevalence ratios increase steeply with advancing age, and the disorder is expected to become correspondingly more common as human life is prolonged. Despite major advances in our understanding of PD, the diagnosis is still made solely on clinical criteria. In the elderly, as in other age groups, attempts must be made to differentiate idiopathic PD (defined by the cardinal features of rest tremor, rigidity, bradykinesia, and postural instability) from other (secondary) causes of parkinsonism. Therapy for PD must be prescribed on an individual basis, taking into account the expectations and needs of the patient, the projected life span, and the presence of co-existing medical conditions. The heightened susceptibility of the elderly to the toxic effects of drugs, particularly anticholinergics, and age-related changes in pharmacokinetics must also be considered when drug therapy for patients with PD is chosen.

PATHOPHYSIOLOGY

Degeneration of Dopaminergic Neurons

Central to the pathology of PD is the degeneration of dopamine-generating neurons, located in the pars compacta of the substantia nigra and ventral tegmental area of the midbrain. These neurons project to the striatum (caudate and putamen) and frontal and limbic brain regions. Clinicopathologic correlations have indicated that clinical deficits emerge when approximately 80% of the nigral cells have been lost, and the course of clinical decline then parallels the degeneration of the remaining nigral neurons.

Differences Between Parkinson's Disease and Normal Aging

Although certain "parkinsonian" features of aging have been attributed to a decline in dopaminergic function, it is clear that PD is not just an exaggeration of "normal" aging. Aging in humans is associated with a slow attrition of nigrostriatal dopaminergic neurons that results in a significant drop in dopamine concentrations in the putamen after the age of 60 years. However, the striatal dopamine loss that occurs with normal aging does not mimic the typical subregional pattern of striatal dopamine loss found in idiopathic PD. Correspondingly, the lateral ventral tier of the substantia nigra is relatively spared in normal aging but is specifically involved in PD. There is evidence, also, of active cell breakdown, phagocytosis, and gliosis in PD but not in age-matched controls or in postencephalitic parkinsonism after years of subsequent "normal aging." These observations, together with the failure of levodopa to affect the mild extrapyramidal impairment of normal elderly subjects,[1] have suggested that PD has a distinct pathobiology.[2]

The Oxidant Stress Hypothesis of Parkinson's Disease

Although the cause of PD remains obscure and may be multifactorial (e.g., toxins, reduced primordial population of nigral dopaminergic neurons, infections, genetic predisposition), toxicity from endogenous and exogenous oxidative mechanisms has been implicated as a fundamental process in the progressive nigral cell loss. In this conceptualization, normal age-related changes may aggravate oxidative stresses on dopaminergic neurons.

In preclinical disease, it has been suggested that the efforts of surviving neurons to compensate with increasing dopamine output may result in enhanced generation of hydroxyl radicals and other potentially toxic by-products of oxidative deamination of dopamine. This process is compounded by a reduced concentration of a number of free radical scavengers, including glutathione, in the substantia nigra and basal ganglia in PD. In mice, experimental glutathione depletion produces morphologic changes in nigral neurons that resemble those seen in both normal aging and the MPTP neurotoxicity model of PD. MPTP (1-methyl-4-phenyl-1,2,5,6-tetrahydropyridine) is highly toxic to neurons in the pars compacta of the substantia nigra and produces clinical and neuropathologic features that closely resemble those of PD in both nonhuman primates and humans. Oxidative biotransformation of MPTP by the enzyme monoamine oxidase B is required for its neurotoxic effect, which is mediated via disruption of mitochondrial functions. Monoamine oxidase B is increased in concentration in the aged brain, and aged animals are more susceptible to the neurotoxic effects of MPTP than younger animals. Such observations have suggested that oxidation of both endogenous and exogenous compounds may predispose to the senescence of dopaminergic neurons in patients with PD, with the further implication that aging may increase their vulnerability to this process.

The Role of Aging in Parkinson's Disease

Despite their appeal and apparent coherence, both the oxidant stress hypothesis of PD and the argument that aging may contribute to dopaminergic cell loss in PD have been challenged.[3, 4] Not all studies have indicated a continuing increase in frequency of PD with age, and some have suggested a decrease in frequency after age 75 to 80. The rate of loss of dopaminergic innervation in the caudate nucleus appears to be similar whether the disease begins before or after 60 years of age. Similarly, neuronal loss in the substantia nigra appears to be no greater and may be less severe in late-onset patients than in early-onset patients despite comparable disease durations. Thus, although aging may contribute an additional risk factor in the development of PD and may clearly alter the expression of symptoms (see later discussion), it may not have a major effect on the degeneration of dopaminergic neurons in this disorder.

CLINICAL ASSESSMENT

The typical presentation of parkinsonism, with initially asymmetrical resting tremor, bradykinesia, and rigidity, may be seen in patients of any age. However, patients with late-onset disease are more likely to present with relatively symmetrical signs, and display at an earlier stage, or to a greater degree, signs of postural instability, gait disorders, frontal lobe symptoms or dementia, and autonomic dysfunction.[5] In addition, more than a third of patients whose parkinsonian symptoms first appear at the age of 75 or older appear to be unresponsive to levodopa despite clinical features that may be otherwise typical. Patients with late-onset disease are also less likely to develop significant "on-off" motor fluctuations,[6] which usually complicate therapy with levodopa in the middle and late stages of the disease. Although use of lower doses of levodopa in older patients may partially account for this observation, age-related changes in the brain (including loss of striatal dopamine receptors), different pathology in some late-onset cases, and other unknown factors may modify the disease course in the elderly.

DIFFERENTIAL DIAGNOSIS OF PARKINSON'S DISEASE

Parkinson's Disease Versus Parkinsonism

In the absence of any available confirmatory diagnostic tests, the diagnosis of idiopathic PD remains a clinical judgment based on a typical history and characteristic neurologic examination. All four of the cardinal clinical signs (see first paragraph of this chapter) need not be present to make the diagnosis, particularly if the patient presents with a characteristic unilateral rest tremor. However, if akinesia and rigidity (even if unilateral) are present in the absence of a rest tremor, the diagnosis of PD is less certain, and other possible causes of parkinsonism must be considered.

After a diagnosis of PD or parkinsonism has been made, attention should be directed toward (1) excluding specific etiologic factors, including drugs (see later discussion), toxins (e.g., manganese, carbon monoxide, carbon disulfide, methanol, and ethanol), anoxic brain injury, and encephalitis (including that due to syphilis and acquired immunodeficiency syndrome (AIDS), and (2) identifying any "unusual" or distinguishing clinical features. These "red flags" include initial bilateral presentation, subacute onset (suggestive of drug-induced or other secondary causes of parkinsonism), lack of response to levodopa, absence of rest tremor, and the presence of nonparkinsonian neurologic deficits, which may suggest a "parkinsonism plus" syndrome.

The "Parkinsonism Plus" Syndromes

"Parkinsonism plus" syndromes are disorders in which the classic features of parkinsonism are combined with other neurologic deficits, particularly autonomic, cerebellar, oculomotor, cortical, and pyramidal dysfunction. The prognosis of these conditions is generally considerably worse than that of idiopathic PD. Although they may be impossible to distinguish from PD early in the course, an absent, limited, or transient response to levodopa, caused by degeneration of striatal or pallidal neurons, should alert the physician to the presence of an atypical syndrome.

The combination of parkinsonism and visual symptoms (unusual in PD), associated with a markedly decreased blink rate and impairment of conjugate eye movements, should suggest the diagnosis of progressive supranuclear palsy (PSP). Early slowing and later limitation of voluntary downgaze may result in difficulties with reading, eating, tying shoes, and walking downstairs. These problems are followed by progressive loss of all voluntary vertical and horizontal eye movements, but oculocephalic reflexes are preserved. There is disproportionate axial rigidity and dystonia, the neck often being held stiffly in extension, as opposed to the flexed posture characteristic of PD. A prominent feature is an early loss of the postural reflexes, which predisposes the person to "log-like" falls, often backward. Pseudobulbar palsy, characterized by dysphagia, dysarthria, and emotional incontinence, may be an early or late finding.

The disorders known as multiple system atrophy (MSA) overlap clinically and pathologically and are best distinguished by their presenting clinical signs. Among these, the Shy-Drager syndrome is notable for prominent dysautonomia, which may be present for up to 3 years before parkinsonian signs appear. Common early features include orthostatic hypotension, syncope, impotence, anhidrosis, and symptoms of neurogenic bladder disturbance (urinary frequency, nocturia, retention, and overflow incontinence). Laryngeal stridor may occur late in the course of the Shy-Drager syndrome and in striatonigral degeneration, a disorder that may be suspected initially on the basis of a levodopa-resistant akinetic-rigid syndrome. In the olivopontocerebellar atrophies (OPCA), parkinsonism is typically associated with cerebellar signs (such as ataxia, intention tremor, and nystagmus), bulbar deficits (dysarthria and dysphagia), and corticospinal signs. Magnetic resonance imaging (MRI) frequently shows atrophy of the brain stem and cerebellum.

Corticobasal ganglionic degeneration is an unusual but readily differentiated syndrome that usually presents in the seventh decade of life and is characterized by extreme rigidity and apraxia, which starts in one limb, often the nondominant upper extremity, and then spreads over a period of a few years to the ipsilateral limb and then to the contralateral limbs. As opposed to the rest tremor characteristic of PD, there is a 6- to 8-Hz action or intention tremor that differs from essential tremor by its myoclonic jerkiness. Associated findings include the "alien limb" syndrome, cortical sensory loss, constructional apraxia, frontal release signs, and, later in the course, cognitive dysfunction or dementia, reflecting the characteristic frontal and parietal cortical pathology.

Drug-Induced Parkinsonism

Because drug-induced parkinsonism is reversible when the offending agent is stopped, it should never be overlooked. Drugs that act presynaptically by inhibiting dopamine synthesis (e.g., alpha-methylparatyrosine), disrupting vesicular storage of dopamine (e.g., reserpine), or producing false neurotransmitters (e.g., alpha-methyldopa) are, fortunately, now relatively uncommon causes of parkinsonism. On the other hand, parkinsonism is still a common complication of drugs that block the central D2 dopamine receptors. Of these, neuroleptic agents such as the phenothiazines (e.g., chlorpromazine) and butyrophenones (e.g., haloperidol) are the most frequently recognized offenders. Parkinsonism may also be a side effect of the tricyclic antidepressant dibenzoxazepine (amoxapine), which has an antipsychotic metabolite, loxapine. However, the most common drug-induced form of parkinsonism seen in the elderly in outpatient settings, and one that is frequently overlooked, is that produced by antiemetics, particularly metoclopramide (Reglan) and prochlorperazine (Compazine).[7, 8] These drugs have the potential to block central as well as peripheral D2 dopamine receptors.

The calcium channel blockers flunarizine and cinnarizine have structural similarities to neuroleptics and are well documented as causes of parkinsonism. Although these drugs are not available in the United States, other commonly used calcium channel blockers, including verapamil and diltiazem, may occasionally cause this complication. The mechanism of this effect is unclear, but blockade of calcium entry into the nigrostriatal neurons and alteration of dopamine release may contribute to it.

Recently, it has been recognized that selective serotonin reuptake inhibitors such as fluoxetine (Prozac), which may be prescribed for depression or obsessive compulsive symptoms, may occasionally induce or aggravate parkinsonism in susceptible individuals. This effect is thought to be mediated by serotonin-induced inhibition of central dopamine systems. Both phenytoin and valproate may rarely produce parkinsonism. Other, less clearly documented causes include lithium (which more commonly causes a postural and action tremor) and captopril.

In general, advanced age predisposes to drug-induced parkinsonism. Age-related loss of nigral dopaminergic neurons or "preclinical" PD in elderly patients could account for this added risk. Female sex is also a predisposing factor. This may be explained by the influence of estrogens and, in the case of neuroleptics, by a higher average per kilogram prescribed dosage in female patients.

Normal Aging

The clinical appearance of the aging process itself bears some resemblance to PD, normal elderly subjects often showing weakness of the voice, motoric slowing, variable increases in muscle tone, particularly in the legs, and a characteristic alteration of posture and gait. The main features of this syndrome are a slightly flexed posture, diminished arm swing, slowness and stiffness in walking, usually on a slightly widened base, and a shortened step (marche a petit pas). Turns are achieved by multiple short steps rather than by a single, fluid movement. Most older individuals adopt this "senile" or "cautious" gait[9] to a greater or lesser degree. In the individual case, it may be a compensation for arthritis, pain, weakness, vestibular inaccuracy, or sensory impairments, including mild proprioceptive loss and age-related visual impairment. Other factors differentiate this condition from PD. Thus, rest tremor is absent in normal aging; there is no festination of gait (a tendency to advance increasingly rapidly, with short steps) and no propulsion or freezing occurs. Furthermore, facial masking is seldom present, micrographia is absent, and slowing of movement is not accompanied by the prominent fatigability (progressive fade and collapse of sequential or repetitive movements) that characterizes true bradykinesia.

Higher-Level Gait Disorders in the Elderly

Adding to the diagnostic difficulties encountered in the elderly, senile gait may be compounded by both fear of falling and other nonparkinsonian neurologic conditions that may produce gait apraxias and "freezing" of various types. The resulting disorder may vary widely in severity and includes sudden "motor blocks" only when the patient is confronted with obstacles, difficulty in initiating gait, with shuffling on the spot ("the slipped clutch"), and, in its most severe form, a total inability to start walking, the feet appearing glued to the floor ("magnetic response"). In the syndrome of "isolated gait ignition failure," the gait has some elements of parkinsonism, with hesitation in starts and turns, shuffling, and freezing, but it is relatively unremarkable once entrained and is marked by upright posture and normal or near-normal equilibrium. The cause of this levodopa-resistant syndrome is unclear, but it may include focal degeneration of the frontal lobes or frontal lobe vascular disease.

A more typical gait in patients with cerebrovascular disease, including those with Binswanger's disease (subcortical arteriosclerotic encephalopathy) combines elements of start and turn hesitation, short steps, and freezing with progressive dysequilibrium and falls. This condition has been termed lower-half or lower-body parkinsonism.[9] Unlike patients with PD, these patients typically walk on a widened base, have an upright trunk and leg posture, and usually do not show festination, propulsion, or retropulsion. Associated findings often include cognitive impairment, pseudobulbar palsy, frontal release signs, paratonia, pyramidal signs, and urinary disturbances. Vascular risk factors, including hypertension, diabetes mellitus, hyperlipidemia, elevated fibrinogen levels, and cardiomyopathy, are often present and should be addressed in an effort to slow the progression of disease. The pathophysiology of this condition may be linked to damage to the reciprocal connections between the frontal lobes and the basal ganglia secondary to subcortical white matter disease. Similar abnormalities of equilibrium and gait have been described in patients with normal pressure hydrocephalus.

Benign Essential (Senile) Tremor

Although rest tremor is absent in normal aging, older persons not uncommonly have a postural-action tremor (a "senile" variant of benign essential tremor), which may be mistaken for a parkinsonian tremor. Essential tremor is frequently a familial condition and is generally inherited as an autosomal dominant trait. It presents as an alcohol-responsive postural and action tremor, affecting the upper limbs, head (as a "no-no" or "yes-yes" movement), and voice, the legs being infrequently affected. This tremor tends to be more symmetrical than the rest tremor of PD. Parkinsonian tremor may involve the lips, tongue, or jaw but usually spares the head and is never associated with vocal tremor. Although other parkinsonian features are absent in essential tremor, between 40% and 50% of patients with PD manifest some postural and action tremor as well as rest tremor. More significantly, a postural-action tremor that is indistinguishable from essential tremor may precede by several years the development of PD in some patients. Elderly patients with apparent essential tremor should therefore be followed closely for emergence of symptoms or signs of PD.

Arthritis and Other Musculoskeletal Conditions

Osteoarthritis of the hips and knees or an old hip fracture may add to postural and gait difficulties in the elderly and sometimes suggests parkinsonism. Conversely, early signs of PD may be missed in elderly arthritic patients in whom painful joints or fixed deformities may hinder accurate assessment of muscle tone, bradykinesia, dexterity, handwriting, or walking. Adding to possible diagnostic confusion, the onset of PD is insidious, and symptoms of stiffness, slow movement, and (occasionally) aching pain may be overlooked or attributed incorrectly to "arthritis" in the elderly. Frozen shoulder may be the first symptom of PD in at least 8% of patients and may occur up to 2 years prior to the onset of more commonly recognized features of parkinsonism. Sciatic-like pain may also occur as an early sign of PD and may lead to unnecessary surgery.

Stroke

Stroke is common in the elderly, and unilateral parkinsonism may sometimes be confused initially with hemiparesis. Attention to certain features of the examination should help in differentiating these conditions. In PD, the patient's increased tone has the characteristics of rigidity ("lead-pipe" resistance throughout the range of movement or "cogwheel"-type resistance when tremor is also present) rather than spasticity (hypertonicity that is direction- and velocity-dependent). A pyramidal tract pattern of weakness should not be present in uncomplicated PD. Similarly, a true Babinski's sign is not a feature of PD, in which even the tonically extended great toe ("striatal toe") should show the normal flexor response to plantar stimulation. Associated findings, including hypophonia, hypomimia (reduced facial expression), and flexed posture on standing, may suggest the correct diagnosis.

Depression

The psychomotor retardation of depression may be mistaken for the bradykinesia and hypomimia of PD, and vice versa. Distinguishing features suggestive of uncomplicated depression are a lack of tremor and rigidity and the presence of vegetative symptoms, such as reduced appetite, weight loss, and insomnia. However, vegetative symptoms and signs are frequently absent in the normal elderly population with depressive symptoms, the majority of whom present with dysphoria rather than major depression. In contrast, symptomatic dysphoria is rare in patients with PD, who are more likely to present with dysthymic disorder, agitated depression (with associated anxiety and panic symptoms), or major depression.

Dementia

Diagnostic difficulties commonly arise when parkinsonism is accompanied by dementia. The prevalence of dementia in patients with PD varies from 20% to 40%, depending on the criteria for diagnosis of dementia and the population surveyed. This figure indicates a risk of dementia that is up to four times greater for parkinsonian subjects than for age-matched controls. Older age, more severe disease, and depression have been found to be predictive of incident dementia in a community population sample of PD patients. In addition to the influences of PD and aging, causes of dementia in a parkinsonian patient include the presence of a parkinsonian plus syndrome (see earlier section), other neurologic conditions, metabolic disorders, and drugs.

Most levodopa-responsive parkinsonian patients who develop dementia have a predominantly "subcortical" dementia syndrome, characterized by cognitive slowing (bradyphrenia), disproportionate impairment in executive skills (including the ability to sustain attention, plan, monitor, and modify behavior appropriately to achieve a particular goal), impaired memory function, and perceptual motor dysfunction. Although there is a relative sparing of language, praxis, and other "higher" cortical functions, a majority of such individuals manifest one or more pathologic correlates of Alzheimer's disease, such as degeneration of cholinergic neurons of the nucleus basalis of Meynert, senile neuritic plaques, and neurofibrillary tangles. Because these patients may experience a worsening of parkinsonism if they are treated with an anticholinesterase drug such as tacrine (Cognex) or donepezil HCl (Aricept), they need to be distinguished from subjects with senile dementia of the Alzheimer's type. The latter patients have a course that is characterized from the onset by a progressive "cortical"-type dementia (typified by such features as aphasia, apraxia, and agnosia, as well as substantial memory impairment), with later development of extrapyramidal signs. In such cases, rigidity may be accompanied by bradykinesia, but true rest tremor should not be present, and there is usually no response to levodopa.

A history of psychosis, vulnerability to levodopa-induced psychosis, sensitivity to neuroleptics, and, occasionally, a positive family history, may suggest a diagnosis of "diffuse Lewy body disease," a pathologic variant of PD in which abundant Lewy bodies (the hallmark of PD) are present throughout the cortex, not just in the substantia nigra compacta. Alternatively, an abrupt onset, stepwise deterioration, or fluctuating course of dementia, presence of vascular risk factors, focal neurologic symptoms or signs, or a history of previous strokes suggests the presence of a vascular dementia, which is likely to be associated with levodopa-resistant "lower-body" parkinsonism (see earlier discussion).

A routine complete blood count, chemistry screen, thyroxine (T_4) and thyroid-stimulating hormone levels, vitamin B_{12} level, and computed tomographic (CT) or MRI scan should exclude common treatable causes of dementia, such as metabolic encephalopathy, normal pressure hydrocephalus, intracranial masses, and multi-infarct state. Finally, even in patients who do not manifest hallucinations or delusions (usually signs of a dopaminergic psychosis) or frank delirium, reduction of unnecessary drugs, particularly those with anticholinergic properties, may improve memory and cognition in the elderly parkinsonian patient.

MANAGEMENT OF PARKINSON'S DISEASE

General Principles

The first step in pharmacologic management of the patient with PD is for the patient and physician to agree on therapeutic goals. Attempts to treat symptoms or signs that are of no importance to the patient will not be useful and may carry the risk of significant adverse effects. Second, it is important in the elderly, who may be very sensitive to drugs, to "start low and go slow" when introducing and titrating medications. Finally, one should explore the effect of dose changes in only one drug at a time.

Management of Parkinsonian Motor Dysfunction

ANTICHOLINERGIC DRUGS AND AMANTADINE

Centrally acting anticholinergic drugs such as trihexyphenidyl (Artane) and benztropine (Cogentin) may be useful for the early treatment of PD in patients 60 years of age or younger in whom resting tremor is the predominant symptom. However, their use is not recommended in older patients or in those with dementia in view of a high incidence of peripheral and central side effects (see later discussion of Psychotoxicity and Its Management).

Amantadine hydrochloride (Symmetrel, Symadine) is an antiviral agent discovered by chance to have antiparkinsonian activity. In addition to possible mild peripheral anticholinergic actions, it is an *N*-methyl D-aspartate (NMDA) receptor antagonist with possible neuroprotective properties (see Psychotoxicity and Its Management), and it promotes release of dopamine from presynaptic terminals, blocks dopamine reuptake, and stimulates dopamine receptors. Amantadine may be used as an initial short-term (1 to 2 years) monotherapy for mild to moderate parkinsonian symptoms. Peripheral side effects include livedo reticularis (a reddish-purple reticular mottling, usually limited to the skin of the ankles and lower legs), ankle edema, dry mouth, constipation, and blurred vision, which are rarely severe enough to limit treatment. However, when amantadine is used in doses of up to 300 mg daily, with or without levodopa, confusion and hallucinations have been found to occur twice as often (47% incidence) in patients over age 65 than in younger patients. The reduced glomerular filtration rate in older patients may account for this phenomenon because amantadine is excreted unchanged from the kidney. In view of the greater risk of toxicity, amantadine should generally be avoided in patients with impaired renal function. In older patients, it is best to titrate amantadine over a 2-week period, preferably using the liquid formulation (50 mg/5 mL), to a maximum of 100 mg bid. If this dose is well tolerated, the capsules (100 mg) can then be substituted. Thereafter, it is necessary to remain vigilant for any emerging adverse effects, which may occur most commonly after 3 to 9 months of treatment.

LEVODOPA

The decision about the timing of the introduction of levodopa, now routinely combined with the peripheral decarboxylase inhibitor carbidopa (in the United States) or benserazide (in other countries), is based entirely on the needs, expectations, and age of the individual patient. In addition, the observed or anticipated response to and the side effects of alternative antiparkinsonian therapies should factor into this judgment and are particularly important considerations in the elderly. Although levodopa remains the most effective treatment for PD, end-of-dose fluctuations (reemergence of parkinsonian signs and symptoms as each levodopa dose wears off) and dyskinesias (abnormal involuntary movements) complicate the course in up to 50% of patients within 5 to 7 years of initiating therapy. However, the available evidence suggests that fluctuations and dyskinesias are likely to take longer to develop after starting levodopa in elderly patients, and when they do develop, they are less likely to be disabling.[6, 10] The elderly patient is more likely to die of unrelated causes before these problems are encountered. When one considers also the heightened susceptibility of the elderly to the toxic effects of alternative medications, such as anticholinergic drugs and amantadine, one can make a strong case for early rather than late introduction of levodopa in this population.

Quality of life and functional status should be the primary factors guiding the decision for initiation of levodopa therapy. Mild bradykinesia or rest tremor, which may produce significant disability for younger patients who are still employed, often does not have the same import for elderly retired individuals. On the other hand, the importance of hobbies or social activities to the psychological well-being of the older patient should not be underestimated. Limitations in these areas, even if there is no significant impact on other activities of daily living, may warrant the introduction of levodopa. Rigidity and bradykinesia that have progressed to the point where social independence is compromised (for example, when difficulties are encountered in such domains as maintenance of personal hygiene, feeding or dressing oneself, getting in and out of bed and chairs, walking, and driving) represent clear indications for levodopa therapy.

In general, plasma concentrations of levodopa are substantially higher in elderly subjects than in younger patients following a given oral dose.[11] Slower gastric emptying in the elderly, with subsequent increased duodenal levodopa absorption, contributes to this phenomenon. In addition, an age-related decrease in first-pass metabolic decarboxylation in the gastrointestinal tract results in levodopa bioavailability in elderly patients that may be as much as 20% greater than that in younger patients. This difference is abolished by the peripheral decarboxylase inhibitor carbidopa.

The systemic clearance and volume of distribution of levodopa, with or without carbidopa, are also reduced in the elderly, probably because of an age-related decline in lean body mass. Regardless of concomitant decarboxylase inhibitor therapy, elderly subjects may therefore require a smaller dose of levodopa than younger patients.[12]

Levodopa is usually best initiated at a dose of half of a 25/100 carbidopa-levodopa (Sinemet) tablet, two or three times daily after a meal and is increased by half a tablet every 4 to 7 days using tid or qid dosing until a satisfactory response occurs. The goal of such therapy should be to eliminate disability rather than to abolish all symptoms or signs of the disease. For the patient with early emerging disability related to PD, an average of 300 to 400 mg of levodopa daily is required to accomplish this goal. With the 25/100 Sinemet tablet, this dose also provides 75 to 100 mg/day of carbidopa, which is normally sufficient to block the peripheral dopamine decarboxylase enzyme, thereby minimizing nausea and other adverse effects of levodopa.

An alternative initial strategy is to begin levodopa with controlled-release (CR) Sinemet at an initial dose of one 25/100 tablet twice a day and then switching to CR 50/200 bid, if this is tolerated. This formulation offers convenience of dosing but is more likely to be associated with confusion or psychosis in patients with preexisting cognitive dysfunction. Other common shortcomings of the CR preparation include inadequate antiparkinsonian effect and a delay in onset of action of the day's first dose. The latter problem can usually be overcome by increasing the first CR dose by half of a 50/200 tablet or supplementing the first CR dose by a tablet of regular Sinemet, 25/100.

The psychiatric complications of levodopa (see section on Psychotoxicity and Its Management) are typically more troublesome in the evening and at night and can often be ameliorated or abolished by discontinuing the evening or bedtime dose. In other cases, however, use of a long-acting dopaminergic drug at bedtime (e.g., Sinemet CR, or a direct dopamine agonist such as bromocriptine or pergolide) may improve not only nocturnal parkinsonian symptoms but also early morning akinesia. The latter symptom is often the first sign of "end-of-dose" deterioration or the "wearing-off" effect of Sinemet.

Wearing-off fluctuations during the day develop later in the course of PD and, similarly, may be effectively managed by switching from regular to controlled-release Sinemet. It is important to realize that the bioavailability of CR averages approximately 70% of that of regular Sinemet. A useful rule of thumb in converting patients to the controlled-release drug is to double each dose of regular Sinemet and administer CR at twice the previous wearing-off interval minus 1 hour. For example, for a patient taking Sinemet 25/100 with wearing-off beginning 3 hours after each dose, the initial CR conversion dose would be 50/200 at twice the wearing-off interval ($2 \times 3 = 6$) minus 1, i.e., every 5 hours.

Alternatively, wearing-off fluctuations can be managed by supplementing regular Sinemet with either a direct dopamine agonist or deprenyl (see next section). In some older patients, however, the resulting prolonged dopaminergic agonism may aggravate side effects, particularly dyskinesias, confusion, and psychosis, and a better overall therapeutic response may be achieved by using monotherapy with smaller, more frequent doses of regular Sinemet.

DEPRENYL

Deprenyl (selegiline, Eldepryl) is an irreversible ("suicide") inhibitor of the type B isoenzyme of monoamine oxidase, which reduces catabolism of brain dopamine. Although some studies have continued to reinforce the earlier hopes of finding a neuroprotective effect of deprenyl, an extension of the DATATOP (deprenyl and tocopherol antioxidant therapy of parkinsonism) study failed to show an enduring benefit of this drug for patients with newly diagnosed disease after 18 months of therapy.[13] Similarly, deprenyl at a dose of 10 mg daily provided no advantage in preventing or postponing complications from levodopa therapy in DATATOP patients.[14]

Disadvantages of deprenyl include its high cost and a generally less favorable risk-benefit ratio in the elderly, especially when it is combined with levodopa. Surprisingly, a recent open randomized study of patients with early PD showed a 60% increase in mortality after 3 to 5 years in patients who received levodopa plus deprenyl compared with those who received levodopa alone.[15] There were several limitations in this study, particularly in regard to accuracy of diagnosis, cause of death, compliance with treatment assignment, and statistical methodology, and "on-treatment" analysis of mortality failed to show a significant difference between treatment groups. The mortality was excessively high, inconsistent with clinical experience, and at variance with findings of 10 previous controlled long-term trials of deprenyl in PD. Nevertheless, the continued use of deprenyl, especially in older patients, merits further study because it has been suggested that we may be using too high a dose for too long.[16]

The combination of deprenyl and selective serotonin reuptake inhibitors (SSRIs) or tricyclic antidepressants may precipitate a potentially serious toxic reaction, the serotonin syndrome. This is characterized by mental status changes (e.g., confusion, altered level of consciousness), motor dysfunction (e.g., rigidity, myoclonus), autonomic disturbance (e.g., fever and tachycardia), and, occasionally, rhabdomyolysis, thus closely resembling the neuroleptic malignant syndrome. Recent evidence suggests that this is a rare reaction and probably complicates combination therapy in less than 0.5% of PD patients. Nevertheless, deprenyl should be used with caution in elderly PD patients and may be best avoided in the presence of concomitant SSRI therapy.

DIRECT DOPAMINE RECEPTOR AGONISTS

Currently, two direct dopamine receptor agonists, both ergot derivatives, are available in the United States: (1) pergolide mesylate (Permax), an agonist at both D1 and D2 dopamine receptors, and (2) bromocriptine mesylate (Parlodel), an agonist at D2 receptors and a mild antagonist at D1 sites. Action at both D1 and D2 receptors appears to be necessary for optimal control of parkinsonism, which perhaps explains the slightly better results obtained with pergolide in studies that have compared the efficacies of the two drugs (see later in this section). Neither drug is as effective as carbidopa-levodopa (Sinemet), and although agonist monotherapy may be sufficient to control emerging symptoms for short periods of time in selected patients with newly diagnosed PD, in general this is not an optimal therapeutic strategy, particularly for elderly subjects.

Later in the course, however, dopamine agonists may be useful as adjunctive medications to prolong the antiparkinsonian effects of levodopa and thereby alleviate end-of-dose deterioration (the "wearing-off" effect). This is particularly true of pergolide, which has a longer duration of action than bromocriptine. At the same time, the addition of pergolide or bromocriptine usually permits a reduction in levodopa dosage, thereby reducing the frequency and severity of peak dose dyskinesias and other adverse effects. Pergolide, often in small doses, may also be effective in reducing pain or dystonia during "off" periods in patients with motor fluctuations and may be similarly effective for painful dystonic cramping that occurs during exercise.

As a general rule, it is recommended that bromocriptine be started at a dose of 1.25 mg at bedtime for several days and then increased by 1.25 mg, in divided doses, every 3 to 7 days until optimal results are achieved. However, a simple three-step method of dose titration (2.5 mg qd for 3 weeks, followed by 2.5 mg tid for 3 weeks and then 5 mg tid) may achieve similar results. No significant difference was noted in efficacy or side effects when this regimen was compared with a more gradual dose titration in elderly subjects.[17] Doses in excess of 15 mg qd in the elderly tend to result in more significant side effects and more frequent drug withdrawal and have marginal if any therapeutic advantage over lower doses.[18]

Pergolide is available in three tablet sizes (0.05 mg, 0.25 mg, and 1.0 mg), 1.0 mg being approximately equivalent to bromocriptine 10 mg. The dose should be increased slowly over several weeks, starting with 0.05 mg qd, advancing to a tid schedule, and then switching to the 0.25-mg tablet once the total daily dose reaches about 0.75 mg. Occasionally, patients may experience a transient worsening of PD symptoms when therapy is initiated; this is attributed to preferential D2 autoreceptor stimulation at low agonist doses. Although the average daily dose of pergolide is 3.0 mg, older patients are more likely to experience adverse effects at doses above 1.5 mg/day. These complications, noted also with bromocriptine, include both hypotension and central effects such as restlessness, hypomania, anxiety, panic attacks, and psychosis, and may be seen even in cognitively intact patients.

Pergolide may be more effective than bromocriptine for longer periods of time[19] and may be effective in ameliorating disability in patients who have experienced a waning response to bromocriptine. While some improvement in antiparkinsonian efficacy relative to bromocriptine may be seen when switches are made, this may be purchased at a cost of increased dyskinesias, which may necessitate a reduction in the dose of levodopa. Two recent reports have suggested that pergolide may slow progression of Parkinson's disease.[19] However, sample bias, ceiling effects, and symptomatic effects of the drug may have contributed to the more benign course observed in these subjects, and further studies are required before firm conclusions can be drawn. A theoretical rationale for considering pergolide in elderly patients is provided by the finding of Felton and colleagues that chronic dietary pergolide administered to aged rats resulted in a reduction in the expected age-related loss of both dopamine cell bodies in the substantia nigra compacta and dopaminergic terminals in the striatum.[19] This effect was attributed to a reduction in the baseline release of dopamine in response to the D2 agonist effect of pergolide at presynaptic autoreceptors (an action shared by bromocriptine), with resulting reduction in toxic metabolites formed by oxidative deamination of dopamine.

Psychotoxicity and Its Management

There is a broad spectrum of psychiatric complications of levodopa, including depression, euphoria, hypomania, hypersexuality, personality changes, confusion, delirium, night terrors, vivid dreams, nightmares, delusions, and paranoid psychosis and hallucinations. Delusions and hallucinations in PD occur more frequently in the elderly, particularly in patients with dementia, and are almost invariably drug-related. The recent observation that hallucinations substantially increase the need for nursing home placement (see later discussion) emphasizes the importance of addressing this complication adequately. Hallucinations associated with levodopa therapy are typically formed, visual, nonfrightening, and stable for each patient, whereas those associated with anticholinergic medications tend to be less formed, multimodal, and threatening and are frequently accompanied by delirium. Both delirium and visual hallucinations have also been observed as side effects of amantadine.

In managing confusion and psychosis in patients with PD, anticholinergics and amantadine should be withdrawn first, followed by selegiline, which potentiates many of the side effects of other dopaminergic drugs. Direct dopamine agonists should then be tapered and if necessary discontinued over a period of several days to avoid the withdrawal hallucinations that may accompany abrupt withdrawal of these drugs. Finally, the dose of levodopa, the most effective antiparkinsonian agent, may have to be cautiously reduced. If troublesome hallucinations persist, or if there is an unacceptable increase in parkinsonism, treatment with clozapine should be considered.[20]

Clozapine is an atypical neuroleptic that acts primarily to block limbic D4 dopamine receptors, its lack of significant D2 receptor blockade accounting for its low incidence of antiparkinsonian side effects. A low starting dose (6.25 mg qd) should be used in older patients, who are more prone to initial sedation. The dose is increased over several weeks according to response, 50 to 75 mg qd usually being sufficient to control symptoms. In view of a small risk of agranulocytosis, weekly white blood cell counts are mandatory for all patients receiving clozapine. This cost, while high, is nevertheless small compared with that of nursing home care.

Olanzapine is another atypical antipsychotic drug, with a high affinity for dopaminergic and serotonergic receptors, that appears promising as a treatment of dopaminergic psychosis in patients with PD, at doses between 1 and 15 mg/day.[21] The clinical profile of olanzapine is comparable to that of clozapine, but it does not produce granulocytopenia.

A variety of anticholinergic drugs may contribute to psychotoxicity in PD, including the tricyclic antidepressants. In selected patients, amitriptyline or imipramine may be useful in low doses at bedtime to improve sleep and anticholinergic-responsive parkinsonian symptoms, such as tremor and dystonic cramping. In older patients with cognitive impairment, an alternative tricyclic with less anticholinergic activity, such as nortriptyline or desipramine, may be preferable. Caution should be used with "peripherally" acting anticholinergics such as oxybutynin and propantheline, which are often prescribed for urinary frequency and urgency in patients with PD (see later section, Urinary Symptoms).

Autonomic Dysfunction and Its Management

CONSTIPATION

Constipation, described by James Parkinson in his original paper, remains one of the most frequent autonomic-related symptoms in patients with PD. The cause is likely to be multifactorial, possible factors including lack of dietary fiber, inadequate fluid intake, diminished physical activity, aging, and the effect of antiparkinsonian medications, particularly anticholinergic agents and amantadine. In addition, primary degeneration of colonic neurons in the myenteric plexus occurs in PD, which results in impaired colonic muscle contraction and slowed stool transit time. Megacolon and sigmoid volvulus may also occur.

In a separate syndrome, some parkinsonian patients, particularly those with more advanced disease, suffer a dyssynergy of pelvic floor muscle contractions (anismus), which prevents rectal emptying. In these patients, attempts to defecate produce contraction rather than relaxation of the striated anal sphincter. The prevalence of this condition is unknown. The powerful dopamine receptor agonist apomorphine (not available in the United States) has been shown to alleviate anismus in some PD patients. Botulinum toxin injection into the anal sphincter has also been suggested as a possible treatment for refractory cases.

In the initial management of constipation, a high-fiber diet (40 to 70 g of fiber per day, contained in raw vegetables such as carrots, cauliflower, and broccoli and in cereals such as oat bran), hydration (drinking at least eight glasses of water each day), an exercise program, and regularly scheduled toileting should be encouraged. Anticholinergics, amantadine, and narcotic analgesics should be avoided. Bulk-forming agents, such as bran and psyllium, with or without stool softeners such as docusates, are effective within 1 to 3 days of intake and should be continued daily. Lactulose, 10 to 20 g/day, may benefit some patients. Glycerin suppositories stimulate defecation by causing retention of fluid in the rectum. They are more effective if given before periods of increased gut motility.

Osmotic laxatives such as milk of magnesia and Fleet enemas can be used on an "as needed" basis to manage constipation, with the awareness that chronic use of magnesium and phosphate salts may induce fluid and electrolyte disturbances. Contact-stimulant laxatives—those containing senna (Senokot), cascara, bisacodyl (Dulcolax), and phenolphthalein (Modane)—should also be used judiciously because regular use of such agents over many years may result in a dilated, atonic "cathartic colon." Mineral oil should probably be avoided in patients with PD, particularly those with more advanced disease, in whom there may be a risk of aspiration.

Cisapride is a relatively new parasympathomimetic agent that has relatively few side effects and may be effective for both gastroparesis (delayed gastric emptying) and constipation in patients with PD. The dose is 10 to 20 mg three times a day before meals.

URINARY SYMPTOMS

Up to 70% of patients with PD experience urinary symptoms. Nocturia, frequency, and urge incontinence are often symptomatic of the autonomic disturbance associated with PD, while more pervasive urinary symptoms, particularly obstructive ones (hesitancy, retention, slowing of stream, postvoid dribbling) require exclusion of prostatic hypertrophy and other neurogenic conditions. It is therefore important for PD patients with urinary dysfunction to have an adequate urologic evaluation. In the individual case, this may require recording of bladder and sphincter pressures, sphincter electromyography, and fluoroscopy.

Urodynamic studies in parkinsonian patients with urinary complaints reveal that 60% to 90% have detrusor hyperreflexia, which is manifested by inappropriate bladder contractions at low bladder volumes. Nocturia is the most common and usually the earliest symptom and can often be alleviated by simply eliminating the intake of liquids after the evening meal. If this intervention is ineffective, peripherally acting anticholinergic agents such as oxybutynin (5 to 10 mg) or propantheline (7.5 to 15 mg) at bedtime can be tried. Similar doses may also be effective on a tid basis for daytime frequency but carry a high risk of side effects in the elderly. If anticholinergics prove ineffective, the parasympatholytic drug hyoscyamine is worth a trial, using a dose of 0.15 to 0.30 mg at night or on a qid schedule. Refractory symptoms may respond to desmopressin, administered as an intranasal spray (DDAVP) at night in incremental doses (usually 10 to 20 μg).

Less commonly, urinary frequency and incomplete bladder emptying occur in patients with PD as a result of weak or absent bladder contraction due to detrusor areflexia or hyporeflexia. Anticholinergic medications may precipitate or aggravate this condition. Non-drug-related detrusor hypoactivity, documented by cystometric studies, may respond to alpha-adrenergic blocking agents such as prazosin or doxazosin, which decrease tone in the bladder neck. Such drugs commonly exacerbate or induce orthostatic hypotension and should be initiated in low doses at bedtime, and blood pressure should be closely monitored. In other patients, urinary hesitancy or retention coincide with motor fluctuations, which usually occur during "off" periods and improve during "on" periods. Treatment with the cholinergic agent bethanechol (at a starting dose of 25 mg every 6 hours) has been recommended for this condition, although evidence of its benefit in controlled studies in PD is lacking. A bedside commode should be provided and a voiding schedule designed to coincide with periods of improved motor function.

There is a subgroup of patients with documented hyperreflexia of the external sphincter for whom drugs that relax striated muscle, such as diazepam, baclofen, or dantrolene, can occasionally be effective. For PD patients with both obstructive symptoms and clinical evidence of prostatic hypertrophy, surgery should be considered only if bladder outlet obstruction can be demonstrated with urodynamic studies because there is a relatively high risk of postsurgical incontinence. Patients with deficient voluntary control of the external urinary sphincter are at especially high risk for this complication.[22] Therapeutic options for incontinence include an external collection device, incontinence pads, or an indwelling catheter.

ORTHOSTATIC HYPOTENSION

Patients with PD tend to have a lower resting blood pressure than the general population and a greater tendency toward orthostatic hypotension. This is likely to be due to a combination of dopaminergic therapy and disease-related factors. Relevant pathologic changes in PD involve the hypothalamus as well as lower levels of the autonomic nervous system, with loss of the preganglionic sympathetic neurons in the intermediolateral column of the spinal cord and Lewy body inclusions in the autonomic ganglia. Prior to the advent of levodopa, however, patients with PD rarely developed orthostatic symptoms. Severe orthostatic hypotension, particularly early in the disease course and in those with relatively mild parkinsonism, should suggest the Shy-Drager syndrome (see earlier section, The "Parkinsonism Plus" Syndromes).

Orthostatic hypotension may be dramatic when dopaminergic therapy is initiated in the parkinsonian patient, particularly in the elderly. This complication can generally be avoided by administering low doses of dopamine agonists at bedtime and then slowly titrating the dose upward. In patients with more advanced PD, symptoms of orthostatic hypotension may be alleviated by reducing the dose of levodopa, dopamine agonists, or selegiline, or by using supplemental carbidopa (Lodosyn, obtained directly from the manufacturer, Merck, Sharpe and Dohme).

In the patient who has an exaggerated increase in pulse with standing, hypovolemia should be suspected and reversible medical causes, such as dehydration, anemia, medication effect (e.g., from diuretics and other antihypertensive agents), and hypoadrenalism excluded. Nonpharmacologic approaches to the management of orthostatic hypotension should include avoidance of hot weather, hot baths, and alcohol, which produce peripheral vasodilatation, and avoidance of large meals, which may redirect blood flow to the splanchnic circulation. It is important to offer advice to patients about techniques of using an adjustment period prior to standing, consisting of sitting up and contracting the muscles of the legs for a few minutes. Regular isotonic exercises and graded physical activity may improve orthostatic tolerance as well as overall fitness. Elastic hip-high stockings prevent pooling of blood in the lower extremities and have been shown to increase venous return but frequently must be applied by a caregiver and may be poorly tolerated, especially in the summer months. Elevation of the head of the bed by 8 to 12 inches at night induces a mild hypotensive stress when the patient is recumbent, reducing renal perfusion and thereby promoting renin release and retention of sodium and water. Dietary salt may have to be liberalized, and this maneuver may be augmented by the use of salt tablets, up to 2 g/day.

When these measures are insufficient, the potent mineralocorticoid fludrocortisone is often helpful for managing orthostatic hypotension. At low doses (0.1 mg qd), fludrocortisone enhances the vasoconstrictor response to norepinephrine, and at higher doses (0.2 to 1.0 mg qd) it promotes retention of sodium, thereby expanding extracellular volume. Potential adverse effects, which necessitate close monitoring, include supine hypertension, congestive heart failure, peripheral edema, and hypokalemia. The prostaglandin inhibitor, indomethacin, at a dose of 25 mg tid, is not as effective as fludrocortisone but is better tolerated.

Management of Sialorrhea

Most common in the later stages of the disease, sialorrhea (drooling) is caused not by an excessive production of saliva but by a reduction in automatic or conscious swallowing, thus representing a hypokinetic phenomenon. Despite their potent effect on other akinetic symptoms, dopaminergic agents are frequently only partially effective in managing sialorrhea. In this situation, low doses of a centrally acting anticholinergic agent may serve the dual purpose of reducing saliva production and ameliorating other parkinsonian symptoms. Benztropine (Cogentin) or trihexyphenidyl (Artane) should be started at doses of 0.5 mg and 1 mg, respectively, at bedtime and gradually increased, using a bid or tid dosing schedule, to a total dose that should generally not exceed 2 and 4 mg, respectively, in older subjects. If these drugs produce unacceptable central side effects, peripherally acting anticholinergic agents such as oxybutynin (5 mg every 8 hours) or propantheline (7.5 to 15 mg every 6 hours) may be tried. The usefulness of these drugs may also be limited, however, by such side effects as constipation, urinary hesitancy or retention, visual blurring (due to impaired pupillary constriction), and tachycardia. In comparison, methscopolamine bromide (Pamine) at a dose of 2.5 mg bid or tid has fewer anticholinergic side effects and may be a useful alternative for some patients. Papaya extract from a health food store may also be tried to decrease saliva production. For extreme cases of sialorrhea that do not respond to drug therapy, a portable suction catheter apparatus may have to be considered.

Management of Seborrhea

Excessive secretion of oil by the sebaceous glands is common in PD. Coal tar or selenium-based shampoos used up to once or twice weekly, may be effective for dandruff as well as for seborrhea affecting the eyebrows and forehead. Daily topical hydrocortisone is also effective, particularly for the face, but its use should be monitored by a dermatologist.

Management of Balance and Gait Difficulties

Just as a variety of strategies other than drugs must be considered in the management of orthostatic hypotension, nonpharmacologic aids are central to the management of certain balance and gait difficulties that emerge later in the course of PD and are poorly responsive or nonresponsive to dopaminergic therapies. Strategically placed rails, particularly in bathrooms and showers, provide support as well as assistance with standing. Physical therapy and gait training may be beneficial and can be aided by certain motor and sensory tricks. Start hesitation, for example, can be ameliorated by encouraging the patient to rock or march in place to initiate gait. The use of another person's foot or an inverted or adapted walking stick[23] (fitted with a low projecting arm) can reduce start hesitation or sudden transient freezing by providing the patient with a visual target over which to step. Parallel stripes marked on the floor provide a similar target and may be particularly useful in frequently traveled areas such as the bedroom and bathroom. In some cases, the mere imagining of a line to step over may be sufficient to interrupt freezing. For patients who experience freezing or balance impairment when turning, the strategy of walking around turns may significantly improve gait and reduce falling. The use of a quadrapod or walker may also help to compensate for postural instability but will not protect against spontaneous retropulsion in the later stages of the disease. The assistance of a caregiver or use of a wheelchair will then be necessary to aid mobility and prevent injury from falls.

INSTITUTIONALIZATION IN PARKINSON'S DISEASE

Based on 1985 utilization statistics in the United States and a survey of 40 Norwegian nursing homes, 2% to 5% of nursing home residents have PD.[24] Neither motor disability nor cognitive impairment are significant risks for nursing home placement, suggesting that these impairments may be managed adequately by community caregivers and other support systems. In contrast, hallucinations represent a significant risk factor for permanent nursing home placement, highlighting the importance of this challenging but potentially treatable complication of advanced PD.[24]

LIFE EXPECTANCY IN PARKINSON'S DISEASE

Epidemiologic studies in both Italy and the United States have shown a change in age-specific mortality for patients with PD in recent decades. There has been a substantial decline in mortality among the middle-aged and a notable increase in mortality in the geriatric age groups (75 years and older). Several factors may contribute to these changes, including a possible reduction in the prevalence of PD in middle life or an increase in the incidence of PD among the elderly, better case ascertainment in the elderly, a decrease in earlier deaths from other competing causes, and improved treatment of PD.

The survival rate of patients with PD improved considerably following the introduction of levodopa in 1967. Indeed, it has been estimated that the median duration of illness, at each stage of the disease, is 3 to 5 years longer in levodopa-treated patients than in those not receiving this medication. Nevertheless, survival of PD patients in the levodopa era is still significantly poorer than that of the general population. After adjusting for age and sex, parkinsonism is associated with a twofold increase in the risk of death, and this risk is strongly related to the presence of a gait disturbance.[25] An important difference from the general population is the higher incidence of death due to bronchopneumonia in PD patients. Other common causes of death in PD patients are atherosclerotic heart disease, malignant neoplasms, stroke, and urinary tract infections.

Improved survival in PD is associated with a higher 10-year expected survival (based on age, gender, and birth year), absence of dementia, diagnosis of idiopathic PD as opposed to other causes of parkinsonism (e.g., progressive supranuclear palsy or multiple system atrophy), and less severe parkinsonism (Hoehn and Yahr stage 1 or 2) at the initial neurologic visit. In addition, a retrospective study has suggested that treatment with amantadine, an antagonist of the *N*-methyl D-aspartate (NMDA) receptor (see earlier section), may be an independent predictor of improved survival in PD.[26] A prospective controlled randomized trial of the effect of amantadine or an alternative NMDA antagonist on PD progression will be required to address this finding definitively.

References

1. Newman RP, LeWitt PA, Jaffe N, Calne DB, Larsen TA: Motor function in the normal aging population: Treatment with levodopa. Neurology 1985;35:571–573.
2. Langston JW, Koller WC, Giron LT: Etiology of Parkinson's disease. *In* Olanow CW, Lieberman AN (eds): The Scientific Basis for the Treatment of Parkinson's Disease. Park Ridge, NJ, The Parthenon Publishing Group, 1992, pp. 33–58.
3. Agid Y: Parkinson's disease: Pathophysiology. Lancet 1991;337:1321–1324.
4. Calne DB: The free radical hypothesis in idiopathic parkinsonism: Evidence against it. Ann Neurol 1992;32:799–803.
5. Broe GA: Antiparkinsonian drugs. *In* Swift C (ed): Clinical Pharmacology in the Elderly. New York, Marcel Dekker, 1987, pp. 473–509.
6. Gibb WR, Lees AJ: A comparison of clinical and pathological features of young and old onset Parkinson's disease. Neurology 1988;38:1402–1406.
7. Friedman JH: Drug-induced parkinsonism. *In* Lang AE, Weiner WJ (eds): Drug-Induced Movement Disorders. Mount Kisco, NY, Futura Publishing, 1992, pp. 41–83.
8. Avorn J, Gurwitz JH, Bohn RL, et al: Increased incidence of levodopa therapy following metoclopramide use. JAMA 1995;274:1780–1782.
9. Nutt JG, Marsden CD, Thompson PD: Human walking and higher-level gait disorders, particularly in the elderly. Neurology 1993;43:268–279.
10. Hoehn MM: Result of chronic levodopa therapy and its modification by bromocriptine in Parkinson's disease. Acta Neurol Scand 1985;71:97–106.
11. Robertson DRC, George CF: Drug therapy for Parkinson's disease in the elderly. Br Med Bull 1990;46:124–146.
12. Yeh KC, August TF, Bush DF, et al: Pharmacokinetics and bioavailability of Sinemet CR: A summary of human studies. Neurology 1989;39 (Suppl 2):25–38.
13. Parkinson Study Group: Impact of deprenyl and tocopherol treatment on Parkinson's disease in DATATOP subjects not requiring levodopa. Ann Neurol 1996;39:29–36.
14. Parkinson Study Group: Impact of deprenyl and tocopherol treatment on Parkinson's disease in DATATOP patients requiring levodopa. Ann Neurol 1996;39:37–45.
15. Lees AJ, on behalf of the Parkinson's Disease Research Group of the United Kingdom: Comparison of therapeutic effects and mortality data of levodopa and levodopa combined with selegiline in patients with early, mild Parkinson's disease. Br Med J 1995;311:1602–1607.
16. MacMahon DG: The use of selegiline in elderly patients: Current indications and future potential. Rev Contemp Pharmacother 1992;3:77–85.
17. MacMahon DG, Overstall PW, Marshall T: Simplification of the initiation of bromocriptine in elderly patients with advanced Parkinson's disease. Age Ageing 1991;20:146–151.
18. The Bromocriptine Multicenter Trial Group: Bromocriptine as initial therapy in elderly parkinsonian patients. Age Ageing 1990;19:62–67.
19. Sage JI, Duvoisin RC: Pergolide. *In* Koller WC, Paulson G (eds): Therapy of Parkinson's Disease, 2nd ed. New York, Marcel Dekker, 1995, pp. 249–259.
20. Friedman JH, Lannon MC: Clozapine in the treatment of psychosis in Parkinson's disease. Neurology 1989;39:1219–1221.
21. Wolters ECh, Jansen ENH, Tuynman-Qua HG,

Bergmans PLM: Olanzapine in the treatment of dopaminomimetic psychosis in patients with Parkinson's disease. Neurology 1996;47:1085–1087.

22. Staskin DS, Vardi Y, Siroky MB: Post-prostatectomy continence in the parkinsonian patient: The significance of poor voluntary sphincter control. J Urol 1988;140:117–118.

23. Dietz MA, Goetz CG, Stebbins GT: Evaluation of a modified inverted walking stick as a treatment for parkinsonian freezing episodes. Mov Disord 1990;5:243–247.

24. Goetz CG, Stebbins GT: Risk factors for nursing home placement in advanced Parkinson's disease. Neurology 1993;43:2227–2229.

25. Bennett DA, Beckett LA, Murray AM, et al: Prevalence of parkinsonian signs and associated mortality in a community population of older people. N Engl J Med 1996;334:71–76.

26. Uitti RJ, Rajput AH, Ahlskog JE, et al: Amantadine treatment is an independent predictor of improved survival in Parkinson's disease. Neurology 1996;46:1551–1556.

Additional Readings

Cohen AM, Weiner WJ (eds): The Comprehensive Management of Parkinson's Disease. Comprehensive Neurologic Rehabilitation, Vol. 8. New York, Demos Publications, 1994.

Nutt JG, Hammerstad JP, Gaucher ST (eds): Parkinson's Disease. One Hundred Maxims in Neurology, Vol. 2. St. Louis, Mosby-Year Book, 1992.

Medical and Surgical Disorders in Geriatric Practice

34 Cardiac Disorders

Donald D. Tresch, M.D.

Iyad Jamali, M.D.

Cardiovascular disease is one of the most common diseases seen in elderly persons, and approximately 50% of persons over 65 years of age have clinical signs of the disease. Not only is the disease common in this age group, but also cardiovascular disease is a major cause of functional impairment and is the principal cause of death in elderly persons. In addition, elderly persons are affected by cardiovascular changes due to normal aging. These normal cardiovascular aging changes usually affect the person's overall function only minimally. However, when cardiovascular disease is present, aging changes accentuate the detrimental effect of the disease and make compensation more difficult for elderly patients.

NORMAL CARDIOVASCULAR AGING CHANGES

Structural Changes

Echocardiographic and autopsy studies have demonstrated an increase in left ventricular wall thickness and mass related to aging.[1, 2] Left ventricular cavity dimensions show little or no change related to aging. Usually the maximum wall thickness is no greater than 13 mm, which is significantly less than that seen in elderly patients with pathologic hypertrophy related to cardiac disorders such as hypertrophic cardiomyopathy, hypertension, or aortic valvular disease. In one autopsy study[2] the ratio of ventricular septal to left ventricular wall thickness increased appreciably with age and often exceeded 1.3 in patients older than 60 years of age. The explanation for the increase in left ventricular wall thickness with aging is unclear, although ventricular hypertrophy may result from the increase in systolic blood pressure and the decrease in aortic compliance that occur with aging. In addition, the increases in myocardial collagen, fibrosis, and lipofusion observed in aging hearts suggest that the increase in wall thickness may represent both cellular hypertrophy and an increase in noncellular components.

Increased left atrial size is another age-related change that is thought to be related to an age-related decrease in left ventricular compliance, resulting in a decreased rate of left ventricular filling.

An age-related increase in valvular circumference has been reported in all four cardiac valves, the greatest changes being observed in the aortic valve; the aortic valvular circumference approaches that of the mitral valve by the tenth decade of life.[2] This increase in valvular circumference related to aging does not appear to be associated with valvular incompetence. Other valvular changes with aging include thickening and calcification of the cusps and leaflets. These changes do not usually cause significant dysfunction, although in some elderly patients, severe aortic valvular stenosis and mitral valvular insufficiency are related to degenerative changes with age (see later in this chapter in the section Valvular Heart Disease).

Cardiac conduction is affected by aging in that the number of pacemaker cells in the sinus node is decreased in advanced age, although the resting heart rate does not appear to be affected by age alone.[3] A less dramatic cellular decrease is noted in the atrioventricular node. Fibrous infiltration of the bundle of His and bundle branches is common, and severe degenerative changes with calcification may occur, which can cause heart block.

Physiologic Changes

Left ventricular systolic function does not appear to be significantly altered by aging. Resting left ventricular ejection fraction is similar in older and younger patients, and animal studies demonstrate that the force of the myocardial contraction is no different in senescent and younger rats.[4] Changes associated with aging include an increase in duration of ventricular contraction,[4] a decreased rate of ventricular filling,[1, 5] and an inability to increase ventricular ejection fraction with exercise to the degree noted in younger subjects.[6]

In contrast to left ventricular systolic function, significant alterations in ventricular diastolic function occur with age.[7] Increased left ventricular stiffness, diminished compliance with resulting prolongation of relaxation, and a reduced rate of early diastolic rapid filling occur with advanced age. Ventricular diastolic function, therefore, is compromised by aging changes, and diastolic filling becomes more dependent on atrial contraction in elderly persons. The degree of ventricular diastolic impairment due to aging alone, however, is not usually severe enough to cause clinical heart failure. Elderly patients are at risk of developing heart failure if hypertension or ischemic heart disease is present even though ventricular systolic function is normal. Some studies have reported that 45% to 55% of patients over 65 years of age with clinical heart failure have normal systolic ventricular function.[8]

The effect of aging specifically on cardiac output remains controversial. Earlier studies reported an age-related decrease in cardiac output, both at rest and with exercise.[9] Other studies, which included highly functional elderly subjects who were extensively screened for silent cardiovascular disease, reported no significant aging changes in cardiac output.[10] Cardiac output was similar in young and older subjects, both at rest and with exercise; a different mechanism, however, was responsible for the increase in cardiac output with exercise in the two age groups. Younger persons markedly increase their heart rate with exercise, whereas elderly persons, instead of accelerating the heart rate demonstrate an increase in stroke volume due to increased end-diastolic volume. This difference in heart rate with exercise in different age groups is thought to be related to a decrease in sympathetic response in elderly persons secondary to aging changes. A decreased sympathetic response due to aging has also been shown to affect myocardial contractility and vasomotor reactivity in elderly persons. The decreased response does not appear to be related to a reduction in serum catecholamines because plasma norepinephrine levels have been found to be higher in elderly persons than in younger persons.

CARDIOVASCULAR DISEASES AND DISORDERS

Coronary Artery Disease

Autopsy studies demonstrate that approximately 70% of persons between 70 and 80 years of age have coronary atherosclerosis. The autopsy findings may be coincidental with the disease, which has been clinically silent throughout the person's lifetime. In other cases, individuals are unaware of having coronary artery disease (CAD) until the advanced age of 75 or 80 years, when they sustain an acute myocardial infarction (MI). At least 40% to 50% of persons over the age of 65 years, however, demonstrate CAD clinically, and many are functionally impaired by the disease. Furthermore, CAD is the number one cause of death in patients older than 65 years.[11]

Women are protected from CAD in their youth and middle years; their coronary deaths from CAD are approximately half those of men in these age groups. After 65 years the mortality from CAD significantly increases in women, and at age 75 coronary mortality is equal in men and women. Statistics show that the majority of MIs in women take place after menopause, and death associated with the initial MI is significantly higher in women than in men.

Despite the high prevalence of CAD, clinical manifestations of the disease are often unrecognized or misdiagnosed in elderly patients. Diagnostic differences in younger and older patients may reflect a difference in the disease process between the two age groups, or may be related to the superimposition of normal physiologic aging changes in older people and the presence of concomitant diseases that mask the usual clinical manifestations.

Because of the high prevalence of CAD in elderly persons and the lack of typical clinical manifestations, it is important that high-risk elderly persons be screened for the disease. Exercise electrocardiography using either a treadmill or a bicycle ergometer is as useful in diagnosing and evaluating elderly patients with suspected or documented CAD as it is in younger patients. Some studies have suggested that exercise electrocardiographic stress testing may be more sensitive in diagnosing CAD in elderly patients than in younger patients, although specificity may be decreased.[12] Exercise stress testing has also been found useful in predicting future coronary artery events in elderly patients with documented CAD, particularly those who have had an acute MI. Exercise stress testing in combination with perfusion scintigraphy may be even more useful than exercise stress testing alone when evaluating elderly persons with CAD.[13]

Because of musculoskeletal disorders or general debilitation many elderly patients are unable to perform exercise stress testing. In such patients pharmacologic stress testing will be necessary. Repeated studies of elderly patients have documented excellent results in the diagnosis of CAD with the use of intravenous dipyridamole-thallium imaging, which has a sensitivity of 85% and a specificity of 75%.[14] Recently, stress tests using dobutamine and dipyridamole echocardiography have been found to be safe and highly sensitive in evaluating CAD in elderly patients.[15, 16] Ambulatory electrocardiography (Holter monitoring) is another noninvasive test that is useful for diagnosing silent myocardial ischemia and predicting future coronary events in elderly persons.[17]

CORONARY ARTERY SYNDROMES

Clinical coronary artery syndromes are usually classified as ischemic episodes (stable angina and unstable angina) and MI. Chest pain is usually the initial and most common clinical manifestation of these syndromes, although in some patients complications secondary to ischemia or infarction, such as heart failure or arrhythmias, including sudden death, may be the initial manifestation.

Myocardial Ischemia

Exertional angina (chest pain) is the most common manifestation of myocardial ischemia in young and middle-aged persons. Because of their more sedentary lifestyle or possibly a difference in pathophysiology, this may not be the case in elderly patients. Instead of exertional chest pain, ischemia may be more commonly manifested as dyspnea in elderly patients. Other elderly patients with CAD are completely asymptomatic, although silent ischemia may be demonstrated by stress testing or Holter monitoring.[17, 18]

Treatment of elderly patients with stable or unstable angina is similar to that for younger patients with these syndromes.[19] Reduction of myocardial oxygen demands, an increase in the myocardial blood supply, and prevention of fibrin clot formation are the initial concerns in all patients regardless of age. Reducing myocardial oxygen demands includes decreasing both physical and emotional stress. Patients with unstable angina require hospitalization and bed rest with close monitoring of their condition, including the heart rhythm. Beta-blockers and vasodilators (nitrates) are considered first-line drug therapy in reducing oxygen demands. Calcium channel blockers may be beneficial in patients whose symptoms are refractory to beta-blockers and nitrates, or who cannot tolerate beta-blockers or nitrates, or whose ischemia is thought to be secondary to coronary vasospasm. Calcium channel blockers are contraindicated in patients with heart failure. Aspirin or heparin (or both) is mandatory unless contraindicated in all patients with angina or unstable angina. The use of interventional therapy (coronary artery bypass grafting [CABG] and percutaneous coronary angioplasty [PTCA]) is usually reserved for high-risk elderly patients with CAD or for those whose angina is refractory to medical therapy (see next section, Acute Myocardial Infarction).

Acute Myocardial Infarction

Myocardial infarction significantly increases with age and is the number one cause of death in elderly patients. In a study from the University of Washington, 28% of all patients hospitalized for acute MI were over the age of 75 years, and 56% were over 64 years.[20] Death rates in elderly MI patients were substantially higher than those in younger patients. Other studies have reported similar results, with hospital deaths in MI patients older than 70 years at least twice those of younger MI patients, and mortality rates for survivors at 1 year approximately three times higher in older patients.[20, 21] Women are more likely to die following an acute MI than men; however, after adjusting for age and other pertinent clinical factors, including left ventricular ejection fraction, most studies have found that gender is not an independent risk factor for long-term outcome.[22]

As with myocardial ischemia, the clinical manifestations of acute MI may be different in elderly and younger patients. The Framingham Study reported that 45% of MIs were silent or unrecognized, and the percentage increased with the patient's age in males.[23] Numerous studies have found that instead of chest pain, elderly patients more commonly complain of dyspnea or have vague symptoms of confusion, abdominal pain, or generalized weakness at the time of acute MI.[24, 25]

Thrombolytic Therapy

It is now well established that fibrin clot in a coronary artery is the final event in the pathophysiology of the great majority of acute MIs. Numerous trials have demonstrated the acute and long-term benefits of thrombolytic agents in treatment of patients with acute Q-wave infarction, and the benefits are as favorable, if not more so, in elderly patients (Table 34–1).[26] Studies have also found that thrombolytic therapy in elderly persons is as cost-effective as other accepted therapies, such as treatment of moderate hypertension.[27]

Despite the overwhelming evidence in favor of thrombolytic treatment for elderly MI patients, this therapy is commonly not used in this age group. The reasons for this underutilization are numerous and include delay in seeking medi-

TABLE 34–1   **ACUTE MYOCARDIAL INFARCTION: EFFICACY OF THERAPY IN YOUNGER VERSUS OLDER PATIENTS[a]**

Therapy	No. Patients	Mortality Rate (%)		Reduction in Mortality	
		Therapy	*Control*	*%*	*p Value*
Thrombolysis					
Early mortality					
Younger patients	26,941	6.2	8.4	25.7	<.0001
Older patients	9841	17.2	20.7	16.9	<.0001
Late mortality					
Younger patients	11,706	9.1	11.2	18.1	.0003
Older patients	6278	26.6	28.6	10.3	.009
Beta-blockers					
Early intervention					
Younger patients	14,687	2.5	2.6	5.0	NS[b]
Older patients	8513	6.9	8.9	23.2	.0005
Late intervention					
Younger patients	4654	5.5	7.6	28.3	.004
Older patients	2462	8.9	14.9	40.0	.0001

[a]Pooled data from major trials. Younger age limit varied from ≤65 to <60 years old; older age range varied from ≥60 to 70, 66 to 75, and >75 years old.
[b]NS, not significant.
Modified from Forman DE, Bernal JL, Wei JY: Management of acute myocardial infarction in the very elderly. Am J Med 1992; 93:315–326.

cal assistance, misdiagnoses due to atypical presentation, increased contraindications, and higher prevalence of non-Q-wave MIs. Also, clinicians are reluctant to use thrombolytics in the aged population for fear of hemorrhage, although most studies show that intracerebral hemorrhage is not significantly increased in elderly MI patients who receive thrombolytics. Only approximately one third of older patients presenting with acute MI have any contraindications to thrombolytic therapy, and less than 5% have absolute contraindications. In regard to patients with non-Q-wave infarction or unstable angina, repeated studies have demonstrated that thrombolytic therapy has no benefits in these patients regardless of age.

In regard to choice of specific thrombolytic agent, initial studies comparing streptokinase (approximate cost $200 per patient) and tissue-type plasminogen activator (approximate cost $2200 per patient) found that both drugs increased the survival rate equally. The Global Utilization of Streptokinase and Tissue Plasminogen Activator (tPA) for Occluded Coronary Arteries (GUSTO)[28] trial, which was designed specifically to compare thrombolytic agents, reported a significant advantage with tPA for the overall study population. Patients over age 75, however, had a significantly higher risk of hemorrhagic stroke when treated with tPA than with streptokinase, and the incidence of death or nonfatal disabling

stroke was not significantly different between the two therapies in this age group. Therefore, streptokinase may be appropriate in patients over the age of 75 years.

Primary Percutaneous Coronary Angioplasty

Even using the most liberal criteria for thrombolytic therapy, there are still many elderly MI patients who cannot be treated with this therapy yet would benefit from opening the clotted coronary artery. Some studies have demonstrated that patients treated with primary PTCA have lower mortality, fewer bleeding complications in the first 30 days, and less left ventricular dysfunction than patients treated with thrombolytic therapy.[29] Elderly patients especially appear to benefit from primary PTCA.

Other subgroups of MI patients in whom primary PTCA may be beneficial are those with evidence of severe left ventricular damage on presentation and those with cardiogenic shock or heart failure. The data consistently show that, even with thrombolytic therapy, the mortality rate in these patients is extremely high. The treatment of choice in this group in essentially all circumstances is primary PTCA, since ensured recanalization of the infarct vessel provides the best hope for survival. Emergency PTCA or CABG in this situation, however, is associated with high morbidity and mortality, especially in elderly patients.[30]

Anticoagulation

The issue of reocclusion following thrombolytic therapy remains a major problem. Anticoagulants have been found beneficial in preventing reocclusion; therefore, intravenous heparin is recommended in all MI patients who receive thrombolytic therapy. In addition, anticoagulation therapy is usually recommended for certain elderly MI patients who are at high risk for thromboembolic events, particularly those with large anterior wall Q-wave MIs and heart failure and those with ventricular thrombus that has been documented echocardiographically.

Aspirin

Aspirin reduces the increased platelet aggregation associated with acute coronary artery syndromes and is beneficial in treating elderly patients with acute MI. In the Second International Study of Infarct Survival (ISIS-2), aspirin given alone (160 mg/day) significantly reduced hospital mortality by 23%, and the combination of aspirin with streptokinase further reduced the mortality rate by 42%.[31] This benefit was independent of the patient's age.

Aspirin is recommended immediately at the onset of an acute MI, with or without thrombolytic therapy. It should be continued indefinitely regardless of the patient's age. The specific dose of aspirin remains controversial, but the usual dose varies from 60 mg to 325 mg/day.

Beta-Blockers

Beta-blockers are beneficial in both the earlier stages of MI (within hours) and as secondary prevention following hospital discharge. As with thrombolytic therapy, many studies have found that beta-blockers have the greatest benefit in the oldest age subgroups (see Table 34–1).[26, 32] Most early studies failed to demonstrate any benefit with the immediate use of beta-blockers in younger MI patients, whereas reductions of as high as 23% in hospital mortality were reported in older MI patients who received beta-blockers early.

Numerous studies have consistently demonstrated the benefits of beta-blockers as secondary preventive therapy in elderly patients with MI. Reduction in overall mortality has been reported to be as high as 48%, and reductions in recurrent MI and sudden death have been 20% and 33%, respectively. The efficacy of beta-blockers has been demonstrated in patients with both Q-wave MIs and non-Q-wave MIs, although the magnitude of benefit may be smaller in the latter.

Angiotensin-Converting Enzyme Inhibitors

It is now well established that therapy with angiotensin-converting enzyme (ACE) inhibitors is useful in the treatment of symptomatic heart failure as well as in prevention in patients with asymptomatic left ventricular dysfunction (see later section, Heart Failure). Recently, studies have investigated the use of ACE inhibitors in the peri-infarction period. The Survival and Ventricular Enlargement (SAVE) trial[33] demonstrated that captopril given 3 to 14 days after MI to patients with left ventricular ejection fractions of 40% or less reduced overall mortality by 19%, clinical congestive heart failure by 37%, and, somewhat surprisingly, reinfarction by 25%. These benefits are mainly related to the favorable effects of ACE inhibitors in retarding left ventricular remodeling and are independent of the patient's age. Other studies using various ACE inhibitors have reported similar benefits when the drug is used early after acute MI (Table 34–2).[34] Issues such as the specific timing of initial administration of the drug following the MI and the need to assess the degree of left ventricular dysfunction remain unresolved.

Calcium Channel Blockers

Despite the popularity of calcium channel blockers in the treatment of hypertension and angina pectoris, these drugs have limited use in the treatment of MI patients. In most studies, mortality was not improved in MI patients who received calcium channel blockers, and in some studies it increased. Diltiazem has been shown to reduce reinfarction and angina in patients with non-Q-wave MI,[35] although an increase in mortality was found in MI patients with heart failure who were treated with diltiazem.[36] A Danish study[37] did report a reduction in mortality and reinfarction with verapamil in patients with MI without left ventricular dysfunction. Therefore, calcium channel blockers may be of value in elderly patients with non-Q-wave MI, in certain patients with Q-wave MI, or in those in whom beta-blockers are strongly contraindicated, but only if there is no congestive heart failure or impaired left ventricular systolic function.

Magnesium

The benefit of the use of magnesium in acute MI patients remains controversial. Results of the

TABLE 34–2   **ANGIOTENSIN-CONVERTING ENZYME INHIBITORS AFTER MYOCARDIAL INFARCTION: SUMMARY OF THE CLINICAL TRIALS**

Trial	Enrollment Criteria	Drug	Initiation Period	Effect on Mortality
SAVE	LVEF ≤40%	Captopril	3–16 days	+
CONSENSUS II	All	Enalapril	<24 hours	–
GISSI 3	All	Lisinopril	<24 hours	+
SMILE	AWMI	Zofenopril	<24 hours	+
TRACE	LVD	Trandolapril	3–7 days	+
AIRE	CHF	Ramipril	3–10 days	+

Abbreviations: +, Significant survival benefit; –, no significant survival benefit; AIRE, acute infarction ramipril efficacy; AWMI, anterior wall myocardial infarction; CONSENSUS II, Cooperative New Scandinavian Enalapril Survival Study II; CHF, congestive heart failure; LVD, left ventricular dysfunction; LVEF, left ventricular ejection fraction; GISSI 3, Gruppo Italiano per lo Studio della Sopravivenza nell'infarcto miocardio; SAVE, Survival and Ventricular Enlargement Trial; SMILE, Survival of Myocardial Infarction Long-term Evaluation; TRACE, Trandolapril Cardiac Evaluation Study.
Modified from Ramahi TM, Lee FA: Medical therapy and prognosis in chronic heart failure. Cardiol Clin 1995;13:5–26.

International Study of Infarct Survival (ISIS) failed to show any benefit for magnesium other than to replete a demonstrated deficiency.[38]

Prehospital Discharge Evaluation

As with younger MI patients, elderly MI patients require risk stratification prior to hospital discharge. Residual ischemia, significant left ventricular dysfunction, and persistent electrical instability are all determinants of poor long-term survival.

A low-level exercise stress test is recommended in most elderly patients before hospital discharge to assess for residual ischemia, functional status, and arrhythmias. Many elderly MI patients, however, have baseline electrocardiographic (ECG) abnormalities that confound interpretation of the exercise ECG, and radionuclide perfusion scanning must be included with the exercise test, an approach that has been proved valid in the elderly. In addition, many elderly patients have co-morbid conditions that prevent them from performing an exercise stress test (e.g., chronic lung disease, amputated limbs, or balance disturbances). In such patients, pharmacologic stress testing, along with nuclear imaging or echocardiography can provide useful information. Intravenous dipyridamole followed by nuclear perfusion scanning with thallium-201 or echocardiography has been found to be beneficial in stratifying elderly MI patients. Dobutamine echocardiography is an alternative to dipyridamole stress testing, and studies in elderly post-MI patients have shown that these tests have excellent predictive accuracy in patients with multivessel disease and that they offer good results in stratifying patients into high- and low-risk groups.

Patients with non-Q-wave infarction, which is more common in elderly patients, require special consideration in regard to stratification prior to hospital discharge. A higher event rate following infarction as well as a high rate of positive results on noninvasive stress testing occurs in patients with non-Q-wave MI compared with those with Q-wave MI. Therefore, many physicians find the noninvasive work-up of limited use in this situation and recommend performing coronary angiography in these patients. Furthermore, pathologically, Q-wave MIs treated with thrombolytics resemble non-Q-wave MIs, and many authorities favor performing coronary angiography during hospitalization in MI patients who are treated with thrombolytics as well as in those with non-Q-wave MIs. Nonetheless, no study has found that routine angiography in MI patients offers a clinical advantage versus noninvasive stratification, and the joint American College of Cardiology/American Heart Association guidelines advocate angiography only in MI patients with demonstrable ischemia either with symptoms or by stress testing.[39]

In addition to noninvasive evaluation for residual ischemia, some determination of left ventricular function, either by echocardiography or by radionuclide ventriculogram (multigated angiography [MUGA]), is necessary for risk stratification prior to hospital discharge of the elderly MI patient. Left ventricular ejection fraction is the most powerful independent predictor of future cardiac events; an ejection fraction of 30% is considered the usual dividing line between low- and high-risk groups.

Elderly MI patients commonly demonstrate ventricular ectopy, which has been shown to be a marker for increased mortality, including sudden death. Elderly patients with nonsustained ventricular tachycardia and poor left ventricular function are the group at highest risk of increased mortality.[40] Patients with left ventricular dysfunction and significant ventricular ectopy can be further stratified using a signal averaged electrocardiogram. If a signal averaged electrocardiogram is abnormal in patients with significant ventricular ectopy and depressed left ventricular function, arrhythmic event rates, including sudden death, have been reported to approach 50% 1 year following myocardial infarction.

Empirical drug therapy for ventricular arrhythmia after MI has not proved beneficial in patients of any age. The Cardiac Arrhythmia Suppression Trial (CAST) actually demonstrated a threefold higher mortality in post-MI patients with asymptomatic ventricular arrhythmias who received flecainide and encainide compared to patients who received placebo.[41] This increased mortality associated with drug therapy was noted in all age groups. Therefore, empirical antiarrhythmic therapy should not be used, and elderly MI patients at high risk for sudden death should be referred for electrophysiologic evaluation. Age alone should not prevent patients from receiving invasive electrophysiologic evaluation plus interventional therapy. Studies have established the benefit and safety of both invasive electrophysiologic testing and interventional therapy, including CABG and defibrillator implantation, in elderly CAD patients with life-threatening arrhythmias.[42, 43] In elderly MI patients who are not candidates for invasive evaluation or interventional therapy, empirical therapy with amiodarone may be considered. The benefits of empirical use of amiodarone remain unclear; numerous multicenter trials are currently underway that ideally will further clarify the use of this drug in post-MI elderly patients.

The role of interventional therapy (PTCA and CABG) requires special consideration when it is used in elderly patients with CAD and is especially pertinent in those with MI. Numerous studies have shown that age alone should not be used to defer interventional therapies in elderly CAD patients. Coronary angioplasty and CABG are associated with excellent results in selected elderly CAD patients, including those 80 years of age or older.[44-46] In one study of nonrandomized very elderly (80 years or older) patients with acute MI, those who had had CABG or PTCA had fewer symptoms and better survival than those who were treated medically.[47] Of course, patient selection and exclusion of those patients with overwhelming co-morbidity are crucial to achieving such outcomes.

Valvular Heart Disease

Valvular heart disorders are not uncommon in elderly persons, although, unlike in younger persons with valvular disorders, the disease process is more often related to a degenerative process rather than to rheumatic or congenital disease.

AORTIC VALVULAR STENOSIS

Aortic valvular stenosis (AVS) is a disorder mainly of the elderly. The disorder is 15 times more prevalent in persons over 60 years of age than in those younger than 30 years. In the general population the disorder is more common in males by 4:1; however, with increasing age, the ratio decreases, and in people over 80 years of age women predominate. Persons with AVS are usually asymptomatic for many years, and the first symptoms may not appear until the eighth or ninth decade. Once symptoms do occur, stenosis is usually severe, and rapid clinical deterioration occurs unless proper therapy is initiated.

Unfortunately, even though the disorder is common, severe AVS is often misdiagnosed in elderly patients, or, if correctly diagnosed, it may be treated inadequately. Symptoms in elderly patients are similar to those experienced by young patients with severe AVS. The classic symptoms of angina, dyspnea, dizziness, or syncope, however, may be misinterpreted in elderly persons.

The physical examination, which is usually considered the hallmark in the diagnosis of severe AVS, can be misleading in the evaluation of elderly patients with the disorder. In a study comparing the autopsy and clinical findings in patients with severe AVS who were older and younger than 65 years of age, striking differences were found in the two age groups.[48] Younger patients usually had congenital bicuspid valves that were calcified with commissural fusion, whereas older patients more often had stenotic, heavily calcified tricuspid valves, thought to be secondary to a "wear and tear" degenerative process, in which commissural fusion was unusual. The rigid calcified bicuspid valve with commissural fusion was thought to be responsible for the ejection sound so commonly audible in younger patients. Such a valve would also be responsible for the classic harsh, rough, grunting systolic ejection murmur, which is loudest at the base and radiates upward into the carotid arteries. In contrast, because of the lack of valvular commissural fusion, elderly patients with AVS commonly have a more blowing, musical systolic murmur related to blood "spraying" across the aortic valve. Consequently, the harsh murmur at the base may be appreciably less intense and comparatively inconspicuous in elderly patients with AVS. Instead, a more blowing, systolic murmur may be heard at the apex, and, because of the location and the quality, the murmur is easily confused with the murmur of mitral valvular incompetence.

In addition to the atypical murmur, elderly patients may have calcification of the mitral annulus with mitral valvular incompetence; therefore, in a certain percentage of elderly patients, both AVS and mitral valve incompetence are present, making the auscultatory findings even more confusing.

Other unusual physical findings may mislead the physician who is evaluating elderly patients with severe AVS. Systemic hypertension is usually never present in younger patients with severe AVS, whereas a narrowed pulse pressure and a slowly rising carotid arterial pulse (parvus et tardus pulse) are usually seen. Such findings may not be present in elderly patients. Systemic hypertension is not uncommon in elderly patients with severe AVS, and, due to the elevated pressure combined with the decreased compliance of the arterial tree, a parvus et tardus carotid pulse may be absent.

Atrial fibrillation, a very rare finding in younger patients with severe AVS, occurs in 25% of elderly patients with this disorder. The combination of atrial fibrillation and the apical systolic murmur may lead the physician further toward the mistaken diagnosis of mitral valvular incompetence in these elderly patients.

Electrocardiographic and chest radiographic findings in elderly patients with severe AVS may be confusing. Younger patients with severe AVS usually have electrocardiographic findings of left ventricular hypertrophy with a strain pattern. Due to an increased chest diameter, the electrocardiographic voltage may not be impressive in many elderly patients with AVS, and, if an intraventricular conduction defect is present, which is often the case in elderly patients, ventricular hypertrophy will be masked.

Chest x-ray findings may not be impressive in elderly patients with AVS. Unless heart failure has occurred, the heart is usually of normal size despite the presence of severe concentric left ventricular hypertrophy. Aortic valvular calcification may be noted, but such calcification may also be seen in elderly patients secondary to aortic valvular sclerosis without severe AVS.

Echocardiography is usually very useful in diagnosing AVS, and some studies have shown that echocardiography is highly accurate in assessing the severity of this disorder.[49] In certain elderly patients, unfortunately, due to chest configuration, a technically adequate echocardiogram is not possible. Cardiac catheterization and angiographic studies, including coronary angiography, are usually performed in most elderly patients

with AVS, who are considered possible candidates for valve replacement.

Once symptoms develop in patients with critical AVS, the clinical course is rapidly downhill. Symptoms and left ventricular dysfunction are progressive, and the average survival is 1½ to 3 years. Prompt therapeutic intervention is mandatory. Digitalis and diuretic therapy will not prevent progressive clinical deterioration, and patients will remain symptomatic. Unloading therapy is contraindicated in patients with severe AVS, and valvular replacement is the therapy of choice. Repeated studies have demonstrated an operative mortality of less than 10% in elderly patients with severe AVS, and long-term survival is excellent; most postsurgical patients have a New York Heart Association functional rating of class I or II.[50] Higher surgical mortality has been reported if coronary artery bypass grafting is necessary at the time of the valve replacement. Operative mortality and morbidity are also significantly increased in elderly patients with severe AVS who have depressed ventricular function, poor functional status, or a need for emergency surgery.[51]

Aortic balloon valvuloplasty may be another option in symptomatic elderly patients with severe AVS. Most studies, however, have reported poor results with this technique, with significant valvular restenosis, recurrent symptoms, and death occurring in 1 year or less following valvuloplasty.[52] Therefore, aortic valvuloplasty is usually recommended only in patients who are not candidates for valve replacement due to the presence of co-morbid conditions or, possibly, in patients with severe clinical deterioration as a bridge to subsequent aortic valve replacement.

When considering the choice of surgical intervention in asymptomatic elderly patients with severe AVS, the main issue is whether the first symptom in such patients will be sudden death. Studies[53, 54] have now documented that sudden death is preceded by a period of symptoms in these patients; therefore, it is recommended that valvular replacement not be offered to asymptomatic elderly patients, even when severe AVS is present. Some authorities do recommend surgery in a small subset of asymptomatic elderly patients with severe AVS who have left ventricular systolic dysfunction at rest or significant ventricular ectopy. All authorities stress the importance of follow-up evaluations in patients with AVS to be certain to recognize the possibility of a denial of symptoms and to realize that the very gradual deterioration seen in some elderly patients may lead to a wrong classification of a symptomatic patient as asymptomatic.

AORTIC VALVULAR INSUFFICIENCY

As with AVS, the prevalence of aortic regurgitation increases with age. Unlike AVS, aortic valvular insufficiency is rarely caused by degenerative aortic valve disease. Acute aortic valvular insufficiency may be due to infective endocarditis, aortic dissection, trauma, or rupture of the sinus of Valsalva. Chronic aortic insufficiency can be caused by valve leaflet disease, including rheumatic heart disease, congenital heart disease, rheumatoid arthritis, ankylosing spondylitis, or myxomatous degeneration. Chronic aortic insufficiency may also be caused by aortic root disease secondary to systemic hypertension, syphilitic aortitis, cystic medial necrosis, ankylosing spondylitis, rheumatoid arthritis, Reiter's disease, systemic lupus erythematosus, Ehlers-Danlos syndrome, and pseudoxanthoma elasticum. Symptoms of aortic valvular insufficiency are the same in older persons as they are in younger ones. Usually the main symptoms are related to heart failure, with exertional dyspnea and weakness being common symptoms. In some elderly patients symptoms of dyspnea and palpitations may be more common at rest than with exertion. Nocturnal angina pectoris, often accompanied by flushing, diaphoresis, and palpitations may occur; this is thought to be related to the slowing of the heart rate and the drop of arterial diastolic pressure. The classic findings of a high-pitched, blowing diastolic murmur and a wide pulse pressure with an abruptly rising and collapsing pulse should make the diagnosis of aortic valvular insufficiency easily recognized in elderly patients.

Aortic valvular replacement is usually performed to control symptoms in patients with chronic aortic valvular insufficiency and will be necessary in most elderly patients with acute severe aortic insufficiency. The use of vasodilator therapy has been shown to be beneficial in postponing valvular replacement in asymptomatic patients with aortic valvular insufficiency.[55] In certain elderly patients with chronic aortic insufficiency, significant left ventricular dysfunction develops before symptoms occur, and in many of these patients the left ventricular damage is irreversible. To perform valve replacement before irreversible ventricular damage occurs in these asymptomatic patients it is necessary to monitor ventricular size and function closely with serial echocardiograms. Once the left ventricular end-systolic dimension reaches 4.5 cm or the left ventricular ejection fraction is less than 50%, the patient should be referred to a cardiologist for further evaluation. Most authorities consider a left ventricular end-systolic dimension of 5.0 to 5.5 cm or greater as a marker of approaching irreversible left ventricular dysfunction and recommend aortic valve replacement even though the patient is asymptomatic. The operative mortality for aortic valve replacement in elderly patients with severe aortic insufficiency is similar to that for patients with aortic valve replacement for AVS. Surgical outcome depends on the degree of left ventricular dysfunction, the presence of associated coronary artery disease requiring bypass surgery, the existence of co-morbid conditions, and the urgency of the surgery.

MITRAL VALVE DISEASE

The mitral valve undergoes structural changes related to aging. Usually aging changes do not produce significant valvular dysfunction. Two degenerative aging processes, mitral valve calcification and mucoid (myxomatous) degeneration of the valve leaflets and chordae tendineae, however, can produce significant valvular insufficiency with clinical manifestations.

Mitral annular calcification is common in elderly persons, especially women. A prevalence of 56% was found in women nursing home residents; the prevalence increased from 18% in women 62 to 70 years of age to 89% in women 91 to 100 years old.[56] In nursing home men over 62 years of age the prevalence was 47%. The amount of calcium may vary from a few spicules to a large mass behind the posterior cusp that often extends to form a ridge or ring encircling the mitral leaflets and occasionally lifts the leaflets toward the left atrium. In some patients, annular calcification can cause improper cooptation of the leaflets during systole, resulting in significant mitral regurgitation. Mitral annular calcification may be diagnosed by chest radiograph, although echocardiography is more sensitive. Besides mitral valvular insufficiency, mitral annular calcification is associated with atrial fibrillation, conduction defects, endocarditis, and cerebrovascular events. In patients with severe mitral valvular insufficiency secondary to mitral annular calcification, mitral valve replacement will be necessary. The mortality and morbidity associated with mitral valve replacement in patients with mitral annular calcification are similar to those reported for mitral valve replacement in patients without annular calcification.

Mitral valve prolapse (MVP), although more prevalent in younger persons, occurs in patients of all ages. In some patients the disease is not diagnosed until they are 75 years old or older. The natural history of the disorder remains unclear, and it is not known whether this entity in the elderly represents a sudden onset of the disorder or whether the disease has progressed to the point where it becomes clinically recognizable. As in younger patients with MVP, the auscultation findings in elderly patients may be variable or completely absent unless they are provoked by maneuvers. Some investigators have found that elderly patients are more disabled by the disorder.[57, 58] The main clinical feature that is different in old and young people with MVP is the occurrence of heart failure in the elderly. The typical patient with MVP who presents with heart failure is an elderly man with a long history of an inconspicuous heart murmur who is completely asymptomatic until heart failure suddenly occurs. Auscultatory findings demonstrate a loud blowing holosystolic murmur characteristic of severe mitral incompetence instead of the mid to late systolic murmur and click typical of MVP. Occasionally, instead of the apical holosystolic blowing murmur, an ejection murmur is present; this is best heard at the upper sternal border and mimics the murmur of aortic valvular stenosis. Atrial fibrillation is not uncommon. Because of the severity of mitral insufficiency, mitral valve surgery is necessary in the majority of these elderly patients with MVP who present with heart failure. At surgery, ruptured chordae tendineae are usually found with a large dilated annulus.[59] In many of these patients mitral valve repair is possible; it is usually associated with low morbidity and mortality and excellent long-term results.

In addition to mitral annular calcification and MVP, other disorders producing mitral valve insufficiency in the elderly are rheumatic heart disease and CAD. Both of these entities can produce severe insufficiency with resultant heart failure, and valvular surgery may be necessary. As in elderly patients with aortic valve insufficiency, many patients with chronic mitral insufficiency may remain asymptomatic even though significant left ventricular dysfunction occurs. Echocardiographic findings of an increasing left ventricular end-systolic dimension of 5.0 cm or a resting left ventricular ejection fraction of less than 50% are two markers commonly used to recommend valvular surgery in symptomatic patients with mitral valve insufficiency. Some authorities recommend obtaining echocardiographic examinations every 6 months in patients with chronic mitral insufficiency.

Mitral valve stenosis is usually rheumatic in origin and is usually diagnosed in the third or fourth decade. In some patients, however, the disorder is not clinically diagnosed until the seventh or eighth decade, at which time the patient may manifest symptoms or signs of heart failure, atrial fibrillation, or stroke. All patients with mitral stenosis and atrial fibrillation, regardless of age, require chronic anticoagulation to prevent embolization.

Mitral valve surgery in elderly patients is associated with higher mortality and morbidity than aortic valve surgery. In selected elderly patients, however, surgery can be gratifying, and even in very elderly patients surgery is a reasonable therapeutic option if medical therapy has failed. Operative mortality from mitral valve surgery varies from 10% to 35% in patients 70 years or older[51, 60] and depends on the urgency of surgery, the presence of coronary artery disease, female gender, and the presence of depressed left ventricular function. Reduced mortality has been reported with mitral valve repair compared with valve replacement. Balloon valvoplasty has been demonstrated to be beneficial in elderly patients with severe mitral stenosis.[61] The majority of elderly patients are functionally improved following valvoplasty and attain New York Heart Association (NYHA) functional class I or II. Many elderly patients with severe mitral stenosis, however, are not candidates for the procedure owing to valve morphology.

Cardiomyopathy

Cardiomyopathies are a group of heart muscle disorders that commonly are of unknown etiology. Clinically, the disorders are usually classified into three types: (1) dilated congestive cardiomyopathy (DCM), in which systolic ventricular dysfunction is the major abnormality; (2) hypertrophic cardiomyopathy, which is characterized by mainly diastolic ventricular dysfunction with usually a small ventricular cavity and hyperdynamic systolic function (hypertrophic cardiomyopathy may be subdivided into an obstructive type with an associated dynamic subvalvular muscular ventricular outflow obstruction [hypertrophic obstructive cardiomyopathy (HOCM)] or a nonobstructive type); and (3) restrictive cardiomyopathy, which may cause mainly right-sided heart failure owing to severe ventricular stiffness and early diastolic dysfunction.

Cardiomyopathies traditionally have been considered disorders of the young and middle-aged; however, it has now been shown that these disorders usually are not diagnosed until patients are older than 60 years of age. One third of all patients with hypertrophic cardiomyopathy are over 60 years of age at the time of diagnosis, and at least 10% of patients with DCM are 60 years or older.

Senile amyloidosis has a different pathologic distribution and immunologic characteristics than primary systemic amyloidosis or secondary amyloidosis. Senile amyloidosis is a common autopsy finding in patients older than 80 years of age, and its clinical significance is related to the extent and severity of myocardial involvement. Extensive myocardial involvement may be associated with cardiac arrhythmias, especially atrial fibrillation, or heart failure, which may be secondary to either systolic or diastolic ventricular dysfunction.

An entity referred to as hypertensive hypertrophic cardiomyopathy of the elderly has been reported.[62] The entity is associated with severe concentric left ventricular hypertrophy with reduced ventricular cavity size, excessive systolic ejection, and impaired diastolic function. Patients are usually over 70 years of age when the disorder is diagnosed, have a history of hypertension, and present with symptoms of heart failure due to diastolic ventricular dysfunction.

Clinical presentation of elderly patients with cardiomyopathies is similar to that of older patients with other cardiac disorders, and symptoms are variable. Heart failure is the most common presentation, although arrhythmias, angina, syncope, arterial embolization, or endocarditis may be the initial manifestation. Prognosis is variable in elderly patients with cardiomyopathies and depends on the clinical type of the cardiomyopathy, the degree of ventricular dysfunction, and the specific etiology of the cardiomyopathy. Some studies have found advanced age to be a powerful independent determinant of adverse prognosis, especially in patients with DCM, whereas a Mayo Clinic study reported a rather benign course in patients 65 years or older with HOCM, with 1- and 5-year survival rates not significantly different from those in patients in an age- and sex-matched control population.[63]

Therapy depends on the symptoms and the type of underlying ventricular dysfunction (see later sections, Heart Failure, and Electrocardiographic Findings and Arrhythmias). Surgical management of elderly patients with HOCM is possible, and symptomatic relief is substantial after surgery. Operative mortality and overall mortality, however, are significantly higher in elderly patients. The Mayo Clinic reported a 15.6% operative mortality in patients 65 years or older compared to a 1.2% mortality in patients younger than 65 years; calculated 6-year survival rates were 63% and 95%, respectively.[64] Because of the high hospital and overall mortality, surgical relief of outflow tract obstruction in elderly patients with HOCM is recommended only in symptomatic patients who have not had a successful response to maximum medical therapy.

Recently, the treatment of patients with HOCM with cardiac pacing and septal preexcitation has been evaluated. Some studies have reported clinical and hemodynamic improvement, although reports of other studies have not been so encouraging. Elderly patients have not been specifically studied, and at this time the use of cardiac pacing in elderly patients with HOCM remains controversial.

Congenital Heart Disease

Congenital heart disease is usually manifested clinically before the patient reaches advanced age, although in some patients congenital cardiac defects may not be manifest or diagnosed until the seventh or eighth decade. Some of these patients are asymptomatic, and the disease is diagnosed by the physical examination or chest x-ray findings. Other elderly patients with congenital heart disease present with a recent onset of symptoms, including heart failure, arrhythmias, or chest pain. In a small percentage of elderly patients, endocarditis is the initial clinical manifestation. Besides AVS, atrial septal defect (ASD) is the most common congenital cardiac defect initially diagnosed in elderly patients. An atrial tachycardia, commonly atrial fibrillation, may be the initial manifestation of ASD in elderly patients. The majority of these patients have a systolic ejection murmur with wide fixed splitting of the second heart sound, and a right bundle branch block (complete or incomplete) is present on the electrocardiogram. The chest radiograph shows the typical radiographic findings of a left-to-right shunt; findings of pulmonary hypertension are present in only a small percentage of elderly patients. An echocardiogram confirms the diagnosis. In the majority of elderly patients surgical correction of the septal defect is possible, although atrial fibrillation persists, and chronic anticoagulation is necessary.

Prophylaxis Against Endocarditis

Prophylaxis against endocarditis is mandatory in elderly patients with valvular heart disease and most types of congenital heart defects. Patients with functional murmurs, such as those with aortic valvular sclerosis in which echocardiographic studies fail to demonstrate a marked thickening of the aortic valve or valvular obstruction, do not require prophylactic antibiotics. In addition, elderly patients with mild mitral insufficiency secondary to coronary artery disease or a DCM do not require endocarditis prophylaxis. In elderly patients with MVP and valvular insufficiency, mitral annular calcification, or HOCM, endocarditis prophylaxis is necessary. The absolute risk of endocarditis in patients with MVP but without clinical or Doppler findings of valvular insufficiency or in patients with ASD is considered so low that prophylactic antibiotics are not necessary in these patients. The American Heart Association guidelines for administration of antibiotics to prevent endocarditis are no different in younger and older patients.

Heart Failure

Heart failure is a common problem, especially in the elderly. In the United States 2 to 3 million patients have a diagnosis of heart failure, and approximately 400,000 new cases occur yearly. Heart failure is the most common reason for hospitalization and recurrent hospitalization in patients over 65 years of age. The Framingham Study found that the prevalence of heart failure rose progressively from 1% in 50- to 59-year-olds to 10% in persons over age 80.[65] Similarly, the incidence of new cases approximately doubled with each decade from age 45 to age 84. After age 85, the incidence of new cases increased four- to sixfold.

Although the causes of heart failure in elderly patients are generally the same as those in younger patients, the clinical presentation may differ in the two age groups. Commonly, elderly patients with heart failure who become mildly symptomatic during exertion tend to curtail their daily activities and become relatively asymptomatic. Therefore, in elderly patients, the diagnosis of clinical heart failure is usually made at a later stage in the disease process than in middle aged and younger patients. Because of the advanced stage of the disorder, stabilization of symptoms is difficult in elderly patients, and hospitalization is usually required. Furthermore, based on the results of recent studies that demonstrated substantial long-term benefits with the use of ACE inhibitors in asymptomatic patients with moderate left ventricular dysfunction, the delay in diagnosing heart failure in elderly patients has other significant implications as well. In these patients, because of the severe left ventricular dysfunction at the time of diagnosis, preventive measures may be impossible; the benefits of therapy are therefore limited to controlling symptoms and are purely palliative. An echocardiogram to screen for moderate to severe left ventricular dysfunction in asymptomatic or moderately symptomatic elderly patients with underlying heart disease may be beneficial in terms of the patient's long-term prognosis and may be cost-effective in preventing hospitalizations and increased medical costs.

Another significant difference between elderly and younger patients with heart failure is the type of ventricular dysfunction found. Approximately 40% to 50% of elderly patients with heart failure have normal left ventricular systolic function with predominantly diastolic dysfunction. Hemodynamically, severe diastolic dysfunction is characterized by an upward shift in the pressure-volume relationship, so that at a normal left ventricular volume, ventricular diastolic pressures are elevated. This elevated pressure is transmitted backward to the atrium and pulmonary veins, resulting in pulmonary congestion. The high prevalence of diastolic ventricular dysfunction in elderly patients with heart failure is partially related to changes occurring with age such as increased ventricular mass, diminished left ventricular compliance, and impaired diastolic filling. In addition, many elderly patients have CAD and left ventricular hypertrophy secondary to long-standing hypertension, which predispose patients to left ventricular diastolic dysfunction. Diastolic dysfunction may also occur in elderly patients with diabetes or any of the infiltrative cardiomyopathies, such as amyloidosis, which is the most common type of infiltrative cardiac disorder in this age group. In elderly patients with hypertrophic cardiomyopathy the most common clinical manifestation is heart failure due to diastolic ventricular dysfunction.

The clinical differentiation between ventricular systolic and diastolic dysfunction in elderly patients with heart failure can be difficult. Generally, elderly patients with cardiomegaly and a history of MI have ventricular systolic dysfunction, whereas those with a normal size heart and hypertension more commonly have ventricular diastolic dysfunction (Table 34–3).[7] The findings, however, are nonspecific, and echocardiography may be necessary to distinguish between the two types of ventricular dysfunction. Therefore, an echocardiogram is recommended in all elderly patients with heart failure. Normal systolic ventricular function is usually defined as an ejection fraction of 48% to 50% or greater. In patients with heart failure who have a left ventricular ejection fraction of 48% or greater, diastolic ventricular dysfunction is considered the cause of the heart failure.

THERAPY

In only a minority of elderly patients with heart failure is a reversible underlying cause found. Nevertheless, reversible causes such as thyrotoxicosis, valvular and pericardial diseases, and acute coronary insufficiency must be considered in all elderly persons with an initial onset of heart failure. Elderly patients in whom heart failure is episodic and left ventricular ejection fraction is greater than 30% to 35% will benefit from stress

TABLE 34–3 **CLINICAL DIFFERENTIATION OF SYSTOLIC VERSUS DIASTOLIC DYSFUNCTION IN PATIENTS WITH HEART FAILURE**

	Systolic Dysfunction	**Diastolic Dysfunction**
Past history	Hypertension Myocardial infarction Diabetes Chronic valvular insufficiency disorders	Hypertension Renal disease Diabetes Aortic stenosis
Presentation	Younger than 65 years Progressive shortness of breath	65 years or older Acute pulmonary edema
Physical examination	Displaced PMI S3 gallop	Sustained PMI S4 gallop
Radiographic findings	Pulmonary congestion Cardiomegaly	Pulmonary congestion Normal size heart
Electrocardiogram	Q waves	LVH
Echocardiogram	Decreased LVEF	Normal or increased LVEF

Abbreviations: LVEF, Left ventricular ejection fraction; LVH, left ventricular hypertrophy; PMI, point of maximum impact.
Adapted from Tresch DD, McGough MF: Heart failure with normal systolic function: A common disorder in older people. J Am Geriatr Soc 1995;43:1035–1042.

testing to identify ischemia as the possible cause of the heart failure.

In the majority of elderly patients with heart failure the primary goal of treatment is to control symptoms, improve maximum functional capacity, and prevent progressive left ventricular dysfunction. Dietary modification with sodium and fluid restrictions is considered one of the most important interventions in treating these patients. In many elderly persons the symptoms of heart failure are exacerbated by excessive sodium intake, and strict adherence to a low-sodium diet may cause the symptoms to resolve.

Pharmacologic management of elderly patients with heart failure is similar to management in younger patients, although renal and hepatic dysfunction related to aging requires downward adjustment of drug doses, with a lower initial dosage and more gradual and judicious increases. Although sodium restriction is important in treating elderly patients with heart failure, compliance is poor, and diuretics are usually necessary to control congestive symptoms. With appropriate diuretic agents, reduction of ventricular pressure with adequate diuresis is possible in most elderly patients. In fact, because of the rapid diuresis, many elderly patients find it difficult to tolerate the depletion of intravascular volume and quickly demonstrate findings of prerenal azotemia. In addition, elderly patients are prone to develop diuretic-induced hypokalemia and hyponatremia, as well as orthostatic hypotension.

The usefulness of digitalis in patients with heart failure has been repeatedly debated. The question of whether digitalis improves long-term survival remains unanswered; however, studies have confirmed its long-term benefits in patients with systolic ventricular dysfunction.[66–68] Digitalis does not appear to be detrimental in terms of long-term survival, and it has been found to reduce hospitalizations. Long-term administration of digoxin, however, is associated with an increased risk of drug side effects in elderly patients. The decrease in skeletal muscle mass in elderly patients reduces the volume of distribution of digoxin, and similar doses of digoxin have been reported to result in blood levels that are twice as high in elderly patients as those seen in younger patients. Due to aging changes, decreased renal function may also contribute to the increased serum concentration of digoxin in elderly patients. Studies have demonstrated that when serum digoxin concentrations are maintained below 1 ng/mL, the risk of overdosage is low, left ventricular performance is improved (as noted by a rise in ejection fraction), and clinical benefits are consistently observed.

Due to the results of numerous studies showing that ACE inhibitors are beneficial in relieving symptoms and preventing progressive ventricular deterioration, it has been suggested that, instead of diuretics, ACE inhibitors should be the initial therapy tried in patients with heart failure. In patients with moderate to severe heart failure due to systolic left ventricular dysfunction, the use of ACE inhibitors alone has not been found to be successful in relieving the signs and symptoms of volume overload. There is no doubt, however, that ACE inhibitors, like digitalis and diuretics, are beneficial in improving the symptoms and prolonging survival in symptomatic patients with left ventricular systolic dysfunction. In the CONSENSUS trial,[69] which demonstrated significant benefits in the use of ACE inhibitors in symptomatic patients, the mean age of the patients was over 70 years, and, at this age, ACE inhibitors were well tolerated. In asymptomatic elderly patients with depressed left ventricular systolic dysfunction, the use of ACE inhibitors is more controversial. The SOLVD trial[70] demonstrated that asymptomatic patients with a depressed left ventricular ejection fraction of less than 35% demonstrated no benefit in survival, although a significant reduction in progression to clinical heart failure with a decrease in hospitalizations was noted. In the SAVE trial,[33] ACE inhibitors were found to be beneficial in improving long-term survival and reducing the development of heart failure and recurrent myocardial infarction in patients with reduced left ventricular systolic function following acute MI, regardless of the patient's age (see earlier section, Coronary Artery Disease).

Despite the benefits of ACE inhibitors, drug side effects are not uncommon in elderly patients, and close monitoring is important. The major limiting side effect is cough, which can be debilitating in elderly patients and may necessitate discontinuing the drug. In these patients, "unloading" with hydralazine and a nitrate is beneficial.[71] The use of the new angiotensin II-blocking agents is another alternative in elderly patients who develop cough with ACE inhibitor I agents; however, specific studies demonstrating the benefits of these agents in heart failure patients have not been performed. Other significant side effects of ACE inhibitors are hypotension and renal dysfunction, which more commonly occur in elderly patients with intravascular volume depletion. In such patients it may be necessary to reduce the dosage of diuretics prior to the initiation of ACE inhibitors, and the initial dosage of the ACE inhibitor should be reduced as well. Elderly diabetic patients and elderly patients taking nonsteroidal anti-inflammatory drugs require especially close monitoring of renal function when ACE inhibitors are used. Elderly patients are also predisposed to hyperkalemia, and therefore potassium-sparing diuretics and potassium supplements should be discontinued or reduced in dosage prior to the initiation of ACE inhibitors. It is important in elderly patients to start ACE inhibitors at a low dosage and slowly titrate the dose to therapeutic levels; a reduction in systolic blood pressure to below 100 mmHg is not a contraindication to increasing the dose if the patient is asymptomatic and stable renal function is preserved.

The management of elderly patients with heart failure secondary to ventricular diastolic dysfunction must be emphasized because the treatment is markedly different from the treatment given for ventricular systolic dysfunction. The clinical manifestation of heart failure in these patients may be recurrent bouts of acute pulmonary edema, and the cornerstone of therapy is adherence to a low-sodium diet plus the use of diuretics. Intravascular depletion, however, is not well tolerated, and prerenal azotemia, because of the dependence of cardiac output on elevated filling pressures, often develops quickly with the use of diuretics in these elderly patients. Vasodilation is also poorly tolerated in elderly patients with severe diastolic dysfunction, and severe hypotension may occur when vasodilator agents are used. Digitalis is not beneficial and may be harmful unless atrial fibrillation is present. In patients with atrial fibrillation, calcium channel blockers such as verapamil or diltiazem or a beta-blocker are usually more advantageous than digitalis. In addition to controlling the heart rate, calcium channel blockers and beta-blockers may be beneficial in improving the symptoms as well as the indices of diastolic dysfunction in patients with hypertrophic cardiomyopathy.

Reduction of left ventricular hypertrophy is another important therapeutic goal in the management of patients with heart failure due to diastolic dysfunction. Calcium channel blockers or ACE inhibitors produce significant regression of left ventricular hypertrophy and may be the appropriate antihypertensive agent in these patients. Some studies have demonstrated improvement in symptoms and survival in elderly patients with heart failure secondary to diastolic dysfunction who were treated with ACE inhibitors. Prevention and control of tachyarrhythmias, especially atrial fibrillation, are important in elderly patients with heart failure secondary to diastolic dysfunction because these patients are prone to develop high intracardiac filling pressures associated with tachycardias and the loss of atrial contraction.

ELECTROCARDIOGRAPHIC FINDINGS AND ARRHYTHMIAS

Abnormal resting ECGs are common in the elderly. The most frequently observed abnormalities in this patient population include nonspecific ST-T-wave changes, atrial fibrillation, premature atrial and ventricular contractions, first-degree atrioventricular block, and left axis deviation.[72, 73] In the absence of structural cardiac disease, these abnormalities, with the exception of atrial fibrillation, have little prognostic value. However, if underlying cardiac disease exists, the corresponding ECG changes are associated with increased morbidity and mortality in the elderly.[74] Duration of the P wave and PR interval increases with age owing to an increase in the left atrium size and conduction time through the atrium and the atrioventricular (AV) node, respectively. First-degree AV block has been reported in 3% to 4% of healthy older volunteers, which is a significantly higher prevalence than that noted in young men.[75] Left axis deviation is one of the most common variations in the ECG seen in the elderly and may reflect the increase in left ventricular mass that occurs with aging. With advanced age, the mean amplitude of the QRS complex decreases despite an increase in the prevalence of other ECG findings of left ventricular hypertrophy. Electrocardiographic findings of left ventricular hypertrophy in elderly patients lack sensitivity but have excellent specificity. Evidence of left ventricular hypertrophy on ECG is an independent risk factor for cardiovascular morbidity and mortality. The prevalence of right and left bundle branch block increases with age; the prevalence of right bundle branch block is reported to be 3.4% in men aged 40 years and older. Left bundle branch block is found less frequently than right bundle branch block in elderly persons; when found, it usually indicates the presence of a cardiovascular disease.[73] Abnormalities involving the ST-T wave have been reported in 16% of subjects aged 70 years and older[73] and were associated with clinical heart disease in the majority of these patients.

Bradyarrhythmias

Bradycardia results from either decreased automaticity of the sinus node or a block in the conduction system. The decline in parasympathetic function that occurs with aging is associated with a reduction in sinus arrhythmias and sinus bradycardia, usually seen after the fourth decade of life. Bradycardias, however, are common after age 60 because of the increased prevalence of ischemic heart disease, degenerative changes of the sinus node and conduction tissue, autonomic and baroreceptor abnormalities, and increased sensitivity to various drugs that affect the conduction system.

Sinoatrial Exit Block

Sinoatrial exit block refers to a failure of the sinus impulse to propagate from the sinus node to the surrounding atrial tissues. This abnormality is fairly common in the elderly owing to autonomic imbalance, degeneration of the sinus node tissue, and the effects of medications (digoxin, calcium channel blockers, beta-blockers, and class I antiarrhythmic preparations). Asymptomatic patients need no specific treatment except for discontinuing the involved medication, although a pacemaker is required in symptomatic patients.

Sick Sinus Syndrome

Sick sinus syndrome comprises a constellation of abnormalities of impulse initiation and conduction, including sinus bradycardia, tachy-bradycardia syndromes, atrial fibrillation with slow ventricular response, sinus arrest or sinus exit block, and combinations of these disorders. Not uncommonly, atrioventricular conduction abnormalities are associated with the sinus abnormalities. Sick sinus syndrome occurs most commonly in the elderly and may be caused by ischemic or rheumatic heart diseases, aging with degeneration and fibrosis of the sinus node, cardioactive drugs, hypothyroidism, and increased vagal tone. Treatment of sick sinus syndrome consists of removing the responsible drug, treating the underlying disease, or permanent pacing. In some patients with the tachy-bradycardia syndrome, administration of drugs that control the tachycardia, such as beta-blockers, calcium channel blockers, or digitalis, may be needed after a permanent pacemaker has been placed. The development of atrial fibrillation is common in elderly patients with sick sinus syndrome and increases in patients treated with permanent ventricular pacing. With atrial pacing, atrial fibrillation develops in a much lower percentage, and atrial pacing is considered the treatment of choice in these patients. Newer dual chamber pacemakers with the capability of detecting supraventricular tachycardia and converting it to ventricular pacing mode have facilitated the management of patients with the tachy-bradycardia syndrome.

Atrioventricular Block

Atrioventricular block is a pathologic delay or complete block of atrial impulse conduction to the ventricle. The blocked atrial impulse that occurs during the ventricular compensatory period should be exempted from this definition. The site of the block can be in the atrium, atrioventricular node, or the His-Purkinje system. The causes of atrioventricular block that are almost exclusive to the elderly include degeneration and calcification of the conduction system. Other conditions that are common but not exclusively present in the elderly include drug effects, ischemic heart disease, amyloidosis, myocarditis, and collagen vascular diseases. The ECG sign of first-degree AV block is prolongation of the PR interval. Second-degree AV block (type I Wenckebach block) produces a gradual prolongation of the PR interval in successive beats with a periodic drop in the QRS complex, whereas second-degree AV block (type II Wenckebach) is manifested by an intermittent QRS drop without antecedent PR prolongation. In third-degree AV block, or complete heart block, there is a complete dissociation between the atrium and the ventricle. The site of the block can be in or below the AV node. In the former, the QRS complexes are usually narrow, and the ventricular escape rate is sufficient to maintain adequate cardiac output and blood pressure. If the block site is below the AV node, the QRS complexes are usually wide and are associated with a slow ventricular rate. Symptomatic patients with AV block should be treated with a permanent pacemaker after excluding an offending drug as a cause of the block.

Tachyarrhythmias

Tachyarrhythmias originate in the atrium or the ventricle from enhanced automaticity, reentry, or triggered activity or any combination of these mechanisms. Enhanced automaticity produces a gradual onset and increase in the rate of arrhythmia followed by a gradual decrease when the arrhythmia terminates. In contrast, arrhythmia caused by reentry usually begins and terminates abruptly. Reentry tachycardias are frequently precipitated, and sometimes terminated, by premature atrial or ventricular complexes. Reentry requires the presence of two electrophysiologically different conduction pathways with a unidirectional block in one of them. Examples of reentry include ventricular and supraventricular tachycardia, atrial flutter, typical and atypical AV node reentry, and sinoatrial reentrant tachycardia.

Triggered activity represents abnormal automaticity in the cardiac tissue. It is commonly caused by drug toxicity such as that due to digoxin or quinidine. Examples of triggered activity include atrial fibrillation, ventricular tachycardia, and probably torsades de pointes.

MULTIFOCAL ATRIAL TACHYCARDIA

Multifocal atrial tachycardia is a rhythm characterized by the presence of at least three P-wave morphologies, variable durations of the PR inter-

val, and an irregular ventricular rhythm. It is commonly seen in elderly patients who have chronic obstructive lung disease. The mechanism that underlies this rhythm is most likely triggered activity. Effective therapies include beta-blockers and verapamil; digitalis may exacerbate the condition.

JUNCTIONAL TACHYCARDIA

Junctional tachycardia is a manifestation of triggered activity and is most commonly encountered in elderly persons following cardiac surgery (especially valvular surgery) or with digoxin toxicity. It is characterized by a supraventricular QRS morphology at a rate ranging from 70 to 200 beats/minute; frequently AV dissociation is present. This disturbance usually resolves with improvement of the primary disorder or discontinuation of the offending drug.

ATRIOVENTRICULAR REENTRY TACHYCARDIA

It is estimated that 60% of patients with supraventricular tachycardia referred for electrophysiologic studies have AV node reentry. This arrhythmia is seen primarily in young and middle-aged patients, although it may present initially in elderly patients. The onset and termination of the tachycardia is abrupt and is frequently followed by sinus tachycardia. Typical AV node reentry is manifested by a short RP interval with retrograde conduction occurring over the rapid pathway and is the most prevalent form. The rare atypical AV node reentry form produces a long RP interval with retrograde conduction over the slow pathway. Acute treatment with carotid massage should be performed carefully in elderly patients and only after ruling out the presence of carotid disease. Pharmacologic treatment includes the use of adenosine, digoxin, verapamil, and class I antiarrhythmic medications. Electrical cardioversion should be carried out promptly in elderly patients who are hemodynamically unstable. Radiofrequency ablation of the reentry pathways is indicated for chronic or frequent AV node reentry tachycardia that is not controlled by medical therapy; this is an effective and safe treatment in elderly patients.[76]

ATRIAL FIBRILLATION

Atrial fibrillation is the most common cardiac arrhythmia in the elderly; it has a prevalence in patients older than 65 that approaches 5% and increases with advancing age. In a study of 2101 unselected nursing home patients with a mean

TABLE 34–4 **EFFECTIVE DRUGS FOR RATE CONTROL IN ATRIAL FIBRILLATION**

Drug	Dosage		Avoid Use	Comments
	Acute Control (IV)	*Maintenance (po)*		
Digoxin	1.0–1.5 mg IV or oral over 24 hours in increments of 0.25–0.5 mg	0.125–0.5 mg daily	WPW, HCM	Loading may take hours to slow rate. Combination with other drugs may be beneficial in slowing heart rate
Diltiazem	0.25–0.35 mg/kg IV followed by 5–15 mg infusion IV per hour	60–90 mg three or four times daily[a]	WPW, severe LV dysfunction[b]	Synergistic with digoxin in slowing rate. Causes peripheral edema, constipation
Verapamil	5–10 mg every 30 minutes or 5 mg/hour	40–120 mg three times daily[a]	Same as diltiazem	Same as diltiazem, but also increases digoxin level
Propranolol	1–5 mg IV (1 mg every 2 minutes)	10–120 mg three times daily[a]	Bronchospastic disease, severe LV dysfunction	Synergistic with digoxin in slowing heart rate
Metoprolol	5 mg every 5 minutes up to 15 mg total	50–200 mg/day[a]	Same as propranolol	Same as propranolol
Esmolol	0.5 mg IV/kg/minute	None	Same as propranolol	Same as propranolol. Very short half-life

[a]Long-acting preparations are available.
[b]Diltiazem has been used intravenously in patients with left ventricular dysfunction.
Abbreviations: HCM, Hypertrophic cardiomyopathy; LV, left ventricular; WPW, Wolff-Parkinson-White syndrome; IV, intravenous.

age of 81 years, the prevalence of atrial fibrillation was found to be 13%.[77] This arrhythmia is an important cause of morbidity and mortality in elderly persons, in whom stroke is a major complication. An estimated 75,000 strokes occur annually in patients with this disease, accounting for one third of embolic events in patients older than 65 years. In the majority of patients with atrial fibrillation there is underlying cardiovascular disease, although valvular heart disease is usually not present. Atrial fibrillation unassociated with underlying heart disease is referred to as "lone atrial fibrillation" and usually occurs in patients under 50 years of age. The disorder is considered benign unless other cardiovascular disorders are present. The mechanism of atrial fibrillation is thought to be either abnormal automaticity in one or more ectopic areas in the atrium or multiple microreentry wavelets presenting simultaneously. Symptoms of atrial fibrillation include palpitations, anxiety, fatigue, dizziness, heart failure, stroke, and syncope.

Treatment of atrial fibrillation should be directed toward achieving the following goals: (1) control of the ventricular rate, (2) restoration and maintenance of the sinus rhythm, and (3) prevention of systemic embolism. Controlling the ventricular response may be achieved by using medications that slow conduction through the AV node including digitalis, beta-blockers, and calcium channel blockers (Table 34–4). Special attention should be given to monitoring the side effects of drugs, and measurement of the digoxin serum level may be beneficial in elderly patients who have a high AV node sensitivity to medications and subnormal renal function. Spontaneous conversion of the atrial fibrillation occurs in 20% of patients, and restoration of sinus rhythm is usually successful in approximately 90% of patients with the use of chemical or electric cardioversion. Prior to an attempted conversion, 3 weeks of anticoagulation therapy is necessary whether the conversion procedure is pharmacologic or electrical. Some authorities do not think that anticoagulation is necessary before an attempt at conversion if the onset of atrial fibrillation occurred 48 hours or less before presentation. The use of transesophageal echocardiography to detect an atrial clot and determine whether anticoagulation is necessary prior to cardioversion remains controversial. The recommendation of the American College of Chest Physicians (ACCP) Consensus Conference on Antithrombolytic Therapies[78] is that echocardiographic findings should not determine the use of anticoagulation therapy prior to cardioversion of atrial fibrillation.

The benefit of antiarrhythmic therapy to prevent recurrence of atrial fibrillation is controversial, and no conclusive study has demonstrated that the risk of death or stroke is decreased with antiarrhythmic drugs. Some studies have actually demonstrated an increased mortality with the use of these drugs in patients with atrial fibrillation. Therefore, antiarrhythmic therapy should be used cautiously and is justified in elderly patients only when the symptoms are prominent and fail to respond to other types of therapy, and when the proarrhythmic effects of the antiarrhythmic drugs are low. The specific antiarrhythmic drug used depends on an individualized assessment of the risks and benefits of therapy and the severity of the underlying heart disease (Table 34–5).[79]

The risk of stroke in patients with nonvalvular atrial fibrillation is more than fivefold higher than that of patients with sinus rhythm. Increased risk of stroke occurs in patients with atrial fibrillation whether the arrhythmia is chronic or paroxysmal. Associated independent risk factors for stroke include advancing age, history of hypertension, diabetes, or a prior stroke or transient ischemic attack (TIA). Other risk factors for strokes considered important in patients with atrial fibrillation are a history of heart failure and the presence of CAD.

In five multicenter randomized studies of patients with nonvalvular atrial fibrillation and a mean age of over 65 years, warfarin decreased the risk of stroke by a mean of 68% (range 50% to 79%) and the risk of death by a mean of 33% (range 9% to 51%).[78, 79] In these studies warfarin therapy was not associated with an increase in incidence of cerebral hemorrhage. Two of the multicenter studies assessed the benefits of aspirin, and in one study a significant reduction in strokes was noted, although no benefit was found in patients over 75 years of age. In another multicenter randomized study, the Stroke Prevention in Atrial Fibrillation II Study (SPAF-II),[80] the use of aspirin was found to be equivalent to that of warfarin in preventing strokes. Also, an increase in significant intracerebral hemorrhage was noted in patients 75 years or older who were treated with warfarin. On close analysis of this study, however, it is evident that 40% of the thromboembolic events in the warfarin group occurred when the patients were either off warfarin or when the international normalized ratio (INR) was below the therapeutic range. Such findings are thought to explain the higher incidence of events in the warfarin group in this study compared to the results of other trials, which favored warfarin. Furthermore, most cases of intracerebral hemorrhage in this study occurred when the patient's INR was elevated above the therapeutic level. Another study, the European Atrial Fibrillation Trial,[81] which was a secondary preventive study, compared warfarin (Coumadin) with aspirin in preventing the occurrence of recurrent stroke or TIA in patients with nonvalvular atrial fibrillation. This study found aspirin to be of no benefit, whereas a reduction

TABLE 34–5 **CONSIDERATIONS IN EVALUATION OF ANTIARRHYTHMIC DRUGS FOR ATRIAL FIBRILLATION**

Agent	Class	Type of Proarrhythmia	Conduction Abnormalities	MI	LV Dysfunction
Quinidine	IA	Torsades de pointes	Caution	Caution	Caution
Procainamide	IA	Torsades de pointes	Caution	Caution	Caution
Disopyramide	IA	Torsades de pointes	Caution	Caution	Avoid
Flecainide	IC	AT or VT, conduction block	Avoid	Avoid	Avoid
Propafenone[a]	IC	VT	Caution	Caution or avoid[b]	Avoid
Sotalol[a]	III	Torsades de pointes, conduction block	Caution	Safe or caution[c]	Avoid
Amiodarone[a]	III	Conduction block	Caution	Safe	Safe

[a]Has beta-blocking properties.
[b]Uncertain of the safety of this IC agent.
[c]Use with caution in patients who have coexisting ventricular arrhythmia after acute MI.
Abbreviations: AT, Atrial tachycardia; LV, left ventricular; MI, myocardial infarction; VT, ventricular tachycardia.
Modified from Blackshear JL, Kopecky SL, Litin SC, et al: Management of atrial fibrillation in adults: Prevention of thromboembolism and symptomatic treatment. Mayo Clin Proc 1996;71:150–160.

TABLE 34–6 **RECOMMENDATIONS FOR ANTICOAGULATION IN PATIENTS WITH ATRIAL FIBRILLATION[a]**

Age	Risk Factors	Recommendations
Age <65	Risk factors[b]	Warfarin INR 2–3
	No risk factors	ASA or nothing
Age 65–75	Risk factors	Warfarin INR 2–3
	No risk factors	Warfarin or ASA
Age >75	Not applicable	Warfarin INR 2–3

[a]Recommendations of the American College of Chest Physicians Consensus Conference.[78]
[b]Risk factors are previous transient ischemic attack or stroke, hypertension, heart failure, diabetes, clinical coronary artery disease, mitral stenosis, prosthetic heart valves, or thyrotoxicosis.
Abbreviations: INR, international normalized ratio. ASA, acetylsalicylic acid.

of 30% was noted with warfarin. The most recent study (SPAF-III),[82] which assessed the benefit of a fixed low-dose warfarin and aspirin combination in elderly patients who were at high risk for stroke, found that the combination therapy was not beneficial in reducing stroke. Therefore, given the information from the many studies available, most authorities favor anticoagulation over antiplatelet therapy in the treatment of elderly patients with nonvalvular atrial fibrillation. More specific guidelines for the management of anticoagulation in patients with atrial fibrillation have been formulated by the ACCP Consensus Conference on Antithrombotic Therapies (Table 34–6).[78]

ATRIAL FLUTTER

Atrial flutter is the second most common supraventricular tachycardia seen in the elderly patients. It is usually associated with organic heart disease and is commonly found in elderly patients with chronic obstructive lung disease and in those who have recently had surgery. Atrial flutter is believed to be a macro-reentry mechanism located in the right atrium. The goals of treatment and the management of patients with atrial flutter are similar to those of atrial fibrillation. In regard to the use of anticoagulation in patients with atrial flutter, the ACCP Consensus Conference on Antithrombotic Therapies[78] recommends following the same guidelines as those used when managing patients with atrial fibrillation.

VENTRICULAR TACHYCARDIA

Ventricular ectopy, including premature ventricular contractions and ventricular tachycardias, are common in the elderly and are associated with increased mortality in patients who have underlying heart disease. In elderly patients without heart disease, as in younger patients, ventricular ectopy is usually a benign finding. Patients at the highest risk for increased mortality are those with nonsustained ventricular tachycardia and abnormal left ventricular function (see earlier section, Acute Myocardial Infarction, for treatment of ventricular arrhythmias).

References

1. Gerstenblith G, Frederiksen J, Yin FCP, et al: Echocardiographic assessment of a normal adult aging population. Circulation 1977;56:273–278.
2. Kitzman DW, Scholz DG, Hagen PT, et al: Age-related changes in normal human hearts during first 10 decades of life. Part II (maturity): A quantitative anatomic study of 765 specimens from subjects 20 to 99 years old. Mayo Clin Proc 1988;63:137–146.
3. Kantelip JP, Sage E, Duchenne-Marullary ZP: Findings in ambulatory electrocardiographic monitoring in subjects older than 80 years. Am J Cardiol 1986;57:398–401.
4. Lakatta EG, Gerstenblith G, Angell CS, et al: Prolonged contraction duration in the aged myocardium. J Clin Invest 1975;55:61–68.
5. Bonow RO, Vitale DF, Bacharach SL, Maron BJ, Green MV: Effects of aging on a synchronous left ventricular regional function and global ventricular filling in normal human subjects. J Am Coll Cardiol 1988;11:50–58.
6. Port S, Cobb FR, Coleman RE, Jones RH: Effect of age on the response of the left ventricular ejection fraction to exercise. N Engl J Med 1980;303:1133–1137.
7. Tresch DD, McGough MF: Heart failure with normal systolic function: A common disorder in older people. J Am Geriatr Soc 1995;43:1035–1042.
8. Aronow WS, Ahn C, Kronszon I: Prognosis of congestive heart failure in elderly patients with normal versus abnormal left ventricular systolic function associated with coronary artery disease. Am J Cardiol 1990;66:1257–1259.
9. Brandfonbrener M, Landowne M, Shock NW: Changes in cardiac output with age. Circulation 1955;12:557–566.
10. Rodeheffer RJ, Gerstenblith G, Becker LC, et al: Exercise cardiac output is maintained with advancing age in healthy human subjects: Cardiac dilatation and increased stroke volume compensate for a diminished heart rate. Circulation 1984;69:203–213.
11. Lerner DJ, Kannel WB: Patterns of coronary heart disease morbidity and mortality in the sexes. A 26-year follow-up of The Framingham Population. Am Heart J 1986;111:383–390.
12. Hlatky MA, Pryer DB, Harrell FE Jr, Califf RM, Mark DB, Rasati RA: Factors affecting sensitivity and specificity of exercise electrocardiography. Multivariate analysis. Am J Med 1984;77:64–71.
13. Iskandrian AS, Heo J, Decoskey D, Askenase A, Segal BL: Use of exercise thallium-201 imaging for risk stratification of elderly patients with coronary artery disease. Am J Cardiol 1988;61:269–272.
14. Lam JY, Chaitman BR, Glaenzer M, Byers S, Fit EJ, Shah Y, Goodgold H, Samuels L: Safety and diagnostic accuracy of dipyridamole-thallium imaging in the elderly. J Am Coll Cardiol 1988;11:585–589.
15. Carlos ME, Smart SG, Tresch DD: Benefits and safety

of dobutamine stress echocardiography in elderly patients. Clin Res 1994;42(3):357A.

16. Camerieri A, Picano E, Landi P, et al: Prognostic value of dipyridamole echocardiography early after myocardial infarction in elderly patients. J Am Coll Cardiol 1993;22:1809–1815.

17. Tresch DD: Diagnostic and prognostic value of ambulatory electrocardiographic monitoring in older patients. J Am Geriatr Soc 1995;43:66–70.

18. Tresch DD, Saeian K, Hoffman R: Elderly patients with late onset of coronary artery disease: Clinical and angiographic findings. Am J Geriatr Cardiol 1992;1:14–25.

19. Olson HG, Aronow WS: Medical management of stable angina and unstable angina in the elderly with coronary artery disease. Clin Geriatr Med 1996;12:121–140.

20. Weaver WD, Litwin PE, Martin JS, Kundenchuk PS, Maynard C, Eisenberg MS, Ho MT, Cobb LA, Lennedy JW, Wirkus MS: MITI Project Group. Effect of age on use of thrombolytic therapy and mortality in acute myocardial infarction. J Am Coll Cardiol 1991;18:657–662.

21. Maggioni AP, Maseri A, Fresco C, Francosi MG, Mauri F, Santoro E, Tognoni G: Age-related increase in mortality among patients with first myocardial infarction treated with thrombolysis. N Engl J Med 1993;329:1442–1448.

22. Vaccarino V, Krumholz HM, Berkman LF, Horwitz RI: Sex differences in mortality after myocardial infarction. Circulation 1995;91:1861–1871.

23. Kannel WB, Abbott RD: Incidence and progress of unrecognized myocardial infarction. An update on the Framingham Study. N Engl J Med 1984;311:1144–1147.

24. Pathy MS: Clinical presentation of myocardial infarction in the elderly. Br Heart J 1967;29:190–199.

25. Bayer AJ, Chadha JS, Farag RR, Pathy MS: Changing presentation of myocardial infarction with increasing age. J Am Geriatr Soc 1986;23:263–266.

26. Forman DE, Bernal JL, Wei JY: Management of acute myocardial infarction in the very elderly. Am J Med 1992;93:315–326.

27. Krumholz HM, Pasternak RS, Weinstein MC, et al: Cost-effectiveness of thrombolytic therapy with streptokinase in elderly patients with suspected acute myocardial infarction. N Engl J Med 1992;327:7–13.

28. The GUSTO Investigators: An international randomized trial comparing four thrombolytic strategies for acute myocardial infarction. N Engl J Med 1993;329:673–682.

29. Michelski B, Yusuf S: Does PTCA in acute myocardial infarction affect mortality and reinfarction rates? A quantitative overview (meta-analysis) of the randomized clinical trials. Circulation 1995;91:476–485.

30. Holland KJ, O'Neill WW, Bates ER, Pitt B, Topol EJ: Emergency percutaneous transluminal coronary angioplasty during acute myocardial infarction for patients more than 70 years of age. Am J Cardiol 1989;63:399–403.

31. ISIS-2 (Second International Study of Infarct Survival) Collaborative Group: Randomized trial of intravenous streptokinase, oral aspirin, both or neither amount: 17,187 cases of suspected myocardial infarction. Lancet 1988;2:349–360.

32. TIMI Study Group: Comparison of invasive and conservative strategies after treatment with intravenous tissue plasminogen activator in acute myocardial infarction. N. Engl J Med 1989;320:618–627.

33. Pfeffer MA, Braunwald E, Moye LA, et al: Effect of captopril on mortality and morbidity in patients with left ventricular dysfunction after myocardial infarction–Results of the Survival and Ventricular Enlargement Trial. N Engl J Med 1992;327:669–677.

34. Ramahi TM, Lee FA: Medical therapy and prognosis in chronic heart failure. Cardiol Clin 1995;13:5–26.

35. Gibson RS, Boden WE, Theroux P, et al: Diltiazem and reinfarction in patients with non-Q-wave myocardial infarction. N Engl J Med 1986;315:423–429.

36. The Multicenter Diltiazem Postinfarction Trial Research Group: The effect of diltiazem on mortality and reinfarction after myocardial infarction. N Engl J Med 1988;319:385–392.

37. The Danish Study Group on Verapamil in Myocardial Infarction: Effect of verapamil on mortality and major events after acute myocardial infarction (the Danish Verapamil Infarction Trial II [DAVIT II]). Am J Cardiol 1990;66:779–785.

38. ISIS-4 (Fourth International Study of Infarct Survival): A randomized factorial trial assessing early oral captopril, oral mononitrate, and intravenous magnesium sulfate in 58,000 patients with suspected acute myocardial infarction. Lancet 1995;345:669–685.

39. American College of Cardiology/American Heart Association Task force on assessment of diagnostic and therapeutic cardiovascular procedures: Guidelines for the early management of patients with acute myocardial infarction: A report of the ACC/AHA task force on assessment of diagnostic and therapeutic cardiovascular procedures. Circulation 1990;82:664–707.

40. Tresch DD, Litzow JT: Management of elderly patients with ventricular arrhythmias. Cardiol Elderly 1993;1:381–390.

41. The Cardiac Arrhythmia Suppression Trial: Preliminary report: Effect of encainide and flecainide on mortality in a randomized trial of arrhythmia suppression after myocardial infarction. N Engl J Med 1989;321:406–412.

42. Tresch DD, Platia EV, Guarneri T, Reid PR, Griffith LS: Refractory symptomatic ventricular tachycardia and ventricular fibrillation in elderly patients. Am J Med 1987;83:399–404.

43. Tresch DD, Troup PJ, Thakur RK, et al: Comparison of efficacy of automatic implantable cardioverter fibrillator in patients older and younger than 65 years of age. Am J Med 1991;90:717–724.

44. Gersh BJ, Kronmal RA, et al: Coronary arteriography and coronary artery bypass surgery. Morbidity and mortality in patients aged 65 years and older. Circulation 1983;67:483–491.

45. Thompson RC, Holmes DR Jr, Gersh BJ, Mock MB, Bailey KR: Percutaneous transluminal coronary angioplasty in the elderly: Early and long-term results. J Am Coll Cardiol 1991;17:1245–1250.

46. Jeroudi MO, Klerman NS, Minor ST, et al: Percutaneous transluminal coronary angioplasty in octogenarians. Ann Intern Med 1990;113:423–428.

47. Krumholz HM, Forman DE, Kungz RE, et al: Coronary revascularization after myocardial infarction in the very elderly: Outcomes and long-term follow-up. Ann Intern Med 1993;119:1084–1090.

48. Roberts WC, Perloff JK, Costantino T: Severe valvular aortic stenosis in patients over 65 years of age. Am J Cardiol 1971;27:497–506.

49. Roger VL, Tajik AJ, Reeder GS, Hayes SN, Mullay CJ, Bailey KR, Seward JB: Effect of Doppler echocardiography on utilization of hemodynamic cardiac catheterization in the preoperative evaluation of aortic stenosis. Mayo Clin Proc 1996;71:141–149.

50. Culliford AT, Galloway AC, Colvin SB, et al: Aortic valve replacement for aortic stenosis in persons aged 80 years and over. Am J Cardiol 1991;67:1256–1260.

51. Freeman WK, Schaff HV, O'Brien PC, Orszulak TA, Naessens JM, Tajik AJ: Cardiac surgery in the octogenarian: Perioperative outcome and clinical follow-up. J Am Coll Cardiol 1991;18:29–35.

52. Block PC, Palacios IF: Clinical and hemodynamic follow-up after percutaneous aortic valvuloplasty in the elderly. Am J Cardiol 1988;62:760–763.

53. Kelly TA, Rothbart RM, Cooper CM, Kaiser DL, Smucker ML, Gibson RS: Comparison of outcome of asymptomatic to symptomatic patients older than 20 years of age with valvular aortic stenosis. Am J Cardiol 1988;61:123–130.

54. Pellikka PA, Nishimura RA, Bailey KR, Tajik AJ: The natural history of adults with asymptomatic, hemodynamically significant aortic stenosis. J Am Coll Cardiol 1990;15:1012–1017.

55. Scognamiglio R, Fasoli G, Ponchia A, Dalla-Volta S: Long-term nifedipine unloading therapy in asymptomatic patients with chronic severe aortic regurgitation. J Am Coll Cardiol 1990;16:424–429.

56. Aronow WS, Schwartz KS, Koenigsberg M: Correlation of atrial fibrillation with presence or absence of mitral annular calcium in 604 persons older than 60 years. Am J Cardiol 1987;59:1213–1214.

57. Tresch DD, Siegel R, Keelan MH Jr, Gross CM, Brooks HL: Mitral valve prolapse in the elderly. J Am Geriatr Soc 1979;27:421–424.

58. Kolibash AJ, Bush CA, Fontana MB, Ryan JM, Kilman J, Wooley CF: Mitral valve prolapse syndrome: Analysis of 62 patients aged 60 years and older. Am J Cardiol 1983;52:534–539.

59. Tresch DD, Doyle TP, Boncheck LI, Siegel R, Keelan MH Jr, Olinger GN, Brooks HL: Mitral valve prolapse requiring surgery. Am J Med 1985;78:245–250.

60. Fremes SE, Goldman BS, Ivanov J, Weisel RD, David TE, Salerno T: Valvular surgery in the elderly. Circulation 1989;80(Suppl 1):77–90.

61. Tuzcu EM, Block PC, Griffin BP, Newell JB, Palacios IF: Immediate and long-term outcome of percutaneous mitral valvotomy in patients 65 years and older. Circulation 1992;85:963–971.

62. Topol EJ, Traill TA, Fortuin NJ: Hypertensive hypertrophic cardiomyopathy of the elderly. N Engl J Med 1985;312:277–307.

63. Fay WP, Taliercio CP, Ilstrup DM, Tajik AJ, Gersh BJ: Natural history of hypertrophic cardiomyopathy in the elderly. J Am Coll Cardiol 1990;16:821–826.

64. Mohr R, Schaff HV, Danielson GK, et al: The outcome of surgical treatment of hypertrophic obstructive cardiomyopathy: Experience over 15 years. J Thorac Cardiovasc Surg 1989;97:666–674.

65. Kannel WB, Belanger AJ: Epidemiology of heart failure. Am Heart J 1991;121:951–957.

66. Captopril-Digoxin Multicenter Research Group: Comparative effects of therapy with captopril and digoxin in patients with mild to moderate heart failure. JAMA 1988;259:539–544.

67. Uretsky BF, Young JB, Shahidi FE, Yellen LG, Harrison MC, Jolly MK, on behalf of the PROVED Investigative Group: Multicenter, double-blind, placebo-controlled randomized withdrawal trial of the efficacy and safety of digoxin in patients with mild to moderate

chronic heart failure not treated with converting enzyme inhibitors. J Am Coll Cardiol 1993;22:955–962.

68. Packer M, Gheorghiade M, Young JB, et al: Withdrawal of digoxin from patients with chronic heart failure treated with angiotensin-converting-enzyme inhibitors. N Engl J Med 1993;329:1–7.

69. The CONSENSUS Trial Study Group: Effects of enalapril on mortality in severe congestive heart failure. Results of the Cooperative North Scandinavian Enalapril Survival Study (CONSENSUS). N Engl J Med 1987;316:1429–1435.

70. The SOLVD Investigators: Effect of enalapril on mortality and the development of heart failure in asymptomatic patients with reduced left ventricular ejection fractions. N Engl J Med 1992;327:685–691.

71. Cohn JN, Archibald DGH, Ziesche S, et al: Effect of vasodilator therapy on mortality in chronic congestive heart failure. Results of a Veterans Administration Cooperative Study. N Engl J Med 1986;314:1547–1552.

72. Rajala S, Haavisto M, Kaltiala K, Mattila K: ECG findings and survival in very old people. Eur Heart J 1985;6:247–252.

73. Mihalic MJ, Fisch C: Electrocardiographic findings in the aged. Am Heart J 1974;87:117–128.

74. Caird FI, Campbell A, Jackson TF: Significance of abnormalities of electrocardiogram in old people. Br Heart J 1974;36:1012–1018.

75. Simonson E: The effect of age on the electrocardiogram. Am J Cardiol 1972;29:64–73.

76. Epstein LM, Chiesa N, Wong MN, et al: Radiofrequency catheter ablation in the treatment of supraventricular tachycardia in the elderly. J Am Coll Cardiol 1994;23:1356–1362.

77. Aronow WS, Ahm C, Gutstein H: Prevalence of atrial fibrillation with prior and new thromboembolic stroke in elderly. J Am Geratr Soc 1996;44:521–523.

78. Laupacis A, Albers G, Dalen J, Dunn M, Feinberg W, Jacobson A: Antithrombotic therapy in atrial fibrillation. Chest 1995;108:352S–359S.

79. Blackshear JL, Kopecky SL, Litin SC, Safford RE, Hammill SC: Management of atrial fibrillation in adults: Prevention of thromboembolism and symptomatic treatment. Mayo Clin Proc 1996;71:150–160.

80. Stroke Prevention in Atrial Fibrillation Investigators: Warfarin versus aspirin for prevention of thromboembolism in atrial fibrillation: Stroke prevention in Atrial Fibrillation II Study. Lancet 1994;343:687–691.

81. EAFT Study Group: European Atrial Fibrillation Trial: Secondary prevention of vascular events in patients with nonrheumatic atrial fibrillation and a recent transient ischaemic attack or minor ischaemic stroke. Lancet 1993;342:1255–1262.

82. Investigators. Adjusted-dose warfarin versus low-intensity, fixed-dose warfarin plus aspirin for high-risk patients with atrial fibrillation: Stroke Prevention in Atrial Fibrillation III randomized clinical trial. Lancet 1996;348:633–638.

35 Hypertension

Mark Andrew Supiano, M.D.

In contrast to the former view that high blood pressure is an expected normal aspect of aging, it is now evident that hypertension in the elderly is a disease state that is associated with significant adverse outcomes. Accordingly, despite an overall age-associated increase in blood pressure, there is no age adjustment to normalize the threshold values defining high blood pressure in the elderly. The classification of high blood pressure outlined, for example, by the Joint National Committee on Detection, Evaluation, and Treatment of High Blood Pressure (Table 35–1) therefore applies equally to older and younger adults.[1]

The National Health and Nutrition Examination Survey II is one of many epidemiologic studies documenting the fact that hypertension is a prevalent condition among older people. In this survey the overall prevalence of hypertension in noninstitutionalized individuals aged 65 to 74 years was 54.3%. According to the definition of hypertension used in this study (an average of three blood pressure readings of at least 140 mmHg systolic and/or 90 mmHg diastolic, or the use of antihypertensive medication), this per-

centage represents the combined prevalence rate for systolic-diastolic hypertension and isolated systolic hypertension. Diastolic blood pressure appears to increase with age up to approximately the age of 60 and then decreases, while systolic blood pressure appears to increase progressively and continuously with increasing age. Isolated systolic hypertension, defined as a systolic blood pressure in excess of 160 mmHg with a diastolic blood pressure of below 90 mmHg, is identified in approximately 20% of men and 33% of women aged 80 and older.

Although common, high blood pressure in the elderly should not be considered benign; the increase in blood pressure is associated with significant morbidity (e.g., coronary heart disease, congestive heart failure, stroke, peripheral vascular disease, and renal disease) and mortality.[2] It is also important to note that for any level of diastolic blood pressure, the risk of these adverse events becomes progressively greater at higher levels of systolic blood pressure.[2] Therefore, the age-associated increase in systolic blood pressure is an important contributor to the morbidity and mortality associated with hypertension in the elderly.[3, 4]

TABLE 35–1 CLASSIFICATION OF BLOOD PRESSURE

Category	Systolic (mmHg)	Diastolic (mmHg)
Normal	<130	<85
High normal	130–139	85–89
Hypertension		
Stage 1 (mild)	140–159	90–99
Stage 2 (moderate)	160–179	100–109
Stage 3 (severe)	180–209	110–119
Stage 4 (very severe)	≥210	≥120
Isolated systolic hypertension	>160	<90

Adapted from Joint National Committee on Detection, Evaluation, and Treatment of High Blood Pressure: The Fifth Report. Arch Intern Med 1993;153:154–183.

PATHOPHYSIOLOGY

A multitude of pathophysiologic mechanisms interact in the dynamic and complex regulation of arterial blood pressure. As is the case in younger individuals, the cause of essential hypertension in older humans remains unknown. Several mechanisms that may contribute to the increase in peripheral vascular resistance, which is one pathognomonic feature of hypertension in the elderly, are listed in Table 35–2. It is important to note that while these mechanisms have not been convincingly proved to be primary age-*associated* changes (i.e., independent of the effects of disease or lifestyle factors), they may be important contributors to hypertension in the elderly. It is also quite possible that the age-associated increase in blood pressure is secondary to age-*related* disease or lifestyle factors, since there are some populations in which the

TABLE 35–2 **PATHOPHYSIOLOGIC ALTERATIONS THAT MAY CONTRIBUTE TO OR ARE ASSOCIATED WITH ELEVATED BLOOD PRESSURE IN AGING**

Increased arterial stiffness
  Increased arterial pulse wave velocity
  Increase in wall-to-lumen ratio
Decreased baroreceptor sensitivity
Increased sympathetic nervous system activity
Decreased alpha- and beta-adrenergic
  responsiveness
Decreased endothelial cell–derived relaxing factor
  function
Salt-sensitivity of blood pressure
Low plasma renin activity
Insulin resistance

Adapted from Supiano MA: Hypertension. *In* Cassell CK, Cohen HJ, Larson EB, et al (eds): Geriatric Medicine, 3rd ed. New York, Springer-Verlag, 1996.

increase in blood pressure with aging is either absent or less marked.

The decrease in sensitivity of the baroreflex with age (perhaps as a manifestation of the decrease in arterial distensibility) illustrates how the approach to therapy of hypertension in the elderly requires an understanding of its pathophysiologic context. The decline in baroreflex sensitivity alters the central nervous system control of sympathetic nervous system (SNS) outflow, resulting in two important manifestations. First, with an insensitive baroreflex a larger change in blood pressure is needed to activate the baroreflex and produce the appropriate compensatory response. Attenuated baroreflex sensitivity is believed to contribute to the greater blood pressure variability seen in older individuals.[5] Second, attenuated baroreflex sensitivity results in enhanced SNS activity for a given level of arterial blood pressure, and this may account in part for the age-associated increase in activity of the SNS.[6]

CLINICAL ASSESSMENT

Measurement Issues

In light of the greater variability in blood pressure among older individuals, making an accurate diagnosis of hypertension poses a challenge. The statement that "hypertension should not be diagnosed on the basis of a single measurement"[1] is especially relevant to older patients. It has been observed that when antihypertensive medication is withdrawn from some older individuals a significant number will not have a blood pressure high enough to be classified as hypertensive. This

suggests that some older people are at risk for overtreatment of their blood pressure. Careful attention to correct measurement of blood pressure (e.g., using the average of two blood pressure measurements separated by at least 2 minutes [more if there is more than a 5-mmHg difference between the first two readings] taken at three separate visits) will minimize the likelihood that older individuals will be misdiagnosed as hypertensive and inappropriately placed on an antihypertensive medication. Although there have been concerns that indirect (cuff) blood pressure measurement overestimates the actual intra-arterial blood pressure of older individuals (due to increased arterial vascular stiffness), indirect blood pressure measurement is as accurate among older people as it is in younger adults. In some individuals the true blood pressure is overestimated by the indirect method owing to incompressibility of the brachial artery, a situation referred to as pseudohypertension. There remains some uncertainty about the frequency of pseudohypertension in the elderly. The possibility of pseudohypertension should be considered in the presence of a discrepancy between the severity of the blood pressure reading and evidence of target organ damage, a wide pulse pressure, and an inadequate response to antihypertensive therapy.

Target Organ Damage and Risk Factor Assessment

Once the diagnosis of hypertension has been appropriately made, the remainder of the evaluation should be directed toward identification of target organ damage, assessment of other cardiovascular risk factors, and identification of comorbid conditions that may influence the therapeutic decision-making process. In older hypertensive patients it may be more difficult to detect the manifestations of target organ damage that are directly attributable to elevated blood pressure in the presence of concurrent age- or disease-associated changes in organ function. The patient should be assessed for any physical signs consistent with coronary artery disease, cardiac failure, cerebrovascular disease (transient ischemic attack or stroke), or peripheral vascular diseases as well as for evidence of hypertensive retinopathy, renal insufficiency, or left ventricular hypertrophy. In addition, an evaluation to determine the presence of hyperlipidemia or diabetes mellitus and information about smoking history, dietary intake of salt and fat, alcohol intake, and level of physical activity should be obtained to aid in a determination of overall cardiovascular risk. This information is also needed to advise the patient about lifestyle modifications that may be recommended as nonpharmacologic approaches to blood pressure control. Finally, knowledge of co-morbid conditions is necessary to identify special clinical situations in which a given class of antihypertensive medication may be either recommended or contraindicated (see Table 35–3).

DIAGNOSIS AND MANAGEMENT

Differential Diagnosis

As is true in younger hypertensive populations, the overwhelming majority (greater than 90%) of older hypertensive patients have essential or primary hypertension. The approach to the evaluation for secondary and potentially reversible factors that may account for the increase in blood pressure in older people is similar to that recommended for younger hypertensive patients. Thus, a standard clinical evaluation consisting of a complete history and physical examination, chemistry profile (to assess electrolytes, renal function, and glucose), electrocardiogram, and chest radiograph is recommended to identify these factors. No further evaluation is normally needed unless abnormal symptoms or signs are elicited from the initial evaluation that would be consistent with renal disease (elevated serum creatinine or abnormal urinalysis), renovascular disease (e.g., presence of an abdominal bruit), hyperaldosteronism (hypokalemia), hypercortisolism (hyperglycemia, cushingoid appearance), hyperparathyroidism (hypercalcemia), or pheochromocytoma (symptoms of headache, palpitations, diaphoresis, and paroxysmal elevations of blood pressure).

Other clinical situations that might lead to an evaluation for secondary hypertension in the older patient include malignant hypertension, abrupt development of diastolic hypertension (which is unusual in light of the general decrease in diastolic blood pressure in persons older than 60 years), worsening of blood pressure control, or blood pressure that remains uncontrolled on

TABLE 35–3 **POTENTIAL ADVANTAGES, DISADVANTAGES, AND SPECIAL CLINICAL CONSIDERATIONS IN THE OLDER HYPERTENSIVE RELATED TO THE MAJOR ANTIHYPERTENSIVE CLASSES RECOMMENDED FOR INITIAL TREATMENT**

Antihypertensive Class	Potential Advantages	Potential Disadvantages	Clinical Situations to Recommend Use	Clinical Situations to Recommend Against Use or That Require Monitoring
Diuretics	• Benefit documented in clinical trials • Produce greater reduction in SBP than DBP • Inexpensive	• Metabolic abnormalities • Urinary incontinence	Systolic hypertension	Glucose intolerance gout, hyperlipidemia
Beta-antagonists	Benefit documented in clinical trials	• May increase peripheral vascular resistance • Metabolic abnormalities • CNS effects	Coronary artery disease and postmyocardial infarction	COPD, peripheral vascular disease, heart block, glucose intolerance, NIDDM, hyperlipidemia, depression
Angiotensin-converting enzyme inhibitors	Absence of CNS or metabolic effects	• Hyperkalemia • Renal insufficiency • Cough	Congestive heart failure, NIDDM	Renal insufficiency or renal artery stenosis
Calcium antagonists	Absence of CNS or metabolic effects	• Peripheral edema • Constipation • Heart block	Coronary artery disease	—
Alpha-1-adrenergic antagonists	Absence of CNS or metabolic effects	Orthostatic hypotension	Prostatism	Orthostatic blood pressure

Abbreviations: SBP, systolic blood pressure; DBP, diastolic blood pressure; COPD, chronic obstructive pulmonary disease; NIDDM, non–insulin-dependent diabetes mellitus; CNS, central nervous system.

Adapted from Supiano MA: Hypertension. *In* Cassel CK, Cohen HJ, Larson EB, et al (eds): Geriatric Medicine, 3rd ed. New York, Springer-Verlag, 1996.

a regimen of three antihypertensive medications. Renal disease and renovascular hypertension are the most frequent causes of secondary hypertension in the elderly; endocrinologic causes are generally less common. The only possible exception is pheochromocytoma, which, although still exceedingly rare (an overall incidence of less than 1% among patients with hypertension), may increase progressively in incidence with age.

General Approach to Therapy

There is now no question that a significant reduction in cardiovascular and cerebrovascular morbidity and mortality results from treatment to reduce blood pressure in older hypertensive patients. Epidemiologic studies have documented the fact that a significant relationship exists between the level of systolic and diastolic blood pressure and cardiovascular morbidity and mortality in the elderly.[2] It is therefore inappropriate to view hypertension in the elderly as benign or a characteristic of normal aging.[7]

Additional support for this point of view is derived from the results of many randomized controlled trials of antihypertensive therapy in older populations. Results from a meta-analysis of six randomized controlled studies (plus three others that did not include a placebo control group), confirm that treatment of hypertension in older people is associated with significant benefits: The treatment group had significant reductions in all-cause mortality (odds ratio 0.88; 95% confidence interval [CI], 0.80 to 0.97), stroke mortality (0.64; CI, 0.49 to 0.82), and morbidity (0.65; CI, 0.55 to 0.76), as well as cardiac mortality (0.75; CI, 0.64 to 0.88) and morbidity (0.85; CI, 0.73 to 0.99).[8] The Systolic Hypertension in the Elderly Program (SHEP) is unique among the studies included in this meta-analysis in its focus on isolated systolic hypertension.[9] The results of the SHEP study provided the first evidence that antihypertensive drug treatment in older patients with isolated systolic hypertension could be accomplished safely and that treatment resulted in a significant (36%) reduction in the incidence of fatal and nonfatal stroke.[9]

Although these studies have convincingly demonstrated the benefits of antihypertensive therapy in the elderly, it is important to tailor the goals of antihypertensive therapy to a given older individual. To this end, the benefits as well as the potential risks of any therapeutic intervention should be balanced to achieve the overall goal of preventing the morbidity and mortality associated with high blood pressure without adversely affecting the patient's functional performance or quality of life. A therapeutic approach directed toward reduction of systolic blood pressure to 135 to 140 mmHg and diastolic blood pressure to 85 to 90 mmHg should be developed using the treatments least likely to produce adverse effects (Fig. 35–1). It is important not to overtreat with an intervention that produces an excessive reduction in blood pressure. It is also unnecessary and perhaps deleterious to attempt rapid reductions in blood pressure to achieve this target level of control. In light of the age-associated pathophysiologic changes that result in impaired blood pressure homeostasis, too rapid a reduction in blood pressure may be associated with development of symptomatic hypotension in some situations (e.g., postural or postprandial hypotension). Likewise, it is advisable not to make dosage adjustments or additions of other therapies too rapidly to avoid overtreatment. Once the patient's blood pressure has been controlled to an optimal level, it is appropriate to reevaluate the need for continued therapy. A

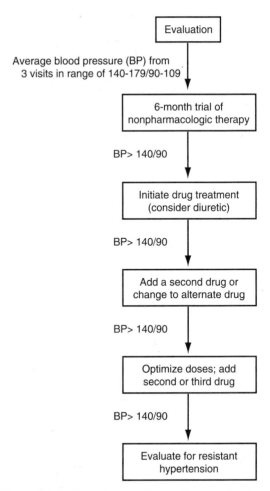

Figure 35–1 General approach to antihypertensive therapy for mild to moderate (stage 1 or 2) hypertension in the elderly.

reduction in dose or, in some cases, a trial period without antihypertensive medication (with close monitoring of the patient's home and office blood pressure) will help to minimize the possibility of overtreatment of blood pressure.

Another general approach to therapy is to assess the patient continuously for the development of treatment-related adverse effects as well as the response to therapy. The development of orthostatic hypotension is an adverse effect that may occur with any antihypertensive medication, although centrally acting agents and vasodilators are more commonly implicated in this regard. The symptoms of orthostatic hypotension may be atypical; rather than eliciting a history of postural unsteadiness, the older patient may cite generalized weakness or fatigue. Since orthostatic hypotension is common in hypertensive patients (its frequency increasing in parallel with the systolic blood pressure level) and its presenting symptoms are often occult, it is imperative to determine the supine and upright blood pressure measurements as part of the routine monitoring of all older hypertensive patients.

Nonpharmacologic Treatment Modalities

There are several reasons to review the role of nonpharmacologic treatment modalities first in discussing treatment of hypertension in the elderly. These modalities may be effective initial therapy for patients with mild to moderate (stage 1 or 2, see Table 35–1) hypertension as well as adjuncts in combination with pharmacologic treatments. Nonpharmacologic treatments may result in concurrent improvements in other cardiovascular risk factors and are associated with minimal risks. The older hypertensive population may in general be characterized as overweight, sedentary, and salt-sensitive. Lifestyle modifications targeted toward these characteristics may therefore be of particular benefit in older hypertensive patients. Weight reduction is recommended for hypertensive individuals who are more than 10% above their ideal body weight; weight loss on the order of 5 kg has been shown to result in small (generally less than 5 mmHg) but significant decreases in blood pressure.[10] The antihypertensive effects of lower extremity aerobic exercise programs are probably additive.[11] Although special considerations apply to older hypertensive patients with regard to screening for the presence of underlying cardiovascular disease and paying attention to the prevention of injuries, the safety and efficacy of aerobic exercise have been demonstrated in studies of older hypertensive individuals.[12] Given the increased prevalence of salt sensitivity of blood pressure among older hypertensive patients, it follows that dietary sodium restriction may be an especially effective nonpharmacologic treatment in this population.

Overview of Pharmacologic Treatments

If a 6-month trial of nonpharmacologic treatment fails to produce the desired reduction in blood pressure in patients with mild to moderate or isolated systolic hypertension (refer to definitions in Table 35–1), pharmacologic therapy should be initiated while nonpharmacologic treatments are continued (see Fig. 35–1). Older patients who present initially with more severe hypertension (stage 3 or 4)[1] almost always require pharmacologic treatment to achieve blood pressure control, and in such patients pharmacologic therapy should be initiated concurrently with nonpharmacologic methods. Since diuretics and beta-antagonists are the only agents that have been documented to decrease morbidity and mortality in clinical trials, the Joint National Committee has advised that one of these classes should be chosen as the initial agent for the treatment of simple hypertension in the absence of conditions in which their use may be relatively contraindicated.[1]

Each of the antihypertensive drug classes has been shown to be effective in reducing blood pressure in the older patient population; in this respect there is no universally preferred agent. Therefore, selection of a particular antihypertensive drug must be an individualized decision for each patient, taking into account the drug's potential advantages and disadvantages (see Tables 35–3 and 35–4). Recently, some reports have suggested the possibility of increased mortality in hypertensive patients who were treated with shorter-acting calcium channel antagonists; for this reason, long-acting calcium channel antagonists are recommended for treating hypertension. Neither direct vasodilators (e.g., hydralazine) nor central- (e.g., clonidine, methyldopa) or peripheral-acting (e.g., reserpine) adrenergic drugs are recommended for initial therapy. Furthermore, these drug classes are usually considered second-line agents in older hypertensives owing to their greater predisposition to develop adverse side effects related to these drugs (e.g., postural hypotension, reflex tachycardia, and CNS effects of sedation, lethargy, or depression). The starting dose of the initially selected agent should be reduced, and dose titration should be done more gradually in older hypertensive patients (see Table 35–4). If the target blood pressure goal is not

TABLE 35–4 **ADMINISTRATION OF INITIAL ANTIHYPERTENSIVE AGENTS**

Class and Agent	Usual Initial Dose and Frequency	Maximum Daily Dose
Diuretics		
Hydrochlorothiazide	12.5 mg qd	50 mg
Furosemide	20 mg qd	1 g
Triamterene	50 mg qd	100 mg
Beta-Antagonists		
Atenolol	25 mg qd	100 mg
Labetalol[a]	100 mg bid	1200 mg
Metoprolol	25 mg qd	200 mg
Propranolol	40 mg qd	240 mg
Angiotensin-Converting Enzyme Inhibitors		
Captopril	12.5 mg qd	150 mg
Enalapril	2.5 mg qd	40 mg
Lisinopril	5 mg qd	40 mg
Calcium Antagonists		
Amlodipine	2.5 mg qd	10 mg
Diltiazem	120 mg qd	360 mg
Nifedipine	30 mg qd	90 mg
Verapamil	120 mg qd	480 mg
Alpha-1-Adrenergic Antagonists		
Doxazosin	1 mg qd	16 mg
Prazosin	1 mg qd	20 mg
Terazosin	1 mg qd	20 mg

[a]Combined alpha and beta antagonist.

obtained at the maximal dose of the initial agent following several months of treatment, either the drug may be switched to a drug from an alternate class or a second drug from another class may be added.

Patient Adherence and Resistant Hypertension

Effective management of hypertension in an older person requires an approach that will promote the patient's adherence to his or her long-term treatment. The role of patient education cannot be overlooked in ensuring that the patient understands the goals of the therapeutic program and the importance of adhering to this program. The interdisciplinary geriatric team (including, for example, nurses, dietitians, pharmacists, and social workers) is well suited to promoting this approach. There are several specific methods that will enhance adherence to the long-term medical therapy of patients with this condition. These include written information describing the

specific treatment and an agreed-upon blood pressure goal, a simpler once-daily regimen, and the use of calendar or pill-box systems. Blood pressure self-monitoring by the patient is another approach that can involve the patient in the management of hypertension and perhaps enhance adherence to therapy.

In patients in whom adequate control of blood pressure fails to occur (i.e., fails to reach a target of 140/90) despite the use of three antihypertensive medications at maximum doses, evaluation for the causes of resistant hypertension should be undertaken. This evaluation should include an assessment of the patient's adherence to the medical therapy, a review focused on potential drug interactions (e.g., nonsteroidal anti-inflammatory agents, corticosteroids, sympathomimetics, and alcohol), and an assessment for volume overload. Other possible explanations to be considered in patients with resistant hypertension are the presence of a secondary cause (renovascular hypertension in particular) or pseudohypertension.

Special Clinical Situations

HYPERTENSIVE URGENCIES AND EMERGENCIES

Hypertensive urgencies and emergencies are defined by the need to reduce blood pressure quickly to prevent target organ damage, not by an absolute blood pressure level. Elevated blood pressure in itself without symptoms or signs of target organ damage does not usually require aggressive therapy. Aggressive blood pressure reduction in a patient who presents with incidentally noted elevated blood pressure is inappropriate in the absence of a true urgency or emergency. It is of particular importance to obtain an accurate blood pressure measurement to avoid overdiagnosis of a hypertensive emergency when none is present (e.g., to consider the possibility of pseudohypertension). Complications such as orthostatic hypotension or coronary or cerebral hypoperfusion syndromes may result from too aggressive treatment of an elderly patient with elevated blood pressure.

Hypertensive urgencies are more common than true hypertensive emergencies.[13] They are defined as situations in which blood pressure should be lowered within 24 hours to prevent the risk of target organ damage, such as accelerated or malignant hypertension without symptoms or evidence of ongoing target organ damage.[1] The majority of these situations can be managed with oral administration of antihypertensive medications (e.g., nifedipine, clonidine, labetalol, or captopril) but generally require a hospitalized setting for frequent blood pressure monitoring. Since no additional benefit has been noted with the use of sublingual administration of any of these agents, and their more rapid onset of action may produce a deleterious reduction in blood pressure unpredictably, the oral dosage forms, which are effective within 15 to 30 minutes, are recommended.

Examples of true hypertensive emergencies in older patients include hypertensive encephalopathy, intracranial hemorrhage, acute heart failure with pulmonary edema, dissecting aortic aneurysm, and unstable angina. These situations present with symptoms and signs of vascular compromise of the affected organs: brain (symptoms of severe headache, altered vision, altered mental status, and severe hypertensive retinopathy including papilledema or focal neurologic signs), heart (symptoms and signs of left ventricular failure or angina), or kidney (presenting as acute renal failure). The goal of treatment in these emergent clinical situations is immediate reduction in blood pressure, although again not necessarily to a normal level. Management of these conditions usually requires an acute care hospital setting to permit parenteral administration of an antihypertensive agent (e.g., nitroprusside) and continuous blood pressure monitoring. In addition, for patients with evidence of fluid overload, parenteral loop diuretics may aid in achieving blood pressure control. Once the hypertensive emergency or urgency has been managed, the next steps are an evaluation to determine the reason for the increase in blood pressure (i.e., a work-up for secondary causes) and development of a plan to achieve effective blood pressure control with appropriate close patient follow-up and monitoring.

HYPERTENSION IN NURSING HOME RESIDENTS

Very little information is available about the unique management of hypertension in residents of nursing homes. This is unfortunate given the prevalence of this condition among this population. While there is perhaps no major difference in the approach to the nursing home patient with hypertension, special considerations are warranted with respect to making the correct diagnosis, defining the goals of therapy and the effects on quality of life in this more frail patient population, and addressing the potential for adverse effects of therapy.

The available data suggest the possibility that blood pressure measurements of nursing home residents obtained by nursing staff may not be accurate; in one study hypertension was misclassified in 20% of nursing home residents.[14] Consideration should be paid to the goals of antihypertensive therapy in this population. The presence of other conditions that limit a patient's life expectancy may dictate a less aggressive approach to treatment of the elevated blood pressure. This benefit-risk approach should also incorporate the probability of adverse effects of antihypertensive therapy in this population. Since one of the most important risk factors for an adverse drug reaction is the total number of medications prescribed, any addition to the list of drugs given a nursing home resident increases the possibility of an adverse drug reaction. Nursing home residents, on average, experience two falls a year, and falls are a major source of morbidity in this population. Therefore, it is imperative that orthostatic blood pressure be carefully monitored in this population to attempt to minimize medication-induced orthostatic hypotension as a causal factor of falls.

References

1. Joint National Committee on Detection, Evaluation, and Treatment of High Blood Pressure: The Fifth Report. Arch Intern Med 1993;153:154–183.
2. Glynn RJ, Field TS, Rosner B, Hebert PR, Taylor JO, Hennekens CH: Evidence for a positive linear relation between blood pressure and mortality in elderly people. Lancet 1995;345:825–829.
3. Nielsen WB, Vestbo J, Jensen GB: Isolated systolic hypertension as a major risk factor for stroke and myocardial infarction and an unexploited source of cardiovascular prevention: A prospective population-based study. J Hum Hypertens 1995;9:175–180.
4. Sutton-Tyrrell K, Alcorn HG, Herzog H, Kelsey SF, Kuller LH: Morbidity, mortality, and antihypertensive treatment effects by extent of atherosclerosis in older adults with isolated systolic hypertension. Stroke 1995;26:1319–1324.
5. Lipsitz LA: Altered blood pressure homeostasis in advanced age: Clinical and research implications. J Gerontol Med Sci 1989;44:M179–M183.
6. Hogikyan RV, Supiano MA: Arterial α-adrenergic responsiveness is decreased and sympathetic nervous system activity is increased in older humans. Am J Physiol 1994;266:E717–E724.
7. Dickerson JE, Brown MJ: Influence of age on general practitioners' definition and treatment of hypertension. Br Med J 1995;310:574.
8. Insua JT, Sacks HS, Lau T-S, et al: Drug treatment of hypertension in the elderly: A meta-analysis. Ann Intern Med 1994;121:355–362.
9. SHEP Cooperative Research Group: Prevention of stroke by antihypertensive drug treatment in older persons with isolated systolic hypertension: Final results of the Systolic Hypertension in the Elderly Program (SHEP). JAMA 1991;265:3255–3264.
10. Cutler JAK: Combinations of lifestyle modification and drug treatment in management of mild-moderate hypertension: A review of randomized clinical trials. Clin Exper Hypertens 1993;15:1193–1204.
11. Kelley G, McClellan P: Antihypertensive effects of

aerobic exercise: A brief meta-analytic review of randomized controlled trials. Am J Hypertens 1994;7:115–119.

12. Hagberg JM, Montain SJ, Martin WH III, Ehsani AA: Effect of exercise training in 60- to 69-year-old persons with essential hypertension. Am J Cardiol 1989;64:348–353.

13. Zampaglione B, Pascale C, Marchisio M, Cavallo-Perin P: Hypertensive urgencies and emergencies; prevalence and clinical presentation. Hypertension 1996;27:144–147.

14. Stoneking HT, Hla KM, Samsa GP, Feussner JR: Blood pressure measurements in the nursing home: Are they accurate? Gerontologist 1992;32:536–540.

36 Oncologic Disorders

Paul P. Carbone, M.D., M.A.C.P., D.Sc.(Hon.)

James F. Cleary, M.B., B.S., F.R.A.C.P.

The risk of developing cancer increases with age. In 1995 the American Cancer Society (ACS) estimated that 1,252,000 new cancers were diagnosed. In addition, there were 120,000 cases of carcinoma in situ, primarily endometrial, cervix, breast, and melanoma, and 800,000 cases of basal and squamous cell skin cancers. Fifty-eight percent of all cancers occur in people over 65. Each year, for every 100 Americans over 65, two are diagnosed with cancer and one will die.[1] For every 100 black males over 65, three will develop cancer.

A high proportion of specific cancers occur in men and women over 65 years of age. For example, 84% of all prostate cancers occur in the over-65 age group. Women over 65 have 61% to 78% of common cancers (colon, lung). Breast and ovarian cancers are about evenly split between those under 65 and those 65 or over (Table 36–1). Between the ages of 20 and 60, the incidence of cancers is about the same in men and women. After age 60 cancer rates in men are 70% higher, and they increase to two times the female rate by age 85 (3381/100,000 in men and 1795/100,000 in women).[2]

Cancer, the second leading cause of death in the United States, caused 547,000 deaths in 1995. The leading causes of cancer deaths in women are lung, breast, colon, and pancreas cancers. In men the major causes are lung, prostate, colorectal, and pancreas cancers. About 22% of all deaths in people over 65 years old are due to cancer. Two thirds of all cancer deaths occur in the over-65 population. The number of cancer deaths has increased in the past 40 years. This increase has occurred predominantly in the population over 65. A large part of the increase can be attributed to lung cancer. Within the U.S. population, individuals of color generally have higher death rates for most cancers. Except for ovarian cancer, Surveillance, Epidemiology and End Results (SEER) program data do not suggest that cancer presents in a more advanced stage in the elderly.

During the last several decades, advances in treatment and early diagnosis have improved the outcome for many patients. However, most of the benefits have occurred in cancers that affect the very young and the population under age 65. Mortality rate changes are shown in Figure 36–1.

TABLE 36–1 **CANCER PATIENTS, SEX, AND AGE**

Cancer site	Men		Women	
	All ages	*≥65 yr (%)*	*All ages*	*≥65 yr (%)*
Lung	100,000	63	72,000	61
Colon	52,000	73	55,000	78
Rectum	23,000	65	19,000	71
Urinary bladder	38,000	70	13,200	74
Stomach	15,000	68	9,000	75
Pancreas	13,000	68	14,000	77
Breast			182,000	50
Ovary			24,000	49
Prostate	200,000	84		

Data from Yancik R, Ries L: Cancer in older persons. Cancer 1994;74:1995–2003.

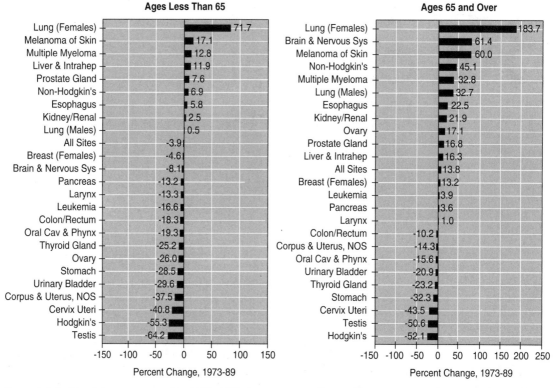

Figure 36–1 Trends in cancer mortality, 1973–1989, by age groups. (From Miller B, Ries L, Hankey B, Kosary C, Edwards B: Cancer Statistics Review 1973–1989. NIH Publication 92-2789. Bethesda, MD, U.S. Department of Health and Human Services, National Institutes of Health, National Cancer Institute, 1992.)

Cancer mortality has decreased (0.2% per year) in the population under 65. In the over-65 age group, mortality has increased by 0.9% per year. For example, lung cancer mortality in the 1973–1989 period increased by 71.7% in women under 65 and by 184% in those over 65. Higher death rates in the elderly have been reported in those with brain tumors (61%), melanoma (60%), non-Hodgkin's lymphoma (45%), multiple myeloma (33%), lung cancer in men (33%), breast cancer (13%), and prostate cancer (17%). When improvements in mortality have occurred, SEER data show that the improvements are less dramatic in the elderly.[3]

SECOND TUMORS

Survivors of one cancer are likely to develop second cancers. These may result from prior exposure to a common carcinogenic factor (cigarette smoking) or treatment (radiation or chemotherapy) or because second cancers increase with age much like the first cancer. Studies in Wisconsin suggest that by age 90 about 15% of patients will have second cancers.[4] This fact is important because a pulmonary nodule may not reflect spread from the first cancer but a treatable and

curable second cancer. Lymph nodes in the retroperitoneal region or neck may represent a lymphoma rather than metastasis from a prior colon cancer.

Second cancers may be the consequence of prior treatment. Radiation for Hodgkin's disease may result in subsequent lung cancer or breast cancer in the treatment field. Patients with one colon cancer may have a second operable colon cancer rather than a recurrence that requires aggressive systemic therapy. Leukemia results from exposure to certain drugs used to cure other malignancies. Myeloma treated with melphalan or leukemia treated with etoposide may be followed by secondary leukemia. These secondary leukemias may have specific chromosome markers. Young women with a strong family history of breast cancer may develop contralateral breast cancers or ovarian cancers.

PATHOPHYSIOLOGY OF CANCER

The relationship between aging and cancer has long been known. The various factors involved in carcinogenesis and their relationship to age are summarized in Table 36–2. As one ages, genetic mistakes accumulate (loss of chromo-

TABLE 36–2 **RELATIONSHIP OF AGING AND CANCER**

Carcinogenesis	Effect	Result	Age Association
Initiation	Genetic mistakes	Loss of chromosomal material, mistakes in DNA repair, DNA amplification	Increases with age
Promotion	Increase in cells with genetic mistakes	Enhanced by smoking, alcohol, hormones, infections, sunlight	Increases with age
Heredity	Genetic predisposition	Rb gene, BRCA1, BRCA2, p53	Not age related
Immunity	Immune surveillance	Allows transformed cells to grow	Decreases with age
Growth factors	Differentiation and cell cycle control	Cells continue to divide, loss of apoptosis	Increases with age
Diet/calories	Unknown	Increased incidence of cancers with increased calories in animals; effect in humans not clear	Not age related

somal material and mistakes in DNA repair) in cells. These cells with genetic changes are numerically enhanced by endogenous or exogenous tumor promoters (hormones, tobacco, alcohol, viruses). The DNA damage may be accentuated as the ability to repair DNA decreases with age. Over time, these events lead to cancers. Added to this carcinogenic pressure are germ line abnormalities. These changes are also related to cancers that occur later in life.

The relationship between aging and cancer has been associated with the increase in exposure to environmental carcinogens with time. However, analyses of age incidence curves indicate that there is no simple explanation for the rise in cancer incidence with age. Age does not explain the shape of the incidence curves. The cancers increase with age but at a decreasing rate. The proliferative rate of a tissue is known to influence the development of cancer. Cells lose this potential with aging. Dix explains the risk of cancer as the difference between the accumulation of genetic and epigenetic changes (increases the risk) and the loss of proliferative potential (decreases the risk). With advancing age the "diminishing force becomes prominent."[5]

Immune System

The immunologic surveillance theory suggests that cancers are eliminated all the time by the body's immune system. As one ages, the activity of the immune system decreases, and therefore cancers start appearing. This theory also implies that cancers grow more rapidly in the elderly. Tumors implanted into older animals grow faster than when they are injected into young mice. The clinical data do not support this concept.

Although cancers present in more advanced stages in the elderly, delay in seeking medical attention and decreased use of screening tools are also operative factors. Survival differences are not seen when stage and treatment are corrected for in both younger and older cancer patients.

Growth Factors

Many cell functions go awry during carcinogenesis. These are often related to the cell cycle. Abnormalities in specific genes cause cells to lose their normal growth controls. They lose the ability to grow old and die. These lost controls include increases in growth factors, mutated oncogenes, loss of suppressor genes, and constitutive activation of receptors. Instead of the cells dividing, maturing, and then dying, they continue to divide. This lack of feedback control results in unfettered growth. These factors all happen more frequently as one ages.

Other Factors

TOBACCO

Prolonged tobacco product use leads to oral, larynx, lung, pancreas, kidney, and bladder cancers. The risk of cancer is related to the duration and intensity of smoking. Smoking is an additive factor for the risk of lung cancers in workers who are exposed to asbestos and uranium ores. The rise in lung cancer mortality is now decreasing in men but is still increasing in women. Not only is smoking an important causative agent, but secondary or passive smoking leads to cancers in the children and spouses of smokers. From the point of view of geriatric risk assessment, former smokers retain a higher incidence of cancer for 20 years after they stop using cigarettes.

ALCOHOL

Alcohol ingestion and smoking are associated with increased oral and other upper airway cancers. Excessive alcohol use leads to cirrhosis of the liver and subsequent liver cancer. Alcohol ingestion is also associated with other cancers (i.e., pancreas, stomach, breast, and bladder cancers).

SUNLIGHT

Skin cancer is a disease of older white populations. About 95% of skin cancers occur in subjects older than 45. Ninety percent of cases are related to ultraviolet light exposure. Host or genetic factors associated with nonmelanoma skin cancers (NMSC) include light eye color, fair complexion, and light hair color. Excessive sun exposure in childhood may be more important than exposure as an adult. Outdoor workers are likely to have more sun exposure and higher rates of skin cancer. A person with one skin cancer has a 30% chance of developing a second skin cancer in the next 5 years.

DIET

The relationship between dietary fat and cancer is more circumstantial than factual. Increased dietary fat is associated with more colon or breast cancer in national population studies. However, in well-designed case-control studies, no relationship is seen.[6] The issue is further complicated by the experimental data, which relate cancer formation to dietary calories rather than to fat content. Certain nutrients such as vitamins C or E or selenium are antioxidants that neutralize the formation of free radicals. An interesting observation has been that colon cancer rates diminish when people move from the northern areas to the southern parts of the United States. It has been suggested that dietary changes may contribute to this reduction.

VIRUSES

There are strong links between viruses and specific human cancers. These include hepatocellular carcinoma (hepatitis B and C), Burkitt's tumor and nasopharyngeal cancer (Epstein-Barr virus), cervix cancer (human papilloma virus [HPV] - 16 and 18), and human T-cell lymphotropic virus (HTLV-1). Kaposi's sarcoma associated with the acquired immunodeficiency syndrome (AIDS) may also be linked with a virus.

FAMILY HISTORY

Most cancers are not associated with strong family histories. In the past, family-related cancers were thought to be found mainly in the pediatric population. However, recent studies suggest that the genetic changes seen in familial cancers are also seen in sporadic cancers. Simultaneous or subsequent breast cancer may occur in the parent of a daughter with early-onset breast cancer.

PREVENTION

Increasing knowledge of the causes of cancers has led to the implementation of strategies to prevent cancer. Very important is the avoidance of known carcinogens. These include radiation, tobacco products, organic dyes, benzene, arsenic, asbestos, and chromium compounds. Important tools that can decrease tobacco-related cancers are tax increases on tobacco products, bans on advertisements for tobacco products, legislation creating more no smoking environments and increased public education about the dangers of second hand smoke.

Sun exposure and skin cancers are linked. Avoiding the burning rays of the sun during the middle of the day in the early years is extremely important. The protective value of sun screens is still controversial. Exposures to toxic metals, asbestos, and pesticides are being reduced during the mining and manufacture of products containing these materials. Vaccination against hepatitis B can limit the development of subsequent liver cancers. Current studies are looking at the use of tamoxifen to prevent breast cancer, finasteride to prevent prostate cancer, and nonsteroidal anti-inflammatory drugs (NSAIDs) to prevent colon cancers. The use of beta-carotene or low-fat diets to prevent lung or breast cancers is still debatable.

SCREENING

Cancer mortality can be decreased by diagnosing the cancers or the precursor lesions earlier. An example of this is the Papanicolaou test for cervical cancer. Mammography decreases breast cancer mortality in women who are over 50 years old. However, few studies have been done in women over 70. Recommendations for the use of mammography are shown in Table 36–3. Table 36–4 summarizes the recommendations for screening for other cancers.

Prostate screening with the digital rectal examination (DRE), transrectal ultrasound (TRU), and prostate specific antigen (PSA) is increasing. Public figures have advocated screening with

TABLE 36–3	**SCREENING RECOMMENDATIONS FOR BREAST CANCER**
Women aged 65–74	Clinical breast examination (CBE) annually, mammogram every 2 years
Women over 75	Those whose life expectancy and general health are good: CBE annually, mammograms every 2 years
Women over 75	Monthly breast self-examination

PSA as a "cure all." However, there is no general agreement on screening men over 50 for prostate cancer, how long to screen, or how often. Unfortunately, screening has led to an enormous increase in incidence of this cancer. Many more men are being treated with surgery or radiotherapy. Despite these treatments, mortality has gone up. The concept of watchful waiting may be appropriate in some patients with small low-grade tumors.

The ACS recommends annual screening for prostate cancer in all men over 50 years old and earlier in African-Americans and those at high risk (men with a family history). Others have advocated no screening in men over 65 or in those in whom the life expectancy is less than 10 years. Resolution of this controversial subject is not possible at this time.

The pathogenesis of colon cancer has been well characterized clinically and molecularly. Early adenomatous polyps are well on the way to cancer. Screening of populations over 50 with sigmoidoscopy and fecal occult blood testing decreases large bowel cancer mortality. In patients with large (1 cm or over) adenomatous polyps or villous adenomas, the entire colon should be examined. The question of when to stop surveillance screening has not been resolved; however, stopping surveillance after two or three normal sigmoidoscopic examinations at 3-year intervals appears reasonable. The value of a full and normal colonoscopic examination may last longer.

Screening for lung cancer in smokers using annual chest radiographs has not been helpful. Repeated testing of the urine for occult blood may detect early treatable bladder cancers. Ovarian cancer screening with CA-125 blood tests and pelvic ultrasound has not been cost-effective. In women with a strong family history of ovarian and breast cancers, BRCA1 and BRCA2 gene mutations can be measured. In these women, prophylactic mastectomy and oophorectomy at an earlier age prevent cancers later in life. Abnormal uterine bleeding in a woman taking tamoxifen or estrogens should be explored further.

Women over 65 who have had repeated normal Pap tests previously have a low risk of developing cervix cancer. Many older women have had a hysterectomy. Pap tests are not sufficiently sensitive to detect endometrial neoplasms. Ovarian masses detected by physical examination should undergo a work-up, particularly in postmenopausal women.

AGING: IMPACT ON DIAGNOSIS AND THERAPY

Older people are less likely to participate in screening programs or seek attention for their

TABLE 36–4	**OTHER SCREENING RECOMMENDATIONS**	
Population with No Increased Risk	**Recommendations**	**Comment**
Prostate cancer	American Cancer Society: Annual digital rectal exam (DRE) and prostate specific antigen (PSA)	No general agreement by other organizations. After age 70 screening may not be appropriate
Colon cancer	Annual DRE starting at age 40, stool occult blood test at 50, and sigmoidoscopy at age 50 every 3–5 years	Positive occult blood or adenomatous polyp needs follow-up with colonoscopy
Lung cancer	No recommendations	
Cervical cancer	Three negative annual Pap tests starting at 20, then every 3 years until age 65	Women over 65 not screened in past 10 years need Pap test
Endometrial cancer	No recommendations	Abnormal bleeding should be followed up with uterine cytology
Ovarian cancer	No recommendations	CA-125 levels may be high in nonmalignant conditions

TABLE 36–5 **MYTHS AND BIASES AFFECTING DIAGNOSIS AND TREATMENT OF THE ELDERLY**

1. The elderly believe that cancer is not preventable and is caused by stress, trauma, or infection (fatalism).
2. Anorexia, weight loss, and fatigue are normal for older people (rationalizing symptoms).
3. The elderly do not feel pain as much as younger patients (undertreatment of pain).
4. Radiation and chemotherapy are too toxic for the elderly (undertreatment).
5. The elderly do not need to see oncologists or be referred to cancer centers (inadequate treatment, underrepresentation in clinical trials).

illnesses. There are many reasons for this lack of attention to healthy living habits. Myths and biases hinder appropriate attempts to seek care in the elderly (Table 36–5). Myths about causation (stress, trauma, contagion), presentation (pain as an early symptom), and co-morbidity (anorexia, fatigue, and weight loss) may mask cancer symptoms.[7] Berkman and colleagues[7] point out that the myth that the elderly do not feel pain leads to analgesia undertreatment. Likewise, myths about the effects of radiation and chemotherapy may cause patients and physicians to defer appropriate treatment.

Women over 65 are less likely to take advantage of mammograms. Cancer Reporting System (CRS) data in Wisconsin have shown that the elderly are more likely to have their diseases diagnosed in smaller hospitals[8] and to receive all their care in small hospitals. CRS data show that the elderly are likely to receive surgical therapy but not adjunctive radiotherapy and chemotherapy as often as younger patients with similar stages of disease. In part, this may be due to social factors such as interference with caregiving, lack of transportation, or concern about toxicity. Table 36–6 lists some of the characteristics of the elderly that may affect appropriate treatment decisions.

Several studies have shown that the elderly are not uniformly infirm and that they tolerate chemotherapy as well as younger patients (those under 70 years old).[9] The elderly (over 70) are excluded from clinical trials. They are not proportionately represented in referrals to cancer centers or clinical trials. Studies by several cooperative groups have shown that the responses and toxicities of treatment are not influenced by age. *Thus, chronologic age should not be a deterrent to entering these patients in trials.* Non-age-related factors in the elderly may also influence selection of therapy or access to trials and treatment. These include impaired access to transportation, low income, ethnicity, and low educational achievement.[10]

Age-related changes influence treatment (see Table 36–6). Many organ systems undergo changes with age; these include decreases in cardiac output, glucose tolerance, glomerular filtration, vital capacity, and maximum breathing capacity. Many chemotherapeutic agents depend on the kidney or liver for metabolism and excretion. Thus, in prescribing certain drugs, specific attention must be paid to both the pharmacokinetics and pharmacodynamics of the agent. In particular, studies have shown that the dosage of methotrexate, which depends on renal clearance, must be modified based on measured renal clearances. Other drugs have specific organ toxicities such as the myocardium for doxorubicin. Underlying cardiac impairment in the elderly may enhance the development of clinical heart failure.

Hematologic toxicities are more likely to be age related. The known pharmacologic disposition of the drugs used (i.e., renal or hepatic clearance) often explains this propensity. While liver enzyme activity does not decrease with age, decreased hepatic blood flow may cause decreases in drug clearances. Other toxicities, such as skin, gastrointestinal, or central nervous system, occur in about the same frequencies in older and younger populations.[9]

TABLE 36–6 **FACTORS INFLUENCING CANCER TREATMENT**

Age-Related Events	Modality	Impact
Co-morbid illnesses	Surgery, radiation, chemotherapy, palliative care	Less than optimal surgery, staging, and treatment
Decreased renal clearances	Chemotherapy, palliative care	Excessive toxicity with agents that are dependent on renal excretion
Polypharmacy	Chemotherapy, palliative care	Inadvertent adverse drug interactions
Caregiving, lack of transportation, low income	Surgery, radiation, chemotherapy, palliative care	Inadequate treatment, low representation in clinical trials

Older people are particularly sensitive to certain drugs such as diazepam, morphine, and the phenothiazines. Morphine clearance is decreased in the elderly, suggesting that the dosing interval may need to be extended in these patients. Unless these changes are considered, the result may be extreme lethargy, constipation, and prolonged drowsiness at the ordinary doses.

Associated Illnesses

Despite the known presence of increasing co-morbid conditions with age, little is known about how these influence diagnosis and management. Arthritis, cardiovascular disease, diabetes, hypertension, chronic obstructive lung disease, and stroke occur in 18% to 55% of cancer patients. These factors do not influence cancer stage at presentation. Specifically, in breast cancer patients Havlik and colleagues found that no differences in stage at the time of presentation were seen in women with up to two, but not in those with three or more, co-morbid conditions. In their report, no difference in stage was observed in patients with and without arthritis and colon cancer or diabetes and bladder cancer.[3]

CLINICAL ASSESSMENT

History

A careful history and follow-up on complaints can lead to a high degree of suspicion for cancer. Generalized symptoms of weight loss, fever, night sweats, jaundice, anorexia, and pain should lead to a high index of suspicion of cancer. Abnormal bleeding or discharges can point to specific organs that need special attention. Neurologic complaints of headache, vision, coordination, and strength should be noted.

An important part of taking any history is the family history and details of social and sexual habits. The history should include questions about occupation and exposures to medications. Occupational exposures to metals, chemicals, and asbestos should be elicited. Use of medications such as estrogen replacement and maternal diethylstilbestrol exposure must be ascertained. Knowledge of the family history may uncover a specific genetic syndrome such as the BRCA1 or BRCA2 breast cancer gene or the Li-Fraumeni or Lynch's syndrome. Information about smoking and ethanol ingestion is important. Exposure to hepatitis may be important in someone with liver cancer. Information about sexual orientation and practices is important in alerting the physician to AIDS-related lymphoma or cervical cancers.

Physical Examination

Together with a detailed history, a targeted physical examination is absolutely imperative for the primary physician. Evidence of jaundice, anemia, petechiae, or weight loss should be noted. Observation and palpation of any skin nodules, ulcerations, and nevi over 5 to 7 mm in size should be done. Skin cancers are likely to occur on sun-exposed surfaces. Melanomas are also likely to be found in the same areas. Careful examination of the back in men and the posterior calves in women should be performed. The mouth should be examined fully for ulcers, leukoplakia, or lumps. Careful palpation of the lymph node areas in the neck, axillae, and epitrochlear and inguinal areas should be performed. Nodes that are 1 cm in size or larger should be considered for biopsy. Inspection and palpation of the breasts in both men and women are important, looking for distortions, masses, or skin changes.

The muscles that are deeper than the subcutaneous tissues should be palpated for any abnormalities in a search for sarcomas. Palpation of the abdomen for organomegaly, renal enlargement, or bladder distention will provide clues to metastatic disease, masses, or obstructions. Splenic enlargement is common with lymphoma or leukemia. Examination of the external and internal genitalia for testicular, vulval, cervical, uterine, or ovarian cancers can detect a variety of cancers that are curable. Finally, a rectal examination is an important part of the physical examination in both men and women.

DIAGNOSIS AND STAGING

Staging implies assessment of the extent of the disease and classification according to specific criteria. The most common classification is the one recommended by the American Joint Committee for Cancer Staging and End Results Reporting, which consists of the tumor, node, metastasis (TNM) classification. Special staging systems have been devised for certain specific tumors. Staging requires additional tests that specify the location or locations of disease. Knowledge of the natural history of the tumor allows the experienced oncologist to order appropriate tests and biopsies to detect disease locations. Before embarking on a comprehensive and expensive series of tests and consultations, the primary physician should consider several questions about the diagnosed cancer.

1. *Is the cancer potentially curable or amenable to worthwhile palliation?* It is unfair to patients and a waste of time and money to investigate a condition

extensively that does not respond to treatment. In the case of an adenocarcinoma of an unknown primary, expensive endoscopic and computed tomographic (CT) tests looking for primary sites are usually futile. One should take the approach of separating treatable cancers (lymphoma, breast, ovarian, prostate, or thyroid cancer) from untreatable cancers (pancreas, stomach, lung). Even if specific diagnoses of these latter tumors can be established, the conditions are often not amenable to therapy. Similarly, an elderly patient with known colon cancer who presents with jaundice and a large liver may not have to undergo extensive tests or a biopsy.

2. *Can the appropriate diagnostic or pathologic examinations be carried out in the community, or is the advice of specialists needed?* The diagnosis of breast cancer or colon cancer does not present a challenge to the local community hospital pathologist. However, a specific cellular diagnosis of lymphoma or leukemia may require special tests including flow cytometry or molecular or cytogenetic studies.

3. *Is the treatment best carried out in the community or at a regional cancer center?* Modern management of many cancers can be done in the community. Clinical trials are also done well in community hospitals. However, some cancers, including pediatric cancers, most acute and some chronic leukemias, recurrent lymphoma, sarcomas, esophageal and head and neck cancers, and brain tumors, require special treatment planning, integrated chemotherapy and radiation, or even experimental approaches. These are best carried out in consultation with regional centers.

TREATMENT

General

Once the right diagnosis has been established and the extent of disease determined, appropriate therapy can be offered. Sometimes staging becomes part of the primary treatment (breast, colon, ovarian cancer). The primary physician should seek consultation with a surgeon experienced in cancer surgery. Organ-sparing techniques to preserve the breast or anus require experience that is not always well developed in the community. Debulking for primary stage 3

ovarian cancer can be a major task that requires special training. Similarly, special equipment may be needed for treatment of brain tumors.

Chemotherapy expertise is widespread in the community. It is usually appropriate to have the patient stay as near home as possible. However, the knowledge of the individual community oncologist and his or her willingness to seek help is important. Consultation is indicated during the terminal phase as well. This may involve consulting with the palliative care specialists at a regional center or with local hospice staff.

Surgery

Surgery is the mainstay of cancer treatment. It has the best chance of cure in most patients with localized disease. Cancer treatment in the elderly regularly includes surgery. There is some evidence that surgeons perform less surgery in the elderly. However, a new dimension has entered the picture. Organ-sparing surgery is performed increasingly often. This involves not only breast conservation but also rectal sphincter sparing, limb sparing, and laparoscopic removal of organs. Often, organ reconstruction is carried out at the same time as the primary surgery. These new approaches require extra training that is found at most major medical centers.

Radiation

Radiotherapy plays a major role in curative therapy and palliation. A good example is the initial treatment of spinal cord compression. This was formerly considered a surgical emergency. However, with the arrival of magnetic resonance imaging (MRI) and CT scanning, diagnoses can be made before paraplegia develops. Radiation can prevent the progression of neurologic symptoms. Specialized treatments with hyperthermia and intraoperative radiotherapy are still experimental but are being used increasingly. Other major roles for radiation involve treatment of prostate cancer and the palliation of bone metastases.

Chemotherapy and Hormone Therapy

Many cancers are either systemic or become metastatic during their clinical course. Many drugs have been developed to treat these cancers. Adjuvant chemotherapy or hormone therapies are effective for a variety of cancers. Significant improvements in survival rates occur in patients with breast and colon cancers with these treatments. Chemotherapy alone has produced cures in patients with Hodgkin's disease and large cell lymphoma. It can significantly prolong survival or induce remissions in patients with leukemia, myeloma, ovarian cancer, small cell lung cancer, and head and neck cancers. Pancreatic cancer, hepatoma, and renal or adrenal cancers are rarely treated successfully with chemotherapy.

The anticipated toxicity of chemotherapeutic agents has deterred the use of chemotherapy in patients over 65. These patients are not entered in trials proportionately and are less likely to be referred to cancer centers. The reasons for denying them this form of therapy are not clearly understood. In part, the reasons may be attributed to the myth that the elderly are more sensitive to the toxic effects of chemotherapy and are less likely to respond to its action. Begg and Carbone analyzed many trials in a cooperative group for response, survival, and organ toxicity.[9] Responses and survivals were no different in elderly patients who were entered in trials for metastatic disease. Except for hematologic toxicity, no major differences were seen in the population under 70 compared to those over 70. Increased hematologic toxicity was associated with specific drugs, especially methotrexate. This outcome might be expected if one recalls that methotrexate is excreted by the kidney. Renal function is known to decrease with age. Prolonged levels of methotrexate increase hematologic toxicity. This study does not suggest that elderly patients should receive chemotherapy for their disease but that physicians should understand that the elderly comprise a heterogeneous population. Those with good performance status and normal physiologic function should receive appropriate treatment.

LEUKOPENIA AND ANEMIA

Chemotherapy affects normal marrow hematopoietic cells as well as cancer cells. There is evidence that the effects of many drugs are the same in older and younger individuals. However, hematologic toxicity has been more prevalent in the elderly. With the use of growth factors, marrow reserve can be maintained. Several studies have shown that hospitalizations are decreased if these growth factors are used. Anemia is another complication of treatment, particularly treatment with cisplatin compounds. Red cell transfusions can be used. Transfusions usually are reserved for individuals in whom the hematocrit levels are less than 30 and are required for those with hematocrits under 25 or those with symptoms. The use of erythropoietin may decrease the need for transfusions.

SPECIFIC TUMORS

Breast Cancer

Breast cancer incidence increases with age. Most women who are diagnosed with breast cancer are over the age of 65. Principles of management of breast cancer are the same as those used with younger patients. Breast cancer in the elderly is diagnosed at more advanced stages, perhaps because of more limited use of mammography in older women.

The diagnosis of breast cancer must be suspected if a palpable mass in the breast is found by either the patient or the physician. Mammography can detect a mass or abnormal clusters of calcifications that need to undergo biopsy. Increasingly, fine needle aspiration biopsy or directed core biopsy can be used to establish a diagnosis of cancer. The patient and the primary physician can seek expert opinion about the appropriate surgery.

Surgery is the primary therapy for breast cancer limited to the breast or regional lymph nodes. Breast-conserving surgery should be offered to the older patient as well the younger woman. Preservation of self-image is as important to older women as it is to younger ones. Women who elect to have a mastectomy may have a reconstructive procedure later. The surgery involves wide excision of the mass and axillary dissection of lymph nodes. Radiotherapy to the breast decreases local recurrences. This procedure has the same outcome as the more traditional modified radical mastectomy.

In the patient who is frail and elderly, simple excision and a regimen of tamoxifen have been used. When the diagnosis is established without excision of the tumor, tamoxifen is used as a systemic treatment. In about 60% of these patients some shrinkage of the tumor will occur. However, recurrences or failure of shrinkage will occur in more than 50% of these patients, and they will then need further surgery.

Adjuvant therapy with tamoxifen, an antiestrogen hormonal therapy, prolongs survival in women over 50. The treatment is more beneficial in tumors that have been documented to have a positive estrogen receptor. Combination chemotherapy should be used in patients who have a more unfavorable prognosis such as multiple positive nodes or large primary tumors. In more recent studies, preoperative chemotherapy has been given to shrink the primary tumor, which increases the chances of performing breast-conserving surgery. Radiotherapy is given with breast-conserving surgery. There is a definite age bias against offering chemotherapy to older women. As mentioned earlier, these patients tolerate chemotherapy as well as the younger patients.

Findings by Greenfield and colleagues clearly add to the growing literature documenting that 70-year-old women and older without co-morbid problems are being treated inappropriately for early-stage disease compared to women between 50 and 69 years of age.[11] They found no differences in stage at presentation in the two populations, but the lymph nodes in the older patients were less likely to have been examined. Their data suggest that women between the ages of 80 and 90 have only a 40% chance of receiving the appropriate treatment for early-stage disease at most hospitals.

A word about the diagnosis of *carcinoma in situ* is in order. These are precancerous lesions characterized as intraductal or lobular. These tumors do not present as a mass but are more likely to be detected by mammography. When such tumors are multifocal, breast-conserving surgery is not recommended. Sometimes areas of infiltration are seen microscopically, and the prognosis is slightly worse. Lymph node involvement is rarely present. The lesions characterized as lobular carcinoma are treated primarily by wide excision. The risk of subsequent cancer is just as likely to appear in the contralateral breast. Local excision and observation are the treatments of choice. Ductal carcinoma in situ, on the other hand, arises in the smaller ducts. Unless it is multifocal or shows evidence of comedo-type, local excision and radiation without axillary dissection are recommended.

Patients with more advanced regional disease (large tumors, palpable lymph nodes, skin ulceration and involvement) require coordinated and aggressive local and regional as well as systemic therapy. These patients have a high probability of recurrence. Treatment must be aggressive. However, high-dose chemotherapy and marrow replacement are not usually offered to those over 55.

The management of metastatic disease is beyond the scope of this chapter. However, older patients need not be treated less intensively than younger patients. Although hormonal therapies are often used, chemotherapy, if needed for visceral progressive disease, is not unreasonable.

Colon and Rectum

Large bowel cancer is a major neoplastic problem in the elderly. More than 150,000 new cases per year are reported. The symptoms masquerade as weakness, anemia, or blood in the stool. Increasingly, lesions are seen in the right side of the colon. The stool is still watery at that location within the bowel, so obstruction does not usually occur. Left-sided lesions more often present as a change in bowel habits or bleeding. Familial colon cancers occur in younger patients. However, patients with adenomatous polyps are more likely to develop subsequent cancers.

Work-up for the geriatric patient in whom colon cancer is suspected is the same as that in the younger patient. A high degree of suspicion should be associated with the patient who presents with anemia, rectal bleeding, or changes in bowel habits. Examinations of the stool for blood and digital examination are simple office procedures. Follow-up studies with fiberoptic endoscopy and biopsy can confirm the diagnosis. If the patient has a complete obstruction, emergency surgery may be needed. Examination of the surgical specimen for bowel wall penetration, lymph node involvement, and liver examination at surgery are essential in assessing the extent of disease.

Surgical treatment has not changed much in the past several decades. New procedures have been introduced to resect low-lying lesions of the rectum. Radiation is used to decrease local recurrences in the rectal area, but there is no evidence that radiation improves survival. Radiation plays a minor role in the management of lesions above the peritoneal reflection.

Adjuvant chemotherapy with fluorouracil and levamisole has been shown to improve survival. More recent studies with other fluorouracil combinations are being tested and may prove to be better. Management of liver metastases is still a challenge. Except in those few patients who have hepatic metastases that are "cured" by resection, systemic management of these patients is mainly palliative.

Patients with extensive colorectal cancer may have bowel obstruction, hepatic failure, or painful pelvic metastases that will challenge the primary physician. Adequate pain control, use of bile duct stents, and surgical or medical relief of bowel obstructions are just some of the challenges whose successful, albeit temporary, management will bring relief to the patient.

Lung Cancer

The rise in lung cancer in both women and men has occurred in the past five or six decades. In the 1930s lung cancer was an uncommon cause of death. Because of the increased use of tobacco since World War II, lung neoplasms have become the most common cause of cancer deaths in both sexes.

Lung cancer may present with either local symptoms (persistent cough, pneumonia, blood in the sputum) or symptoms of distant spread (bone pain, seizures, or stroke). The diagnosis is supported by an abnormal chest radiograph. The diagnosis usually is established by bronchoscopy or biopsy of a superficial mass. Rarely is the primary lesion resectable. Radiation with or without chemotherapy is used to control the primary lesion, relieve obstructive symptoms, decrease cerebral pressure, or relieve pain.

Lung cancer is classified into small cell and non–small cell types. The former type is often widespread at diagnosis. It may involve the brain, bone marrow, or central nervous system. Treatment rarely involves surgery. These tumors do respond to combination chemotherapy but are rarely curable. Non–small cell cancer is more often limited in extent and may benefit by resection of the primary. When it involves the mediastinal lymph nodes, surgical resection is not usually appropriate. Local radiotherapy may be indicated for control of local symptoms. Systemic chemotherapy is less able to control the disease compared to treatment of small cell cancer.

Prostate Cancer

Cancer of the prostate is now the leading type of cancer in males and the second leading cause of death. Despite the use of PSA tests, mortality has not improved. The greatest increase in incidence is in men over 70, in whom the benefits of early diagnosis and aggressive treatment may be counterbalanced by a risk of complications.[12] The factors that are useful for planning treatment are the pathologic stage of disease and the degree of differentiation of the tumor. Even with PSA screening and digital rectal examination, 30% to 50% of the cancers detected have already spread beyond the capsule.[13] Disease that has spread to the seminal vesicles or lymph nodes is not appropriate for radical surgery or radiation therapy. In contrast, patients with moderately or well-differentiated tumors that are limited in volume (less than 0.5 mL) are unlikely to die of their disease. The 10-year disease-free survival for patients with minimal disease is 87%, close to the natural life expectancy for normal elderly men. Patients with undifferentiated tumors have only a 34% survival.

Complications that may occur following local therapies are not insignificant and include impotence, incontinence, urethral stricture, and mortality. These problems are seen with surgery or radiation. Unfortunately, well-designed clinical trials comparing the two treatments in the same study have not been done. The appropriate therapy for early, low-grade prostate cancer is controversial. Decisions must be made in older men over 70. Factors that must be considered include the anticipated gain in life expectancy, the likelihood of toxicity, and the chances of developing metastasis. In some circumstances watchful waiting is most appropriate.[14]

Metastatic disease is likely to be present in 25% to 30% of men at presentation. Many of those treated for localized disease develop metastatic disease. The treatment is usually androgen withdrawal by means of orchiectomy or medical androgen block. Additional treatment with radiation for painful bone lesions is important. Unfortunately, unlike the situation in breast cancer, sequential hormonal therapy has shown little benefit. Chemotherapy also has a very limited ability to improve symptoms or survival.

Cervical, Ovarian, and Endometrial Cancers

These cancers of the female reproductive tract account for about 65,000 new cases annually and 23,000 deaths. About 25% of all invasive cervical cancers and 41% of all deaths due to cervical cancer occur in the over-65 age group. Black women over the age of 65 have a higher incidence and a poorer survival. Once the disease has been detected, management of these patients is unlikely to be different from that used for younger women. However, because of the advanced stage of disease at the time of presentation, the use of chemotherapy and radiation may be limited because of the patient's age. The challenge for the future is to clarify the association of this disease with the human papilloma virus and to overcome the social and age-related barriers to screening.

Most deaths resulting from cancers of the female reproductive organs are due to ovarian cancer. About half of ovarian cancers occur in the age group over 50. Ovarian cancer is more likely to be in an advanced stage at presentation in older women. About 75% of all cancers diagnosed as stages 3 and 4 are seen in women aged 65 to 74. Surgery is the primary modality of treatment, used as either a curative or debulking procedure before systemic chemotherapy. The drug cisplatin has been the mainstay of treatment, but unfortunately this drug has renal toxicity. This must be taken into account during the design of appropriate therapy. The treatment of advanced disease is rarely curative. The relationship of this disease to heredity and the definition of appropriate screening approaches are future challenges.

Patients with endometrial cancer most often present with abnormal uterine bleeding. There is a clear relationship of this disease to unopposed estrogen use. Histologically, 95% of these cancers are of the adenocarcinoma type. Survival of patients with endometrial cancer becomes poorer as the age at diagnosis increases. Black women have lower incidence rates but poorer survival. These cancers are treated by surgery with or without postoperative radiation therapy. Many patients may be obese and elderly, but surgery is not often curtailed for these reasons. The use of chemotherapy for metastatic disease is only partially successful.

Brain Tumors

Brain tumors, while uncommon, have been increasing since 1973. In the population over 65 the increase has been about 3% per year, and there is a corresponding increase in mortality. Survival rates are poorer in the elderly. Some of the increase in diagnosis of these tumors may have resulted from better imaging techniques using MRI or CT. Before these imaging approaches became common, brain tumor diagnoses may have been missed.[3]

Non-Hodgkin's Lymphoma

The incidence of this tumor type has increased by 60% since 1973. The most rapid increase has occurred in males under 65 years old, due in part to the increase in AIDS-related lymphoma. However, an increase of 56% has also been noted in the population over 65. Mortality in this age group has also increased by 45% (see Fig. 36–1). Both the incidence and mortality of patients with Hodgkin's disease, both over and under 65 years of age, have decreased by about 50%.

Skin Cancers

Skin cancers are the most common cancers in humans. Melanoma is also increasing in frequency. Physicians must examine carefully all sun-exposed areas of the skin and perform biopsies of all suspicious lesions. Major age-related problems are that these cancers continue to appear, and patients with one skin cancer are likely to have others. When such cancers occur around the eyes, ears, lips, and nose they may cause difficult cosmetic problems. Beyond excision, the Mohs' chemosurgery technique limits the amount of normal tissue that has to be resected. Superficial radiographs are also being used. Melanomas, although appearing on the skin, often progress to become a more aggressive disseminated disease. In both circumstances, early detection and prompt treatment offer the best hope for cure.

Leukemia

About 50% of all acute nonlymphocytic leukemias occur in patients over 60 years old. The prognosis is generally less favorable in the elderly, who have many treatment-related deaths. The likelihood of survival in adults over 60 is less than 20% after treatment. Less intensive and less adequate therapy, however, increase the mortality by decreasing the chance of remission.

Chronic lymphocytic leukemia is the most common form of leukemia in Western countries. Only 10% of these cancers occur in patients under the age of 50. These patients can be easily managed with a variety of medications that control the signs and symptoms of the disease. These signs include bulky adenopathy, splenomegaly, and anemia. In addition to progression of disease, these patients are subject to hemolytic anemias and an increased incidence of infections that require diligent and rapid treatment. A small percentage (5% to 10%) of these cancers progress into a more aggressive form of lymphoma, the large cell type. This disease, unlike the chronic form, moves quickly and is marked by rapid lymph node enlargement, marrow failure, and fever.

Chronic myeloid leukemia is associated in most cases with a specific chromosome abnormality, the Philadelphia (Ph) chromosome. It is a result of transposition of genetic material from chromosomes 22 and 9. The disease usually presents in a chronic form with granulocytosis but most often progresses into a blastic or acute phase. Therapeutic options have increased in the past decade with the use of interferons and allogeneic and autologous bone marrow transplantation. The longest remissions occur when the Ph chromosome cells are eliminated from the bone marrow.

CLINICAL TRIALS

Although most cancers afflict patients over 65 years of age, in a study of 30,000 patients entered in 500 therapeutic trials, only 39% of the men and 26% of the women were over 65. The discrepancies were most marked for breast cancer in women and leukemia in men.[15] The differences were least marked in prostate cancer trials. If one uses the over-75 population as a reference point and then compares the incidence of these patients in the SEER data base and those in National Cancer Institute (NCI)-supported clinical trials, the discrepancies are more pronounced. Whereas those over 75 constitute about 29% of all cancer patients, only 5% of subjects in clinical trials are in that age group. Several reasons for this difference in representation can be postulated. The elderly population has more second cancers and co-morbid conditions that prevent them from entering trials. They are also more likely to present with advanced disease and have a lower level of education and medical awareness. There are physician-related reasons as well. Physicians are not as willing to suggest appropriate therapy for the elderly as they are for younger patients. To make more trials available, the NCI has encouraged specific trials for the elderly and eliminated age restrictions on all protocols.

PALLIATIVE CARE

The importance of a team approach in the management of pain and other symptoms is vital for optimal care. Hospice and home care nurses are often well versed in the concepts of adequate symptom control, and they should be considered part of the health care team. During the last stages of life, hospice services may assist physicians in providing comfort and palliation to patients. However, relief of symptoms and palliation should be a primary objective for all patients with cancer throughout their illness. Further reference to the work of hospice and the Hospice Medicare benefit is found in Chapter 12.

Pain

Pain is often underreported by patients and undertreated by health care professionals. As many as 50% to 70% of patients have cancer pain. Tumor invasion of nerves, bones, or internal organs causes pain. In a third of patients pain is associated with cancer treatment. Peripheral neuropathies, oral ulcers, radiation fibrosis, and infections are legitimate causes of pain. The appropriate therapy requires assessing the cause and treating the underlying cause. For those conditions that cannot be effectively relieved, adequate pain management requires the use of analgesic drugs. This means the appropriate use of aspirin or NSAIDs together with opiates such as codeine and morphine. Opiates can be given orally, intravenously, rectally, or transdermally. The major concepts that must be kept in mind are the biologic disposition of the drugs, their equivalency, and listening to the patient. Adequate pain control may require high doses of opioids. Combinations of agents are also important, as is the judicious use of radiation therapy. Single large-fraction dosing may be just as effective as more protracted daily treatments.

Older patients are often reluctant to take prescribed analgesics and may take lower doses than those recommended. Polypharmacy may complicate the use of drugs with inadvertent combinations that synergize or antagonize analgesics. Older patients may be more reluctant to tolerate side effects such as constipation, sleepiness, and dryness of the mouth. Elderly, minority women with cancer are the patients who are most unlikely to receive adequate pain management.[16] Undertreatment of pain results from an inadequate understanding of the use of pain medications as well as myths about tolerance and sensitivity of the elderly to pain. Training of oncologists and primary physicians in pain management has been lacking. The management of pain and other symptoms such as fatigue, anorexia, and dyspnea are discussed in detail in Chapter 12.

References

1. Miller B, Ries L, Hankey B, Kosary C, Edwards B: Cancer Statistics Review 1973–1989. NIH Publication No. 92-2789. Bethesda, MD, U.S. Department of Health and Human Resources, National Institutes of Health, National Cancer Institute, 1992.
2. Yancik R, Ries L: Cancer in older persons. Cancer 1994;74:1995–2003.
3. Havlik R, Yancik R, Long S, Ries L, Edwards B: The NIA and the NCI SEER collaborative study on comorbidity and early diagnosis of cancer in the elderly. Cancer 1994;74:2101–2106.
4. Carbone P, Begg C, Moorman J: Cancer in the elderly: Clinical and biologic considerations. *In* Pullman B, Tso P, Schneider E (eds): Interrelationship Among Aging, Cancer and Differentiation. Dordrecht, The Netherlands, D. Reidel Publishing, 1985 pp. 313–324.
5. Dix D: The role of aging in cancer incidence: An epidemiological study. Biol Sci 1989;9:10–18.
6. Hunter D, Spiegelman D, Adami H, Beeson L, Willet W: Cohort studies of fat intake and the risk of breast cancer—a pooled analysis. N Engl J Med 1996;334:334–336.
7. Berkman B, Rohan B, Sampson S: Myths and biases related to cancer in the elderly. Cancer 1994;74:2004–2008.
8. Phillips J: Aging and cancer. Health Data Rev 1991;5:1–6.
9. Begg C, Carbone P: Clinical trials and drug toxicity in the elderly: The experience of the Eastern Cooperative Oncology Group. Cancer 1983;52:1986–1992.
10. Goodwin J, Hunt W, Samet J: Determinants of cancer therapy in elderly patients. Cancer 1993;72:594–601.
11. Greenfield S, Aronow H, Ganz P, Elashoff R: The effect of age in the management of elderly cancer patients. *In* Yancik R, Yates J (eds): Cancer in the Elderly—Approaches to Early Detection and Treatment. New York, Springer, 1989 pp. 55–70.
12. Chodak G: The role of conservative management in localized prostate cancer. Cancer 1994;74:2178–2181.
13. Bruskewitz R, Carbone P: Management dilemmas in prostate cancer. Hosp Pract 1996;31:79–86.
14. Albertson PC, Fryback DG, Storer BE, Kolon TF, Fine J: Long term survival among men with conservatively treated localized prostate cancer. JAMA 1995;274:626–631.
15. Trimble E, Carter C, Cain D, Freidlin B, Ungerleider

R, Friedman M: Representation of older patients in cancer treatment trials. Cancer 1994;74:2208–2214.

16. Cleeland C, Gonin R, Hatfield A, Edmundson J, Blum R, Stewart J, Pandya K: Pain and its treatment in outpatients with metastatic disease. N Engl J Med 1994;330:592–596.

37 Hematologic Disorders

Marc Gautier, M.D.,

Jeffrey Crawford, M.D.

Harvey Jay Cohen, M.D.

Hematologic disorders in the elderly individual often present difficult diagnostic and therapeutic dilemmas to the practitioner. One is frequently faced with laboratory abnormalities generated from screening studies or during the evaluation of other problems. The practitioner must decide whether these results represent a true disease state and how aggressively they should be pursued. On the other hand, many of the symptoms of hematologic disorders are relatively nonspecific and may be quite vague. Thus, the tendency to ascribe such changes to "getting older" must be avoided lest correctable disease states be missed.

Vigorous diagnostic efforts in the elderly patient must be tempered by the functional status of the patient, the benefit-risk ratio of the diagnostic intervention, and the potential of the outcome to influence management of the patient in a meaningful way. Co-morbid diseases, not age alone, may limit the value of an aggressive diagnostic work-up. Evaluation for reversible causes of anemia may be warranted in almost all elderly patients to try to prevent the consequences of falls, confusion, or ischemic events. However, an exhaustive search for occult gastrointestinal bleeding in the bedridden, severely demented elderly patient may be inhumane.

CHANGES IN NORMAL HEMATOPOIESIS WITH AGE

Red blood cells, granulocytes, monocytes, platelets, lymphocytes, and plasma cells are produced in the bone marrow from a common stem cell. Estimations of the normal senescence of the bone marrow are complicated by its diversity and are at this point quite imperfect. Although they show a great deal of individual variation, anatomic studies of bone marrow suggest that, overall, bone marrow cellularity decreases by approximately one third during adult life, and bone marrow scans using iron labeling of erythroid elements also indicate a decline in marrow activity with advancing age.[1]

Studies of murine bone marrow suggest that the number of stem cells is similar in young and old mice, but the number of committed stem cells at a more advanced stage of differentiation may be higher.[2] These cells have an enhanced proliferative capacity, which may be the result of a compensatory mechanism to ensure production of a normal number of peripheral blood cells. These observations are also consistent with the inverse correlation between bone marrow cellularity and myeloid progenitor cell numbers in humans.[3] The clinical corollary of these laboratory observations is that elderly patients may not respond to infection with the same degree of leukocytosis or to bleeding with the same degree of reticulocytosis as younger patients. Whether these blunted responses in humans are secondary to aging alone or to co-morbid diseases has not been rigorously studied.

A number of studies have suggested that the mean hemoglobin value is 1 g% lower in elderly females and 2 g% lower in elderly males, with a much wider standard deviation.[4] However, most of these studies are flawed by cross-sectional design and by lack of a clear distinction between healthy and unhealthy individuals. One longitudinal study does suggest that a modest decline in hemoglobin occurs with advancing age; in both men and women followed from age 70 to 81 this decline could not be explained by factors other than age.[5] The mechanism of this decline is not clear, although some investigators have implicated erythropoietin, the major hormone of red blood cell production. Direct investigations of the endogenous erythropoietin response to blood loss have not revealed any age-dependent changes in this system.[6] Other changes in the red cells are age related and may include slight increases in red cell size and membrane viscosity, a shortened red blood cell life span, and slight decrements in enzyme content and metabolic activity. However, from a clinical standpoint, whether or not slight defects in production or destruction rates exist, if a significant decline in hemoglobin below the normal adult range occurs in an elderly individual, one must assume that a pathologic process is present until proved otherwise.

Longitudinal studies suggest that no significant alteration in leukocyte numbers occurs with aging.[7] The leukocytes present in elderly individuals may, however, be less readily mobilized by a stressful challenge, such as bacterial pyrogen and steroid hormone. This is of considerable clinical relevance because infection in some older people may not be recognized if the physician relies on the white blood cell count. Studies of granulocyte function in healthy older donors have demonstrated mildly abnormal functional activity, most notably in the ability to amplify the respiratory burst. While this blunted response is demonstrable in the laboratory, it has not been clinically relevant.[8] Further, defects in migration, such as impaired in vivo delivery of neutrophils into skin abrasions, have been identified.[9] These defects may be associated with an age-related decrease in chemotactic peptide receptor expression and an altered state and function of actin in the membranes of granulocytes in the elderly.[10]

Peripheral blood lymphocyte numbers appear to be maintained throughout life, although cross-sectional studies have suggested that T-cell numbers may decrease, though the ratio of helper to suppressor cells may increase. Functional impairment has been documented by the fact that lymphocytes from elderly individuals fail to respond appropriately to mitogenic stimuli. For example, in vitro phytohemagglutinin-stimulated cultures reveal a decrease in T-cell response and an exaggerated B-cell response, which mimic the immune dysregulation characteristic of aging.[11] Platelet counts appear to be maintained in a normal range throughout the age span.

Another area of confusion has been the erythrocyte sedimentation rate (ESR) in the aged. While previous studies have suggested that an increase in the ESR above the normal range occurs in 20% to 40% of the elderly, the cause of this increase may be more related to the presence of co-morbid disease than to advancing age. In an elderly population with a low prevalence of anemia and hypoalbuminemia, age per se had no influence on the ESR.[12] In a recent study of 1-year mortality in elderly people, an ESR of greater than 50 was associated with both a significant diagnosis in nearly all patients and a minimum increase in 1-year mortality of three- to fourfold.[13] Thus, an elevated ESR should not be assumed to be part of the natural aging process.

CLINICAL PROBLEMS OF THE HEMATOPOIETIC SYSTEM

Anemia

Anemia is the most frequently encountered hematologic problem in the elderly. It must be remembered that anemia is not a disease but simply a sign of an underlying problem of either a primary or a secondary nature.[14] The definition of the "limits of normal" for the elderly population with respect to hemoglobin and hematocrit has been controversial. The normal adult values used routinely in hematology cite a mean of 15.5 g/100 mL percent (13.3 to 17.7) for men and 13.6 (11.7 to 15.7) for women. The World Health Organization (WHO) established the criteria for anemia as a hemoglobin level of less than 13 g/100 mL in men and 12 g/100 mL in women. In surveys of presumably well ambulatory patients, 12% to 20% of the population had hemoglobin levels below the usual limits. Such low values are even more common in surveys of nursing home populations and people over age 75, which may be at least partially explained by the increased prevalence of chronic diseases in these groups. In Lipschitz and colleagues' study of 222 presumably healthy individuals over the age of 65, more than 25% of the group were found to be in the anemic range. Specific causes of the anemia could be demonstrated in very few, even following a therapeutic trial of iron, prompting the authors to use the term "anemia of senescence."[15] The low socioeconomic status and unknown nutritional status of these patients raise other possibilities, however. Another study of 292 elderly ambulatory patients also found that 25% had hemoglobin levels in the anemic range.[16] However, in the subgroup evaluated for anemia, a cause was determined in the majority of cases. In summary, the majority of healthy elderly people maintain hemoglobin values in the normal adult range. Those who do not should undergo evaluation for possible reversible causes of anemia.

The classic signs and symptoms of pallor, weakness, and fatigue may be present in the anemic elderly patient. However, unlike the situation in younger patients, the initial manifestations may be those of specific end-organ dysfunction. Thus, behavioral changes and confusional states, ischemic chest pain, congestive heart failure, pulmonary decompensation, syncope, or falls may all be initial presenting complaints of anemia in the older patient. A relatively small improvement in hemoglobin level may produce dramatic symptomatic improvement in such patients, a fact that provides additional impetus toward appropriate evaluation of anemia in the elderly.

When anemia is diagnosed, initial information to be obtained should include the hemoglobin, hematocrit, red cell indices, white blood cell and platelet counts, peripheral blood film, and reticulocyte count. Multiple causes of anemia may exist in the same individual, so a careful description and analysis of the anemia is important. An elevated reticulocyte count represents an appropriate response to anemia by the bone marrow and should suggest a hemolytic process, blood loss, or recent recovery from a toxin or nutritional deficiency. However, failure to mount an appropriate reticulocyte response may be due to complicating diseases and does not exclude the former possibilities. By definition, a hypoproliferative anemia is accompanied by a low reticulocyte count. The anemia can be further categorized morphologically as microcytic, normocytic, or macrocytic.

MICROCYTIC ANEMIAS

Iron deficiency anemia and the anemia of chronic disease are commonly microcytic but may be normocytic in the earlier phases. Serum iron and total iron-binding capacity are not reliable tests for iron deficiency in the elderly because of their wide fluctuations in disease states and a tendency for serum iron to decrease with age in the absence of true iron deficiency. On the other hand, a low serum ferritin level is diagnostic of iron deficiency. It may be falsely raised into the normal range by liver disease or inflammation. One study suggests that a serum ferritin level of 45 pg/liter may be a better method of detecting iron deficiency in the elderly than currently used values.[17] If the serum ferritin is nondiagnostic, iron stores can be directly assessed by bone marrow aspiration.

A diagnosis of iron deficiency requires identification of a cause for this deficiency. Absorption of iron decreases in the elderly, perhaps because of an age-related increase in gastric achlorhydria. However, dietary iron deficiency is rare except in strict vegetarians. Overwhelmingly, iron deficiency in the elderly is a result of blood loss, most often from the gastrointestinal tract. Many drugs, such as aspirin and other nonsteroidal anti-inflammatory agents, can frequently produce low-grade gastrointestinal blood loss. Peptic ulcer disease, colon carcinoma, diverticulitis, and vascular abnormalities must be considered. Past history should be assessed because many patients may have had a prior partial gastrectomy, resulting in abnormal iron absorption secondary to achlorhydria.

Treatment of the iron deficiency per se can generally be accomplished with ferrous sulfate, 300 mg tid for 6 months. However, increased gastric sensitivity in elderly individuals may produce many complaints, leading to failures in compliance. One 300-mg tablet per day, if taken compulsively, can result in adequate correction of anemia.[18] This dosage may require a longer period of therapy to replete iron stores. Use of a pediatric liquid suspension of ferrous sulfate is an alternative approach.

Some symptoms of iron deficiency such as fatigue may result from iron depletion at the tissue level in addition to the changes brought about by anemia per se. In such patients one may see a symptomatic improvement before the hemoglobin rises 10 days to 2 weeks following initiation of therapy. The reticulocyte response or hemoglobin level can be followed to ensure adequacy of response. If a complete response is not obtained, compliance should be evaluated and other causes of anemia reconsidered.

The anemia of chronic disease, also known as simple chronic anemia or secondary anemia, can be difficult to distinguish from iron deficiency anemia.[19] When mild, it may be normocytic, but often it may be microcytic and somewhat hypochromic. This anemia is due in part to a block in the release of iron from the reticuloendothelial system, creating an abnormality in iron utilization that simulates an iron-deficient state in the developing red blood cell precursors. This failure of iron reutilization may be due to direct effects on the monocyte-macrophage by interleukin-1 and other lymphokines released as part of an inflammatory response. The anemia of chronic disease is quite common in the elderly population because of the high incidence of chronic inflammatory diseases in this age group. Serum iron and total iron capacity do not reliably distinguish the anemia of chronic disease from iron deficiency. A normal serum ferritin level makes iron deficiency less likely. However, an unequivocal diagnosis can only be established by bone marrow examination to document iron stores and to exclude other causes of hypoproliferative anemia. This anemia may be responsible for some of the diagnoses of "anemia of senescence" in elderly individuals. Once the diagnosis has been made, correction of underlying problems such as chronic inflammatory states, infections, neoplastic disorders, and so on can result in improvement of the anemia. Generally, this form of anemia is mild and well tolerated and requires no specific therapy.

Another microcytic anemia that may present initially in older age is thalassemia minor. This group of disorders, characterized by genetically determined imbalances in globin chain synthesis resulting in decreased hemoglobin production, is compatible with long life and very mild symptoms in the heterozygous state. This type of anemia may escape detection until the patient develops another illness or disease in later life that leads to exacerbation of the anemia or to screening blood studies. The blood film in such instances is quite similar to that seen with iron deficiency anemia, although it sometimes shows basophilic stippling of red cells. Unlike iron deficiency, hemoglobinopathies may show severe microcytosis when the anemia is mild and are often accompanied by reticulocytosis. The diagnosis can be confirmed by studying family members. Distinguishing this disorder from iron deficiency anemia is of some importance because iron overload can result from inappropriate iron treatment and is to be avoided.

The fourth anemia that may be microcytic is sideroblastic anemia, or refractory anemia. These anemias are seen with increasing frequency in elderly individuals but are uncommon in younger people. They are characterized by the presence of increased serum iron and increased saturation of iron-binding capacity, or an elevated serum ferritin level. Bone marrow aspiration and examination are necessary for diagnosis, since the characteristic finding is that of iron-laden mitochondria in the red cell precursors, or ringed sideroblasts. Sideroblastic anemia may be secondary to drugs, alcohol, or pyridoxine deficiency, but more frequently in the elderly it occurs as an acquired idiopathic form. It may be accompanied by thrombocytopenia or leukopenia. Sideroblastic anemia is often considered a preleukemic syndrome that may develop into a form of acute granulocytic or monomyelocytic leukemia in 10% of patients and in some instances into multiple myeloma. Once the diagnosis has been made, treatment is symptomatic, which often requires transfusion therapy. Accurate diagnosis allows one to avoid iron therapy, which could be further damaging to such patients.

MACROCYTIC ANEMIAS

In the elderly, macrocytic anemias resulting from megaloblastic erythropoiesis are most frequently produced by a deficiency of folic acid or vitamin B_{12}. Blood film findings include macrocytosis and macro-ovalocytes in the red cells with cell size variation and hypersegmentation of the neutrophils. Bone marrow examination should confirm the presence of megaloblastic changes with delay in nuclear maturation of red cell, white cell, and platelet precursors. While these changes can be due to an intrinsic marrow disorder such as myelodysplasia, generally such abnormalities can be distinguished by additional abnormalities in the marrow. The distinction of folate deficiency from vitamin B_{12} deficiency, however, requires a careful history, physical examination, and additional laboratory studies.

Nutritional folic acid deficiency is probably found more often than vitamin B_{12} deficiency in the elderly population. The dietary source of folic acid is predominantly green vegetables and fresh fruit. Elderly individuals may fail to meet the daily requirement of 0.50 mg of folic acid if they markedly decrease their intake of such foodstuffs. Body stores of folate are limited and may be exhausted by a deficient diet within weeks to months. Moreover, folate metabolism may be adversely affected by alcohol ingestion, and the continuing and often unsuspected problem of alcoholism in the elderly is being recognized more frequently as a contributing factor in such a problem. In addition to macrocytic anemia, thrombocytopenia and leukopenia may be seen. Clinical symptoms are nonspecific, although they may include glossitis. Serum folate levels are not helpful. Red cell folate levels are a more reliable criteria of tissue folate deficiency but are not widely available. Deficiency of vitamin C in elderly undernourished patients may further complicate the situation, since vitamin C is necessary to reduce folic acid to its metabolically active form. Folic acid deficiency is readily corrected by the administration of 1 mg of folic acid per day orally unless a malabsorptive process is present.

Vitamin B_{12} deficiency in the elderly can be caused by pernicious anemia, a failure of absorption of vitamin B_{12} due to a lack of intrinsic factor normally produced by the gastric parietal cells. This lack of intrinsic factor is secondary to chronic atrophic gastritis, an idiopathic disease that increases in frequency with age. In the absence of this type of malabsorptive defect or others to be described later, the very large body stores of vitamin B_{12} (predominantly in the liver) and the high content of vitamin B_{12} in much of the American diet make it unlikely that this deficiency is produced by lack of dietary intake. In the elderly, however, other forms of malabsorption, including previous total gastrectomy or disease of the terminal ileum (final site of absorption of vitamin B_{12}), can also produce vitamin B_{12} deficiency.

The initial approach to diagnosis involves serum B_{12} measurement (normal range, 200 to 900 pg/mL). Unfortunately, the specificity of the serum B_{12} measurement is low, due in part to the intracellular location of B_{12} and the complex protein carrier system. Additional serum markers of true tissue vitamin B_{12} deficiency have evolved during the past several years. Methylmalonic acid (MMA) and homocysteine (Hcys) have been well correlated with B_{12} deficiency even when serum B_{12} levels have been normal. Both of these molecules are related to substrates for the enzymatic reactions involving B_{12} and build up in individuals with B_{12} deficiency. They appear to be most helpful when the B_{12} level is in the low to low-normal range. Further diagnostic evaluation includes a Schilling's test. The patient is given radiolabeled vitamin B_{12}, and the 24-hour urinary excretion of this compound is determined. Normal individuals excrete at least 8% of the administered dose, whereas patients with pernicious anemia excrete less than 2% to 3% in the absence of intrinsic factor, and normal amounts when intrinsic factor is supplied. Failure of B_{12} absorption at the ileal site can also be determined by this test.

The elderly appear to be particularly vulnerable to vitamin B_{12} deficiency. Using the newer metabolically sensitive assays, a 14.5% prevalence of B_{12} deficiency was detected in a group of elderly outpatients.[20] The serum level of B_{12} was more than 200 pg/mL in about half of the patients with B_{12} deficiency, which again argues for paying close attention to patients with B_{12} levels in the low-normal range. The clinical presentation of B_{12} deficiency can be subtle, especially in patients with other co-morbid conditions.

Vitamin B_{12} deficiency can produce a variety of neurologic changes including paresthesias, dysesthesias, difficulty in proprioception, and personality changes. A low serum level of B_{12} may exist with minimum signs or symptoms of anemia or macrocytosis in the presence of neuropsychiatric symptoms and vice versa.[21] A trial of B_{12} in this situation, paying careful attention to changes in hematologic and neuropsychiatric abnormalities, may be warranted. Screening older populations for B_{12} deficiency is currently being advocated in the hope of reversing some early neuropsychiatric changes before they become permanent.[22]

The treatment of vitamin B_{12} deficiency can generally be accomplished with the use of intramuscular injections of vitamin B_{12}. Initially, weekly doses of 1000 μg are given, and mainte-nance therapy of 1000 μg/month is quite adequate. A brisk reticulocyte response can generally be seen within 5 to 7 days following initial therapy. The same time course of response is generally seen in treatment of folic acid deficiency with oral folic acid.

One note of caution concerning nutritional deficiency in the elderly individual is especially pertinent. It is not uncommon to see combined nutritional deficiencies involving both vitamin B_{12} and folic acid or a megaloblastic process complicated by iron deficiency. Thus, a patient with documented B_{12} deficiency may appear to respond initially to therapy, but the therapy then fails to correct the situation. In some instances, there may have been limited iron present in the bone marrow prior to therapy; this iron is used during the initial burst of red cell production, resulting in a subsequent state of iron lack. Such patients require iron replacement to complete the hematologic response. In addition, once this phenomenon is revealed, the previously described approach to determining the cause of the iron deficiency should be followed.

NORMOCHROMIC NORMOCYTIC ANEMIAS

Blood loss must always be suspected first in patients with normochromic normocytic anemia. The physician cannot depend on the elderly patient to report melena. There is no substitute for several negative tests for occult blood in the stool. Beyond this, the blood film and reticulocyte count are essential in subclassifying these anemias because most anemias may present with normal indices. Early iron deficiency anemia or anemia of chronic disease may be normocytic. Vitamin B_{12} and folate deficiencies may not be associated with macrocytosis if iron deficiency coexists. A dimorphic population of cells is helpful in diagnosing the latter, as is sideroblastic anemia.

A blood film with microspherocytes should suggest the presence of autoimmune hemolytic anemia. Warm antibody autoimmune hemolytic anemia, both idiopathic and drug-induced, increases in frequency in the older population. Moreover, the occurrence of autoimmune hemolytic anemia in patients with chronic lymphocytic leukemia (to be described later) contributes to the high incidence of this disorder in the elderly population. In elderly patients with other chronic illnesses, the absence of a marked reticulocytosis should not blunt further inquiry when hemolysis is suspected, and a Coombs' test should be performed. The test should be performed to detect both IgG and C3 on the surface, since in some instances of cold agglutinin hemolysis the only remaining evidence of hemolysis is the presence of C3 on the red blood cells. Chronic cold agglutinin disease, characterized by both agglutination and hemolysis due to cold-reacting IgM antibodies, is predominantly a disease of the elderly. Since red cell destruction is often complete in cold agglutinin hemolysis, the blood film may be normal. However, signs of hemolysis often exist, including increased reticulocyte count, bilirubin, and urinary hemoglobin-hemosiderin levels.

The possibility of a mild hereditary anemia that has escaped attention until old age must always be considered. Hereditary spherocytosis may mimic autoimmune hemolytic anemia on a blood film but can be differentiated by a negative Coombs' test result, a positive family history, and the presence of splenomegaly. Glucose-6-phosphate dehydrogenase (G6PD) deficiency is generally associated with acute self-limited hemolysis in the presence of an oxidant stress, generally drug-related. The blood film may be normal, but the signs of intravascular hemolysis noted earlier for cold agglutinin disease are generally present.

A normocytic hypoproliferative anemia with a normal blood film may be the initial clue to a coexisting renal or endocrine disease. Renal insufficiency is common in the elderly and may be associated with decreased erythropoietin. Endocrine disease, particularly hyperthyroidism and hypothyroidism and other endocrine insufficiency states, are commonly associated with anemia.

PANCYTOPENIA

When anemia is accompanied by leukopenia and thrombocytopenia, other diagnostic considerations should be included. An elevated reticulocyte count in this situation suggests peripheral destruction of cells, as might occur with splenomegaly of any cause. Less commonly, immune pancytopenia may occur. More often, the reticulocyte count is low, and the pancytopenia is secondary to a lack of production. While this may be due to a nutritional deficiency of vitamin B_{12}, folate, or even iron, intrinsic bone marrow failure must be considered. Aplastic anemia is uncommon but increases in frequency with age.[23] The presence of immature red cell or white cell precursors on the blood film should suggest the possibility of a myeloproliferative or myelodysplastic process, or cancer or other infiltrative disease. Bone marrow aspirate and biopsy are essential in this situation. The myeloproliferative and myelodysplastic syndromes are discussed in a subsequent section.

In summary, anemia is common in the elderly, and the differential diagnosis is large. By using basic laboratory data, history, and physical examination, the work-up can be directed simply, inexpensively, and generally noninvasively. Evaluation is often rewarded by finding a reversible cause. In other patients, transfusions may be necessary on an acute or chronic basis. In elderly patients with symptomatic anemia, appropriate studies should be performed and transfusions initiated to avoid a major ischemic event or fall. Each unit of packed red cells should be transfused over 3 to 4 hours to avoid precipitation of angina or congestive heart failure. If these symptoms already exist, careful transfusion should reverse them.

Myeloproliferative Disorders

POLYCYTHEMIA

The elderly patient with primary or secondary polycythemia generally presents with vague symptoms such as dizziness, headaches, or thrombo-occlusive events. Elevated hemoglobin and hematocrit levels are noted. Absolute erythrocytosis may be confirmed by measurement of the red cell mass, and plasma volume can be confirmed by radioisotopic techniques, but these formal studies are not generally necessary. Attempts to identify a "spurious" polycythemia can be made by looking at the history to find causes of a decreased plasma volume, such as hypertension, use of diuretics, or cigarette smoking. Secondary polycythemia is most frequently associated with cigarette smoking combined with an elevated carbon monoxide level, or chronic pulmonary disease associated with a decreased arterial oxygen saturation. Less commonly, secondary polycythemia may be associated with renal tumors, cysts, or hydronephrosis, hepatomas, or ovarian or cerebellar tumors.

Primary polycythemia, or polycythemia vera, is a proliferative disorder involving the red cells, granulocytes, and platelets. Unlike secondary polycythemia, splenomegaly, leukocytosis, and thrombocytosis are frequently present in patients with primary polycythemia. Symptoms may include those created by the elevated blood viscosity as well as the paradoxical association of thromboembolic and bleeding events produced by the increased number of platelets that are functionally defective. The clinical course of polycythemia vera follows typical stages. There is an initial asymptomatic phase followed by a more marked polycythemic period of active disease. Eventually, an inactive phase followed by a post-polycythemic phase similar to that seen in myeloid metaplasia may develop.

Treatment of secondary polycythemia depends on accurate diagnosis and treatment of the primary illness. When the primary problem, such as chronic pulmonary disease, is not correctable, consideration should be given to lowering the hematocrit because hematocrits above 60% are associated with reduced cerebral blood flow, to which the elderly patient may be most susceptible. Thus, cautious, staged phlebotomy with the goal of maintaining the hematocrit below 50% is indicated.[24]

The treatment of polycythemia vera has undergone shifts in emphasis during the past few years. Common therapies have included P32, chlorambucil, or phlebotomy alone. However, the first two therapies increase the rate of leukemic transformation, and the last is associated with a high incidence of thrombotic events, presumably resulting from uncontrolled thrombocytosis. Aspirin has not been effective in reducing this risk and in fact may increase the risk of hemorrhage. Hydroxyurea has the advantage of being nonleukemogenic and may reduce the platelet count as well as the red cell mass. Alpha-interferon may also be a useful antiproliferative agent for polycythemia vera.[25] All elective surgical procedures should be delayed in a patient newly diagnosed with polycythemia vera until the hematocrit has been brought under control for several months. As noted, many patients with polycythemia vera ultimately exhibit a "burned out" or "spent" phase in which myelofibrosis supervenes and hepatosplenomegaly and marked cytopenias become the major problems. It is ironic that such patients who earlier required phlebotomy may now require transfusion therapy. At this stage of the disease cytotoxic therapy does not appear to be very useful.

AGNOGENIC MYELOID METAPLASIA WITH MYELOFIBROSIS

Patients with myeloid metaplasia with myelofibrosis frequently present with symptoms of anemia, hepatosplenomegaly, and lymph node enlargement. Leukocytosis with variable platelet counts is frequently present. The peripheral blood film characteristically has teardrop-shaped erythrocytes and immature granulocyte precursors, though less than in acute leukemia. The bone marrow may be hypercellular with marked fibrosis. This disorder may overlap with other myeloproliferative disorders including polycythemia vera, essential thrombocytosis, chronic granulocytic leukemia, and acute myelogenous leukemia. In general, this disorder is treated symptomatically, paying attention to specific cy-

topenias. Thus, folic acid deficiency or iron deficiency, when they exist, may be corrected, and blood transfusions may be used when anemia is predominant. Chemotherapy should be used judiciously, since such patients are often in a precarious balance, and therapy has the potential to do more harm than good. Splenectomy may be useful when this organ is the source of major complications such as splenic infarction, portal hypertension, or severe cytopenia. Because this disease may be indolent for long periods of time, a cautious approach is generally warranted.

CHRONIC GRANULOCYTIC LEUKEMIA

Although often considered a disease of middle age, chronic granulocytic leukemia (CGL), like all leukemias, continues to increase in incidence with advancing age. In the early stages, patients have minimal symptoms including fatigue and occasionally symptoms related to splenomegaly. The blood film characteristically shows a leukocytosis consisting of granulocytes and myelocytes without blasts. Occasionally, thrombocytosis may be prominent, causing confusion with essential thrombocytosis. The bone marrow picture often cannot be distinguished from the appearance of a benign increase in myeloid activity except by chromosomal studies, which reveal the presence of a Philadelphia chromosome in 95% of cases. The Philadelphia chromosome involves a translocation between chromosomes 9 and 22. Using molecular techniques, the breakpoint on chromosome 9 has been identified as the abl oncogene. This breakpoint cluster region (bcr) can be identified in virtually all cases of CGL and is involved in the pathogenesis of the disease.[26]

CGL has a standard triphasic course characterized by an initial chronic phase followed by an accelerated phase and ultimately a terminal blast phase. The goal of treatment in the chronic phase and accelerated phase is control of the elevated granulocyte counts and is best achieved with intermittent alkylating agents such as melphalan or hydroxyurea. The terminal phase of CGL, or blast crisis, is heralded by a fall in peripheral granulocyte counts, rapid splenic growth, fever, or marked systemic symptoms and a conversion of the bone marrow to acute leukemia, often accompanied by further chromosomal abnormalities. The median time from CGL to blast crisis is 3 years, and there is a mean survival of 2 months after the blast crisis. Approximately 20% of patients with CGL in blast crisis respond to treatment for acute lymphoblastic leukemia with vincristine and prednisone. High-dose chemotherapy, bone marrow transplantation, and other experimental protocols are being evaluated for other patients with acute myeloblastic leukemia arising from CGL.

Alpha-interferon has recently been shown to be an effective therapy for CGL. Aside from controlling the peripheral counts in the chronic phase, interferon selectively depresses the CGL clone and may delay the progression to blast phase. Survival was better in one study for interferon-treated patients than for those treated with hydroxyurea (72 months versus 52 months).[27] Unfortunately, few elderly people can tolerate full doses of interferon because side effects occur that are similar to the flu. Bone marrow transplantation has been curative for patients under the age of 50 but is not an option for older individuals because of the high mortality associated with this intensive treatment.

ACUTE MYELOBLASTIC LEUKEMIA

Acute myeloblastic leukemia (AML) poses one of the most difficult problems in clinical decision making for elderly patients.[28] Although AML constitutes only a small proportion of neoplastic diseases in the elderly, it is often one of the more dramatic events and has a rapid clinical course and a short survival when untreated. Over half of all patients with AML are over the age of 60 years. Acute leukemia in the elderly may present with large numbers of circulating myeloblasts. However, more commonly, elderly patients present with nonspecific symptoms including fatigue, anorexia, weakness, loss of weight, and so on. On examination of the peripheral blood, cytopenia with few or no characteristic myeloblasts may be noted. In such a situation, the index of suspicion must be high because the only way to establish the diagnosis is through bone marrow aspiration or biopsy. In this circumstance, the marrow is generally hypercellular and is marked by extensive replacement by immature myeloid cells, especially myeloblasts. Such patients often have the rapid and severe course characteristic of acute leukemia.

Another presentation may be similar to that just described but the bone marrow contains a lower percentage of blast cells and a less severe cytopenia. Such patients may have indolent or smoldering leukemia. Finally, there is a group of elderly patients with AML, perhaps as high as one third, who have a preleukemic phase. Such patients may have a previous history of cytopenias, refractory anemia, sideroblastic anemia, or other so-called myelodysplastic syndromes that, although sometimes characterized by slightly increased numbers of myeloblasts or other immature myeloid cells, are not fully consistent with the diagnosis of acute leukemia. Such patients may have chromosomal abnormalities as well as other qualitative abnormalities of the myeloid cells but may continue in a fairly stable situation for a period of years before they develop a more characteristic picture of acute leukemia. Once again, only careful clinical follow-up can be used as the guideline for appropriate treatment for such patients.

Given these variabilities in presentation, treatment decisions are difficult. In general, it is suggested that most patients with indolent or smoldering leukemia or the "preleukemic" myelodysplastic syndrome who do not have life-threatening complications be carefully followed with symptomatic treatment including blood transfusions. In such situations, attempts to use cytotoxic chemotherapy in the presence of decreased total marrow reserve may be fraught with considerable difficulty. On the other hand, when the patient clearly develops overt acute leukemia or the clinical situation suggests that a prolonged or indolent course is not likely, a decision to treat with chemotherapy must be faced. The usual approach to chemotherapy for acute leukemia in younger individuals involves a combination of agents generally including cytosine arabinoside and an anthracycline (either Adriamycin or daunomycin). The goal is to achieve complete bone marrow aplasia and then allow cellular regrowth in the hope that normal myeloid elements will repopulate the marrow to the exclusion of the previous leukemic cells. With this approach and with currently available supportive and ancillary therapy, 50% of patients can expect to achieve a complete remission, which is associated with an increase in overall survival for such patients.[29]

Earlier clinical series had suggested that older patients (over 50 years) with acute leukemia had remission rates ranging from 20% to 40%. Many older patients were unable to tolerate prolonged bone marrow aplasia and succumbed to infection and other complications during the initial phases of treatment. With correct treatment and supportive care, the response rate has improved, but it remains lower than that for younger individuals. Alternative treatments include low-dose cytarabine, which results in less marrow aplasia but also a lower response rate. A comparison of this approach with more intensive chemotherapy in the elderly resulted in similar overall survival.[30] Colony-stimulating factors have been demonstrated to reduce the duration and morbidity of chemotherapy-induced neutropenia. A colony-stimulating factor as an adjunct to induction chemotherapy has been evaluated prospectively in elderly patients with AML. Although the duration of neutropenia was significantly shorter, there was no improvement in overall survival.[31] Thus, despite the tendency toward decreased marrow reserve and the more precarious homeostatic balance of elderly patients, in appropriately selected individuals intense chemotherapeutic regimens can be successful.

The patient's physiologic status rather than the chronologic age should be especially considered in this situation, and other organ systems (cardiovascular, pulmonary, and so on) should be carefully assessed before final decisions are made. This is an area in which a specialist and physicians experienced in dealing with geriatric patients can form a fruitful collaboration. For example, an awareness of the potential alterations in renal function that may affect chemotherapeutic drug excretion in patients in this age group would have a major impact on the design of appropriate therapy for such patients. When the patient has major physiologic deficits that may seriously compromise the patient's ability to deliver or recover from therapy, alternative approaches involving less intense therapy may be needed. Such decisions should involve discussions with the patient and the family. Optimal care is best provided by a team of health professionals who can work to maintain the functional level of the elderly patient during treatment.

Lymphoproliferative Disorders

ACUTE LYMPHOBLASTIC LEUKEMIA

Acute lymphoblastic leukemia (ALL) is a disorder that has two peaks of incidence at the extremes of age. These may represent two considerably different disorders, although both are characterized by a proliferation of blastic cells of similar morphology, generally null cell, but occasionally B, T, or pre-B cell phenotypes may be present, and myeloid antigens may be coexpressed.[32] The clinical presentation of ALL in the elderly is similar to that described for acute myeloblastic leukemia. This disorder is less responsive than acute lymphocytic leukemia of childhood, and advancing age is a poor prognostic factor; this may be related to an age-related increase in poor prognostic factors with reference to the biology of the disease rather than to age per se.[33] This disorder can be treated with a combination of vincristine and prednisone without necessarily producing complete bone marrow aplasia. It is, thus, important to establish whether acute leukemia in an elderly patient is lymphoblastic or myeloblastic using currently available enzymatic, histochemical, morphologic, and immunologic techniques.

CHRONIC LYMPHOCYTIC LEUKEMIA

The most prevalent lymphoid neoplasias in the elderly are those of B lymphocyte origin. Most characteristic among these is chronic lymphocytic leukemia (CLL), which occurs generally in patients over the age of 60.[34] The high prevalence of CLL is due to the increasing population over 60 in the United States and the long median survival associated with this disease. CLL is characterized by the accumulation of large numbers of mature-appearing small B lymphocytes in the bone marrow, peripheral blood, and other lymphoid organs. These are abnormal cells both qualitatively and quantitatively, and they result in hypogammaglobulinemia, cytopenias, and frequent association with Coombs' positive hemolytic anemia. Patients with stage I and II disease, which predominantly involves cellular accumulation in the peripheral blood, lymph nodes, and bone marrow without cytopenias, have a good prognosis. They can expect many years of good quality survival, often without specific therapy. On the other hand, patients with advanced disease, generally with bone marrow involvement sufficient to produce cytopenias, have a median survival of less than 3 years and need treatment. This generally involves an alkylating agent such as chlorambucil, frequently given in combination with prednisone. This approach has been well tolerated, and complete responses or partial control of disease can often be obtained. In some instances, radiation therapy, splenectomy, and leukapheresis can be helpful adjuncts for specific symptomatic problems. Newer therapies including fludarabine, pentostatin, and 2-chloro-deoxyadenosine have shown promising activity in CLL for patients who are resistant to chlorambucil as well as for initial therapy.[35] For many patients with CLL, recurrent infections are a major source of morbidity and mortality. Prompt attention to infections with liberal use of antibiotics is the mainstay of supportive treatment. Replacement therapy with intravenous immunoglobulin (IVIG) can improve hypogammaglobulinemia and decrease the incidence of serious infections.[36]

Other variants of CLL including prolymphocytic leukemia, hairy cell leukemia, and lymphosarcoma cell leukemia are less common but also occur predominantly in the elderly population. These disorders are characterized by proliferation of lymphoid cells presumed to be of different B-cell subtypes or differentiation stages. Cells have characteristic morphologic and surface immunoglobulin fluorescence features that can aid in diagnosis. Lymphosarcoma cell leukemia is derived most often from a previously existing tissue-phase lymphoma, whereas hairy cell leukemia is often dominated by marked splenomegaly and peripheral cytopenia. Currently, the hematologist has several effective treatments for hairy cell leukemia including splenectomy, which usually produces a transient improvement. Alpha-interferon works in 80% of cases, but relapses are common once therapy is halted. Most recently, deoxycoformycin (DCF) and chlorodeoxyadenosine (2-CDA) have shown remarkable activity, and some patients may be cured after a single cycle of 2-CDA.[37]

LYMPHOMA

The non-Hodgkin's lymphomas are predominantly B-cell tumors of the elderly. Nodular or follicular lymphomas occur frequently and may follow a relatively indolent course. In many such elderly patients initial therapy can be withheld until the pace of the disease has been determined. When treatment is warranted, a single alkylating agent is suggested. Diffuse large cell lymphomas, on the other hand, are more aggressive and require earlier therapy. Paradoxically, the chance for cure is higher in these "intermediate-grade" lymphomas than in the "low-grade" lymphomas. In the earlier stages a combination of chemotherapy and radiation therapy may be curative in 80% of patients regardless of age.[38] In more advanced stages, the 5-year survival of patients over 60 is lower (28% to 34%) than for patients under 60 (47% to 62%), which may be a function of a lower complete response rate and a less durable response as well as a higher mortality due to co-morbid diseases.[39] An international prognostic index has been formulated for patients with intermediate-grade lymphoma that includes age, stage, serum LDH level, involvement of extra nodal sites, and patient performance status.[40] This index can be used in both intermediate-grade and low-grade lymphomas. Intensive chemotherapy has been thought to be superior to standard multiagent treatment such as CHOP (cyclophosphamide, doxorubicin, vincristine, prednisone), but a recent randomized trial demonstrated that standard-dose CHOP was as effective as more toxic regimens.[41] A great deal of experience using CHOP in elderly patients has been gained, and it should be the standard for intermediate-grade lymphoma in patients who can tolerate chemotherapy.

Hodgkin's disease, which is usually considered characteristic of the young population, has a bimodal incidence with a second peak occurring in the elderly population. In general, the response rate and survival of patients in the older group with Hodgkin's disease are worse than response and survival in the younger population. This may be partially explained by differences in stage at presentation of Hodgkin's disease in the elderly. In addition, older patients are also less likely to undergo the same staging procedures, such as lymphangiogram and laparotomy, as younger patients. Therefore, they may be understaged, and treatment may be less than optimal. Treatment of early stage, localized disease consists of radiation therapy, and disseminated disease is treated with multiagent chemotherapy. Even when one corrects for stage, B symptoms (e.g., fever, sweats, or weight loss), and histologic type, the 5-year survival rate for patients over 50 is less than 40% compared to more than 70% for patients aged 15 to 34.[42]

MONOCLONAL GAMMOPATHIES

These disorders also show a striking relationship of age to incidence and range from benign to malignant clonal proliferations of plasma cells that produce protein of a single immunoglobulin class, which can be detected by serum or urine protein electrophoresis and immunoelectrophoresis. The most common of these diseases is an age-related monoclonal gammopathy that occurs with a frequency of 1% in people over age 50 and 10% over the age of 80.[43] Although this disease is initially asymptomatic, in more than a third of patients it evolves into a malignant disorder such as multiple myeloma, amyloidosis, or lymphoma. The evolution may occur within a year of diagnosis or not for 15 to 20 years. Unfortunately, there are no reliable criteria to determine prospectively when the disease will progress and when the patient will remain asymptomatic for prolonged periods of time.

Multiple myeloma is characterized by marked proliferation of plasma cells in the bone marrow and occasionally in extramedullary organs, resulting in bone destruction and bone pain, anemia and other cytopenias, hypercalcemia, renal failure, and an increased tendency toward infection.[44] In such patients one must be careful not to dismiss the weakness and aches and pains as simply symptoms of "old age." Serum and urine protein electrophoresis demonstrate the monoclonal protein abnormality in approximately 99% of such patients. Bone marrow aspiration and demonstration of plasma cell proliferation are then confirmatory. The abnormal protein is most frequently IgG or IgA. Approximately 20% of patients with multiple myeloma produce only free light chains (Bence-Jones proteins). Thus, even in the absence of an obvious serum protein abnormality, urine light chains should be sought first by a sulfosalicylic acid precipitation test of the urine (light chain immunoglobulins are not detected on dipstick) and then by urine protein electrophoresis. Although most of the symptoms of this disease are produced by the malignant plasma cell proliferation, the serum proteins themselves may produce abnormalities in the form of the hyperviscosity syndrome.[45] The latter can be treated symptomatically by plasmapheresis, but ultimately control of the cellular proliferation must be achieved with specific chemotherapy. Elderly patients with multiple myeloma can be treated with combination chemotherapy, which results in responses and survival equivalent to those seen in younger patients with little increase in toxicity.[46] Supportive care can maintain good control of otherwise debilitating symptoms and allows elderly patients to retain a high level of function. Recent advances in supportive care for patients with multiple myeloma include treatment with pamidronate, which prevents bone pain, fractures, and hypercalcemia.[47] Erythropoietin therapy can improve anemia for many patients who otherwise would be dependent on transfusions.

Waldenström's macroglobulinemia is a clinical syndrome more related to the lymphomas with organomegaly and lymphoid enlargement accompanied by a monoclonal IgM serum protein abnormality. Because of the higher intrinsic viscosity of IgM, hyperviscosity may be particularly problematic, especially in the elderly patients with a tenuously balanced microcirculatory system. Since plasma volume expansion occurs in this situation, elderly patients with reduced cardiovascular reserve may be more prone to congestive heart failure and may require earlier symptomatic therapy. For ultimate control of the proliferative process, therapy with alkylating agents has been used most frequently and appears to be well tolerated in the elderly patient.

Disorders of Hemostasis

PURPURA

The most frequent clinical disorder of hemostasis in the elderly is senile purpura, which occurs in 10% to 20% of geriatric patients. The purpura occurs as purple-red lesions, generally on the extensor surfaces of the forearms and hands. The presumed mechanism is related to the age-related loss of subcutaneous fat and weakening of the supporting structure of small blood vessels, often with no history of trauma. Qualitative platelet dysfunction may also exist in the elderly patient owing to drug usage and other causes and must be considered if the distribution of purpura

is not consistent with a diagnosis of senile purpura.[48]

Steroid purpura may have the same appearance as senile purpura. Thus, the clinician must always be aware of the other manifestations of Cushing's syndrome. Purpura secondary to thrombocytopenia or vasculitis can often be suspected by the coexistence of petechiae or dot-like hemorrhages. The purpura of vasculitis is often palpable and is accompanied by other clinical or laboratory features.

THROMBOCYTOPENIA

Thrombocytopenia may be one of the presenting signs of a myeloproliferative, myelodysplastic, or lymphoproliferative disorder, but it may also exist independently. Immune thrombocytopenia occurs in the elderly but does not occur as an acute event as frequently as it does in younger people.[48] Its onset appears to be somewhat more insidious and its course more chronic when it does occur. Depending on the older patient's physiologic status, however, the approach would be similar to that used in younger individuals, and splenectomy, steroid treatment, IVIG, or cytotoxic therapy should be considered.[49] Because of the hazards of prolonged steroid therapy in the elderly, splenectomy should be considered in patients in whom a complete response is not achieved within 4 to 6 weeks of prednisone therapy.

Drug-induced thrombocytopenia is of special concern in elderly patients and should always be considered, since many of the drugs known to cause thrombocytopenia are in common use in the elderly population. Moreover, these drugs are often used simultaneously and present especially difficult diagnostic situations. Thus, such drugs as barbiturates, quinidine, diuretics, digoxin, and many others are frequently being taken by elderly patients who present with thrombocytopenia. Whenever possible, such drugs should be discontinued to determine whether they played a role in the process, and they should be restarted only if they are specifically required or if alternative drugs are not available. Discontinuation of drugs is the only practical way to establish the diagnosis because assays for drug-associated antiplatelet antibodies are not yet widely available.

THROMBOCYTOSIS

Thrombocytosis is most often secondary to iron deficiency, chronic inflammatory and infectious disorders, and malignancies, all of which occur frequently in the elderly population. The level to which the platelet count rises may be indistinguishable from that seen in essential thrombocytosis or other myeloproliferative disorders. Patients with the latter disorders may have thrombotic or bleeding complications, but those with secondary thrombocytosis have normal platelet function. Evidence of iron deficiency should be sought, since treatment of this disorder can readily reverse the associated thrombocytosis.

COAGULATION DISORDERS

Clotting factors, like other elements of the hematopoietic system, do not vary to a major degree with age in the absence of associated disease states. Congenital factor deficiencies are generally detected at an early age, with the possible exceptions of a mild factor XI deficiency and von Willebrand's disease. The latter condition is associated with a decreased factor VIII level and/or abnormal platelet function, manifested by a prolonged bleeding time or impaired platelet aggregation with ristocetin in vitro. A coagulation inhibitor may be suggested by a prolonged partial thromboplastin time that does not correct after the sample is mixed with normal plasma. In addition to the usual spectrum of acquired clotting factor deficiencies, factor V or VIII deficiency can occur secondary to the presence of spontaneous antibody-like inhibitors. This occurs in the aged and in postpartum women. Inhibitors, such as the lupus anticoagulant, also occur more frequently in the elderly. The lupus anticoagulant affects phospholipid-dependent coagulation in clotting assays and is not associated with bleeding. Paradoxically, however, it is associated with a thrombotic tendency.[48]

Thrombosis is common in the geriatric population because of the high prevalence of venous stasis and insufficiency as well as limited mobility. Studies of fibrinopeptide A and protein C activation have suggested that an acquired prethrombotic state occurs with advancing age.[50] Anticoagulation, although necessary for patients with deep venous thrombosis above the calf or pulmonary embolism, is associated with increased bleeding complications in the elderly owing to their altered vascular integrity and complicating drug regimens, which may make therapeutic control difficult. The list of drug interactions is extensive, but nonsteroidal anti-inflammatory agents, antibiotics, and barbiturates are major offenders. In addition, the problem of falls as well as cerebrovascular accidents in the elderly leads to a potential for life-threatening central nervous system bleeding. However, in the elderly patient with a well-documented thrombotic event, age should not be a barrier to anticoagulation as long as it is accompanied by careful clinical and laboratory monitoring.

SUMMARY

The diagnosis and treatment of hematologic disorders in the elderly patient presents major challenges to the practitioner. Using currently available clinical and laboratory tools, most of the diagnostic challenges can be met without undue risk or expense to the patient. Furthermore, by working together with the patient and family, the therapeutic dilemmas can be resolved by individualizing the approach to the elderly patient.

References

1. Lipschitz DA, Udupa KB, Milton KY, et al: Effect of age on hematopoiesis in man. Blood 1984;63:502–509.
2. Sharp A, Zipori D, Toledo J, et al: Age related changes in hemopoietic capacity of bone marrow cells. Mech Ageing Dev 1989;48:91–99.
3. Resnitzky P, Segal M, Barak Y, et al: Granulopoiesis in aged people: Inverse correlation between bone marrow cellularity and myeloid progenitor cell numbers. Gerontology 1987;33:109–114.
4. O'Rourke MA, Cohen HJ: Anemias. *In* Richard JH (ed): Geriatric Medicine Annual 1987. Oradel, NJ, Medical Economics, 1987; pp. 237–266.
5. Nilsson-Ehle H, Jagenburg RJ, Landahl S, et al: Decline of blood haemoglobin in the aged: A longitudinal study of an urban Swedish population from age 70–81. Br J Haematol 1989;71:437–442.
6. Goodnough LT, Price TH, Parvin CA: The endogenous erythropoietin response and the erythropoietic response to blood loss anemia: The effects of age and gender. J Lab Clin Med 1995;125:57–64.
7. Nagel JE, Pyle RS, Chrest FJ, et al: Oxidative metabolism and bactericidal capacity of polymorphonuclear leukocytes from normal young and aged adults. J Gerontol 1982;37:529–534.
8. Lipschitz DA: Aging of the hematopoietic system. *In* Hazzard WR, Bierman EL, Blass JP, Ettinger WH, Halter JB (eds): Principles of Geriatric Medicine and Gerontology. New York, McGraw-Hill, 1994; pp. 733–739.
9. MacGregor RR, Shalit M: Neutrophil function in healthy elderly subjects. J Gerontol 1990;45:M55–M60.
10. Rao KM, Currie MS, Padmanabhan J, et al: Age-related alterations in actin cytoskeleton and receptor expression in human leukocytes. J Gerontol 1992;47:B37–B44.
11. Crawford J, Oates S, Wolfe LA, et al: An in vitro analogue of immune dysfunction with altered immunoglobulin production in the aged. J Am Geriatr Soc 1989;37:1140–1146.
12. Crawford J, Eye-Boland MK, Cohen HJ: Clinical utility of erythrocyte sedimentation rate and plasma protein analysis in the elderly. Am J Med 1987;82:239–246.
13. Stevens D, Tallis R, Hollis S: Persistent grossly elevated erythrocyte sedimentation rate in elderly people: One year follow-up of morbidity and mortality. Gerontology 1995;41:220–226.
14. Scott RB: Common blood disorders: A primary care approach. Geriatrics 1993;48:72–80.

15. Lipschitz DA, Mitchell CO, Thompson C: The anemia of senescence. Am J Hematol 1981;11:47–54.

16. Freedman ML, Marcus DI: Anemia and the elderly: Is it physiology or pathology? Am J Med Sci 1980;280:81–85.

17. Patterson C, Turpie ID, Benger AM: Assessment of iron stores in anemic geriatric patients. J Am Geriatr Soc 1985;33:764–767.

18. Fulcher RA, Hyland CM: Effectiveness of once daily oral iron in the elderly. Age Ageing 1981;10:44–46.

19. Damon LE: Anemias of chronic disease in the aged: Diagnosis and treatment. Geriatrics 1992;47:47–57.

20. Pennypacker LC, Allen RH, Kelly JP, et al: High prevalence of cobalamin deficiency in elderly populations. J Am Geriatr Soc 1992;40:1197–1204.

21. Stabler SP, Allen RH, Savage DG, et al: Clinical spectrum and diagnosis of cobalamin deficiency. Blood 1990;76:871–881.

22. Stabler SP: Screening the older population for cobalamin (vitamin B_{12}) deficiency. J Am Geriatr Soc 1995;43:1290–1297.

23. Bottiger LE, Bottiger B: Incidence and cause of aplastic anemia, hemolytic anemia, agranulocytosis and thrombocytopenia. Acta Med Scand 1981;210:475–479.

24. York EL, Jones RL, Menon D, et al: Effects of secondary polycythemia on cerebral blood flow in chronic obstructive pulmonary disease. Am Rev Respir Dis 1980;121:813–818.

25. Silver R: Interferon alpha$_{2b}$: A new treatment for polycythemia vera. Ann Intern Med 1993;119:1091–1092.

26. Kantarjian HM, Deisseroth A, Kurzrock R, et al: Chronic myelogenous leukemia: A concise update. Blood 1993;82:691–703.

27. Tura S, Baccarani M, Zuffa E, et al: Interferon alpha-2a as compared to conventional chemotherapy for the treatment of chronic myelogenous leukemia. N Engl J Med 1994;330:820–825.

28. Ballaster O, Moscinski LC, Morris D, et al: Acute myelogenous leukemia in the elderly. J Am Geriatr Soc 1992;40:277–284.

29. Lowenberg B: Treatment of the elderly patient with acute myeloid leukaemia. Bailliere's Clin Haematol 1996;9:147–159.

30. Tilly H, Castaigne S, Bordessoule D, et al: Low-dose cytarabine versus intensive chemotherapy in the treatment of acute nonlymphocytic leukemia in the elderly. J Clin Oncol 1990;8:272–279.

31. Dombret H, Chastang C, Fenaux P, et al: A controlled study of recombinant human granulocyte colony-stimulating factor in elderly patients after treatment for acute myelogenous leukemia. N Engl J Med 1995;332:1678–1683.

32. Sobol R, Mick R, Royston I, et al: Clinical importance of myeloid antigen expression in adult acute lymphoblastic leukemia. N Engl J Med 1987;316:1111–1117.

33. Hoelzer D, Thiel E, Loffler H, et al: Prognostic factors in a multicenter study for treatment of acute lymphoblastic leukemia in adults. Blood 1988;71:123–131.

34. Foon KA, Rai KR, Gale RP: Chronic lymphocytic leukemia: New insights into biology and therapy. Ann Intern Med 1990;113:525–539.

35. Obrien S, del Giglio A, Keating M: Advances in the biology and treatment of B-cell chronic lymphocytic leukemia. Blood 1995;85:307–318.

36. Cooperative Group for the Study of Immunoglobulin in Chronic Lymphocytic Leukemia: Intravenous immunoglobulin for the prevention of infection in chronic lymphocytic leukemia: A randomized controlled clinical trial. N Engl J Med 1988;319:902–907.

37. Saven A, Piro L: Newer purine analogues for the treatment of hairy-cell leukemia. N Engl J Med 1994;330:691–697.

38. Jones SE, Miller TP, Connors JM: Long-term follow-up and analysis for prognostic factors for patients with limited-stage diffuse large-cell lymphoma treated with initial chemotherapy with or without adjuvant radiotherapy. J Clin Oncol 1989;7:1186–1191.

39. Vose JM, Armitage JO, Weisenburger DD, et al: The importance of age in survival of patients treated with chemotherapy for aggressive non-Hodgkin's lymphoma. J Clin Oncol 1988;6:1838–1844.

40. Shipp MA: Prognostic factors in aggressive non-Hodgkin's lymphoma: Who has "high-risk" disease? Blood 1994;83:1165–1173.

41. Fisher RI, Gaynor ER, Dahlberg S, et al: Comparison of a standard regimen (CHOP) with three intensive chemotherapy regimens for advanced non-Hodgkin's lymphoma. N Engl J Med 1993;328:1002–1006.

42. Walker A, Schoenfeld E, Lowman J, et al: Survival of the older patient compared with the younger patient with Hodgkin's disease. Cancer 1990;65:1635–1640.

43. Crawford J, Eye MK, Cohen HJ: Evaluation of monoclonal gammopathies in the "well" elderly. Am J Med 1987;82:39–45.

44. Gautier M, Cohen HJ: Multiple myeloma in the elderly. J Am Geriatr Soc 1994;42:653–664.

45. Crawford J, Cox ED, Cohen HJ: Evaluation of hyperviscosity in monoclonal gammopathies. Am J Med 1985;79:13–22.

46. Cohen HJ, Bartolucci A: Age and the treatment of multiple myeloma. Am J Med 1985;79:316–324.

47. Berenson JR, Lichtenstein A, Porter L, et al: Efficacy of pamidronate in reducing skeletal events in patients with advanced multiple myeloma. N Engl J Med 1996;334:488–493.

48. Mansouri A, Bradford US, Lipschitz DA: Acquired hemostatic abnormalities in the elderly. J Am Geriatr Soc 1990;38:809–816.

49. George JN, Woolf SH, Raskob GE, et al: Idiopathic thrombocytopenic purpura: A practice guideline developed by explicit methods for the American Society of Hematology. Blood 1996;88:3–40.

50. Bauer K, Weiss L, Sparrow D, et al: Aging-associated changes in indices of thrombin generation and protein C activation in humans. J Clin Invest 1987;80:1527–1534.

38 Infections

Mira Cantrell, M.D.

Dean C. Norman, M.D.

EPIDEMIOLOGY

Infections have a major impact on the elderly, particularly those who are more disabled and institutionalized. Many infections occur more frequently in the elderly, and most of these have greater morbidity and mortality rates in the old than in the young (Tables 38–1 and 38–2).[1–3] Since many of these illnesses are preventable or curable, it is imperative that geriatricians have a good understanding of the diagnosis, treatment, and prevention of infection in aging adults.

PATHOGENESIS OF INFECTION IN THE ELDERLY

The risk and severity of infection are directly related to the virulence and inoculum of the pathogen and inversely related to the integrity of the host defenses.

$$\text{Infection} = \frac{\text{Virulence} \times \text{Inoculum}}{\text{Host defenses}}$$

Virulence

Approximately 40% of acute care hospital beds are occupied by patients in the geriatric age category, and 5% of elderly patients reside in long-term care institutions. Thus, the risk of exposure to nosocomial pathogens such as gram-negative bacilli is increased in this population. In the acute care setting it has been established that the risk per day of hospitalization among older acute care patients for developing a nosocomial infection is 1.5 times that of the young.[4] Similarly, the risks of developing a nosocomial urinary tract infection (threefold increase), bacteremia (fivefold increase), pneumonia (threefold increase), or wound infection (twofold increase) increase with age.[5] The risk of colonization and infection with gram-negative bacilli is also high in the nursing home population.[6, 7] Moreover, the widespread and in some cases inappropriate use of antimicrobial agents, along with often inadequate infection control procedures has had a dramatic impact on the microbial flora. For example, studies demonstrate that patients treated with antibiotics in a nursing home may become colonized by *Clostridium difficile* (the pathogen most often associated with antibiotic-associated colitis).[8, 9] Methicillin-resistant *Staphylococcus aureus* (MRSA) infections also occur in long-term care facilities, and vancomycin-resistant *Enterococcus* (VRE) poses a new threat.

Inoculum

Older adults are more likely to be exposed to higher inocula (quantity) of pathogens for a variety of reasons. For example, in the case of bacterial pneumonia the elderly are more likely to aspirate oropharyngeal flora secondary to central nervous system disorders, oversedation, or placement of feeding nasogastric tubes; pressure sores remove skin, which is an important physical barrier against bacterial colonization; and the use

---

TABLE 38–1 **MORTALITY RATE OF INFECTIONS IN ELDERLY COMPARED TO YOUNG**

Infection	Mortality Rate in Elderly Compared to Young[a]
Pneumonia	3×
Upper urinary tract infection	5–10×
Sepsis	3×
Appendicitis	15–20×
Cholecystitis	2–8×
Tuberculosis	10×
Infective endocarditis	2–3×
Bacterial meningitis	3×

Adapted from Yoshikawa TT, Norman DC (eds): Aging and Clinical Practice: Infectious Diseases: Diagnosis and Treatment. New York, Igaku-Shoin Medical Publishers, 1987, pp. 3–267.

[a]Excess mortality rate is especially significant for older persons residing in long-term care facilities. They account for the most frequent reasons for transfers to acute care facilities.[7]

TABLE 38–2   **EXCESS MORBIDITY OF INFECTIONS IN ELDERLY**

Infection	Morbid Event(s)
Pneumonia	Bacteremia; prolonged resolution; poor gas exchange
Urinary tract infection	Bacteremia; recurrence
Intra-abdominal infection	Perforation; gangrene; abscess; sepsis
Herpes zoster	Postherpetic neuralgia
Infective endocarditis	Stroke; heart failure
Tuberculosis	Reactivation; dissemination

Adapted from Yoshikawa TT, Norman DC (eds): Aging and Clinical Practice: Infectious Diseases: Diagnosis and Treatment. New York, Igaku-Shoin Medical Publishers, 1987, pp. 3–267.

of chronic indwelling bladder catheters allows colonization of the lower urinary tract with potential pathogens.

Host Defenses

As alluded to earlier, the skin and mucosal epithelial lining are important physical barriers to infection. The epidermis thins with age, and this thinning is exacerbated by chronic diseases and malnutrition. Other important changes in the skin include decreases in Langerhans cells, interleukin-1 production, and production and response to epidermal thymocyte-activating factor. These changes, coupled with poor perfusion, further increase the risk of damage to the skin and the subsequent development of soft tissue infection such as cellulitis and infected decubitus ulcers. Mucosal surfaces are also adversely affected by age, disease, and lifestyle (e.g., cigarette smoking with loss of the ciliary action of the epithelial cells of the upper respiratory tract and possibly reduction of secretory immunoglobulins).

Primary immunity (also called natural immunity) consists of phagocytosis, complement, and natural killer cells. Age in itself may have little effect on this form of immunity, which does not depend on prior exposure to pathogens (antigens) to be effective (hence the term primary). However, acute and chronic diseases, especially malnutrition, may compromise these defense mechanisms.

Secondary immunity (also called acquired immunity) refers to immune function that is activated only after prior exposure to a pathogen (antigen). This arm of the immune system requires a complex interaction between thymus-

derived cells (T lymphocytes or T cells), bursa-derived cells (B lymphocytes or B cells), and antigen-presenting macrophages. T cells are most adversely affected by aging, during which there is a qualitative loss of function that parallels the involution of the thymus and the reduction of thymic hormones, which occurs by middle age. Two subsets of T cells, the CD45RO$^+$ and the CD45RA, change most dramatically with age. The first is a predominantly naive subset, while the second consists predominantly of memory cells. With advancing age, the percentage of memory cells increases in relation to naive cells as the naive cells undergo a transition to memory cells. This altered ratio contributes to age-related changes in T-cell function including a decreased proliferative response to mitogens, production of and response to interleukin-2 and anti-CD-3 monoclonal antibody. T cells are necessary to enhance B-cell function. Although B cells are the cells responsible for antibody production, the diminished antibody response to vaccines that is observed with aging is due to defects in helper T-cell function and possibly B-cell function. Secondary immunity is also compromised by chronic diseases, malnutrition, and immunosuppressive agents.[10]

Other factors leading to increased morbidity and mortality for infectious diseases in the elderly include low physiologic reserve, presence of chronic underlying diseases, delays in diagnosis due to atypical clinical presentations leading to therapeutic delays, higher rates of adverse antibiotic and other drug interactions, and complications resulting from invasive diagnostic procedures.

FACTORS PECULIAR TO INFECTIONS IN THE ELDERLY

Etiology

Pathogens infecting older persons are different and more diverse than those infecting younger adults. Community-acquired pneumonia in young persons is most often due to *Mycoplasma pneumoniae* and *Streptococcus pneumoniae*. However, in aging adults, *Mycoplasma* is uncommon, and although *S. pneumoniae* causes 40% to 60% of cases of pneumonia, a variety of bacterial organisms including *Staphylococcus aureus, Klebsiella pneumoniae, Escherichia coli, Branhamella catarrhalis,* and *Haemophilus* sp as well as mixed flora (including anaerobes) account for many cases of lower respiratory infection in this population. A variety of *Legionella* sp cause a variable number of cases of pneumonia in the elderly depending on geographic location and immune status; *Chlamydia pneumoniae* causes a still undefined number of pneumonias in the elderly.

Urinary tract infections (UTIs) in the general population occur almost exclusively in sexually active women and are caused by *Escherichia coli* in over 85% of cases. In contrast, UTIs occur frequently in both elderly women and men, and the cause is frequently uropathogens other than *E. coli* (e.g., *Klebsiella* sp, *Proteus* sp, and *Enterococcus* sp). Moreover, polymicrobial bacteriuria is common in patients with indwelling bladder catheters.

The elderly are more likely to be in institutions and account for an increasing percentage of acute care hospital inpatients. They are therefore more likely to be exposed to nosocomial pathogens such as aerobic gram-negative bacilli and *S. aureus* as well as to multidrug-resistant pathogens including MRSA and VRE.

Viral illnesses also have a major impact on the elderly. Although rhinovirus infection (the "common cold") decreases with age, respiratory viruses such as influenza virus cause very high morbidity and mortality in older adults, and there is a risk of hospitalization of about 1 per 300 and a risk of death of 1 per 1500 during influenza outbreaks.[11] Respiratory syncytial virus[12, 13] as well as influenza virus may cause outbreaks of respiratory illness in nursing homes. Varicella-zoster virus is another important pathogen that is manifest in the elderly in the form of herpes zoster. This infection carries with it the dreaded potential complication of postherpetic neuralgia, which also occurs almost exclusively in the geriatric age group (see later)

Diagnosis

CLINICAL MANIFESTATIONS

The diagnosis and therapy of infections in the elderly present unique problems that are reviewed here briefly. Aside from prevention, early diagnosis with rapid institution of antimicrobial therapy is the mainstay of treatment for reducing the appallingly high morbidity and mortality of infection in the aged. Unfortunately, infection may present in an atypical manner in a significant number of cases (e.g., blunted or absent fever response in 20% to 30% of patients). This is particularly true in the old-old (i.e., persons 75 years old or older) and in long-term care institutions, in which residents are typically frail, suffer from multiple diseases, and are cognitively impaired.

There are basically four factors that contribute to the atypical presentation of infection in the elderly compared to the young. These include *underreporting of illness*, which may cause delay in bringing an elderly patient to medical attention, and *different pathogens* (which was discussed earlier). Underreporting of illness is an important problem in the cognitively impaired elderly patient, who may not complain or may be unable to communicate information about symptoms. Furthermore, even noncentral nervous system infections may result in compromising cognition in elderly patients. The presence of *coexisting diseases* such as chronic bronchitis, which may mask acute pneumonia, or rheumatoid arthritis, which can confound the presence of septic arthritis, may compound difficulties in making the diagnosis of infection. Finally, *altered physiologic responses* to infection, or for the manner to any acute illness, are due to many factors including the decremental biologic changes of normal aging, which may be exacerbated by lifestyle. For example, age-related changes in chest wall expansion and lung tissue elasticity, which may be made worse by smoking, contribute to a diminished cough reflex. A weakened cough has the double negative effect of contributing to a decline in pulmonary host defenses and making the diagnosis of respiratory infection more difficult.

Another example of an altered physiologic response to infection in older persons that deserves special mention is the often-observed blunted fever response.[14, 15] Although fever is the cardinal sign of infection, the traditional definition of fever (oral temperature of 100.4° to 101°F or 38° to 38.3°C) may not be sensitive enough to diagnose infection in elderly patients. We have found in a nursing home population that baseline body temperatures are approximately 1°F below those of a normal young person and that with infection, despite a rise in temperature comparable to that seen in the young, the maximum temperature may be below the traditional definition of fever. However, we also found that a temperature of 100°F (37.8°C) *coupled* with a decline in functional status is highly indicative of infection in this population.[16, 17]

The presence or absence of fever—aside from facilitating or inhibiting the diagnosis of infection—has other implications. The presence of fever (as defined by an oral temperature of 101°F) is highly specific for the presence of a serious, usually bacterial, infection.[18, 19] Moreover, when the syndrome of fever of unknown origin (FUO) occurs in elderly persons, it typically signifies a treatable condition such as intra-abdominal infection, infective endocarditis, temporal arteritis, or other rheumatologic condition.[20, 21] A blunted fever response to infection frequently portends a poor prognosis.[22] This may be relevant to the mounting evidence that fever may play an important role in host defenses.[15, 23]

In summary, an acute infection in the elderly may present with either typical clinical manifestations or subtle findings. Signs and symptoms pointing to a specific organ system infection may be lacking. Thus, an infection should be sought in any elderly person with an unexplained acute to subacute (days to weeks) decline in functional status.

LABORATORY TESTS

It is more difficult and hazardous to perform invasive diagnostic tests in the elderly, particularly if they are frail and unable to cooperate. Furthermore, waning cellular immunity with age makes skin testing less reliable (e.g., for tuberculosis), whereas increased nonspecific immunoglobulin production may give false-positive serologic test results (e.g., positive rheumatoid factor). Also, radiologic procedures may be difficult to interpret in older adults because of biologic changes with age and age-related disorders (e.g., changes secondary to chronic congestive heart failure or obstructive pulmonary disease may confound the diagnosis of pneumonia). Finally, colonization of normally sterile sites by bacteria such as the age-related gastric colonization by *Helicobacter pylori* may make it difficult to assess the role of this pathogen in gastrointestinal disease in the elderly.[24] Similarly, colonization of the bladder in elderly persons who are often completely asymptomatic may make it difficult to assess the clinical significance of a positive urine culture.

Still, basic laboratory studies such as a white blood cell (WBC) count with a differential remain the cornerstone of laboratory diagnosis. A high WBC count with a left shift, regardless of a patient's hydration status, is highly suggestive of a developing infectious process.

Antimicrobial Therapy

PHARMACOLOGY

A detailed description of the pharmacology of antibiotics is beyond the scope of this chapter, and the reader is referred to a more comprehensive review.[25] Briefly, oral absorption, tissue penetration, hepatic metabolism, and volume of distribution are either minimally or variably affected by age. In the pharmacology of antibiotics age affects mainly renal clearance. This is not a trivial effect because the majority of antibiotics are cleared predominantly by this mechanism.

Therefore, drugs that are cleared predominantly by the kidneys, such as the aminoglycosides and vancomycin, require serial monitoring of the patient's clinical status, renal function, and serum drug levels because they are associated with low therapeutic indices and potential serious adverse side effects (i.e., nephrotoxicity and ototoxicity). It has been demonstrated that reliance on simple serum creatinine measurements or formulas predicting creatinine clearance based on serum creatinine levels are inadequate in seriously ill elderly patients with an infection.[25, 26]

SPECIFIC DRUGS

Table 38–3 lists some of the antibiotics more frequently used for treating infection in the elderly as well as their spectrum of action and potential indications. The list is not exhaustive and summarizes only some of the antibiotics believed by the authors to be particularly relevant for use in the elderly.

GENERAL APPROACH TO THE MANAGEMENT OF INFECTION IN THE ELDERLY

The diagnostic approach should take into consideration the setting in which the infection occurs. Community-acquired infections are more likely to be found in the respiratory tract, urinary tract, or abdomen. More than 80% of infections in nursing homes are pneumonias, urinary tract infections, and soft tissue infections (acronym, PUS). Hospital-acquired infections commonly comprise aspiration pneumonia involving nosocomial flora, catheter-associated urinary tract infections, and intravenous catheter-associated septic thrombophlebitis.

Empirical therapy with broad-spectrum antibiotics is often indicated pending culture results in seriously ill frail elderly patients with an infection. In general, this therapy should include a broad-spectrum beta-lactam antibiotic. The more toxic aminoglycosides should be avoided in the elderly unless the risk of death from sepsis outweighs the risk of ototoxicity and nephrotoxicity. Therapy should be altered to more narrow-spectrum agents based on the culture data.[27, 28] Because of cost considerations, patients should be switched to oral antibiotics as soon as possible.

Home intravenous antimicrobial therapy may be given to *selected* elderly patients who have stable infections if they and their caregivers are motivated to participate in this form of therapy.[29]

Despite some questions about cost-effectiveness and reimbursement for this kind of treatment, a significant number of infected elderly

TABLE 38–3   **SOME IMPORTANT ANTIBIOTICS FOR INFECTION IN THE ELDERLY**

Drug	Antimicrobial Spectrum	Primary Indications
Ampicillin (PO, IV)	Streptococci, *E. coli, Proteus*	UTI, bronchitis
Amoxicillin-clavulanate (PO)	Streptococci, staphylococci, *E. coli, Proteus, Klebsiella,* anaerobes	UTI, bronchitis, pneumonia, soft tissue infections
Ticarcillin-clavulanate (IV)	Same as amoxicillin-clavulanate plus *Pseudomonas aeruginosa*	UTI, bronchitis, pneumonia, soft tissue infections, intra-abdominal infections
Ampicillin-sulbactam (IV)	Same as amoxicillin-clavulanate	Same as ticarcillin-clavulanate
Cefazolin (IM, IV)	Streptococci, staphylococci, *E. coli, Proteus, Klebsiella*	Soft tissue infections, UTI
Cefuroxime (PO, IM, IV)	Streptococci, staphylococci, *H. influenzae, E. coli, Proteus, Klebsiella*	Pneumonia, UTI
Cefoxitin or cefotetan (IV)	Streptococci, anaerobes, *E. coli, Proteus, Klebsiella*	Pneumonia, soft tissue infections, intra-abdominal infections
Ceftizoxime (IM, IV)	Streptococci, most gram-negative bacteria	Pneumonia, UTIs, meningitis, sepsis
Ceftriaxone (IM, IV)	Same as ceftizoxime	Same as ceftizoxime
Ceftazidime (IM, IV)	Same as ceftizoxime except improved *Pseudomonas aeruginosa*	Severe infections when *P. aeruginosa* is suspected
Aztreonam (IV)	Most gram-negative bacilli	UTIs, sepsis
Imipenem-cilastatin (IV)	Streptococci, staphylococci, most gram-negative bacilli, anaerobes, *Listeria*	Reserved for multiresistant organisms in serious infections
Vancomycin (IV, oral for *C. difficile*)	Streptococci, staphylococci, *Clostridium difficile*	Antibiotic-associated colitis, methicillin-resistant staphylococcal infection, penicillin-allergic patients
Trimethoprim-sulfamethoxazole (PO, IV)	Streptococci, *E. coli, Proteus, Klebsiella*	UTIs
Ciprofloxacin and other quinolones (PO, some IV)	Staphylococci, some streptococci, most gram-negative bacilli	UTIs, pneumonia, sepsis, soft tissue infections
Metronidazole (PO, IV)	Anaerobes including *C. difficile*	Intra-abdominal infections, brain abscess, soft tissue infections, antibiotic-associated colitis

Abbreviations: UTI, urinary tract infection

patients may benefit from this therapeutic option. Broad-spectrum cephalosporins with long half-lives and limited toxicity such as ceftriaxone are the antibiotics most frequently used in home intravenous therapy.

Specific Infections

PNEUMONIA

Pneumonia or influenza is the leading infectious cause of mortality in the elderly and the fourth leading cause of mortality in those over age 75. Moreover, compared with younger adults, the elderly have a five- to tenfold increased risk of developing pneumonia. One study showed that the risk was highest in those with coexisting alco-holism, followed in order by chronic obstructive pulmonary disease, immunosuppressive therapy, cardiovascular disease, and institutionalization.[30]

The majority of pneumonias are secondary to micro- or macroaspiration of oral pharyngeal flora in patients with compromised host defenses (e.g., diminished cough reflex, waning cellular immunity). The causes of pneumonia differ significantly from those in the young depending on the clinical setting (see earlier section on etiology). Data on the etiology of pneumonia in long-term care facilities are limited, and the available information is based primarily on sputum culture results, which are not definitive in establishing the actual etiologic pathogen.[31] Nevertheless, it is estimated that, compared to community-acquired pneumonia, of which 40% to 60% of cases are caused by *S. pneumoniae*, pneumonia occurring in the nursing home frequently results from mixed causes. Moreover, in nursing homes there is an increased likelihood of isolating aerobic gram-negative bacilli such as *Klebsiella* sp and *E. coli* from the sputum. Fortunately, multiple drug-resistant pathogens such as *Pseudomonas aeruginosa* are infrequently found as respiratory pathogens unless the patient has recently been in an acute care facility or has been taking broad-spectrum antibiotics. Hospital-acquired pneumonia in the elderly is more likely to be caused by mixed flora, usually oral aerobic and anaerobic flora. In people over the age of 65, the risk of oropharyngeal colonization by staphylococci and aerobic gram-negative bacilli increases with decreasing functional status and increasing level of care.[32] Therefore, it is not surprising that a significant proportion of cases involve these pathogens, again usually in mixed infections.

The diagnosis of pneumonia in debilitated elderly patients may be difficult.[28] Cough and fever may be diminished or absent. Tachypnea and tachycardia are sensitive but not specific findings. Older patients may present simply with altered mental status or a decline in functional status. Physical examination usually does not reveal signs of consolidation and may be confusing in aging patients with coexisting congestive heart failure or chronic obstructive pulmonary disease. The chest radiograph along with the history and physical examination are important in establishing a diagnosis of pneumonia in the elderly patient. The chest radiograph typically shows a patchy pattern of bronchopneumonia but may be initially negative or difficult to interpret in patients with coexisting pulmonary disease. Following hospitalization, the pulmonary infiltrates may become worse in approximately half the patients. Moreover, resolution of the infiltrates typically takes longer in elderly patients than in younger ones.

Higher mortality rates for pneumonia in the elderly should not discourage aggressive therapy given that in one large study of community-acquired pneumonia (excluding nursing home cases) 2-year mortality rates for pneumonia patients discharged from the hospital were similar in both old and young.[33] Management of pneumonia in the elderly requires hospitalization in most cases because of the higher mortality and more frequent complications, difficulties in establishing both the diagnosis and the precise cause, severity of the illness (which may be masked by the clinical presentation), and the need to monitor therapy. Pneumonia in nursing home patients with mild to moderate illness may be managed in the nursing home only if suffi-cient resources are available (e.g., staff, laboratory support, administration of intravenous fluids and antibiotics).

In all cases, an effort should be made to obtain sputum for a Gram's stain smear and bacterial culture, and for a smear and culture for mycobacteria if tuberculosis is suspected. Older patients may be unable to provide an optimal sputum specimen (less than 10 epithelial cells and more than 25 polymorphonuclear cells per low-power field), but more invasive procedures such as transtracheal aspiration, shielded bronchoscopy, and transbronchial biopsy should be reserved for patients who are at high risk of unusual or opportunistic infections (e.g., those with immunosuppressed status) or who fail to respond to initial antimicrobial therapy and show clinically deteriorating signs. Other routine laboratory tests, including blood cultures (positive in about 5% to 10% of cases), serum electrolytes, complete blood count, and renal function tests, should also be performed. Monitoring of arterial blood gases is important for assessing adequate gas exchange and acid-base balance. At a minimum, measurement of oxygen saturation with a pulse oximeter should be performed, and an electrocardiogram should be obtained initially to evaluate any potential cardiac complications of pneumonia. Additionally, skin testing for tuberculosis and, in certain geographic areas, assessment for fungal infection (e.g., coccidioidomycosis) should be performed in elderly patients with pneumonia. Finally, diagnostic thoracocentesis for pleural fluid smear, culture, pH, leukocytes, glucose, protein, and cytologic examination as well as pleural biopsy should be considered in patients who have no coagulopathy and who can cooperate with the procedure. This is especially appropriate for patients who have large pleural effusions or in whom the effusion does not improve with therapy.

Antimicrobial therapy for pneumonia in the elderly should be based on the results of the tests just mentioned. In view of the severity of the illness, early empirical therapy with broad-spectrum antibiotics is advised for most older patients with pneumonia; adjustments are made when the culture data become available.[28] It is the authors' recommendation that for *clinically stable* elderly patients with community-acquired pneumonia, treatment should be started according to the Gram's stain results. If the sputum specimen is of "poor" quality, empirical therapy with any one of the following antibiotics should be considered: parenteral second- or third-generation cephalosporin, ampicillin-sulbactam, or ticarcillin-clavulanate. In mildly ill patients, oral ciprofloxacin, with or without ampicillin to ensure adequate coverage of *S. pneumoniae,* may be considered. *Clinically unstable* patients—those with nosocomial-acquired pneumonia, who have recently begun taking antibiotics or who are immunosup pressed—should receive empirical therapy consisting of a parenteral third-generation cephalosporin plus either aztreonam, quinolone, or an aminoglycoside. Aminoglycosides should be avoided if possible. Erythromycin should be part of the therapeutic regimen if Legionnaire's disease is suspected.

The prevention of pneumonia is best accomplished by reducing the risk of aspiration whenever possible (e.g., avoiding sedating medications, alcohol, and nasogastric tubes [Table 38–4]). Vaccination with the current pneumococcal vaccine is now strongly recommended despite some past questions about its efficacy. Influenza vaccination is very important in preventing influenza pneumonia as well as secondary bacterial pneumonia (see next paragraph).

INFLUENZA

Although other respiratory viruses such as respiratory syncytial virus are capable of infecting

older persons, influenza has had the greatest impact by far, and much of the excess morbidity and mortality ascribed to influenza outbreaks has occurred in people at the extreme ends of the age scale.[11] It should be kept in mind that in addition to damaging respiratory epithelial cells, decreasing the effectiveness of cell-mediated immunity, and causing upper and lower viral respiratory infection and secondary bacterial bronchitis and pneumonia, influenza may exacerbate and worsen chronic underlying medical conditions. This activity accounts in part for the high hospitalization rates of the elderly observed during influenza outbreaks in the community.

The virus undergoes antigenic changes (usually "drift," although an actual "shift" occurs about every 10 years), and manufacturers of vaccines must take these changes into account annually. Thus, vaccinations must be given yearly. The precise efficacy of the influenza vaccine has not been established in the elderly, but it appears to be at least 60% effective in reducing the incidence of influenza infection. In addition to patients with special health problems and health care professionals who interact regularly with patients at high risk for influenza, the vaccine is recommended for all persons aged 65 and older. Amantadine and presumably rimantadine are effective for the early treatment of influenza (within 48 hours of exposure) and for prophylaxis against influenza A (*not* influenza B). The efficacy of amantadine is better established in the literature than that of rimantadine. Both are usually given in a reduced dosage of 100 mg orally per day in elderly persons. However, in the case of amantadine, which is cleared by the kidneys, even this dose may be too high for some debilitated elderly persons, and the dose must be adjusted downward based on creatinine clearance.[7, 34]

TABLE 38–4   **PREVENTION OF PNEUMONIA**

- Avoid increasing gastric pH (may increase gastric colonization)
- Initiate early nutritional intervention
- Reduce duration of surgical procedures and mechanical ventilation
- Order swallowing assessment if indicated[a]
- If enteral feeding is indicated, continuous enteral feeding may reduce risk of reflux and macroaspiration. Bolus feeding should be done with patient sitting upright. Gastric tubes do not appear to be better than nasogastric tubes in reducing risk of aspiration pneumonia
- Prevent viral infection (with vaccination, amantadine, isolation)
- Aviod sedatives but use short-acting drugs if necessary
- Avoid cigarettes because they decrease mucociliary host defenses and lead to chronic obstructive pulmonary disease, which increases lower airway colonization with bacteria

---

[a]Speech pathology videofluorographic evaluation of swallowing may yield useful recommendations about posture and food consistency to improve swallowing function and reduce the risk of aspiration (e.g., turning head to the damaged side and using liquids and thinner foods in some patients with unilateral pharyngeal paresis). No hard evidence points to decreased risk of aspiration pneumonia with continuous as opposed to bolus feeding, but the authors believe that bolus feeding leads to an increased risk of reflux with possible secondary aspiration complications.

TUBERCULOSIS

Mycobacterium tuberculosis infection occurs disproportionately in the older population and is associated with higher mortality rates in this population. Among all cases of tuberculosis in the United States, 26% occur in people over the age of 65, in whom the morbidity rate is 60%. Although the majority (80%) of all cases are diagnosed in community dwellers, the incidence rate is three to four times higher in those residing in nursing homes. The association between the tuberculous pathogen and the aged may exist in part because the majority of elderly people have been exposed to tuberculosis at an earlier age (when tuberculosis infection was quite common in the general population) but were able to eliminate or control the infection at that time. However, the waning of cell-mediated immunity with age as well as the presence of coexisting chronic illnesses, which may further compromise host defenses, may allow for "reactivation" of this infection in the geriatric age group. Although reactivation of preexisting infection is the usual pathogenesis of tuberculosis in the elderly, it should be emphasized that outbreaks of primary infection with active pulmonary tuberculosis have been well described in long-term care institutions.[7, 35]

The diagnosis of tuberculosis should be considered in any elderly individual who has a cough, chronic fatigue, night sweats, unexplained fever, weight loss, or gradual or subacute decline in functional status. Unfortunately, a proper diagnosis may be difficult to ascertain because of subtle or unusual clinical features and atypical chest x-ray findings are common. Moreover, skin testing for tuberculosis is often unreliable in the elderly because reactivity to the tuberculin antigen (purified protein derivative [PPD]) wanes with age. Nevertheless, elderly patients with unexplained pulmonary infiltrates should undergo skin testing with PPD as well as with control antigens to exclude cutaneous anergy, and multiple sputum specimens for acid-fast bacteria smears and mycobacterial culture should be collected. In patients with significant pleural effusion, a pleural biopsy and culture should be attempted, and in patients with suspected miliary tuberculosis, a transbronchial biopsy and culture may be indicated.

Uncomplicated (drug-susceptible) pulmonary tuberculosis can be treated with 6 months of isoniazid 300 mg/day and rifampin 600 mg/day plus pyrazinamide 30 mg/kg/day for the first 2 months (intensive phase) of treatment, or, alternatively, 9 months of daily isoniazid (300 mg) and rifampin (600 mg) can be given. If the sputum smear and culture remain negative and drug resistance is unlikely, therapy can be shortened from 9 to 4 months. Elderly patients should also receive 25 mg/day of pyridoxine to reduce the risk of peripheral neuropathy associated with isoniazid.[35]

Due to a substantial increase in the incidence of multidrug-resistant tuberculosis (MDR-TB), the Centers for Disease Control recently published new recommendations for treatment of tuberculosis. In persons with a high likelihood of acquiring multidrug-resistant tuberculosis, the recommendations for treatment include three treatment options with four drug regimens consisting of isoniazid, rifampin, pyrazinamide, and ethambutol or streptomycin. However, most elderly patients do not require this type of treatment because of the low risk of drug resistance in this population group.

PRESSURE SORES

Pressure sores develop from the interaction of external factors with the patient's own internal factors. Major external factors are pressure, shearing forces, friction, and moisture. Major internal factors include the patient's overall skin condition, mobility, nutritional state, and underlying medical or surgical condition. Most patients with pressure sores are in the geriatric age group, and those over the age of 70 account for two thirds of all patients with bed sores. Although the prevalence of pressure sores is highest in patients residing in long-term care facilities, the incidence is highest in patients in acute care hospitals. More than 60% of patients with pressure sores develop them in hospitals, 18% in nursing homes, and another 18% at home. It is significant that the majority of pressure sores develop during the first 2 weeks of hospitalization.

Since pressure sores are wounds that are chronically contaminated, lowering the bacterial count may facilitate healing. Healing wounds typically show no anaerobic bacteria, whereas nonhealing wounds show the highest counts of both aerobic and anaerobic organisms.[36]

A local bactericidal effect can be achieved by using conservative measures consisting of cleansing, disinfection, and debridement. The use of topical antibiotics for this purpose remains controversial. Although they may lower bacterial counts, they penetrate poorly through devitalized tissue. Topical antibiotics can cause localized tissue sensitivity and promote the relatively rapid emergence of resistant organisms (especially the *Pseudomonas* species).

When cellulitis, osteomyelitis, or sepsis is present, treatment with systemic antibiotics directed against a mixed population of aerobic and anaerobic bacteria is mandatory. The most commonly found bacteria are *S. aureus*, gram-negative rods, and *Bacteroides fragilis*. A combination of clindamycin or metronidazole (for anaerobic coverage) with a quinolone, an aminoglycoside, a third-generation cephalosporin, or aztreonam (for coverage of gram-negative bacilli) provides an effective treatment. Ticarcillin-clavulanic acid and ampicillin-sulbactam also provide good coverage for the variety of organisms found in pressure sores. A decision about the use of antibiotics for infections associated with pressure sores frequently must be made empirically pending the results of meaningful cultures (blood cultures, tissue biopsy). Swab cultures of the necrotic debris are of little value. If the exact wound microbiology is sought, a biopsy of the viable tissue interface should be performed.

Sepsis associated with pressure sores carries a mortality rate of approximately 50%. It is even higher in patients over the age of 60 and in those who have multiple ulcer sites. Wound debridement may be associated with transient bacteremia but appears to have no serious consequences. Osteomyelitis occurs in 26% of patients with nonhealing pressure sores; the diagnosis should be confirmed by radionuclide scintigraphy of the bone and bone biopsy.[37] Septic arthritis may also be seen and is frequently associated with a sinus tract leading from an ulcerous lesion.

The possibility of tetanus infection should be considered in patients with deep necrotic lesions that are becoming progressively larger and are resistant to local and systemic treatment. Because many elderly patients have not received adequate tetanus immunization, administration of tetanus toxoid should be considered.

URINARY TRACT INFECTIONS

Urinary tract infections (UTIs) are the most common type of infection and the most frequent cause of gram-negative bacillary sepsis in the elderly.

The frequency of bacteriuria in ambulatory patients over the age of 65 is 10% to 30% in women and 5% to 10% in men. These figures increase to 15% to 20% in elderly men and 25% to 50% in elderly women residing in long-term care facilities. Bacteriuria in the elderly is typically caused by a variety of gram-negative organisms. *E. coli* is responsible for the majority of episodes, but organisms such as *Proteus, Klebsiella, Pseudomonas* species, and, less frequently, *Citrobacter* and *Providentia* species are increasing in importance. Bacteriuria, especially when it is associated with chronic indwelling catheter use, is polymicrobial and often includes group D streptococcus (*Enterococcus* sp).[38]

Asymptomatic bacteriuria in the elderly is a well-described phenomenon. It is defined by a finding of 10^5 or more colony-forming units (CFU)/mL bacteria in urine, is not associated with clinical signs and symptoms of infection, and is frequently transient or intermittent. Often pyuria is lacking as well. The available data on the long-term sequelae of asymptomatic bacteriuria are conflicting. However, there is general agreement among clinicians that in the absence of chronic urinary obstruction, asymptomatic bacteriuria in aging adults should not be treated with antibiotics.[39, 40]

An uncomplicated, symptomatic community-acquired UTI can present with fever, dysuria, frequency, and urgency, or, less typically, as weakness and fatigue, anorexia, or change in mental status. Once the diagnosis has been made, the choice of antimicrobial agent will depend on the urine bacteriology, clinical status of the patient, and pharmacokinetic properties of the agent chosen as well as patient tolerance of the drug. The antimicrobials most commonly used today are as follows: trimethoprim-sulfamethoxazole (TMP/SMZ); first-generation cephalosporins such as cephradine, cefazolin, cefadroxil, and cephalexin; quinolones; and clavulanic acid combinations with amoxicillin or ticarcillin. Ampicillin and amoxicillin provide good coverage for enterococcal infections. Treatment is usually given for 7 to 14 days with the goal of alleviating the symptoms and sterilizing the urine. Single-dose treatment of uncomplicated urinary tract infections in the elderly is not recommended because it carries an unacceptably high relapse rate.

Complicated UTIs are associated with structural or functional abnormalities of the urinary tract. These infections are frequently caused by organisms that are resistant to different antibiotics. Hence, culture and sensitivity data are essential for the appropriate management of a complicated UTI. Empirical therapy requiring parenteral antibiotics for these infections should include third-generation cephalosporins, aztreonam, quinolones, or aminoglycosides. Complicated UTIs may be recurrent because of either relapse or reinfection and may require prolonged treatment of 4 to 6 weeks, usually with an oral agent such as quinolone, TMP-SMZ, or a cephalosporin.[41–43]

Patients with chronic indwelling urinary catheters invariably have infected urine and often present with polymicrobial bacteriuria. The rate of acquisition of bacteria after the catheter has been inserted is 7% to 8% per day. After a period of 3 to 4 weeks, virtually 100% of patients become bacteriuric. Characteristically, the microbial flora changes during the period of catheterization, averaging 2.0 species changes per month. However, antimicrobial treatment is reserved only for patients who develop clinical signs of infection. About 20% of these patients develop symptomatic urinary tract infection within 1 year. Routine surveillance of urine cultures in patients with indwelling urinary catheters is not necessary or cost-effective. Urine cultures should be obtained in all patients with indwelling catheters who show clinical signs of infection or changes in mentation or functional status. When a urine sample is to be obtained from a patient with an indwelling catheter, it should be done by using a needle and syringe, aspirating the specimen through the aspiration port after the port has been thoroughly cleaned with an iodophor agent. Treatment of catheter-associated infections in patients who are clinically stable can be accomplished by using oral quinolones, TMP/SMZ, or amoxicillin-clavulanic acid. In unstable patients who have a septic presentation, a combination of parenteral ampicillin with either aztreonam, a third-generation cephalosporin, quinolone, or an aminoglycoside, or imipenem plus cilastatin provides good coverage for most polymicrobial flora.[44, 45]

References

1. Yoshikawa TT, Norman DC (eds): Unique aspects of infection in older adults. *In* Antimicrobial Therapy in the Elderly Patient. New York, Marcel Dekker, 1994, pp. 1–8.
2. Yoshikawa TT, Norman DC (eds): Aging and Clinical Practice: Infectious Diseases: Diagnosis and Treatment. New York, Igaku-Shoin Medical Publishers, 1987, pp. 3–267.
3. Crossley KB, Peterson PK: Infections in the elderly. Clin Infect Dis 1996; 22:209–215.
4. Saviteer SM, Samsa GP, Rutala WA: Nosocomial infections in the elderly. Increased risk per hospital day. Am J Med 1988; 84:661–666.
5. Haley RW, Mouton TM, Culver DM, et al: Nosocomial infections in U.S. hospitals. Estimated frequency by selected characteristics of patients. Am J Med 1981; 70:947–959.
6. Norman DC, Castle SC, Cantrell M: Infections in the nursing home. J Am Geriatr Soc 1987; 35:796–805.
7. Yoshikawa TT, Norman DC: Approach to fever and infection in the nursing home. J Am Geriatr Soc 1996; 44:74–82.
8. Thomas DR, Bennet RG, Laghon BE, Greenough WB, Bartlett JG: Postantibiotic colonization with *Clostridium difficile* in nursing home patients. J Am Geriatr Soc 1990; 38:415–420.
9. Walker KJ, Gilliland SS, Vance-Bryan K, et al: *Clostridium difficile* colonization in residents of long-term care facilities: Prevalence and risk factors. J Am Geriatr Soc 1993; 41:940–946.
10. Castle S: Age-related changes in host defenses. *In* Yoshikawa TT, Norman DC (eds): Antimicrobial Therapy in the Elderly Patient. New York, Marcel Dekker, 1994, pp. 9–22.
11. Couch RB, Kasel A, Glezen WP, et al: Influenza: Its control in persons and populations. J Infect Dis 1986; 153(3):431–440.
12. Osterweil D, Norman DC: An outbreak of an influenza-like illness in a nursing home. J Am Geriatr Soc 1990; 38:659–662.
13. Wald TG, Miller BA, Shult P, et al: Can respiratory syncytial virus and influenza A be distinguished clinically in institutionalized older persons? J Am Geriatr Soc 1995; 43:170–174.
14. Norman DC, Toledo SD: Infections in elderly persons. An altered clinical presentation. Clin Geriatr Med 1992; 8:713–719.
15. Norman DC, Yoshikawa TT: Fever in the elderly. Infect Dis Clin North Am 1996; 10:93–100.
16. Castle SC, Norman DC, Yeh M, et al: Fever response in elderly nursing home residents: Are the older truly colder? Clin Res J Am Geriatr Soc 1991; 39:853–857.
17. Castle SC, Yeh M, Toledo S, et al: Lowering the temperature criterion improves detection of infections in nursing home residents. Aging Immun Infect Dis 1993; 4:67–76.
18. Keating MJ III, Klimek JJ, Levine, DS, Kierman FJ: Effect of aging on the clinical significance of fever in ambulatory adult patients. J Am Geriatr Soc 1984; 32:282–287.
19. Wasserman M, Levinstein M, Keller E, Yoshikawa TT: Utility of fever, white blood cell, and differential count in predicting bacterial infections in the elderly. J Am Geriatr Soc 1989; 37:534–543.
20. Knockaert DC, Vanneste LJ, Bobbaers HJ: Fever of unknown origin in elderly patients. J Am Geriatr Soc 1993; 32:282–287.
21. Berland B, Gleckman RA: Fever of unknown origin in the elderly: A sequential approach to diagnosis. Postgrad Med 1992; 92:197–210.
22. Weinstein MP, Murphy JR, Reller RB, Lichtenstein KA: The clinical significance of positive blood cultures: A comprehensive analysis of 500 episodes of bacteremia and fungemia II. Clinical observations with special reference to factors influencing prognosis. Rev Infect Dis 1983; 5:54–70.
23. Kluger MJ, Kozak W, Conn C, et al: The adaptive value of fever. Infect Dis Clin North Am 1996; 10:1–20.
24. Graham DY, Malaty HM, Evans DJ, et al: Epidemiology of *Helicobacter pylori* in asymptomatic populations in United States: Effect of age, race and socioeconomic status. Gastroenterology 1991; 100(6):1495–1501.
25. Ljungberg B, Nilsson-Ehle I: Pharmacology of antimicrobial agents with aging. *In* Yoshikawa TT, Norman DC (eds): Antimicrobial Therapy in the Elderly Patient. New York, Marcel Dekker, 1994, pp. 33–45.
26. Zaske DE: Aminoglycosides. *In* Yoshikawa TT, Norman DC (eds): Antimicrobial Therapy in the Elderly Patient. New York, Marcel Dekker, 1994, pp. 183–235.
27. Yoshikawa TT: Empiric antimicrobial therapy. *In* Yoshikawa TT, Norman DC (eds): Antimicrobial Therapy in the Elderly Patient. New York, Marcel Dekker, 1994, pp. 469–477.
28. Yoshikawa TT, Norman DC: Treatment of infections in elderly patients. Med Clin North Am 1995; 79:651–661.
29. Nagami PH, Landis SA: Home intravenous antibiotic therapy. *In* Yoshikawa TT, Norman DC (eds): Antimicrobial Therapy in the Elderly Patient. New York, Marcel Dekker, 1994, pp. 505–519.
30. Koivula I, Stein M, Makela PH: Risk factors for pneumonia in the elderly. Am J Med 1994; 96:313–319.
31. Crossley KB, Thorn JR: Nursing home-acquired pneumonia. Semin Respir Infect 1989; 4(1):64–72.
32. Valenti WM, Trudell RG, Bentley DW: Factors predisposing to oropharyngeal colonization with gram negative bacilli in the aged. N Engl J Med 1978; 298:1108–1111.
33. Brancati FL, Chow JW, Wagener MM, Vacarello DD, Yu VL: Is pneumonia really the old man's friend? Two-year prognosis after community-acquired pneumonia. Lancet 1993; 342:30–33.
34. Gomolin IH, Leib HB, Arden NH, Sherman FT: Control of influenza outbreaks in the nursing home: Guidelines for diagnosis and management. J Am Geriatr Soc 1995; 43:71–74.
35. Dutt AK, Stead WW: Tuberculosis. Clin Geriatr Med 1992; 8(4):761–775.
36. Sapico FL, Ginunas VJ, Thornhill-Joynes M, et al: Quantitative microbiology of pressure sores in different stages of healing. Diagn Microbiol Infect Dis 1986; 5(1):31–38.

37. Darouiche RO, Landon GC, Klima M, et al: Osteomyelitis associated with pressure sores. Arch Intern Med 1994; 154:753–758.

38. Nicolle LE: Urinary tract infections in the elderly. J Antimicrob Chemother 1994; 33(S):99–109.

39. Zhanel GG, Harding GKM, Guay DRP: Asymptomatic bacteriuria: Which patients should be treated? Arch Intern Med 1990; 150:1389–1396.

40. Mims AD, Norman DC, Yamamura RH, Yoshikawa TT: Clinically inapparent (asymptomatic) bacteriuria in ambulatory elderly men: Epidemiological, clinical and microbiological findings. J Am Geriatr Soc 1990; 38:1209–1214.

41. Nicolle LE: Urinary tract infections in the elderly. How to treat and when? Infections 1992; 4S:261–265.

42. Yoshikawa TT: Chronic urinary tract infections in elderly patients. Hosp Pract 1993; June 15, 28:103–118.

43. Stamm WE, Hooton TM: Management of urinary tract infections in adults. N Engl J Med 1993; 329(18): 1328–1334.

44. Breitenbucher RB: Bacterial changes in the urine samples of patients with long-term indwelling catheters. Arch Intern Med 1984; 144:1585–1588.

45. Warren JW: Catheter-associated bacteriuria. Clin Geriatr Med 1992; 8(4):805–819.

39 Musculoskeletal Disorders

Evan Calkins, M.D.

Adrian O. Vladutiu, M.D., Ph.D., F.A.C.P.

CLASSIFICATION AND PATHOPHYSIOLOGY

Aches and pains in the musculoskeletal system constitute the most frequent complaints of older persons (Fig. 39–1) and account for a very significant segment of the practice of primary care physicians caring for patients in this age group. The causes of these complaints fall into three categories: (1) the classic rheumatic diseases, (2) conditions not generally regarded as rheumatic in nature whose clinical manifestations are expressed in the musculoskeletal system, and (3) a wide range of musculoskeletal disorders, primarily localized in nature, that fall under the general category of "soft tissue rheumatism." The process of aging is accompanied by an increased frequency of conditions in all three of these categories.

Among the classic rheumatic diseases, certain entities, such as Still's disease, Reiter's disease, and new-onset ankylosing spondylitis, occur ex-clusively among young people and do not need to be considered in the differential diagnosis in older persons. In contrast, many other conditions, such as polymyalgia rheumatica, giant cell arteritis, Sjögren's syndrome, and calcium pyrophosphatase deposition disease, are rarely seen among young persons and occur primarily or exclusively in the older population.[1] Rheumatoid arthritis and gout occur in persons at many stages of life but are seen with increasing frequency in the later years. While osteoarthritis has its origins in early life (through genetic determinants, developmental problems affecting posture, and traumatic injuries), it rarely emerges as a significant clinical problem in persons under 40 years of age. However, it affects an estimated 80% of people aged 70 and older. Thus, there is a close interface between many of the classic rheumatic diseases and the process of aging.

At all stages of life, but especially among older patients, a number of disorders, not usually regarded as rheumatic in nature, are manifested

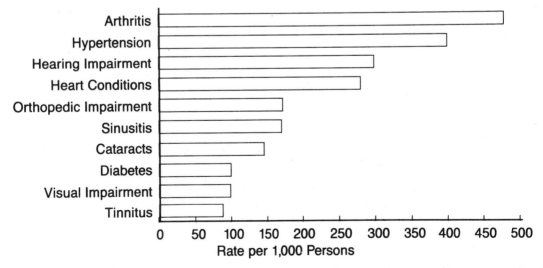

Figure 39–1 Morbidity from top ten chronic conditions among the elderly. Relative frequency of most common chronic conditions among persons aged 65 and older. (From National Center for Health Statistics: Current estimates from the National Health Interview Survey: United States, 1986. Vital and Health Statistics Series 10, No. 164, 1987.)

by musculoskeletal symptoms or accentuate the symptoms of coincidental rheumatic disorders. Some of these, osteoporosis and Paget's disease, for example, are disorders of the musculoskeletal system. Others, such as metastatic carcinoma and multiple myeloma, involve the skeletal system secondarily. Still others are disorders of the endocrine system. In addition to causing loss of skeletal calcium, hyperthyroidism is often associated with constitutional manifestations resembling rheumatoid arthritis and accentuates the symptoms, especially the constitutional symptoms, of the latter disease. Similarly, in a person with long-standing rheumatoid arthritis who exhibits progressive slowing of the locomotor system and gruffness of the voice, it is all too easy to attribute these symptoms to the rheumatoid process, failing to recognize the simultaneous presence of myxedema, treatment of which almost always yields significant improvement in the symptoms of rheumatoid arthritis.

Finally, and of special importance, there is the range of localized entities such as bursitis, tendonitis, muscle strain, fasciitis, fibromyalgia, and the various conditions leading to low back pain, all of which occur with increasing frequency in the older age group. Indeed, it is surprising that anyone can live out his allotted years without being afflicted by one condition or another that leads to musculoskeletal pain.

The multiplicity of musculoskeletal disorders, often in multiples, that afflict almost all older people lends a quality of nonspecificity to musculoskeletal symptoms among older patients that is rarely seen in the young. When young people present with pain in the joints, the problem is apt to fall within the framework of either a traumatic injury or one of the classic rheumatic disorders. When an older person complains of soreness and stiffness of the bones and joints, the cause is as apt to be metastatic carcinoma, osteoporosis, Paget's disease, an endocrinopathy, or a neurologic disorder such as Parkinson's disease as it is a classic rheumatic disease. If one adds the range of problems that are secondary to efforts to treat these conditions, and the influence that these disorders have on the functional capacity, independence, and emotional well-being of older people, one gains a perspective on the importance and complexity of musculoskeletal symptoms and disorders in the older segment of one's practice.

CLINICAL ASSESSMENT

History

Even in a busy primary care office, it is preferable to obtain a history with the patient fully clothed and sitting in a comfortable chair rather than perched on an examining table. The history of the present illness should start with the patient's earliest experience with musculoskeletal symptoms. These initial manifestations may prove more helpful in establishing a diagnosis than more recent symptoms because the latter are influenced by a variety of secondary processes.

As one attempts to differentiate a local or structural abnormality in the musculoskeletal system from a systemic condition, it is important to inquire carefully about the presence of constitutional symptoms such as fatigue, weight loss, and vasomotor instability resembling Raynaud's phenomenon, which are characteristic not only of many of the classic rheumatic diseases but also of metastatic carcinoma and multiple myeloma. One would not expect to encounter these symptoms in patients with osteoarthritis or gout unless they were due to an independent co-morbid systemic disease. It is particularly important to inquire specifically about the presence and duration of morning stiffness. Stiffness lasting for several hours or throughout the day is highly characteristic of rheumatoid arthritis, polymyalgia rheumatica, and remitting seronegative symmetrical synovitis with pitting edema (RS$_3$PE) syndrome. It is not characteristic of osteoarthritis, septic arthritis, or gout.

Physical Examination

After obtaining a history, it is important to watch the patient as he or she rises from the chair and walks around the room a bit, wearing shoes. Following this, the patient can undress as appropriate and climb onto the examining table. Rather than attempting to help, it is useful to watch the patient to obtain important information about the patient's functional status. For a patient with diffuse musculoskeletal symptoms it is important to carry out a complete physical examination including examination of the skin, lymph nodes, breasts, abdomen, and rectum plus a basic neurologic examination.

Laboratory Tests

In interpreting the laboratory data,[2] two points should be kept in mind. First, the process of aging itself yields values in some tests that would be regarded as abnormal in a younger person. For example, the erythrocyte sedimentation rate (ESR) reaches values of 30 to 35 mm in 1 hour in many healthy persons aged 80 or older.[2] Both rheumatoid factor (RF) and antinuclear antibodies (ANA), in low titer, are present in many persons aged 70 or older, including those with no rheumatic or other symptoms of definable illness.[2] Thus, the presence of RF in a titer of 1:64 (1280 IU) or ANA in a titer of less than 1:120 has no diagnostic or prognostic significance in a person aged 75 or older. In persons with slightly higher values in these tests, the interpretation should be made in the light of the clinical symptomatology, as discussed later in this chapter.

It is important to order laboratory procedures judiciously and properly. For example, for optimal interpretation of radiographs of the knee, it is essential to request specifically that the anteroposterior (AP) view be obtained with the patient standing so that the space between the surfaces of the femur and the tibia can be interpreted correctly as indicative of the depth of the interposed cartilage. To request an AP view of the knee without specifying the standing position will result in a radiograph that is of little or no value to a consulting rheumatologist or orthopedist and will almost surely have to be repeated. The lateral view of the knee, obtained to evaluate the patellofemoral interface, should be obtained in a supine position. The standing position is also helpful when obtaining AP views of the hips.

SPECIFIC CLINICAL ENTITIES

Osteoarthritis

Osteoarthritis (OA) is by far the most common musculoskeletal disorder of older people. Osteoarthritis of the hands, especially the distal interphalangeal joints but also the proximal interphalangeal joints, carpometacarpal joint of the thumb and wrists, and osteoarthritis of the hips, knees, and spine are all seen with increasing frequency in persons of advanced age, but may occur independently of each other. Although there is general agreement that the focal point of the osteoarthritic process is the joint cartilage, we still do not have a clear understanding of the pathogenetic mechanisms. Although patients frequently have a history of repeated trauma or overuse of a given joint, an abnormality in the joint cartilage, sometimes occurring as a familial tendency, is an important contributing factor.

Once it has set in, osteoarthritis, especially arthritis of the knee or hip, is a seriously disabling disorder that is associated with several patterns of pain. With osteoarthritis of the knees, for example, some people experience pain with every step they take, while others complain of crampy pain in the leg muscles after walking a short distance—a few hundred yards. Many patients with osteoarthritis of the knees experi-

ence pain at night. This may consist of severe boring pain in the knees themselves or diffuse cramps in the adjacent muscles.

Physical examination of the knee in severe cases reveals any or all of the following: bony thickening, decreased range of motion, crepitus on motion, weakness of the quadriceps muscles, flexion deformity, malalignment (subluxation) of the joint, lateral instability, synovial thickening, and, at times, effusion, with warmth and tenderness. The joint fluid exhibits decreased viscosity and a low white cell count (usually less than 5000/mm³). The process in the hip, shoulder, ankle, and wrist follows a generally similar pattern. In the wrist, the synovial thickening is constricted by the carpal ligaments, resulting, in many cases, in carpal tunnel syndrome.

TREATMENT OF OSTEOARTHRITIS

Analgesic Drugs. Treatment of osteoarthritis of the large joints involves use of analgesic drugs, basic modalities of physical therapy, additional support through use of a cane or walker and, at times, surgery.[3, 4] The mainstay of pharmacologic therapy is acetaminophen. The dose must be individualized, with lower doses prescribed for persons with any form of renal disease. Although the drug may be given in doses as high as 4000 mg/day, we usually limit it to 2000 mg/day in older people because higher doses may produce a sense of grogginess and an increased potential for renal toxicity.[5] Tinnitus does not occur. Blood urea nitrogen and serum creatinine determinations should be obtained every 3 or 4 months. In patients who do not obtain sufficient relief from acetaminophen, the dose can be reduced slightly and a small dose of propoxyphene added.

Most of the nonsteroidal antirheumatic drugs are also effective in reducing the pain and inflammation of osteoarthritis. However, especially in older persons, use of these drugs is frequently associated with gastropathy, often leading to upper gastrointestinal bleeding, which may be life-threatening.[6, 7] Unfortunately, screening for occult blood does not provide a warning of possible major blood loss; many patients in whom the Hemoccult test has been negative on several occasions suddenly develop an abrupt and unheralded upper gastrointestinal bleed. Similarly, one cannot count on upper gastrointestinal symptoms to provide a warning of an impending bleed.

The likelihood of nonsteroidal anti-inflammatory drug (NSAID) gastropathy can be reduced substantially if one seeks to identify and strictly avoid use of these drugs in patients at high risk for this complication. The risk factors include old age, multiple chronic diseases (such as heart disease, chronic obstructive pulmonary disease [COPD], and/or diabetes mellitus), and a history of a previous duodenal ulcer or upper gastrointestinal bleed.[8] In the absence of these contraindications, use of these agents in a moderate dose, such as ibuprofen 400 mg three times a day, naproxen 375 mg twice daily (or, at most, 500 mg bid), or other NSAIDs in moderate doses taken with meals, carries a considerably reduced risk of upper gastrointestinal bleeding. In patients who are at high risk for gastropathy whose pain cannot be controlled by acetaminophen with, perhaps, small doses of propoxyphene added, one can consider several alternative approaches. While simultaneous administration of H_2 blockers or sucralfate has little effect in inhibiting NSAID-induced gastric disease, misoprostol in a dose of 200 μg qid with meals and on retiring has been shown to be effective in this regard.[9] Misoprostol also has a suppressive effect on NSAID-induced duodenal disease, but its effectiveness in this case is minimal and is no greater than that achieved by H_2 blockers or sucralfate. Unfortunately, misoprostol is expensive and has a tendency to lead to diarrhea. Commencing therapy with a smaller dose, such as 100 μg two or three times daily, may alleviate this problem.

In patients in whom the symptoms are localized primarily in a single joint, intra-articular administration of a corticosteroid drug often yields relief that may last 3 or more months. These injections should not be repeated more frequently than three or four times a year, and the total series should not extend for more than a year and a half. In some patients administration of small doses of acetaminophen with codeine No. 3 may be indicated despite the risk of habituation. Surgical joint replacement may actually provide a better prognosis for life than use of NSAIDs in some of these high-risk patients with advanced osteoarthritis.

Exercise. A very important additional approach to providing symptomatic relief for patients with OA involves varied modalities of physical therapy, especially exercise.[10] Several patterns of exercise have proved quite effective. One emphasizes active muscle contraction against resistance.[11] For the quadriceps muscle, this can be accomplished by sitting on the edge of a firm table and raising the lower leg into the horizontal position using ankle weights. The weights, ranging between 1 and 7 pounds, are prescribed individually for each patient. We usually suggest 18 contractions, followed by a period in which the patient holds the knee horizontally extended for as long as possible; after a rest, the entire sequence is re-

peated over a period of 10 to 15 minutes. This process, which should be carried out within the limits of pain, should be repeated daily. Because exercises of this sort strengthen the muscle at the length at which the exercise is carried out, they should be performed with the patient in two positions, sitting vertically and lying horizontally with the lower legs dropped over the edge of the exercise table. An alternative approach, which is more difficult to monitor, is achieved by performing quadriceps setting exercises, in which the patient clenches the muscle vigorously but does not move the knee. This exercise should also be done in both sitting and lying positions. A 2 to 3 month exercise program, if conscientiously pursued, often results in significant increases in strength, decreased pain, and improvement in overall function. In our experience these benefits are particularly evident in patients who have experienced a crampy feeling in the legs after walking or at night.

The problem with a home-based exercise program is that it is extremely boring, and few patients will carry it out by themselves without frequent review and encouragement. Use of an exercise bicycle or rowing machine provides a more entertaining mode of exercise and is reasonably effective if it is carried out conscientiously. As an alternative, a group approach to exercise may be employed, with classes of approximately 20 patients supervised by a physical therapist and one assistant.[12] Such a program should include patient education and social support. Results have shown significant benefits in relief of pain, increase in function, and enhancement of the patient's sense of control over his or her disease.

An important aspect of management of patients with osteoarthritis is decreasing the level of stress on the joint as well as on the whole person. For individual patients, this may involve use of a cane or walker and, for obese people, loss of weight. Social and psychological support are also important elements of good care.[13, 14] Controlled trials have shown that programs of health education and continuing telephone contact with patients yield improved functional status and decreased overall costs.[15–17]

Surgery. Improved surgical intervention in patients with osteoarthritis, especially joint replacement, is one of the major advances that have occurred in rheumatology during the past 50 years. The attitude of the patient is an important determinant of success. A patient who is determined to regain full activity and does so quickly will achieve a far better result than the dependent "show me" type of person. Prior to surgery, the patient should be informed about the importance of appropriate follow-up, together with the need to receive prophylactic antibiotics in conjunction with dental and rectal procedures, which is similar to the recommendation for patients with artificial cardiac valves.

Rheumatoid Arthritis

The second most frequent rheumatic disease among the older population is rheumatoid arthritis (RA). Despite the life-limiting impact of RA and its treatment,[18, 19] the majority of patients who develop the disease in early or midlife live on to old age and present to their physicians problems of reduced physical function, decreased resistance to infection, and, in many, severe osteoporosis secondary to long-term prednisone therapy. In addition, since the incidence of rheumatoid arthritis increases with age,[20] a number of older patients with new-onset disease will be encountered as well.

The manifestations and course of RA in old people are slightly different from those in younger persons. Several clinical presentations have been described.[21] Approximately one fourth of patients have an acute onset of disease, manifested by swelling, tenderness, and pain on motion of the hands, wrists, elbows, knees, and ankles. The disease occurs over the course of several days or even overnight and is often accompanied by severe morning stiffness and constitutional symptoms. Most of these patients experience a complete remission in time.[22] In another group, possibly 25%, the pain, tenderness, and stiffness are focused primarily in the shoulders, hips, and wrists, sparing the hands. These patients have symptoms closely resembling those of polymyalgia rheumatica, including, in some, a markedly elevated ESR value, and their disease may bear a relationship to this disorder.[23] Although, for the most part, patients with late-life onset have a somewhat better outcome in terms of the likelihood of remission than is true for patients with onset earlier in life, there is a small percentage of older patients who have a high titer of RF and have the same adverse course that prevails in younger persons with seropositive disease.

Differentiation of rheumatoid arthritis from osteoarthritis is extremely important and is often more difficult than it is in younger individuals. While the classic differential characteristics may be present in persons at midlife, this is frequently not the case in older patients. For example, osteoarthritis may involve the proximal interphalangeal joints more than the distal interphalangeal joints. Osteoarthritis of the large joints often

leads to joint effusion and synovial thickening accompanied by warmth and sometimes tenderness, closely resembling the symptoms one sees in rheumatoid arthritis. While osteoarthritis does not lead to constitutional symptoms, older people frequently have coincidental diseases that can cause these symptoms. Many, possibly most, older patients experiencing new-onset RA have considerable osteoarthritis as well, which is enhanced in time by the sequelae of the rheumatoid process. The fact that both the ESR and RF values reach levels in many older people that would be significant in younger persons lessens the diagnostic value of these determinations in the older population. Thus, the differentiation between these common entities in many older people is by no means easy.

Synovial fluid examination often provides a reliable clue to the correct diagnosis. In patients with rheumatoid arthritis the fluid is watery in consistency, and the white cell count is almost always increased—in the range of 5000 to 25,000/mm³. In patients with osteoarthritis the fluid is viscous, and the white cell count is low. Synovial fluid should also be examined under polarized light for crystals of uric acid or calcium pyrophosphate. Calcium pyrophosphate deposition (CaPPD) disease often occurs in the presence of osteoarthritis and provides an additional explanation of the inflammatory manifestations that may be seen with this condition.[24]

The differential diagnosis between rheumatoid arthritis and osteoarthritis is important for therapy. Some patients with rheumatoid arthritis derive considerable relief from aspirin, coated or buffered, in a dose of 2.6 to 3.9 g/day (8 to 12 tablets) with meals. Use of higher doses, often recommended in younger persons, is rarely attempted in older people because of their increased sensitivity to the auditory and gastrointestinal side effects. Salsalate, 750 mg bid, provides a more convenient mode of administration of salicylate and has fewer gastrointestinal side effects. Determination of the blood salicylate level will confirm that the agent is in fact being absorbed. A concentration of 15 to 20 mg/dL is the desired level. In patients in whom salicylate provides inadequate relief, a trial with a NSAID is usually justified. The potential hazards of NSAID therapy and the precautions that should be taken have already been mentioned. Examples of commonly used NSAIDs include ibuprofen, 400 mg tid, sulindac (Clinoril) 150 mg bid, and naproxen 375 mg two or three times daily. Acetaminophen is seldom of value in patients with rheumatoid arthritis. It is rarely if ever justifiable to use codeine or other narcotic agents in patients with rheumatoid arthritis except in those in whom the symptoms focus in a single joint, such as the hip or knee, and a decision has already been made to undertake joint replacement. Joint injection with a corticosteroid preparation (usually given, for a large joint, in a dose of 40 mg of corticosteroid diluted in 3 to 4 mL of 1% lidocaine) almost always provides considerable symptomatic relief that may last for 2 to 4 months. These injections may be repeated two or three times during the course of a year. It is believed that larger series of injections exert an adverse effect on the articular tissues.

Simultaneously with the use of these agents, it is important to place the patient on a good conservative regimen, including rest and exercise. Rheumatoid arthritis is a constitutional disease, and carefully monitored rest is an important component of therapy. Rest should be prescribed in specific terms and with the same care one would take in prescribing a potentially toxic drug. As a rule, patients should achieve the degree of rest necessary to avoid fatigue. Complete bed rest, however, should never be prescribed for an older person for fear that the patient may lose the ability to walk. Even older patients with active arthritis should be encouraged to walk every day, often with the help of a walker, to the bathroom and meal table.

If an older patient fails to show symptomatic improvement during the course of about 6 to 8 weeks on this program, a more effective antirheumatic agent should be prescribed. Indeed, there is an increasing consensus that introduction of a second-line antirheumatic drug early in the course of the disease may attenuate the destructive changes of the disease.[25] Although sulfasalazine and hydroxychloroquine have been extensively studied[26] and have been shown to be valuable, especially in younger patients, their usefulness as sole second-line therapy in older patients remains questionable. As one describes the possibility that hydroxychloroquine may accumulate in their eyes and may affect the retina, many older patients become fearful and do not welcome the prospect of slit lamp and retinal examinations before and at intervals during therapy. A recently developed antirheumatic agent, tenidap, shows promise as an effective and relatively nontoxic alternative to NSAIDs,[27] but little experience with it has yet been achieved in older patients.

In patients who do not respond to a 6- to 8-week trial of the conservative program outlined earlier, the addition of methotrexate, a folic acid antagonist, may offer additional benefit. To prevent secondary folic acid deficiency, patients receiving this drug should also be given folic acid, either 1 mg po qd or 5 mg 1 day per week.

This does not interfere with the antirheumatic effectiveness of the methotrexate. Although severe pancytopenia has been described early in the course of methotrexate therapy,[28] and guidelines clearly indicate the importance of obtaining complete blood cell counts at 1- to 2-month intervals throughout the course of treatment, this is a rare complication. The most common side effect, abnormalities in liver function, requires tests of the alanine aminotransferase (ALT) level at similar intervals. Since a decline in serum albumin concentration often precedes an elevation in the ALT level, it is a good practice to measure the serum ALT, serum albumin, and total protein ("liver profile") as well as the complete blood cell count every 4 to 6 weeks. Alcohol should be strictly forbidden. The initial dose of methotrexate, 7.5 mg po 1 day per week, may be increased to twice that level if the initial response is not satisfactory.[29] If gastrointestinal symptoms ensue, the drug may be given intramuscularly, watching the serum chemistry values and complete blood cell count carefully. Elevations of ALT to twice the upper levels of normal is not a cause for alarm, but higher values may require discontinuation of the drug. Since pulmonary fibrosis is an occasional but serious complication of methotrexate therapy, chest films should be obtained prior to initiation of treatment, at intervals of 1 to 1½ years afterwards, or if the patient develops chronic cough or dyspnea. The drug should be stopped immediately if pulmonary sequelae ensue.

Methotrexate is a highly effective agent in older people,[30] especially in patients whose disease is accompanied by marked synovial thickening. Benefit is not achieved, however, until after about 2 months of treatment. If a satisfactory response is not obtained, even with an increased dosage, the addition of a second remittive drug, such as sulfasalazine or hydroxychloroquine, can be considered.[31] In patients with seropositive rheumatoid arthritis, methotrexate therapy may be accompanied by an increase in the size of the nodules, an effect that may be attenuated by the addition of hydroxychloroquine. Once a satisfactory response has been achieved and the patient's condition has stabilized, the dose should be tapered gradually, watching for signs of increased disease activity.

In patients in whom methotrexate, possibly in combination with another second-line agent, is not effective or is deemed inappropriate, and in patients in whom an immediate symptomatic improvement is mandated by their social situation or serious malnutrition and "failure to thrive," the most practical alternative is low-dose prednisone therapy.[32] Although the adverse implications of this approach, in terms of initiation or exacerbation of diabetes mellitus, hypertension, or osteoporosis, are not to be taken lightly, these sequelae are infrequently seen when doses are limited to not more than 8 mg/day (i.e., one 5-mg tablet and three 1-mg tablets, all taken together in the morning). It is prudent not to start therapy in patients with rheumatoid arthritis with doses greater than 10 mg/day. Reductions in dose should be undertaken extremely slowly. By restoring the capacity for enhanced physical activity to a patient who would otherwise be bed- or chair-bound, the benefits of the activity counterbalance to a considerable extent the negative effects of the drug on the osseous skeleton.

Osteoporosis constitutes an important threat for older patients with rheumatoid arthritis, especially those who are receiving maintenance prednisone therapy, even in low doses. Such patients should be given estrogen replacement therapy, if tolerated, and also supplemental calcium, with vitamin D, to yield a total intake of 1500 mg of calcium per day. Patients who are at high risk for osteoporosis, who cannot tolerate or will not accept estrogen replacement or in whom it is contraindicated, should receive alendronate, 10 mg per day, po, taken 45 minutes before breakfast, with the patient sitting erect.[33] For patients with severe osteoporosis and fractures, a combination of estrogen and alendronate is probably indicated. Whether alendronate treatment should be continued for longer than 3 years has not yet been determined. Guidelines have recently been developed for prevention and management of steroid-induced osteoporosis in patients with rheumatoid arthritis.[34]

Continued treatment with methotrexate or prednisone or both does not relieve the patient from the need to continue all elements of the conservative program, including periods of rest, exercise (within the limits of pain), local heat or ice, as required by symptoms, and continued strides toward functional independence.

Gout

The frequency of gout increases with age, especially in postmenopausal women, in whom the frequency of acute attacks is equal to that of men of comparable age. Diagnosis is suspected on clinical grounds (which are slightly different in the older population)[35] and is confirmed by the demonstration of urate crystals in synovial fluid. The treatment is more effective the earlier it is begun. Patients with recurrent gouty attacks can usually anticipate an attack by noting very minor symptoms. When these occur, prompt administration of 0.6 mg of colchicine, two or three tablets throughout the first day, followed by one tablet daily for 3 or 4 days, often aborts the attack. When full-blown gouty arthritis occurs, treatment with the classic regimen of colchicine (0.6 mg po every 2 hours until relief or diarrhea occurs) is not recommended in older patients. Short courses of a NSAID such as indomethacin, 100 mg the first day, 75 mg daily for 2 or 3 days, 50 mg for 2 or 3 days, 25 mg for 2 days, and then stop, are usually effective but may carry a high risk of gastropathy, as previously discussed. Prednisone in an initial dose of 20 mg/day is effective in some patients but disappointing in others. For gout in large joints, intra-articular injection of a corticosteroid may be effective and avoids the hazards of systemic therapy. It has recently been shown that a former mode of therapy, adrenocorticotropic hormone (ACTH), given in doses of 40 or 80 units intramuscularly three times a day with subsequent tapering over 3 or 4 days, is an effective mode of therapy in older patients with co-morbid disease.[36] Colchicine, 0.6 mg/day, should be started at the midpoint of any of these regimens to decrease the likelihood of flare-up after the initial drug has been discontinued.

Patients with gout that has been inactive for a considerable period of time, either spontaneously or because of small doses of colchicine, may have an acute attack during periods of hospitalization for coincidental disease. It is important to anticipate and prevent this occurrence by continuing the colchicine or reestablishing it during the period of hospitalization. Gout is an eminently treatable condition. In managing an older patient with chronic or acute gout one should not be content with anything less than a perfect or close-to-perfect result.

Pseudogout (CaPPD Disease)

Accumulation of calcium pyrophosphate crystals in joint cartilage of the knees and, less frequently, shoulders, metacarpal phalangeal joints, elbows, hips, metatarsal phalangeal joints, and wrists is a common concomitant of aging and occurs in as many as 20% of women aged 75 and older and less frequently in men.[24] In approximately one fourth of these patients this condition, chondrocalcinosis, is accompanied by pain and inflammatory symptoms resembling those seen in acute gout.[37] The treatment of pseudogout is similar to but less effective than that for gout. Accumulation of crystals in the shoulder joint may lead to the so-called Milwaukee shoulder, accompanied by severe pain, limitation of motion, and damage to the joint.[38]

Septic Arthritis

In a patient with long-standing chronic arthritis, either osteoarthritis or rheumatoid arthritis, the existence of inflammatory changes—pain, swelling, redness, and tenderness—in a single joint that are out of proportion to the findings in other joints should lead to a suspicion not only of gout but, more importantly, of a septic process. Joint aspiration should be undertaken, cultures obtained, and the synovial fluid examined for crystals. Treatment with intravenous antibiotics should be undertaken. Joint aspiration should be carried out daily to facilitate drainage and permit assessment of the response.

Polymyalgia Rheumatica and Giant Cell Arteritis

The frequency of polymyalgia rheumatica in older patients approximates that of rheumatoid arthritis. Clinical features include severe aching and stiffness, absence of objective inflammation of the large joints, and, in most cases, a strikingly elevated ESR.[39] Rapid response to a test dose of prednisone, 15 mg/day for 2 or 3 days, supports the diagnosis. Treatment with low-dose prednisone, 7 or 8 mg/day, is almost always effective in relieving symptoms. While the condition often subsides during the course of 1 or 2 years, the symptoms may continue in some patients indefinitely, flaring up as the dose of prednisone is gradually decreased.

Temporal arteritis occurs in approximately 8% to 10% of patients with polymyalgia rheumatica.[40] Visual difficulties, such as zigzag lines in a visual field or a general dimness of vision, soreness or claudication of the masseter muscles, and tenderness over the temporal artery are important clues to the presence of this disorder. Once the condition is seriously suspected the patient should be started immediately on prednisone in a dose of 70 or 80 mg/day. Gradual lowering of the dose is guided by symptoms; serial determinations of the ESR may be helpful but are by no means an infallible guide.

Failure to recognize temporal arteritis in its earliest stages and initiate prompt treatment may result in permanent blindness. Biopsy of the temporal arteries is usually undertaken in suspected cases to confirm the diagnosis. Nevertheless, the process of obtaining the biopsy should not be permitted to delay initiation of prednisone therapy because of the very real hazard that the patient will develop blindness while one is awaiting the results of the biopsy. Since the histologic change in the artery is often spotty in nature, the biopsy does not always show the charac-

teristic lesions, even in the presence of active disease. No significant change in the histologic appearance of the artery occurs after the initial few days of prednisone therapy, and the biopsy may be undertaken after the drug has been initiated.

Remitting Seronegative Symmetrical Synovitis with Pitting Edema Syndrome (RS₃PE)

Analogous, in some ways, to polymyalgia rheumatica, this syndrome is characterized by a sudden onset of symmetrical tenderness, redness and swelling of the hands, wrists, forearms, and, at times, pretibial areas and feet, accompanied by striking morning stiffness, which often lasts up to 6 hours.[41] Involvement focuses primarily in the tendon sheaths. Laboratory studies show a markedly elevated ESR and a disproportionate increase in the percentage of the HLA-B7 haplotype. Radiographs show no evidence of articular involvement. Of the 30 cases described to date, men outnumber women by a factor of two; mean age of onset is 75 years. Treatment with prednisone, in dosages resembling those used for polymyalgia rheumatica, is usually effective.

Use of Immunologic Tests in Older Patients

Although systemic lupus erythematosus (SLE) has been described in persons of far-advanced age, even in their nineties, this is an extremely rare occurrence. Of all patients with SLE, only approximately 2% are 70 or older. In contrast, older persons frequently present manifestations that suggest the possibility of SLE, such as fever, arthralgia, fatigue, weight loss, pleural chest pain, rashes of various sorts, and Raynaud's phenomenon. Most of these symptoms are also characteristic of entities that are much more common in older patients than SLE. The primary care physician, concerned about the possibility that these symptoms may indeed reflect SLE or one of the other connective tissue diseases, is faced with the need to determine which of the variety of available serologic studies should be obtained in a cost-effective work-up. Table 39–1 provides guidance in this regard (see also references 42 to 49).

An ANA screening test is the most appropriate first step. In most laboratories, if the test is positive in a dilution of 1:40 it will be followed by a quantitative titration. In older patients, a titer of 1:160 or above is clinically significant. This occurs in more than 95% of patients with SLE or drug-induced lupus, 95% of those with mixed connec-

TABLE 39–1 **PREVALENCE OF THE MOST COMMONLY TESTED ANTIBODIES ASSOCIATED WITH SYSTEMIC RHEUMATIC DISEASES**

Antibody	RA (%)	SLE (%)	Drug-Induced Lupus (%)	PSS (%)	CREST Syndrome (%)	MCTD (%)	PM/DM (%)	Sjögren's Syndrome (%)
IF-ANA	30–50	>98	>95	80–90	80–90	95	30–40	70–90
Anti-dsDNA	—	50–70°	>1	—	—	—	—	—
Anti-histone	<20	60–70	>95°	—	—	>80	—	—
Anti-Sm	—	15–30°	—	—	—	—	—	—
Anti-U1-RNP	—	35–40	—	15–20	5–20	>95°	5	<5
Anti-SS-A/Ro	5–10	30–50	—	—	—	—	<5	80–95
Anti-SS-B/La	—	15–20	—	—	—	—	—	70–95°
Anti-Scl-70	—	—	—	30–60°	15–20	—	—	—
Anti-centromere	—	—	—	10–15	70–90°	—	—	—
Anti-PM-1 and Jo-1	—	—	—	—	—	—	30–60°	—

Abbreviations: RA, rheumatoid arthritis: SLE, systemic lupus erythematosus; PSS, progressive systemic sclerosis; CREST, variant of scleroderma; MCTD, mixed connective tissue disease; PM/DM, polymyositis/dermatomyositis; IF-ANA, antinuclear antibodies as detected by immunofluorescence assay.
°High diagnostic value of the antibodies.

tive tissue disease, and a high percentage (more than 70%) of those with progressive systemic sclerosis, the CREST syndrome (calcinosis, Raynaud's phenomenon, esophageal dysmotility, sclerodactyly, and telangiectasias), and Sjögren's syndrome. It is also positive in many patients with rheumatoid arthritis, in occasional patients with polymyositis, periarteritis nodosum, and Waldenström's macroglobulinemia and in about 50% of patients with myasthenia gravis. Thus, a positive ANA test result is not in itself diagnostic of systemic lupus. Different patterns of nuclear fluorescence, visualized in the ANA test, are often reported. The homogeneous and speckled patterns are very nonspecific. The peripheral pattern, which is thought to correspond to antibodies directed to DNA or DNA histones, is predominantly seen in SLE. The nucleolar pattern is seen in patients with systemic sclerosis or Sjögren's syndrome, while the centromere pattern is characteristic of the CREST syndrome.

In patients with symptoms suggestive of SLE, the next test to be obtained, following the ANA test, is an anti-double stranded or native DNA (dsDNA) test. A positive reaction provides strong confirmation of the diagnosis and is also useful in following patients with SLE. Another autoantibody test that is characteristic of SLE is the anti-Sm antibody. Although ANAs are present both in SLE and in drug-induced lupus, antibodies to dsDNA and Sm (by enzyme-linked immunosorbent assay [ELISA] IgG, the method currently employed) are specific for SLE and are not found in drug-induced lupus. Conversely, the antihistone antibodies, which are frequently present in drug-induced lupus, are not seen in SLE. The anti-SS-A/Ro and anti-SS-B/La antibodies are not necessary to confirm the diagnosis of SLE. The chief value of these antibodies is to identify the presence of Sjögren's syndrome, either as an independent entity or in association with SLE or RA. In patients in whom progressive systemic sclerosis is suspected, the detection of anti-Scl-70 will prove useful.

Systemic Lupus Erythematosus

Considerable interest has been shown in the question, Do the clinical manifestations of this disease, occurring in an older population, differ from those seen in patients with early-onset disease, and if so, how? Because of the rarity of this disorder among persons aged 70 and older, the demarcation between "young" and "old," in the various series, ranges from age 40 to age 60. There is general agreement that the patient with late-onset illness has an increased frequency of interstitial pulmonary disease, serositis, and symptoms suggestive of Sjögren's syndrome and a decreased frequency of fever, Raynaud's phenomenon, lymphadenopathy, and psychiatric illness.[50-52] Nephritis, arthritis, rash, photosensitivity, myalgia, leukopenia, and thrombocytopenia occur in patients with older-onset disease in the same frequency as that seen in younger individuals. Serologic studies show a greater frequency of the anti-SS-B/La antibody in the older age group, while hypocomplementemia and rheumatoid factor are frequently seen in patients with early-onset disease. Prednisone is the most frequently used therapeutic agent in older patients with SLE; methotrexate may be added in patients who do not respond. In patients with mild disease, especially if photosensitivity is present, hydroxychloroquine is sometimes effective.

Drug-Induced Lupus

In contrast to SLE, the syndrome of drug-induced lupus occurs with increasing frequency in older patients owing, at least in part, to the large number of drugs consumed by many of these patients. Procainamide and hydralazine are most often implicated and lead to the development of ANA in 50% to 70% of cases. Other commonly used drugs that may lead to this syndrome include isoniazid, sulfonamides, diphenylhydantoin, penicillin, and tetracycline.[53] The predominant ANA is antihistone. Antibodies to dsDNA, Sm (by ELISA IgG), SS-A/Ro, and SS-B/La are negative. Only one third of patients who develop ANA have symptoms. Fever, arthralgia, swelling, and tenderness of many peripheral joints, often accompanied by severe morning stiffness, are the most common symptoms. Pleuritis and parenchymal involvement of the lung, sometimes accompanied by hemoptysis, may also occur. Hepatosplenomegaly and pericarditis are present in fewer than 10% of cases. Manifestations common in SLE but rarely observed in drug-induced lupus include rash, alopecia, hemolytic anemia, thrombocytopenia, leukopenia, and renal involvement. Most patients with procainamide-induced lupus are males; the majority of those with hydralazine-induced disease are females. The disorder is rare among African-Americans. The duration of therapy prior to appearance of clinical manifestations varies and depends in part on the genetically controlled activity of drug acetylation in the liver.[54] Persons with reduced acetylation activity have a higher frequency of drug-induced lupus than rapid acetylators and develop the clinical manifestations after a shorter period of drug therapy (an average of 12 months compared to 48 months for the fast-acetylators). Treatment involves discontinuation of the lupus-inducing agent. If manifestations continue for a period of 2 months or more thereafter, the possibility of underlying SLE should be considered.

Sjögren's Syndrome

In sharp contrast to the low frequency of SLE among the elderly, Sjögren's syndrome (SS) is one of the most frequent rheumatologic entities found in this age group and has a frequency of approximately that of rheumatoid arthritis. The classic sicca syndromes, xerostomia and xerophthalmia, occur in 15% to 25% of otherwise normal older people.[55] These symptoms should be differentiated from those associated with true SS, a constitutional illness, in which xerostomia and xerophthalmia are accompanied by a range of systemic manifestations that may include fatigue, depression, migraine headaches, hoarseness, difficulty in swallowing, achlorhydria, nephritis, Raynaud's syndrome, vasculitic skin eruptions, enlargement of the lacrimal glands, and occasionally chronic pulmonary insufficiency, peripheral neuropathy, Bell's palsy, epilepsy, and stroke.[56, 57]

Sjögren's syndrome is present in 10% to 20% of patients with rheumatoid arthritis and in up to 38% of patients with late-onset SLE. It has also been encountered among patients with systemic sclerosis and mixed connective tissue disease. It occurs as an independent entity in about a third of the cases. In patients in whom xerophthalmia is suspected, a Schirmer's test provides effective and inexpensive confirmation. To perform the test, a piece of Whatman's No. 41 filter paper, 0.25 cm wide and 3 cm long, is folded, and one end is placed in the lower eyelid. In the presence of normal tears, at least 1.5 cm of the paper will be saturated in 5 minutes. In patients with keratoconjunctivitis sicca the moistening covers 0.5 cm or less of the paper. Another procedure for confirming the presence of keratoconjunctivitis sicca involves slit lamp examination following intraocular instillation of rose bengal dye. Anti-SS-A/Ro and anti-SS-B/La antibodies, if present, are also helpful in supporting the clinical diagnosis. Although for practical purposes the disorder can usually be diagnosed on the basis of its clinical manifestations and immunologic reactions, full confirmation requires biopsy, usually obtained from the lip. Demonstration of diffuse lymphocytic infiltration of the mucosal glands confirms the presence of SS.

Between 5% and 10% of patients with longstanding SS eventually develop B-cell lymphoma. Others develop renal tubular dysfunction. Most patients, however, do not show these complications and have good survival rates but continue to grapple with extremely troublesome symptoms. Keratoconjunctivitis sicca, if improperly treated, may lead to permanent loss of vision. Loss of normal salivary function is often associated with severe dental problems.

Treatment of SS is predominantly symptomatic. Artificial tears without preservatives and lemon-and-glycerine mouth rinses are the backbone of therapy. Corticosteroid eye medications should not be used because they may cause further damage to the cornea. Systemic corticosteroids in low doses may be helpful in patients with enlarged tender salivary glands and severe constitutional symptoms. The effect of corticosteroid therapy on other manifestations of chronic

SS has not been studied adequately. The Sjögren's Syndrome Foundation provides extremely effective support services. These include a monthly publication, The Moisture Seekers, an excellent book (*The Sjögren's Syndrome Handbook*), and a support network for patients and families. All patients with this syndrome should be given access to this extremely helpful source of information. The foundation can be reached at 333 North Broadway, Jericho, NY (telephone [516] 933–6365).

Progressive Systemic Sclerosis (Scleroderma)

This syndrome occurs primarily in late middle age.[58] It is seen occasionally in patients aged 65 or older, either as a new entity or in patients who have grown old with their disease. The characteristic clinical changes are thickening and atrophy of the skin of the hands and often subtle changes in the face as well. When the condition is first seen in old persons, the close resemblance of its manifestations, especially changes in facial expression, to those of normal aging is such that the diagnosis is easily overlooked. As the disease progresses, the hand changes take on the characteristics of sclerodactyly, with limited motion of the interphalangeal joints and marked thickening and atrophy of the skin. The fingertips show loss of the normal pulp and frequently pits or scars that tend to become infected. X-ray films may show loss of bone from the distal phalanges. The skin changes frequently extend into the forearms and anterior chest, where the skin appears to be bound to the rib cage more tightly than normal. Esophageal dysmotility is frequently present. Progressive fibrosis or vascular changes are often seen in the lung, gastrointestinal tract, heart, and kidney, and sometimes lead to chronic pulmonary fibrosis or severe hypertension.

Two other clinical syndromes are either closely related to or are variants of scleroderma. These are the CREST syndrome[59] and the so-called mixed connective tissue disease. The latter entity is characterized by edema of the hands, Raynaud's phenomenon, esophageal dysmotility, and, at times, pulmonary changes.[60]

Treatment of scleroderma and its related disorders includes supportive measures, such as the use of thermal gloves, down slippers or boots, emollients for the skin, and antibiotic treatment of infected ulcers on the fingertips. Patients should stop smoking. Calcium channel blocking agents, alpha-adrenergic blocking agents, or catecholamine-depleting agents such as reserpine may be helpful in the treatment of Raynaud's phenomenon. Penicillamine has been recommended for patients who are beginning to show changes in the lung or gastrointestinal tract.[61] Treatment should be started early in the disease in a dose of 250 to 500 mg/day and should be continued for at least 2 to 4 years. Penicillamine-related myasthenia symptoms are seldom encountered. Cyclophosphamide may prove helpful in patients with pulmonary fibrosis and active alveolitis. As a last resort, short courses of prednisone, in a dose of 20 to 60 mg/day, may be employed in patients with active disease, although some investigators are concerned that this may increase the likelihood of renal crisis. If acute hypertensive crisis occurs, it often responds well to the use of potent antihypertensive agents, especially inhibitors of angiotensin-converting enzyme, such as captopril. Renal dialysis may be necessary.

Fibromyalgia

One of the more common entities encountered in a primary care practice is a syndrome of chronic tiredness, often accompanied by diffuse muscle aching, stiffness, sharply localized sites of deep tenderness (so-called tender points), and sleeplessness. Although some clinicians regard these symptoms as nonspecific sequelae of chronic anxiety, depression, or overwork, there is increasing recognition of the concept that the syndrome does represent a specific entity known as fibromyalgia and that this is one of the more common musculoskeletal disorders.[62] Key to the diagnosis is the demonstration of sharply localized areas of deep tenderness, which frequently occur at the base of the neck, posterior aspect of the shoulders, upper portion of the chest, presacral area, and adjacent to the elbows or knees. If carefully sought, one can detect these tender points in as many as 12 loci in a given patient. Four such points are regarded as a requisite for the diagnosis. Fibromyalgia may exist independently of other musculoskeletal conditions or it may accompany other disorders, especially rheumatoid arthritis and SLE.

Many theories have been advanced concerning the pathophysiology and pathogenesis of the disorder, but no agreement has yet been reached. The treatment most commonly used, antidepressants and muscle relaxants, is only modestly effective. Recent attention has been paid to the overlap between many characteristics of fibromyalgia and those of another common but puzzling disorder, chronic fatigue syndrome.[63] A new and promising approach to the treatment of the latter disorder[64] may provide a new approach to the issue of fibromyalgia as well. Information for patients with fibromyalgia is provided in the

Fibromyalgia Network News Letter, obtainable from the Fibromyalgia Network, PO Box 31750, Tucson, Arizona 85751 (telephone [602] 290-5508).

Paget's Disease of Bone

Although not regarded as one of the rheumatic diseases, Paget's disease of bone is a common cause of disability among older patients.[65-67] This is a localized disorder of bone characterized by an increase in osteoclastic mediated bone resorption and accompanied by osteoblastic mediated new bone formation. Due to the chaotic nature of the newly created bone, it is architecturally inferior, leading to a propensity for fractures and, in advanced cases, to skeletal deformities including bowing of the legs and an enlarged skull. Thought to be triggered initially by a virus, the disease has a prolonged course, lasting many decades from the earliest symptoms to advanced manifestations. The predominant symptom is pain. This may arise from the bone itself, in which case it occurs predominantly at night when the patient is lying in bed. The pain may also be due to osteoarthritic changes in the joints secondary to the abnormal stresses caused by bone deformity. Many patients with Paget's disease also suffer from gouty arthritis, thought to be due to the increased turnover of nucleotides in the highly vascular lesions. Approximately one third of patients have calcific periarthritis. Other symptoms are due to pressure on neurostructures by the deformed bone, leading to deafness, neuropathy, and occasionally visual changes, even blindness. Warmth of the skin over the involved lesions, a roaring noise through the ears, and occasionally general lassitude or even cognitive deficiency may be present owing to the shunting of blood through the vascular pagetic lesions, which robs key organs of their share of blood. Although the disease itself is not fatal, it occasionally evolves into an osteosarcoma or other mesenchymal tumor.

For many years, the most effective treatment for Paget's disease was salmon or human calcitonin. Although usually effective, this agent has the disadvantage that it must be given either by injection or by nasal spray. In addition, formation of antibodies, especially with the salmon preparation, frequently leads to unresponsiveness. More recently, the use of the bisphosphonates has gained favor because of the greater ease of administration and decreased frequency of resistance. Etidronate, if given with care, usually leads to a good response of clinical manifestations and biochemical parameters. More recently developed bisphosphonates[33] provide several advantages, including a decrease in propensity for development of osteomalacia and effectiveness in patients who are resistant to etidronate.

SOFT TISSUE RHEUMATISM: MEDICAL ORTHOPEDICS

The largest segment of musculoskeletal complaints among older people relates, not to the systemic rheumatic diseases such as those mentioned earlier, but to a range of localized conditions involving tendons, bursi, muscle sheets, and muscles themselves, which fall under the general heading of soft tissue rheumatism.[68]

The diagnosis of these disorders rests primarily on a careful history and a well-informed physical examination. An example of such a diagnosis can be illustrated by a consideration of pain in the shoulder. Inflammation of the shoulder joint itself is only one cause of shoulder pain. The pain may also be referred from the C5 cervical roots, from intrathoracic conditions such as an apical lung tumor or pleural disease, from the heart as a result of myocardial ischemia, or from subdiaphragmatic irritation due to gallbladder disease, abscess, or tumor. Even when the symptoms are due to structures in the shoulder region, they may reflect inflammation of or damage to the tendon sheaths or bursi surrounding the shoulder, or inflammation of any of the three joints involved.

One of the characteristics of musculoskeletal pain is the extent to which it is perceived, not at the site of origin but in a more remote area. Referred pain of this sort is of two types. The more commonly encountered type is that due to the shared innervation of many connective tissues with specific areas of the skin (dermatomes). A structure inflamed in a dermatome may cause pain anywhere along the dermatome. Thus, pain due to inflammation of a shoulder joint may be manifested by aching in the upper arms rather than in the shoulder itself. Pain due to inflammation of the hip is often perceived as pain in the knee.

A second type of referred pain occurs when the lesion causing the pain results in irritation of a nerve root due to interference with the root at its point of exit from the vertebral canal or to irritation as the nerve trunk passes by an inflamed structure such as a sacroiliac joint. As noted previously, pain in the shoulder may result from osteoarthritis in the neck; arthritis of the lumbosacral spine may be evidenced by pain or numbness in a sharply demarcated area in the foot.

An examination for the cause of shoulder pain should address not only the extent and location of swelling, weakness, and tenderness and possible crepitus on motion of the shoulder structures themselves and their surrounding tissues, but also the status of the neck, cervical and axillary lymph nodes, and abdomen. An effort should be made to determine the precise maneuvers that most clearly reproduce the pain. For example, patients with arthritis of the shoulder show discomfort and resistance not only on abduction but especially on external and internal rotation. While the pain of bursitis is usually accentuated by passive motion, that due to tendonitis or myositis is accentuated, not by passive motion, but by active motion against resistance.

Treatment of localized disorders of the shoulder involves local applications of heat, limitation of activity, gentle exercises to maintain range of motion, and judicious use of NSAIDs, being careful to limit or avoid use of these agents in patients at high risk for the development of gastropathy. Localized injections into the shoulder joint, tendon sheaths, or bursi often result in symptomatic improvement lasting many months.[69, 70] Following an explanation to the patient of the goals, benefits, and risks involved, instillation of 20 to 40 mg of triamcinolone hexacetonide in 2 to 3 mL of 1% lidocaine often provides relief. Care should be taken to inject the material into the joint space, bursi, or tendon sheath. Injection into the tendon or, nonspecifically, into the surrounding soft tissue may result in weakening or atrophy of the tissue. Two or three injections may be performed at intervals of 4 to 8 weeks. More than three injections during a year are seldom indicated.

If localized musculoskeletal pain continues for a number of months, it begins to become self-perpetuating, i.e., it leads to the chronic pain syndrome. Although this syndrome is resistant to therapy, use of acupuncture, relaxation therapy, or psychological therapy may be of benefit. In some cases, actual nerve block may be necessary.

SUMMARY

Musculoskeletal complaints constitute the most common array of symptoms presented by older persons. The range of entities that underlie these symptoms is extremely wide and includes not only the classic connective tissue diseases but also a variety of conditions, many with serious implications, that are not usually regarded as rheumatic in nature. An equally wide spectrum of localized disorders may also give rise to musculoskeletal symptoms.

To address these issues effectively, the physician must be equipped with a well-tuned array of clinical skills, including the techniques of local injections, physical therapy, and psychosocial support. Many of these topics receive little attention in the curriculum of medical schools or residency training programs. As with other aspects of medicine, the patient is one's best teacher. Most of these entities respond to appropriate treatment as long as the physician has the patience and interest in providing it.

References

1. Lawrence RC, Hochberg MC, Kelscy JL, McDuffie FC, Medsger TA Jr, Felts WR, Shulman LE: Estimates of the prevalence of selected arthritic and musculoskeletal diseases in the United States. J Rheumatol 1989;16:427–441.
2. Hayes GS, Stinson IN: Erythrocyte sedimentation rate and age. Arch Ophthalmol 1976;94:939–940.
3. Hochberg MC, Altman RD, Brandt KD, Clark BM, Dieppe PA, Griffin MR, Moskowitz RW, Schnitzer TJ: Special article: Guidelines for the medical management of osteoarthritis, Part I. Osteoarthritis of the hip. Arthritis Rheum 1995;38:1535–1540.
4. Hochberg MC, Altman RD, Brandt KD, Clark BM, Dieppe PA, Griffin MR, Moskowitz RW, Schnitzer TJ: Special article: Guidelines for the medical management of osteoarthritis, Part II. Osteoarthritis of the knee. Arthritis Rheum 1995;38:1541–1546.
5. Perneger TV, Whelton PK, Klag MJ: Risk of kidney failure associated with use of acetaminophen, aspirin and nonsteroidal antiinflammatory drugs. N Engl J Med 1994;331:1675–1679.
6. Griffin MR, Piper JM, Dougherty JR, Showden M, Ray WA: Nonsteroidal anti-inflammatory drug use and increased risk for peptic ulcer disease in elderly persons. Ann Intern Med 1991;114:257–263.
7. Liechtenstein DR, Syngal S, Wolfe MM: Nonsteroidal anti-inflammatory drugs and the gastrointestinal tract: The double edged sword. Arthritis Rheum 1995;38:5–18.
8. Jenssen M, Dijkman BAC, Lamers CBHW, Zwonderman AH, Vandenbroucke JP: A gastroscopic survey of the predictive value of risk factors for nonsteroidal anti-inflammatory drug-associated ulcer disease in rheumatoid arthritis patients. Br J Rheumatol 1994;33:449–454.
9. Silverstein FE, Graham DY, Senior JR, Davies HW, Struthers BJ, Bittman RM, Geis S: Misoprostol reduces serious gastrointestinal complications in patients with rheumatoid arthritis receiving nonsteroidal anti-inflammatory drugs. A randomized double-blind placebo-controlled trial. Ann Intern Med 1995;123:241–249.
10. Minor MA: Exercise in the management of osteoarthritis of the knee and hip. Arthritis Care Res 1994;97:198–220.
11. Fisher NM, Pendergast GR, Gresham GE, Calkins E: Muscle rehabilitation: Its effect on muscular and functional performance of patients with knee osteoarthritis. Arch Phys Med Rehabil 1991;72:367–374.
12. Gunther JS, Taylor M, Calkins E, Karuza J: Outcomes of dynamics system exercise class for older adults with arthritis. Gerontologist 1996;36 (special issue 1):331.
13. Lichtenberg PA, Swenson CH, Skehan MW: Further investigation of the role of personality, lifestyle and arthritic severity in predicating pain. J Psychosom Res 1986;30:327–337.
14. Keefe FJ, Caldwell DS, Queen KT, Gil KM, Martinen

S, Crisson JE, Ogden W, Nunley J: Pain coping strategies in osteoarthritis patients. J Consulting Clin Psychol 1987;55:208–212.

15. Long KR, Mazonson PD, Holman HR: Evidence suggesting that health education for self-management in patients with chronic arthritis has sustained health benefits while reducing health care costs. Arthritis Rheum 1993;36:439–446.

16. Weinberger M, Tierney WM, Booker P, Katz BP: Can the provision of information to patients with osteoarthritis improve functional status? A randomized clinical trial. Arthritis Rheum 1989;32:1577–1583.

17. Weinberger M, Tierney WM, Cowlser PA, Katz BP, Booker PA: Cost effectiveness of increased telephone contact for patients with osteoarthritis: A randomized control trial. Arthritis Rheum 1993;36:243–246.

18. Girdwood RH: Death after taking medicaments. BMJ 1974;1(906):501–504.

19. Pincus T, Callahan LF: Taking mortality in rheumatoid arthritis seriously—predictive markers, socioeconomic status and comorbidity. J Rheumatol 1986;13:841–845.

20. Linos A, Worthington JW, O'Fallon WN, Kurland LT: The epidemiology of rheumatoid arthritis in Rochester, Minnesota. A study of incidence, prevalence, and morbidity. Am J Epidemiol 1980;111:87–98.

21. Deal CL, Meenan RF, Goldenberg DL, Anderson JJ, Sack B, Pastan RS, Cohen AS: The clinical features of elderly-onset rheumatoid arthritis. A comparison with younger-onset disease of similar duration. Arthritis Rheum 1985;28:987–994.

22. Corrigan AB, Robinson RG, Terenty TR, Dick-Smith JB, Walters D: Benign rheumatoid arthritis of the aged. Br Med J 1974;1:444–446.

23. Healey LA, Sheets PK: The relation of polymyalgia rheumatic to rheumatoid arthritis. J Rheumatol 1988;15:750–752.

24. Wilkens E, Dieppe P, Maddison P, Evison G: Osteoarthritis and articular chondrocalcinosis in the elderly. Ann Rheum Dis 1983;42:280.

25. Ward JR: Earlier intervention with second-line therapies. J Rheumatol 1990 (Suppl);25:18–23.

26. Felson DT, Anderson JT, Meenan RI: The comparative efficacy and toxicity of second-line drugs in rheumatoid arthritis: Results of two meta-analyses. Arthritis Rheum 1990;33:1449–1461.

27. Blackburn WD Jr., Prupus HM, Silverfield JC, et al: Tenidap in rheumatoid arthritis. A 24-hour double-blind comparison with hydroxy-chloroquine-plus-piroxicam and piroxicam alone. Arthritis Rheum 1995;38:1447–1456.

28. Doolittle GC, Simpson KM, Lindsley HP: Methotrexate-associated early onset pancytopenia in rheumatoid arthritis. Arch Intern Med 1989;149:1430–1431.

29. Furst DE, Koehnke R, Burmeister LF, Kohler J, Cargill I: Increasing methotrexate effect with increasing dose in the treatment of resistant rheumatoid arthritis. J Rheumatol 1989;313:320.

30. Wolfe F, Cathey MA: The effect of age on methotrexate efficacy and toxicity. J Rheumatol 1991;18:973–977.

31. Paulus HE: The use of combinations of disease-modifying antirheumatic agents in rheumatoid arthritis. Arthritis Rheum 1990;33:113–120.

32. Harris ED, Emkey RD, Nichols TE, Newberg A: Low-dose prednisone therapy in rheumatoid arthritis: A double-blind study. J Rheumatol 1983;10:713–721.

33. Liberman UA, Weiss SR, Broll J, Minne HW, et al: Effect of oral alendronate on bone mineral density and the incidence of fractures in post-menopausal osteoporosis. N Engl J Med 1995;333:1437–1443.

34. American College of Rheumatology Task Force on Osteoporosis Guidelines: Recommendations for the Prevention and Treatment of Glucocorticoid-Induced Osteoporosis. Arthritis Rheum 1996;39:1791–1801.

35. Campbell SM: Gout: How presentation, diagnosis, and treatment differ in the elderly. Geriatrics 1988;43:71–77.

36. Ritter J, Kerr LD, Valeriano-Marcet J, Spiera H: ACTH revisited: Effective treatment for acute crystal-induced synovitis in patients with multiple medical problems. J Rheumatol 1994;21:696–699.

37. Fam GA, Topp JR, Stein HB, Little AH: Clinical and roentgenographic aspects of pseudogout: A study of 50 cases and a review. Can Med Assoc J 1981;124:545–551.

38. Halverson PB, McCarty DJ, Cheung HS, Ryan LM: Milwaukee shoulder syndrome: Eleven additional cases with involvement of the knee in seven (basic calcium phosphate crystal deposition disease). Semin Arthritis Rheum 1984; 14:36–44.

39. Chuang TY, Hunder GG, Ilstrup DM, Kurland LT: Polymyalgia rheumatica. A ten-year epidemiologic and clinical study. Ann Intern Med 1983;97:672–680.

40. Faunchald P, Rygvold O, Oystese B: Temporal arteritis and polymyalgia rheumatica. Clinical and biopsy findings. Ann Intern Med 1972;77:845–852.

41. McCarty DJ, O'Duffy JD, Pearson L, Hunter JB: Remitting seronegative symmetrical synovitis with pitting edema: RS3PE syndrome. JAMA 1985;254:2763–2767.

42. Shiel WC Jr, Jason M: The diagnostic associations of patients with antinuclear antibodies referred to a community rheumatologist. J Rheumatol 1989;16:782–785.

43. Fields RA, Toubbeh H, Searles RP, Bankhurst AD: The prevalence of anticardiolipin antibodies in a healthy elderly population and its association with antinuclear antibodies. J Rheumatol 1989;16:623–625.

44. Ruffatti A, Rossi L, Calligaro A, Del Ross T, Lagni M, Marson P, Todesco S: Autoantibodies of systemic rheumatic diseases in the healthy elderly. Gerontology 1990;36:104–111.

45. Juby A, Johnston C, Davis P: Specificity, sensitivity and diagnostic predictive value of selected laboratory generated autoantibody profiles in patients with connective tissue diseases. J Rheumatol 1991;18:354–358.

46. Condemi JJ: The autoimmune diseases. JAMA 1992;268:2882–2892.

47. Thomas C, Robinson JA: The antinuclear antibody test: When is a positive result clinically relevant? Postgrad Med 1993;94:55–58, 63, 66.

48. Homburger HA: Cascade testing for autoantibodies in connective tissue diseases. Mayo Clin Proc 1995;70:183–186.

49. Grigolo B, Mazzetti L, Borzi RM, Melicorni R, Origgi L, Scorzo R, Facchin A: Comparison of different methods for the detection of autoantibodies in autoimmune diseases. Nat J Clin Lab Res 1995;25:205–210.

50. Ward MM, Polisson RP: A meta-analysis of the clinical manifestations of older onset systemic lupus erythematosus. Arthritis Rheum 1989;32:1226–1232.

51. Hochberg MC, Boyd RE, Ahearn JM, Arnett FC, et al: Systemic lupus erythematosus: Review of clinico-lab features and immunogenetic markers in 150 patients with emphasis in demographic subsets. Medicine 1985;64:285–295.

52. Cervera R, et al: Systemic lupus erythematosus: Clinical and immunologic patterns of disease. Expression in a cohort of 1000 patients. Medicine 1993;72:113–124.

53. Solinger AM: Drug-related lupus, clinical and etiologic

considerations. Rheum Dis Clin North Am 1988;1:187–202.

54. Woodley RL, Draye DE, Redenberg MM, Nies AS, Carr K, Oats JA: Effects of acetylator phenotype on the rate at which procainamide induces antinuclear antibodies and lupus syndrome. N Engl J Med 1978;298:1157–1160.

55. Strickland RW, Tesar JT, Berne HH, Hobbs BR, Lewis DM, Welton RC: The frequency of sicca syndrome in the elderly female population. J Rheumatol 1987;14:766–771.

56. Strand V, Talal N: Advances in the diagnosis and concept of Sjögren's syndrome (autoimmune exocrinopathy). Bull Rheum Dis 1979–1980;30: 1046–1052.

57. Kaplan JG, Rosenberg R, Reinitz E, Buchbinder S, Schaumbers HH: Invited review: Peripheral neuropathy in Sjögren's syndrome. Muscle Nerve 1990;13:570–579.

58. Sebold JR: Scleroderma. *In* Kelly WN, Harris ED, Reddy S, Slege DB (eds): Textbook of Rheumatology. Philadelphia, WB Saunders, 1989, pp. 1215–1244.

59. Hodkinson HM: Scleroderma in the elderly with special reference to the CREST syndrome. J Am Geriat Soc 1971;19:224–228.

60. Alarcon-Segovia D, Cardiel MH: Comparison between the diagnostic criteria for mixed connective tissue diseases. Study of 593 patients. J Rheumatol 1989;16:328–334.

61. Black CM: Systemic sclerosis: Is there a treatment yet? Ann Rheum Dis 1990;49:735–737.

62. Goldenberg DL: Fibromyalgia syndrome. An emerging but controversial condition. JAMA 1987;257:2782–2787.

63. Buchwald D, Garrity D: Comparison of patients with chronic fatigue syndrome, fibromyalgia and multiple chemical sensitivities. Arch Intern Med 1994;154:2049–2053.

64. Boh-Holaigah I, Rowe PC, Kan J, Calkins H: The relationship between neurally medicated hypotension and the chronic fatigue syndrome. JAMA 1995;274:961–967.

65. Hamdy RC, Moore S, LeRoy J: Clinical presentation of Paget's disease of the bone in older patients. South Med J 1993;86:1097–1100.

66. Kaplan FS: Paget's disease of bone: Orthopedic complications. Semin Arthritis Rheum 1994;23:250–252.

67. Siris ES: Extensive personal experience: Paget's disease of bone. J Clin Endocrinol Metab 1995;80:335–338.

68. Sheon RP, Moskowitz RW, Goldberg VM: Soft Tissue Rheumatic Pain. Recognition, Management, Prevention, 2nd ed. Philadelphia, Lea & Febiger, 1987.

69. Doherty M, Hazleman BL, Hutton CW, Maddison PH, Perry JD: Rheumatology: Examination and Injection Techniques. Philadelphia, WB Saunders, 1992.

70. Dorman TA, Ravin TH: Diagnosis and Injection Techniques in Orthopedic Medicine. Baltimore, Williams & Wilkins, 1991.

40 Orthopedic Disorders

Thomas P. Sculco, M.D.

The impact of musculoskeletal disorders on the geriatric population is immense. It is estimated that by the year 2030, 21% of the United States population will be over the age of 65. Today 30% of all hospitalized individuals are elderly.[1] In addition to the medical risks and disabilities produced by musculoskeletal diseases, these conditions may significantly alter the ability of geriatric patients to maintain independent function. This is most commonly seen in elderly patients who fall and fracture a hip. The need for hospitalization and rehabilitation is difficult and frightening for these patients, but just as worrisome is the possible loss of autonomy that may ensue as a result of such injuries. Aside from trauma, osteoporosis and arthritic afflictions are also major causes of functional disability in the elderly leading to loss of independence. The myriad medical diseases that exist concomitantly in this population compound the loss of function from musculoskeletal problems and may be devastating physically and psychologically. Once these conditions weaken the physical well-being of geriatric patients, their will to persevere emotionally weakens, and a downward spiral may begin that can lead to their demise.

Prevention of loss of ambulatory and independent functioning is the cornerstone of musculoskeletal care in the geriatric population. Conditioning and exercise programs to maintain the strength and mobility of joints is vital. Additionally, bone density is best maintained by exercise, which helps to maintain mineral bone by muscle forces acting on bone. Balance dysfunction and poor coordination affect gait and severely affect the elderly. Falls may ensue with fracture or failure to walk because of fear, greatly weakening the muscles necessary to promote ambulation and aggravating osteoporosis.

In this chapter the major orthopedic problems seen in the geriatric patient are reviewed. These include fractures, osteoporosis, and arthritis. An approach to the patient with these conditions, as well as their medical and surgical management, is also described.

TRAUMA AND FRACTURE MANAGEMENT

Fractures occur commonly in geriatric patients for a number of reasons. First, most patients, particularly postmenopausal females, have significant osteopenia. Reduction in bone mineral frequently leads to fractures of the femoral neck, wrist, and spine. Falls in these patients occur because of poor balance and proprioception; vision may also be impaired.[2] Even a minor impairment in walking ability can lead to unexpected events, which in weakened bone can produce significant fractures. Additionally, bone may be so compromised in elderly patients that stress fractures in the femoral neck may occur, in fact precipitating a fall rather than the fall leading to a fracture.[3] Many elderly people take multiple medications, which may impair balance and lead to injury. Furthermore, particularly at night, episodic confusion may develop, possibly resulting in traumatic injury and fracture.

Hip Fracture

A common and devastating fracture in the older patient is a fracture of the upper femur. In 1990 there were 1.66 million hip fractures globally, more than half of them in the United States and Europe. This number is expected to rise significantly to 6.26 million in the year 2050.[4] Although the term commonly used is hip fracture, these fractures do not actually involve the hip joint itself but are located in either the femoral neck or the intertrochanteric area of the upper femur. Femoral neck fractures are often displaced, the head of the femur being shifted into an inferior position on the neck of the femur and the lower extremity shortened and externally rotated (Fig. 40–1). Intertrochanteric fractures

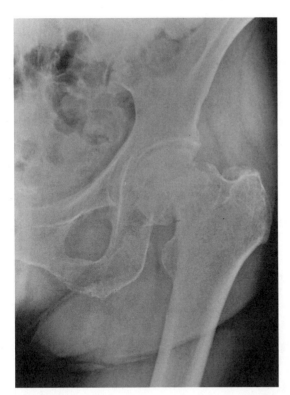

Figure 40–1   Left femoral neck fracture with displacement of the femur.

occur through the lesser and greater trochanter and generally do not produce as much shortening or limb rotation.

Whenever an elderly patient falls and is unable to rise and bear weight on the injured lower limb, a fracture of the upper femur must be suspected. These patients should be made comfortable and should not be moved because further displacement of the fracture may occur. The limb should be splinted, and the patient brought to an emergency room for confirmatory radiographs.

Depending on the location of the fracture, internal fixation, a femoral head replacement, or total hip replacement is needed. In severe fractures of the femoral neck, the shaft of the femur migrates proximally and the femoral neck essentially collapses posteriorly and medially. Because of the tenuous blood supply to the femoral head that enters through the capsule of the hip joint, femoral neck fractures that are displaced can violate this circulation and jeopardize the viability of the femoral head. Reduction in blood flow to the fracture site by this injury can also lead to non-union of these femoral neck fractures even after internal fixation has been performed. For these reasons, subsequent avascular necrosis to the head of the femur and non-union of the

fracture may occur in 40% to 50% of patients. Excision of the fractured femoral neck and head and replacement with a prosthetic head is therefore the treatment of choice in these patients[5] (Fig. 40–2). If the femoral neck fracture is minimally displaced, the blood supply is generally preserved, and internal fixation with multiple pins may be performed.

Intertrochanteric fractures tend to be more complex and are not easily amenable to replacement. These fractures involve the lesser and greater trochanters and are below the femoral neck. They are generally treated by internal fixation with screw or blade devices that transfix the fracture; plates are incorporated into these devices and are attached to the femoral shaft with multiple screws (Fig. 40–3). Avascular necrosis and non-union are uncommon in intertrochanteric fractures because the fracture is below the neck of the femur and the hip capsule and does not compromise the blood supply to the femoral head.

The goal of management of intertrochanteric or femoral neck fractures is stabilization of the fracture (or replacement of the involved bone) and early mobilization of the patient. Rapid and

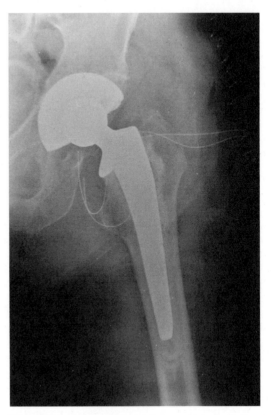

Figure 40–2   Left femoral neck fracture treated with femoral neck excision and replacement with a prosthetic femoral head and acetabulum.

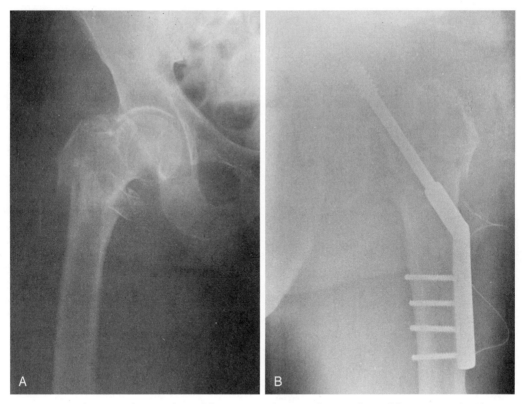

Figure 40–3 *A*, Right intertrochanteric femoral fracture. *B*, Left intertrochanteric femoral fracture treated with an internal fixation device.

aggressive rehabilitation of the patient is crucial if a return to ambulatory status is to be accomplished. Medical problems develop quickly in geriatric patients who cannot be mobilized from bed. Atelectasis, pneumonia, decubitus ulcer, urinary retention, ileus, and confusion are all seen in postoperative geriatric patients after fracture of the upper femur, and these complications can seriously compromise recovery. It is imperative for the orthopedic surgeon to obtain stabilization of the fracture so that the patient can be transferred comfortably from bed, and rehabilitation can begin immediately. Comprehensive geriatric-orthopedic care has been demonstrated to improve outcomes in elderly patients with hip fractures.[6, 7]

Rehabilitation should include ambulation with assistive devices, depending on the strength of the patient. Most patients begin with a walker and advance to a cane when weight-bearing is permitted. When a prosthetic replacement is performed, weight-bearing can begin immediately, and the patient can advance as tolerated. In patients with fractures that have been internally fixed, weight-bearing may be delayed, progressing as healing at the fracture site is demonstrated on radiographs. Generally, these patients remain on a walker for 6 weeks and use a cane or crutches for an additional 6 to 8 weeks. Because of other associated conditions that may influence the patient's ability to ambulate safely, a cane is often needed outdoors for walking. This practice should be encouraged in patients who have poor balance and are prone to falls. Most patients do return to ambulatory status after a hip fracture although they are not as independent as they were before the fracture. Koval and colleagues reported in a review of 336 patients with hip fractures that by 1 year after hip fracture 41% of patients had regained their prefracture ambulatory ability, 40% remained ambulatory but required assistive devices, 12% regressed from community to household ambulation, and 8% became nonfunctional ambulators.[8]

Many elderly patients with hip fractures present in a poor nutritional state, which may lead to delayed postoperative wound healing. Wound drainage postoperatively due to fat necrosis of subcutaneous tissue, superficial and deep infection, and wound breakdown are all more common in geriatric patients. Physiologic reserves are lower in geriatric patients, and should a major medical or surgical complication occur, their recovery potential is markedly impaired. In turn, this may lead to a series of additive problems that aggravate and prolong recovery and may in fact become life threatening. Careful proactive medical management and nutritional supplementation is important in these patients.

Aside from the myriad medical complications that can ensue after surgical treatment of fractures of the upper femur, the patient may not be able to return to independent functioning in the home after discharge. A period of time at a rehabilitation center is routinely recommended for these patients, and a home care program is necessary when they are able to return home. Often these patients have been living marginally alone and have adapted their home setting to make it possible to remain independent and fairly self-sufficient. When admission to a hospital is necessary for stabilization of a fracture, the fragile nature of the home situation becomes more problematic. Although many vigorously demand to return to their previous living arrangements, rehabilitation from a hip fracture may be slow and arduous and may reduce their ability to return to their previous accommodations. Most patients fear being sent to a nursing home or institution, but the traumatic event of the musculoskeletal injury has decreased their ambulatory function, and an unsupervised existence is unsafe. This situation may severely affect the patient psychologically, leading to depression, which can compromise rehabilitation efforts.

Pelvic Fracture

Aside from fractures involving the hip joint and upper femur, fractures of the pelvis, usually the pubic rami, occur commonly in the elderly. These fractures may result from trivial trauma, or, in a severely osteoporotic patient, simply rolling over in bed may precipitate a stress fracture of the pubic rami. The patient complains of groin pain that is exacerbated by walking or rising from a seated position. These fractures tend to be quite stable and heal with no problems. Pain with weight-bearing may persist for 6 to 8 weeks, however, and this severely limits the ability of the patient to be independent. This immobility may lead to a series of complications resulting from bed rest that are often far more life-threatening than the pelvic fracture itself. Treatment is symptomatic, and the patient should be encouraged to ambulate with a walker as soon as he or she is comfortable. Early mobilization from bed is necessary to avoid the systemic complications associated with bed rest. Most pelvic fractures heal within 6 to 8 weeks.

Lower Extremity Fractures

Aside from fractures of the hip, the femoral shaft, knee joint, tibia, and ankle may be fractured in older people. Ambulatory function is immediately curtailed once these injuries occur, and the primary goals of treatment are restoration of fracture stability and return to ambulation. Prolonged periods of immobility produced by these injuries will lead to marked muscle atrophy, joint contracture, and failure to regain the ability to walk. For these reasons, nonsurgical treatment with plaster immobilization and traction methods are employed infrequently. When appropriate, immobilization for management of a fracture is best performed using the newer synthetic bracing materials, which tend to be lighter in weight and are better tolerated in the elderly. These braces can be removed for observation of the skin, which is fragile in the elderly and is prone to breakdown. Impaired sensation can also produce skin ulceration beneath immobilizing devices; if this is undetected, infection may occur that may threaten the viability of the limb. Early discontinuation of immobilization is preferred in the management of all fractures if function is to be recovered.

In addition to problems related to the soft tissues encased beneath a cast, the limb must be constantly observed for swelling, and the patient should be encouraged to elevate to the leg. Plaster, because of its weight, makes transferral from a seated position more difficult and ambulation often impossible, and therefore it is now used infrequently.

Open surgical reduction of the fracture fragments and internal fixation with various newer devices can produce immediate stability of the fracture, allowing early joint mobilization and ambulation. Difficulty with fracture fixation in osteoporotic bone persists as a problem, and this can compromise fracture position and healing. In fractures of the lower limb in which the joint is involved, constant passive motion devices are used to allow early joint motion. Bracing is used to supplement fracture fixation externally when the bone is of poor quality and additional support is needed for fracture healing. Protected weight-bearing with a walker, crutches, or a cane is generally necessary after a fracture of the lower extremity. Crutches are often difficult for geriatric patients to master, and therefore a walker is recommended to improve support and assist balance.

Early return to ambulation is the essential outcome of any fracture of the lower extremity, and management of these fractures must be directed at this end result. Complications of fractures in the elderly include non-union, malalignment after fracture healing, delayed wound healing, and infection. Should any of these problems develop, further surgical intervention is often necessary, leading to increased morbidity.

Upper Extremity Fractures

The concepts of fracture management in the upper extremity are similar to those of lower extremity fractures. The goal is to effect fracture healing and maintain function. Early return of motion is especially important in the upper extremity, and this dictates early removal of immobilization devices and physical therapy for active and passive range of motion and strengthening exercises.

The most common fractures of the upper extremity in the geriatric patient are Colles' fractures (fracture of the distal part of the radius at the wrist joint) and shoulder fractures involving the neck of the humerus. These fractures result from a fall in which the patient lands directly on an outstretched hand or on the shoulder. In one series of patients with Colles' fractures, 75% of patients were noted to have osteoporosis.[9] Such fractures are usually characterized by swelling and deformity about the wrist, or, in shoulder fractures, an inability to move the shoulder. Treatment for both wrist and shoulder fractures is usually nonsurgical. In patients with Colles' fractures, if displacement has occurred, reduction by an orthopedic surgeon is necessary as well as application of a splint that immobilizes the wrist but leaves the hand free. The splint is generally removed 4 to 5 weeks after the injury, and early wrist and hand motion is started. While the splint is on, careful attention must be given to the fingers, which may become edematous. Sensation and capillary refill, therefore, must be checked frequently, especially during the first week after fracture.

Fractures involving the surgical and anatomic neck of the humerus are best managed with a simple sling, which may be wrapped with an elastic bandage to the patient's torso if pain is severe. Reduction, as a rule, is not necessary if displacement is not marked because these fractures tend to heal without problem. Shoulder motion is universal, and therefore some offset at the fracture site does not significantly affect function. The sling should be removed as soon as possible, based on the patient's comfort, and certainly within 2 to 3 weeks after fracture. At that point, physical therapy is necessary to achieve return of motion of the shoulder. This may be slow because of the hemarthrosis that

occurs in the shoulder joint with these fractures and the tendency for fibrosis and scarring to occur in the capsule of the shoulder joint. Most patients achieve satisfactory recovery of motion within 2 to 3 months after fracture.

Acute Management of Long Bone Fractures

When a geriatric patient is injured and a long bone fracture is suspected, the patient should be made comfortable by splinting the involved area with available pillows or cushions. If the limb is obviously displaced, gentle manipulation to a more normal alignment may make the patient more comfortable. Neurovascular examination of the distal limb should be performed to identify nerve or vessel injury. If the fracture is in the upper extremity, the area should be splinted with a sling wrapped around the torso to prevent movement of the limb away from the plane of the body. If the fracture is at the wrist, a splint can be fabricated from a piece of plywood and the limb wrapped with an Ace bandage applied loosely.

Long bone fractures of the lower extremity should be splinted with the limb in a comfortable position. Displacement of the fracture generally occurs with the initial injury, and further fracture displacement can be avoided by using fracture frames, which immobilize the patient and prevent limb rotation. Analgesics should be administered as needed to make the patient comfortable until appropriate radiographs have been obtained and transfer to an emergency room has been arranged.

Spinal Fracture

Vertebral compression fractures are common in the elderly, particularly in postmenopausal women. These fractures may occur without trauma and may be associated with a sudden movement in bed or after lifting objects. Patients with these fractures complain of severe pain in the lower or midback. Usually these fractures involve the thoracic or upper lumbar vertebrae (Fig. 40–4). On radiographs a compression fracture secondary to poor quality bone is usually wedged anteriorly. In the most severe cases of osteoporosis spinal fractures may be multiple and may involve the entire vertebral body. As a rule, however, involvement or collapse that is strictly posterior may indicate a malignant process within the vertebrae and a pathologic fracture. Vertebral fractures tend to heal without surgical intervention, but because they may be extremely painful

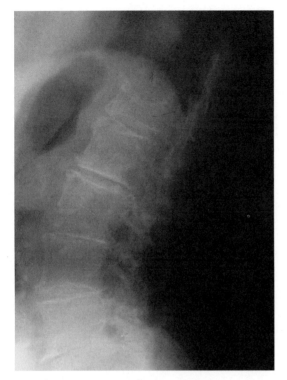

Figure 40-4 Upper lumbar vertebral fracture.

they limit the function and ambulation of the patient. Fortunately, these fractures generally stabilize quickly. A reduction in activity is recommended until the patient is comfortable, but a rapid return to the prefracture activity level is encouraged. A fitted thoracolumbar corset may be used in patients with ongoing pain and multiple compression fractures.

Dislocations

The shoulder is the most commonly dislocated joint in the geriatric patient. Generally, this injury is related to a fall on the shoulder. The patient experiences severe pain and is unable to use his or her arm. On physical examination an obvious depression is seen in the lateral shoulder. The humeral head may be palpable anterior to the glenoid. Shoulder dislocations are treated by reduction after an intravenous analgesic has been administered. A short period of immobilization in a sling is used after reduction. Early return of motion may occur with avoidance of external rotation and abduction movements for at least 6 weeks after the dislocation.

OSTEOPOROSIS

Osteoporosis is reviewed in detail in Chapter 21, but recommendations to prevent or ameliorate

this disease must be constantly reinforced in affected patients. Dietary calcium supplementation remains important in all elderly patients, as is adequate vitamin D intake. Maintenance of activity and exercise programs, particularly those with weight-bearing stress, are vital to preserve bone mass.[10-14] In patients with more severe osteoporosis, especially postmenopausal women, more vigorous pharmacologic management may be necessary. Estrogen or the use of biphosphonates is indicated in many of these women. Complications can occur with the use of all these agents, and therefore the patient must be appraised of potential hazards and must be monitored closely.

MANAGEMENT OF ARTHRITIS IN GERIATRIC PATIENTS

Arthritic afflictions of the skeleton are common in the elderly and often produce disabling pain and severe limitation of function.[15] Osteoarthritis is the most prevalent type of degenerative disease, although rheumatoid arthritis, which is considered a disease of young women, does occur in older patients as well. Osteoarthritis may affect any of the synovial joints but is most common in the spine and the small joints of the hand, particularly the distal interphalangeal joints, and the knee, hip, ankle, and shoulder. When the upper extremity joints are affected, activities of daily living are compromised. Simple activities such as holding an object, putting on a coat, buttoning a shirt, or turning a key may become problematic. When the lower extremity joints are involved in osteoarthritis, the major functional result is a decreased ability to ambulate, climb and descend stairs, and arise from a seated position.

Further discussion of the pathogenesis and management of osteoarthritis is found in Chapter 39. In evaluating the patient with osteoarthritis, the entire complex of soft tissue, joint, and bone involvement should be considered. All of these structures are involved and can lead to pain, loss of motion, and dysfunction of the joint. Conservative and surgical treatment of osteoarthritis in the older patient is predicated on management of all anatomic structures involved in the arthritic process. Early in the disease when synovitis is most marked, medical management may be successful, but as joint destruction progresses, the mechanical component becomes predominant, and surgical correction or replacement of the joint must be performed to relieve patient pain and improve function.

Conservative Management of Osteoarthritis

Conservative management of arthritis in the geriatric population can be divided into two main categories: rehabilitative and pharmacologic. Rehabilitative treatment is directed at reducing the load to the arthritic joint and maintaining joint mobility and strength. Weight reduction that decreases the load on the joint significantly reduces pain in arthritic patients in whom the weight-bearing joints are involved. Avoidance of activities, particularly running or overhead sports in those with shoulder arthritis, will also reduce the load on the affected joint and relieve pain. However, although rest for a painful arthritic joint is helpful in the short term, prolonged periods of inactivity will lead to the more serious problem of immobility in the geriatric patient. The use of a cane will significantly reduce joint forces in all lower extremity joints and allow continuation of a walking program. The patient will rapidly modify his or her activities to lessen the load on an arthritic joint. Stair climbing will be avoided or will be performed one step at a time. Shopping will be done only as necessary. In patients with upper extremity arthritis, modifications will be made to reduce the need for overhead activities.

Exercise programs are important to maintain joint motion and strength in an arthritic joint. Both passive and active exercises should therefore be encouraged. Because pain may be aggravated if resistance is excessive in these exercise programs, resistance should be avoided. Simple antigravity exercises without weight-bearing are generally well tolerated. The shoulder quickly loses motion when arthritis develops, and, passive range of motion exercises of the shoulder must be maintained even if some pain occurs. This is best done by grasping a segment of a broomstick with both hands and using the uninvolved upper extremity to move the affected shoulder through a full range of motion.

A formal physical therapy program is recommended for the geriatric patient with osteoarthritis. A therapist can provide the full exercise program to the patient and determine which exercises exacerbate the pain. These exercises can then be modified immediately to allow strengthening of the intended muscle group without causing patient discomfort. Repetitive instruction in the correct method of performing the exercise and positive reinforcement improve compliance. Confusion about the type of exercise needed, the method, and the number of exercises performed can be avoided if the program is supervised and these questions are constantly addressed. Aside from strengthening exercises, a therapist can work with the patient to increase joint range of motion. This may be painful if the joint is badly destroyed and should be done only in a gently passive and assisted active manner. The patient should be encouraged to limit all attempted range of motion exercises if pain is significant. Joint inflammation becomes more marked, and effusion may ensue, leading to increased fibrosis and further joint contracture if continued painful range of motion exercises are pursued. In the patient with lower extremity involvement, the physical therapist can instruct the patient in the proper use of a cane and size it appropriately. Assistive devices such as modified eating utensils and buttoning hooks can also be provided by the therapist to improve upper extremity function.

Pharmacologic treatment is accomplished primarily with nonsteroidal anti-inflammatory medications and analgesics. Anti-inflammatory medications are particularly effective in the early stages of the disease when there is a significant inflammatory component and synovitis exists. As the disease progresses and joint incongruity becomes more severe, these medications tend to be less effective. Medical management is further highlighted in Chapter 39.

Hydrocortisone intra-articular injections are often efficacious in reducing joint inflammation and swelling. As with anti-inflammatory medications, these injections work best when they are used before severe mechanical joint changes have occurred. Depo-Medrol 40 to 80 mg is usually administered with 2 to 3 mL of 1% lidocaine after the skin has been prepared with Betadine. Joint contamination and infection is a catastrophe, and all injections into a joint must be performed in accordance with strict sterile technique as a minor surgical procedure. Intra-articular injections should not be performed more than three or four times yearly because damage to the joint surfaces may occur.

Surgical Treatment of Osteoarthritis

Surgical treatment is indicated in severely arthritic joints that are unresponsive to conservative treatment. Joint replacement is the procedure most commonly indicated when the joint has lost its articular cartilage surfaces. Joint replacement can now be performed in most peripheral joints including the shoulder, elbow, wrist, hand, hip, knee, and ankle. Hip and knee replacements are the procedures most often performed because of the frequency and disabling nature of arthritis that affects these two major weight-bearing joints. At the Hospital for Special Surgery in New York, for example, 2500 hip and knee replacements are performed yearly, but the combined number of other joints replaced is less than 100. The concept of joint replacement is to resurface the arthritic joint with a prosthetic surface that is usually made of metal and plastic (ultra-high molecular weight polyethylene). In geriatric patients these implants are generally fixed to bone with an acrylic cement called methylmethacrylate. Because soft tissue investments and ligamentous structures tend to be incorporated in the arthritic process, these structures must be balanced to provide joint stability, particularly in knee replacements. Bone loss may also be corrected by grafting excised bone into bony defects and supporting the implant on these grafted surfaces (Fig. 40–5). More options are available today in terms of augmentation of implants to deal with specialized areas of ligament instability and bone loss in the patient undergoing revision knee replacement (Fig. 40–6).

Operative technique and implant materials have improved dramatically during the past decade. Joint replacement is performed under regional anesthesia routinely with only light sedation. This is particularly important in geriatric patients, who do not tolerate general anesthesia well.[16–19] Most procedures are completed within 2 hours. Blood loss from raw bony surfaces tends to continue even after the wound has been closed, and therefore blood levels can drop and transfusion may be required. Autologous blood donation programs are used routinely for most joint replacement procedures, and even geriatric patients tend to tolerate providing their own blood for these procedures.

Patients are usually hospitalized for 5 to 6 days until ambulation is possible in patients with a lower extremity joint replacement and when motion has begun in those with an upper extremity replacement. Physical therapy programs in the home are arranged after discharge, or the patient is sent to a rehabilitative center for more intense therapy. Recovery from joint replacement surgery, barring a complication, progresses rapidly, and most patients are ambulatory without assistive devices 2 to 3 months after the surgery.

Overall long-term results of joint replacement have been excellent. In patients with hip and knee replacements 10- to 15-year results show continued success rates in the 90% range[20–23] (Fig. 40–7). The most common causes of failure of joint replacement are related to breakdown of fixation of the device with time or to excessive polyethylene wear, which can lead to inflamma-

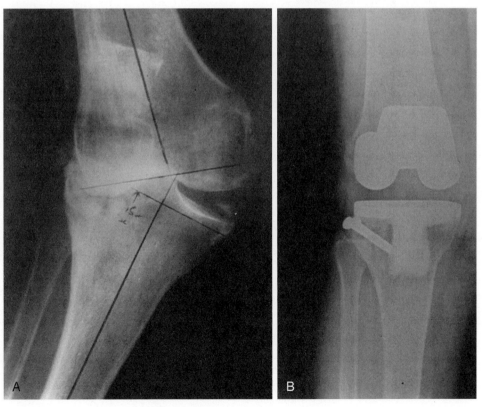

Figure 40–5 *A,* Advanced osteoarthritis of right knee. *B,* Postoperative view of right knee with prosthetic joint in place.

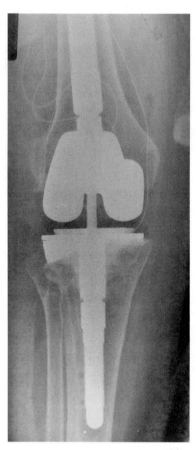

Figure 40–6 Augmented prosthetic joint of right knee.

tory cell production with release of osteolytic enzymes. Improvements in materials and techniques have lessened the incidence of both of these problems. Infection remains the most catastrophic complication that can occur after joint replacement. Deep periprosthetic infection involving the bone-cement-implant interface can be eradicated only by removing the implant and administering parenteral antibiotics for 6 weeks. The device is then reimplanted if there is no evidence of persistent infection. Use of this protocol at the Hospital for Special Surgery in over 400 cases has produced a success rate of 90% in patients with hip joint infections and 95% in those with knee replacement infections.

Bone quality is poor in geriatric patients, and periprosthetic fractures may occur after a fall. The principles of management of these fractures are similar to those of fractures described earlier, with internal fixation devices being used to stabilize the bone around the implant. If fixation of the implant has been altered by the fracture, the implant can be revised and the fracture stabilized at the same time.

Spinal Arthritis

Osteoarthritis may involve the spinal synovial articulating joints as well as the peripheral joints. In the spine, however, because of the close proximity of the neural structures, distal manifestations of the primary spinal arthritis may be seen. Therefore, paresthesias, numbness, and weakness may be secondary to nerve root compromise centrally. In the assessment of any spinal disorder it is important to perform a careful neurological examination. The presence of neurological loss is a significant finding and may lead to early decompression of either the nerve root or the spinal cord, depending on the location of the neural compression.

Osteoarthritis that affects the facets of the apophyseal joints in the spine leads to the same pathological progression of symptoms as that seen in the peripheral joints. Articular cartilage is lost as the load on the articulating bony surfaces increases. The biological response to these altered joint loads leads to the production of reparative tissue in the form of new bone and fibrous and cartilaginous tissue. These osteophytes then tend to limit joint motion further as their overgrowth further locks in the joint. These osteophytes and the degeneration of the intervertebral disk that is anterior to the nerve root lead to

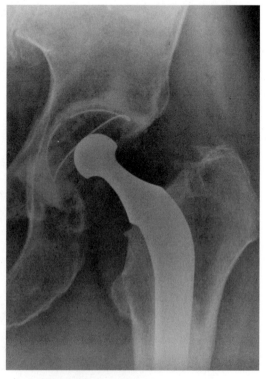

Figure 40–7 Left total hip replacement.

compression of the neural foramen through which the nerve passes. In the most severe form of the disease, the neural foramen is compromised and central narrowing of the neural canal occurs, causing possible compression of the spinal cord (above L1–L2) and cauda equina (below L1–L2). The full composite picture of disk degeneration and severe osteoarthritic facet joint involvement with neural compression is called spinal stenosis.

The most common complaints of patients with osteoarthritic involvement of the spine are pain, stiffness, and radicular symptoms (paresthesias, numbness, and weakness). The radicular component of the disease tends to be more common in patients with cervical spondylosis (arthritis affecting the apophyseal joints) because of the proximity of the nerve root to the arthritic apophyseal and uncovertebral joints. Symptoms of paresthesias and pain radiating into the shoulder and upper extremity are common in persons with cervical arthritic disease, and these must be differentiated from primary problems affecting the shoulder, wrist, and hand. Spinal stenosis affecting the lumbar spine may lead to the development of bilateral buttock and posterior leg pain (often burning in nature) as well as dysesthesias, numbness, and weakness. Radicular symptoms are related to nerve root compression and tend to be present when the main area of stenosis is in the lumbar canal below the cauda equina. In severe cases the patient has specific neurologic abnormalities that are related to the particular nerve roots compromised. In patients with compressive syndromes of spinal stenosis with spinal cord involvement in the lower thoracic or upper lumbar area more severe parapareses may be present, and bladder and bowel dysfunction may be seen in the most severe cases. In the most advanced cases spasticity of the lower extremities may be noted.

In classic spinal stenosis of the lower lumbar area pain is generally aggravated by walking and is relieved by rest and forward flexion of the lumbar spine. The flexed position increases the space in the neural canal and relieves the compression of the nerve structures, thereby reducing pain.

The neural canal of the cervical spine is considerably smaller than that in the lumbar area, and severe arthritic involvement may lead to compressive syndromes of the nerve roots or, in the most severe form, cervical myelopathy. The onset of myelopathy may be extremely subtle. Patients may have difficulty in walking, may drop objects from their hands, or experience a general lack of coordination. Frank weakness and quadriplegia tend to be relatively uncommon until the later stages of myelopathy. Physical examination may reveal only mild weakness with no sensory changes. Patients with myelopathy generally have hyperreflexia, and abnormal reflexes consistent with spinal cord compression may be present.

The diagnosis is best confirmed on radiographic evaluation. Standard radiographs of the involved area should be obtained, including anteroposterior, lateral, and oblique views. These films document the extent of disease both in severity and in localization of vertebral involvement. A computed tomographic (CT) scan or magnetic resonance imaging (MRI) film can be performed to demonstrate more definitively the degree of stenosis and compression of the neural canal and foramina. In patients with cervical myelopathic findings an MRI should be obtained to define the extent and degree of spinal cord compression. CT scans tend to be better for bone and joint findings, whereas MRI is better for demonstrating soft tissue impingement (Fig. 40–8). A neurologic evaluation and electrodiagnostic studies are also useful when objective evidence of neurologic dysfunction is needed.

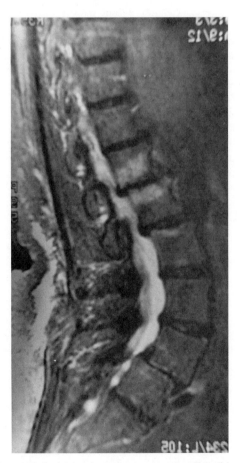

Figure 40–8 Magnetic resonance imaging film of lower spine (lateral view) in a patient with spinal arthritis.

Treatment for spinal arthritis is similar to that for arthritic disease in the appendicular skeleton. Exercises are important to maintain strength and mobility in the cervical, thoracic, and lumbar spine. Pain should not be exacerbated during the performance of exercises, and often a therapist is needed to supervise the onset of an exercise program and instruct the patient in the proper way to perform the exercises without provoking pain. Anti-inflammatory medications can be used, although they may be poorly tolerated. Epidural hydrocortisone injections can be administered in patients with lumbar spinal stenosis, and these often provide significant relief of pain and dysesthesias. Relief tends to be short, however, and repeated injections are usually necessary. Corsets and braces provide some symptomatic improvement also, but if they are cumbersome and heavy they are not well tolerated in the elderly.

If compression of the neural elements is severe in patients with spinal stenosis (cervical or lumbar), conservative measures are frequently unsuccessful. Spinal decompression of the neural foramina and lamina may be necessary to remove pressure on the nerve root by osteophytes and synovial and ligamentous tissue. In the most severe cases there may be associated instability of the vertebrae with spondylolisthesis (forward slippage of a vertebral body on another), which may require fusion with internal fixation devices. If decompression must be augmented by a fusion procedure the magnitude of risk increases significantly in the elderly patient, as does the morbidity. Results of surgical treatment can be quite dramatic, however, with marked relief of symptoms of neurogenic claudication and recovery of neurologic function. Return to a more mobile and ambulatory existence is possible after surgical decompression in patients with spinal stenosis, and the overall physical state of geriatric patients benefits tremendously when independent function is restored.

SUMMARY

Musculoskeletal disease is one of the most common and disabling of all afflictions in the geriatric population. These conditions are devastating not because they are life threatening but because they limit function, independence, and autonomy. The immobility produced by many of these conditions, particularly those discussed in this chapter, can lead to a cascade effect of medical maladies that may jeopardize the independent existence of the older patient. Newer techniques of dealing with fractures, osteoporosis, and ar-

thritic conditions all have concentrated on rapid mobilization of the patient to a functional state. Rapid recovery of function must always be of prime concern because once the older patient has lost function, be it ambulatory or use of the upper extremity, it is difficult to master such functions again. Hippocrates, in the fifth century BC, noted that if the body is used actively it will age slowly and function will be maintained. It is to this end that all orthopedic care of the geriatric patient must be directed.

References

1. Sculco TP: Orthopedic Care of the Geriatric Patient. St. Louis, Mosby, 1985.
2. Meunier PJ: Prevention of hip fractures. Am J Med 1993;95(5A):75S–78S.
3. Tountas AA: Insufficiency stress fractures of the femoral neck in elderly women. Clin Orthop 1993;292:202–209.
4. Melton LJ 3d: Hip fractures: A worldwide problem today and tomorrow. Bone 1993;14 Suppl 1:S1–8.
5. Malhotra R, Arya R, Bhan S: Bipolar hemiarthroplasty in femoral neck fractures. Arch Orthop Trauma Surg 1995;114(2):79–82.
6. Hempsall VJ, Robertson DR, Campbell MJ, Briggs RS: Orthopaedic geriatric care—is it effective? A prospective population-based comparison of outcome in fractured neck of femur. J R Coll Physicians Lond 1990;24(1):47–50.
7. Zuckerman JD, Sakales SR, Fabian DR, Frankel VH: Hip fractures in geriatric patients. Results of an interdisciplinary hospital care program. Clin Orthop 1992;274:213–225.
8. Koval KJ, Skovron ML, Aharonoff GB, Meadows SE, Zuckerman JD: Ambulatory ability after hip fracture. A prospective study in geriatric patients. Clin Orthop 1995;310:150–159.
9. Dias JJ, Wray CC, Jones JM: Osteoporosis and Colles' fractures in the elderly. J Hand Surg 1987;12(1):57–59.
10. Galindo-Ciocon D, Ciocon JO, Galindo D: Functional impairment among elderly women with osteoporotic vertebral fractures. Rehabil Nurs 1995;20(2):79–83.
11. Gutin B, Kasper MJ: Can vigorous exercise play a role in osteoporosis prevention? A review. Osteoporos Int 1992;2(2):55–69.
12. Nguyen TV, Kelly PJ, Sambrook PN, Gilbert C, Pocock NA, Eisman JA: Life-style fractures and bone density in the elderly: Implications for osteoporosis prevention. J Bone Miner Res 1994;9:1339–1346.
13. Preisinger E, Alacamlioglu Y, Pils K, Saradeth T, Schneider B: Therapeutic exercise in the prevention of bone loss. Am J Phys Med Rehabil 1995;74:120–123.
14. Voorrips LE, Lemmink KA, van Heuvelen MJ, Bult P, van Staveren WA: The physical condition of elderly women differing in habitual physical activity. Med Sci Sports Exerc 1993;25:1152–1157.
15. Abyad A, Boyer JT: Arthritis and aging. Curr Opin Rheumatol 1992;4:153–159.
16. Gustafson Y, Brannstrom B, Berggren D, Ragnarsson JI, Sigaard J, Bucht G, Reiz S, Norberg A, Winglad B: A geriatric-anesthesiologic program to reduce acute confusional states in elderly patients treated for femoral neck fractures. J Am Geriatr Soc 1991;39:655–662.
17. Hole A, Terjesen T, Breivik H: Epidural versus general anaesthesia for total hip arthroplasty in elderly patients. Acta Anaesthesiol Scand 1980;24:279–287.

18. Pargger H, Scheidegger D: Surgical risk and anesthesia in geriatric patients. Orthopade 1994;23:16–20.

19. Sculco TP, Ranawat C: Spinal anesthesia and total hip replacement. J Bone Joint Surg 1975;66A:202–208.

20. Dunlop WE, Rosenblood L, Lawrason L, Birdsall L, Rusnak CH: Effects of age and severity of illness on outcome and length of stay in geriatric surgical patients. Am J Surg 1993;165:577–580.

21. Levy RN, Levy CM, Synder J, Digiovanni J: Outcome and long-term results following total hip replacement in elderly patients. Clin Orthop 1995;316:25–30.

22. Newington DP, Bannister GC, Fordyce M: Primary total hip replacement in patients over 80 years of age. J Bone Joint Surg 1990;72:450–452.

23. Pitson D, Bhaskaran V, Bond H, Yarnold R, Drewett R: Effectiveness of knee replacement surgery in arthritis. Int J Nurs Stud 1994;31:49–56.

41 Otologic Disorders

Bradford S. Patt, M.D., F.A.C.S.

Otologic disorders can affect the aged in many ways, causing problems that involve the external auditory canal, the middle ear, and the inner ear. Sensorineural hearing loss and aural rehabilitation are two other areas that have significant ramifications in the aged.

EXTERNAL AUDITORY CANAL

Anatomy

Changes in the auditory canal associated with aging are better understood in the light of knowledge of the normal anatomy of the ear. The external canal extends from the opening of the ear laterally to the tympanic membrane medially (Fig. 41–1). The skin of the outer or lateral portion of the canal is thick and contains numerous hair follicles and sebaceous and cerumen glands. It also includes well-developed dermal and subcutaneous layers. The skin of the medial portion, in contrast, overlies the periosteum and is thin; it is firmly attached to the underlying bone and has few hair follicles and glands.[1]

Age-Related Changes

Two kinds of hair grow within the external auditory canal. Minute vellus hairs cover almost all of the ear canal, while larger tragi hairs are laterally situated in the external canal. The tragi hairs are a secondary sex characteristic and become coarser, larger, and more noticeable in the third or fourth decades of life. The tragi are also found on the auricle but only in males.[1]

Cerumen glands are actually modified apocrine sweat glands. In the ear canal they are responsible for the distinctive odor of cerumen. Cerumen glands open onto the skin or into hair follicles just external to the opening of sebaceous gland ducts. In the hair follicle, sebum, apocrine secretions, and desquamated epithelial cells combine to form wet or dry cerumen depending on a person's phenotype. Cerumen glands atrophy in the ear canals of the elderly, leading to an increased impaction of wax in the older male population.

Impactions

Cerumen impactions occur more often in elderly men because of the large tragi in the external ear canal that trap the drier wax secondary to atrophy of the cerumen glands. Impactions can be remedied in several ways. If the wax is soft, gentle irrigation of the canal with warm water may be attempted. Dry, firm wax may be softened with ceruminolytic agents (e.g., Debrox or Ceruminex) and then irrigated. Wax that remains after irrigation should be carefully extracted using a curette and an otoscope or microscope. It is important to avoid trauma to the skin of the canal because it can lead to bleeding, hematoma, or infection.[2]

Dermatitis

Itching in the external auditory canal is also due to atrophy of the glands in the canal. Dermatitis presents as a constant itching in the canal, and a cycle of itch-scratch-itch ensues, leading to desquamation of the canal.[3] Occasionally a normal appearing canal can itch, but normally the lack of cerumen in the canal is a good clue to the onset of dermatitis.

Treatment is aimed at adding moisture to the external ear using lubricating agents such as glycerin or mineral oil. Overuse of alcohol-based mixtures should be avoided because these tend to dry the ear further. Instillation of steroid-based creams in the external canal with a syringe may be effective in more resistant cases. Always be aware that itching can be a sign of early infection, and a complete examination of the canal is warranted before initiating any treatment.

Infections

Aging is associated with an increased incidence of fungal infections in the external canal due to the aforementioned age-related changes in the canal. Fungal otitis is caused by increased moisture in the external canal resulting from hearing aid use or trapped moisture due to cerumen impaction. Unlike bacterial infection, fungal oti-

449

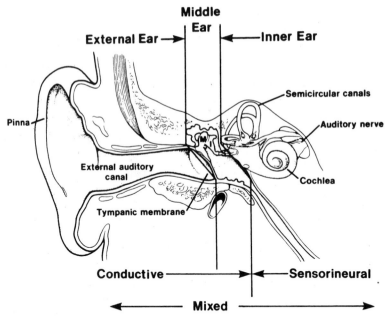

Figure 41–1 Types of hearing loss. This cross section demonstrates the external, middle, and inner regions of the ear. The type of hearing loss is also classified according to the region of the ear involved. M = malleus; I = incus; S = stapes.

tis presents as persistent itching without acute pain, although some tenderness may be present. There is usually some discharge or odor from the external canal. Treatment consists of debridement of the discharge within the ear, culture of the discharge, and use of antifungal medication. Because the most common organisms involved are *Candida* and *Aspergillus* species, clotrimazole (Lotrimin) drops, usually mixed with a steroid-type liquid, are used to resolve the infection.[3] Other drops used include those based on acetic acid or boric acid (e.g., Otic Domeboro or Vo-Sol Otic ear drops); antifungal creams may also be used. Fungal infections can be recalcitrant to any treatment, and frequent debridement of the canal may be the only way to resolve the problem. Systemic treatment is not warranted in most cases of fungal otitis.

Bacterial otitis externa presents as acute pain of the ear canal associated with tragal tenderness, canal erythema and edema, and foul discharge.[2, 3] Treatment includes thorough cleansing of the canal and the instillation of antibiotic and steroid-based drops (e.g., Cortisporin Otic). Severe swelling of the canal may require intubation of the canal with a cotton or Merocel wick to allow medication to enter the canal. Persistent symptoms may require systemic antibiotics and culture of the canal. Antibiotics used should cover gram-negative organisms, especially *Pseudomonas aeruginosa*. If pain continues despite these measures, or if the patient is diabetic or other-

wise immunocompromised, malignant otitis externa should be suspected.

Tumors

Tumors involving the external canal usually involve the auricle and include actinic keratosis, basal cell carcinoma, and squamous cell carcinoma. These lesions present most commonly in patients 50 to 60 years old. Any nonhealing lesion in the elderly should undergo biopsy. Treatment in the early stages involves excision with adequate margins and immediate reconstruction. In patients with larger lesions excision with delayed reconstruction or radiation therapy may be required.

MIDDLE EAR

Anatomy

The middle ear includes the tympanic membrane, the tympanic cavity, two muscles (the tensor tympani and the stapedius), and three bony ossicles (malleus, incus, and stapes).

Age-Related Changes

The middle ear undergoes senile changes that affect the ossicles and their respective articulations. Erosive changes within the joint capsule may range from mild to severe and can occasionally lead to narrowing of the joint space between the ossicles. Severe changes may lead to calcification of the joint capsule, diffuse calcification of the articular cartilages and disk, and obliteration of portions or all of the joint space. All individuals over 70 years of age show moderate to severe degeneration of the middle ear. Fortunately, even complete obliteration of the joint space within the ossicles causes no identifiable loss of sound transmission through the middle ear. Aging does not directly affect the conductive hearing mechanism.

INNER EAR

Anatomy

The inner ear is encased in a dense capsule, which includes the vestibule, three semicircular canals (balance organs), the cochlea (hearing organ), and the cochlea and vestibular aqueduct.[4] The common denominator of function of the vestibule and cochlea is the hair cell. Degeneration of the hair cells in the vestibular and cochlear systems causes loss of function in these areas, leading to vertigo and hearing loss, respectively.

VERTIGO

Dizziness, disequilibrium, and vertigo are common complaints of the elderly. By age 65, 90% of adults have listed imbalance as the primary reason for visiting the doctor.[5] An estimated 13 million persons over age 65 in the United States are significantly affected by vertigo or some type of balance disturbance. To understand the management of vertiginous patients, it is important to understand the general principles of balance control. Loss of balance is a common denominator in many elderly patients' complaints of dizziness.

Balance is maintained by the accurate and rapid integration of three primary sensory inputs—visual, vestibular, and somatosensory—within the brain, leading to the delivery of appropriate task-specific motor signals to the eye, trunk, and limb musculature. A sense of imbalance, therefore, can come from (1) an absence of two or more sensory inputs, (2) an orientationally incorrect sensory input, (3) poor central nervous system integration of sensory information, or (4) faulty motor signal or motor response.[6, 7] In patients with dizziness resulting from altered sensory information, imbalance does not occur until either the sensory input from vision and proprioception is reduced and vestibular cues are faulty, or the conflict between different sensory cues

cannot be resolved quickly enough to produce the correct motor response. In contrast, central causes of dizziness imply an improper integration of normal yet conflicting sensory information and the production of appropriate muscle action. The treatment of balance disorders must not be limited solely to the role of the inner ear taken in isolation but should also focus on the interaction with sensory inputs from the central nervous system and proprioception.[7, 8]

Another issue is the symptoms created by acute inner ear dysfunction versus those generated by either abnormal visual and somatosensory cues or problems with the resolution of sensory conflicts. Acute unilateral dysfunction presents as true vertigo (a false sense of motion). Defective sensory selection or conflict resolution between the senses leads to persistent feelings of disequilibrium rather than episodic illusions of motion. Vertigo, therefore, is the most distinct sensation and is most likely created by paroxysmal changes in eighth cranial nerve function. The problem with evaluating a patient with vertigo is the nervous system's remarkable ability to compensate for peripheral (eighth cranial nerve) vestibular disease. In many instances, vertigo experienced by the patient produces a paucity of physical findings on examination. In many cases, longitudinal follow-up and repeated examinations are necessary to document changes in vestibular function.[8]

Evaluation of the Dizzy Patient

HISTORY

Seventy-five percent of dizzy patients can be diagnosed on the basis of a complete history using a live interview and a written questionnaire. The questionnaire should include six major categories: (1) A description of the dizzy sensation without using the word dizzy. In most cases of vertigo, the patient has no trouble in describing the illusion of motion. In all other forms of dizziness or disequilibrium, the patient usually struggles to describe what he or she experiences. (2) Direct questions about the history of vertigo. Questions may include those about the sensations the patient experiences during the dizzy spells or what initiates the attacks of vertigo. (3) Typical accompanying symptoms of peripheral vestibular disease. The presence of distinct attacks, nausea, worsening of symptoms with movement, and a duration of vertigo from seconds to hours are all clues that support a diagnosis of a peripheral etiology of vertigo. (4) Typical accompanying symptoms of central vestibular disease. Associated neurologic deficits, syncope, and altered mentation all indicate the presence of posterior fossa–cerebellar disease. (5) Typical hearing complaints. Unilateral tinnitus, fullness, or hearing loss are important lateralizing symptoms. (6) General history, including the use of habit medications. Sedative medications, caffeine, tobacco, alcohol, and stress all play a potential role in the dizzy patient.[5, 6]

Based on the history alone, patients with distinct attacks of vertigo and episodic unilateral auditory complaints are likely to have a disorder of the eighth cranial nerve. Patients with vertigo with auditory symptoms may still have neuronitis or benign paroxysmal vertigo (BPV) or a variety of extralabyrinthine problems. Patients with unilateral auditory complaints without vertigo may have either a nonvestibular disease or a slowly compensating unilateral disease (e.g., acoustic neuroma). Finally, patients without vertigo or unilateral auditory complaints belong to a large group of patients with either partially compensated vestibular disease, diffuse central, metabolic, or vascular disorders, or psychogenic disorders.[6]

PHYSICAL EXAMINATION

Every dizzy patient requires a full medical evaluation, including blood pressure and cardiac and pulmonary examinations as well as neurologic and neuro-otologic examinations. General medical causes of vertigo, including hypertension, hypotension, and cardiac arrhythmias, must be excluded. Furthermore, vision checks are important to rule out simple problems with acuity.

The otologic examination focuses on tympanic membrane and middle ear abnormalities and on the presence of vertigo or nystagmus with pneumatic otoscopy. In the neuro-otologic examination one looks for cranial nerve deficits as well as the presence of nystagmus. Nystagmus may be spontaneous, positional, or gaze-related or may be present on headshake. Cerebellar tests of the upper and lower extremities are performed to detect dysmetria. Finally, the Romberg test and gait testing are used to evaluate the patient's static and dynamic postural control.

LABORATORY TESTS

Vestibular function tests are performed to quantify the degree to which a person is affected by vertigo and may identify the source of the problem. Unfortunately, these tests can show great variability in results, especially in the elderly population. Vestibular testing is used to determine the primary source of the disorder, whether peripheral or central, and whether the disorder is unilateral or bilateral. Quantitative testing includes electronystagmography (ENG) with caloric stimulation, rotary chair testing, and computerized posturography. Magnetic resonance imaging (MRI) with gadolinium is an important test that is used to rule out vascular loops, tumors, or other central nervous system problems (e.g., multiple sclerosis, infarcts).[9]

DIFFERENTIAL DIAGNOSIS

Vertigo can be related to acute unilateral peripheral dysfunction, acute central dysfunction, or secondary peripheral involvement with a systemic process.

Acute Unilateral Dysfunction

Acute unilateral dysfunction generates vertigo by sending asymmetrical labyrinthine signals to the vestibular nuclei; this asymmetry is misinterpreted as motion, which the patient senses. In such cases, the duration of the spell gives a clue to the cause. Vertigo lasting seconds frequently implies the presence of benign paroxysmal positional vertigo (BPPV). Vertigo lasting minutes to hours may accompany a hydrops attack or mild neuronitis. Spells lasting up to 24 hours with constant vertigo frequently imply neuronitis. Rarely does acute labyrinthine dysfunction cause constant vertigo lasting for days. Other, less common causes are a perilymph fistula (which causes Valsalva-related vertigo and fluctuating hearing loss), labyrinthitis (which causes hearing loss and vertigo), and acoustic neuroma (which rarely presents with vertigo).[6, 7]

Acute Central Dysfunction

Acute central dysfunction generates vertigo by interrupting vestibular-related brain stem or cerebellar connections at the pontomedullary junction. Most commonly, ischemia resulting from significant small vessel disease or even a full-blown transient ischemic attack (TIA) causes vertigo that lasts for seconds to minutes and is frequently produced or exacerbated by antigravity movements. Demyelination plaques may also affect the brain stem pathways, causing vertigo as well as other symptoms of multiple sclerosis. Tumors of the cerebellopontine angle rarely cause acute attacks of vertigo because of their slow growth and gradual compensation of the brain stem. Infarcts of the brain stem or cerebellum generate severe vertigo and gait ataxia, which can be confused with the vertigo of peripheral origin. Finally, migraine-induced vertigo may take a variable course and can mimic peripheral vertigo.[5]

Secondary Labyrinthine Involvement

Labyrinthine dysfunction may occur with systemic diseases that impair either the circulation or metabolism or that directly attack the membranous labyrinth. Hypertension, hypercholesterolemia, diabetes mellitus, and advanced atherosclerosis all affect oxygen delivery to the labyrinth and can sometimes produce vertigo. In some patients with systemic connective tissue disease, autoimmune-mediated hearing loss and vertigo may occur.[6]

Generally speaking, symmetrical bilateral labyrinthine dysfunction (ototoxicity, presbycusis [age-related hearing loss]), slowly progressive unilateral dysfunction (acoustic neuroma), and diffuse CNS disease produce disequilibrium rather than vertigo. Disorders of sensory conflict resolution belong in this category also, as described earlier.

THERAPY

Acute Vertigo

The CNS compensates rapidly for an isolated episode of acute vertigo or peripheral vertigo within days to weeks after the spell, given adequate visual and proprioceptive activity. Thus, the elderly may have a more prolonged recovery with an attack of acute vertigo. In such instances, treatment consists of vestibular suppressants and antiemetics for the acute episode only, along with encouragement for activity and reassurance. As an initial regimen, prochlorperazine (Compazine) suppositories, 25 mg per rectum every 6 hours, and meclizine (Antivert), 25 mg by mouth three times a day for 48 to 72 hours, are often sufficient to control vomiting and vertigo. In recalcitrant cases, diazepam (Valium), 2 to 10 mg by mouth every 6 hours, may help but carries a significant risk of sedation and addiction. In certain patients dehydration occurs, and the patient requires intravenous resuscitation along with diazepam, 5 to 10 mg intramuscularly, droperidol, 2.5 mg intramuscularly, or ondansetron (Zofran), 4 mg intravenously, to successfully control emesis. In patients in whom neuronitis is suspected, tapering doses of oral or intravenous steroids appear to shorten the attack and lessen its severity. Early ambulation and regular exercise tend to hasten full recovery. Minor episodes of dizziness may occur months after an initial episode, but routine use of vestibular suppressants is not warranted and may in fact delay recovery.

Recurrent Vertigo

Treatment of recurrent vertigo depends on the cause of the attack. For instance, BPV is treated effectively with repeated head-positioning exercises with no need for prolonged medication use.[8] Endolymphatic hydrops attacks, however, require adequate sedation and antiemetics during the severe episodes but no suppressants between attacks. As in isolated cases of acute vertigo, the use of steroids during hydrops attacks has been successful. Recalcitrant cases of vertigo secondary to hydrops may require surgical intervention.

Central Vertigo

Vertigo of central origin can be difficult to manage depending on the location and extent of the injury in relation to the central balance center. For patients with diffuse small vessel cerebrovascular disease, cessation of smoking, increased exercise, control of blood pressure and cholesterol, and antiplatelet aspirin therapy have proved useful. In patients with demyelination, high-dose steroid therapy seems to lessen the severity of the symptoms. Of course, tumors of the CNS require surgical removal. Postoperatively, the patient's balance may in fact become worse and may require extensive formal balance retraining and medication.

Vestibular Rehabilitation

Patients with nonfluctuating, poorly compensated, unilateral peripheral disease, bilateral vestibular disease, limited central disease, head trauma, and disorders of sensory conflict resolution are excellent candidates for formal vestibular rehabilitation therapy. Using this approach, a specially trained physical therapist designs an exercise program consisting of progressively more challenging oculomotor and postural tasks that are learned by the patient and incorporated into daily life. Patients learn to augment existing vestibular cues, substitute vision and proprioception for lost vestibular input, resolve sensory conflict among visual, vestibular, and proprioceptive input, and avoid tasks that are deemed beyond their balance capability.[8] It is important to note that there is no place for rehabilitation training in patients with acute peripheral vertigo because the brain cannot adjust to changing peripheral input by repetition and habituation.

AUDITORY DYSFUNCTION

Types of Hearing Loss

Hearing impairment is classified as conductive, sensorineural, or mixed. Conductive hearing loss may be caused by anything that precludes the normal transmission of sound energy through the external auditory canal, tympanic membrane, or middle ear. Various conditions that frequently result in conductive hearing loss include impacted cerumen, tympanic membrane perforation, otitis media, and discontinuity or fixation of the ossicles (e.g., otosclerosis). Sensorineural hearing loss results when the inner ear, auditory nerve (eighth cranial nerve), brain stem, or cortical auditory pathways do not function properly. A mixed hearing loss is a conductive hearing loss superimposed on a sensorineural hearing loss.

Presbycusis

Presbycusis, a sensorineural form of hearing loss, is the most common form of hearing loss in the elderly. Studies have indicated that approximately 25% of people between 65 and 74 years of age and 50% of people 75 years of age or older experience hearing difficulties.[10] The cause of hearing loss due to presbycusis remains unclear. Studies have attempted to link the effects of diet, metabolism, arteriosclerosis, noise, stress, and heredity on hearing, but no clear correlation has emerged. Presbycusis remains a diagnosis of exclusion, and other causes of bilateral progressive sensorineural hearing loss must be ruled out before the diagnosis is made. Some research has correlated long exposure to environmental noise with presbycusis, but it would be overly simplistic to assume that noise is the only etiologic factor. Research has yet to elucidate the exact cause of presbycusis, but it probably has many sources, including degeneration of the cochlea and disorders in central auditory processing that occur with increasing age.[10]

Presbycusis is not a simple entity but a complex disorder involving a wide range of problems varying from loss of speech processing to decreased word intelligibility. The elderly require careful explanations of their problem to help prevent the isolation and frustration that may result from progressive hearing loss. Auditory rehabilitation plays an important role in keeping the older person with a hearing deficit from withdrawing from society.

To develop an optimum rehabilitation plan it is necessary to look beyond the standard audiogram. Multiple factors, acoustic and nonacoustic, influence a person's success in the rehabilitation process. Intervention decisions should be based on a careful study of the elderly patient's auditory and nonauditory performance. The need for patient counseling is an important element of the rehabilitation process.

Audiologic Evaluation

The audiologic evaluation involves obtaining an objective picture of a patient's hearing deficit. It helps to identify the possible cause of a person's hearing loss. Initial evaluation begins with a complete head and neck examination. An adequate history is taken to further elucidate the source of the hearing loss. An audiogram is performed to identify the nature and degree of hearing impairment. An audiogram, however, does not provide information about the effect of the hearing loss on the patient's ability to function. Because each person responds to a loss of hearing in a different manner, assumptions should not be made about a patient's hearing handicap based solely on interpretation of the audiogram. A self-assessment hearing handicap scale can be used to fully evaluate the actual hearing handicap an elderly patient is experiencing.[10] A number of self-assessment scales are available for clinical use. These scales can provide information about the difficulties experienced by hearing-impaired people in a variety of listening conditions, the impact of hearing loss on psychosocial function, and the self-perception of the hearing-impaired person.[11, 12]

Amplification Selection

A number of amplification options are available to the elderly person who is hearing impaired. Levitt in 1987[13] suggested that we refer to this group of devices as rehabilitation technology for the hearing impaired. He divided the technology into four categories: (1) sound enhancement technology, (2) television enhancement technology, (3) telecommunication technology, and (4) signal-alerting technology.[13, 14]

Sound enhancement technology refers to amplification systems that are used to assist in the reception of sound. Included in this group are traditional and programmable hearing aids, assistive listening devices such as hardware, infrared, and frequency modulation (FM) systems, and cochlear implants.

Television enhancement technology refers to equipment used to improve the auditory perception of television. Included in this group may be sound enhancement technology such as infrared or FM systems and closed caption decoding devices.

Telecommunication technology refers to systems that improve the ability to communicate over the telephone. Included in this group are specific devices such as amplified telephone handsets, portable strap-on telephone amplifiers, and the telephone device for the deaf (TDD).

Signal-alerting technology refers to equipment used to alert a hearing-impaired person to the presence of sound by using either a visual or tactile signal. Included in this group are lights that flash in the presence of sound, vibrating alarm systems, and hearing ear dogs.

A complete assessment of a hearing-impaired person's needs must be done to determine the appropriate choice for amplification. All areas of communication should be considered when making this decision.

Hearing aids (Fig. 41–2) are the sound enhancement device most commonly recommended for hearing-impaired patients. In addition to the degree and configuration of the hearing loss, many nonacoustic factors, such as motivation, financial ability, manual dexterity, cognitive ability, and cosmetic concerns, may influence the patient's choice of a hearing aid. A number of choices are available; however, it must be stressed that no hearing aid can improve communication ability if the hearing-impaired patient is unable to use it.

The growing complexity of hearing aid devices increases the need for hearing aid orientation. The type of hearing aid prescribed depends on the needs and capabilities of the patient and the exact nature and configuration of the hearing loss.[15, 16] In general, binaural aids are more useful than single aids in the bilaterally hearing-impaired person. Contralateral routing of signal (CROS) aids can be used for people who perceive a need for bilateral input when only a unilateral loss exists. Smaller in-the-ear or in-the-canal aids may be cosmetically appealing, but they provide only limited amplification and require considerable dexterity on the part of the patient to use. Eyeglass hearing aids are limited by the ability of the dealer to adjust the aid without causing the patient to lose the use of the glasses temporarily.

A hearing aid alone may not offer sufficient help to enable a hearing-impaired person to hear in the presence of background noise, in a highly reverberating environment, or over the telephone. Many assistive listening devices are effective in such adverse conditions. Success with these devices is due to the increased signal-to-noise ratio, which helps to reduce the perception of background noise.

The clinician should possess an understanding of an elderly person's communication needs and should determine the most effective plan to meet those needs.[15–18] This plan may include a prescription for either short- or long-term counseling. Cooperation among hearing-impaired patients, their families, the clinician, and the audiologist allows optimum auditory rehabilitation.

References

1. Perry ET: The Human Ear Canal. Springfield, IL, Charles C Thomas, 1957, pp. 57–70.
2. Glasscock ME III, Shambaugh GE Jr: Surgery of the Ear, 4th ed. Philadelphia, WB Saunders, 1990.
3. Senturia BH, Marcus MD, Lucente FE: Diseases of the External Ear: An Otologic-Dermatologic Manual. New York, Grune & Stratton, 1980.
4. Maceri DR: Sensorineural hearing loss: Sudden, fluctuating, and gradual. *In* Meyerhoff WL, Rice DH (eds): Otolaryngology: Head and Neck Surgery. Philadelphia, WB Saunders, 1992.
5. Sloane P, Baloh RW: Persistent dizziness in geriatric patients. J Am Geriatr Soc 1989;37:1031–1038.
6. Gacek RR, Ham R: A clinical approach to the management of geriatric disequilibrium. Ear Nose Throat J 1989;68:958–960.
7. Baloh RW, Honrubia V: Clinical Neurophysiology of the Vestibular System. Philadelphia, FA Davis, 1990.
8. Barber HO, Sharpe JA: Vestibular Disorders. Chicago, Mosby-Yearbook, 1988.
9. Baloh RW, Sakala SM, Yee RD, et al: Quantitative vestibular testing. Arch Otolaryngol Head Neck Surg 1985;92:145–156.
10. Meyerhoff WL: Diagnosis and Management of Hearing Loss. Philadelphia, WB Saunders, 1984.
11. American Speech-Language and Hearing Association: Definition of and competencies for aural rehabilitation. ASHA 1984;26:37–41.
12. High W, Fairbanks C, Glorig A: Scale of self-assessment of hearing handicap. JSHD 1964;29:215–230.
13. Malinoff R, Weinstein B: Measurement of hearing aid benefit in the elderly. Ear Hear 1989;10:354–356.
14. Schow R, Nerbonne M: Communication screening profile: Use with elderly clients. Ear Hear 1980;3:135–148.

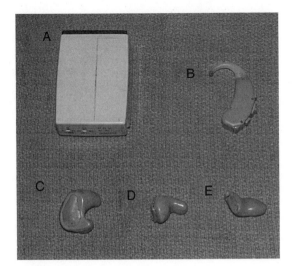

Figure 41–2 Types of hearing aids. *A,* Bone-conduction aid. *B,* Behind the ear (BTE). *C,* In the ear (ITE). *D,* In the canal (ITC). *E,* Completely in canal (CIC).

15. Ventry I, Weinstein B: The hearing handicap inventory for the elderly: A new tool. Ear Hear 1982;3:128–134.

16. Traynor R: Hearing aid counseling and orientation. *In* Hull R (ed): Rehabilitative Audiology. New York, Grune & Stratton, 1982.

17. Shumway-Cook A, Horak FB: Rehabilitation strategies for patients with vestibular deficits. Neurol Clin 1990;8:441–457.

18. American Academy of Otolaryngology and American Council of Otology: Guidelines for evaluation of hearing handicap. JAMA 1979;241:2055–2059.

42 Ophthalmologic Disorders

Carol R. Kollarits, M.D.

Blindness is the disability feared most by elderly Americans. This fear is rational, since 3% of the patients studied in the mobile population of the Framingham Study cohort were found to be legally blind.[1] In a study of geriatric patients confined to nursing homes, more than 25% were found to be legally blind.[2]

This chapter acquaints the physician caring for geriatric patients with his or her responsibilities in the early diagnosis of potentially blinding eye diseases. In addition, it outlines the elements of emergency management of ocular trauma and the management of common ocular complaints

of the elderly. Common surgical techniques and medications used by ophthalmologists are described briefly, since geriatric physicians are often called on to diagnose symptoms arising from interactions and side effects of ocular medications or advise patients about the need for certain types of eye surgery.

ANATOMIC REVIEW

Figure 42–1 represents a vertical cross-section through a human eye and orbit. The upper lid is elevated by the action of the levator muscle

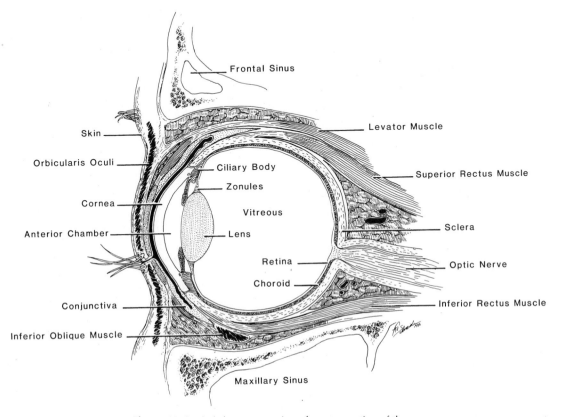

Figure 42–1 Artist's representation of a cross-section of the eye.

(innervated by the third cranial nerve). The lids are closed by contraction of the subcutaneous orbicularis muscles (seventh cranial nerve) in both the upper and lower lids. The inner surfaces of the lids are lined with conjunctiva. The conjunctiva forms a continuous lining from the inner surfaces of the lids over the sclera up to the limbus (the junction of the sclera with the cornea). The tear film is composed of mucus from conjunctival goblet cells, aqueous tears secreted by the lacrimal gland, and oil from glands opening at the lid margin. The tear film lubricates the movement of the lids over the cornea.

The cornea is the clear "watch glass" covering of the front of the eye. Its composition is similar to that of the white sclera except that its collagen fibers are arranged more regularly. It is covered by five layers of epithelial cells on its anterior surface. Posteriorly, it is lined by a single layer of endothelial cells that actively pump fluid from the corneal stroma, maintaining the clarity of the cornea.

The anterior chamber is filled with aqueous humor produced by the ciliary body behind the clear lens. The lens is attached to the ciliary body by collagen fibers called zonules. The ciliary body contains muscles that, when contracted, cause the lens to increase its anteroposterior diameter, bringing the eye into focus on near objects.

The central portion of the eye is filled with vitreous humor, a matrix of collagen fibrils interspersed through a gel composed of hyaluronic acid. The retina is 10 cell layers thick and extends from the optic nerve to the edge of the ciliary body. The choroid is a vascular layer that underlies the retina. The tough white outer coat of the eye is the sclera. The optic nerve consists of axons from the nerve fiber layer of the retina. These axons form synapses in the lateral geniculate body on second-order neurons whose axons proceed to the occipital cortex.

The six extraocular muscles insert into the sclera to move the eye. The lateral rectus muscle is innervated by the sixth cranial nerve. The superior oblique muscle is innervated by the fourth cranial nerve. The medial rectus, inferior rectus, inferior oblique, and superior rectus, as well as the previously mentioned levator muscle, are innervated by the third cranial nerve. The sphincter muscle of the iris is innervated by parasympathetic fibers carried in the third cranial nerve. The dilator muscle of the pupil is innervated by sympathetic fibers.[3]

EYE EXAMINATION

The screening area of every physician's office should be equipped with a well-illuminated Snel-

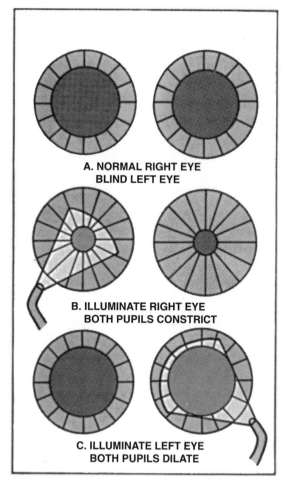

A. NORMAL RIGHT EYE BLIND LEFT EYE

B. ILLUMINATE RIGHT EYE BOTH PUPILS CONSTRICT

C. ILLUMINATE LEFT EYE BOTH PUPILS DILATE

Figure 42–2 Swinging flashlight test for a Marcus Gunn afferent pupillary defect. In dim illumination, the blind left eye has the same size pupil as its normal fellow eye (*A*). Illumination of the normal eye causes both pupils to constrict equally (direct and consensual pupillary miosis), as shown in *B*. Swinging the flashlight over to illuminate the blind eye is followed by dilation of the pupil because the pupil of the blind eye dilates consensually in response to loss of illumination of the normal eye (*C*). (From Mehelas TJ, Kollarits CR: Pupillary clues to neuro-ophthalmic diagnosis. Postgrad Med 71:199, 1982.)

len chart for estimating visual acuity at a distance of 20 feet. The examiner should obtain the best corrected visual acuity of each eye separately using the patient's current spectacles. Pupil light responses should be checked with a flashlight, including use of the "swinging flashlight test" for every patient (Fig. 42–2). Ophthalmoscopy is accomplished more easily if the patient's pupils are dilated. One drop of 2.5% phenylephrine hydrochloride (Neosynephrine) in each eye will dilate the pupils of most eyes with blue irises within 15 to 20 minutes, usually without elevating blood pressure. More darkly pigmented eyes require two to three sets of drops, given at 5-

minute intervals. The only contraindications to pupillary dilation are recent head injury, a history of angle-closure glaucoma, or previous admonition by an ophthalmologist that the patient's pupils should not be dilated.

COMMON OCULAR PROBLEMS

Presbyopia

The most common ocular complaint of Americans over 40 years old is a diminished ability to focus clearly at normal (less than arm's length) reading distances. This is presbyopia. It is caused by thickening (increased anteroposterior diameter) of the lens within the eye as a result of continued growth of the lens fibers. In the young eye, focusing on a near object is accomplished by contracting the muscles in the ciliary body, which reduces the tension of the zonules and elastic capsule of the lens. The resulting increase in thickness of the anteroposterior lens is allowed to continue until the desired focal distance is reached. In the older eye, the already thickened lens responds more slowly to changes in tension of the elastic capsule. Some individuals notice that they can, with some effort, focus clearly for reading but then when they look up, their distance vision is blurred for several seconds to a few minutes as the lens very slowly resumes its previous anteroposterior diameter. These symptoms are relieved by the use of reading glasses or the addition of bifocal segments to the patient's distance spectacle correction.

Second Sight

After being presbyopic for many years, some individuals find that they can once again focus clearly for reading without using their bifocals. This "second sight" phenomenon is caused by acquired myopia (nearsightedness) secondary to increasing lens thickness. The protein composition of the lens may change at this time, causing lens opacities (cataract formation).

Ocular Injuries

If the patient experiences pain following an injury, a drop of topical anesthetic can be carefully instilled by gently pulling down the lower eyelid and placing the drop on the conjunctival surface of the lid. The examiner's fingers should be placed well below the lash margin, and the lid should be pulled away from the eye by rolling the skin over the inferior orbital rim rather than pushing the lid downward. Pushing the lid may transmit pressure to the injured eye, causing pain

and prolapse of the vitreous and retina through a corneoscleral laceration. Once the anesthetic drop has been instilled, patients with superficial injuries feel nearly complete relief from pain. Deeper injuries are usually still painful despite the topical anesthetic.

If a corneal abrasion is suspected, it can often be more readily identified by placing a fluorescein strip in the tear film just long enough to color the tears yellow. After the patient blinks, the abraded area of the cornea will stain bright yellow, making it more readily distinguishable from the normal nonstaining corneal surface. Corneal abrasions can be treated by instilling an antibiotic ointment and applying a patch firmly. The lids should be patched tightly enough so that they cannot open under the patch and allow the patch to further abrade the cornea. Use of a patch for 24 hours will permit most corneal abrasions to heal.

If a penetrating ocular injury is suspected on the basis of an irregular pupil, or if an obvious laceration is evident on inspection, the eye should not be patched; rather, a metal shield should be taped over the eye to prevent further damage while the patient is transported to an ophthalmologist for definitive surgical management.

Sudden Visual Loss

In patients who report a sudden loss of vision, visual acuity should be checked with the Snellen chart and recorded. Pupil responses should be examined carefully. In a patient with monocular visual loss resulting from a retinal or optic nerve problem, a Marcus Gunn afferent pupillary defect will be present in that eye when the swinging flashlight test is performed (see Fig. 42–2). If the Marcus Gunn pupil is not present in the affected eye, visual loss is due to an opacity of the media (cataract or vitreous hemorrhage), or there is no visual loss (the patient is hysterical or malingering). If the pupils are normal, confrontation visual field testing should be performed to rule out a homonymous hemianopia due to a stroke, because many patients interpret the loss of the right half of the visual field of each eye as blindness of the right eye.

The most common causes of sudden monocular painless visual loss in the elderly are (1) subretinal hemorrhage (macular degeneration), (2) central retinal artery or vein occlusion, (3) ischemic optic neuropathy (caused by atherosclerosis or giant cell arteritis), (4) retinal detachment, and (5) vitreous hemorrhage resulting from diabetic retinopathy or retinal hole formation. Central retinal artery occlusion can seldom be reversed in time to allow recovery of vision, but the patient requires a work-up for sources of emboli such as atheromatous plaques at the carotid bifurcation or a diseased mitral valve.[4] Patients with central retinal vein occlusion also have a poor prognosis for visual recovery. Patients with a branch retinal vein occlusion have a much better chance of recovery of useful vision, but some will require laser treatment. Patients with venous occlusive disease must be evaluated for systemic hypertension, chronic simple glaucoma, and any disease that increases blood viscosity. These include polycythemia, leukemia, the coagulopathies, and macroglobulinemia.

Patients with sudden visual loss in one eye should be examined by an ophthalmologist on an emergency basis. Binocular sudden visual loss is most commonly caused by bilateral occipital lobe infarcts. The pupil responses are normal if the visual loss is a result of occipital infarction.

Gradual Visual Loss

Progressive, unrelenting visual blurring occurring over months or years is most often due to cataracts. Visual loss due to macular degeneration often has an intermittent downhill course. Untreated chronic simple glaucoma results in progressive peripheral visual field loss that the patient may not notice until the central vision is threatened. Gradual visual loss may also be caused by optic nerve atrophy.

Every patient with optic atrophy (pallor of the optic disk) and gradual visual loss should be evaluated for tertiary syphilis, diabetes mellitus, pernicious anemia and other anemias, brain tumor, and poor nutrition (possibly associated with chronic alcoholism and cigarette smoking — "tobacco-ethanol amblyopia").

Patients with ischemic optic neuropathy may present with optic atrophy in one eye and an apparently edematous disk in the other eye. This is the classic Foster Kennedy syndrome, often ascribed to sphenoid ridge meningioma. However, the most common cause is not meningioma but atherosclerosis or giant cell arteritis. Work-up of the patient with ischemic optic neuropathy should include skull films, determination of erythrocyte sedimentation rate (ESR), and temporal artery biopsy. If the ESR is normal and the skull films are interpreted as normal, a computed tomographic scan of the brain should be obtained to rule out an intracranial tumor. Acute visual loss, whether due to atherosclerosis or giant cell arteritis, should be treated with 100 mg of prednisone by mouth daily for 3 to 5 days. If a diagnosis of giant cell arteritis is made, oral corticosteroids should be continued until the ESR is reduced to normal even if vision is not improved, since patients with this disorder have an increased mortality rate from myocardial infarction if the problem is left untreated. In desperate situations, when steroid therapy has failed to restore vision in the patient's only remaining eye, transient blood pressure elevation with intravenous levo-norepinephrine may be considered.[5]

Hereditary causes of progressive optic nerve or retinal degeneration usually become apparent prior to age 50 and will have been diagnosed previously. In the absence of observed ocular abnormalities, unexplained visual loss should be considered the result of a brain tumor until proved otherwise by appropriate studies.

Tearing and Irritation

Many older people are troubled by irritation, the sensation of a foreign body in the eye, or excessive tearing. All these can be symptoms of a "dry eye syndrome." If no foreign body or trichiasis (misdirected lashes rubbing on the cornea) is found after inspection of the eye with fluorescein staining of the tear film, a presumptive diagnosis of dry eye syndrome can be made. Treatment consists of an artificial tear preparation containing a long-chain polymer that mimics the action of the mucus that is often deficient in the tears of the elderly. Tears II, HypoTears, or a similar preparation should be used at least four times daily and especially before reading or other activities that require frequent eye movements. If the artificial tear preparation does not relieve the excessive tearing, an ophthalmologist should evaluate the patient for dysfunction of the nasolacrimal duct or abnormal lid position.

Drooping Lids

Irritation may be caused by malposition of the lower lid. Entropion (turning in) and ectropion (turning out) are both caused by laxity of the orbicularis muscle and require surgical procedures that tighten this muscle. Laxity of the orbicularis muscle over the upper lid results in blepharochalasis, the development of an extra lid fold, which often contains herniated orbital fat. This lid fold may hang down on the upper lashes, making it difficult for the patient to elevate the lids sufficiently to see. In true ptosis of the upper lid, the entire lid droops downward over the cornea, and the lid fold disappears. This is usually caused by dehiscence of the levator muscle, but myasthenia gravis and Horner's syndrome should be ruled out.

Horner's syndrome may cause minor ptosis of both upper and lower lids, making the affected eye appear smaller because of the narrowed lid fissure. The pupil is smaller in the affected eye than in the other eye, and the skin on the same side of the face produces less sweat. If the patient has no other neurologic signs, a chest film with apical lordotic views should be obtained to rule out the presence of a Pancoast tumor or tuberculosis of the apex of the lung, which affects the sympathetic pathway to the pupil. If the radiographic results are negative and the patient develops no other neurologic symptoms, no further work-up is necessary.

Light Flashes, Floaters, and Visual Hallucinations

Flashing lights that the patient can localize to one eye (rather than half of the visual field in both eyes) are usually due to a vitreous detachment. When the vitreous detaches from the optic nerve, a circular condensation of collagen fibers may float free just in front of the macula and will be seen as a nearly transparent "doughnut" by the patient. Other floaters may be described as "wiggly lines," "worms," or "fishnets" that move when the eye moves and continue to move across the patient's visual field for a short time after the eye stops moving. These floaters are usually no cause for alarm, but floaters appearing as a "swarm of gnats" in the field of one eye usually represent red blood cells from a retinal tear. Since retinal tears may result from vitreous detachment and can cause retinal detachment, a patient with this complaint should be examined by an ophthalmologist. Most elderly patients experience the symptoms of a vitreous detachment, but only 1 in 10,000 develop a retinal detachment.

Brain tumor or cortical ischemia may cause visual hallucinations. When a lesion affects the temporal lobe, the patient may have the sensation that he or she is seeing a movie of some past episode in his or her life. A lesion of the occipital cortex causes unformed hallucinations, such as flashing lights or zigzag lines. The most common example is the visual aura of migraine, which is not necessarily accompanied or followed by a migraine headache. Formed hallucinations, often described as "wallpaper patterns," sometimes occur in patients who have combined central and peripheral visual loss in both eyes (for example, macular degeneration and glaucoma).

Diplopia

Paralysis of the third, fourth, or sixth cranial nerve may cause diplopia (double vision) that is troublesome to the patient in the field of gaze of the affected extraocular muscle or muscles. Patching the affected eye may be necessary to allow the patient to recover from a cerebral vascular accident or head trauma without the added distraction of diplopia. Corrective muscle surgery is usually not done for 6 months following a head injury or stroke because spontaneous recovery is possible in that time. The young patient who complains of diplopia with one eye covered is usually hysterical, but the elderly individual who describes monocular diplopia often is suffering from a (double focus) cataract. Visual acuity may be quite good with such a cataract, but the diplopia may be sufficiently annoying to justify cataract removal.

Intermittent vertical diplopia is a common sign of basivertebral artery insufficiency in the elderly. Double vision or ptosis that occurs only in the evening is most likely due to myasthenia gravis. If symptoms are not present during a morning examination, another examination should be carried out as late in the day as possible. If double vision or ptosis can be documented at this time, an edrophonium chloride (Tensilon) test may alleviate the symptoms and confirm the suspected diagnosis of myasthenia gravis.

Purulent Discharge and Lid Crusting

Bacterial conjunctivitis is characterized by a purulent discharge that often mats the lids shut when the patient wakes up in the morning. This disorder is not accompanied by pain and should be relieved within 3 to 4 days by frequent use of antibiotic drops.

Infection of the lid margins (marginal blepharitis) is manifest by greasy crusts around the bases of the lashes and swelling and redness of the underlying skin. Warm, moist compresses should be applied to the affected lids four times daily, followed by gentle scrubbing of the lid margins with lid scrub pads or cotton-tipped applicators dipped in baby shampoo. After the lids have been gently dried, a drop of antibiotic solution such as Neosporin should be applied to the inferior cul-de-sac. The common sty (hordeolum) can be treated similarly.

Painless watery discharge, accompanied by conjunctival hyperemia and symptoms of fullness of the lids, is most likely due to a viral or chlamydial conjunctivitis. Topical antibiotics should be used in the same way as for treatment of bacterial conjunctivitis to prevent a bacterial superinfection in these conditions. Sulfonamide eye drops may be used in patients with suspected viral or chlamydial conjunctivitis, but they are not effective in the average case of bacterial conjunctivitis because of the large amount of para-aminobenzoic acid present in purulent discharge.[6] If the symptoms last more than 1 week or if the patient complains of pain, an ophthalmologist should be consulted.

Redness, watery discharge, and itching are most commonly caused by allergy. A decongestant-antihistamine preparation (such as Albalon-A or Naphcon-A) should be applied, one drop four times daily. Topical steroid drops should not be used by a physician other than an ophthalmologist because of the danger of potentiating a viral infection and inducing glaucoma. Alomide or Crolom drops prevent histamine release from mast cells in the conjunctiva and are useful for chronic allergic conjunctivitis.

Subconjunctival hemorrhage presents as a dramatic bright red infiltration over the sclera. No treatment other than reassurance should be given, and no work-up is required if the patient has no cutaneous petechial hemorrhages and no history of recent easy bruising or bleeding suggesting a platelet deficiency.

Painful Red Eye

A patient with a red painful eye that has an apparent corneal ulcer (white spot on the cornea) should be referred to an ophthalmologist as an emergency. No antibiotic drops or ointment should be instilled prior to referral, since this may suppress growth of organisms cultured from corneal scrapings. Bacterial corneal ulcers are usually painful, whereas ulcers caused by herpes simplex may not be very painful.

In addition to bacterial or viral corneal ulcers, a red painful eye may be caused by angle-closure glaucoma or iritis. In angle-closure glaucoma the pupil of the affected eye is dilated compared with the pupil of the normal eye, and the eye has a significantly increased intraocular pressure that can easily be detected by finger palpation or tonometry. In iritis, the pupil of the affected eye is smaller than that of the normal eye, and the pressure can be quite low. For either condition, the patient should be referred to an ophthalmologist for definitive management.

Glaucoma

At least 2% of the population over the age of 40 have chronic simple glaucoma. In its early stages, this is an asymptomatic disease that, unlike the much rarer acute angle-closure glaucoma, causes no pain. Gradual loss of vision due to prolonged elevation of intraocular pressure is often unnoticed by the patient until a significant amount of the visual field is gone. Patients with optic disk pallor, hemorrhage on the disk, or a progressive increase in the cup-disk ratio over a period of years should be referred to an ophthalmologist for evaluation for possible chronic simple glaucoma. A family history of glaucoma should prompt earlier referral. Glaucoma is the leading cause of irreversible blindness in American blacks. The prevalence of glaucoma in blacks is four to six times higher than that in whites. Other risk factors for glaucoma besides family history and race include diabetes mellitus, cardiovascular disease, and myopia. Patients with these risk factors should have annual examinations by an ophthalmologist.

Most of the medications used to treat glaucoma produce significant side effects. Pilocarpine produces blurring of vision because of induced spasm of accommodation in young patients, and decreased vision because of the decreased pupil size, which in turn reduces the amount of light entering the eye. This may severely reduce vision in an eye with a cataract. Timolol maleate and other beta-blocking drops have been known to precipitate status asthmaticus, congestive heart failure, and psychosis. Epinephrine drops can cause conjunctival redness, browache, and cardiac arrythmias, as well as deposition of pigment in the conjunctiva. The carbonic anhydrase inhibitors acetazolamide (Diamox) and methazolamide (Neptazane) are prescribed to manage severe glaucoma when combinations of eye drops have failed to control the intraocular pressure sufficiently to prevent continued visual loss. Diamox is chemically similar in structure to the sulfonamides and may cause blurred vision, decreased appetite, a metallic taste in the mouth, dizziness, and renal stones. These side effects are less frequent with Neptazane but are not entirely absent. Dorzolamide hydrochloride [Trusopt] is a new topical carbonic anhydrase inhibitor that usually causes no systemic side effects but sometimes causes allergic reactions in patients with a history of allergy to sulfa drugs. Other topical medications for glaucoma include alpha-adrenergic agonists (apraclonidine [Iopidine] and brimonidine tartrate [Alphagan]) and a prostaglandin analogue, latanoprost.[7, 8] Since the different classes of glaucoma medications lower intraocular pressure by different mechanisms, several of these medications may be combined in a regimen designed specifically for each patient.

The argon laser may be used to treat the trabecular meshwork of eyes in patients with chronic simple glaucoma and progressive visual field loss. If laser trabeculopexy is not successful in lowering intraocular pressure, a surgical trabeculectomy or another fistulizing procedure can be performed.

A recent study of patients with primary open-angle glaucoma showed that argon laser trabeculoplasty used as the initial therapy (instead of topical drops) may be more effective in preventing visual field loss. Because 30% of glaucoma patients have significant side effects from eye drops and the current cost of eye drops for glaucoma may be almost $60 for a single month's supply of one medication, argon laser trabeculoplasty is likely to be performed in a higher percentage of glaucoma patients in the near future.[9]

Angle-closure glaucoma is much less common than chronic simple glaucoma, but it is less likely to be neglected because its most common symptom is severe pain. The pain results from abrupt elevation of intraocular pressure due to blockage of the trabecular meshwork by the peripheral iris. In addition to pain, the elevated pressure causes corneal edema, creating colored halos around lights observed with the affected eye. The angle closure can be relieved by creating an iridotomy (hole in the iris) with the argon laser or neodynium YAG laser or by surgical iridectomy.

Periocular Pain

The most common cause of periocular pain is sinus disease. Because of the proximity of the sinuses to the orbit (see Fig. 42–1) and common innervation of these structures by the fifth cranial nerve, sinus pain is often referred to the eye. In the absence of decreased vision, elevated intraocular pressure, or redness, most complaints of ocular pain deserve a trial of oral decongestant therapy.

The lancinating pain of tic douloureux and the throbbing pain of migraine may also involve the eye. Tic douloureux responds well to carbamazepine (Tegretol), whereas migraine may be reduced in frequency by the use of propranolol hydrochloride (Inderal). For patients with frequent debilitating migraine, Inderal 40 mg/day should be tried. This dose may have to be reduced if it produces orthostatic hypotension. Some patients who experience a definite warning aura 15 to 30 minutes prior to the onset of the headache can abort the headache by taking one 10-mg tablet of Inderal and one 5-grain tablet of aspirin as soon as they notice the warning migraine aura. Oral or intramuscular sumatriptan (Imitrex) may be used in patients who do not respond to Inderal.

Pain in the distribution of the ophthalmic division of the trigeminal nerve may be caused by herpes zoster. Often pain may be noted when combing the hair up to 10 days before the appearance of the vesicles. No specific ocular therapy is indicated unless vesicles develop on the tip of the nose on the same side as the "shingles."

When this occurs, the eye is usually severely inflamed, often resulting in chronic pain and accelerated cataract formation. As in any elderly person with herpes zoster, systemic evaluation should be done for leukemia, lymphoma, and other diseases affecting the immune system. Postherpetic pain may be severe and may last for a period of several months. Tegretol is often useful in the management of this pain. Oral acyclovir (Zovirax), 800 mg five times daily for 10 days, or famciclovir (Famvir), 500 mg three times daily for 7 days during the acute attack, may reduce the severity and duration of postherpetic pain.

The cause of throbbing pain accompanied by an ipsilateral paralysis of the third cranial nerve (upper lid ptosis, dilated pupil, eye displaced down and laterally) should be considered an intracranial aneurysm until a normal arteriogram has been obtained. Painful ophthalmoplegia caused by the Tolosa-Hunt syndrome may be treated with steroids after aneurysm and diabetes mellitus have been ruled out. Paralysis of the third cranial nerve caused by diabetes mellitus does not involve the pupil and usually is not accompanied by the severe pain seen in patients with aneurysm or Tolosa-Hunt syndrome. If caused by diabetes, the paralysis will disappear spontaneously within 90 days.

Cataracts

Any decrease in transparency or alteration of the optical homogeneity of the lens is called a cataract. Cataract formation begins in everyone over 30 years of age but progresses at varying rates in different individuals. Total opacification of the lens, resulting in a white, "mature," or "ripe" cataract, actually occurs in very few people.

Compared with a normal lens, a cataractous lens has different water and ionic concentrations and protein constituents. Some of these changes in lens chemistry may result from exposure to ultraviolet light or other unknown toxic environmental influences. Cataract formation is more common in diabetics because of the increased hydration resulting from the presence of excessive sorbitol and fructose in the diabetic lens. Inhibition of the enzyme aldose reductase reduces sorbitol accumulation in the lens and may retard the development of cataracts in diabetics. Unfortunately, use of topical aldose reductase inhibitors and other eye drops have not reversed cataract changes. For most patients with cataracts, surgical extraction is the only alternative to progressive visual loss.

CATARACT SURGERY

Cataract extraction is the most commonly performed operation in the United States today, with approximately 1 million being performed each year. The risk of visual loss as a result of cataract surgery is less than 5%.

Cataract phacoemulsification (use of ultrasonic fragmentation of the nucleus) with implantation of a synthetic intraocular lens in the remaining capsular bag is the cataract procedure most commonly performed today because it can be performed through a smaller incision than intracapsular or other types of extracapsular surgery. In phacoemulsification, an opening is made in the anterior capsule. The nucleus of the lens is then fragmented ultrasonically and aspirated, care being taken to avoid damage to the corneal endothelium. The softer cortical material can then be aspirated and peeled away from the remaining capsule before the intraocular lens is implanted. The final spectacle lens for the pseudophakic eye is usually prescribed about 6 weeks following cataract surgery. Accurate intraocular lens power calculation allows the pseudophakic eye to see well with a much thinner spectacle lens than would have to be prescribed for the aphakic eye, eliminating the magnification and distortion produced by "old-fashioned" thick cataract glasses.

In many pseudophakic eyes, the posterior capsule behind the intraocular lens implant opacifies because of proliferation of residual cortical lens fibers across the posterior capsule. If this capsular opacification (secondary cataract or secondary membrane formation) interferes with vision, a neodynium YAG laser can be used to create a clear opening in the posterior capsule, restoring vision. This laser treatment can be done with topical anesthetic drops in a few minutes and often results in restoration of good vision within hours.

If the patient has been advised to have cataract surgery but does not believe that vision is compromised sufficiently to justify surgery, near vision should be checked with the patient wearing current bifocals. If the patient can read newsprint with the affected eye, surgery can usually be deferred. Sometimes the patient is eager to have cataract surgery, but the ophthalmologist may recommend that no surgery be done, often because macular degeneration, diabetic retinopathy, or chronic simple glaucoma has reduced the patient's vision so much that cataract surgery may provide little or no visual improvement. When other intraocular diseases coexist with a cataract, the timing of cataract surgery becomes a matter of careful judgment by the ophthalmologist.

SIDE EFFECTS OF OCULAR MEDICATIONS

Instillation of a drop of medication in the conjunctival cul-de-sac is equivalent to giving the same amount of medication intravenously. It should be apparent that systemic anaphylactic reactions can occur just as easily as local allergic responses to the active pharmaceutical agent, its vehicle, or the preservative added to the drug and its vehicle. Some patients may complain of dryness of the mouth and flushing of the skin while taking atropine drops. This is a true pharmacologic side effect rather than an allergic reaction. Any of the topical antibiotic drops can cause a local allergic reaction and are capable of causing anaphylaxis in patients with a history of prior exposure to the drug. Chloramphenicol eye drops have (rarely) been associated with aplastic anemia. Topical corticosteroid-containing eye drops cause elevation of intraocular pressure in a third of the normal population. Corticosteroid drops may potentiate herpes simplex or fungal keratitis. In addition, patients with tissue antigen HLA-A1 are likely to develop corticosteroid-induced cataracts whether the steroid is given topically or systemically.[10]

SURGERY

Retinal Surgery

The argon laser is most commonly used in the treatment of diabetic retinopathy and macular degeneration. Diabetic patients with decreased vision resulting from macular edema or exudates may show improvement following focal laser therapy of the leaking blood vessels that are responsible for the edema or exudates. Diabetics with normal vision may receive laser panretinal ablation to prevent future loss of vision if they have neovascularization (growth of new blood vessels) of the disk, neovascularization elsewhere, or vitreous hemorrhage.

Patients with macular degeneration may complain of distorted images (a "kink" in telephone poles or a "bend" in lines on the road). They should undergo fluorescein angiography, a procedure performed to detect abnormal blood vessels entering the subretinal space from the underlying choroid. If these vessels are not directly under the foveal avascular zone or the nerve fiber bundle connecting the macula and the optic disk, they can sometimes be ablated with argon laser therapy. This may result in stabilization of vision and prevention of future visual loss; however, it is relatively rare for a patient to regain normal vision. Retinal pigment epithelial detachments can sometimes be sealed, resulting in improvement in visual acuity. Unfortunately, only 10% of patients with macular degeneration have "wet" lesions such as leaking blood vessels that are suitable for laser treatment. The remaining patients have "dry" macular degeneration with progressive atrophy of the macular tissues.

The argon laser may be used to seal retinal holes; however, it is often not useful in the treatment of retinal detachment because the detached retina is nearly transparent. Most retinal detachments (85% to 90%) can be repaired by applying cryotherapy to the causative retinal hole and temporarily occluding the hole with a slowly absorbing bubble of gas (such as C3F8) injected into the vitreous cavity, or, alternatively, by indenting (buckling) the sclera overlying the hole with an external silicone band or explant. The scleral buckle places the detached retina closer to its original position against the choroid. If the cryoretinopexy has created sufficient inflammation, the retinal hole will seal shut on the buckle, and the subretinal fluid will be reabsorbed.

Corneal Surgery

Corneal transplants may be performed for corneal decompensation following cataract surgery or for primary corneal endothelial failure (Fuchs' endothelial dystrophy). Corneal decompensation may be painful as well as visually debilitating. Corneal transplantation (penetrating keratoplasty) for this indication has a success rate of at least 85%. Corneal surgery for the correction of refractive errors (to eliminate the need for wearing spectacles) is still in evolution. The use of the Excimer laser to sculpt the cornea has now been approved by the Food and Drug Administration (FDA) for correction of myopia (between −1.00 and −7.00 diopters of near-sightedness). Myopic geriatric patients who enjoy reading without glasses should be advised that they will need reading glasses after refractive surgery.

Enucleation

If total blindness affects an eye (i.e., the patient experiences no perception of light when exposed to the brightest illumination available) and the eye is free of pain and cosmetically acceptable, it should be left alone. If a blind eye becomes painful because of corneal degeneration, neovascular glaucoma, or other ongoing intraocular pathologic process, it should be enucleated. Either a silicone sphere is buried under the extraocular muscles or a hydroxyapatite implant is sutured to the cut ends of the extraocular muscles. In about 6 weeks, the patient's conjunctiva

is usually healed sufficiently to permit fitting of a cosmetically acceptable prosthesis. The prosthesis can be removed and cleaned as needed, but it can often be left undisturbed for months because of the cleansing action of the lids.

Periocular Surgery

True ptosis (drooping of the upper lid) interferes with vision. It is most commonly caused by dehiscence of the aponeurosis of the levator muscle in the upper lid. After myasthenia gravis and congenital and inherited causes of ptosis have been ruled out, an incision in the upper lid can be made, the detached levator tendon identified, and the tendon sutured to the tarsal plate. This procedure is usually done under local anesthesia (with conscious sedation, if necessary), so that the patient can open and close his or her lids to permit assessment of adequate lid elevation. Excessive upper lid skin (dermatochalasis) and orbital fat that has herniated through an age-attenuated orbital septum into the lid can be excised (upper lid blepharoplasty) at the same time. Ptosis repair and upper and lower lid blepharoplasties should be performed only if the patient has refrained from taking warfarin (Coumadin) and platelet inhibitors long enough to have regained normal clotting functions, since there is a risk of blindness from orbital hemorrhage following any incisional lid procedure. This risk may be reduced by making the incisions with an ultrapulsed carbon dioxide laser instead of a steel blade. Laser skin resurfacing for periocular rhytids and dermatochalasis requires no incision and probably carries little or no risk of hemorrhage.[11]

BLINDNESS AND LOW VISION

In most states, legal blindness is defined as a visual acuity of 20/200 or worse in the better eye with the aid of the best possible spectacle or contact lens correction. A person may be legally blind with a visual acuity of better than 20/200 if the visual field is constricted to less than 20 degrees in the eye with the larger visual field. The terms low vision, legal blindness, and total blindness are not synonymous. A legally blind patient may be able to read with proper low vision aids, and a patient with low vision (20/50 to 20/200) may benefit immensely from low vision aids.

PREVENTION OF VISUAL LOSS

The most common causes of visual loss in the aging population are cataracts, glaucoma, diabetic retinopathy, and macular degeneration. Early detection and appropriate treatment reduce the risk of blindness from glaucoma and diabetic retinopathy.

Progression of visual loss from cataract and macular degeneration may be slowed by the use of ultraviolet filter coatings on spectacle lenses and sunglasses to protect the lens and retina from photodynamic damage.[12] Free radical scavengers or antioxidants such as selenium, beta-carotene, vitamin C, and vitamin E may limit the extent of photodynamic damage. Daily oral supplementation with 80 mg of elemental zinc may retard the progression of macular degeneration.[13] Since zinc given without copper may cause a reversible anemia, a nutritional supplement such as Ocuvite (which contains zinc, copper, vitamin C, vitamin E, beta-carotene, and selenium) should be recommended for patients with macular degeneration and patients with visible macular drusen. A low-fat diet rich in yellow and green leafy vegetables may be more effective than dietary supplementation for prevention of macular degeneration.[14]

References

1. Leibowitz HM, Krueger DE, Maunder LR, et al: The Framingham eye study monograph. An ophthalmological and epidemiological study of cataract, glaucoma, diabetic retinopathy, macular degeneration, and visual acuity in a general population of 2631 adults, 1973–1975. Surv Ophthalmol 1980;24:335–338.
2. Mehelas TJ, Kiess RD, Kollarits CR, et al: Visual loss in geriatric residents of Northwestern Ohio nursing homes. Ohio State Med 1984;80:235–237.
3. Mehelas TJ, Kollarits CR: Pupillary clues to neuro-ophthalmic diagnoses. Postgrad Med 1982;71:199–201.
4. Kollarits CR, Lubow M, Hissong S: Retinal strokes: Incidence of carotid atheromata. JAMA 1972;222:1273–1275.
5. Kollarits CR, McCarthy RW, et al: Norepinephrine therapy of ischemic optic neuropathy. J Clin Neuro-ophthalmol 1981;1:283–288.
6. Havener WH: Ocular Pharmacology, 4th ed. St. Louis, C.V. Mosby, 1978.
7. Gharagozloo NZ, Relf SJ, Brubaker RF: Aqueous flow is reduced by the alpha-adrenergic agonist, apraclonidine hydrochloride (ALO2145). Ophthalmology 1988;95:1217–1220.
8. Camras CB, the United States Latanoprost Study Group: Comparison of latanoprost and timolol in patients with ocular hypertension and glaucoma. Ophthalmology 1996;103:138.
9. Charters L: Treating glaucoma. Ophthalmology Times 1996;Feb 12–18:8.
10. Kollarits CR, Swann ER, Shapiro RS, et al: HLA-A1 and steroid-induced cataracts in renal transplant patients. Ann Ophthalmol 1982;14:1116–1118.
11. Seckel BR: Aesthetic Laser Surgery. Boston, Little, Brown, 1996.
12. Young RW: Solar radiation and age-related macular degeneration. Surv Ophthalmol 1988;32:252–259.
13. Newsome DA, Schwartz M, Leone NC, et al: Oral zinc in macular degeneration. Arch Ophthalmol 1988;106:192–198.
14. Seddon J, Ajani U, Sperduto R, et al: Dietary carotenoids, vitamins A, C, and E and advanced age-related macular degeneration. JAMA 1994;272:1413–1420.

Additional Reading

Cataract Management Guideline Panel: Cataracts in Adults: Management of Functional Impairment. Clinical Practice Guideline, No. 4. AHCPR Pub. No. 93-0542. Rockville, MD, U.S. Department of Health and Human Services, Public Health Service, Agency for Health Care Policy and Research, 1993.

43 Skin Disorders

Randy Berger, M.D.

Barbara A. Gilchrest, M.D.

Skin is the interface between people and their environment that protects the other organs of the body from excessive temperature changes, mechanical injury, ultraviolet irradiation, toxic chemicals, and microbial pathogens. It is also a tactile organ through which individuals receive pleasurable stimuli and assess their physical surroundings. With age, the skin performs each of these vital functions less well. Skin is also readily visible and hence of great psychological and social as well as physiologic importance. For these reasons, the morphologic changes that accompany aging in the skin often affect an individual as much as the functional changes.

Dermatologic problems are exceedingly common, especially among the elderly, and are frequently among the chief complaints that bring geriatric patients to the physician. It has been estimated that 6% of all physician visits are prompted by disorders of the skin.[1] Moreover, examination of more than 20,000 noninstitutionalized Americans revealed that 40% of those over the age of 65 suffered from a dermatologic disease sufficiently severe, in the opinion of the consulting dermatologist, to justify at least one physician visit, and that the average affected individual had 1.5 such disorders.[2] These figures do not include the nearly universal "cosmetic" changes characteristic of aging skin, which may lower self-esteem and may have a measurable negative impact on society's perception of the elderly.[3]

Morphologic and probably even physiologic age-associated cutaneous changes are most pronounced in fair-skinned individuals, in whom sun damage is superimposed on intrinsic aging. The major stigmata of aging in the skin—wrinkling, "dryness" (roughness), uneven pigmentation, and cancer—are indeed virtually restricted to habitually sun-exposed areas. However, these sun-induced changes, which have dominated the public and even medical perception of cutaneous aging, are only one aspect of a subtle but undoubtedly biologically significant process that gradually alters the function of normal skin and its response to a large number of disease states. The following sections review the age-associated changes now recognized in normal skin and discuss selected disorders of the skin with special relevance to the elderly.

PATHOPHYSIOLOGY: AGE-ASSOCIATED CHANGES IN NORMAL SKIN

Histologic features associated with aging in human skin are shown schematically in Figure 43–1. The most striking and consistent change is flattening of the dermoepidermal junction, with effacement of both the dermal papillae and the epidermal rete pegs. Ultrastructurally, there is also a decrease in villous cytoplasmic projections of the epidermal basal cells into the dermis.[4, 5] This results in a considerably smaller contiguous surface between the two compartments, presum-

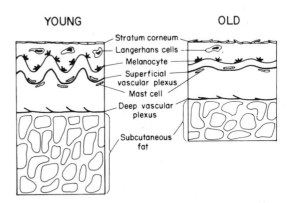

Figure 43–1 Histologic changes in aging normal skin. Schematic drawings emphasize the age-associated flattening of the dermoepidermal junction (basement membrane zone [BMZ]): loss of dermal and subcutaneous mass; shortened capillary loops; and reduced numbers of melanocytes, Langerhans' cells, and mast cells. Note that the average thickness of the stratum corneum (barrier layer) and viable epidermis (area above BMZ) does not vary with age. In most body areas, epidermal thickness is approximately 0.1 mm; dermal thicknesses range from 1.0 to 4.0 mm, depending on body site. Melanocyte densities range from 1000/mm² to 2000/mm² surface area in most body areas; Langerhans' cell density is approximately 500/mm². (From Gilchrest BA: Age-associated changes in the skin. J Am Geriatr Soc 30:139–143, 1982.)

TABLE 43–1 **PHYSIOLOGIC PARAMETERS IN HUMAN SKIN THAT DECLINE WITH AGE**

Growth rate	Immunosurveillance
Injury response	Vascular responsiveness
Barrier function	Thermoregulation
Chemical clearance rates	Sweat production
Sensory perception	Sebum production
Mechanical protection	Vitamin D synthesis

Adapted from Gilchrest BA: Age-associated changes in the skin. J Am Geriatr Soc 1982;30:139–143.

ably less "communication" and nutrient transfer, and less resistance to shearing forces. Loss of dermal thickness approaches 20% in elderly individuals and may account for the paper-thin, sometimes nearly transparent quality of their skin. The remaining dermis is relatively acellular and avascular. Precise histologic concomitants of wrinkling, if any, are unknown, although age-related loss of normal collagen and elastin fibers is probably a contributory factor. Table 43–1 lists the major functions of the skin that decline with age.[4] Many of these functions are necessarily interrelated or overlapping.

An age-associated decrease in epidermal turnover rate of approximately 30% to 50% between the third and eighth decades has been determined by a study of desquamation rates for corneocytes (cells of the stratum corneum) at selected body sites; other investigators have reported a corresponding 100% prolongation of the stratum corneum replacement rate in old men as opposed to young men. The repair rate in injured skin likewise declines with age.[6] In vitro studies of cultured keratinocytes and fibroblasts demonstrate a diminished responsiveness to mitogens and an enhanced sensitivity to growth inhibitors in adult compared with newborn cells. These findings are even more marked in cells from older adults.[7-9] In general, as cells age, they become less responsive to signals in their environment. Linear growth rates of hair and nails also decrease by approximately 30% to 50% between early and late adulthood.

Although stratum corneum thickness and degree of compaction remain constant, an age-related decrease in surface barrier function, as measured by percutaneous absorption of at least some substances, has been reported. This increased absorption is accompanied by a decreased dermal clearance rate for the materials, possibly increasing the risk of an irritant or allergic contact dermatitis.[10]

Decreased sensory perception has been documented in elderly skin using the techniques of optimal stimulus in grams for light touch, vibratory sensation, and corneal sensation. Pacinian and Meissner's corpuscles, the cutaneous end-organs responsible for pressure perception and light touch, progressively decrease to approximately one-third their initial average density between the second and ninth decades of life.[11]

Early studies demonstrated that eccrine sweating is markedly impaired with age. Spontaneous sweating in response to dry heat, measured on digital pads, is reduced by more than 70% in healthy elderly subjects compared with young control subjects. The response is attributable primarily to a decreased output per gland, although the number of eccrine glands also decreases by approximately 15% during adulthood in most body sites.[11]

Decreased vascular responsiveness in the normal skin of old versus younger individuals has been documented by measuring vasodilation and transudation after application of standardized chemical irritants and exposure to a standardized ultraviolet dose. The decreased erythematous response is probably in part attributable to the striking age-associated loss of dermal venules, although decreased responsiveness of individual vessels may also be responsible. Compromised thermoregulation, which predisposes the elderly to hypothermia and possibly to heat stroke, may be due in part to reduced vasoconstriction or vasodilation of dermal arterioles, in part to decreased eccrine sweat production, and in part to loss of subcutaneous fat, all of which occur with advancing age.[4]

Dermoepidermal separation has been reported to occur more readily in the elderly under experimental conditions, as might be anticipated from the histologic finding of reduced interdigitation between the dermis and the epidermis. The poor adhesion between these two cutaneous compartments undoubtedly explains the propensity of elderly people to show "torn" skin and superficial abrasions following minor trauma, such as removal of bandages, and to form bullae in edematous sites. It may also contribute to the increased prevalence of certain bullous dermatoses in the elderly.[11]

An age-associated decrease in delayed hypersensitivity reactions in human skin is manifested by a relative inability of healthy older subjects to develop sensitivity to dinitrochlorobenzene. Similarly, elderly subjects have a lower rate of positivity for standard test antigens compared with young adult controls. This decrease undoubtedly partly reflects the well-documented loss of circulating thymus-derived lymphocytes and their decreased responsiveness to standard mitogens. Additionally, with age there is decreased elaboration of interleukin-1, interleukin-2, and other cytokines.[12] Also implicated is the nearly 50% reduction in morphologically identifiable epidermal Langerhans' cells (the cell population believed to be responsible for immunosurveillance in the skin) that occurs between early and late adulthood. The further loss of Langerhans' cells in skin habitually exposed to the sun is postulated to predispose it to skin cancer.

Cutaneous manifestations of immediate hypersensitivity also decrease with age. In one well-controlled epidemiologic study of over 3000 subjects, the percentage of people with at least one positive wheal-and-flare reaction to a standard battery of potential allergens fell from 52% at age 20 years to 16% at age 75 years. Smaller groups of subjects with at least 3, 7, or 11 positive test results showed parallel reductions with advancing age. Investigators were unable to determine the relative contributions of systemic versus local cutaneous changes in this decline.[13] Another study demonstrated an approximately 50% reduction in mast cells (the source of histamine in the skin) in the papillary dermis of buttock skin in old adults; this was associated with a corresponding reduction in stimulated histamine release.

A decrease in sebum production of approximately 60% accompanies advancing age in both men and women. This has been attributed to the concomitant decrease in production of gonadal or adrenal androgens, to which sebaceous glands are exquisitely sensitive. The clinical effects of decreased sebum production, if any, are unknown. There is no direct relationship to xerosis or seborrheic dermatitis.

One endocrine function of human skin that is thought to decline with age is vitamin D production. In response to sun exposure, the epidermis converts 7-dehydrocholesterol to previtamin D, which is further metabolized and ultimately hydroxylated in the liver and kidneys to the active form responsible for regulation of calcium homeostasis. Between early and late adulthood, the level of epidermal 7-dehydrocholesterol decreases by approximately 75%, suggesting that the lack of an immediate precursor may limit vitamin D production in the elderly.[14] These concerns are reinforced by studies that have shown occult osteomalacia (bone loss due to vitamin D deficiency) as determined by bone biopsy in 20% to 30% of women and in up to 40% of men presenting with hip fractures; other laboratory evidence of vitamin D deficiency or secondary hyperparathyroidism has been found in 48% of homebound elderly.[15] It is thus postulated that in elderly individuals already compromised by osteoporosis, reduced vitamin D synthetic capacity, compounded by insufficient sun exposure, sunscreen use,[16] or poor dietary intake of vitamin D, may cause osteomalacia and hence further increase the risk of trabecular bone fracture.

CLINICAL ASSESSMENT

When evaluating a patient for a dermatologic complaint, it is essential to take a complete medical history, paying particular attention to the medications being taken. It is important to inquire what topical treatments, either prescribed or self-determined, the patient is employing. Over-the-counter topical anesthetics, cosmetics, or isopropyl alcohol, for example, can each exacerbate various skin conditions. Bathing habits and exposures to harsh detergents and other irritants should be discussed. The duration of a complaint, response to various treatments, and the presence of close contacts with a similar condition can suggest diagnostic possibilities.

Ideally, the entire cutaneous surface should be examined with adequate lighting. Often physical findings in areas other than those mentioned by the patient can give clues to the diagnosis. For example, genital lesions, about which the patient may not necessarily complain, can help make a diagnosis of scabies. A full skin examination also allows detection of cutaneous malignancies or other significant conditions of which the patient may not be aware. Finally, as mentioned earlier, owing to blunted vascular and immune responses, the skin findings may be more subtle in elderly patients than in younger ones with similar disorders, which often makes diagnosis more challenging in this population.

DISEASES—DIAGNOSIS AND MANAGEMENT

The following discussion expands on the diagnosis and management of selected topics in dermatology. Most of the disorders included are particularly prevalent in the geriatric population, and a familiarity with them will aid in their recognition when caring for such patients. Pruritus and xerosis are among the most frequent dermatologic complaints of the elderly. Seborrheic dermatitis, while less troublesome symptomatically, is commonly seen among geriatric patients and may be associated with concomitant disorders in this population. The elderly are particularly likely to be taking a multiplicity of medications, putting them at risk for adverse drug reactions. When caring for such patients, it is important to recognize both the more common and less severe drug eruptions as well as the uncommon, life-threatening ones. Bullous pemphigoid, while not particularly common in the general population, is seen with significantly higher frequency in the geriatric population and is presented here as a prototype of autoimmune bullous disease.

Infections of all types are common in the elderly, and two infections involving the skin are discussed in this chapter. Herpes zoster is a frequent viral infection of the skin that rises in incidence with increasing age. It is responsible for significant morbidity in some patients. Scabies, while not restricted to the elderly, is often more challenging to diagnose in geriatric patients and, if overlooked, can lead to marked discomfort and widespread infestation among nursing home residents and health care workers. Finally, skin cancer is an important dermatologic condition that especially affects the elderly owing to their many years of ultraviolet irradiation. Early diagnosis and treatment can significantly affect morbidity and mortality in this population.

Pruritus

Elderly people often experience localized or generalized pruritus. For some it is a minor annoyance; for others it leads to extensive, slow-healing excoriations or loss of sleep with associated irritability and impaired mental function.

Many patients presenting to the physician because of pruritus in fact have an eruption that is responsible for the symptom,[17] although its other manifestations may be so subtle that the patient or even the physician does not notice the rash. Because inflammatory responses may be muted in the elderly, a careful history and physical examination are necessary before primary disorders of the skin such as eczema, early bullous pemphigoid, urticaria, scabies, or pediculosis are excluded. Proper identification of a causative dermatosis leads to effective treatment in most patients and allows the patient to avoid the hematologic, radiographic, and other laboratory procedures that constitute the work-up for unexplained generalized pruritus.

Table 43–2 lists the most common systemic disorders associated with generalized pruritus. Among all patients seeking medical attention for pruritus, the prevalence of underlying systemic disease has been reported as 10% to 50%,[18] the percentage depending on patient selection, diagnostic evaluation, and period of follow-up. Numerically, perhaps the most important known cause of persistent generalized pruritus is chronic renal failure. However, the degree of renal failure necessary to cause pruritus is unknown, complicating interpretation of this symptom in the elderly patient with mild to moderate renal insuf-

TABLE 43–2 SYSTEMIC DISORDERS SOMETIMES ASSOCIATED WITH PRURITUS IN THE ELDERLY

Renal	Chronic renal failure
Hepatic	Extrahepatic biliary obstruction
	Hepatitis
	Drug ingestion
Hematopoietic	Polycythemia vera
	Hodgkin's disease
	Other lymphomas and leukemias
	Multiple myeloma
	Iron deficiency anemia
Endocrine	Hyperthyroidism
	Diabetes mellitus
Miscellaneous	Visceral malignancies
	Opiate ingestion
	Drug ingestion
	Psychosis
	Acquired immune deficiency syndrome

Adapted from Gilchrest BA: Pruritus: Pathogenesis, therapy and significance in systemic disease states. Arch Intern Med 1982;142:101–105. Copyright 1982, American Medical Association.

ficiency. From a practical viewpoint, it is probably unwise to attribute pruritus to otherwise asymptomatic renal failure or to renal insufficiency not requiring specific therapy for metabolic imbalance.

Pruritus is probably the most distressing and consistent symptom of chronic cholestasis, which underlies all the hepatic disorders listed in Table 43–2. Overall, pruritus occurs in approximately 20% to 25% of jaundiced patients, but it is rare in those with hepatic disease lacking cholestasis. Drugs that can cause pruritus by inducing cholestasis include phenothiazines, tolbutamide, erythromycin estolate, anabolic hormones, estrogens, and progestins.[19] Other drugs that can result in considerable pruritus without cholestasis are opiates.

Approximately 30% to 50% of patients with polycythemia vera and up to 20% of patients with Hodgkin's disease experience pruritus.[18] The incidence and significance of pruritus in other lymphomas and leukemias are unknown, but the occasional association cannot be disputed. Generalized pruritus has been reported as an initial symptom in patients with multiple myeloma, Waldenström's macroglobulinemia, and benign gammopathies. Iron deficiency anemia has been reported as the cause of generalized pruritus in more than 50 patients,[20] including six with polycythemia,[21] although this association is apparently rare. Pruritus attributable to endocrine or specific "miscellaneous" causes is rare, and many elderly people experience generalized pruritus for which there is no apparent explanation. Hence, one must either accept a higher incidence of idiopathic pruritus with advancing age or infer the existence of "senile pruritus." Physiologic factors that may contribute to this hypothetical entity include age-associated alterations in the skin, peripheral nerve endings, and dermal neuropeptide release. Alterations in the barrier function of the skin, which possibly facilitate low-grade irritant dermatitis, include decreased keratohyalin granule formation in the epidermis, decreased skin surface hydration,[22] diminished stratum corneum lipids, and a slower rate of stratum corneum barrier repair.[23] In addition, altered sensory thresholds of C-fiber neurons as well as modifications in the synthesis, release, and clearance of dermal neuropeptides, such as substance P, histamine, neurokinin A, calcitonin gene-related peptide, and other mediators with opiate activity,[24] may also play a role.

The appropriate laboratory evaluation for the patient with unexplained generalized pruritus remains a matter of opinion because cost-benefit ratios for individual procedures have not been determined. Measurement of serum creatinine, blood urea nitrogen, bilirubin, and hepatic enzymes with a complete blood count and urinalysis seem to constitute a reasonable survey; a chest radiograph may also be justified as a screening test for malignancy. Physical examination should include examination of the lymph nodes, liver, and spleen. Additional tests may be suggested by the history, review of systems, or physical examination.

The pathophysiology of pruritus associated with systemic disease is incompletely understood, and the optimal therapy is the same as that for the underlying disease whenever possible. Specific approaches to the treatment of the pruritus itself are available in a few instances, but for most patients nonspecific therapies must be employed.[25] Often it is worthwhile to prescribe an emollient, even in the absence of clinical xerosis, because minimal or intermittent "dryness," present in virtually all elderly individuals, may notably exacerbate pruritus of another cause. Patients should be cautioned specifically against topical application of alcohol or hot water (both of which may temporarily relieve but ultimately exacerbate pruritus) or excessive washing, especially with soap. Topical application of menthol and camphor in an emollient base, such as in Sarna lotion, may provide considerable temporary relief; other topical anesthetics can be used only at the risk of allergic sensitization. Oral antihistamines are widely prescribed for pruritus of all causes, although their efficacy is slight in most instances, even when combinations of H_1 and H_2 blockers are used. The use of antihistamines by the elderly may result in additional problems of urinary retention, paradoxical restlessness, or significantly impaired psychomotor function. Newer nonsedating antihistamines pose fewer problems in terms of neurologic side effects; however, care must be taken to avoid potential drug interactions.

Xerosis

Xerosis is the term used to describe the "dry" or rough quality of skin that is almost universal among the elderly. The condition may be generalized but is especially prominent on the lower legs and is exacerbated by the low-humidity environments classically found in overheated rooms during cold weather. The term xerosis is a misnomer; the initial assumption that the disorder results from a lack of water in the skin overall has been disproved.[26] In vivo and in vitro measurements demonstrate diminished hydration of the superficial portion of the stratum corneum, but the deeper portion maintains normal hydration.[27] The occasional classification of xerosis as a disorder of the sebaceous (oil) glands is similarly without experimental basis.[2] Xerosis probably reflects minor abnormalities in epidermal maturation that in turn result in an irregular surface of the stratum corneum.[24] Xerotic skin in the elderly is often pruritic and may show evidence of inflammation, probably due to defects in the stratum corneum, with secondary entry of irritating substances into the dermis. The resulting condition, called erythema craquelé or winter eczema, responds promptly to topical corticosteroid ointment or emollients, although these preparations do not correct the xerosis itself.

Frequent, regular use of a topical emollient makes dry skin more attractive and more comfortable and prevents the complications discussed previously. Emollients are most effective when applied to already moistened skin (e.g., immediately after the bath or shower). "Heavy," frankly greasy emollients have the additional property of perceptibly coating the skin, producing a smooth surface film, and they are usually better barriers against evaporation than are more cosmetically elegant preparations. Preparations containing ammonium lactate[28] or other alpha-hydroxy acids are especially effective in restoring skin barrier function and improving xerosis. Finally, it should be noted that emollients applied to the skin immediately after bathing retain water more effectively than gels or oils added to the bath water that coat the bathtub as well as the skin, producing a dangerously slippery surface that is difficult to clean.

Seborrheic Dermatitis

Seborrheic dermatitis is a common dermatologic condition in the geriatric population.[29-31] Clinically, it presents as erythema and greasy-appearing scales in what is referred to as a seborrheic distribution, namely, the scalp, ears, central face (particularly the eyebrows, glabella, perinasal area, nasolabial folds, and beard area), and the central chest and interscapular areas. When present in the scalp, it is referred to in lay terms as dandruff. Seborrheic dermatitis is found with greater frequency among patients with underlying neurologic conditions, such as Parkinson's disease, facial nerve injury, spinal cord injury, poliomyelitis, and syringomyelia, as well as in patients taking neuroleptic medications with parkinsonian side effects. Human immunodeficiency virus (HIV) infection has also been associated with severe seborrheic dermatitis.

The role of resident lipophilic yeast, *Pityrosporum ovale*, is controversial, although studies have shown that the organism is present in greater number in patients with seborrheic dermatitis. Treatment is directed at either killing the pityrosporum yeast with antifungal preparations, such as ketoconazole cream, or directly suppressing inflammation by means of low-potency topical steroids. It should be noted that topical ketoconazole also has some anti-inflammatory properties. In a double-blinded study comparing 2% ketoconazole cream with 1% hydrocortisone cream, a therapeutic response was noted in 80.5% of subjects using ketoconazole and 94.4% of those using hydrocortisone, demonstrating a somewhat higher efficacy of hydrocortisone, although establishing ketoconazole as an effective, steroid-sparing alternative.[32] For hair-bearing regions, shampoos containing ketoconazole, selenium sulfide, salicylic acid, zinc pyrithione, or tar are effective.

Drug Eruptions

Adverse cutaneous reactions to medication include expected, usually dose-related, side effects such as acneiform eruptions following corticosteroid administration or xerosis following retinoids, and unexpected, immune-mediated, allergic reactions. These latter reactions typically occur within 3 days to 2 weeks of challenge and persist for up to 2 weeks after the drug has been discontinued. Rechallenge results in a more rapid onset of the eruption. Less commonly, a patient may have an adverse reaction to a medication after weeks, months, or, rarely, years of use. Although any medication can cause a drug eruption, certain medications are statistically more likely to do so. In two studies surveying separately over 22,000 and 15,000 inpatients, the Boston Collaborative Drug Surveillance Program identified the following drugs as having the highest incidences of drug eruption: amoxicillin, ampicillin, penicillin, semisynthetic penicillins, trimethoprim-sulfamethoxazole, transfused blood, cephalosporins, gentamicin sulfate, acetylcysteine, allopurinol, quinidine, and dipyrone. Conversely, digoxin, antacids, meperidine, promethazine, and acetaminophen were among the medications administered to more than 1000 patients with no reported cutaneous eruptions.[33, 34]

Central to management of a drug eruption is discontinuation of the culprit medication. This is particularly essential in patients with the more serious and potentially life-threatening reactions. Midpotency topical steroids, antihistamines, and antipruritic lotions provide symptomatic relief.

The most common form of drug eruption is the morbilliform or exanthemous eruption, sometimes referred to as a maculopapular eruption. It is characterized by discrete and coalescing erythematous macules and papules symmetrically distributed on the trunk and extremities. The most common causative agents are those listed in the previous paragraph. Morbilliform eruptions typically begin within 1 week of exposure, except in the case of penicillins, which may cause eruptions beginning 2 weeks or longer after the initial exposure.[35]

Other forms of drug eruption include photosensitivity, as is seen with doxycycline or thiazides; a lichenoid or lichen planus-like eruption, seen with gold and phenothiazines; and urticaria, often associated with penicillin or iodine-containing contrast media. A fixed drug eruption is manifest by one or few, red to violaceous, round plaques that recur in the same location if the patient is rechallenged. These lesions resolve with hyperpigmentation, which becomes more pronounced with each episode. Drugs that cause a fixed drug eruption include tetracyclines and nonsteroidal anti-inflammatory drugs.[36] Vasculitis, presenting as palpable purpura, can occur as the result of a hypersensitivity reaction to a medication, among many other possible causes. Immune complex formation can lead to a serum sickness reaction, characterized by an urticarial eruption, fever, arthritis, nephritis, and sometimes neurologic symptoms. Penicillins, sulfonamides, and streptomycin are among the causative agents.[35]

Some of the less common reactions are important because of their life-threatening nature. These include hypersensitivity reactions, anaphylaxis, exfoliative erythroderma, erythema multiforme major (Stevens-Johnson syndrome), and toxic epidermal necrolysis (TEN). These conditions often require hospitalization with intensive supportive care as well as discontinuation of the causative agent. Hypersensitivity reaction was first described with phenytoin and is now recognized with drugs other than anticonvulsants, particularly sulfonamides. It is a multisystemic response manifested by a cutaneous eruption, which may be of any type, in conjunction with fever, adenopathy, hematologic abnormalities, and hepatitis.[37] It should be noted that phenytoin, carbamazepine, and phenobarbital cross react with each other, and all three agents are contraindicated in patients sensitive to any of them. Anaphylaxis occurs in a spectrum of IgE-dependent reactions including urticaria, bronchospasm, laryngeal edema, and hypotension. Penicillins are the most common drugs associated with anaphylaxis, and the reaction is more likely to occur with intravenous administration.[35] Exfoliative erythroderma presents as diffuse erythema and scaling. Temperature, fluids, electrolytes, and nutrition must be carefully monitored. Erythema multiforme is recognized by the presence of pathognomonic target lesions with an erythematous periphery and a dusky center, which sometimes progress to a central blister or erosion. When the mucous membranes are involved the eruption is classified as the Stevens-Johnson syndrome. When large areas of skin are sloughed it is termed toxic epidermal necrolysis. TEN is characterized by skin tenderness and a positive Nikolsky's sign, along with shearing off of the epidermis with lateral force, which may appear de novo or may evolve from severe erythema multiforme. Again, fluid and electrolyte management and the avoidance of sepsis are crucial. The mortality rate for TEN is 30% to 50%, and patients are best managed in a burn unit.[38]

Bullous Pemphigoid

Bullous pemphigoid (BP) is an idiopathic, antibody-mediated disease, which can be differentiated clinically, histologically, and immunologically from the much less common pemphigus vulgaris. The elderly are affected most commonly, and, conversely, BP is the most common immune-mediated blistering disease affecting older patients. Untreated, this disease varies in severity from mild to disabling, and the prolonged loss of

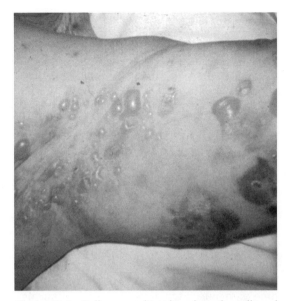

Figure 43–2 Bullous pemphigoid involving the axilla and medial arm. Note numerous tense bullae and scattered hemorrhagic erosions. (Courtesy of K. Arndt, M.D.)

an effective cutaneous barrier may be fatal. The disease is self-limited, lasting months to years, but recurrences follow disease-free periods in a minority of patients.[39]

Bullous pemphigoid is characterized clinically by tense bullae arising on either erythematous or normal-appearing skin (Fig. 43–2). Preceding or accompanying pruritus is common and may be intense. Crusted erosions and urticarial wheals may coexist with intact bullae, and hemorrhagic bullae are not unusual. Lesions occur most often on the trunk and proximal extremities and show a predilection for flexural surfaces; approximately one third of patients have oral blisters, although, unlike the situation in pemphigus vulgaris, the mouth is rarely the initial site of involvement. In some patients, bullae remain localized to one area for several months, and in a few, the lesions never become widespread. The diagnosis is confirmed by skin biopsy. Immunofluorescent staining of perilesional skin, which is virtually pathognomonic, shows linear deposition along the basement membrane zone of C3 (third component of complement) in all patients and of IgG in most. Indirect immunofluorescent studies demonstrate anti-basement membrane zone antibodies of the IgG class in approximately 70% of patients.[39]

A 230-kD protein and a 180-kD protein, referred to as the bullous pemphigoid antigen 1 and the bullous pemphigoid antigen 2, respectively, are implicated as the targets for antibody binding in patients with BP. These two antigens are components of the hemidesmosome,[40] which attaches the basal keratinocyte to the basement membrane. Thus, when this attachment is disturbed, dermoepidermal separation and blister formation ensue.

Corticosteroids are the gold standard of therapy. In mild or localized cases, topical or intralesional steroid application may control the lesions, but almost all patients require systemic treatment at least initially. Patients with extensive or rapidly progressive disabling disease should begin therapy with prednisone, 60 to 100 mg daily (some authors recommend two to three times this dose). Patients should be reevaluated at weekly intervals and the prednisone dose progressively reduced once new blisters have ceased forming and clinical remission has been achieved. An immunosuppressant, such as azathioprine, cyclophosphamide,[39, 41] or methotrexate,[42] may be added to the regimen initially or at the time of remission to reduce the eventual maintenance level of prednisone. Six to eight weeks are required for full expression of the steroid-sparing effect. In patients with less severe disease therapy may be initiated with 40 to 60 mg of prednisone on alternate days and/or an immunosuppressant. Drug dosages are decreased gradually to zero over many months, provided the disease remains in remission. Sulfapyridine or sulfones may be valuable alternative therapies for patients with major contraindications to systemic steroids. Recently, investigators have reported successful therapy with high-dose tetracycline (500 mg four times a day) and nicotinamide (500 mg three times a day).[43] In most patients prolonged remissions are achieved, and in at least half, treatment ultimately can be discontinued without recurrence of lesions. However, frequent exacerbations of bullous pemphigoid and potential complications of therapy require close monitoring of all patients throughout the course of their disease.

Herpes Zoster

Herpes zoster, or "shingles," is a familiar vesicular dermatomal eruption that is due to reactivation of latent varicella virus in the dorsal sensory ganglia. More than two thirds of cases occur in patients older than 50 years. Age-adjusted annual incidence rates per 1000 population are less than 1 from birth to 10 years, approximately 2.5 at age 20 to 50 years, and more than 10 at age 80 years.[44] It has been estimated that by age 85 an individual has a 50% risk of having had at least one attack of herpes zoster and a 10% risk of having had two attacks. Immunosuppressed patients have an annual incidence of herpes zoster

20 to 100 times that of the general population and often have much more severe disease.

Herpes zoster usually begins with dysesthesia or paresthesia of the involved dermatome. These symptoms persist for days but rarely longer than a week before vesicles appear. Depending on the dermatome affected, prodromal symptoms may mimic angina, spinal cord compression, renal or biliary colic, muscle sprains, or many other disorders. Constitutional symptoms are rare.

The rash of herpes zoster is virtually pathognomonic (Fig. 43–3). Clusters of vesicles, usually superimposed on erythematous plaques, erupt in a dermatomal distribution. In 98% of patients, the eruption is unilateral, and lesions do not cross the midline, although occasional individual vesicles can be found outside the affected dermatome. The diagnosis of herpes virus infection may be confirmed by a Tzanck test of material scraped from the base of an intact vesicle. A positive test is indicated by the appearance of multinucleated giant cells characteristic of herpetic infection, though this test cannot distinguish herpes simplex from herpes zoster. The initially clear vesicles may become pustular or, especially in the elderly, hemorrhagic within a few days. New lesions continue to appear for several days, often progressing distally along the dermatome. Widespread dissemination, if it occurs, usually does so during this period. Pain and hyperesthesia are frequently prominent during the first days of the eruption, although their severity is unrelated to either the risk or the severity of postherpetic neuralgia in individual patients. Vesicles usually begin to crust in the second week and resolve within 4 weeks in most patients; the eruption tends to persist longer and to be more severe in the elderly. Vesicle fluid is

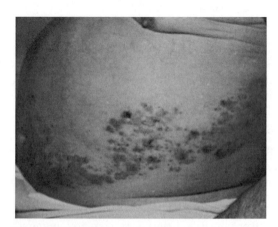

Figure 43–3 Herpes zoster involving the left T10 dermatome. Eruption consists of clear grouped vesicles and hemorrhagic crusts superimposed on erythematous plaques. Note sharp cutoff at the umbilicus.

contagious, but the attack rate (cases of varicella) in susceptible household contacts is much less than that for chickenpox (primary varicella infection).

The course of herpes zoster infection in young and old adults differs primarily in the incidence and severity of postherpetic neuralgia. This problem occurs in approximately 10% of patients overall, but there is a notable increase in incidence correlated with increased age. Although postherpetic neuralgia is uncommon in patients less than 40 years of age, it occurs in more than half of patients aged 60 or over and in more than three quarters of patients aged 70 or more.[45] The increases in severity and duration of postherpetic neuralgia with age are even more marked than the increase in incidence. Persistent pain is especially common in patients with trigeminal involvement (10% to 15% of reported cases) or immunosuppression. Although they are less debilitating than other complications of herpes zoster, persistent hyperpigmentation and true scarring of the involved skin are also more common in the elderly.

During the acute phase of the infection, some patients require narcotic analgesics for adequate relief of pain. These agents should be prescribed cautiously in the elderly to avoid overmedication and adverse systemic effects. Early skin lesions are best treated with local compresses of Burow's solution (1:20 in cool water) or other hypertonic soaks for 10 minutes, three to four times daily, followed by gentle washing with Hibiclens or other antibacterial soap to hasten drying and prevent bacterial superinfection. A topical antibiotic such as mupirocin ointment may be applied two to three times daily to already crusted lesions. While systemic treatment of herpes zoster is not mandatory in the immunocompetent host, studies have shown that patients treated with antiviral therapy experience faster healing, a shortened duration of viral shedding, and a decrease in severity and duration of acute pain.[46] Treatment should be started within 72 hours of the onset of symptoms to be effective. Currently three antiviral drugs are approved for the treatment of herpes zoster: acyclovir, 800 mg five times a day for 7 to 10 days, famciclovir, 500 mg three times a day for 7 days, and valacyclovir, 1000 mg three times a day for 7 days.

Although antiviral therapy has definite proven benefit for the treatment of acute zoster, its role in the prevention of postherpetic neuralgia is less definite. While some studies have concluded that treatment of acute herpes zoster does not affect the outcome of postherpetic neuralgia, others have shown that some benefit does occur. In one study acyclovir 800 mg five times a day for 10 days decreased the incidence of postherpetic neuralgia from 16.7% in the placebo group to 4.2% in the treated group during the first 3 months.[46] From 4 to 6 months, the groups did not differ statistically in the prevalence of neuralgia. The patients in these groups averaged 55 and 59 years of age, respectively, and more than 70 persons aged 50 years or older were in each group, but data for the more elderly cohorts were not analyzed separately. However, no reduction in incidence of postherpetic neuralgia was detected in a second study of 364 patients aged 60 years or older,[47] using a very similar design in which acyclovir was administered for only 7 days. Neither study found medically significant side effects of acyclovir. In a separate double-blind controlled study of herpes zoster ophthalmicus, acyclovir 600 mg five times a day for 10 days was found to reduce the rate of ocular complications such as keratitis and uveitis when treatment was initiated as late as 7 days after the appearance of lesions.[48] Treatment with systemic corticosteroids is likewise controversial. A randomized, controlled study of 349 subjects comparing 7- and 21-day treatments of acyclovir alone or in addition to prednisolone revealed that a longer course of acyclovir or the addition of steroids provided only minimal benefit, although an increase in adverse events (31 versus 13 patients) was reported in the group treated with steroids.[49]

Treatment of already established postherpetic neuralgia can be frustrating. Often topical therapy is initiated as a first-line treatment owing to its safety compared with other modalities. In one study, capsaicin, which exerts its effects through the local depletion of substance P and other neuropeptides, was applied as a 0.75% cream three to four times a day for 6 weeks; it decreased the pain of postherpetic neuralgia by at least 40% within 6 weeks of therapy in the majority of patients compared to only 6% of patients treated with a vehicle control.[50] However, transient stinging and burning at the time of application and the requirement for frequent indefinite treatment may decrease patient acceptance of this modality. Other topical treatments that have been used include topical anti-inflammatory agents, such as formulations containing aspirin or indomethacin, and topical anesthetics, such as eutectic mixture of local anesthetics (EMLA), though data on the long-term efficacy of these agents are limited.[45]

Despite trials and anecdotal use of numerous systemic agents for the treatment of postherpetic neuralgia, antidepressants such as amitriptyline remain the most consistently effective.[51] Often doses lower than those needed for antidepressant action are effective. A variety of nonmedical therapies, such as nerve blocks, transcutaneous electrical nerve stimulation, and deep brain stimulation, have also been employed.

Scabies

Scabies is a severely pruritic infestation by the *Sarcoptes scabiei* mite. Symptoms are due to a hypersensitivity reaction to the mite, which may explain why pruritus can persist for days to weeks following adequate treatment. While the male mite remains on the surface of the skin, the female burrows through the stratum corneum to lay her eggs. In an average infested host, only 10 to 12 live female mites are present at one time. Transmission occurs through person-to-person contact, and epidemics can arise among institutionalized patients, necessitating widespread treatment of patients, staff, and visitors.

The hallmark lesion of scabies is the burrow, a linear ridge that often ends with a tiny vesicle (Fig. 43–4). Other cutaneous manifestations are papules, vesicles, nodules, and excoriations. Lesions are concentrated in the interdigital web spaces, axillae, umbilicus, volar wrists, and genitalia. Diagnosis can be confirmed by scraping the contents of the burrow onto a slide with mineral oil and examining it microscopically. The presence of a mite, eggs, or feces confirms the diagnosis, but this evidence is not essential to making the diagnosis if clinical suspicion is high. In some elderly or disabled patients a nonspecific pruritic eruption may be the only sign of scabies.[52] In immunocompromised patients or those who have an impaired ability to scratch, a severe, hyperkeratotic eruption involving thousands of mites on a single patient may ensue.[53]

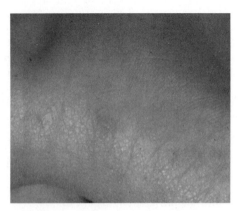

Figure 43–4 A classic burrow of scabies. This hallmark lesion appears as a superficial linear ridge. Newer lesions may have a tiny vesicle at one end with a minute black dot that represents the *Sarcoptes scabiei* mite. In older lesions the burrow begins to desquamate and appears more scaly. (Courtesy of A. Kurban, M.D.)

Treatment consists of application of antiscabietic creams or lotions. The two most widely used medications are lindane and permethrin. Permethrin lacks the neurologic toxicity sometimes seen with lindane, and it has the advantage of being able to kill the scabies eggs as well as the mites; thus, in theory only one application is necessary. For successful treatment, all household and other close contacts must be treated at the same time as the affected patient even if they are asymptomatic because newly infested individuals develop pruritus only when they have been allergically sensitized, often after a delay of 2 weeks or more. The medication is applied from the neck down, paying particular attention to the subungual area and the genitalia. The medication is then washed off in 8 hours. At that time all clothing and linens should be washed in hot water, dry cleaned, or placed in a hot dryer. One week later, the entire process is repeated to kill any larvae that have hatched since the first treatment. It is essential to avoid application of lindane immediately after a hot bath, as increased absorption has been reported to cause seizures in some elderly individuals. Residual pruritus can be managed with topical steroids or antihistamines. However, if pruritus continues for more than a few weeks or if new lesions appear, treatment failure, reinfestation, or misdiagnosis may be indicated.

Malignancy

Malignant neoplasms are strongly age associated in most organ systems, including the skin, for which there is an almost 20-fold increase in incidence in individuals aged 70 or older compared with those aged 35 to 40.[2] This section briefly reviews the clinical features of the most common cutaneous malignancies: basal cell carcinoma (BCC), squamous cell carcinoma (SCC), and malignant melanoma. Actinic keratosis, a common precursor lesion to SCC, is also discussed. Skin cancers account for perhaps half of all cancers in the United States and are increasing in incidence. Estimates of the incidence of nonmelanomatous skin cancers range from 800,000[54] to 1,200,000 cases per year compared with 480,000 in 1978.[55] Such dramatic increases have led many authorities to describe skin cancer as an epidemic—one that particularly affects the elderly.

Ultraviolet irradiation, particularly the ultraviolet B or sunburn spectrum, is the major causative agent of skin cancer. The incidence rates of BCC and SCC rise with increased cumulative ultraviolet exposure, whereas melanoma is correlated more specifically with intense intermittent exposures such as those causing blistering sunburns.[56] Other risk factors include male gender and the interrelated features of fair skin, freckling, blue or light-colored eyes, red or light-colored hair, and a tendency to sunburn rather than tan.[57] Cigarette smoking is also statistically associated with an increased risk of skin cancer.[58]

Unlike most malignancies, virtually all skin cancers can be recognized early in their course because of their visibility on the skin's surface. Cutaneous malignancies that are detected and treated at an early stage are nearly always curable, particularly in nonmelanoma skin cancers, whereas malignancies that are left untreated are associated with a greater incidence of cosmetic disfigurement, functional impairment, metastasis, and fatal outcome.

BASAL CELL CARCINOMAS

The great majority of skin cancers are BCCs. Typical early lesions are asymptomatic, firm, opalescent or "pearly" papules with fine surface telangiectases. Ninety percent occur on the face and neck (Fig. 43–5). BCCs enlarge very slowly, and patients frequently insist that 4-mm lesions have been present for years. The classic neglected "rodent ulcer" is much less common today but can still be identified by its firm, opalescent, telangiectatic, rolled border. Differential diagnosis includes dermal nevi, which are flesh-colored but not as firm, and sebaceous hyperplasia, which is also less firm and is characterized by a slightly yellow color and a central punctum,

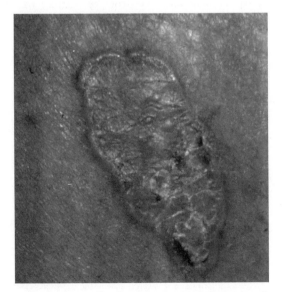

Figure 43–5 Basal cell carcinoma (epithelioma) on the midback of an elderly woman. The center is flat and scaly, but the firm, rolled, telangiectatic border is diagnostic.

the sebaceous orifice. Subtypes include nodular BCC, described earlier; superficial or multicentric BCC, which appears as a scaly pink macule or thin papule; morpheaform BCC, which appears sclerotic and scarlike and can often extend far beyond its clinically apparent borders; and pigmented BCC, with black, brown, and gray pigmentation, which is often mistaken for a melanoma or seborrheic keratosis.[57]

BCCs have an extremely low incidence of metastasis, and thus mortality is low. The morbidity, however, can be great if the lesion is left untreated owing to its ability to erode into the adjacent structures, causing considerable local destruction. A variety of treatment modalities exist. These include simple excision, micrographic surgery, electrodesiccation and curettage, cryotherapy, and irradiation with X-rays. Five-year recurrence rates vary from 1% to 10%, the lowest overall recurrence rate being associated with micrographic surgery.[59] The choice of treatment depends on numerous factors, such as the location of the lesion, histologic variant, size, whether the tumor is primary or recurrent, the general health of the patient, and cosmetic considerations.

SQUAMOUS CELL CARCINOMAS

Squamous cell carcinomas (SCCs) occur in the same fair-skinned patient population, primarily in habitually sun-exposed areas such as the head, neck, and upper extremities, but occasionally in sites of chronic ulceration or other skin damage. Early lesions are asymptomatic, firm, red papules or plaques, usually with scale; more advanced lesions are often ulcerated (Fig. 43–6). Differential diagnosis includes premalignant actinic keratoses and viral warts, in patients with verrucous lesions. Biopsy of suspect lesions is always warranted.

Again, most SCCs are only locally invasive. However, the risk of metastasis, 2% to 10%,[57, 60] is not insignificant. Factors that predispose to a greater risk of metastasis are location on the lip or in areas of chronic inflammation, tumors arising within scars or sites of prior ionizing irradiation, size greater than 1 cm in diameter and 4 mm in thickness, and the presence of immunosuppression.[57] The best treatment is excision or micrographic surgery. There is also a role for radiation therapy in some cases.

ACTINIC KERATOSES

Actinic keratoses (AKs) are SCC precursor lesions. They are commonly found in the same distribution, namely, the head, neck, dorsal

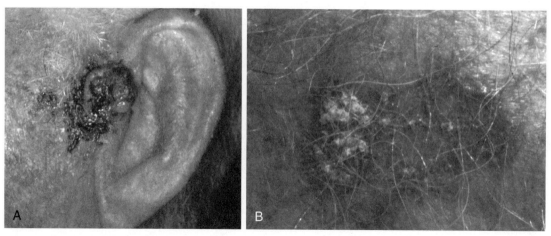

Figure 43–6 *A,* Squamous cell carcinoma of the preauricular area. Central ulceration and hemorrhage are present. *B,* Squamous cell carcinoma in situ (Bowen's disease). The lesion is a thin, pink, scaly plaque.

hands, and arms. Clinically, they appear as rough, scaly, pink-red, poorly circumscribed macules. Identification is sometimes easier by palpation than by visualization. Induration of a suspected lesion may be a sign of progression to SCC or simply a manifestation of inflammation, and such lesions require biopsy to exclude malignancy. Multiple lesions are common and are a marker for cumulative ultraviolet damage and skin cancer risk. The rate of malignant transformation for individual AKs is difficult to ascertain; estimates range from less than 1:1000 to 20%, although the true rate is probably closer to the former. An estimated 10% to 36% of these lesions regress spontaneously,[61] particularly with avoidance of sunlight.[62] Lesions are usually treated with cryotherapy or topical chemotherapy with fluorouracil or masoprocol cream. In some patients, observation alone is an acceptable alternative. Nevertheless, all patients with actinic keratoses should be monitored at least annually for the development of skin cancer.

MALIGNANT MELANOMA

Malignant melanoma is rare compared with nonmelanoma skin cancer, but it is now more common than Hodgkin's disease or thyroid carcinoma,[54] and its incidence is increasing faster than that of any other cancer in the United States.[63] An estimated 38,300 new cases of invasive melanoma were predicted for 1996, the last year for which statistics are available.[54] Others believe that the statistics for melanoma are greatly underestimated and estimate that the combined number of invasive and in situ melanomas was approximately 800,000 in 1992.[64] Depending on the subtype, the peak incidence occurs in the fifth to eighth decade of life, and statistically

higher mortality occurs among older men.[65] Even more than with other cutaneous malignancies, successful treatment depends on early recognition. Clinical criteria for the diagnosis of melanoma have been extensively reviewed and include: diameter greater than 6 mm, variation in color (red, white, and blue areas within a brownblack lesion), irregular border, and irregular surface topography (Fig. 43–7). The extremely common seborrheic or senile keratoses can usually be differentiated by their "stuck on" quality, their even brown pigmentation, and their "regularly irregular" surface. Any change or rapid growth in an existing nevus or new pigmented lesion arising in an elderly individual should be suspected. Reports indicate that between 18% and 85% of melanomas arise from preexisting nevi.

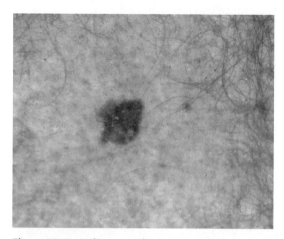

Figure 43–7 Malignant melanoma, superficial spreading type, on the trunk. The asymmetrical location, irregular notched borders, and variations in color raise a suspicion of malignancy. Lighter areas represent foci of regression. (Courtesy of T. Rohrer, M.D.)

The presence of atypical nevi or multiple nevi, particularly in conjunction with a personal or family history of melanoma, is a marker of increased risk for the development of melanoma.[66]

As is the case with basal cell carcinomas, there are several clinical subtypes of melanoma. The most common is the superficial spreading type, which accounts for approximately 70% of cases. Lentigo maligna melanoma, which arises from its slow-growing precursor, lentigo maligna, usually has a larger diameter and a varied pigmentation and occurs on sun-exposed surfaces, usually the face. Nodular melanomas are rapidly growing lesions that lack a radial growth phase and tend to invade deeply early in their course, resulting in a poor prognosis. Acrolentiginous melanoma occurs on the hands and feet, is often periungual, and is the most common form of melanoma in blacks and Asians. A variant of this type of melanoma occurs on the mucosal surfaces. Finally, the rare amelanotic melanoma poses a particular diagnostic challenge because of its lack of pigmentation.

The most important prognostic indicator in melanoma is the Breslow tumor thickness. Lesions with a thickness of less than 0.76 mm have a 5-year survival of 96%, and those between 0.76 and 1.49 mm have an 87% 5-year survival; these figures decline to 75%, 66%, and 47% for lesions 1.5 to 2.49 mm, 2.5 to 3.99 mm, and greater than 4 mm, respectively. In general, older patients have a worse prognosis than younger ones.[66]

Surgical excision is the mainstay of treatment, the recommended margins of excision increasing with tumor thickness. The benefits of elective lymph node dissection or adjuvant therapy (or both) in patients with medium-thickness or medium to thick melanomas, respectively, are controversial at this point.[67] Recently, however, alpha-interferon has been shown to improve survival in thick (more than 4 mm) melanomas.[68] Patients in whom melanoma has been diagnosed must be closely monitored for recurrence, metastasis, and development of a second primary melanoma.

References

1. Woodwell DA, Schappert SM: National Ambulatory Medical Care Survey: 1993 Summary. Advance data from Vital and Health Statistics, No. 270. Hyattsville, MD, National Center for Health Statistics, 1995.
2. Johnson MLT, Roberts J: Prevalence of Dermatologic Disease Among Persons 1–74 Years of Age: United States. Advance data No. 4. Washington, DC, U.S. Department of Health, Education and Welfare, 1977.
3. Lutsky NS: Attitudes toward old age and elderly persons. *In* Eisdorfer C (ed): Annual Review of Gerontology and Geriatrics. New York, Springer, 1980, pp. 287–336.
4. Gilchrest BA: Age-associated changes in the skin. J Am Geriatr Soc 1982; 30:139–143.
5. West MD: The cellular and molecular biology of skin aging. Arch Dermatol 1994;130:87–95.
6. Gerstein AD, Phillips TJ, Rogers GS, Gilchrest BA: Wound healing and aging. Dermatol Clin 1993;11(4):749–757.
7. Garmyn M, Yaar M, Boileau N, Backendorf C, Gilchrest BA: Effect of aging and habitual sun exposure on the genetic response of cultured keratinocytes to solar-simulated irradiation. J Invest Dermatol 1992;99:743–748.
8. Gilchrest BA: Cellular and molecular changes in aging skin. J Geriatr Dermatol 1994;2:3–6.
9. Reenstra WR, Yaar M, Gilchrest BA: Effect of donor age on epidermal growth factor processing in man. Exp Cell Res 1993;209:118–122.
10. Harvell JD, Maibach HI: Percutaneous absorption and inflammation in aged skin: A review. J Am Acad Dermatol 1994;31:1015–1021.
11. Gilchrest BA: Skin and Aging Processes. Boca Raton, FL, CRC Press, 1984.
12. Sauder DN: The immunology of aging skin. J Geriatr Dermatol 1994;2:15–18.
13. Barbee RA, Lebowitz MD, Thompson HC, Burrows B: Immediate skin-test reactivity in a general population sample. Ann Intern Med 1976;84:129–133.
14. MacLaughlin J, Holick MF: Aging decreases the capacity of human skin to produce vitamin D_3. J Clin Invest 1985;76:1536–1538.
15. Gloth FM, Gundberg CM, Hollis BW, Haddad JG, Tobin JD: Vitamin D deficiency in homebound elderly persons. JAMA 1995;274:1683–1686.
16. Matsuoka LY, Wortsman J, Hanifan N, Holick MF: Chronic sunscreen use decreases circulating concentrations of 25-hydroxyvitamin D: A preliminary study. Arch Dermatol 1988;124:1802–1804.
17. Klecz RJ, Schwartz RA: Pruritus. Am Fam Physician 1992;45:2681–2686.
18. Gilchrest BA: Pruritus: Pathogenesis, therapy and significance in systemic disease states. Arch Intern Med 1982;142:101–105.
19. Thorne EG: Coping with pruritus: A common geriatric complaint. Geriatrics 1978;33:47–49.
20. Lewiecki MEM, Rahman F: Pruritus: A manifestation of iron deficiency. JAMA 1976;236:2319–2320.
21. Salem HH, van der Weyden MB, Young IF, Wiley JS: Pruritus and severe iron deficiency in polycythemia vera. Br Med J 1982;285:91–92.
22. Potts RO, Buras EM, Chrisman DA: Changes with age in the moisture content of human skin. J Invest Dermatol 1984;82:97–100.
23. Ghadially R, Brown BE, Sequeira-Martin SM, et al: The aged epidermal permeability barrier: Structural, functional, and lipid biochemical abnormalities in humans and a senescent murine model. J Clin Invest 1995;95:2281–2290.
24. Gilchrest BA: Pruritus in the elderly. Semin Dermatol 1995;14:317–319.
25. Fleischer AB: Pruritus in the elderly: Management by senior dermatologists. J Am Acad Dermatol 1993;28:603–609.
26. Kligman AM: Perspectives and problems in cutaneous gerontology. J Invest Dermatol 1979;73:39–46.
27. Tagami H: Quantitative measurements of water concentration of the statum corneum *in vivo* by high-frequency current. Acta Dermatol Venereol 1994; 185(Suppl):29–33.
28. Vilaplana J, Coll J, Trullas C, Pelejero C: Clinical and non-invasive evaluation of 12% ammonium lactate emulsion for the treatment of dry skin in atopic and non-atopic subjects. Acta Dermatol Venereol 1992;72:28–33.

29. Beauregard S, Gilchrest BA: A survey of skin problems and skin care regimens in the elderly. Arch Dermatol 1987;123:1638–1643.

30. Johnson MLT: Aging of the United States population: The dermatologic implications. Dermatol Clin 1986;4:371–377.

31. Tindal JP: Skin changes and lesions in our senior citizens: Incidences. Cutis 1976;18:359–362.

32. Stratigos JD, Antoniou C, Katsambas A, et al: Ketoconazole 2% cream versus hydrocortisone 1% cream in the treatment of seborrheic dermatitis. J Am Acad Dermatol 1988;19:850–853.

33. Arndt KA, Jick H: Rates of cutaneous reactions to drugs: A report from the Boston Collaborative Drug Surveillance Program. JAMA 1976;235:918–922.

34. Bigby M, Jick S, Jick H, Arndt K: Drug-induced cutaneous reactions: A report from the Boston Collaborative Drug Surveillance Program on 15,438 consecutive inpatients, 1975 to 1982. JAMA 1986;256:3358–3363.

35. Wintroub BU, Stern R: Cutaneous drug reactions: Pathogenesis and clinical classification. J Am Acad Dermatol 1985;13:167–179.

36. Goldstein SM, Wintroub BU: A Physician's Guide—Adverse Cutaneous Reactions to Medication. New York, CoMedia, 1994.

37. Shear NH, Spielberg SP: Anticonvulsant hypersensitivity syndrome: In vitro assessment of risk. J Clin Invest 1988;82:1826–1832.

38. Roujeau JC, Stern RS: Severe adverse cutaneous reactions to drugs. N Engl J Med 1994;331:1272–1285.

39. Mutasim DF: Bullous pemphigoid: Review and update. J Geriatr Dermatol 1993;1:62–71.

40. Ishiko A, Shimizu H, Kikuchi A, Ebihara T, Hashimoto T, Nishikawa T: Human autoantibodies against the 230-kD bullous pemphigoid antigen (BPAG1) bind only to the intracellular domain of the hemidesmosome, whereas those against the 180-kD bullous pemphigoid antigen (BPAG2) bind along the plasma membrane of the hemidesmosome in normal human and swine skin. J Clin Invest 1993;91:1608–1615.

41. Fine JD: Management of acquired bullous skin diseases. N Engl J Med 1995;333:1475–1484.

42. Paul MA, Jorizzo JL, Fleischer AB, White WL: Low-dose methotrexate treatment in elderly patients with bullous pemphigoid. J Am Acad Dermatol 1994;31:620–625.

43. Fivenson DP, Breneman DL, Rosen GB, Hersh CS, Cardone S, Mutasim D: Nicotinamide and tetracycline therapy of bullous pemphigoid. Arch Dermatol 1994;130:753–758.

44. Oxman MN, Alani R: Varicella and herpes zoster. *In* Fitzpatrick TB, Eisen AZ, Wolff K, et al (eds): Dermatology in General Medicine, 4th ed. New York, McGraw-Hill, 1993, pp. 2543–2572.

45. Lee JJ, Gauci CAG: Postherpetic neuralgia: Current concepts and management. Br J Hosp Med 1994;52:565–567, 570.

46. Huff JC, Bean B, Balfour HH, et al: Therapy of herpes zoster with oral acyclovir. Am J Med 1988;85(Suppl 2A):84–89.

47. Wood MJ, Ogan PH, McKendrick MW, Care CD, McGill, JI, Webb EM: Efficacy of oral acyclovir treatment of acute herpes zoster. Am J Med 1988;85(Suppl 2A):79–83.

48. Cobo M: Reduction of the ocular complications of herpes zoster ophthalmicus by oral acyclovir. Am J Med 1988;85(Suppl 2A):90–93.

49. Wood, MJ, Johnson RW, McKendrick MW, Taylor J, Mandal BK, Crooks J: A randomized trial of acyclovir for 7 days or 21 days with and without prednisolone for treatment of acute herpes zoster. N Engl J Med 1994;330:896–900.

50. Bernstein JE, Korman NJ, Bickers DR, Dahl MV, Millikan LE: Topical capsaicin treatment of chronic postherpetic neuralgia. J Am Acad Dermatol 1989;21:265–270.

51. Rowbotham MC: Treatment of postherpetic neuralgia. Semin Dermatol 1992;11:218–225.

52. Parish LC, Witkowski JA, Millikan LE: Scabies in the extended care facility: Revisited. Int J Dermatol 1991:30:703–706.

53. Estes SA, Estes J: Therapy of scabies: Nursing homes, hospitals, and the homeless. Semin Dermatol 1993;12:26–33.

54. Parker SL, Tong T, Bolden S, Wingo PA: Cancer statistics, 1996. CA Cancer J Clin 1996;46:5–27.

55. Miller DL, Weinstock MA: Nonmelanoma skin cancer in the United States: Incidence. J Am Acad Dermatol 1994;30:774–778.

56. Elmets CA, Mukhtar H: Ultraviolet radiation and skin cancer: Progress in pathophysiologic mechanisms. Prog Dermatol 1995;30(1):1–16.

57. Preston DS, Stern RS: Nonmelanoma cancers of the skin. N Engl J Med 1992;327:1649–1662.

58. Karagas MR, Stukel TA, Greenberg ER, Baron JA, Mott LA, Stern RS: Risk of subsequent basal cell carcinoma and squamous cell carcinoma of the skin among patients with prior skin cancer. JAMA 1992;267:3305–3310.

59. Rowe DE, Carroll RJ, Day CL: Long-term recurrence rates in previously untreated (primary) basal cell carcinoma: Implications for patient follow-up. J Dermatol Surg Oncol 1989;15:315–328.

60. Salasche SJ, Cheney ML, Varvares MA: Recognition and management of the high-risk cutaneous squamous cell carcinoma. Curr Probl Dermatol 1993;5:141–192.

61. Frost CA, Green AC: Epidemiology of solar keratoses. Br J Dermatol 1994;131:455–464.

62. Thompson SC, Jolley D, Marks R: Reduction of solar keratoses by regular sunscreen use. N Engl J Med 1993;329:1147–1151.

63. Ries LAG, Miller BA, Hankey BF, Kosary CL, Harras A, Edwards BK (eds): SEER Cancer Statistics Review, 1973–1991: Tables and Graphs. NIH Publication No. 94-2789. Bethesda, MD, National Cancer Institute, 1994, pp. 287–299.

64. Salopek TG, Marghoob AA, Slade JM, et al: An estimate of the incidence of malignant melanoma in the United States. Dermatol Surg 1995;21:301–305.

65. Geller AC, Koh HK, Miller DR, Mercer MB, Lew RA: Death rates of malignant melanoma among white men: United States, 1973–1988. MMWR 1992;41:20–21, 27.

66. Koh HK: Cutaneous melanoma. N Engl J Med 1991;325:171–182.

67. Johnson TM, Smith JW, Nelson BR, Chang A: Current therapy for cutaneous melanoma. J Am Acad Dermatol 1995;32:689–707.

68. Kirkwood JM, Strawderman MH, Ernstoff MS, Smith TJ, Borden EC, Blum RH: Interferon alpha-2b adjuvant therapy of high risk resected cutaneous melanoma: The Eastern Cooperative Oncology Group Trial EST 1684. J Clin Oncol 1996;14:7–17.

Additional Readings

Gilchrest BA: Geriatric dermatology. Geriatric Clin 1989;5(1):1–257.

Gilchrest BA: Photodamage. Cambridge, MA, Blackwell Science, 1995.

Marks R: Skin and Skin Diseases in Old Age. London, Martin Dunitz, 1986.

44 Dental and Oral Disorders

Kenneth Shay, D.D.S., M.S.

Oral disease is extremely common in advanced age. In the United States, nearly one third of adults over age 65 have no teeth at all (Fig. 44–1). Although over 90% of edentulous adults use dentures, most denture wearers complain of pain, inadequate function, or some other shortcoming associated with their oral prostheses. Essentially all older adults who retain some or all of their natural teeth have lost some measure of the bony support around the teeth, and a majority at any point in time suffer from active destructive periodontal disease. Dental decay (caries) is as prevalent in older adults as it is in younger ones, and decay of the roots of the teeth is more common in advanced age than at any other time in life.[1] Oral disease can be particularly pronounced in institutionalized and dependent elderly, in whom oral care has declined or disappeared along with other daily self-care behaviors.

Yet oral diseases may be unrecognized or untreated in older people for several reasons. Symptoms of dental decay (sensitivity to hot, cold, and sweets; acute, spontaneous tooth pain) decline and disappear with age. Oral problems may be dismissed by patients or their caregivers as unavoidable or unimportant consequences of aging. The expenses of dental treatment can represent a large part of the fixed or shrinking income of an elder and are not covered by Medicare. Knowledge of a suitable dentist or ability to travel to the dental office can be a significant barrier for a homebound elder or one with limited mobility.[2]

Oral health is strongly linked to overall health and the quality of an older person's life. Eating ability and enjoyment of food as well as interpersonal relationships can be strongly impaired by oral disease that affects the functions of chewing, swallowing, tasting, and olfaction. Oral pathogens can significantly impair general health through direct extension of disease or its spread to heart, lungs, joints, or other sites. Finally, many of the nonoral diseases prevalent in advanced age, as well as their treatments, are themselves expressed in the oral cavity through exacerbation of existing conditions or the onset of new ones.[3]

Physicians who treat older adults must appreciate the importance of oral health to their patients' general well-being. They must recognize the difference between the few true age changes that affect the mouth and the common diseases or environmental effects that are subject to prevention or treatment. They should encourage the inclusion of preventive dentistry as part of their older patients' preventive regimens and

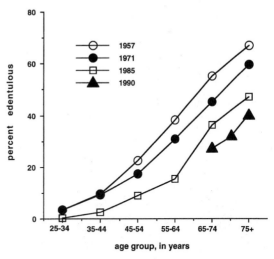

Figure 44–1 Toothlessness rates in older Americans as reported in 1957, 1971, 1986, and 1993. Data are derived from the following sources: (1) National Center for Health Statistics: Edentulous persons, United States, 1971. Data from the National Health Survey, Vital and Health Statistics 1974, Series 10, No. 89. U. S. Department of Health and Human Services Publication No. (HRA) 74-1516. (2) Miller AJ, Brunelle JA, Carlos JP, et al: Oral Health of United States Adults. NIH Publication No. 87-2868. Washington, DC, U.S. Department of Health and Human Services, National Institutes of Health, 1987. (3) Brunell JA, Marcus SE, Winn DM, Brown LJ: Trends in oral health status of the elderly 1971–1991. J Dent Res 75 (special issue):41, 1996 (Abstract, 192). (4) Douglass CW, Jette AM, Fox CH, et al: Oral health status of the elderly in New England. J Gerontol 48:M39–M46, 1993.

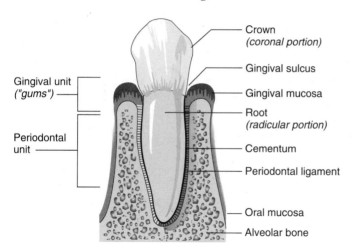

Figure 44-2 Terminology of structures of the tooth and periodontium. (From Shay K, Ship JA: The importance of oral health in the older patient. J Am Geriatr Soc 43:1414–1422, 1995.)

include appraisal of the mouth in the geriatric assessment. Finally, they should be familiar with common medical questions asked by dentists who treat their older patients.

ORAL TISSUES IN THE AGED PATIENT

The modifications undergone by parts of the oral cavity due strictly to advancing age are relatively minor compared with those that result from accumulated diseases, traumatic incidents, and the management of both.

Periodontal Diseases

The periodontium[4] is the complex of tissues surrounding the teeth (Fig. 44–2). Colonies of aerobic and anaerobic microorganisms that develop on the teeth near the gum line release endotoxins and stimulate an immune response resulting in a local inflammation, termed gingivitis. Gingivitis is a reversible, edematous, erythematous change localized to the gum tissue near the teeth. Patients may complain of gingival bleeding or minor pain or itching of the gums. Daily removal of the bacterial colonies by brushing or professional debridement normally remedies this condition in a matter of days. In patients taking phenytoin, cyclosporin, or a calcium channel blocking agent, gingivitis may be made worse by a prolific hypertrophic response to the bacterial plaque (Fig. 44–3), in which case surgical reduction of the enlarged gingiva may be required.

Under certain host conditions, particular organisms within the gingival sulcus may trigger a host response that stimulates osteoclast activation. While this process is active, pus may be expressed from the sulcus. If this process occurs repeatedly, the bony support of the affected

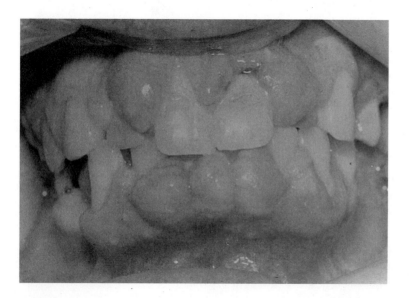

Figure 44-3 Gingival overgrowth due to nifedipine. This 69-year-old male had been taking 20 mg of nifedipine TID for 4 months.

tooth or teeth becomes affected clinically. Over 95% of Americans aged 65 or over display indications of some present or past periodontitis. The teeth appear to be longer and may be somewhat loosened or may gradually shift position in the mouth. Active periodontal disease is managed by a combination of removal of hopelessly affected teeth, professional scaling, surgical resection of gum tissue to promote easier self-care, and optimal daily oral hygiene.

Periodontal diseases have significant interactions with systemic health. Gingivitis and periodontitis become worse with psychological stress. These oral conditions are often more exaggerated, advanced, and difficult to control in patients with diabetes. It is believed that the chronic infection of periodontitis may interfere with blood glucose control in diabetics with poor glycemic control. Periodontal pathogens are known to colonize the oropharynx and have been implicated in gram-negative pneumonia.

Dental Caries

More than 98% of the dentate population carries the organism *Streptococcus mutans* in the oral cavity. *S. mutans* metabolizes simple sugars into lactate, resulting in local dissolution of tooth mineral. Dental caries[5] occurs in areas where this process has been repeated so often that the dissolution invades the tooth. Older adults experience the same rates of decay of the crowns of teeth as do younger adults, although a greater proportion of this decay affects existing dental restorations rather than previously undiseased surfaces. Due to a lifetime of exposure to periodontal pathogens, most older adults with teeth have parts of the roots exposed to the oral environment, resulting in an increase in root caries with advancing age.

Dental caries appears as light to dark brown, softened spots on the teeth, usually between the teeth, adjacent to the gum, or next to a restoration. As the lesion progresses, frank holes appear, or perhaps a piece of the tooth or filling is actually missing. In older adults, dental caries is seldom accompanied by pain; one true normative age change that affects the oral cavity is the progressive diminution in size and decreased neuronal component of the dental pulp. Epithelial cells lining the dental pulp constantly elaborate an osteoid-like tissue, and the volume of the dental pulp therefore declines with age. Pulp consists of vascular, neuronal, lymphatic, and connective tissues. Aged pulps are characterized by an increase in connective tissue relative to neuronal tissue. The result of these changes is a delayed or omitted report of the oral symptoms

of early caries (such as sensitivity or spontaneous pain) that might be more regularly reported by younger patients.

Prevention of dental caries requires daily toothbrushing and is enhanced by exposure to fluoride ion, usually in toothpaste or a fluoride mouth rinse. Management of dental caries consists of removal of the diseased tissue and replacement with a wear-resistant material—a filling or crown. If the caries has progressed to affect the pulp, the pulp chamber must be debrided and filled (a "root canal" treatment) if the tooth is to be retained.

Tooth Loss

Teeth are lost because of a combination of dental and nondental factors. Periodontal disease can so compromise the support structures of the teeth that extraction is inevitable. Yet although dental caries can destroy the oral component of a tooth, root canal treatment and surgery to expose more of the root area to the oral cavity may allow its restoration. But the considerable expense and elapsed time needed for this approach often result in a decision to extract such a tooth. The fate of a carious tooth is thus the result of the biomedical prognosis and the financial, emotional, and temporal priority that the patient places on it.

Retention of teeth into advanced age is increasingly common. Today's elders are far more likely than their predecessors to have been exposed to preventive dental practices earlier in life so that they now carry a larger portion of their natural dentitions into their advanced years. This change is not entirely without problems because the preservation of teeth brings with it the need for their daily care, an obligation that becomes more difficult if skills that depend on visual and manual dexterity are declining.

The absence of a tooth is not a static event. If other teeth remain, extraction is usually followed by a slow anterior migration of the tooth or teeth posterior to the lost one. In some cases, the tooth that opposed the lost one migrates toward the opposite jaw (Fig. 44–4). Areas of the alveolar processes that lack teeth gradually undergo bony resorption. This loss of bone is of most concern to those who lack all their teeth. In such people dentures become progressively more ill-fitting over a period of months or years. Improved fit of the dentures may be possible by modifying the fitting surfaces or by fabricating a new prosthesis, but either option may result in a lower level of function than was possible when the patient possessed a more intact anatomic configuration. Increasingly, those who have lost their

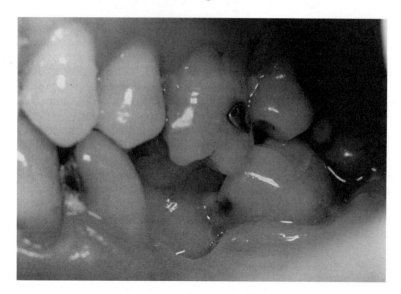

Figure 44–4 When a tooth is lost, the tooth opposing it and the tooth next to it may migrate into the space left behind.

teeth and have the means to afford it obtain osseointegrated titanium implants, wherein metallic posts in the edentulous jaws securely anchor a dental prosthesis.

Oral Mucosal Disease

There are three distinct varieties of oral mucosa: the keratinized, tightly bound mucosa surrounding the teeth (gingiva) and covering the hard palate; the loose, parakeratinized alveolar mucosa that covers the inside of the cheeks and lips, floor of the mouth, and ventrum of the tongue; and the specialized mucosa of the dorsum of the tongue. These sites in older persons are subject to a variety of conditions, the most prevalent of which are discussed here.

Traumatic ulceration caused by the use of removable dentures results from food entrapment or eventual poor fit due to the bony resorption described earlier (Fig. 44–5). In extreme cases, an ill-fitting denture can evoke a proliferative tissue response, in which folds of hyperplastic mucosa develop at the border of the denture. Removal of the denture is the most effective management for denture sores; referral to a dentist for assessment and management of the condition must follow to prevent recurrence.

Candidiasis results from local or disseminated pathogenic colonization by a commensal oral yeast. The lesion is most common on the denture-bearing tissues of the maxilla and may be asymptomatic or can present as a persistent unpleasant taste or a burning or itching sensation.

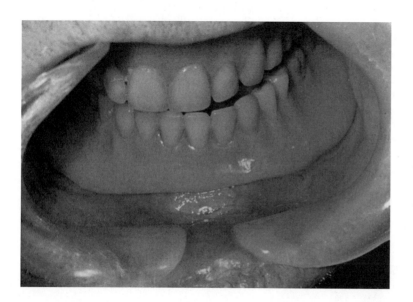

Figure 44–5 Severe denture ulcer due to resorption of the mandibular alveolar ridge and subsequent impingement on the insertion of the mentalis muscle. The denture has been adjusted so that it no longer traumatizes the affected area.

The affected mucosa may be diffusely erythematous or may feature small (less than 1 mm) areas of redness or curd-like white plaques that can be removed with gauze, leaving behind a reddened, denuded surface. The condition seems to be due to one or more of the following: ill-fitting dentures; poor denture hygiene; altered salivary flow; or impaired immune response. In many cases, improved daily hygiene and removal of the dentures during sleep is sufficient to resolve the condition. In persistent or recurring cases an antifungal agent such as nystatin, clotrimazole, or fluconazole may be necessary; the denture may also require modification by a dentist. Candidal infection that occurs independent of the use of dental prostheses may indicate a recent shift in the oral microflora (e.g., following a course of antibiotic) or a change in salivary composition due to a medication side effect. Infection that persists despite excellent hygiene and dental and pharmacologic interventions is probably due to an altered host response.

Squamous cell carcinoma of the oral cavity accounts for approximately 3% of new cancers and 2% of cancer deaths annually in the United States. It affects males twice as frequently as females, and 90% of diagnoses are made in patients aged 50 years or older. Smoking, alcohol, and particularly the combination of the two are strong risk factors. Cancerous and precancerous oral lesions appear as asymptomatic white, red, or white and red patches or ulcerations, most commonly on the lip, floor of the mouth, lateral border of the tongue, and oropharynx (Fig. 44–6). Lesions of this description that are not attributable to another obvious cause (such as recent or chronic trauma that resolves when the source of the trauma is removed for 7 to 14 days) must be submitted to biopsy. Five-year survival and degree of morbidity are dramatically improved by early detection and treatment. For this reason, a thorough oral mucosal evaluation must be a routine part of the assessment of every geriatric patient, especially those who are smokers or heavy drinkers.[6]

Aphthous stomatitis affects the alveolar mucosa with isolated painful ulcerations that disappear within 7 to 10 days (Fig. 44–7). Aphthous ulcers have been linked to psychogenic (stress), chemical (usually acidic), and traumatic (e.g., a new toothbrush) stimuli. Herpetic ulcers appear as isolated fluid-filled blisters that burst and coalesce into irregular, denuded, painful patches on the attached tissues of the mouth (Fig. 44–8) and at the vermilion border of the lip. Resolution occurs without treatment in 7 to 10 days but may be accelerated by the use of a topical antiviral agent such as acyclovir. Topical steroid or viscous lidocaine (Xylocaine) agents applied to aphthous or herpetic ulcerations may make eating less uncomfortable.

ORAL FUNCTION IN THE AGING PATIENT

The oral cavity is involved in alimentation, host protection, and communication. Although perfect oral health is not essential for these functions, various disease states may impair a person's ability to perform them, leading to the further detriment of general health.

Chewing

With advancing age, people with intact dentition need to chew for a longer period of time and

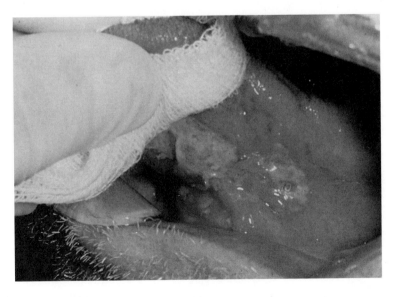

Figure 44–6 Squamous cell carcinoma of the lateral border of the tongue. Note the use of gauze to aid retraction and visualization.

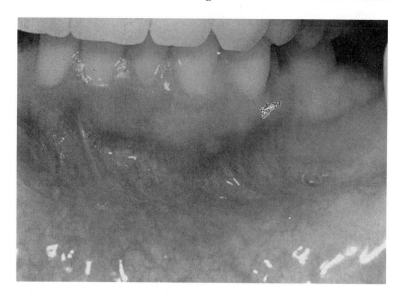

Figure 44–7 Aphthous ulcer of the alveolar mucosa of the vestibule that arose after the patient ate fresh pineapple.

with an increasing number of chewing strokes to achieve the same level of food maceration as they did when they were younger.[7] As the number of natural teeth in the dentition declines, the duration and number of chewing strokes continue to increase, and the achievable level of food reduction can no longer match the level attained with an intact dentition. This is true even if missing teeth are replaced with removable dental prostheses. In a person with no natural teeth and complete dentures, chewing efficiency is, on average, about one-sixth that of the intact natural dentition. Numerous studies have demonstrated a correlation between the number of food types avoided and the degree of debility of an individual's dentition. It may be concluded that persons with symptomatic oral disease or chew-

ing status compromised by tooth loss are at increased risk of inadequate nutritional intake. It does not follow, however, that replacement of the missing teeth will resolve a person's weight loss or eating disorder.

Swallowing

The duration of the swallowing[8] sequence increases with age, although aspiration episodes do not seem to increase in prevalence owing to age alone. Yet disease states that are known to affect swallowing and protection of the airway profoundly, such as stroke and Parkinson's disease, are more prevalent in the elderly. Studies demonstrate a significant correlation between impaired chewing ability and frequency of aspira-

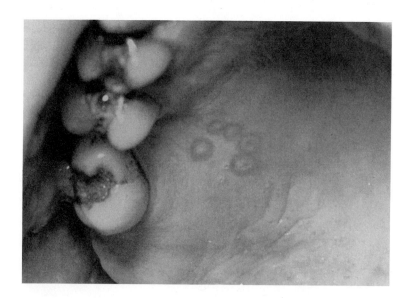

Figure 44–8 Early stage of *Herpes simplex* lesion of the hard palate. The blisters will burst and coalesce into a single denuded ulcer.

tion of oral contents. It is prudent to regard patients with neuromuscular disease and oral disability as having an increased risk of aspiration.

Chemosensory Function

The ability to discern the difference between distilled water and water with an extremely diluted salt, sweet, bitter, or sour component ("taste threshold") remains essentially intact with increasing age.[9] Suprathreshold response—the degree of perceived "saltiness" for a given salt stimulus (and likewise for sour, sweet, and bitter)—does diminish with age, raising questions about the role this change may play in one person's habit of oversalting food or another's growing fondness for sweets. Taste perception may also be affected by the use of a maxillary denture, which physically covers the palatal taste pores. Numerous medications have potential side effects involving disruption of taste (Table 44–1). Many others can cause diminution of salivary flow (Table 44–2), which interferes with the taste function owing to blocked taste pores or inadequate fluid available for dissolving tastant molecules. Finally, an older person's complaint of taste impairment may be due to disruption of some other oral sensation, inasmuch as the "flavor" of a food is derived not only from its taste but also from its smell, texture, and temperature.

Olfactory function undergoes demonstrable decline with advancing age. Like taste, olfaction may be further affected by medications. It is also impaired by poor oral hygiene and improves if oral hygiene (particularly that of the tongue) improves.

Salivary Function

Saliva is essential for the maintenance of oral health.[10] It neutralizes acid that promotes caries and remineralizes areas of incipient dissolution. Saliva contains specific antifungal agents and reduces intraoral bacteria through dilution, aggregating factors, and microbicidal enzymes. In the absence of saliva, caries becomes rampant (Fig. 44–9). Salivary mucins reduce intraoral trauma by lubricating the hard and soft tissues and aiding swallowing by facilitating bolus formation.

Reduced salivary flow is a common complaint of older adults. Longitudinal studies, however, have established that salivary flow from the parotid is essentially unchanged with advancing age. There are conflicting findings about submandibular and minor salivary gland output as a function of advancing age, but it is safe to assert that a patient who complains that his mouth has

TABLE 44–1 DRUGS THAT INTERFERE WITH TASTE AND SMELL

Drugs That Interfere with the Gustatory System	
Acetazolamide	Glipizide
Allopurinol	Gold
Amiloride	Griseofulvin
Amphetamine	Hextidine
Amphotericin B	Hydrocortisone
Ampicillin	Idoxuridine
Azathioprine	Iron sorbitex
Baclofen	Levadopa
Bamifylline hydrochloride	Levamisole
	Lincomycin
Bleomycin	Lithium carbonate
Captopril	Methimazole
Carbamazepine	Methotrexate
Carbimazole	Methylthiouracil
Carmustine	Metronidazole
Cefamandole	Nifedipine
Chlormezanone	Niridazole
Chlorpheniramine maleate	Nitroglycerine patch
	Oxyfedrine
Clofibrate	Phenformin
Colchicine	Phenindione
D-Penicillamine	Phenylbutazone
Dexamethasone	Phenytoin
Diazoxide	Propyluracil
Diltiazem	Sulfasalazine
Dipyridamole	Tetracyclines
Doxorubicin	Thiouracil
Enalapril	Trifluoperazine
Ethacrynic acid	Vincristine sulfate
Ethambutol hydrochloride	Vitamin D
Etidronate	
5-Thiopyridoxine	
Drugs That Interfere with the Olfactory System	
Allicin	Methyluracil
Amitriptyline	Morphine
Amphetamine	Nifedipine
Carbimazole	Phenmetrazine
Codeine	Propyluracil
Diltiazem	Streptomycin
Hydromorphone hydrochloride	Tyrothricin
Methimazole	

After Schiffman SS: Drugs influencing taste and smell perception. *In* Getchell TV, et al (eds): Smell and Taste in Health and Disease. New York, Raven Press, 1991, pp. 845–850.

recently become dry is not experiencing a normal change of aging.

Probably the most prevalent cause of a dry mouth is a side effect of one or more medications (see Table 44–2). Management of psychiatric disorders, incontinence, hypertension, cardiac disease, Parkinson's disease, and pain all commonly

TABLE 44–2 **AGENTS AMONG THE 200 MOST COMMONLY PRESCRIBED DRUGS REPORTED TO HAVE XEROSTOMIA AS A SIDE EFFECT, AND REPORTED XEROSTOMIA PREVALENCES FOR AGENTS FOR WHICH SUCH DATA ARE AVAILABLE**

Agent	Prevalence (%)	Agent	Prevalence (%)
Albuterol	<1	Ketoprofen	<1
Alprazolam	19.7–32.8	Ketorolac	<1
Amitriptyline	C[a]	Lisinopril	0.3–1
Astemizole	5.2	Lorazepam	1–10
Atenolol	N[b]	Lovastatin	0.5–1
Beclomethasone	1–10	Metoprolol	1
Bumetanide	0.1	Nabumetone	1
Buspirone	3	Nicotine topical	1–3
Captopril	0.5–2	Nifedipine	<3
Carbamazepine	1–10	Nitroglycerin	C
Carbidopa/levodopa	C	Nizatidine	1.4
Cefixime	1–11	Norfloxacin	0.3–1
Ciprofloxacin	<1	Nortriptyline	C
Phenylpropanolamine	C	Ofloxacin	1–3
Clonazepam	N	Omeprazole	<1
Codeine/acetaminophen	C	Oxycodone/acetaminophen	C
Cromolyn sodium	C	Penicillin VK	C
Cyclobenzaprine	27	Pentoxifylline	<1
Diazepam	1–10	Phenylpropanolamine	N
Diclofenac	<1	Piroxicam	<1
Diltiazem	<1	Prednisone	1–10
Enalapril	0.5–2	Prochlorperazine	C
Etodolac	<1	Promethazine	C
Famotidine	N	Propoxyphene/acetaminophen	C
Fluoxetine	1–10	Propranolol	N
Flurbiprofen	<1	Pseudoephedrine	21.7
Furosemide	N	Sertraline	16.3
Gemfibrozil	N	Sucralfate	<0.5
Guanfacine	<54	Temazepam	1.7
Hydrochlorothiazide (HCTZ)	1–10	Terazosin	1
Hydrocodone/acetaminophen	C	Terfenadine	2.3–4.8
Ibuprofen	<1	Timolol	N
Indapamide	<5	Triamcinolone acetonide	N
Ipratropium bromide	2.4	Triamterene/HCTZ	1–10
Isosorbide	C	Triazolam	<0.5
Isradipine	0.5–1	Verapamil	1

[a]Common (expected and sometimes inevitable). [b]No prevalence reported.
 After Smith RG, Burtner P: Oral side effects of the most frequently prescribed drugs. Spec Care Dent 1994;14:96–102.

involve medications that are xerogenic. Severe salivary gland hypofunction results from therapeutic irradiation given for tumors of the head and neck. Xerostomia may develop from secretions blocking the nasal passages, resulting in mouth breathing. One to three million Americans suffer from Sjögren's syndrome (see Chapter 39), of which xerostomia is a sentinel symptom. A decrease in saliva has been associated with Alzheimer's disease, depression, and other diseases as well.

Management of xerostomia begins with its recognition as a potentially reversible disorder. Dental referral is imperative to institute an optimal preventive regimen that includes frequent recall, dietary counseling, and daily application of fluoride. Elimination of redundant or excessive medications should be followed by attempts to substitute other drugs for potentially xerogenic agents. If manipulation of the drug regimen is impossible or does not solve the problem, some palliation may be possible through the use of salivary substitutes (over-the-counter, aqueous surfactants taken ad lib). In patients with xerostomia due to a nonpharmacologic cause, a prescription of oral pilocarpine may be helpful for those who do not object to the side effects of perspiration and lacrimation. Sugarless hard candies and gum, or frequent sips of water and artificially sweetened drinks are also alternatives. Patients must

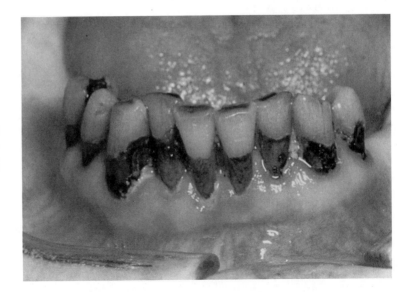

Figure 44–9 In the absence of adequate saliva, there is little natural defense against dental caries, which then rampantly destroys the teeth.

be educated not to sip sucrose-containing drinks or use sugar-containing gum or candy, which brings about rapid destruction of teeth in a dry mouth (see Fig. 44–9).

PREVENTIVE DENTISTRY FOR OLDER PATIENTS

Most oral problems are related to disease or its treatment and in many cases are preventable wholly or in part. Prevention of oral diseases is a focus of the dental profession, but economic and other barriers may impede many elders, particularly the oldest and most infirm, from seeking needed dental care. The close connection between oral and general health is a compelling reason for physicians to have a working knowledge of preventive dentistry, so they can encourage their older patients to practice these effective and necessary preventive behaviors.

Patients with any number of natural teeth must brush them thoroughly at least daily, ideally after each meal, and always before going to bed (salivary flow is at a minimum during sleep). A soft-bristle brush, directed at a 45-degree angle to the tooth, should be used with a fluoride-containing toothpaste on all surfaces of each tooth and pointed toward the gum line. Dental floss or specialized brushes for cleaning between the teeth are excellent daily adjuncts for patients who can manage them.

Dietary sugar is not in itself deleterious to teeth, but in the presence of plaque each ingestion results in a 20-minute pulse of intraoral acidity. Thus, frequent sweet or starchy snacks, regardless of size, are worse for the dentition than the sum of those foods eaten at once. Frequency of eating is irrelevant to oral health if the mouth is cleaned promptly after each ingestion.

Patients who have a removable denture should keep the prosthesis out of the mouth for at least 6 hours daily to maintain the health of the mucosa. Prostheses should be removed and rinsed after each meal and should be scrubbed with a suitable brush at least daily. They should be soaked in an antimicrobial rinse (either a commercially available agent or a dilute solution of household bleach) for at least 20 minutes several times per week.

Everyone should see a dentist at least twice annually. Patients with one or more natural teeth need to have their teeth thoroughly examined and cleaned professionally. Those at high risk for caries (e.g., those with salivary dysfunction or impaired self-care abilities) may have to be seen at more frequent intervals. Patients who no longer have their natural teeth should receive a mucosal examination and an evaluation of their prosthesis at least annually; those at high risk for oral malignancy (smokers and drinkers) should have a mucosal evaluation performed twice annually.

Because of the importance of regular mucosal evaluation for older patients and because many elders either do not seek or cannot afford dental care, the following section describes the procedure used for oral evaluation.

ASSESSMENT OF THE ORAL CAVITY

Assessment of the oral cavity should begin with a systematic examination of the oral mucosa.[11] An easy sequence to remember begins with the lips and cheeks, then the vestibular areas and alveolar ridges, the tongue and floor of the mouth, and finally the hard and soft palates. The examination should be conducted with a strong light, one or two tongue blades, and a gauze sponge for retraction of the tongue. Performed properly, the examination need take no longer than 90 seconds and can easily be quicker for an edentulous patient. The clinician should be alert for areas of ulceration, induration, inflammation, whitening, or reddening of the mucosa.

In examining the lips, the clinician should pay close attention to the vermilion border, where herpetic and malignant lesions are seen most commonly. A cracked, weeping lesion at the corner of the mouth is most commonly due to *Candida albicans* or riboflavin deficiency. Bluish vascular lesions of the lip are common elsewhere throughout the mouth as well and generally require no treatment. A small (2 to 6 mm) fleshy protuberance high on the inside of the cheek is the duct for the parotid gland.

The vestibules and alveolar ridges cannot be adequately examined until any dentures have been removed. Reddened or ulcerated denture-bearing areas are most likely due to trauma from the denture, and the patient should be urged to seek dental attention. The denture should be kept out of the mouth for at least 72 hours and the area then reexamined; if the lesion has not resolved in this time period it should be biopsied. In the presence of teeth, circular papules on the alveolar ridge that are 1 to 2 mm in diameter may be fistulous tracts from teeth with necrotic pulps—a sign of abscess. Smooth but prominent bony protuberances on either side of the mandible (Fig. 44–10) or maxilla or along the palatal suture are benign osteomas and are no cause for concern.

Examination of the tongue requires its retraction. The gauze sponge should be held on the patient's lower lip and the patient instructed to stick out the tongue. The tongue is then firmly grasped with the gauze and retracted. Switching hands and rotating the tongue to the opposite side will complete the tongue examination. Discrete white, red, or mixed red and white lesions require biopsy if they are not attributable to an obvious cause (e.g., candidal infection or trauma from a sharp tooth). When the lateral borders have been examined, the tongue is released, and the patient is instructed to place the tip of the tongue against the back of the front teeth, allowing visualization of the areas covered by gauze as well as the floor of the mouth. The dorsum is examined last; a depapillated appearance may indicate vitamin B_{12} deficiency (Fig. 44–11).

In denture wearers, the hard palate is commonly reddened owing to candidiasis. In some patients a disseminated papillary growth is displayed on the palate; this is also due to fungi but requires resection for resolution.

When the mucosal surfaces of the mouth have been examined, the teeth and gums can be assessed for signs of disease: deposits, inflammation, purulence, and mobility. Food debris and bacterial deposits (either hard or soft) are signs of inadequate oral hygiene and must be removed to determine whether dental decay and periodontal disease are present beneath them (Fig. 44–12).

QUESTIONS FREQUENTLY RAISED BY DENTISTS

As more older Americans retain their teeth, dentists find a growing proportion of their practices devoted to seniors. These older patients gener-

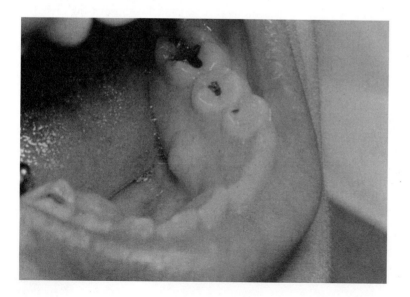

Figure 44–10 Common benign osseous tumor of the lingual mandible: "torus mandibularis."

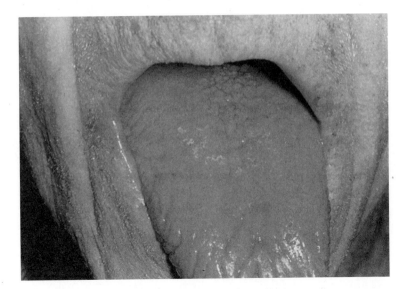

Figure 44–11 Depapillated tongue and angular cheilitis due to vitamin B_{12} deficiency.

ally take more medications and are afflicted by more chronic diseases than dentists' other patients. Dentists are encouraged to seek guidance from physicians in conjunction with providing dental treatment to patients who have and are being treated for certain medical conditions. The following section addresses three questions frequently asked of physicians by dentists.

Is Antibiotic Prophylaxis Necessary for This Patient?

Bacteremia results from a variety of dental procedures, including tooth extraction, subgingival cleaning, and periodontal surgery (Table 44–3). For several decades it has been recognized that the beta-hemolytic streptococci of the oral cavity are responsible for more than 30% of cases of endocarditis. Patients at risk for bacterial endocarditis because of congenital or acquired cardiac malformations or dysfunction should receive 2.0 g of amoxicillin 1 hour prior to dental treatment that is likely to induce bacteremia.

In patients with major joint arthroplasty, it is now recognized that the risk of bacteremia-induced late joint infection is limited in general. However, antibiotics should still be considered for certain high-risk groups: insulin-dependent diabetics, rheumatoid arthritics, patients taking corticosteroids, and those whose arthroplasty is less than 2 years old. A cephalosporin or amoxicillin regimen has been recommended. Indications for coverage are less clear for xenogenic implants about which there have been no case

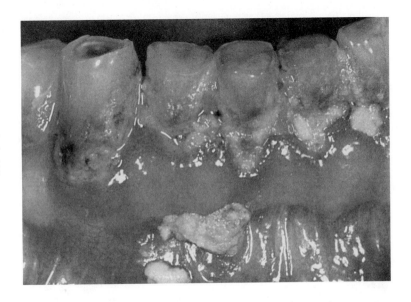

Figure 44–12 Debris and bacterial deposits impede effective examination of the teeth and gums, and disease is likely to be found beneath.

TABLE 44–3 **PREVENTION OF BACTERIAL ENDOCARDITIS IN DENTAL PATIENTS**

Cardiac Conditions for Which:	Dental Treatments for Which:	Standard Antibiotic Prophylaxis Regimen
Prophylaxis **IS Recommended**	*Prophylaxis* **IS Recommended**	*Standard Regimen*
Prosthetic cardiac valves	Dental extractions	Amoxicillin 2.0 g orally 1 hour before procedure
Prior history of bacterial endocarditis	Periodontal procedures, including surgery, root planing, scaling, and probing	*Unable to Take Oral Medications*
Surgically constructed systemic-pulmonary shunts	Dental implant placement and reimplantation of avulsed teeth	Ampicillin 2.0 g IM or IV within 30 minutes before procedure
Cyanotic congenital cardiac disease	Endodontic (root canal) treatment beyond the tooth apex	*Allergic to Amoxicillin*
Acquired valvular dysfunction	Subgingival placement of antibiotic fibers or strips	Clindamycin 600 mg orally 1 hour before procedure
Hypertrophic cardiomyopathy	Subgingival rubber dam clamp placement	*or*
Mitral valve prolapse with valvular regurgitation	Initial placement of orthodontic bands but not brackets	Cephalexin[a] or cefadroxil[a] 2.0 g 1 hour before procedure
Prophylaxis **IS NOT Recommended**	Intraligamentary local anesthetic injections	*or*
Previous coronary artery bypass graft surgery	Prophylactic cleaning of teeth or implants where bleeding is expected	Azithromycin or clarithromycin 500 mg 1 hour before procedure
Mitral valve prolapse without valvular regurgitation	*Prophylaxis* **IS NOT Recommended**	*Allergic to Penicillin and Unable to Take Oral Medications*
Physiologic, functional, or innocent heart mumurs	Restorative dentistry (without retraction cord)	Clindamycin 600 IV within 30 minutes before procedure
Previous rheumatic fever without valvular dysfunction	Local anesthetic injections (nonligamentary)	*or*
Previous Kawasaki disease without valvular dysfunction	Intracanal endodontic treatment, including post placement and build-up	Cefazolin[a] 1.0 g IM or IV within 30 minutes before procedure
Cardiac pacemakers and implanted defibrillators	Placement of rubber dams	
Isolated secundum atrial septal defect	Postoperative suture removal	
Surgical repair without residual dysfunction of secundum atrial septal defect, ventricular septal defect, or patent ductus arteriosus	Making impressions	
	Intraoral radiography	
	Removable prosthodontic and orthodontic appliances	

[a]Should not be used in patients with immediate-type hypersensitivity reaction to penicillins.

reports of complications—arteriovenous shunts, ventriculoperitoneal shunts, vascular grafts and filters—and for which there are no published recommendations for antibiotic prophylaxis.

There is also no standard recommendation for treatment of diabetic patients in oral surgery. Empirically, diabetics suffer in a more exaggerated fashion from mucosal and periodontal problems and are more prone to postoperative infections than are nondiabetics. There are no published clinical trials for guidance, but a loading dose (2 g) of amoxicillin (or the equivalent of erythromycin for the penicillin-allergic patient) given 1 hour prior to the procedure is a common prophylactic approach for the historically infec-

tion-prone diabetic patient undergoing oral surgery.

Is It Safe to Use Epinephrine-Containing Local Anesthetic for This Patient?

Dentists routinely anesthetize their patients prior to restorative, endodontic, and surgical procedures. The most commonly used local anesthetic solution is 2% lidocaine with 1:100,000 epinephrine, injected from an aspirating syringe in 1.8-mL cartridges. Dentists are cautioned that extreme care should be taken in administering epinephrine to a patient with a history of coronary artery disease or hypertension. An epinephrine dose limit that has received general acceptance is 50 μg per appointment for these patients, which suggests that slightly less than three full cartridges of anesthetic be used in a single sitting.

Elimination of the epinephrine from the anesthetic solution is not generally advised because of the risk of inadequate analgesia. Most authorities agree that endogenous epinephrine release due to breakthrough pain or even preoperative anxiety is a greater risk to the patient than the amount given in a properly administered anesthetic; with an aspirating injection technique, a bolus dose of epinephrine is avoided in any case.

Can This Patient Safely Undergo Dental Treatment So Soon After a Heart Attack (or Stroke)?

A widely disseminated but unsupported guideline within the dental profession is that elective dental treatment should not be performed within 6 months of a patient's myocardial infarction or stroke. Retrospective investigations suggest that a history of recent myocardial infarction is less relevant to perioperative risk than a multifactorial assessment that also accounts for signs of continued cardiac dysfunction such as unstable angina, pulmonary edema, or underlying valvular disease. Studies of coronary artery disease patients undergoing dental procedures show no greater incidence of electrocardiographic findings indicative of ischemia or threatening arrhythmia than those observed in age- and sex-matched normals.

The 6-month recommendation for stroke patients is due to the greater likelihood of cardiac co-morbidity in these patients. There are thus no strong data supporting this 6-month limit; the reader is referred to the suggestion in the previous paragraph to guide risk assessment. A second, independent question concerns the likelihood that a post-stroke patient may be taking an anticoagulant, necessitating adjustment of the warfarin (Coumadin) regimen prior to dental treatment. The current recommendation is that most dental and oral surgical treatment can be safely performed if a patient's International Normalized Ratio (INR) is at or below 2.0.

SUMMARY

Oral health is inseparable from general health. The past quarter century has seen the stereotype of the toothless older person fade before the reality of seniors retaining their teeth into advanced age. Yet the multiplicity of diseases and accumulated disabilities among the elderly complicates both the delivery of restorative dental treatment and the maintenance of oral health. The physician's commitment to optimize his or her older patients' health and well-being should include recognition of the importance of oral health and efforts to assist patients to maintain it.

References

1. Shay K, Ship JA: The importance of oral health in the older patient. J Am Geriatr Soc 1995;43:1414–1422.
2. Lloyd P, Shay K: Dental pain in the elderly. AGE 1987;10:70–80.
3. Ship JA: Oral sequelae of common geriatric diseases, disorders, and impairments. Clin Geriatr Med 1992;8:483–497.
4. Ellen RP: Considerations for physicians caring for older adults with periodontal disease. Clin Geriatr Med 1992;8:599–616.
5. Berkey DB, Shay K: General dental care for the elderly. Clin Geriatr Med 1992;8:579–597.
6. Fedele DJ, Jones JA, Niessen LC: Oral cancer screening in the elderly. J Am Geriatr Soc 1991;39:920–925.
7. Wayler AH, Muench ME, Kapur KK, Chauncey HH: Masticatory performance and food acceptability in persons with removable partial dentures, full dentures, and intact natural dentition. J Gerontol 1984; 39:284–289.
8. Robbins J, Hamilton J, Lof G, Kempster G: Oropharyngeal swallowing in normal adults of different ages. Gastroenterology 1992;103:823–829.
9. Ship JA: Gustatory and olfactory considerations: Examination and treatment in general practice. J Am Dent Assoc 1993;124:55–62.
10. Atkinson JC, Fox PC: Salivary gland dysfunction. Clin Geriatr Med 1992;8:499–511.
11. Gordon SR, Jahnigen DW: Oral assessment of the dentulous elderly patient. J Am Geriatr Soc 1986;34:276–281.

45 Pulmonary Disorders

William John Hall, M.D., F.A.C.P.

All primary care physicians are aware on a daily basis of the impact of respiratory illnesses on the care of older adults. National studies confirm that acute respiratory symptoms are among the most common reasons for older persons to seek medical attention. In addition, the clinical manifestations of the more chronic respiratory diseases play a major role in the reduced function, acute hospitalizations, and increased mortality seen in older persons.[1] In this chapter the prognostic and clinical significance of age-related changes in respiratory function itself is emphasized, and some of the altered clinical manifestations of common acute and chronic respiratory diseases that are especially pertinent to the modern and effective primary care of older persons are selectively reviewed.

AGE-RELATED CHANGES IN IMMUNE RESPONSE

Definite but not well understood alterations in host defense are associated with aging. Mucociliary clearance in both the upper and lower airways is probably diminished, but the effect of aging is hard to isolate from other age-related changes such as swallowing difficulties and relative malnutrition. Age-related changes in immune function represent a complex series of events that lead to imbalances in the immune system.[2] Thymic involution and loss of thymic hormones are thought to be important primary events in age-related changes in immunity. Lymphocyte function declines with age, as evidenced by diminished proliferative responses to a variety of mitogens and antigens. Other changes include alterations in lymphocyte subpopulations, decreased secretion of interleukin-2, and functional alterations in cytotoxic lymphocytes and natural killer cells.

While the most dramatic changes occur in cellular immunity, aging also affects humoral immunity. Immunoglobulin levels generally do not change with age, although antibody levels to specific pathogens may decline. Response to immunization is diminished in aging individuals. From a practical standpoint, age-related changes in the immune system predispose the lung to attack from respiratory viral infections, while at the same time, reliable responses to protective measures, such as influenza vaccine administration, are blunted.

PHYSIOLOGIC AND ANATOMIC CHANGES IN THE LUNG WITH AGING

Despite decades of research in the fields of respiratory physiology and lung biology, there is still difficulty in isolating age-related changes in lung structure and function from the many other confounding risk factors encountered by most individuals during 70 or more years of living. These uncertainties should perhaps not be surprising. The current cohort of persons over age 65 was born and raised in the preantibiotic era, when the devastating effects on lung development of then common childhood respiratory viral infections such as pertussis and measles were rampant. Tuberculosis was the most common cause of death during the teens and early adulthood of this cohort, and exposure as measured by tuberculin testing was nearly 100%. As a whole, there has probably been a higher prevalence of cigarette smoking in the generation born between 1910 and 1930 than at any time in the history of the human race. As adults in the post-World War II era, they have had the longest potential exposure to ambient levels of air pollution ever experienced. Finally, until recent decades, studies intended to develop normative standards for lung function have been largely cross-sectional in design and predominantly excluded persons older than 65 on the flawed assumption that projections from regression equations accurately reflect the aging effects on lung function.

However, accurate characterization of the age-

494

related changes in respiratory function is more important clinically now than ever before. From a variety of epidemiologic studies it is now known that evidence of impaired lung function, especially diminution in expiratory flow rates, is predictive of higher mortality rates, not only from lung disease but also from heart disease and most of the other leading causes of death in both men and women.[3] Impaired lung function may even be predictive of cognitive disorders in aging adults. As the population of older persons increases, and older individuals seek permission and guidelines from their physicians to pursue a more active lifestyle, measurement of respiratory function has even been suggested as an important global "biomarker" of successful aging and quality of life. The subsequent discussion briefly summarizes the available data pertinent to age-related changes in the mechanics of lung function, gas exchange, control of ventilation, and exercise capacity.

Age-Related Changes in the Lung and Chest Wall

A common observation made on physical examination of older persons is that the chest configuration often appears "abnormal," a finding that is actually far more attributable to changes in muscle mass and thoracic spine configuration than to actual changes in the physical properties of the lung. The actual changes in lung capacity instead represent a redistribution of the classic subdivisions of lung volume. Both the lung and the chest wall have rubber band-like elastic properties. Thus, the lung at the end of inspiration has a natural tendency to collapse, while the chest wall has a tendency to recoil outward, thus serving as an opposing force to the retractive properties of the lung itself. This elastic recoil pressure for the lung decreases with age, the classic assumption being that changes occur in the amount and composition of the lung connective tissue components (elastin, collagen, proteoglycans), although more recent data have questioned this assumption. Simultaneously, the chest wall itself stiffens with age. The net effect of these changes is a decrease in compliance (change in volume, change in pressure) of the total respiratory system, which in turn increases the work of breathing. Simultaneously, there is a diminution in the mass and efficiency of the respiratory muscles. The net result is that a 70-year-old has to work nearly twice as hard to compensate for age-related compliance changes as he or she did at the age of 20. The age-related changes in lung volumes follow from these alterations in compliance.[4]

Static Lung Volumes

While the total lung capacity (TLC) remains constant with age, some of the lung subdivisions demonstrate age-related changes. One of the most reliable measures of lung volume, the so-called functional residual capacity (FRC), is slightly elevated as a function of age. The FRC is determined by the balance between the natural tendency of the lung to collapse and the opposing tendency of the chest wall to expand outward, forces that are fairly evenly matched with aging. The vital capacity is slightly reduced owing to an increase in the residual volume (RV), the amount of air remaining in the lungs after maximum expiration. The increase in RV is a reflection of the changes in the elastic properties of the lung. In summary, these so-called static lung volumes do not change appreciably with age, and any alterations suggest a pathologic process. Accurate documentation of lung volumes is important to avoid mislabeling older persons as having lung disease when none is present, particularly in overreading a chest radiograph. For example, the combined changes in lung and chest wall properties and the increased kyphotic curve of the spine with aging may result in a clinical and radiologic appearance of an increased anteroposterior (AP) diameter, sometimes referred to as "senile emphysema." This is certainly a misnomer from the physiologic point of view. There is some degree of airspace enlargement with aging, and possibly some decline in the absolute number of alveoli, but the other more progressive and destructive aspects of emphysema are not seen solely as a function of advanced age. These individuals have normal lung volumes.

Expiratory Flow Rates

Both respiratory muscle function and the elastic recoil of the lung contribute to flow rates as measured by the classic forced expiratory maneuver, which is the basis of the commonly used clinical spirometry measurement. During the forced flow maneuver, assuming maximum expiratory effort, expiratory flow rates are determined mainly by the elastic recoil of the lung. Since recoil is diminished with age, compression of the airways occurs earlier during the expiratory maneuver in older persons. In addition to explaining the age-associated reduction in forced flow rates, this decrease of flow in smaller airways has several important implications. First, diminished expiratory flow rates may result in a less effective cough, and the premature closure of small airways may lead to gas exchange abnormalities, most notably hypoxemia. As a general approximation, males experience a drop of 14 to 30 mL/year in forced vital capacity (FVC), and a drop of 23 to 32 mL/year in 1-second forced vital capacity (FEV_1). Comparable values for women are 14 to 24 mL/year (FVC) and 19 to 26 mL/year (FEV_1).[5] Recent longitudinal studies of older persons strongly indicate that decline in expiratory flow rates is a nonlinear phenomenon characterized by accelerated decline after age 50.[6] Also, there is in all studies tremendous variability, reflecting the heterogeneous nature of aging effects in the lung as in virtually all other organs. The reasons for this variability is not known. European studies comparing lung function in sets of older identical twins living together or separated at an early age suggest that between a half and two thirds of the variability seen in pulmonary function can be attributed to genetic factors.[7]

Gas Exchange

Many studies have documented a linear age-related drop in P_aO_2 with no change in P_AO_2 or P_aCO_2. (Throughout this chapter the subscript A refers to alveolar gas partial pressures, while the subscript a designates partial pressures of respiratory gases in arterial blood.) In absolute terms, there is a linear deterioration of about 0.3% P_aO_2/year, or a drop of about 4 mmHg per decade.[8] The most likely reason for these changes is increased heterogeneity in ventilation-perfusion matching throughout the lung and premature airway closure.

Control of Ventilation

Classic teaching suggests that rather remarkable age-related changes occur in the ventilatory response to both hypoxia and hypercapnia, both responses decreasing with age. Sophisticated studies using mouth occlusion pressure techniques have documented a decrease of approximately 50% as measured by P_{100} in response to isocapneic hypoxia and hyperoxic hypercapnia compared to young subjects. These changes are almost certainly due to central neural mechanisms and possibly diminished muscle strength and coordination rather than to any alteration in the lungs.[9] The obvious clinical implication of these age-related blunted responses is that in selected situations, symptoms of breathlessness will be lacking despite clinically significant alterations in arterial blood gases.

Exercise Capacity

Maximum oxygen capacity (VO_{2max}) is influenced by age, but any substantial diminution is much more a reflection of reduced muscle mass, cardiac function, and overall level of conditioning. It is very unlikely that age-related changes in pulmonary function play a major role in exercise limitation in older age groups.

Pulmonary Function Tests

For clinical purposes, pulmonary function data obtained through clinical spirometry are the mainstay of clinical practice, and a working knowledge of testing and age-related changes is of practical importance. Two important principles bear emphasis. First, given normal levels of comprehension and adequate neuromuscular coordination, spirometric measures, including evaluation of bronchodilator responsiveness, have the same degree of accuracy in older persons as in younger ones. Adequacy of testing is usually verified by the direct observations made at the time of pulmonary function testing and by establishing the reproducibility of repeated measurements. Consequently, serial comparisons in the same individual are highly predictive in older persons, just as they are in younger cohorts. Second, caution must be exercised in the use of "normal" standards for the various spirometric indices. The usual way to describe normative values is to construct regression equations based on spirometric results from cross-sectional surveys of nonsmoking individuals. These equations are usually expressed as a function of height and age for males and females. The major applicability of these normal values, of course, is to identify individuals outside the normal range and, in the case of older subjects, to differentiate age-related changes from disease states. As is true with many other normative standards, the populations tested to derive the standards include a paucity of older persons and may not reflect the actual age-related changes that would be evident from longitudinal measurements made over years in the same subjects. Recently, a number of longitudinal studies on lung function have been done, and regression equations derived from these studies are probably more representative of the aging process.[5] In general, these studies indicate a more substantial effect of age on lung function than was previously predicted from cross-sectional data. Moreover, they demonstrate a nonlinear, accelerated decline in function after the fifth decade. These data are replacing the older cross-sectional normals used in most software programs and commercially available prediction charts.

Even when the most contemporary normal values are available, the primary care physician must still interpret the clinical significance of any change in pulmonary function. By convention, individual values within 80% of predictive values have been considered "normal" in younger populations. Given the tremendous individual variability in most volume and flow rate changes with age, use of the 80% range may give spurious results. Most experts recommend using the 95% confidence intervals in applying normal ranges.

PULMONARY ASSESSMENT OF OLDER PERSONS

Evaluation of respiratory symptoms can be difficult and frustrating in older patients. The presence of co-morbidity in the form of cardiovascular and arthritic disease is confusing. Patients at times cannot reliably perform pulmonary function and exercise studies. There is some information about respiratory sensation and aging that is relevant to an accurate clinical evaluation. Studies examining psychological recognition of increasing resistive and elastic loads have demonstrated that older subjects have decreased sensation of these loads, which seems to occur at the level of central nervous system (CNS) processing.[10] The authors have already commented on the decreased perception of chemical stimuli (hypoxia, hypercapnia). Putting all this together, there is suggestive evidence that older persons may not develop dyspnea or breathlessness until a substantially later stage of their clinical illness compared to younger people. This phenomenon is surely apparent to anyone who cares for older persons with pneumonia, who present with subtle symptoms and very abnormal arterial blood gas measurements. A very common response of the older patient who experiences dyspnea with exertion is to simply become less active, often under the mistaken impression that the complaints are an expected concomitant of age. Thus, when questioned by the physician about dyspnea, these patients legitimately answer in the negative. Evaluation of older persons with pulmonary disease should always include some assessment of change in activity. Conversely, complaints of breathlessness should always be taken very seriously in the older patient, since this symptom may indicate a more advanced stage of disease. Some practical suggestions: In the great majority of cases, these evaluations are no different from those in younger adults. However, when the diagnosis is more perplexing, the physician should try to quantitate the symptoms of dyspnea and breathlessness. One of the most reliable ways to do this is by using a variety of quantitative scales (e.g., Borg's scale), which have demonstrated remarkable validity in older persons. Second, one can be more imaginative in "testing." For example, taking an older patient for a walk up a flight of stairs accompanied by a pulse oximeter almost invariably allows the astute clinician to characterize the disorder. This maneuver cannot be delegated to a lab technician or a nurse.

The well-described blunting of the immune system may also mask some of the more commonly observed signs and symptoms of respiratory disease, especially acute respiratory tract infections. Thus, blunted febrile response and diminished sputum production are common manifestations of pneumonia in older patients.

OBSTRUCTIVE AIRWAYS SYNDROMES IN OLDER PATIENTS

Chronic Obstructive Pulmonary Disease

The health impact of chronic obstructive pulmonary disease (COPD) in elderly patients is enormous. Compared with the general population, older patients with COPD are twice as likely to rate their health as fair or poor, nearly twice as likely to report limitations in their usual activities, and visit physicians for medical care more frequently. For at least the past 25 years, there has been a steady increase in age-adjusted office visits, hospitalizations, and mortality for COPD in both men and women. Several factors may explain why COPD is increasing as a health problem for the elderly. First, as previously mentioned, the current generation of older persons were the generation with the highest prevalence of heavy cigarette smoking in the history of the world. Even people who have previously smoked but have now stopped may experience an accelerated decline in respiratory function late in life.[11] This decline, combined with the age-related decline in expiratory flow rates, may lead to signs and symptoms of COPD at an advanced age. As previously emphasized, these patients are often not detected early, since the development of breathlessness is considered by the patient to be due to "old age." Standard physiologic measures used to evaluate older patients with COPD (e.g., spirometry, arterial blood gases, pulse oximetry) have the same validity as in younger cohorts. Increasingly, however, it has been realized that various clinical parameters may be of more value in assessing the severity of COPD and the response to treatment in older persons. Use of the previously cited Borg scale and the baseline dyspnea index score predict general health status to a greater extent than physiologic measurements in older patients with COPD.

Reversible Airways Obstruction

Although the previous literature describes asthma as a disease of childhood or early adult life, more current data strongly suggest that asthma is a very common and especially serious disease in older persons. Various studies cite an asthma prevalence rate of 4% to 8% in persons over age 65. Rates of hospitalization for asthma are highest in the age groups over age 65. Asthma death rates also rise dramatically with advancing age. Although many older patients with asthma have a clear lifelong clinical history of symptomatic bronchospasm, there is growing appreciation that asthma may commonly become manifest after age 65. In a recent report of older asthmatics attending a pulmonary referral clinic, 48% had developed asthma after age 65. Early- and late-onset asthmatics had similar clinical manifestations of wheeze and cough and notable paroxysms of dyspnea at night.[12] There are at least two reasonable conclusions from these studies. First, individuals with asthma can survive to an older age. In these studies, asthma did not "burn out" with age as folk wisdom suggests. Second, reversible airways obstruction can develop in older persons, in which case certain less common causes should be evaluated. In particular, when elderly patients present with new symptoms of wheeze and cough, a diagnosis of gastroesophageal reflux should be considered. Failure to do this may lead to a potentially dangerous course of therapy for "asthma" with little likelihood of causing anything other than (occasionally fatal) side effects. Typical symptoms of gastroesophageal reflux in older persons are more often respiratory symptoms than heartburn. In the acute hospital setting, it has been noted that patients who have a fall in oxyhemoglobin saturation as measured by pulse oximetry when swallowing water are often experiencing occult aspiration.[13] Respiratory viral infections, especially those due to influenza and respiratory syncytial virus, are the most common precipitating agents of new asthma in older persons and regularly produce by far the most serious and prolonged episodes of bronchospasm.[14] Subsequent episodes can be substantially prevented with the use of influenza vaccination each fall. Presently, less than 50% of eligible persons over age 54 receive a yearly flu shot.

Special Therapeutic Considerations in Obstructive Airways Syndromes

The pharmacologic management of obstructive airways disease does not differ substantially in principle from standard treatment regimens. However, older persons are unequivocally more prone to the side effects of these agents, most of which can be avoided or attenuated if they are anticipated by the primary care physician. In addition, it is increasingly important to maintain vigilance against the untoward effects of various drug combinations. Some of these considerations are outlined in the following section.

SYMPATHOMIMETICS

Inhaled beta-2 agonists are the most important class of drugs for the treatment of bronchospasm in all age groups. Their rapid onset of action, relatively low incidence of side effects, and lack of interaction with other agents make them ideal for use in older patients as well. These agents are not without drawbacks. Studies of older COPD patients who underwent 24-hour Holter monitoring during nebulized beta-agonist therapy have reported an increase in asymptomatic arrhythmias. Metered-dose inhaler (MDI) administration can often "fail" because of the inherent difficulties many older persons encounter in using these devices. At a minimum, patients must have adequate comprehension, hand-eye coordination, and use of wrist and fingers, and must be able to perform a sustained vital capacity maneuver for 5 to 10 seconds.[15] A major reason for the failure of MDI administration in older persons is a lack of proper instruction in their use. When MDIs cannot be used, several "user friendly" mechanical aids can be tried that, along with spacers, improve the feasibility and efficacy of this form of treatment. When older patients cannot successfully use MDIs, a traditional nebulizer powered by a small air compressor can often be used very effectively instead. Anticholinergic therapy, usually with quaternary ammonium compounds such as ipratropium bromide, are effective in the treatment of COPD.[16] These compounds have the advantage of being poorly absorbed and tend not to produce anticholinergic side effects such as confusion, thickened secretions, and urinary retention, even when used improperly. While no specific studies of the clinical use of these agents in older patients have been done, most reported series do include substantial numbers of patients in their seventies and eighties. There have been a few case reports of precipitation of acute angle-closure glaucoma related to improper use of ipratropium by MDI.

STEROID THERAPY

Given the sometimes unrelenting clinical course of bronchospastic disease in older persons, the use of corticosteroids is a necessity at times.

Specific guidelines for the use of systemic steroids are not available. However, as with many other medications, steroid use carries special hazards for older persons. There is a higher incidence of the familiar complications of chronic steroid use, including cataracts, hypertension, glucose metabolism, muscle wasting, and osteoporosis. In particular, older persons are much more prone to the adverse effects of steroid administration on bone metabolism. All older persons (the majority of whom are women) should take ample calcium supplementation (2 g/day) and vitamin D (800 IU/day), and, in most instances, women should take estrogen replacement. Newer bisphosphonate preparations (e.g., alendronate) should often be prescribed. Aerosolized steroids are probably effective for the modulation of bronchospasm in older patients. Although some of the more serious side effects of systemic steroid therapy can be avoided by the use of aerosolized steroids, the same issues previously described in connection with the use of beta-agonists by MDI are relevant. If used improperly, substantial steroid absorption can take place through the oral mucous membranes. In addition, older persons are probably more prone to develop oral thrush, given the fact of age-related immune suppression.

THE USE OF METHYLXANTHINES

Theophylline clearance is not altered by age, but clinical confounders that do alter clearance (e.g., congestive heart failure [CHF], liver disease, erythromycin, ciprofloxacin, cimetidine administration) are all much more common in the elderly. Chronic theophylline toxicity, as opposed to acute theophylline intoxication, is associated with clinical differences, including a lower frequency of vomiting and a greater frequency of seizures and cardiac arrhythmias. Moreover, there is a striking lack of correlation of the peak serum theophylline concentrations with the clinical course. Recent studies have confirmed that chronologic age is a greater influence than peak theophylline concentration on the likelihood that clinical manifestations of theophylline poisoning will occur. The influence of advancing age is perhaps not surprising. The elderly patient with airway obstruction often has secondary cardiac disease that may be subclinical. Longstanding cardiovascular disease compounded by the vasoconstrictive effect of theophylline on the cerebral vasculature may lead to impaired cerebral blood flow. In summary, elderly patients have an inordinately greater risk of experiencing a life-threatening event with theophylline toxicity than younger persons. Peak serum theophylline concentration

cannot predict which patients with chronic theophylline intoxication will experience one of these events.[17] Given the many other therapeutic choices, there is very little reason to use this class of agents in the management of older persons with obstructive airways syndromes.

DRUG INTERACTIONS

Most older patients with obstructive airways disease have substantial co-morbidity because of the increased prevalence of other chronic illnesses such as cardiovascular disease, hypertension, musculoskeletal disorders, cataracts, urinary retention, and osteoporosis. At times, treatment options for disease in one organ system are restricted or contraindicated because of a concomitant disorder in another organ system. For example, beta-blockers are commonly used for the treatment of coronary artery disease and hypertension, but they exacerbate bronchospasm in older patients. Likewise, cough induced by ACE inhibitors may be confusing in patients undergoing therapy for asthma because cough is such a dominant symptom in older persons with asthma. Eye drops often contain beta-blockers and nonsteroidal anti-inflammatory drugs (NSAIDs), which may exacerbate asthma. The use of some H_2 blockers prolongs the metabolism of theophylline preparations. In summary, the recognition and therapy of obstructive airways disease in older persons is an important aspect of medical management. Proper selection of drugs is challenging and is a very good test of a physician's clinical skills.

LUNG CANCER

Lung cancer is responsible for 18% of all cases of cancer in men and 12% in women. Of all deaths related to cancer, approximately 34% in men and 22% in women are attributable to lung cancer. Half of all cases of lung cancer occur in patients 65 years of age and older, the peak incidence occurring at about age 75.[18] The increased importance of this neoplasm with age in both sexes is attributable mainly to cigarette smoking and possibly to an age-related diminution in immunologic surveillance. The approach to diagnosis does not differ in older persons. Tissue confirmation and evidence of metastases can usually be obtained relatively noninvasively by the use of sputum cytology, fiberoptic bronchoscopy, and computed tomographic (CT) imaging. Decisions about treatment must take life expectancy and the presence of co-morbid conditions into careful consideration. However, age per se is not a contraindication to resectional surgery or participation in chemotherapy and radiation therapy protocols.

SMOKING CESSATION IN THE OLDER PATIENT

The current generation of older persons grew up in an era when there was far more societal approval of smoking than is currently the case in the United States. In fact, national surveys have documented that the highest prevalence of smoking in men occurs in the cohort born between 1910 and 1930, that is, those individuals currently between the ages of 65 and 85. Given the well-known reduced life expectancy of smokers, there are fewer smokers in the ranks of the elderly, and there has been some speculation that these individuals are relatively "immune" from the adverse effects of smoking. In fact, continued cigarette smoking after age 65 remains a major risk factor for death and a reduced quality of life. A male smoker in the age range of 60 to 64 who can stop smoking reduces his risk of dying of a smoking-related illness in the next 15 years by 10%. The relative risk of death from all causes in both older males and females is approximately double that of individuals who have never smoked. Rates of life-threatening influenza and pneumonia are reduced in former smokers. Recent studies have documented an improvement in expiratory flow rates and markedly reduced prevalence of respiratory symptoms in cohorts over age 65.[11] In addition, smoking cessation has well-documented beneficial effects on the morbidity and mortality of many of the chronic diseases most closely associated with aging (e.g., cardiovascular disease, cancer, and osteoporosis). Given these data, it is puzzling that efforts at smoking cessation seem to play such a minor role in the primary care of older persons. The key to successful intervention hinges very much on the role of the primary care physician. Older persons tend to be much more respectful and adherent to strong advice given by their physicians than younger cohorts. Perhaps the most important factor in the success of smoking cessation is the advice and encouragement given by the primary care provider. As in younger cohorts, nicotine gum and transdermal nicotine patches can be successful adjuncts to a program centered around strong physician advocacy and group support through a variety of community agencies.

THROMBOEMBOLISM

Pulmonary embolization is a major cause of morbidity in older persons, especially among the more sedentary and bedbound. A number of factors predispose older persons to deep venous thrombosis. There is a higher frequency of factors contributing to venous stasis, such as congestive heart failure and general immobility. There is also increasing evidence that older persons frequently have a hypercoagulable state, as evidenced by increased fibrinogen concentrations and other clotting factors, and a decrease in the activity of the fibrinolytic system. Hypercoagulable states, such as those following myocardial infarction or even viral respiratory illnesses, may be transient. Pulmonary embolism has been thought to be particularly difficult to diagnose because its common symptoms, such as dyspnea and hemoptysis, may be absent. Angiography has been avoided in older patients and has been thought by some to be relatively contraindicated in this age group. When the diagnostic features of acute pulmonary embolism are evaluated and the characteristics among younger and older patients are compared, surprisingly few differences are observed.[19] Clinical syndromes characterized by either pleuritic pain or hemoptysis, isolated dyspnea, or circulatory collapse are observed with comparable frequency in all age groups. Furthermore, these nonspecific manifestations are quite frequent in patients over the age of 70. Among these patients with documented pulmonary embolism, dyspnea or tachypnea occurs in 92%, dyspnea, tachycardia, or pleuritic pain in 94%, and dyspnea, tachypnea, or radiographic evidence of atelectasis or parenchymal abnormality in 100%. In various trials, complications of pulmonary angiography were not more frequent in patients over age 70.

The clinical approach to thromboembolism does not differ in older patients. The use of Doppler flow studies seems particularly well suited to the diagnosis of deep venous thrombosis in older persons. There is no evidence that the operating characteristics of perfusion lung scanning differ with age. Lung scans are often not obtained in older persons because of the mistaken impression that age per se will produce "false positives." Therapy for thromboembolic states does not differ in older persons, and heparin therapy remains the mainstay of acute therapy. Older persons, especially women, seem to have an increased incidence of bleeding. It is unknown whether this is a factor of age per se or the effect of concomitant hepatic or renal disease. Continuous intravenous infusion of heparin may be more controllable in older persons than the use of intermittent dosing. Warfarin therapy has become much more precise with the introduction of the international normalized ratio (INR) as the standard of adequate anticoagulation. Contemporary studies suggest that oral warfarin therapy is not inherently associated with more bleeding complications in older people than in younger patients.

INTERSTITIAL PULMONARY FIBROSIS

Interstitial pulmonary fibrosis (IPF) encompasses an extremely heterogeneous group of disorders whose discussion is well beyond the scope of this chapter. Several points bear emphasis. These are not predominantly diseases of the young. In fact, in carefully performed studies of the clinical course of IPF, the most common age group experiencing onset of symptoms attributable to IPF is the 60- to 65-year-old age group. Fully a third of IPF patients have no clinical manifestations before age 65. Among the many known and unknown etiologic factors in IPF, idiosyncratic drug reactions are notable. In addition to some well-described associations (e.g., bleomycin and nitrofurantoin), some of the newer cardiac antiarrythmic agents (e.g., amiodarone) have been associated with IPF. The approach to diagnosis and treatment is not altered in older persons. A increasingly common form of "restrictive" lung disease is caused by the effects of severe osteoporosis in older women. Compression fractures of the vertebral column result in thoracic kyphosis with a resultant diminution in vital capacity.[20]

PNEUMONIA

When Sir William Osler called pneumonia "the special enemy of old age," he could scarcely have anticipated the status of lower respiratory tract infection among the elderly in the last half of the twentieth century. Despite sophisticated diagnostic techniques and new therapies, respiratory infections remain important maladies among the elderly. Compounding this picture of increased incidence, mortality, and difficulties in diagnosis are the therapeutic problems associated with the altered metabolism of pharmacologic agents among the elderly. Ironically, in later years Osler changed his assessment of pneumonia, calling it "the friend of the aged" several years before he himself succumbed to this infection at age 70.

Pneumonia and influenza currently rank as the fourth or fifth most common cause of death in those over age 65 in the United States.[21] Influenza virus infection is perhaps the most dramatic example of the importance of respiratory infection in these age groups. Despite the enormous clinical importance of influenza infection among older persons and the availability of safe, inexpensive immunization, annual rates of vaccine administration among persons over age 65 in

most American communities is around 30%. It is well known that influenza immunization is associated with reductions in rates of hospitalization by 50% and reductions in mortality of 40% to 55%. Increasing the frequency of annual immunization in persons over age 65 is perhaps the most cost-effective practice that primary care physicians can bring to their older patients.

Community-acquired pneumonia remains a very common and serious disorder. Most experts currently recommend that the empirical choice of antibiotic therapy take age into consideration. The American Thoracic Society has published guidelines for the initial evaluation and therapy of pneumonia in both younger and older patients.[22]

TUBERCULOSIS

It is now well recognized that tuberculosis is not a vanishing health problem and has special importance for older persons. In 1953, 14% of new tuberculosis cases occurred in persons aged 65 or older. However, by 1980 this percentage had risen to 29%, a rise that could not be explained simply by the increased number of persons over the age of 60.[23] Prior to the initiation of effective control of tuberculosis, approximately 80% of persons in the early 1900s were infected with *Mycobacterium tuberculosis* by age 30. The survivors of this cohort comprise the majority of cases of tuberculosis found today in the elderly population. In 1985, a study of cases from 29 states performed by the Centers for Disease Control (CDC) showed an incidence of 21.5 cases per 100,000 population in persons over age 65. The national incidence rates of tuberculosis at that time were approximately 9.1 cases per 100,000. During the same time frame, the tuberculosis rate in nursing home residents was 39.2 cases per 100,000. Based on two-stage tuberculin skin tests on admission to chronic care facilities, a positive reaction can be documented in 29% to 51% of all residents. The majority of active cases of tuberculosis found in nursing homes are, therefore, in persons who acquired the infection before entering the chronic care facility. It has been known for some time that the mortality rate for tuberculosis is highest in persons age 65 or older. In fact, this group accounts for over 60% of all the deaths from tuberculosis. The primary care physician is the "line of first defense" in terms of diagnosing tuberculosis in older persons, and it is a diagnosis that should almost always be at least considered in older persons with unexplained pulmonary infiltrates, including involvement of the middle and lower lobes, locations not considered "classic" for tuberculosis.

SLEEP DISORDERS

Sleep-related problems among older persons are extremely common.[24] In most instances, these complaints lead to an evaluation focused predominantly on the respiratory system, which is why they are considered here. A knowledge of the pathophysiology and clinical significance of these disorders is important for both the primary care provider (who must decide when to refer) and the pulmonologist, who may be required to unravel these often puzzling clinical presentations. Laboratory assessment of sleep correlates information gained simultaneously from electroencephalographic (EEG), electromyographic, and electro-oculographic studies. Sleep is characterized as either REM (rapid eye movement) or non-REM (NREM) sleep on the basis of data from the sources just listed. NREM sleep is further subdivided into four stages, characterized by increasing frequency of slow wave and delta activity on the EEG. Most subjects appear calm during NREM sleep, with slow, even respirations. They may be difficult to arouse. REM sleep represents a dramatic change, which is reflected in all measurements. The EEG suddenly resembles that observed during wakefulness, rapid eye movements appear, and there is a profound decrease in muscle tone. The commonly held belief that older persons sleep less may in fact be valid. In many instances, however, total sleep time over 24 hours is unchanged, but patterns shift to less nocturnal sleep with more daytime napping. Sleep efficiency (ratio of sleep to total time in bed) drops, but the time needed to fall asleep (sleep latency) is unchanged. Older persons experience REM sleep more rapidly (thus the observation of dreaming even during short episodes of sleep) and experience a decrease in sleep of stages 3 and 4. Daytime sleep latency also decreases (easy to nod off during the day). The significance of these changes is that these sleep patterns mimic the patterns often cited as pathognomonic of sleep disorders.

Sleep-Disordered Breathing in the Elderly

Three types of abnormalities bear mentioning: sleep apnea, periodic leg movements of sleep in the elderly, and REM sleep behavior disorders. Snoring is very common in the elderly. Sleep apnea in older men is also common and seems to increase with advancing age. Prevalence figures of 10% to 75% have been cited. Although the data are mixed, it is likely that these episodes are of clinical significance in at least a subset of individuals, probably when transient hypoxemia is associated with these episodes. Studies have suggested an adverse impact on cognitive functioning and possibly an increase in cardiovascular mortality. However, the great majority of older persons with sleep apnea experience no adverse consequences of these episodes. The usual first-line therapy begins with a careful, common sense clinical evaluation to rule out occult congestive heart failure (especially diastolic dysfunction) and adverse effects of drug administration, especially hypnotics and benzodiazepines. Periodic leg movements of sleep (PLMS) is a geriatric syndrome characterized by periodic episodes of repetitive limb movements and wakefulness. Most patients have an uncontrollable urge to move their legs as they are falling asleep. Prevalence figures suggest that 25% to 60% of older persons may have manifestations of PLMS. Patients are often brought to medical attention by their spouses or well-meaning care givers who mistake the movements for seizure activity. Many medications have been associated with this disorder, especially tricyclic antidepressants, and elimination of all potentially psychoactive drugs should be the first therapeutic approach. In REM sleep behavior disorders, the usual sharply reduced motor tone characteristic of REM sleep is replaced by a tendency to act out dreams, sometimes in very dramatic fashion. As opposed to sleepwalking, which occurs in sleep stages 3 and 4, when individuals are very hard to arouse, patients with REM disorders remember the dream content, which is often very frightening. Not surprisingly, these episodes can be mistaken for manifestations of dementia. Clonazepam at bedtime has been successfully used to treat this condition.

CRITICAL CARE MANAGEMENT OF THE OLDER PATIENT

Outcomes as a Function of Age

In our present era of cost constraints, consideration is being given to rationing expensive medical resources according to age. In the past few years several studies have documented that age per se is not a strong predictor of outcome of intensive care unit (ICU) intervention.[25] This generalization pertains to various definitions of outcome including mortality, hospital discharge, neurologic condition, and functional state. The care of older persons in the critical care setting is perhaps one of the greatest tests of clinical skill and judgment in all of contemporary medicine.

Withdrawal of Life Support

Considerable attention has been paid in the past 5 years to understanding the issues surrounding end-of-life decisions and the withdrawal of critical measures of life support when there is virtually no hope for restored function. More often than not, these decisions involve older patients. The most prominent decision nodes usually focus on withdrawal of ventilator and nutritional support. More and more often, issues of withdrawal of respiratory support are becoming more routine and more accepted by patients, families, and physicians. Withdrawal of nutritional and fluid support, however, is still very controversial. Since survival is rarely in doubt, the real issue rests with concepts of avoiding pain and suffering. Are food and water forms of medical intervention, or are they rather the "stuff of life," and thereby out of the realm of physician decision making? Most legal and religious bodies have agreed that nutrition and hydration may at times be considered unnecessary forms of therapy. Less attention, however, has been paid to the clinical significance of these decisions not to initiate the use of artificial nutrition in terminally ill patients. While there is a widespread intuitive assumption that the physical and emotional well-being of patients, especially those who retain mental capacity for decision-making, is enhanced by artificial nutrition and hydration, few objective data exist to substantiate these beliefs. In fact, there is some evidence that the reverse might be the case. Unwanted nutritional support and hydration through intravenous or enteral routes may not only be ineffective in reducing morbidity in patients with advanced cancer and other terminal illnesses, it may also be associated with an increase in medical complications and a reduction in the quality of life. One recent study asked if limiting food and fluids to only those requested by a terminally ill patient wishing comfort and care had had an adverse effect on the quality of remaining life.[26] Most subjects never experienced any hunger or thirst. In all patients, symptoms of hunger, thirst, and dry mouth could be alleviated, usually with small amounts of food, fluids, or application of ice chips and lubrication to the lips. Attempts at forced feeding more often than not resulted in abdominal pain and vomiting. The authors concluded that, from a clinical point of view, food and fluid administration beyond the specific requests of the patient may play a minimum role in providing comfort to a terminally ill patient.

References

1. Hospitalizations for the leading causes of death among the elderly—United States, 1987. MMWR 1990;39:777–779.
2. Gyetko MR, Toews GB: Immunology of the aging lung. Clin Chest Med 1993;14:379–392.
3. Sorlie PD, Kannel WB, O'Connor G: Mortality associated with respiratory function and symptoms in advanced age: The Framingham Study. Am Rev Respir Dis 1989;140:379–384.
4. Turner JM, Mead J, Wohl ME: Elasticity of human lungs in relation to age. J Appl Physiol 1968;25:664–671.
5. Ware JH, Dockery DW, Louis TA, Xiping X, Ferris BG, Speizer FE: Longitudinal and cross-sectional estimates of pulmonary function decline in never-smoking adults. Am J Epidemiol 1990;132:685–700.
6. Enright PL, Adams AB, Boyle PJR, Sherrill DL: Spirometric and maximal respiratory pressure references from healthy Minnesota 65- to 85-year-old women and men. Chest 1995;108:663–669.
7. McClearn GE, Svartengren M, Pedersen NL, Heller DA, Plomin R: Genetic and environmental influences on pulmonary function in aging Swedish twins. J Gerontol 1994;49:M264–M268.
8. Crapo RO, Jensen RL, Berlin SL: PaO2 in healthy subjects at 1500m altitude are well predicted by meta analysis. Chest 1991;100:96S.
9. McConnell AK, Davies CTM: A comparison of the ventilatory responses to exercise of elderly and younger humans. J Gerontol 1992;47:B137–B141.
10. Leitner J, Cherniack NS: Effects of age and respiratory efforts on the perception of resistive ventilatory loads. J Gerontol 1983;40:147–153.
11. Bosse R, Sparrow D, Rose CL, Weiss ST: Longitudinal effect of age and smoking cessation on pulmonary function. Am Rev Respir Dis 1981;123:378–381.
12. Braman SS, Kaemmerlen JT, Davis SM: Asthma in the elderly: A comparison between recently acquired and long-standing disease. Am Rev Respir Dis 1991;143:336–340.
13. Zaidi NH, Smith HA, King SC, Park C, O'Neill PA, Connolly MJ: Oxygen desaturation on swallowing as a potential marker of aspiration in acute stroke. Age Aging 1995;24:267–270.
14. Hall WJ, Hall CB: Bacterial and viral infections in the etiology of asthma. In Weiss EB, Stein M (eds): Bronchial Asthma: Mechanisms and Therapeutics, 3rd ed. Boston, Little Brown, 1993, pp. 564–576.
15. Allen SC, Prior A: What determines whether an elderly patient can use a metered dose inhaler correctly? Br J Dis Chest 1986;80:45–49.
16. Braun SR, Levy S, Grossman J: Comparison of ipratropium bromide and albuterol in chronic obstructive disease: A three center study. Am J Med 1991;91:28s–32s.
17. Shannon M, Lovejoy FH Jr: The influence of age vs peak serum concentration on life-threatening events after chronic theophylline intoxication. Arch Intern Med 1992;150:A763.
18. Lee-Chiong TL, Matthay RA: Lung cancer in the elderly. Clin Chest Med 1993;14:453–478.
19. Stein PD, Gottschalk A, Saltsman HA, Terrin ML: Diagnosis of acute pulmonary embolism in the elderly. J Am Coll Cardiol 1991: 8:1452–1457.
20. Culham EG, Jiminez HA, King CE: Thoracic kyphosis, rib mobility, and lung volumes in normal women and women with osteoporosis. Spine 1994;19:1250–1255.
21. McBean AM, Babish JD, Warren JL: The impact and cost of influenza in the elderly. Arch Intern Med 1993;153:2105–2111.
22. Niederman RD, Bass JB, Campbell GD, Fein AM, Grossman RF, Mandell LA, Marrie TJ, Sarosi GA, Torres A, Yu VL: Guidelines for the initial management of adults with community acquired pneumonia:

Diagnosis, assessment of severity, and initial antimicrobial therapy. Am Rev Respir Dis 1993;148:1418–1426.

23. Yoshikawa TT: Tuberculosis in aging adults. J Am Geriatr Soc 1992;40:178–187.

24. Webb WE: Age-related changes in sleep. Clin Geriatr Med 1989;5:275–288.

25. Tresch D, Heudebert G, Kutty K, et al: Cardiopulmonary resuscitation in elderly patients hospitalized in the 1990s: A favorable outcome. J Am Geriatr Soc 1994; 2:137–141.

26. McCann RM, Hall WJ, Groth-Junker A: Comfort care for terminally ill patients: The appropriate use of nutrition and hydration. JAMA 1994;272:1263–1266.

46 Gastroenterologic Disorders

Reza Shaker, M.D.

Kulwinder S. Dua, M.D., M.B., B.S., M.R.C.P., DNB

Timothy R. Koch, M.D.

PHARYNGEAL AND ESOPHAGEAL DISORDERS

Dysphagia

Swallowing is a highly coordinated event that involves sequential and overlapping contractions of the facial, cervical, oral, pharyngeal, laryngeal, and esophageal muscular apparatus. It results in transit of ingested material and saliva from the mouth into the stomach. For descriptive purposes, swallowing can be divided into four consecutive phases: (1) preparatory, (2) oral, (3) pharyngeal, and (4) esophageal phases. These phases merely represent the anatomic regions traversed by the bolus.

During the preparatory phase, the bolus remains for the most part in the oral cavity, undergoing physical and some chemical changes. Through the act of mastication and mixing with saliva it develops suitable physical qualities that prepare it for transit through the aerodigestive tract. During the oral phase, sequential squeezing of the tongue against the hard and soft palates generates a peristaltic pressure wave that propels the bolus from the oral cavity into the pharynx. During the pharyngeal phase, the pharynx, upper esophageal sphincter (UES), and larynx are elevated, and three of the four routes connected to the pharynx—namely, the nasal cavity, oral cavity, and larynx—are sealed off while the fourth route, the UES, opens and the bolus is transported into the esophagus by rapid forceful posterior tongue movements as well as by peristaltic contractions of the pharyngeal constrictors. During oropharyngeal swallowing, the nasopharynx is sealed by the contraction of the superior pharyngeal constrictor and elevation of the soft palate and its contact with the posterior pharyngeal wall. During oropharyngeal swallowing, the UES transiently relaxes and subsequently is pulled upward and forward by the contraction of the same suprahyoid muscles that displace the larynx. Oropharyngeal swallowing begins with the closure of the vocal cords,[1] signifying the activation of airway protection, and ends when the cords return to their resting positions. During this time respiration is reflexively inhibited. During the esophageal phase of swallowing the bolus is transported further into the esophagus and stomach.

Oropharyngeal dysphagia (OPD) may develop when either the efficacy or the coordination of either the transport or protective aspects of oropharyngeal swallowing are compromised. The true prevalence of OPD is not known. However, studies have shown that it has a 50% to 60% prevalence in nursing homes and a 10% to 30% prevalence in general medical wards.[1, 2]

Except for silent aspiration, which presents with frequent episodes of pneumonia, most patients with OPD seek help because of symptoms. These symptoms reflect abnormalities in the transport or protective functions of oropharyngeal swallowing (Table 46–1). Dysphagia symptoms are highly specific and should not be labeled psychogenic. A frequently reported symptom is a sensation of inadequate clearance of the bolus from the pharynx: "food sticks in the throat." This sensation, although it may be caused by the presence of a large residue in the piriform sinus or valleculae, may also be a referred sensation resulting from obstruction of the distal esophagus. Strictures of the proximal esophagus may also present with cervical symptoms. For this reason, in patients with complaints of cervical symptoms evaluation of the esophagus must be part of the dysphagia work-up. Because inflammation, abrasion, or tumors of the hypopharyngeal area may produce the same sensation, a careful examination by direct visualization of this area must be included in the work-up. Swallow-related coughing or choking due to misdirection of the bolus into the airway is another common complaint. Predeglutitive aspiration occurs when the bolus is lost from the mouth into the

---

TABLE 46–1 **SYMPTOMS OF ORAL AND PHARYNGEAL DYSPHAGIA**

Inability to keep bolus in the oral cavity
Difficulty in gathering bolus in the back of the tongue
Hesitation or inability to initiate swallowing
Food sticking in the throat
Nasal regurgitation
Inability to propel food bolus caudad into pharynx
Difficulty in swallowing solids
Frequent repetitive swallowing
Frequent throat clearing
Gargly voice after meal
Hoarse voice
Nasal speech and dysarthria
Swallow-related cough: before, during, or after swallowing
Avoidance of social dining
Weight loss
Recurrent pneumonia

---

hypopharynx prematurely when swallowing has not yet been triggered and the airway is still open. This condition is commonly seen in post-cerebrovascular accident (CVA) dysphagic patients. Deglutitive aspiration results from incompetent or absent closure of the glottis during the swallowing sequence, allowing the bolus to invade the airway while being transported through the hypopharynx. Postdeglutitive aspiration occurs when bolus transport is incomplete and a large residue remains behind in the piriform sinus or valleculae at the end of the swallowing sequence; it is seen in patients with parkinsonism, postcerebrovascular accident, myasthenia gravis, and multiple sclerosis.

Because of the variety of organs involved in oropharyngeal swallowing, dysphagia results from a large number of causes that may affect the muscular apparatus of the oropharynx or their related neuromuscular plates and the peripheral as well as the central nervous systems. These diseases may affect oropharyngeal transport, deglutitive airway closure, or both (Table 46–2). Neuromuscular diseases are responsible for approximately 80% of cases, while local structural lesions of the oropharynx account for the rest. OPD has been reported in approximately 25% of adults following head injury, of which 94% have been reported to recover in about 3 months. OPD also poses a significant clinical problem in post-CVA patients. Malignancies of the head and neck account for approximately 10% of all the cancers occurring in North America. The total number of newly diagnosed cases of head and neck cancer in the United States, excluding skin

cancer, is estimated at 78,000. The age-specific incidence increases markedly after age 50, and the male-to-female ratio is 3:1. Surgical resection or radiation therapy in these patients can result in OPD, leading to difficult management problems.

TABLE 46–2 **CAUSES OF ORAL OR PHARYNGEAL DYSPHAGIA**

Peripheral and Central Nervous System
Amyotrophic lateral sclerosis
Bulbar poliomyelitis
Central nervous system tumor
Cerebrovascular accident
Disorders of the central nervous system (e.g., Alzheimer's disease)
Familial dysautonomia
Friedreich's spastic ataxia
Head injury
Huntington's chorea
Multiple sclerosis
Parkinson's disease
Peripheral neuropathies
Post-traumatic causes
Tabes dorsalis

Muscular or Neuromuscular
Alcoholic myopathy
Inflammatory muscle diseases
    Dermatomyositis
    Inclusion body myositis
    Polymyositis
Kearns-Sayre syndrome
Metabolic myopathy (thyroid-associated myopathy)
Muscular dystrophies (myotonic oculopharyngeal)
Myasthenia gravis

Local Structural Lesions
Cricopharyngeal abnormalities
    Achalasia
    Fibrosis
Extrinsic compression
    Enlarged thyroid gland
    Senile ankylosing hyperostosis of the cervical spine
Laryngeal carcinoma
Oropharyngeal carcinoma
Proximal esophageal webs and rings
Radiation injury
    Neuromuscular damage
    Salivary gland damage
Rheumatoid cricoarytenoid arthritis
Surgical resection of oropharynx or larynx
Zenker's diverticulum

Pharmacologic Agents
Anticholinergics
Antihistamines
Phenothiazines

Primary neurogenic cricopharyngeal (CP) muscle dysfunction includes cricopharyngeal achalasia and discoordination of UES relaxation and opening, with pharyngeal peristalsis due to neurogenic causes such as cerebrovascular hemorrhage and Parkinson's disease. Primary myogenic CP dysfunction is due to loss of elasticity as well as fibrotic changes of the UES. A variety of causes, including gastroesophageal reflux and aging, have been suggested. Causes of laryngeal paralysis include insults to the recurrent or superior laryngeal nerve due to a variety of surgical, inflammatory, or central nervous system diseases.

Because of the proximity to the pharynx, structural abnormalities of the most proximal portion of the esophagus may present with symptoms of cervical dysphagia. These abnormalities include proximal esophageal rings, which are usually reflux induced. Dysphagia usually is associated with solid food. Cervical symptoms and choking develop when bolus impaction occurs. Reflux symptoms such as heartburn may be minimal. Proximal esophageal webs, as seen in the Plummer-Vinson or the Paterson-Brown-Kelly syndrome, occur in the upper 2 to 4 cm of the esophagus and are associated with iron deficiency anemia. Proximal esophageal strictures may develop from lye ingestion, nasogastric tube placement, or reflux disease. However, isolated involvement of the proximal esophagus is rare. Malignant strictures of the proximal esophagus induced by squamous cell carcinoma or adenocarcinoma in the presence of Barrett's esophagus present with symptoms of cervical dysphagia and should be included in the differential diagnosis of an esophageal stricture.

Diagnostic modalities in the majority of cases will identify a specific derangement in the oral or pharyngeal phase of swallowing, although they rarely help in determining causative factors. The approach to the dysphagic patient must be systematic, starting with a detailed history of the problem and followed by physical and neurologic examinations. Special attention should be given to concomitant disorders that may be responsible for OPD. A history of recurrent pneumonia, weight loss, water and sour brash, regurgitation, and heartburn must be sought, and a careful account of the use of medications, including tranquilizers and ulcer and cancer agents, must be taken. Because some symptoms of OPD such as hoarseness may be due to either unilateral paralysis of the cords or inflammation of the glottis resulting from frequent aspiration of food, correct diagnosis requires a thorough laryngologic examination.

Until recently, barium studies were the only modality used for evaluation of OPD patients.

During the past decade, several other modalities such as manometry, endoscopy, ultrasonography, and scintigraphy have been introduced to this field. Intense research in various disciplines is ongoing, making the approach to the OPD patient a dynamic and improving phenomenon. Currently, videofluoroscopic recording of a modified barium swallow is the diagnostic modality of choice. During this study, recordings of a variety of boluses with different consistencies and volumes are made for subsequent analysis, and these recordings are also used for future comparisons to evaluate progress. Although the use of intraluminal strain gauges for pharyngeal manometry has resulted in a significant increase in our knowledge of pharyngeal pressure phenomena, this modality remains mainly a research tool.

Only a minority of patients with OPD are amenable to medical or surgical therapy. The majority, however, require retraining and practice in the use of various swallowing maneuvers and techniques to achieve an adequate and safe swallow. Cricopharyngeal dilatation and myotomy have been performed for a variety of neurogenic and myogenic causes of OPD with variable results. In general, myotomy yields good results in CP achalasia owing to primary CP muscle involvement. The results are less predictable for disease due to primary neurogenic causes if other parts of the swallowing apparatus are also involved. Recently, endoscopic transmucosal botulinum toxin injection into the CP muscle has been tried in patients with CP achalasia. However, the close proximity of the injection area to the vocal cords raises special concern about possible respiratory complications. Surgical treatment of Zenker's diverticulum has evolved with advances in the understanding of its pathophysiology. Transcutaneous extramucosal cricopharyngeal myotomy with or without diverticulectomy or diverticulopexy traditionally has been the treatment of choice depending on the size of the diverticulum; it yields excellent results in over 90% of cases.

In patients with an inadequate deglutitive glottal closure mechanism such as that seen after partial laryngectomy due to malignancy or in patients with Parkinson's disease or amyotrophic lateral sclerosis, the deglutitive airway closure could be improved by injecting a nonabsorbable material such as Teflon into the posthemilaryngectomy pseudo–vocal cords or lateral thyroarytenoid muscle. Injection of Teflon results in bulk formation in the injection site and displaces the true cord or surgically constructed pseudo-cord toward the midline. The majority of OPD patients, however, require specialized rehabilitation of their swallowing function. Maintaining adequate nutrition during this period is essential; otherwise, the vicious cycle of malnutrition, OPD complications, and further malnutrition will become self-perpetuating.

Several therapeutic maneuvers have been used to improve oropharyngeal bolus transport and airway safety. A change in bolus size or consistency is helpful in some patients, while in others swallowing with the head in a specific position may help to ensure safe passage of the bolus through the hypopharynx. Flexion of the head by displacing the larynx under the epiglottis reduces the chances of aspiration, and rotating the head toward the weaker side causes relative closure of this side and improves pharyngeal transit. Similarly, tilting the head toward the weaker side directs the bolus laterally and may improve pharyngeal bolus transit and prevent aspiration. In summary, a multidisciplinary approach is needed, not only to identify the cause or causes of OPD but also to direct its management. The disciplines involved may include gastroenterology, otolaryngology, neurology, and speech-language pathology. Speech therapists with a special interest in swallowing problems are needed to participate in the treatment of these patients.

Gastroesophageal Reflux

Entry of the gastric contents into the esophagus (i.e., gastroesophageal reflux) occurs in varying degrees in symptomatic as well as asymptomatic individuals. Depending on a variety of factors including but not limited to the frequency of reflux episodes and the composition of the refluxed material, the effectiveness of the esophageal clearance mechanism, and the esophageal mucosal resistance and regeneration capability, gastroesophageal reflux events may lead to inflammation, mucosal disruption, ulceration, stricture, bleeding, and a premalignant condition marked by gastric metaplasia of the esophageal mucosa (Barrett's esophagus). The term gastroesophageal reflux disease (GERD) is commonly used to describe any symptomatic clinical condition or histologic changes that result from a backward flow of the gastric contents into the esophagus. Symptomatic GERD is the most common disease of the esophagus. Heartburn (pyrosis) is the cardial symptom of GERD and is reported to occur in 10% to 20% of the population. Four to seven percent of the population are reported to experience heartburn daily.

A multitude of airway and aerodigestive disorders have been attributed to GERD. The most common clinical symptom of GERD, however, is heartburn or pyrosis, described as a retrosternal burning sensation or discomfort. Heartburn may be absent in a substantial percentage of GERD patients with esophageal injury as well as in those with supraesophageal complications of GERD. Severe heartburn may not be accompanied by any detectable macroscopic changes. Therefore, the severity of various symptoms of reflux disease varies widely among patients and may not correlate closely with the degree of severity of esophageal injury. There is wide variation in the clinical course of reflux symptoms; in some patients they undergo spontaneous remission, whereas in others they become intractable and are accompanied by complications.

Other symptoms of GERD include regurgitation, hypersalivation (water brash), sour taste (sour brash), frequent belching, and epigastric pain. GERD-induced odynophagia is uncommon, and the presence of this symptom should prompt investigation for infectious esophagitis such as that induced by *Candida*, herpes simplex, or cytomegalovirus infection of the esophagus. Gastrointestinal blood loss due to esophagitis generally presents as occult gastrointestinal blood loss, but occasionally esophagitis may induce frank upper gastrointestinal bleeding.

Distal esophageal stricture presents with gradually developing solid food dysphagia. With formation of a stricture, reflux symptoms may abate. In severe cases, liquid dysphagia may be present. In reflux patients without heartburn, solid food dysphagia due to stricture formation may be the presenting symptom. Although peptic esophageal strictures are nearly always located in the distal esophagus, they may occur in the proximal esophagus and present as cervical dysphagia.

The pathogenesis of GERD is believed to be multifactorial. These factors include (1) those affecting the antireflux mechanism (such as lower esophageal sphincter tone, frequency of inappropriate lower esophageal sphincter [LES] relaxation, angle of the esophagogastric junction, and presence or absence of hiatal hernia), (2) volume of gastric content (balance between intake and gastric secretion against gastric emptying), (3) composition and potency of refluxed material (presence of acid, pepsin, bile salts, pancreatic enzyme, byproducts of digestion, and so on), (4) efficiency of the esophageal clearance mechanism (primary and secondary esophageal peristalsis, saliva and its bicarbonate content), and (5) esophageal mucosal resistance to injury and its reparative abilities. Each of these factors or a combination of them may play a predominant role in inducing reflux injury in a given patient. Other conditions that may predispose a patient to reflux by reducing LES tone, provoking LES relaxation, or impairing the esophageal clearance mechanism include unconsciousness, head injury, mental retardation, and nasogastric intubation. Systemic sclerosis especially predisposes the patient to reflux injury and its complication of stricture because of the negligible LES tone, impaired esophageal peristalsis, and decreased salivary production associated with this disease. Pill-induced esophageal lesions (due to potassium tablets, tetracycline, vitamin C, or quinidine) must be considered.

Recent clinical observations indicate that the extent of reflux injury is not limited to the esophagus, and supraesophageal complications of reflux disease are more prevalent than was previously thought. GERD is becoming a disease attended by physicians of various disciplines. About 10% of patients with severe reflux esophagitis develop peptic stricture during the course of their disease. About 40% of all peptic strictures are accompanied by Barrett's esophagus.

Barrett's esophagus is defined as replacement of the esophageal squamous cell epithelium by metaplastic columnar-type epithelium due to reflux injury. Because of its malignant potential, development of Barrett's esophagus is clinically significant and must be followed closely. About 10% to 20% of patients with reflux esophagitis develop Barrett's epithelium. The true incidence of adenocarcinoma arising from Barrett's esophagus is unclear. The risk has been reported to be between 5% and 10%, and it is commonly seen in patients older than 40 years of age. Barrett's ulcer develops most often on the posterior or posterolateral esophageal wall and may result in significant bleeding or perforation. Stricture may also develop in patients with Barrett's esophagus. Transformation of the columnar epithelium in Barrett's esophagus into the stages of mild dysplasia, then severe dysplasia, and eventually frank adenocarcinoma is a time-dependent process. An estimated 5% to 10% of all esophageal malignancies are thought to be due to adenocarcinoma developed in Barrett's esophagus. Adenocarcinoma in Barrett's epithelium may be multifocal and is well advanced at diagnosis.

Extreme caution must be exercised in attributing chest pain to reflux disease even when the results of a conventional cardiac work-up such as angiography are reported normal because abnormalities of the microvascular cardiac circulation that escape detection by conventional methods may exist.

Most patients with simple heartburn, especially that of a mild nature and transient or short duration, do not require any diagnostic tests and are easily managed medically. However, patients with severe or long-standing heartburn, dysphagia, atypical symptoms such as chest pain, GI bleeding, and supraesophageal complaints require one or more diagnostic tests to determine the extent and severity of the disease and to tailor their therapy. Endoscopy with or without biopsy is the diagnostic modality of choice. It helps to determine the presence or absence of Barrett's mucosa, significant stricture, and the extent and severity of the mucosal injury.

A barium esophagram is helpful in selected patients with dysphagia in whom it is possible that a distal esophageal ring exists as well as for preoperative evaluation. Atypical symptoms of GERD, such as chest pain and pressure and wheezing, can be elicited by the Bernstein test (intraesophageal acid-saline infusion, with patient unaware of sequence of infusion). Manometry can help in the evaluation of reflux-associated dysphagia, since dysphagia may be caused by abnormal esophageal motor function induced by gastroesophageal reflux disease. Manometry is also useful in preoperative evaluation of esophageal peristaltic function. Concurrent ambulatory pH monitoring of the esophagus and pharynx aids in the detection of pharyngeal acid reflux. It also helps in evaluating the correlation between reflux episodes and the patient's atypical symptoms and has been used to assess the efficacy of acid suppressive or surgical therapy.

Treatment must be tailored to the disease of each patient. In most patients, reflux symptoms respond favorably to aggressive therapy but recur soon after therapy is stopped. In a minority of patients, reflux symptoms are refractory to treatment and may require surgical therapy.

General precautionary measures include elevating the head of the bed (6 to 8 inches) and dietary measures such as avoidance of fatty foods, chocolate, alcohol, cigarettes, peppermint, and caffeine, which are known to decrease the LES resting pressure. Another measure is weight loss. Since reflux episodes occur most frequently 1 to 3 hours after a meal, refraining from eating for 2 to 3 hours prior to retiring will be helpful. However, these measures are not usually sufficient by themselves to remedy moderate to severe reflux symptoms. Although dietary discretion may reduce the frequency of symptoms, it is ineffective in treating esophagitis.

Antacid and algenic acid work primarily by their capacity to neutralize acids, but this effect is temporary. Large doses of antacid (½ and 3 hours after meals and at bedtime) have been used to treat GERD. Algenic acid, which is present in some aluminum hydroxide antacids, acts as a mechanical barrier by forming a highly viscous solution that floats over the gastric contents and may reduce the number of reflux episodes. Acid-suppressive agents, either H_2 receptor antagonists such as ranitidine, nizatidine, or famotidine, or proton pump inhibitors such as omeprazole or lansoprazole comprise the mainstay of the medical management of gastroesophageal reflux disease. Mild to moderate esophagitis responds favorably to H_2 receptor antagonists in 75% to 90% of cases. In patients with severe disease, H_2 receptor antagonists tend to be less effective. Proton pump inhibitors have been shown consistently to be superior to H_2 receptor antagonists in healing reflux esophagitis and relieving symptoms. In patients with severe reflux esophagitis, a proton pump inhibitor such as omeprazole (20 to 40 mg po bid for 8 to 12 weeks) is frequently needed for efficacy.

One of the characteristics of moderate to severe reflux disease is its tendency to recur. More than 80% of esophageal mucosal lesions recur within 6 months of the termination of pharmacologic antireflux therapy. For this reason, maintenance therapy is needed to sustain healing. Maintenance therapy requires full doses of therapeutic agents. Prokinetic agents such as cisapride (Propulsid), 10 mg po qid or 20 mg po bid, in combination with acid-suppressive therapy may improve results in selected cases by enhancing esophageal motility, LES tone, and gastric emptying.

Surgical therapy (conventional or laparoscopic fundoplication) is reserved for patients who fail to respond to medical management such as young patients in whom lifetime therapy is undesirable or patients with supraesophageal manifestation of reflux disease such as asthma and laryngitis that do not respond adequately to acid-suppressive therapy.

DISORDERS OF THE STOMACH, DUODENUM, PANCREAS, AND LIVER

Gastritis

An erosion is a break in the mucosa that appears as a whitish lesion with an erythematous halo on endoscopy. Hemorrhagic gastritis, on the other hand, appears as red streaks, patches, or petechiae. Because of the high use of aspirin and other nonsteroidal anti-inflammatory drugs (NSAIDs) in the geriatric population, erosive and hemorrhagic gastritis should always be considered in old patients presenting with nausea, abdominal discomfort or symptoms of anemia secondary to chronic blood loss. Some may present with acute upper gastrointestinal bleeding. Therapy with synthetic prostaglandins (e.g., misoprostol) reduces NSAID-induced mucosal injury. Enteric-coated NSAIDs have also been shown to reduce the incidence of gastritis. These patients

may also benefit by using a newer generation of prostaglandin-sparing NSAIDs (e.g., nabumetone).

In patients with atrophic gastritis, there is variable gland loss, often accompanied by intestinal metaplasia. The gastric antrum may show an increase in the number of gastrin cells when hypochlorhydria or achlorhydria is associated with gastric atrophy. Serum gastrin levels are raised. Hyperplasia of the enterochromaffin-like cells may also occur. Many studies have shown that a high proportion of asymptomatic people over the age of 60 years have atrophic gastritis. However, there is no relation between age and degree of atrophy.[3] In one study, no one over the age of 60 with an initially normal gastric mucosa developed gastric atrophy during follow-up for 10 years.[4] Thus, gastric atrophy is not a normal part of aging but rather is the result of some specific abnormal mechanisms. Basal and peak gastric acid output appear to decrease with increasing age; however, if one corrects for the presence of *Helicobacter pylori* and atrophic gastritis, there may be no change in acid production with aging. Pepsin secretion does not change with age. Severe atrophic gastritis can result in diminished production of intrinsic factor leading to vitamin B_{12} malabsorption.

Helicobacter pylori is a gram-negative, wavy-shaped rod. In the developed countries, *H. pylori* infection is uncommon before the third decade of life; thereafter, it shows an age-related rise in prevalence. Seropositivity peaks at around 40% to 50% after the age of 50 years. Although *H. pylori* is a frequent cause of nonerosive nonspecific gastritis, its role in the pathogenesis of gastric atrophy and hypochlorhydria is also now well established. More than 80% of patients with pernicious anemia have antibodies to *H. pylori*. Because the prevalence of *H. pylori* rises with age, it is possible that age-related changes in the histology and function of the stomach could be secondary to *H. pylori* infection.[5]

Peptic Ulcer Disease

Peptic ulcers can develop in the esophagus, stomach, duodenum, and jejunum (after gastrojejunostomy) and in areas with ectopic gastric mucosa. Although there is an implied pathogenic association with acid and pepsin, present data suggest that there are two common types of peptic ulcers: ulcers associated with NSAIDs and those associated with the *H. pylori* organism. The incidence of peptic ulcer has risen with age, possibly because of the increased use of NSAIDs and the increased prevalence of *H. pylori* in the elderly.

NSAID therapy is associated with a three- to fivefold increased risk of hospitalization for ulcers or their complications. Gastric ulcers are more common than duodenal ulcers, and rarely, NSAIDs can also induce small bowel or esophageal ulcers. Ulcers related to NSAIDs can be categorized into three types[6]: (1) small mucosal ulcers that develop acutely, probably secondary to topical contact and involving the fundus more than the antrum. These ulcers heal rapidly and can be prevented by using prostaglandin cytoprotection or enteric-coated NSAIDs; (2) 3- to 5-mm ulcers that develop over days to months of NSAID use and involve the antrum more than the fundus. These ulcers probably develop secondary to topical or systemic effects of NSAIDs and therefore may or may not be prevented by using enteric-coated pills, but they can be prevented by using prostaglandin cytoprotection; and (3) chronic, large, deep ulcers, mainly in the antrum and probably related to the systemic effects of NSAIDs. These ulcers may cause complications such as bleeding and perforation and may not be prevented by taking enteric-coated pills or by using prostaglandin cytoprotection.

The risk of NSAID-induced ulcer complications increases in patients over the age of 60 years who have cardiovascular disease, take high or multiple doses of NSAIDs, and take concomitant corticosteroid therapy. Prostaglandin analogs (misoprostol) significantly reduce the incidence of gastric as well as duodenal ulcers induced by NSAIDs. NSAID-induced ulcers can heal with the use of proton pump inhibitors despite the continuous use of NSAIDs.

Helicobacter pylori shows an age-related rise in prevalence. About 40% to 50% of individuals are *H. pylori* seropositive by the age of 50 years. *H. pylori* prevalence reaches 95% in those with duodenal ulcers and 65% in those with gastric ulcers. The mechanism by which this bacteria leads to ulceration is not known. The organism, or factors released by it, might weaken mucosal defenses. Infected individuals also show elevated levels of gastrin and pepsinogen. Several tests are available for diagnosing *H. pylori* infection. Tests using the urease activity of the bacteria are the ^{13}C breath test (90% to 95% sensitivity) and the *Campylobacter*-like organism (CLO) test (90% to 98% sensitivity) on gastric biopsy specimen. Serum antibodies against *H. pylori* (95% sensitivity) cannot differentiate present from past infection unless follow-up titers show a rise. Other methods to diagnose *H. pylori* infection include histology or culture (70% to 95% sensitivity).

Elderly patients with peptic ulcer disease usually present with nonspecific abdominal discomfort or marked weight loss, or they may be asymptomatic. Many present for the first time with complications such as bleeding, perforation, or symptoms of obstruction. Some with chronic blood loss present with cardiac symptoms such as angina or cardiac failure. The presence of systemic diseases like chronic obstructive pulmonary disease (COPD), cardiopulmonary diseases requiring aspirin or anticoagulation for therapy, chronic renal failure, or chronic liver diseases predispose the elderly to peptic ulcer disease and its complications. Complications are seen in about 50% of patients over 70 years. Bleeding is most common and has a higher mortality rate than it does in young patients.

Esophageal and gastric cancers also present frequently in the elderly, and therefore all esophageal and gastric ulcers need endoscopic evaluation, including biopsies and follow-up documentation of healing.

Peptic ulcer disease in the elderly patient is treated using the same guidelines as for the young. However, because many old patients receive drugs for other systemic conditions, one should also be aware of drug interactions and side effects. For example, inhibition of hepatic microsomal cytochrome P450 by cimetidine will raise serum levels of drugs like warfarin, theophylline, and phenytoin. Almost all H_2-receptor antagonists can cause nondose-related central nervous system (CNS) effects such as confusion, disorientation, lethargy, and somnolence. Eradication of *H. pylori* requires combination therapy (Table 46–3). Frail elderly people with multiorgan diseases who are high surgical risks, those who have had complications, those who have had ulcer disease and need anticoagulation, and those who have frequent recurrences of ulcers despite avoiding NSAIDs or eradicating *H. pylori* can be given a H_2-receptor antagonist at bedtime for prophylaxis. Patients requiring NSAIDs can be given enteric-coated ones, or concurrent administration of misoprostol can be tried. A new generation of prostaglandin-sparing NSAIDs (e.g., nabumetone) is also being tried in some of these patients.

Upper Gastrointestinal Bleeding

Table 46–4 lists some of the causes of upper gastrointestinal bleeding. More than 90% of upper gastrointestinal bleeds are secondary to peptic ulcer disease, erosions, varices, and Mallory-Weiss tears. In the elderly, one should also consider upper gastrointestinal malignancies, vascular anomalies like Dieulafoy's anomaly, and aortoenteric fistulas. Increasing use of NSAIDs and systemic conditions like COPD, chronic re-

TABLE 46–3   **TREATMENT OPTIONS FOR**
Helicobacter pylori **WITH >90%**
SUCCESS RATE

	Drug	Mg	Tabs	Dose	Days
I	B		2	qid	7–14
	T	500		qid	7–14
	M	250		tid	7–14
	H₂RA/PPI	Usual		Usual	7–14
II	B		2	qid	14
	T	500		qid	14
	C	500		tid	14
	H₂RA/PPI	Usual		Usual	14
III	A	750		tid	14
	C	500		tid	14
	H₂RA/PPI	Usual		Usual	14
IV	O	20		bid	14
	A	1000		bid	14
	C	500		bid	14
V	O	20		bid	7–14
	M	500		bid	7–14
	C	250		bid	7–14

B, bismuth subsalicylate; T, tetracycline; M, metronidazole; H₂RA, histamine-2-receptor antagonist; PPI, proton pump inhibitor; C, clarithromycin; A, amoxicillin; O, omeprazole.

Modified from Spring 1997 Treatment Options for *H. pylori* Gastritis, G.I. Supply, 200 Grandview Avenue, Camp Hill, PA 17011–1706.

nal failure, and chronic liver disease predispose the elderly to bleeding from ulcer disease.

Upper gastrointestinal bleeding can be overt (e.g., hematemesis or melena), or it can be occult. If severe, it can present as hematochezia. Because of associated systemic disease, acute bleeding may not be as well tolerated by the elderly as by the young. Similarly, chronic occult bleeding leading to anemia may present as worsening cardiac failure or exacerbation of angina.

Mortality from upper gastrointestinal bleeding has remained at around 10% for the past 45 to 50 years despite advances in endoscopy, surgery, and intensive care units. This constant rate may be related to the fact that high-risk patients like the elderly are now living longer and constitute the 10% of patients who die from bleeding.[7, 8] In one study, of 1098 cases admitted to a specialized bleeding unit, 52% had severe upper gastrointestinal bleeding, of which two thirds were over 60 years of age.[9] Thirty-day bleeding-related mortality was around 4%, and all these were elderly patients. The National American Society of Gastrointestinal Endoscopy survey on upper gastrointestinal bleeding revealed that the mortality rate was 13.4% in those over 60 years, whereas it was 8.7% in those below 60 years.[10] Preexisting congestive heart failure and arrhythmias, stroke, encephalopathy, liver disease, neoplasms, COPD,

pneumonia, and renal disease all were associated with higher mortality rates. A recent study showed that age, shock, co-morbidity, major endoscopic stigmata of recent hemorrhage, and rebleeding were all independent predictors of mortality.[11]

General principles of management of gastrointestinal bleeding are similar in the young and the old. The need for blood transfusion is largely dictated by the presence of ongoing bleeding, hemodynamic instability, and the presence of preexisting conditions that decrease the patient's tolerance to blood loss. Those without volume depletion but requiring transfusion (e.g., severe anemia precipitating congestive heart failure) can be given packed red cells and monitored closely for volume overload. The timing of diagnostic procedures depends on the urgency of the need for therapeutic intervention. Endoscopy is accurate, rapid, and relatively safe and allows therapeutic intervention. Endoscopic evidence of active bleeding, visible blood vessels, and fresh clots on an ulcer base indicate a high risk of continued or recurrent bleeding. These features in an elderly patient merit active therapeutic intervention including early surgery, because rebleeding significantly increases mortality in the elderly. In 5% to 10% of cases, endoscopy does not identify the bleeding site. In these patients, angiography can be considered if bleeding is ongoing or recurrent. Elderly patients with variceal bleeding should be treated aggressively because the survival rate in patients with variceal bleeding is similar in the young and the old.

Pancreatic Diseases

Several structural and functional changes occur in the pancreas with increasing age. The diame-

TABLE 46–4   **CAUSES OF UPPER GASTROINTESTINAL BLEEDING**

Esophagus	**Duodenum**
Varices	Ulcer
Esophagitis	Neoplasm
Ulcer	Vascular anomalies
Neoplasm	**Jejuno-Ileum**
Stomach	Vascular anomalies
Erosion	Ulcer
Mallory-Weiss tear	Neoplasm
Ulcer	Crohn's disease
Varices	Infarction
Neoplasm	Aortoenteric fistula
Congestive gastropathy	Varices
Vascular anomalies	**Systemic Conditions**
Liver	Coagulopathies
Hematobilia	Thrombocytopenia
	Swallowed blood

ter of the pancreatic duct increases,[12, 13] and there is strong evidence of impaired pancreatic function in older people.[14] Although the clinical consequences of these changes remain unclear, they must be taken into account when interpreting radiographs obtained during endoscopic retrograde pancreatography and in evaluating pancreatic function in elderly individuals.

ACUTE PANCREATITIS

Alcohol use and gallstones account for 80% of cases of acute pancreatitis observed in the general population. About 10% to 15% of cases are idiopathic. When causes of pancreatitis are stratified by age, ischemia is seen to be an important cause of acute pancreatitis in the elderly. In one study, 27% of patients developed pancreatitis following coronary bypass.[15] The incidence of gallstone pancreatitis is significantly higher in older people than in younger ones. As much as 55% of all cases of pancreatitis in those over 60 years of age are due to biliary tract disease, whereas alcohol accounts for only 20% of cases.[16] There is also a higher incidence of idiopathic pancreatitis in the elderly. Some of these cases may be secondary to biliary microlithiasis. Drugs such as diuretics and steroids can also cause pancreatitis. Pancreatic cancer should be suspected in all elderly patients presenting with pancreatitis for the first time.

Acute pancreatitis frequently presents atypically in those over 60 years of age. Absence of typical abdominal pain and the presence of multiorgan failure, shock, hypothermia, and hyperglycemia are some of the clinical presentations. Unfortunately, in many cases the diagnosis is made at autopsy. Pancreatic necrosis is frequently observed in these cases. Acute pancreatitis should be strongly considered in elderly patients who present with unexplained systemic complications, especially during the postoperative period. Diagnostic investigations, including amylase-lipase levels, computed tomography (CT) of the abdomen, and, when appropriate, endoscopic retrograde cholangiopancreatography (ERCP) should be done.

Treatment guidelines in the elderly are similar to those used in younger individuals. However, patients presenting with acute severe nonresolving gallstone pancreatitis should undergo urgent ERCP and sphincterotomy for stone removal.[17, 18] Those with idiopathic pancreatitis should be evaluated for biliary microlithiasis, and, if these are present, these patients should also undergo sphincterotomy. Another option includes the use of ursodeoxycholic acid. Rarely, manometry of the sphincter of Oddi may be required to diagnose papillary stenosis as a cause of idiopathic pancreatitis requiring sphincterotomy. Other obstructive causes, such as adenomas and carcinomas, should also be considered in these cases.

CHRONIC PANCREATITIS

Although some cases of chronic pancreatitis are idiopathic, most are secondary to alcohol consumption. Obstructive chronic pancreatitis should always raise the suspicion of an ampullary neoplasm or pancreatic carcinoma. These patients usually have a dilated pancreatic duct and do not show the typical pancreatic calcification seen in those with alcohol or idiopathic pancreatitis. Rarely, pancreatic stones are noted in the pancreatic duct in asymptomatic elderly subjects.[19]

Pain is less severe in older patients with chronic pancreatitis, and many may never experience any pain. Disease progression is also slower in the elderly than in the young, and therefore few, if any, show evidence of endocrine or exocrine insufficiency or require intervention for complications.

PANCREATIC NEOPLASMS

Most patients with ductal adenocarcinoma of the pancreas are over the age of 60 years. Patients with chronic pancreatitis from any cause have a higher risk of developing pancreatic carcinoma.[20, 21] The chances of developing pancreatic carcinoma in patients with chronic pancreatitis are directly related to increasing age.

Brushings for cytologic examination obtained during ERCP, endoscopic ultrasonography with fine-needle aspiration, and analysis of cystic fluid may provide further help in diagnosis. In selected cases, angiography and laparoscopy may be required.

The only hope for cure in patients with pancreatic adenocarcinoma is surgery. Surgery is also the preferred treatment for mucinous ductal ectasia and cystic neoplasms because some of these tumors may be either malignant or premalignant. Evidence of biliary obstruction in patients with pancreatic carcinoma generally implies advanced disease except in those with ampullary carcinoma, in whom biliary obstruction can occur early. Palliative therapy includes modalities such as placement of biliary endoprostheses to relieve biliary obstruction, radiotherapy, and pain control, which may involve celiac ganglion block.

Liver Diseases

Several age-related changes have been described in liver structure and function. With aging, there is a decline in liver volume.[22] On histologic examination, using postmortem tissue from individuals over 60 years, fewer but larger hepatocytes were seen. Similar age-related alterations have been reported in the mitochondria.[23] Although hepatic blood flow declines with age, studies have failed to show any significant deterioration in liver function tests with aging. However, with increasing age, the bile becomes more lithogenic as bile acid synthesis declines and cholesterol secretion increases. There is indirect evidence in humans of an age-related decline in hepatic regeneration ability following liver resection surgery.[24] Although there is no evidence of any decline in cytochrome P450-dependent metabolism with aging, reduced liver volume and blood flow contribute to reduced clearance of some drugs, thereby possibly predisposing elderly individuals to adverse drug-induced diseases.

The mortality rate from chronic liver disease is highest among patients over 65 years. Some of these diseases develop in the young who survive to older age, whereas others develop in old age. In one national study, the incidence of toxic hepatitis, primary biliary cirrhosis, and nonalcoholic cirrhosis peaked in patients between 70 and 79 years, whereas alcoholic cirrhosis peaked at 50 to 59 years.[25] Liver can be affected by systemic conditions such as cardiac failure. Some rare diseases such as the Budd-Chiari syndrome and idiopathic hemochromatosis can also present in the elderly.

GALLSTONE DISEASE

Decreased bile acid production, increased cholesterol saturation of bile, reduced gallbladder sensitivity to cholecystokinin, and increased prevalence of duodenal diverticula are some of the factors that predispose to formation of gallstones in the elderly. By 70 years of age, about 35% of women and 20% of men have gallstones. Although many are asymptomatic, some may present with biliary pain, cholecystitis, pancreatitis, cholangitis, or obstructive jaundice. Gallbladder cancer, also found predominantly in the elderly, can present with several of the same clinical features. As in younger patients, diagnostic investigations include liver function tests, ultrasound or CT scans of the abdomen (or both), and ERCP examination. In interpreting abnormal liver function test results, one should keep in mind that an isolated rise in alkaline phosphatase levels in the elderly can be secondary to bone disease. With advances in anesthesia and surgical techniques, urgent cholecystectomy in elderly patients presenting with acute cholecystitis has a mortality rate similar to that seen in the young.

Laparoscopic cholecystectomy is becoming increasingly popular and is particularly useful in treating symptomatic cholelithiasis in the frail elderly. If clinical and biochemical test results raise a suspicion of common bile duct stones, patients scheduled for laparoscopic cholecystectomy should undergo ERCP evaluation prior to surgery. Extremely ill elderly patients considered to be at high risk for surgery and not responding to conservative treatment can be treated by ultrasound-guided percutaneous cholecystostomy. Patients with gallstones in the common bile duct and those with gallstone pancreatitis require ERCP with sphincterotomy and stone extraction using a basket or a balloon. Larger stones can be removed by crushing them with a lithotriptor. In a subset of cases, biliary endoprostheses with regular exchanges can be used for long-term management of nonretrievable common bile duct stones.

BILIARY OBSTRUCTION

Obstructive jaundice in the elderly is more commonly secondary to malignancy than to choledocholithiasis. Adenocarcinoma of the pancreas accounts for most of these cases. Other malignancies include ampullary, gallbladder, bile duct, duodenal, and metastatic cancers. Most of these patients present with painless jaundice with or without a palpably enlarged gallbladder. Benign biliary strictures can result from cholangitis, bile duct injuries, or radiotherapy. Primary sclerosing cholangitis is rare in persons over 65 years of age.

Malignant biliary obstruction usually requires palliative treatment because most of these obstructions are secondary to advanced diseases or the frail elderly patient is too ill to undergo extensive surgical resection. Diagnosis can be made by obtaining samples from ERCP brushings or biopsies or by CT-guided or endoscopic ultrasound-guided fine-needle aspiration. Biliary decompression is generally achieved by ERCP sphincterotomy or placement of an endoprosthesis. In tumors involving the hepatic hilum, multiple endoprostheses may be required to decompress the right and left hepatic systems. Endoscopic biliary decompression is as successful in relieving obstruction as surgery is, but it requires a shorter hospital stay and is less expensive. It should therefore be the preferred treatment modality, especially in the elderly. Percutaneous biliary decompression (external or internal) is another alternative. Complications of this method include hemorrhage, infection, peritonitis, and catheter displacement. It should therefore be considered if the ERCP technique fails.

ALCOHOL LIVER DISEASE

Alcohol liver disease should always be considered in the differential diagnosis when an elderly person presents with hepatic dysfunction. In one study from the United States, presentation with alcohol liver cirrhosis peaked in the seventh decade.[26] Clinical features of alcohol liver disease in the elderly are similar to those seen in younger patients. However, older patients are more likely to present with severe disease than younger subjects.[27] Elderly patients with alcohol liver disease also have a higher mortality rate.[28]

DRUG-INDUCED LIVER DISEASE

Decreased hepatic volume and decreased blood flow with increasing age may result in altered pharmacokinetics and predispose the elderly to drug-related diseases. Unfortunately, many old patients are taking multiple medications. Not surprisingly, adverse drug reactions have an increased prevalence in the elderly. In a Danish study, the incidence of toxic hepatitis reached 50 per million person-years in 70- to 79-year-old people compared to an overall incidence of 20 per million person-years.[25] Elderly patients are particularly likely to develop toxic hepatitis with certain drugs. For example, isoniazid-induced hepatitis occurs in more than 2% of patients over 50 years old but is virtually unknown under the age of 20 years. An anti-inflammatory drug, benoxaprofen, had to be withdrawn from use following fatal hepatotoxicity that occurred predominantly in elderly women. Halothane reexposure in patients with previously known halothane-induced injury results in more severe hepatotoxicity in elderly patients than in young ones. Whereas several drug-related hepatic injuries are idiosyncratic reactions and therefore are unpredictable, many are dose-related and require dose adjustments. For example, amiodarone toxicity requires dose adjustment in the elderly. Drug-induced liver disease may present like hepatitis with increased transaminase levels (acetaminophen, isoniazid, methyldopa), or like cholestatic hepatitis with raised transaminases and alkaline phosphatase levels, mimicking cholangitis (phenytoin, quinidine, nitrofurantoin, erythromycin), or with a primarily cholestatic picture (estrogens, chlorpromazine, chlorpropamide, anabolic steroids).

HEPATIC MALIGNANCY

Although the peak incidence of hepatocellular carcinoma worldwide occurs in early to middle adulthood, this cancer is predominantly a disease of the elderly in Europe and North America. Some of the common predisposing factors are liver cirrhosis, previous hepatitis B infection, and hemochromatosis.

Metastases to the liver, especially from the gastrointestinal tract, form another important group of hepatic malignancies seen in the elderly. Anorexia, weight loss, malaise, abdominal pain, jaundice, hepatomegaly, and ascites are some of the clinical features. These patients usually have raised alkaline phosphatase levels, and those with hepatocellular carcinoma may have raised alpha-fetoprotein levels. Diagnosis generally requires liver biopsy, usually CT-guided. Surgical resection, regional chemotherapy, cryoablation, and alcohol injection into the tumor are some of the treatment options.

LIVER ABSCESS

More than 50% of cases of liver abscess in the developed countries occur in those over 60 years of age. Most of these cases are secondary to ascending cholangitis. High fever, rigors, and other classic features of sepsis are generally lacking in the elderly, most of whom present with nonspecific symptoms such as epigastric pain, weight loss, or confusion. Alkaline phosphatase levels are usually raised in these patients. Due to the potential lethal nature of this condition, especially in the elderly, early intervention by percutaneous or surgical drainage may be necessary.

OTHER LIVER DISEASES

Viral hepatitis should always be considered in the differential diagnosis of any elderly patient presenting with anorexia, jaundice, and elevated transaminase concentrations. In patients who are admitted with episodes of hypotension and grossly elevated transaminase levels, one should consider ischemic hepatitis. Fluctuating liver function test results are seen in patients with heart failure. Mild increases in transaminase levels may be associated with alcoholism, chronic hepatitis, and fatty liver in patients with obesity, hyperlipidemia, and diabetes mellitus. Primary biliary cirrhosis and chronic active hepatitis may also occur in the elderly. Although with the availability of serologic markers for hepatitis C, the diagnosis of cryptogenic cirrhosis had to be revised in several cases, a study from the Mayo Clinic reported that a higher incidence of cryptogenic cirrhosis occurs in the elderly, raising the possibility that there may be a specific form of senile cirrhosis.[29] Variceal bleeding secondary to portal hypertension should be treated aggressively because the survival rate following variceal bleeding is similar in the old and the young. In a confused old individual, one should always consider hepatic encephalopathy in the differential diagnosis.

LIVER TRANSPLANTATION AND THE ELDERLY

Advances in surgery and immunosuppressive treatment have greatly improved the results of liver transplantation. In a retrospective analysis, Pirsch and colleagues found excellent graft and patient survival in liver transplant recipients over 60 years of age compared to those under 60 years.[30] Old age alone, therefore, should not be a contraindication to liver transplantation.

DISORDERS OF THE SMALL AND LARGE INTESTINES

There is little evidence that a generalized age-related loss of absorptive function occurs in the small intestine. Age-related declines in specific enzymes such as lactase have been reported. There has been more interest in studies of intestinal motor activity in the elderly. Abnormal motility could be related to the aging process or to underlying diseases that are increasingly prevalent in older patients.

Small intestinal motility, as measured by manometric tubes passed into the intestine, does not appear to change with age, showing only minor changes in amplitude of contractions. Studies have consistently shown that fasting and postprandial small intestinal contractions are similar in young and elderly subjects. Individuals who have symptoms consistent with abnormal small intestinal transit, such as abdominal distention or diarrhea, should be evaluated to exclude an underlying disease as an explanation. A small intestinal barium x-ray study is a useful screening test for evaluating symptoms related to small intestinal transit. Findings of abnormal small intestinal transit, dilatation, or diverticulosis may suggest a reason for the patient's symptoms. Small intestinal transit can be altered by autonomic neuropathic disorders. Rapid small bowel transit can induce diarrhea. Dilatation of the small bowel may be due to malabsorption syndromes, and small intestinal diverticulosis and slow intestinal transit can result in small bowel bacterial overgrowth that causes diarrhea.

Many studies have been designed to define the prevalence of intestinal symptoms in young and old patients. These studies have included inpatient and outpatient diagnoses in individuals seeking medical care as well as surveys of defined populations of individuals who have not necessarily consulted a physician. One of the proposed gastrointestinal motility disorders is irritable bowel syndrome (IBS), which can be defined by the presence of three or more Manning criteria (briefly summarized as follows: (1) pain relieved by defecation, (2) looser stools during pain, (3) more frequent stooling during pain, (4) abdominal distention, (5) a feeling of incomplete evacuation, and (6) passing mucus through the rectum). The prevalence of IBS in a population of individuals not necessarily seen by a physician has been estimated as 11% among individuals 65 years old or older.[31]

Chronic constipation is another common chronic gastrointestinal disorder in the United States.[32] The prevalence of constipation is 4.5% among individuals 65 to 74 years old and 10.2% among individuals 75 years old or older. Constipation affects three times as many women as men. An estimated 4.5 million individuals in the United States have constipation, and they visit a physician an estimated 2.5 million times yearly for evaluation of this symptom.

The development of fecal incontinence is an important factor in considering future requirements for nursing home care of elderly individuals. Incontinence of liquid fecal material is most common. Fecal incontinence is more common in men than in women.

The effects of aging on neural and intrinsic muscular control of gastrointestinal smooth muscle are poorly understood. Principal theories of the process of senescence include two main hypotheses: (1) chronic exposure to toxins results in an age-related neuropathic or myopathic process, or (2) genes involved in the normal functioning of neurons or smooth muscle undergo gradual changes in expression that eventually result in "aging." In the first proposed mechanism, potential exposures include chronic ingestion of exogenous neurotoxins or chronic production of endogenous neurotoxins such as tissue free radicals. In examination of the second mechanism, studies of gene expression in senescence have led to the concept of genetic instability, in which changes in DNA and chromatin occur with aging. It is not yet known whether genetic instability results in changes in intestinal function.

Motility of the intestine is regulated by endocrine and neural systems. Extrinsic nerve fibers (preganglionic parasympathetic and postganglionic sympathetic fibers) communicate with nerve cell bodies in intestinal nerve plexuses. Disruption of extrinsic innervation (due to central nervous system damage or spinal cord injury) alters enteric nervous system function and results in altered motility. There is little evidence to support the idea of an age-related change in extrinsic nerve input to intestinal nerve plexuses, but this is an important disease-related consideration.

Intrinsic intestinal nerves provide both excitatory and inhibitory input to smooth muscle cells. Age-related changes may include a loss of nerve input (either inhibitory or excitatory) from enteric neurons that innervate the intestinal smooth muscle cells. Multiple studies have supported the concept of an age-related loss of enteric neurons, and recent work using human colon has revealed that an age-related loss of inhibitory nerve input to colonic circular smooth muscle may occur. Loss of inhibitory nerve input could change colonic motility by diminishing the normal descending relaxation of the colon or by decreasing the normal inhibition of nonpropagating colonic contractions. Opiates, for example, induce constipation by increasing the occurrence of nonpropagating contractions in the distal gut.

To induce normal relaxation or contraction of smooth muscle cells, receptors for specific excitatory or inhibitory neurotransmitters must be present on the smooth muscle cell, and the contractile apparatus of the myocyte must be functional. There is little evidence in humans at present to support the idea that an age-related myopathic disorder may cause abnormalities in intestinal motility.

Evaluation and Treatment of Specific Intestinal Disorders

LOWER INTESTINAL BLEEDING

Bleeding from the lower gut may present as outlet bleeding (bright red blood during or after defecation), suspicious bleeding (blood mixed with or streaked on stool), acute hemorrhage, or occult bleeding (anemia, iron deficiency, or positive results on stool occult blood test).

The differential diagnosis remains complex. Outlet bleeding is commonly thought to be due to an anal fissure, hemorrhoids, distal colorectal neoplasia, or proctitis. It has been suggested that a flexible sigmoidoscopy should be performed for simple uncomplicated outlet bleeding.

The available studies support a recommendation for total colonoscopy for evaluation of suspicious bleeding, acute hemorrhage (when the patient is stable), and occult bleeding.[33] Causes of acute hemorrhage, in descending order of occurrence, include diverticular bleeding (often from right-sided diverticula), angiodysplasia, inflammatory bowel disease, ischemic colitis, and, less likely, infectious colitis, colorectal neoplasia, solitary rectal ulcer syndrome, and radiation colitis. There are many unusual origins of acute

lower intestinal hemorrhage. Poor visualization of the colon during an acute hemorrhage may lead to performance of visceral angiography as an additional diagnostic study. In patients with occult bleeding, a common finding is colorectal neoplasia; angiodysplasia is less likely, and ischemic colitis and occult inflammatory bowel disease are unlikely.

INFLAMMATORY BOWEL DISEASE

Epidemiologic studies of inflammatory bowel disease (IBD) have shown a second peak in occurrence in patients over the age of 60. The etiology of colitis can be complex in elderly patients. Several other conditions must be considered during evaluation of an elderly patient who presents with a colitis-like disorder.

Two types of infectious colitis may be overlooked in elderly patients. Because of the use of many antibiotics, patients can develop a pseudomembranous colitis that can mimic the picture of toxic megacolon. Overgrowth of *Clostridium difficile* is thought to be the main pathogenic factor, and a stool test may show the presence of a *C. difficile* toxin. On endoscopy of the lower intestine, patchy but multiple cream-yellow plaques or membranes may be seen in the left colon more commonly than in the right colon. Treatment regimens include oral metronidazole or oral vancomycin. Recurrent pseudomembranous colitis can be treated by changing the oral antibiotic regimen, treating for a longer period (4 weeks), or adding therapy to potentially bind the bacterial toxin (cholestyramine). In a second type of atypical infectious colitis, cancer chemotherapy is associated with development of a cytomegalovirus-induced colitis. At colonoscopy, discrete ulcers are seen in the colon, and colonic mucosal biopsies will aid in the diagnosis.

Three types of noninfectious colitis should be considered in evaluating elderly patients. Colitis induced by the use of NSAIDs can mimic the signs of mild ulcerative colitis. Following radiation therapy, especially in men with adenocarcinoma of the prostate, lower endoscopy may reveal rectal telangiectasias consistent with a diagnosis of radiation proctitis. Medical therapies are often ineffective in this condition, but laser therapy has been useful in selected patients to reduce blood loss. Ischemic colitis is more common in elderly patients, and it has been reported especially often following aortoiliac reconstructive surgery. At colonoscopy, findings include deep linear ulcers, edema, diffuse petechiae, and a sharp demarcation proximal to the splenic flexure of the colon; the finding of necrotic colon requires rapid surgical intervention.

TABLE 46–5 MEDICAL MANAGEMENT OF IDIOPATHIC INFLAMMATORY BOWEL DISEASE

Sulfasalazine
5-Aminosalicylic acid compounds (oral or enema)
Corticosteroids (oral or enema)
Antibiotics
  Metronidazole
  Ciprofloxacin
Nutritional therapy
Newer immunosuppressive therapy
  6-Mercaptopurine
  Cyclosporine
  Methotrexate

When no specific cause of colitis can be identified after tests that include appropriate stool cultures for pathogenic bacteria and stool examinations to exclude ova and parasites, treatment is designed to improve symptoms. Medical therapy for idiopathic IBD should begin with the safest and most cost-effective treatment, and progression to increasingly complex treatments should be based on the patient's response. Medical treatment of idiopathic IBD is summarized in Table 46–5. Distal colitis or proctitis may respond initially to treatment with enemas (containing a corticosteroid or a 5-aminosalicylic acid compound).

Mildly or moderately active colitis is often treated with sulfasalazine. The lowest effective dose should be used, and folic acid should be given simultaneously as a supplement. In patients who cannot tolerate the side effects of sulfasalazine and in selected patients who are allergic to sulfa drugs, compounds derived from the active moiety of sulfasalazine (Azulfidine), 5-aminosalicylic acid, are now available. 5-Aminosalicylic acid compounds are no more effective than sulfasalazine.

Moderately active to severely active colitis may require oral corticosteroid therapy, usually for periods of at least 2 to 3 months. Low doses of corticosteroids are no more effective than placebo for maintenance. Long-term high-dose corticosteroid therapy is associated with significant complications. Antibiotic therapy appears to be more effective in patients with Crohn's disease, especially for fistulous disease or treatment of perineal Crohn's disease. Nutritional therapy is not effective for primary therapy of ulcerative colitis, and nutritional treatment of Crohn's disease requires a liquid diet that many patients do not find acceptable. Although a polymeric diet or an elemental diet may diminish the corticoste-

roid dose needed in Crohn's disease, its benefit is lost after it has been discontinued.

Immunosuppressive therapy should not be considered simply a substitute for surgical therapy and should be used by physicians with the appropriate experience. 6-Mercaptopurine does not appear to be effective as a single agent but can diminish the corticosteroid dose needed. Cyclosporine and methotrexate are both toxic medications and should probably be reserved for treatment of Crohn's disease. Long-term maintenance therapy of IBD includes use of sulfasalazine, 5-aminosalicylic acid compounds, metronidazole, or 6-mercaptopurine (in combination with low-dose corticosteroid therapy).

CONSTIPATION

Constipation, a subjective term describing the symptom of unsatisfactory defecation, is a common chronic digestive disorder.[32] Most patients with a complaint of constipation are seen by general practitioners and general internists. Constipation represents different problems to different individuals. It may be described as infrequent defecation or straining, passage of firm or small-volume fecal material, pain with defecation, or a discrepancy between expected output and actual results.

The cause of age-related constipation is presently incompletely understood. Conventional proposals of causation include chronic disease processes (e.g., diabetes mellitus), intake of opiates or medications that have anticholinergic side effects, or insufficient exercise or water-fiber intake. None of these proposals has been convincingly supported by available studies. Colon transit studies have repeatedly shown an increase in the number of retained markers in the rectosigmoid region, suggesting that constipated elderly individuals have slow left-sided colorectal transit.

To understand the causes of constipation it is important to consider the mechanisms of defecation. The process of defecation requires four major mechanisms: (1) an anorectal sensation of an urge to defecate following rectal distention, (2) reflex relaxation of the internal anal sphincter, (3) colorectal motility, chiefly manifested by propagating contractions, and (4) an increase in intra-abdominal pressure by Valsalva's maneuver to produce perineal descent.

Constipation can be caused by many different diseases (Table 46–6). Known causes of constipation include neuropathic disorders such as Hirschsprung's disease and Chagas' disease, myopathic disorders such as scleroderma and amyloidosis, and mechanical or functional obstruction, such as that due to adenocarcinoma of the

---

TABLE 46–6 DIFFERENTIAL DIAGNOSIS OF CONSTIPATION

Neurogenic Disorders	**Myopathic Disorders**
Parkinson's disease	Scleroderma
Multiple sclerosis	Amyloidosis
Cerebral infarction	**Metabolic and**
Tabes dorsalis	**Endocrine**
Mechanical	**Disorders**
Obstruction	Diabetes mellitus with
Postsurgical	autonomic
abnormalities	neuropathy
Strictures: postischemic	Uremia
or diverticular	Hypothyroidism
Rectocele	Hypokalemia
Internal rectal prolapse	Hypercalcemia
Endometriosis	
Neoplasia	
Drug Therapy	
Opiate analgesics	
Anticholinergic agents	
Calcium channel	
antagonists	
Calcium-containing	
supplements	
Aluminum-containing	
antacids	
Metallic intoxication	
(e.g., lead, mercury,	
and arsenic)	
Vinca alkaloids	

---

rectum, anal fissures, rectocele, and internal prolapse. Other causes are metabolic and endocrine disorders, such as hypokalemia and hypothyroidism, and toxins or drugs. In many patients, the cause of constipation remains unknown.

At the initial visit, evaluation of a complaint of constipation begins with a proper history and physical examination. This includes an estimate of the frequency of stooling, length of time symptoms have been present, and associated symptoms such as straining, abdominal pain, abdominal distention, and fullness or bloating. Recent onset of constipation, especially in older patients, suggests a need to exclude mechanical obstruction. Imaging of the colon and rectum by endoscopy or barium colon radiography should then be performed. To exclude endocrine causes of colonic dysmotility, fasting serum glucose, serum calcium, potassium, creatinine, and thyroid-stimulating hormone levels should be measured. Constipation may be associated with beginning a new medication or increasing the dosage of an existing medication, especially calcium channel antagonists, opiate agonists, anticholinergic medications, and aluminum-containing antacids.

Other historical factors that must be addressed are the possible habitual use of laxatives for the purpose of purgation and an onset of constipation following an episode of anal pain.

In many patients, the cause of the symptoms may remain unclear. A primary differentiation that must be made is whether the patient has normal transit constipation (probably irritable bowel syndrome) or abnormal colorectal transit. A simple test to distinguish these two categories is a Sitzmarks colonic transit study. Commercially prepared gelatin capsules containing 24 radiopaque rings are available (Sitzmarks, Lafayette Pharmacal, Inc., Fort Worth, Texas). The movement of nonabsorbable markers through the colon is followed by exposing flat plate abdominal radiographs. Before performing this test, it may be necessary to evacuate the patient's colon. It is necessary during the study for patients to refrain from taking laxatives, enemas, suppositories, and medications that cause constipation. The presence of retained markers (defined as greater than 20% of the total ingested) throughout the colon at day 5 is consistent with constipation due to so-called colonic inertia, while markers retained within the rectosigmoid region are consistent with constipation due to rectosigmoid dysmotility or a rectal outlet obstruction. The term spastic pelvic floor syndrome should be reserved for patients who have difficulty in initiating defecation and in whom insufficient relaxation of the levator ani muscle can be demonstrated.

As summarized in Table 46–7, optimal treatment of constipation would be a specific therapy designed to correct an underlying condition. In many patients no specific cause can be identified, and instruction about a high-fiber diet remains

---

TABLE 46–7 MEDICAL MANAGEMENT OF CHRONIC CONSTIPATION

At presentation:	Specific therapy
	Instruction about a high fiber diet
	Instruction about the gastrocolonic response
Secondary therapy:	Low fiber diet
	Osmotic laxatives: magnesium salts or nonabsorbable sugars such as lactulose or sorbitol
	Prokinetic agents: bethanechol chloride or cisapride
	Suppositories: glycerin, bisacodyl, or carbon dioxide-producing
	Polymeric liquid diet
	Biofeedback techniques

the simplest initial therapy for patients who have normal transit constipation (irritable bowel syndrome). To increase dietary fiber intake, patients should be instructed to increase daily consumption of raw fruits, raw vegetables, and whole grain products. In addition, instruction in methods of initiating the gastrocolonic response may be beneficial. The patient is instructed to eat a warm meal or to drink a warm fluid after arising in the morning. The patient should then spend time attempting to initiate defecation while sitting on the toilet and use Valsalva's maneuver for continuous periods of no longer than 5 to 10 seconds.

If these initial measures are not helpful, patients with constipation and documented abnormal results on a marker study may experience symptomatic improvement by consuming a low-fiber diet. A small group of patients with severe colorectal dysmotility obtain relief from abdominal pain through colonic cleansing, but they cannot maintain colonic evacuation. If additional medical therapy is required, there are three major categories of laxatives that may be used. Irritant or stimulant laxatives include anthraquinone compounds, which are active ingredients in extracts of senna, aloe, cascara, or rhubarb. Many available herbal tea preparations include an anthraquinone compound. Other over-the-counter stimulant chemicals include phenolphthalein and bisacodyl. *These agents generally should not be prescribed for the long term because increasing doses will be necessary over time to initiate defecation, and older patients may develop fecal incontinence as well as potential colonic nerve toxicity.*

Osmotic agents tend to increase the water content of fecal material. The use of mineral oil is not recommended because reflux of this material can cause lipid pneumonia. Magnesium salts such as citrate of magnesia have been extensively used and are relatively safe. Patients receiving these agents should have periodic screening of renal function and serum magnesium level. In patients with decreased renal function, poorly absorbed sugars such as lactulose and sorbitol may be beneficial. The use of sorbitol 70% syrup may be preferable because it is less expensive.[34] Among other similar agents, available studies have found that wetting agents or surfactants such as docusate calcium or docusate sodium produce no consistent benefit.

The third major class of laxatives includes drugs that function as neurotransmitter agonists. In general, use of these compounds has been disappointing. Bethanechol chloride is a cholinergic agonist that increases phasic contractions in human colon. Neostigmine bromide can decrease metabolism of endogenous acetylcholine, which in normal individuals increases phasic contractions. Its use may induce severe side effects. Cisapride releases acetylcholine at the level of the nerve plexus and seems to be helpful in inducing phasic colonic contractions. Cisapride may be ineffective in long-term therapy and has been associated with development of prolonged QT syndrome.

Regular use of suppositories (two to three mornings a week) may be beneficial in maintaining rectal evacuation in patients with constipation due to a rectal outlet obstruction. Carbon dioxide–producing suppositories distend the rectum and may initiate descending relaxation of the circular smooth muscle. In selected patients with the spastic pelvic floor syndrome and in patients with neurologic diseases affecting the external anal sphincter, biofeedback techniques designed to teach the patient to relax the external anal sphincter may be helpful.[35] These methods require good patient compliance, are time-consuming, and require a specialist for instruction.

Among potential complications, there is evidence that chronic constipation can lead to fecal impaction, overflow fecal incontinence, sigmoid volvulus, and stercoral (pressure) colonic ulcerations. Chronic therapy may be helpful in preventing these problems. There is little evidence that hemorrhoids, melanosis coli, or colon cancer are caused by constipation. Identification of melanosis coli is not helpful because there is no correlation between the occurrence of melanosis coli and the presence of abnormal colorectal transit or the frequency of bowel movements.

ACUTE MEGACOLON

Acute dilatation of the colon (Ogilvie's syndrome) can be related to multiple causes including surgery or trauma (spinal surgery, hip fracture), use of medications (narcotic analgesics, anticholinergic medications), endocrine disorders (hypothyroidism), or electrolyte imbalance (hypokalemia or hypercalcemia). An increased risk of colonic perforation is thought to be associated with a transverse colonic or cecal diameter of more than 9 cm on an abdominal flat plate radiograph. Management is often hotly debated. If a specific cause is identified, it should be corrected. If an endocrine origin, electrolyte imbalance, or medication-induced origin cannot be rapidly reversed, a decision must be made about whether the patient needs lower endoscopy to decompress the colon or a conservative management plan that includes repositioning the patient and passing a short-term nasogastric decompression tube and a soft rectal decompression tube. Cautious use of intravenous neostigmine methylsulfate while the patient is under cardiac monitoring is suggested in the literature. A suspicion of colonic perforation requires consideration of surgical intervention. Treatment of each patient must be tailored to the individual.

SIGMOID VOLVULUS

Sigmoid volvulus is a poorly studied colonic disorder. Development of megacolon is believed to be a major risk factor for the formation of a sigmoid volvulus. Patients in the United States with sigmoid volvulus have a mean age of approximately 70, whereas in African nations in which a high-fiber diet is consumed, the mean age of patients with sigmoid volvulus is at least 20 years younger. Symptoms may be very poorly localized in patients who present with sigmoid volvulus. Physicians must maintain a high level of suspicion, especially in older individuals who present with abdominal distention, a change in bowel habits, or poorly localized abdominal discomfort. On an abdominal flat plate radiograph, classically there are multiple dilated loops of ahaustral bowel that stop abruptly at the pelvic inlet. Colonic perforation is a major complication that is to be feared in this disorder. Initial management includes acute decompression of the volvulus by lower endoscopy or, less commonly, radiologically through use of a gentle Gastrografin enema. If the situation recurs, the surgical literature supports sigmoid colon resection before the patient is discharged from the hospital.

DIVERTICULOSIS

Diverticulosis is an interesting but very poorly understood colonic disorder. There is good evidence that the prevalence of diverticulosis increases with age. In Western countries, diverticulosis is more common in the sigmoid colon, while in East Asian countries it is more common in the right colon. Radiologic studies have initiated an understanding that diverticulosis is often a clinically insignificant finding. Theories of formation have focused on diverticula as hernias related to a combination of high intracolonic pressure or an inherent weakening of the colonic wall. In the older literature there was speculation that this disorder was caused by constipation, straining at stool, or flatulence (all discounted at this time). It has been proposed more recently that a low-fiber diet leads to increased intracolonic pressure. Simultaneously, classic advice had focused on avoiding certain high-fiber foods (containing seeds and similar fiber-rich items) in the hope that this could prevent episodes of diverticulitis.

Among complications of diverticulosis, it is commonly believed that right-sided colonic diverticula are more likely to present as hematochezia, whereas left-sided colonic diverticula are more likely to present as diverticulitis. Diverticulitis as a clinical diagnosis remains a concern in patients who present with a change in bowel habits, a new onset of lower abdominal pain, fever, or leukocytosis. Many unusual fistulas have been reported in patients with diverticulitis. If there is a suspicion of an intra-abdominal abscess, a CT scan of the abdomen may be helpful. Uncomplicated diverticulitis has been treated with oral antibiotic therapy designed to provide coverage for anaerobic bacteria and coliform bacteria. Patients require a follow-up study to image the colon and rectum to exclude a neoplasm. The surgical literature has proposed segmental sigmoid colonic resection for patients who have had two documented episodes of diverticulitis.

FECAL INCONTINENCE

Incontinence of liquid or solid stool has been called the "unvoiced symptom" because many individuals with this disorder have not discussed their problem with a physician.[36] This suggests that physicians must specifically inquire about this disorder. Maintenance of fecal continence involves coordination of the internal and external anal sphincters. Incontinence occurs when rectal pressure exceeds the combined anal canal pressure. There are few controlled studies of the epidemiology of fecal incontinence. There does appear to be an age-related increase in the prevalence of this disorder, although different studies provide conflicting evidence about potential gender differences. Evidence in many studies shows that the overall prevalence of fecal incontinence in individuals over age 65 appears to range from 3% to 18%.

It is not entirely clear whether the increased prevalence of incontinence in the elderly is due to age-related changes in anal sphincter function or to an increased prevalence in the elderly of diseases that affect the anal sphincter. Physiologic studies of the anal sphincteric muscles demonstrate age-related declines in resting anal canal pressure (associated with internal anal sphincter pressure) as well as maximal squeeze pressure (associated with external anal sphincter pressure). It has been proposed from histologic studies that sclerosis of the internal anal sphincter is an age-related process. However, among patients with fecal incontinence, 40% have normal anal canal pressures, and it has been estimated that 80% of patients with fecal incontinence have a neurologic disease, diabetes mellitus, cognitive impairment, inflammatory bowel disease, or prior trauma or surgery involving the perineum.

In the individual patient with fecal incontinence, the physician must consider these possible explanations: presence of liquid stool in the rectum (diarrhea-related such as diabetic diarrhea), an inadequate rectal reservoir (poor rectal compliance), poor rectal sensation (a common problem in spinal cord injury patients), or anal sphincteric dysfunction related to pelvic muscle or nerve damage (common after childbirth). History and physical examination should be useful in distinguishing patients with fecal incontinence related to a neurologic disorder, such as a spinal cord lesion or cerebral infarction, or to previous trauma such as anal surgery or vaginal delivery. A major differentiation that must be made in patients with fecal incontinence is whether there is overflow incontinence induced by a rectal impaction or loss of anal sphincter function. Patients with overflow incontinence often present with diarrhea and should respond to rectal evacuation. A commonly used method of examination of fecal incontinence is anorectal manometry. This test allows measurement of anal canal pressure, rectal sensation, and rectal compliance. During the test, perianal sensation is examined to exclude the presence of a spinal cord lesion.

Treatment options include intermittent fecal disimpaction, a trial of nonflatus-producing fiber supplements (calcium polycarbophil or methylcellulose), loperamide hydrochloride (interferes with propagating contractions and increases anal sphincter pressure), or a trial of a bile acid-binding agent (such as cholestyramine). Recently reported successes in the use of anorectal neuromuscular retraining by biofeedback for treatment of fecal incontinence encourage the performance of anorectal manometry in patients with fecal incontinence that is potentially related to loss of anal sphincter function.

References

1. Shaker R. Oropharyngeal dysphagia: Practical approach to diagnosis and management. Semin Gastrointest Dis 1992; 3(3):115–128.
2. Shaker R, Lang IM. Effect of aging on the deglutitive oral, pharyngeal, and esophageal motor function. Dysphagia 1994; 9(4):221–228.
3. Bird T, Hall MR, Schade RO. Gastric histology and its relation to anaemia in the elderly. Gerontology 1977; 23:309–321.
4. Ihamaki T, Kekki M, Sipponen P, et al. The sequelae and course of chronic gastritis during a 30- to 34-year bioptic follow-up study. Scand J Gastroenterol 1985; 20:485–491.
5. Lovat LB. Age related changes in gut physiology and nutritional status. Gut 1996; 38:306–309.
6. Soll AH. Gastric, duodenal, and stress ulcer. *In* Sleisenger MH, Fordtran JS (eds): Gastrointestinal Disease. Pathophysiology/Diagnosis/Management, 5th ed. Vol. 1. Philadelphia, W.B. Saunders, 1993, pp. 596–597.
7. Crook JN, Gray LW Jr, Nance FC, et al. Upper gastrointestinal bleeding. Ann Surg 1972; 175:771.
8. Logan RFA, Finlayson NDC. Death in acute upper gastrointestinal bleeding. Can endoscopy reduce mortality? Lancet 1976; 1:1173.
9. Masson J, Bremley P, McKnight G, et al. Specialized bleeding units are the logical way forward in the management of upper gastrointestinal hemorrhage: A two year prospective study. Gut 1995; 37:A162.
10. Silverstein FE, Gilbert DA, Tedesco FJ, et al. The national ASGE survey on upper gastrointestinal bleeding II. Clinical prognostic factors. Gastrointest Endosc 1981; 27:80–93.
11. Rockall TA, Logan RFA, Devlin HB, et al. Risk assessment after acute upper gastrointestinal hemorrhage. Gut 1996; 38:316–321.
12. Anand BS, Vij JC, Mac HS, et al. Effect of aging on the pancreatic ducts: A study based on endoscopic retrograde pancreatography. Gastrointest Endosc 1989; 35:210–212.
13. Jones SN, McNeil NI, Lees WR. The interpretation of retrograde pancreatography in the elderly. Clin Radiol 1989; 40:393–396.
14. Vellas B, Balas D, Moreau J, et al. Exocrine pancreatic secretion in the elderly. Int J Pancreatol 1988; 3:497–502.
15. Fernandez-del Castillo C, Harringer W, Warshaw AL, et al. Risk factors for pancreatic cellular injury after cardiopulmonary bypass. N Engl J Med 1991; 325:382–387.
16. Browder W, Patterson MD, Thompson JL, et al. Acute pancreatitis of unknown etiology in the elderly. Ann Surg 1993; 217:469–475.
17. Neoptolemos JP, London NJ, James D, et al. Controlled trial of urgent endoscopic retrograde cholangiopancreatography and endoscopic sphincterotomy versus conservative treatment for acute pancreatitis due to gallstones. Lancet 1988; 1:979–983.
18. Fan ST, Lai ECS, Mok FPT, et al. Early treatment of acute biliary pancreatitis by endoscopic papillotomy. N Engl J Med 1993; 328:268–279.
19. Nagai H, Ohtsubo K. Pancreatic lithiasis in the aged. Gastroenterology 1984; 86:331–338.
20. Lowenfels AB, Maisonneuve P, Cavallini G, et al. Pancreatitis and the risk of pancreatic cancer. N Engl J Med 1993; 328:1433–1437.
21. Bansal P, Sonnenberg A. Pancreatitis and the risk of pancreatic cancer. Gastroenterology 1995; 109:247–251.
22. Wynne HA, Cope LH, Mutch W, et al. The effect of age upon liver volume and apparent liver blood flow in healthy man. Hepatology 1989; 9:297–301.
23. Tauchi H, Sato T. Age changes in size and number of mitochondria of human hepatic cells. J Gerontol 1968; 23:454–461.
24. Fortner JG, Lincer RM. Hepatic resection in the elderly. Ann Surg 1990; 211:141–145.
25. Almdal TP, Sorensen TIA, and the Danish Association for the Study of the Liver. Incidence of parenchymal liver disease in Denmark, 1981 to 1985: Analysis of hospitalization registry data. Hepatology 1991; 13:650–655.
26. Garagliana CF, Lillenfeld AM, Mendelhof AI. Incidence of liver cirrhosis and related diseases in Baltimore and selected areas of the United States. J Chronic Dis 1979; 32:543–554.
27. Potter JR, James OFW. Clinical features and prognosis of alcoholic liver disease in respect of advancing age. Gerontology 1987; 33:380–387.

28. Bouchier IAD, Hislop WS, Prescott RJ. A prospective study of alcoholic liver disease and mortality. J Hepatol 1992; 16:290–297.

29. Ludwig J, Baggenstoss AH. Cirrhosis of the aged and senile cirrhosis—Are there two conditions? J Gerontol 1970; 25:244–248.

30. Pirsch JD, Kalayoglu M, D'Alessandro AM, et al. Orthotopic liver transplantation in patients 60 years of age and older. Transplantation 1991; 51:431–433.

31. Talley NJ, Zinsmeister AR, Van Dyke C, Melton LJ III. Epidemiology of colonic symptoms and the irritable bowel syndrome. Gastroenterology 1991; 101:927–934.

32. Sonnenberg A, Koch TR. Epidemiology of constipation in the United States. Dis Colon Rectum 1989; 32:1–8.

33. Barry MJ, Mulley AG, Richter JM. Effect of workup strategy on the cost-effectiveness of fecal occult blood screening for colorectal cancer. Gastroenterology 1987; 93:301–310.

34. Lederle FA, Busch DL, Mattox KM, West MJ, Aske DM. Cost-effective treatment of constipation in the elderly: A randomized double-blind comparison of sorbitol and lactulose. Am J Med 1990; 89:597–601.

35. Van Baal JG, Leguit P, Brummelkamp WH. Relaxation biofeedback conditioning as treatment of a disturbed defecation reflex. Dis Colon Rectum 1984; 27:187–189.

36. Madoff RD, Williams JG, Caushaj PF. Fecal incontinence. N Engl J Med 1992; 326:1002–1007.

47 Gynecologic Disorders

Marsha Smith, M.D.

In every adult age group, females now outnumber males, reversing the ratio at the beginning of the twentieth century. For generations the average age at menopause has remained stable at 50 years while women's life expectancy in the United States has increased.[1] At age 65 a woman may anticipate living an additional 18 years, and a 75-year-old woman may expect to live to age 85.[2] At present one third of American women are postmenopausal and will be postmenopausal for a third of their lifetime. Today 20% of the female population of the United States are aged 65 years or older; at the end of the twentieth century, 60% of the United States population aged 65 and over will be women, and they will account for 70% of a primary physician's practice. Appropriate care for this population requires an understanding of medical problems related to aging in general and female endocrine decline in particular, a combination of both geriatric and gynecologic knowledge.

Women are more frequent utilizers of the health care system than their male counterparts.[3] Of women over age 65, 88% saw a physician during the past 12 months[3]; 75% of women in this age group visit a physician an average of five times a year; and 85% see general internists and family practitioners rather than gynecologists for their routine gynecologic care.[3]

Older women commonly fail to undergo routine gynecologic examination and screening procedures, and when a gynecologic problem is diagnosed, they have been symptomatic for an average of 8.3 months and have had no pelvic examination for an average of 4.5 years.[4]

Only recently has there been consensus regarding recommendations for the periodic gynecologic examination of women. Medicare first began coverage for Papanicolaou (Pap) smear screening for cervical cancer in 1990.[5, 6] The National Cancer Institute (NCI) set a goal of 80% to 90% participation by women in triennial Pap screening by the year 2000. In 1988, NCI, American Cancer Society (ACS), American Med-

ical Association (AMA), and American College of Obstetricians and Gynecologists (ACOG) published a consensus recommendation of triennial Pap smear screening with no age limit after two negative sequential Pap smears. An annual pelvic examination as part of a periodic health examination permits evaluation of pelvic organs for which effective screening modalities do not exist. At present, between 50% and 80% of American women aged 65 years and older have had inadequate Pap screening according to these consensus criteria.[7, 8]

The present population of American women over age 65 may represent a unique cohort. These women were born prior to the emergence of gynecology as a recognized medical specialty, were post–reproductive age when Pap smear cytologic screening as part of an annual gynecologic examination became routine, and were postmenopausal when estrogen replacement therapy was introduced. The present cohort never established the habit of regular gynecologic care and hesitate to accept hormone replacement therapy.

The older female patient has medical problems resulting in morbidity and disabilities that negatively impact quality of life. Many of these problems have an underlying gynecologic etiology and, with appropriate attention to gynecologic history and examination, can be prevented or diagnosed and treated. Up to 30% of postmenopausal women have undiagnosed gynecologic problems.[9]

AGE-RELATED CHANGES OF THE FEMALE REPRODUCTIVE SYSTEM

The female endocrine system is the only endocrine system with a physiologically discernible decrease in function. This age-related change occurs at three levels: the ovarian or endocrine organ level, the estrogen or circulating hormone level, and the target organ level. Both intrapelvic and extrapelvic target organs are affected. Decreased ovarian function and decreased circulating estrogen result in short-term acute symptoms and long-term chronic disease. There is now abundant epidemiologic and clinical evidence to suggest that menopause induces specific deficiencies that can be alleviated or even prevented by appropriate estrogen replacement therapy.

Atrophic changes secondary to a decrease in circulating estrogen occur in all tissues with estrogen receptors. This change, characterized by a decrease in vascular and adipose tissue and an increase in fibrous tissue, results in smaller target organ size. A loss of follicle number and responsiveness occurs in the ovary, and the sclerotic ovary atrophies to a size of $1.5 \times 1.0 \times 0.5$ cm on average, which is not palpable. Physiologic enlargement and functional cysts should not be present in postmenopausal ovaries.

The vagina becomes pale, shortened, and narrowed, with weakened walls. Vaginal tissues become thin, dry, and shiny, with scant discharge and decreased lubrication. Decreased glycogen deposition in the superficial vaginal epithelium results in a decrease of lactic and acetic acids, and the vaginal pH changes from acidic (3.8–4.2) to alkaline (6.5–7.5). Recognizable mucosal layers (basal, intermediate, and superficial) are lost, as demonstrated by a vaginal maturation smear. A combination of disuse and estrogen deprivation results in introital stenosis.

The vulvar skin becomes thin, and there is increased keratinization and sparse hair growth. The vulvar mucosa decreases in thickness, with atrophy of the subcutaneous fat, loss of vascularity, and decreased secretion by the vestibular glands. The uterus reverts to the cervical-to-fundal childhood ratio of 2:1 and decreases in overall size until it is no longer palpable in women over age 75. The flattened, retracted, and pale cervix is often difficult to isolate and identify, and the squamocolumnar junction recedes within the stenosing cervix. The bladder and urethral mucosa, of embryologic origin similar to that of other female genital organs, contain estrogen receptors and also undergo atrophic changes.

Estrogen-dependent tissues outside the pelvis are also affected. Estrogen receptors have been identified in the skin, which becomes thin with decreased collagen; hair follicles; and sebaceous and sweat glands, resulting in dryness and decreased resilience due to estrogen deprivation. Estrogen receptors are present in bone, and decreased estrogen availability results in a negative calcium balance and increased bone resorption. The estrogen receptor–rich breasts lose connective tissue, and adipose tissue replaces the glandular breast tissue. Decreased estrogen levels are associated with increased levels of lipoproteins, particularly cholesterol and low-density lipoproteins, and estrogen receptors have been identified in vascular endothelium. There also appears to be a direct as well as an indirect central nervous system response to decreased estrogen, resulting in insomnia, depression, and possibly some cognitive decline.

Postmenopausally there is increased peripheral conversion of androgen into estrone, a weak estrogen. Estrogen levels fall to approximately 20% of the reproductive level, and progesterone levels fall by 60%. The androgen-to-estrogen ratio shifts in favor of the androgenic steroids.

CLINICAL APPROACH

A lifetime plan of health care for women should be established prior to menopause and should anticipate these changes. Good gynecologic care of the elderly patient requires documentation of relevant medical and gynecologic history, adequate examination, and recommendation of appropriate screening.

History

Special problems make it difficult to obtain a gynecologic history from the older patient, further emphasizing the advantage of adequate earlier medical records. Medical records may be inaccessible and family members may not know relevant gynecologic history when an older patient is unable or unwilling to recount her history owing to cognitive decline or generational modesty. A history of complicated or uncomplicated pregnancy and delivery, prior gynecologic disease and surgery, and hormonal or radiation therapy should be sought. Prior to 1960, subtotal or supracervical hysterectomy was common, and 30% of women reporting "total hysterectomy" are found to have remaining cervical stumps.[10] From 30% to 70% of women reporting "hysterectomies" have an intact cervix and/or ovaries. Many women received radium therapy for control of abnormal uterine bleeding in the early twentieth century.

Prior Pap smear screening and mammography should be recorded. Family history, particularly of endocrine-related malignancy, may be contributory. Symptoms such as dyspareunia, incontinence, bleeding, discharge, or itching may direct attention to particular gynecologic problems.

Examination

The periodic gynecologic visit should include measurements of height, weight, blood pressure, and pulse, and examination of the thyroid, breast, abdomen, pelvis, and rectum. It is often necessary to persuade the older woman of the benefit of the pelvic examination. Adjustments must be made in the approach and equipment used for a gynecologic examination. A regular examination table with stirrups can be used for the majority of patients, but the traditional lithotomy position may be uncomfortable or impossible for some patients owing to arthritis, osteoporosis, or lack of cooperation or assistance. An automated examination table facilitates positioning, and examination may be adequately performed in the left lateral decubitus or Sims position. Necessary equipment includes proper-sized specula; a narrow 1.0- to 1.5-cm bivalve Pedersen speculum; and small, medium, and large Graves specula. A clear plastic anoscope is an appropriate alternative. A 2× to 4× magnifying glass improves vulvar examination. Atrophic change and a narrowed introital opening may preclude introduction of the narrowest speculum.

The bladder must be emptied. Examination of the pelvis begins with visual examination and palpation of the external perineal and vulvar tissues with the gloved hand. Descriptive mention should be made of the appearance of the mucosal tissues and the presence and location of any lesions. Separation of the labia may reveal the presence of a urethral caruncle, a benign erythematous protrusion of the urethral mucosa through the external urethral orifice, which is usually asymptomatic and requires no treatment. Any discharge can be sampled. Since lubricating gel compromises the cellular integrity of the cytologic specimen, warm water is used to facilitate introduction of an appropriate-sized speculum.

The speculum is inserted with closed blades parallel to the vaginal opening and gently turned while keeping pressure directed toward the rectum. When the speculum is opened the cervix will be in view unless narrowing of the vagina prevents adequate insertion. Despite introital narrowing and cervical stenosis in the postmenopausal female, over 90% of older women tolerate speculum examination and Pap screening. In older women the cervix is atrophic or friable and the os is stenotic.

When the transformation zone is visible, either a moistened cotton applicator or a plastic or wooden spatula may be used to obtain the cervical sample; without a visible transformation zone, a moistened cotton applicator, glass pipette, or Cytobrush should be used. A digitally directed "blind" Pap smear can be done. A saline-moistened cotton-tipped applicator can be inserted and an adequate Pap sample obtained without cervical trauma or bleeding. In the absence of a history suggesting cervical disease or a visible lesion, a single sampling of the squamocolumnar junction is adequate. Cervical cytology should

always be attempted, especially if prior sampling has been inadequate. The smear made on the microscope slide should be neither too thick nor too sparse to ensure accurate reading, and fixative should be applied immediately.

Rotate and remove the speculum slowly while viewing the entire vagina and especially the posterior wall. The vagina should be inspected for signs of atrophic vaginitis such as mucosal friability, petechiae, telangiectasia, and vaginal erosions. A cytologic maturation index showing 100% parabasal cells confirms atrophy, although not necessarily atrophic vaginitis.

Bimanual examination is adapted to the adequacy of the introitus. The uterus should be small, and the ovaries should not be palpable. The visible or palpable presence or absence of the cervix is recorded. Pelvic muscle laxity may cause a cystocele, enterocele, rectocele, or uterine prolapse. Using the examiner's finger that is inserted in the vagina, a single speculum blade, or a tongue blade, the physician should apply support sequentially to the anterior and posterior vaginal walls and ask the patient to cough or strain. Bulging of the anterior wall when the posterior wall is stabilized indicates a cystocele. Conversely, bulging of the posterior wall indicates a rectocele and/or enterocele. Rectovaginal examination permits evaluation of the thickness and condition of the rectovaginal septum, the presence of disease, and assessment of the cul-de-sac. Rectal examination is often the only means of assessing the pelvic organs. Stool should be tested for occult blood. Assessment for incontinence, bladder capacity, and post-void residual quantity may be done if indicated.

An integral part of adequate gynecologic care is careful discussion of the examination findings, recommendations for therapy, referral for specialized evaluation, and scheduling for follow-up and periodic examinations and screening procedures with the patient and involved family members.

BENIGN GYNECOLOGIC DISEASE

Eighty percent of gynecologic problems in women over 60 years of age are related to postmenopausal bleeding, vulvovaginal inflammations or infections, genital prolapse, or alterations in bladder function. Common gynecologic problems in older women include:

O Osteoporosis
V Voiding problems
A Atrophic change
R Relaxation of pelvic structures
I Inflammation and infection
A Abnormal bleeding
N Neoplasia

Atrophic Change

Atrophic changes occur during menopause in all tissues with estrogen receptors. Loss of rugae, thinning, pallor, and loss of elasticity are the common atrophic changes in the vaginal mucosa of aging women. Vulvar changes become apparent months or years after vaginal atrophy is first observed. The labia minora shrink in thickness and length and may be difficult to identify. The introitus may become narrow and rigid so that intercourse is painful or impossible. Decreased maturation of vaginal mucosal epithelium can lead to atrophic vaginitis with symptoms of burning, itching, bleeding, leukorrhea, and dyspareunia. Locally applied conjugated vaginal estrogen cream in a standard dose of 0.625 mg/g (1 to 4 g daily) is systemically absorbed. Lower doses of topical estrogen, 0.5 mg every third day, may provide relief with fewer systemic effects. Alternative regimens include 0.3 mg vaginal estrogen daily for 3 months, combined with periodic progesterone; a water-based lubricant; and dilute acetic or boric acid douches to restore an acidic vaginal pH. Estrogen deprivation can result in atrophy of bladder and urethral tissue, producing dysuria, urinary frequency, urgency, and incontinence. These symptoms also respond well to low-dose systemic and vaginal estrogen therapy. Restoration of genitourinary tissue function usually requires months of treatment.

Inflammations or Infections

An increased incidence of infection and vaginitis in older women is related to the higher vaginal pH and decreased structural resistance to infectious agents. The bacterial and fungal causes of vaginitis are similar to those in younger women and the evaluation and management are also essentially the same. Topical estrogen treatment alone or in combination with antibacterial or antifungal creams will reestablish a more resistant vaginal epithelium. Trichomoniasis is uncommon in postmenopausal patients, but monilial vulvovaginitis is more frequent, especially in the diabetic patient or one recently treated with antibiotics. Ascending pelvic infections and abscess formation are rare. Vulvovaginitis, simultaneous involvement of both vaginal and external vulvar tissues, is common, and combined therapy is most effective. Any dermatologic condition, such as psoriasis or seborrheic and contact dermatitis, may involve the vulva.

Abnormal Bleeding

Eighty percent of postmenopausal vaginal bleeding has a benign cause. Evaluation requires pelvic examination with Pap screening and endometrial sampling. Endometrial atrophy is found in 70% of these cases, endometrial hyperplasia in 15%, polyps in about 9%, and uterine sarcoma or other lesions in about 1% of cases.[11]

Relaxation of Pelvic Structures

The endopelvic fascia, uterosacral and cardinal ligaments, and levator ani muscles, which support the pelvic organs, become weakened owing to obstetric trauma, obesity, strenuous activity, and atrophic change, resulting in relaxation of pelvic structures. Uterine prolapse is described according to the degree of descent of the uterus. The cervix presents at the introitus in first-degree prolapse, the cervix and half of the uterus protrude through the introitus with second-degree prolapse, and the entire uterus is exposed and the vaginal walls everted in third-degree prolapse or procidentia. Symptoms of prolapse are a sensation of pelvic heaviness or vaginal mass, back pain, urinary incontinence, or bleeding of the exposed mucosal tissues. Mild relaxation may be treated with Kegel exercises to increase the muscle tone of the pelvic floor.

Vaginal surgery is the usual therapy for complete uterine prolapse, but when surgery is medically contraindicated a trial of a pessary for support is practical. A ring or doughnut pessary treats prolapse by applying pressure in all directions on the vaginal wall and lifting the uterus into the pelvis and holding it there. Inflatable pessaries are easier to insert and remove. After insertion of a pessary, the patient must be reexamined within 24 hours to assess proper placement and effectiveness and to rule out discomfort or urinary obstruction or retention. Mucosal tissues may be protected by intermittent vaginal application of estrogen cream. Pessary care includes periodic removal and cleansing, pelvic examination, and replacement with a new pessary as needed.

Cystocele or prolapse of the bladder commonly accompanies or precedes uterine prolapse. Symptoms include a sensation of vaginal fullness or a palpable mass protruding from the vagina. Recurrent cystitis due to incomplete bladder emptying, urinary incontinence, or vaginal ulceration due to exposed mucosal tissues may necessitate surgical repair. Urethrocele or eversion of the urethral mucosa with inflammation or bleeding may occur at the same time as the cystocele. Symptomatic urethroceles may benefit from topical application of estrogen. A large rectocele or bulging of the posterior wall of the vagina may result in incomplete stool evacuation.

Voiding Problems

There is an increased incidence of urinary tract infection in older women due to increased vulnerability of atrophic tissues to bacterial invasion and to an increase in residual urine after voiding. Symptoms include frequency and pain or burning with urination. When recurrent urethritis occurs without a dominant causative organism, local estrogen therapy may be helpful.

Women over age 65 commonly suffer incontinence (see Chapter 18). Incontinence may exist without a cystocele; likewise, pelvic floor muscle laxity, even when present, may not be the cause of incontinence. Stress incontinence is best assessed with a provocative stress test. With a full bladder, the standing patient provides a single, vigorous cough. The patient is monitored for urine leakage. A false-negative result may occur if the patient does not relax, if the bladder is not full, if the cough is not strong, or if the test is conducted in the upright position in a woman with a large cystocele. In the last case, the test should be repeated in the supine position with the cystocele reduced. Urethrovesical pressure dynamic studies indicate that the mechanism of continence in significant uterovaginal prolapse is urethral obstruction.

Doughnut pessaries used to replace the prolapse may cause the previously continent patient to become incontinent. The doughnut replaces a prolapsed uterus but gives no support to the proximal urethra. Lever pessaries applied behind the pubic arch support the proximal urethra. Smith and Hodge–type pessaries promote increases in the functional length and closing pressure of the urethra without causing obstruction. Pessaries may be used as temporizing measures prior to surgical vaginal repair or as definitive treatment when surgery is contraindicated. The aged, the frail, and the disabled are unfortunately also those most likely to develop complications from pessary use, such as embedment, incarceration, and, rarely, fistulae from poorly fitted, infrequently monitored, or forgotten pessaries.

MALIGNANT GYNECOLOGIC DISEASE

At the 1995 American Cancer Society National Conference on Gynecologic Cancers significant progress was noted in overall diagnosis and treatment during the past 25 years; however, there was a relative lack of progress for older patients.[12] The incidence of all gynecologic cancers increases with increasing age.[4, 13] Twenty-seven percent of cervical cancer, 45% of endometrial cancer, and 43% of ovarian cancer occur over age 65.[13] Forty-four percent of breast cancer,[14] 65% of vulvar cancer,[13] and 57% of vaginal cancer[13] also occur in this age group.

Cancer Detection

The most common gynecologic malignancies in older women are similar to those in the general population. Cancer of the corpus uteri is the most common,[15] with cancers of the ovary and cervix following second and third, respectively. Surveillance, Epidemiology, and End Results (SEER) data show that 81% of gynecologic cancers in elderly women originate in the uterine corpus or ovary, making these two malignancies by far the most common gynecologic malignancies for this age group.[4, 13] The risk of a woman over age 65 developing ovarian, endometrial, or cervical cancer compared with women aged 40 to 65 is nearly three times as high for ovarian cancer, nearly twice as high for uterine cancer, and 10% higher for cervical cancer.[16]

Diagnosis of gynecologic cancer in the elderly occurs at a more advanced stage. Early-stage ovarian cancer has few symptoms and is very difficult to diagnose, so the majority of patients present with advanced-stage disease. At present the bimanual pelvic examination remains the most cost-effective means of diagnosis, but it is not sensitive enough for the detection of early disease. Two diagnostic modalities are under active investigation: tumor marker CA-125 and sonography.[11] Annual endometrial sampling or transvaginal ultrasound for screening asymptomatic women for endometrial cancer is not cost-effective either, although it may identify women at increased risk.[11, 17]

Cervical cytology (Pap smear) screening, introduced over 50 years ago, is effective in detecting preinvasive disease and has resulted in a dramatic decrease in the incidence and mortality of invasive cervical cancer. Owing to regular pelvic examinations with Pap screening, there has been a 70% decrease in age-adjusted cancer death rates for carcinoma of the cervix in the last 30 years. The Pap smear false-negative rate of 20% may be higher in elderly women because of the difficulty encountered in adequately sampling the squamocolumnar junction within the endocervical canal. Forty percent of elderly women in this country have never had a Pap smear,[18] and older women who have Pap smear screening have two to three times the number of abnormal smears.[18] Because of the cervix's unique accessibility, 90% of cervical cancer can and should be detected early with a Pap smear.

Endometrial Cancer

Carcinoma of the endometrium is the most common gynecologic cancer in elderly women. About 45% of cases are diagnosed over age 65, and 36% over age 75. Adenocarcinoma of the endometrium occurs along a continuum from cystic hyperplasia to adenomatous hyperplasia to atypia to early carcinoma to frank carcinoma. Adenomatous hyperplasia is known to antedate adenocarcinoma in 25% to 30% of cases. Women at risk include those with a family history of genital cancer and those exhibiting the characteristics of Saint's triad of obesity, hypertension, and diabetes mellitus. Other associations are persistent anovulatory bleeding, chronic liver disease, pelvic irradiation for benign conditions, nulliparity, and late menopause.

The initial symptom, postmenopausal bleeding, occurs early in the spectrum of the disease. Almost all have abnormal vaginal bleeding—serosanguineous to frank bleeding—with pyometra and hematometra if a stenosed cervical canal obstructs uterine drainage. Up to 50% of endometrial carcinoma is picked up on Pap screening. Pain occurs late with advanced disease. Diagnosis is made by endometrial sampling and dilation and curettage (D&C), and endocervical curettage is performed to determine tumor extent. From 85% to 90% of cases will still be confined to the uterus at the time of diagnosis. Prognosis is encouraging because of early diagnosis and precise treatment selection. Although accounting for 50% of all new female genital cancer, endometrial carcinoma is responsible for only 23% of gynecologic cancer deaths because its diagnosis is usually made early. The age-adjusted death rate has decreased 50% over the past 30 years.

The etiologic role of estrogen in the development of adenocarcinoma of the endometrium is established. While the source of estrogen may be polycystic ovarian disease or hormone-producing ovarian tumors (granulosa cell/thecoma), the most common source in postmenopausal women is unopposed exogenous estrogen. An increased incidence of endometrial adenocarcinoma was noted in the early 1970s among women receiving estrogen replacement therapy. We now recognize that unopposed estrogen replacement therapy increases the risk of endometrial cancer by two to ten times, the increase in risk directly related to dosage and duration of therapy and continuing for up to 10 years after discontinuation.[19] Lower estrogen dosage and the addition of cyclic progestogens significantly reduce this risk. Progestational agents reverse adenomatous hyperplasia and carcinoma in situ and may also be used in advanced disease to control vaginal bleeding and decrease metastasis. Estrogen replacement therapy has been prescribed without increasing the recurrence rate after treatment of Stage I adenocarcinoma of the endometrium.[17, 20]

Cervical Cancer

The incidence of all cervical cancers increases up to the last decade of life[15]; the increased incidence in older women reflects diagnosis in symptomatic women rather than screening in asymptomatic women. About 27% of cases of carcinoma of the cervix occur after the age of 65 years; 25% of new diagnoses of invasive cervical cancer are made in women over age 65 years, and of these, 65% had never had Pap smear screening.[21] Only 37% of women over age 65 had a Pap smear within 12 months,[10] and slightly more than 50% of women aged 65 and older have had a Pap smear within the past 3 years.[5]

Ninety-five percent of cervical carcinoma is of squamous cell type arising in the transformation zone. Similar to endometrial carcinoma, squamous cell carcinoma develops along a spectrum from cervical dysplasia to in situ to invasive disease. Forty percent progress from carcinoma in situ to invasive carcinoma within 1 to 20 years (average, 10 years). It is not known if the conversion rate increases with age. Women at highest risk have included those younger than age 18 at first coitus, those with multiple sex partners or a partner with multiple partners, smokers, and those with a history of sexually transmitted disease, particularly human papillomavirus or herpes simplex.

Early disease is asymptomatic; the first sign is commonly an abnormal Pap smear. There may be vaginal spotting, usually postcoital, or discharge with early invasion; pain rarely occurs until spread to the vagina or secondary infection occurs. Frequency, urgency, rectal tenesmus, or rectal bleeding are late manifestations. Low back pain and leg pain result from compression of lumbosacral nerves.

Carcinoma of the cervix is the only gynecologic cancer preventable by screening. The frequency of screening and the age at which to discontinue screening are subjects of controversy. Following two negative smears there is low risk for at least 5 years, while screening every three years between the ages of 25 and 64 provides 95% maximal protection. There have been no prospective trials of cervical cancer screening examination in the elderly, but Pap smear sensitivity is unaltered by age. False-positives may be due to atrophic change. Before age 65 an abnormal smear indicates invasive cervical cancer in 1 of 30 positive smears; after age 65 this rate increases to 1 of 5.[21]

Five-year survival for Stage I cervical carcinoma treated with surgery or irradiation is 85% to 90%; there is no difference in survival by stage among older women. From 1973–1974 to 1986–1987, mortality from carcinoma of the cervix decreased 17% in women over age 50 and decreased 43% in women under age 50.

Ovarian Cancer

Ovarian carcinoma accounts for 52% of all gynecologic cancer deaths, and the age-adjusted death rate has remained stable for the past 30 years.[22, 23] Fifty percent of cases are diagnosed after age 65 and 12% after 75 years of age.[11] Three distinct hereditary patterns have been described: ovarian cancer alone, ovarian and breast cancers, and ovarian and colon cancers. However, 90% to 95% of ovarian cancer is of sporadic occurrence. Signs and symptoms are vague gastrointestinal discomfort and abdominal swelling, pelvic pressure, mild constipation, abdominal mass, weakness, and weight loss.

Ovarian cancer should be suspected in 40- to 69-year-old women with persistent undiagnosed gastrointestinal symptoms. Often asymptomatic in the early stages, most patients have widespread disease at the time of diagnosis. About 75% of cases are diagnosed late[10, 24]; 75% present with an abdominal mass and 50% with ascites. The annual pelvic examination of asymptomatic women yields one early ovarian carcinoma per 10,000 routine pelvic examinations. A finding of adenocarcinoma cells on Pap screening, with negative evaluation of vulva, vagina, cervix, and endometrium, indicates ovarian, tubal, or other intra-abdominal carcinoma. Routine ultrasound is helpful in the obese or uncooperative patient.

Postmenopausal palpable ovarian syndrome (PPOS) is a term applied to palpable ovaries on bimanual pelvic examination of postmenopausal women, especially after the age of 70 years. The high risk of malignancy in this age group requires immediate investigation; however, only 10% of patients with PPOS subjected to oophorectomy may have malignant ovarian neoplasm.[25] It has been recommended that all perimenopausal women have bilateral oophorectomy at the time of pelvic surgery for benign disease. The five-year survival rate for ovarian carcinoma is 25% and has been unchanged for decades. The death rate increases with age, with peak mortality occurring at ages 80 to 84 years.

Vulvar Cancer

Vulvar dystrophies as well as vulvar neoplasia increase in frequency with advancing age. Any woman with perineal complaints should undergo careful inspection of the vulva, followed by a biopsy of any suspicious lesion. Until histologically proven otherwise, all vulvar lesions must be suspected of being malignant. Lesions may be pigmented or white and vary in appearance depending on local factors such as excoriation and hygiene. White lesions were previously called "leukoplakia," erroneously implying premalignant or malignant disease; the whiteness, however, indicates hyperkeratotic skin with loss of skin pigment and decreased vascularity. Atypia occurs in only 5%; nevertheless, all should be biopsied. All dark lesions must be excised to detect atypia and melanoma.

At the time of presentation, approximately 3% to 5% of women with vulvar lesions have invasive carcinoma. A 1% aqueous solution of toluidine blue dye fixes to cell nuclei. A 1% aqueous acetic acid solution applied 3 minutes after the dye decolorizes unbound dye. Since there are no surface nuclei on normal vulva, no blue stain remains on normal skin surface. Nuclei may be present, however, in both benign and malignant lesions. Toluidine blue–directed biopsies may be done following local infiltration of 1% lidocaine, using a Keyes dermal punch or disposable Baker's biopsy punch. Local hemostasis is achieved with silver nitrate.

The lesion of lichen sclerosus with its thinned epithelium is distinct from that of hyperplastic dystrophy. In patients with lichen sclerosus the lesions appear as white to pale pink flat macules, often coalesced into plaques, and the skin is dry and scaly with many fine wrinkles. Approximately 30% of patients with lichen sclerosus have mixed dystrophies with foci of hyperplastic dystrophy. At the time of the initial biopsy, nuclear atypia is observed in 4% to 8% of the dystrophic areas. These lesions should be completely excised because they are associated with premalignant potential. A helpful distinction is between itching and burning. Pruritus or itching represents atrophic change secondary to decreased estrogen, infection, or lichen sclerosus. Burning represents hypertrophy, atypia, in situ carcinoma, or Paget's disease. Hyperplastic dystrophy is treated with corticosteroids to promote dermal atrophy. The treatment of choice for lichen sclerosus is topical testosterone propionate 1% or 2% applied two to three times daily for 6 weeks or until pruritus is relieved. Until proven otherwise, an enlargement of the Bartholin gland should be considered malignant.

Vulvar carcinoma is most frequent in the 60- to 70-year-old age group and peaks at age 85. Sixty-five percent of cases occur over age 65 and 19% of cases over age 75. Elderly women may be embarrassed and thus delay evaluation, eventually presenting with bleeding and foul discharge. The majority (90%) of vulvar carcinoma is squamous cell[26]; melanoma, sarcoma, and Paget's disease of the vulva occur less frequently. In 20% to 30% of patients with Paget's disease there is associated invasive adenocarcinoma of sweat glands, and women with this disease are at high risk for adenocarcinoma of the breast, colon, cervix, and uterus. Risk factors for vulvar carcinoma include chronic vulvar irritation; vulvar dystrophies, especially with atypia; granulomatous disease of the vulva; venereal disease; and preinvasive or invasive cancer of the cervix. Early symptoms include pruritus, a persisting lump, a nonbleeding ulcer, or burning with urination. Late symptoms are pain and bleeding. There appears to be a 20-year interval between preinvasive and invasive disease of the vulva, a slower progression than in vaginal or cervical neoplasia.

Other Cancers

Fifty-seven percent of cases of vaginal cancer occur after age 65 and 7% of cases after age 75. Primary vaginal carcinoma is rare and occurs most often in the upper half of the vagina, usually involving the posterior vaginal wall; 19% of these are missed on initial examination. Most vaginal cancer is metastatic carcinoma by direct invasion from bladder, vulva, or cervix or by blood and lymphatic spread from the uterus or, rarely, kidney, breast, or colon. Preinvasive vaginal cancer is asymptomatic. Early invasive cancer causes vaginal bleeding or foul vaginal discharge. A large infected lesion causes rectal or bladder pain; a lesion near the bladder or urethra causes urinary tract symptoms. The average duration of symptoms before diagnosis is 7.4 months, and 68% of lesions are greater than 2 cm when diagnosed. Diagnosis is made by a Pap smear of the vagina, colposcopy, or biopsy. Risk factors include low socioeconomic status, papilloma, early hysterectomy, previous abnormal Pap, and prior radiation therapy.

Fallopian tube carcinoma is the least common gynecologic cancer. Undiagnosed abnormal bleeding in the absence of endometrial disease may indicate this rare cancer. Tubal obstruction leads to crampy unilateral lower abdominal pain with a watery or blood-tinged discharge. The differential diagnosis of a palpable or sonographic adnexal mass includes fallopian tube carcinoma.

Cancer Management

Four factors determine gynecologic cancer outcome in elderly patients: the relationship of age to provision of gynecologic care, the relationship of age to the stage of cancer at time of diagnosis, the relationship of age to the first course of cancer treatment, and the relationship of age to mortality rate.

Elderly women receive less gynecologic care.[10] Leventhal reported women over age 65 had fewer clinical breast examinations, and only 16% of mammograms were performed in women over age 60.[27] Mammographic screening of elderly women, which is covered by Medicare, could potentially decrease breast cancer mortality by as much as 30%. There is a documented age-related decrease in routine gynecologic examination[4, 18] as well as recommendation of Pap screening and mammography among all physicians providing care to women.[7, 27, 28] The percentage of tumors localized at diagnosis decreases significantly with advancing age for uterine, ovarian, and cervical cancers.[10, 29, 30, 31]

Treatment modality is related to the site of origin of the gynecologic cancer and the stage of disease at diagnosis. Thirty-seven percent of women over 75 years of age had therapy modified by age or medical condition.[4] SEER data show that 76% of women receiving no therapy for ovarian cancer were aged 65 or older, and these patients were more likely to be treated with single rather than multiple modality therapy.[32] Ninety percent of older women could have standard surgical procedures with similar minor postoperative complication rates, similar mean inpatient statistics, and the same morbidity, mortality, and 5-year survival rates; therefore, surgery should not be withheld based on age alone.[33] Those at greatest surgical therapy risk are often referred for radiation therapy, which carries significant morbidity. Many elderly patients receive less than optimal chemotherapy or radiotherapy owing to the misconception that they cannot tolerate such treatment (see Chapter 36). The elderly are also less likely to be included in investigational drug programs and more likely to have dosage modification or to receive palliative rather than curative therapy. Subjects aged over 70 years have been excluded from prospective randomized studies.

Survival probability is also related to the site of origin of the gynecologic cancer and the stage of disease at diagnosis. As age increases, survival within stage was found to decrease in cancers in all sites.[37] The National Cancer Institute reported a decline in cancer mortality in those women under age 54 years but an increase in mortality in those over age 65.[16] Mortality statistics showing an increased risk of gynecologic cancer–related deaths in older women cannot be explained on the basis of increased incidence alone.[10] Mortality-to-incidence ratios for each of these malignancies rises with age, suggesting that prognosis is worse. Women aged 65 years and older have a 50% greater risk of dying of their disease, and for those over 85, the mortality-to-incidence ratio is 0.9.[16]

ESTROGEN REPLACEMENT THERAPY

Hormone replacement therapy has been tried since the ancient Egyptians used "glandular therapy." Estrogen was isolated in the 1920s, and diethylstilbestrol (DES) was synthesized in the 1930s. Unopposed estrogen use in the 1970s led to an unanticipated increase in endometrial carcinoma. Current estrogen replacement is at lower doses on an intermittent schedule, with progesterone added for endometrial protection.

Indications for hormone replacement therapy (HRT) are related to signs and symptoms of estrogen deficiency, such as atrophy of genitourinary tissues; osteoporosis prophylaxis and treatment; and prevention of cardiovascular morbidity and mortality. Estrogen benefit for atrophic change has been discussed. Cardiovascular disease in older women results in morbidity and mortality similar to that in older men but with a 10-year delay in coronary heart disease and a 20-year delay in myocardial infarction[38] because of premenopausal advantages of higher high-density lipoprotein levels and lower low-density lipoprotein levels.[39]

Risks of HRT are hypertension because of estrogen's effect on the renin/angiotensin system; thromboembolic disease due to increased clotting factors V, VII, and VIII (prothrombin and partial prothrombin time are not affected); increased gallbladder disease; and an increased incidence of endometrial carcinoma. The effect on breast tissue is still controversial. The largest case-control study from the Centers for Disease Control and Prevention (CDC), the Cancer and Steroid Hormone (CASH) study, and the largest cohort study, the Nurses' Health Study, failed to find a link between breast cancer and the use of estrogen for up to 20 years.[40, 41] Absolute contraindications to estrogen replacement are thromboembolic disease, undiagnosed vaginal bleeding, abnormal liver function tests, hormone-dependent tumor, and an acute vascular event. Relative contraindications are obesity, hypertension, fibrocystic disease, uterine fibroids, migraine, familial hyperlipemia, gallbladder disease, endometriosis, and smoking. Side effects include nausea, mastalgia, and bleeding.

Oral estrogen preparations are not physiologic. Estradiol is metabolized in the gut and converted to estrone and does not restore the premeno-pausal estradiol-to-estrone ratio. The "first-pass effect," as the hormone passes via the portal vein to the liver, results in 35% to 95% of hormone conversion to estrone 3-glucuronide, which is inert. Transdermal administration overcomes both poor absorption and the hepatic first-pass effect while achieving higher plasma levels of hormone. Of women using the transdermal route, 30% report skin rash and 2% experience nausea.

Decisions on dosage level and route of administration must be individualized. There is no evidence that one form of estrogen is superior to another. More important are the duration and dose and the presence or absence of progestin. Combinations of estrogens and progestins may be used (e.g., 0.625 mg conjugated estrogen or 1 mg micronized estradiol with 2.5 mg medroxyprogesterone acetate or 0.35 mg norethindrone).[42] A 10-day minimum usage of the progestogen is essential for endometrial protection. Unopposed estrogen replacement therapy increases the risk of adenocarcinoma of the endometrium two- to tenfold.[42] With the addition of progestogen, no woman who received 10 or more days of progestogen developed hyperplasia, and no cases of adenomatous hyperplasia or cancer were reported. After 4 to 6 months, most biopsies show atrophic endometrium, and bleeding ceases in 80% to 90%.[42] This continuous approach maintains a beneficial lipoprotein pattern and increases the bone density in the spinal column. Relative potencies for bone conservation are:

> Estradiol: 2 mg daily
> Transdermal: 50 µg daily placed twice weekly
> Conjugated: 0.625 mg daily

Data indicate that the preventive health benefits of estrogen replacement therapy persist as long as use continues, but compliance statistics are disappointing. In one study, only 30% of the women complied with their prescribed estrogen regimen.[43] If all eligible women used estrogen, myocardial infarctions could be reduced as much as 45%,[42] with a 46% reduction in death from stroke.[44]

CONCLUSION

Cancer screening guidelines recommend annual clinical breast examinations, pelvic examination by bimanual palpation, digital rectal examination with stool guiac, and mammography. Triennial Pap smear cytology is adequate screening after three or more consecutive satisfactory annual normal examinations. An annual pelvic examination separate from the Pap test is recommended because, although new detection procedures are being evaluated, bimanual palpation of the ovaries is the only examination that currently meets the American Cancer Society's criteria of feasibility, practicality, reasonable cost, and low risk for evaluation of the adnexae.

Gynecologic examinations and Pap smears are the principal reasons for a decline in physician visits with advancing age, although significant morbidity and mortality continue owing to gynecologic disease. Physician failure adequately to address the gynecologic problems of women seen for other medical reasons represents missed opportunities to affect a woman's health and quality of life positively. Criteria appropriate for younger patients may not be suitable in the elderly, for whom effective stabilization of disease, a partial remission, or a complete remission of short duration may be sufficient to achieve worthwhile prolongation of life with an acceptable quality of life.

References

1. McKinlay SM, Brambilla DJ, Posner JG: The normal menopause transition. Maturitas 1992;14:103–115.
2. United States Bureau of the Census: Projections of the population of the United States—1977 to 2050. Current Population Reports Series P–25, No 704.
3. Mossey JM, Shapiro E: Physician use by the elderly over an eight-year period. Am J Public Health 1985;75:1333–1334.
4. Kennedy AW, Flagg JS, Webster KD: Gynecologic cancer in the very elderly. Gynecol Oncol 1989;32:49–54.
5. Power EJ: Cervical cancer screening in elderly women. JAMA 1990;263:2996.
6. Murata PJ, Li JE: Relationship between Pap smear performance and physician ordering a mammogram. J Fam Pract 1992;35:644–648.
7. Robie RW: Cancer screening in the elderly. J Am Geriatr Soc 1989;37:888–893.
8. Mayer JA, Slymen DJ, Drew JA, et al: Breast and cervical cancer screening in older women: The San Diego Medicare Preventive Health Project. Prev Med 1992;21:395–404.
9. Denny MS, Koren ME, Wisby M: Gynecological health needs of elderly women. J Geront Nurs 1989;15:33–38.
10. Grover SA, Cook EF, Adam J, et al: Delayed diagnosis of gynecologic tumors in elderly women: Relation to national medical practice patterns. Am J Med 1989;86:151–157.
11. McGonigle KF, Lagasse LD, Karlan BY: Ovarian, uterine, and cervical cancer in the elderly woman. Clin Geriatr Med 1993;9:115–130.
12. American Cancer Society: National Conference on Gynecologic Cancers, Washington, DC. Cancer (10 Suppl)1995;76:1883–2180.
13. Baranovsky A, Myers MH: Cancer incidence and survival in patients 65 years of age and older. CA 1986;36:26–41.
14. Miller CB: Screening the "well elderly." CA 1986;36:318–319.
15. Boring CC, Squires TS, Tong T: Cancer statistics. CA 1992;42:19–38.
16. National Cancer Institute: Annual Cancer Statistics Review, Including Cancer Trends: 1950–1985. Bethesda, MD, National Institutes of Health, 1989.
17. American College of Obstetricians and Gynecologists: Report of task force on routine cancer screening. ACOG Committee Opinion 68, Washington, DC, American College of Obstetricians and Gynecologists, 1989.
18. Mandelblatt J, Gopaul I, Wistreich M: Gynecological care of elderly women: Another look at Papanicolaou smear testing. JAMA 1986;256:367–371.
19. Paganini-Hill A, Ross RK, Henderson BEW: Endometrial cancer and patterns of use of estrogen replacement therapy: A cohort study. Br J Cancer 1989;59:445–447.
20. Creasman WT, Henderson D, Hinshaw W, et al: Estrogen replacement therapy in the patient treated for endometrial cancer. Obstet Gynecol 1986;67:326–330.
21. Parazzini F, Negri E, La Vecchia C, et al: Screening practices and invasive cervical cancer risk in different age strata. Gynecol Oncol 1990;38:76–80.
22. Edmonson JH, Su J, Krook JE: Treatment of ovarian cancer in elderly women. Cancer (2 Suppl) 1993;71:615–617.
23. American Medical Association Council on Scientific Affairs: Societal effects and other factors affecting health care for the elderly: Report of the Council on Scientific Affairs. Arch Intern Med 1990;150:1184–1189.
24. Tottolero-Luna G, Mitchell MF, Rhodes-Morris HE: Epidemiology and screening of ovarian cancer. Obstet Gynecol Clin North Am 1994;21:1–22.
25. Barber HR: Perimenopausal and Geriatric Gynecology. New York, Macmillan, 1988, pp. 87–96, 169–177.
26. Farias-Eisner R, Berek JS: Current management of invasive squamous carcinoma of the vulva. Clin Geriatr Med 1993;9(1):131–143.
27. Leventhal EA: The dilemma of cancer in the elderly. Front Radiat Ther Oncol 1986;20:1–13.
28. American Cancer Society 1989 Survey of Physicians' Attitudes and Practices in Early Cancer Detection. CA 1990;40:77–101.
29. Yancik R, Ries LG: Cancer in the aged: An epidemiologic perspective on treatment issues. Cancer 1991;68:2502–2510.
30. Goodwin JS, Samet JM, Key CR, et al: Stage of diagnosis of cancer varies with the age of the patient. J Am Geriatr Soc 1986;34:20–26.
31. Holmes FF, Hearne E: Cancer stage-to-age relationship: Implications for cancer screening in the elderly. J Am Geriatr Soc 1981;29:55–57.
32. Yancik R, Ries LG, Yates JW: Ovarian cancer in the elderly: An analysis of surveillance, epidemiology, and end results program data. Am J Obstet Gynecol 1986;154:639–647.
33. Levrant SG, Fruchter RG, Maiman M: Radical hysterectomy for cervical cancer: Morbidity and survival in relation to weight and age. Gynecol Oncol 1992;45:317–322.
34. Lawton FG, Hacker NF: Surgery for invasive gynecologic cancer in the elderly female population. Obstet Gynecol 1990;76:287–289.
35. Kinney WK, Egorshin EV, Podrate AC: Wertheim hysterectomy in the geriatric population. Gynecol Oncol 1988;31:227–232.
36. Matthews CM, Morris M, Burke TW, et al: Pelvic exenteration in the elderly patient. Obstet Gynecol 1992;79:773–777.
37. Kosary CL: FIGO stage, histology, histologic grade, age and race as prognostic factors in determining survival for cancers of the female gynecological system. Semin Surg Oncol 1994;10:31–46.

38. Kannel WB: Metabolic risk factors for coronary heart disease in women: Perspective from the Framingham Study. Am Heart J 1987;114:413–419.

39. Soler JT, Folsom AR, Kaye SA, et al: Associations of abdominal adiposity, fasting insulin, sex hormone binding globulin and estrogen with lipids and lipoproteins in post-menopausal women. Atherosclerosis 1989;79:21–27.

40. Wingo PA, Layde PM, Lee NC, et al: The risk of breast cancer in postmenopausal women who have used estrogen replacement therapy. JAMA 1987;257:209–215.

41. Colditz GA: Epidemiology of breast cancer: Findings from the Nurses' Health Study. Cancer (Suppl)1993;71(4):1480–1489.

42. Speroff L: Menopause and hormone replacement therapy. Clin Geriatr Med 1993;9:33–55.

43. Ravnikar VA: Compliance with hormonal therapy. Am J Obstet Gynecol 1987;156:1332–1334.

44. Paganini-Hill A, Ross RK, Henderson BE: Postmenopausal estrogen treatment and stroke: A prospective study. BMJ 1988;297:519–522.

48 Prostate Gland Disease

Jay B. Hollander, M.D.

Ananias C. Diokno, M.D.

The prostate is the site of two of the most common clinical problems facing the elderly male: benign prostatic hyperplasia (BPH) and prostatic carcinoma. BPH develops in virtually every male if he lives long enough, and although few suffer significant morbidity, the majority of men over 60 will have some symptoms of prostatism. Similarly, prostate cancer is now the most commonly diagnosed cancer in the United States and the second most common cancer causing death from malignancy in American males.

This chapter is devoted to updating the geriatric caregiver about BPH and prostate cancer. It is hoped that information contained in this chapter will be of practical use in better managing and counseling men with BPH and in approaching the topic of prostate cancer in a primary care setting.

ANATOMY AND PATHOPHYSIOLOGY

The prostate can be divided into a number of different regions of importance to anatomists, pathologists, radiologists, and urologists. For the purposes of the primary caregiver it is important to understand some of these terms because they have day-to-day clinical importance and can help with communication, examinations, and understanding reports. The narrowest portion of the "triangular" prostate is first encountered on digital rectal examination and is referred to as the apex. As the digital examination proceeds, the prostate widens superiorly to the portion adjacent to the bladder outlet. This is referred to as the base of the prostate. On each side of the midline sulcus the prostate tends to bulge normally with a smooth rubbery consistency. These bulges are referred to as the right and left lobes of the prostate.

The prostatic parenchyma is composed of glandular tissue within a fibromuscular stroma.

Two zones of the prostate are of particular interest (five have been identified): the peripheral zone and the transition zone. The peripheral zone is located posteriorly and represents most if not all of the surface of the prostate that is palpated through the rectal mucosa. It is thought to be the site of origin of most (but not all) prostate cancers. The transition zone is very small in the young man and surrounds the proximal two thirds of the prostatic urethra. It is therefore not normally palpable in the young male.

The glands and fibromuscular stroma of the transition zone undergo a remarkable change with aging. A true hyperplasia of these elements occurs that appears to be hormonally sensitive. In eunuchs who have very low levels of testosterone, BPH does not develop. Moreover, with androgen deprivation some hyperplastic glands undergo involution. The clinical significance of BPH is related to the fact that the bulk of the enlarging prostate gland encroaches on the lumen of the prostatic urethra or bladder outlet, causing obstructive or irritative voiding symptoms, urinary tract infections (UTIs), retention of urine, hydronephrosis, and even renal failure in its most severe form.

In addition to their hormonal sensitivity, the smooth muscle components of the prostate are responsive to nervous stimulation. Alpha-adrenergic stimulation can cause contraction of smooth muscle within the prostate and the adjacent bladder neck with narrowing of the bladder outlet and prostatic urethra. Blocking such stimulation may, therefore, relax the smooth muscle and possibly improve voiding despite the presence of BPH. The androgen and alpha-adrenergic sensitivity of the prostate allows various methods of medical management of BPH, which will be discussed later.

Prostate cancer, which is similarly a disease of aging, is also hormonally sensitive. Although most cancers arise within the peripheral zone, cancers can arise anywhere in the prostate. Why prostate cancer develops is still unknown. It arises from the prostatic glandular elements and is, therefore, an adenocarcinoma.

INCIDENCE AND PREVALENCE

Benign Prostatic Hyperplasia

Benign prostatic hyperplasia is so common in the geriatric population that its presence should be expected and considered normal for any man over the age of 60. If prostate biopsies performed for the purpose of looking for prostate cancer are reviewed, evidence of BPH will be found in the majority whether or not the biopsies are positive for cancer. Some symptoms of prostatism can be elicited in most men over 60 even though many may not be bothered by the symptoms or require any work-up or therapy. The problem is still so large that the transurethral resection of the prostate (TURP) was one of the most commonly performed operations in the United States prior to the advent of effective medical modalities.

Prostate Cancer

Prostate cancer is now the most common visceral malignancy of men. It is the second most frequent cause of death from cancer in men in the United States. The incidence of prostate cancer has risen dramatically during the last decade. This increase is no doubt related to the fact that more biopsies are performed because there is greater public awareness of the importance of screening, greater physician awareness, and, most important, newer screening modalities such as prostate-specific antigen (PSA). Of major importance, however, is the fact that the prevalence of prostate cancer is extremely high. Autopsy studies have repeatedly shown evidence of local prostate cancer in more than 50% of men over the age of 70 who die for other reasons. The probability of finding prostate cancer is directly related to age, and the older one gets, the more

likely it is that a cancer is hidden somewhere in the prostate. At least 80% of 90-year-old men harbor adenocarcinoma somewhere in the prostate. Despite the high incidence of prostate cancer (cancer diagnosed while the patient is alive) and the high death rate relative to other cancer death rates, the fact is that most men with prostate cancer die of other causes with no symptoms from prostate cancer or knowledge that it ever existed. Emphasis of this fact is important when one is dealing with patients who, because of age or other medical conditions, have a projected life span of less than 10 years.

INITIAL EVALUATION

History

Clinical assessment of the prostate begins with the history and physical examination. All men in the geriatric age range should be questioned routinely in the urologic review of systems about obstructive or irritative symptoms, urinary tract infection, or hematuria. Incontinence can be a sign of a prostate problem. Table 48–1 lists various voiding symptoms and signs that may be related to prostate disease. Not infrequently, however, patients are not bothered by or are unaware that their voiding patterns have changed because the process has been gradual and is accepted as normal for their age. The history alone is very unreliable in determining who would benefit from further work-up or therapy unless it can be discovered from the patient how bothersome the symptoms are.

The American Urological Association (AUA) symptom index is a self-administered questionnaire that has been validated as a reasonable tool for assessing symptom severity (Table 48–2).[1] The questionnaire contains seven questions about urination and grades of symptom severity. The result is a numerical total that grades overall symptom severity, that is, 0 to 7 mild, 8 to 19 moderate, and 20 to 35 severe symptoms of prostatism.

The patient's medications can play a role in that they may be responsible for a worsening of

TABLE 48–1 **SIGNS AND SYMPTOMS OF PROSTATISM**

Obstructive Symptoms	Irritative Symptoms	Signs
Decreased force of stream	Urgency	Bacteriuria
Hesitancy	Frequency	Large gland
Intermittency	Nocturia	High residual postvoid
Strain to void	Dysuria	Trabeculated bladder
Incomplete emptying	Urge incontinence	Poor observed stream

TABLE 48–2 **AMERICAN UROLOGICAL ASSOCIATION (AUA) SYMPTOM INDEX**

Questions To Be Answered	Not At All
1. Over the past month, how often have you had a sensation of not emptying your bladder completely after you finished urinating?	0
2. Over the past month, how often have you had to urinate again less than 2 hours after you finished urinating?	0
3. Over the past month, how often have you stopped and started again several times when you urinated?	0
4. Over the past month, how often have you found it difficult to postpone urination?	0
5. Over the past month, how often have you had a weak urinary stream?	0
6. Over the past month, how often have you had to push or strain to begin urination?	0
7. Over the past month, how many times did you most typically get up to urinate from the time you went to bed at night until the time you got up in the morning?	0 (None)
Sum of seven circled numbers (AUA symptom score): _____	

Data from Barry MJ, Fowler FJ Jr, O'Leary MP, Bruskewitz RC, Holtgrewe HL, Mebust WK, Cockett ATK: AUA Measurement Committee: The American Urological Association symptom index for benign prostatic hyperplasia. J Urol 1992a;148:1549–1557.

the symptoms. Diuretics, for instance, when given in the evening, may predispose the patient to nocturia, and over-the-counter cold medicines that contain alpha-adrenergic agonists such as phenylpropanolamine may exacerbate obstructive symptoms. Dietary history can also be revealing. Fluid intake alone may be responsible for urinary frequency or urgency, as in the case of an elderly male who drinks too much coffee without being aware of its relation to his voiding symptoms. Local symptoms of prostate cancer are similar to those of BPH and thus nonspecific. The review of symptoms, in general, may elicit a history of weight loss or bone pain that should place possible prostate cancer high in the differential diagnosis of any elderly male. The family history may also be very revealing in that men with siblings, fathers, or sons with prostate can-

cer are at increased risk for developing the disease.[2]

Physical Examination

The physical examination is essential in the initial assessment of the prostate. The examination should include a careful abdominal examination with palpation and percussion of the suprapubic region because gross bladder distention can be present without any acute symptoms. If bladder distention is suspected, a postvoid residual urine may be obtained by catheterization or bladder ultrasound. The external genitalia should be examined to rule out such common findings as phimosis, balanitis, or epididymitis that might be associated with the patient's voiding complaints or predispose him to problems. The rectal examination, however, is the only portion of the physical examination that gives information directly about the prostate.

The gland is palpated from apex to base with the pad of the index finger, paying attention to symmetry, size, indurated areas, nodules, and surface irregularities. The size of the gland should be noted, but size has poor correlation with the presence or absence of clinical symptoms or pathology in most cases as long as the examination is otherwise benign with no suspicion of tumor.

Clinical Testing

URINALYSIS

Both BPH and prostate cancer can predispose to urinary tract infection and hematuria. In many cases asymptomatic bacteriuria or microhematuria may be the only sign of a potentially significant prostate lesion. Although abnormal microscopic findings are not specific and may be caused by an abnormality anywhere in the urinary tract, the urinalysis is critical to certain management decisions. Glucosuria may be a source of voiding symptoms, and proteinuria or an abnormal sediment may be a sign of renal disease.

SERUM CREATININE

Testing of any new patient with symptoms of either prostate cancer or BPH should include a serum creatinine measurement because both conditions can affect renal function. Outlet obstruction can cause chronic retention and may be unnoticed by the patient. Such "silent retention" may ultimately result in renal insufficiency secondary to hydronephrosis. Prostate cancer, if advanced, can also cause ureteral obstruction due to a locally advanced tumor or metastatic nodal involvement.

PROSTATIC-SPECIFIC ANTIGEN

The PSA is a study that can be used to screen for prostate cancer and help with its management. The AUA recommends that it be ordered in men over 50 who wish to be screened for prostate cancer provided that if a tumor is found the patient would be a candidate for some form of therapy. In African-American men and men with a family history of prostate cancer, screening should start at 40 years of age because these groups have an increased risk of prostate cancer. Elevations in PSA may be due to BPH and an enlarged prostate gland, prostatitis, trauma (i.e., Foley catheter or cystoscopy), urinary tract infection, or cancer. Judgment is required in ordering a PSA in very old men or those who have a life expectancy of less than 5 years. In these individuals, if the history and physical examination are not suspicious for prostate cancer, a PSA is likely to be of little use and might prompt unnecessary biopsies and cause unnecessary anxiety for patient and family. The PSA has no role in the management of BPH other than in helping to rule out the presence of prostate cancer.

Summary of Initial Evaluation

A careful history and physical examination along with three simple laboratory tests—the urinalysis, serum creatinine, and PSA—should suffice to evaluate most elderly men in a manner that can detect most clinically significant prostate problems due to BPH or cancer. Abnormalities may prompt further action such as imaging studies, biopsies, or referral to a urologist. Treatment may be offered, or expectant management plans can be discussed. The balance of this chapter is devoted to discussing these and other issues related to BPH and prostate cancer.

BENIGN PROSTATIC HYPERPLASIA—MANAGEMENT

The initial assessment of a patient's prostate status may indicate that further management may be appropriate. If a patient has no voiding complaints or history that might suggest a problem with the urinary tract and the physical examination, urinalysis, and serum creatinine are normal, no further work-up is required for the geriatric patient being screened for BPH. A serum PSA may be indicated for screening purposes only as will be discussed later in the section on prostate

cancer. The primary care physician may elect to proceed directly with medical or expectant management programs, if indicated, without further diagnostic testing or referral. If the patient has symptoms that do not respond to medical management or if the physician is uncomfortable in instituting medical therapy, referral for urologic evaluation should be made.

Urologic Evaluation

The peak urinary flow rate can be measured and computed by means of nomograms to determine how the patient's stream compares with that of a normal patient his own age. Postvoid residuals can be measured by bladder ultrasound examination or directly with catheterization. Further information can be obtained with cystoscopy and urodynamic testing. These studies are most productive in patients who have had prior lower urinary tract procedures, have symptoms that do not correlate with uroflow findings, or have predominantly irritative symptoms rather than obstructive symptoms. Finally, upper urinary tract imaging may be indicated in patients in whom postvoid residuals are very high and renal insufficiency exists. Similarly, upper urinary tract evaluation should be considered if the urinalysis shows evidence of infection or hematuria.

Indications for Treatment

The Agency for Health Care Policy and Research (AHCPR) has developed guidelines for the management of prostatism.[1] Following extensive literature reviews, the AHCPR panel found that the frequency of serious complications resulting from untreated BPH was poorly understood and likely to be small. The guidelines recommend that treatment of BPH be directed at improvement of symptoms rather than prevention of complications. As such, patients with mild prostatism (AUA symptom score of less than 8) can be managed by watchful waiting and follow-up only. This alternative can apply to any symptomatic individual as long as he has not had a complication such as a urinary tract infection, retention, or obstructive uropathy.

Treatment Options

MEDICAL TREATMENT OF BPH

At this time two major medical treatment options are available for the management of BPH—5-alpha-reductase inhibitors and alpha-adrenergic blocking agents. The use of these medications is now widespread, and doubtless new agents will become available in the future.

5-Alpha-Reductase Inhibitors

Finasteride was approved for treatment of BPH by the Food and Drug Administration in 1992. This drug was engineered specifically to block the conversion of testosterone to dihydrotestosterone by the enzyme 5-alpha-reductase. Dihydrotestosterone is the major intraprostatic androgen, and deprivation of intraprostatic androgen can result in reduction in the size of the prostate. Finasteride, when taken daily at a dose of 5 mg, may improve symptoms of BPH by reducing the size of the prostate. Unfortunately, the drug has limited efficacy for most patients. Long-term studies confirm that the drug is extraordinarily safe and has no dangerous side effects or need for clinical or laboratory monitoring.[3] Dosage does not have to be adjusted in the elderly. The most common side effect, impotence, occurs in less than 5% of patients. Although the drug can reduce the size of the prostate by approximately 30%, it may take more than a year for this to occur. Moreover, although the actual volume of the prostate may be reduced, this reduction may not result in any symptom improvement. Only a third of patients show any objective improvement in urinary flow or ability to empty the bladder. It takes months and up to 1 year to determine whether the drug is of any benefit. Patients must be aware that the drug will not work quickly, and it has no role in the treatment of acute obstructive symptoms. Finally, patients and their physicians must be aware that finasteride affects the PSA, reducing the true value by an average of 50%. A normal PSA in a patient taking finasteride may in fact be worrisome depending on the patient's age and prior PSA values.

Alpha-Adrenergic Antagonist Drugs

Alpha-adrenergic antagonists were developed for the treatment of hypertension. Vascular smooth muscle relaxation is thought to be the mechanism of action. Similarly, smooth muscle in the prostate and nearby bladder neck can be relaxed by these medications, providing relief of obstructive symptoms in many individuals. The two most often prescribed preparations of this category are terazosin and doxazosin. Both have been studied extensively for the treatment of BPH and overall are similar in dose, efficacy, and toxicity profile. As with finasteride, neither drug is effective in every patient or even in most patients for relief of prostatism. Nevertheless, a significant number of patients benefit from this type of medical therapy, which may be offered as a trial to determine whether other more invasive options such as surgery can be avoided or delayed.

Both preparations are prescribed in a once daily dose that is best taken at bedtime. During the first month of use the dosage must be increased gradually to the target dose (5 to 10 mg terazosin or 4 to 8 mg doxazosin) for the safest prescription. The most common side effects are asthenia, dizziness, and postural hypotension, which occur in 5% to 10% of patients. These problems may be more pronounced in the elderly, and a lower target dose should be considered in the very old or infirm. There are some potential benefits of alpha-blockers compared with 5-alpha-reductase inhibitors. Symptomatic improvement should occur if it is going to occur within the first month or two of dose titration. If the medication is not effective, it should be discontinued at that time and should not be tried for 3 to 6 months as recommended for finasteride. The antihypertensive effect may also be beneficial to the patient if he has hypertension. Alpha-blockers will not affect the PSA measurement. A recent cooperative study clearly shows that alpha-blockers are preferable to finasteride for the treatment of benign prostatic hyperplasia.[4]

SURGICAL TREATMENT OPTIONS

Medical treatment of BPH can be considered initially for patients desiring treatment for chronic symptoms. If medical management is unsuccessful, or if symptoms worsen or become acute (i.e., urinary retention), surgical treatment must be considered. Surgical options have increased dramatically during the last 10 years, but at this time there is no clear-cut choice for the relief of outlet obstruction due to BPH. The risks and benefits of each procedure must be discussed with the patient, and the decision is best left to the patient and his urologist. Current common surgical treatment options for BPH are summarized in Table 48–3.

TREATMENT OF THE HIGH-RISK GERIATRIC PATIENT

In the alert, healthy ambulatory geriatric patient treatment of BPH should be undertaken provided that the indications are clear and treatment is desired. Options should be presented to the patient so that he can weigh the risks and benefits with the guidance of his physician. Watchful waiting must be one of the options unless an absolute indication for treatment exists such as urinary retention with postrenal insufficiency. In older infirm or high-risk surgical patients, treatment options must be tailored to the individual. There is no question that the complication rate

---

TABLE 48–3 **CURRENT COMMON SURGICAL TREATMENT OPTIONS FOR BPH**

Transurethral Resection of the Prostate (TURP)

Tissue removed by electrosurgical resection

Pros

Most effective procedure for improving urinary flow and improving symptoms (to date)

Cons

10% complications
Incontinence <1%
Impotence <5%
Bleeding in up to 2% of patients requires transfusion
Requires full anesthetic
1- to 2-day hospital stay

Transurethral Incision of the Prostate (TUIP)

Electrosurgical cuts open prostatic urethra (no tissue removed)

Pros

Can yield results similar to TURP in selected patients
Can be performed as an outpatient
Less bleeding than TURP

Cons

Less effective in large glands
Requires full anesthetic
Bleeding can still occur

Laser Prostatectomy

Laser energy ablates or causes coagulative necrosis of periurethral prostatic tissue

Pros

Can be performed with intravenous sedation
Usually bloodless
Can be performed as an outpatient
Proven objective improvement

Cons

Efficacy not as good as TURP, especially in large glands
Irritative symptoms postoperatively
Limited long-term follow-up
Requires Foley catheter 3 to 5 days postoperatively

Transurethral Electrovaporization of the Prostate (TUEP)

Electrosurgical vaporization of prostate to ablate periurethral tissue in newly developed technique

Pros

Can be performed as an outpatient
Less bleeding than TURP

Cons

Full anesthetic needed
No long-term follow-up
Less effective in large glands

Transurethral Microwave Thermotherapy

Microwave probe is passed transurethrally to heat the prostate deep to the urethra

Pros

Bloodless
Minimal or no anesthesia
Can be performed as an outpatient
Improved symptoms

Cons

May have irritative symptoms postoperatively
Flow improvement less than TURP
Limited long-term follow-up

---

for TURP is higher in patients over 80 years old and that the risks increase with the number of additional medical problems and the size of the prostate gland, as mentioned earlier. The less invasive treatment options that have been developed during the last decade have therefore been quite useful in this group of patients. In addition, a chronic urethral or suprapubic indwelling catheter and clean intermittent catheterization may also have a role in some patients in whom outlet obstruction must be relieved but the patient's medical status dictates against surgical intervention.

Attention should also be paid to quality-of-life issues. In the demented, bedridden institutionalized male there may not be any benefit from TURP compared with chronic Foley catheterization for urinary retention even if the procedure is uncomplicated and relieves the obstruction.

Incontinence may become a problem, and if a condom catheter or pads are unsatisfactory, a Foley catheter may still be required. In high-risk individuals who are not candidates for any invasive form of treatment, medical management can be considered while a Foley catheter or clean intermittent catheterization is used temporarily, thus giving the medical trial time to work.

PROSTATE CANCER

The initial assessment of the prostate gland, as previously described, should be sufficient to screen for the presence of prostate cancer. If the initial evaluation suggests that the patient might be at increased risk for prostate cancer, further testing may be indicated. If a diagnosis of prostate cancer is confirmed, staging may be indicated to decide on management alternatives.

This section discusses the diagnosis and management of prostate cancer.

Diagnosis

HISTORY AND PHYSICAL EXAMINATION

Prostate cancer causes few symptoms in its early stages, and unfortunately it is only in the early stages that it is most successfully treated. Most men presenting with voiding symptoms have something other than prostate cancer such as BPH or urinary tract infection as a source of the problem. In its advanced stages, prostate cancer may present with voiding symptoms, hematuria, anemia, weakness, weight loss, and bone pain, most commonly in the bony pelvic region or back. Despite this, many men with metastatic prostate cancer may be totally free of symptoms. The history is, therefore, an unreliable indicator of prostate cancer. The family history, however, can be very significant. If a patient has a first-degree relative with prostate cancer, he may have a twofold risk of harboring the disease. If the patient has more than one first-degree relative with prostate cancer the risk may be as much as fivefold higher than the risk in the general population.[2] African-Americans are also at increased risk for developing prostate cancer. The American Cancer Society and the American Urological Association recommend that screening for prostate cancer should begin at age 50, but for those at increased risk screening should be initiated at age 40. The rectal examination, as previously described, is an essential part of the evaluation. Even though the PSA is available as a blood test to screen for prostate cancer, the rectal examination cannot be ignored. Although there are a number of conditions that can cause an abnormal prostate (i.e., prostatic calculi, inflammation, nodular BPH, prostatic infarction), any nodule or induration found should be considered suspicious for malignancy until it is proved otherwise. A prostate nodule found on digital rectal examination has a 30% to 50% chance of being malignant.

DIAGNOSTIC TESTING

Prostate-Specific Antigen

Prostate-specific antigen is a glycoprotein specifically made in the prostate gland and found in the circulation of men with prostatic tissue. As such, it is not detectable at any significant level in females or in men who have had the prostate totally removed and have no subsequent evidence of prostate disease (i.e., prostate cancer

that has metastasized or recurred). Prostate-specific antigen can be elevated in patients with abnormal prostate conditions such as prostate cancer, BPH, or inflammatory conditions of the prostate. Unexplained elevated levels, however, should alert the examiner to the possibility of prostate cancer, and prompt referral for prostate ultrasound and possible biopsy should be done, assuming that the patient is a candidate for treatment of the disease or is interested in knowing that he has prostate cancer. If a PSA level obtained for screening purposes is abnormally elevated, the patient should be referred for prostate ultrasound and possible biopsy. If the digital rectal examination raises a suspicion of tumor, the patient should be referred to a urologist because biopsy will probably be indicated. Referral for possible biopsy is indicated if a prostate nodule is found regardless of the PSA level or even the presence of normal results on prostate ultrasound examination.

Prostate Ultrasound

Endorectal ultrasound probes specifically designed to image the prostate have enhanced our diagnostic abilities with respect to prostate cancer. The study should not be used as a screening tool as the PSA has been but rather as a diagnostic tool to target biopsies when prostate cancer is suspected either by abnormal digital rectal examination, abnormal PSA level, or a history that is highly suggestive of prostate cancer such as the presence of new bony metastasis in an elderly male with no apparent cause.

Prostate Biopsy

The indications for prostate biopsy are best understood by physicians who frequently deal with prostate cancer. The following guidelines are mentioned to assist with appropriate referral.

1. Abnormal prostate that raises suspicion of prostate cancer on digital rectal examination.
2. Abnormal PSA level unrelated to inflammation or unexplained by prostatic enlargement.
3. Abnormal prostate ultrasound that raises suspicion of prostate cancer.
4. Metastatic prostate cancer suspected in a patient with no prior history of prostate cancer.

Does everyone with an elevated PSA need a prostate biopsy? Does every geriatric male need a PSA? Judgment is very important in managing the topic of prostate cancer to avoid unnecessary biopsies and the anxiety or dilemmas that may arise as a result of such biopsies. In the very elderly or those with significant medical problems in whom life expectancy is estimated at less than 10 years, a diagnosis of prostate cancer may not result in any therapeutic action if the patient is asymptomatic and the disease is localized. In such a patient, a PSA measurement may be of no value if the digital rectal examination is normal. Mild elevations of PSA do not always require a biopsy. Urologists have developed tools that can assist with the decision about whether or not a biopsy of the prostate is needed because of an abnormal PSA. Age-specific PSA ranges have been suggested and can assist in making this decision (Table 48–4);[5, 6] new PSA measurements are being developed that may also be of assistance. PSA can be measured in its free form as opposed to its total amount, much of which may be bound to certain serum carriers.[6] The percentage of free PSA may suggest the need for a biopsy because malignant states may be associated with less free PSA. Clearly, other techniques will be developed that will help in screening for prostate cancer or in determining when to order a biopsy. For now, the primary physician can follow the guideline that if prostate cancer is suspected either by digital rectal examination or by PSA measurement, referral for possible biopsy is indicated if confirmation of prostate cancer would alter the management plan.

PROSTATE CANCER GRADING—THE GLEASON SCORE

Prostate cancer is reported by the pathologist in terms of its potential to be aggressive (high-grade or poorly differentiated) or slow growing (low-grade or well-differentiated). The most common way of conveying this information is by patho-

logic evaluation of the architectural patterns that prostate cancer can present with. The patterns are graded from 1 to 5 and the two most prevalent patterns are added, for an overall score referred to as the Gleason score in honor of the pathologist who devised the system.[7] Therefore, the Gleason score may range from 2 to 10, with the most aggressive or poorly differentiated cancers having the highest scores.

STAGING

Prostate cancer is staged clinically by rectal examination combined with the results of the prostate biopsy. High-grade and large tumors that extend beyond the capsule of the prostate are more likely to be metastatic. The pelvic lymph nodes and axial skeleton are the most common sites of metastasis. If metastasis is suspected, further staging studies such as bone scans and pelvic computed tomographic (CT) scans may be indicated. In general, these studies have a very low yield if the cancer is believed to be confined to the prostate, the PSA is less than 10, and the Gleason score is under 7 (not high grade). Table 48–5 shows an abbreviated version of the currently accepted staging systems. The tumor-node-metastasis (TNM) system is now clearly preferred by the scientific community, and the modified Jewett system is of historical significance. More detailed staging systems exist but are beyond the scope of this text. In general, prostate cancer is very difficult to treat if it is not confined to the prostate (i.e., stage T3 [stage C] or greater).

Treatment

The treatment of prostate cancer is best approached by understanding that in very few instances is there a uniformly accepted correct treatment modality. Rather, there are usually a number of options available to the patient, and the decision is best made by properly informing the patient of the risks versus benefits of each option. This is best done by those who have experience in treating prostate cancer, that is, urologists, oncologists, or radiation oncologists.

LOCALIZED PROSTATE CANCER

Standard Treatment Options—Surgery versus Radiation

There should be no argument that if a low-grade, completely confined tumor is removed by radical prostatectomy the cure rate is high. The fact that nonoperative treatment options exist makes

| TABLE 48–4 | **SERUM PROSTATE-SPECIFIC ANTIGEN AND PATIENT AGE** |

Age Range (years)	Median Value (ng/mL)	Interquartile Range[a] (ng/mL)	Reference Range[b] (ng/mL)
40–49	0.7	0.5–1.1	0.0–2.5
50–59	1.0	0.6–1.4	0.0–3.5
60–69	1.4	0.9–3.0	0.0–4.5
70–79	2.0	0.9–3.2	0.0–6.5

[a]25th to 75th percentile.
[b]Upper limit defined by the 95th percentile.
Data from Oesterling JE: Current thoughts on the detection of prostate cancer. Bull Am Coll Surg 1996;81(2):33–39.

TABLE 48–5 **STAGING OF PROSTATE CANCER**

Clinical Findings	Stage	
	TNM	*Modified Jewett*
Prostate examination normal	T1	A
Tumor palpable but confined to prostate	T2	B
Tumor extends beyond prostate	T3–4	C
Tumor spread to lymph nodes	N+	D1
Tumor spread to bone	M+	D2

Abbreviations: TNM, tumor-node-metastasis.

decision-making difficult for patients. The younger and healthier the patient, the more often surgery is chosen, both because the patient is a better surgical candidate and because longer-term cure may be easier to attain. The prostate that has been removed has no chance of developing cancer in the future unless cancer cells were left behind at the time of surgery. Moreover, the PSA should be undetectable if the procedure was successful, and follow-up is simplified as long as the PSA remains undetectable. With radiation therapy, prostate tissue remains, and unfortunately cancer can continue to develop despite proper treatment. In addition, the PSA often varies during follow-up, and minor elevations of low values may be significant and problematic for both patient and physician. Although recurrence after radiation can occur, it may take years for such a recurrence to appear and even longer to become clinically symptomatic. In many cases, the patient's normal life expectancy may be realized, and death may be caused by conditions other than prostate cancer. This being the case, radiation therapy is chosen more often than surgery in patients over 70, and surgery is chosen more often in patients under 60. Both options should be given to any patient seeking treatment for local prostate cancer.

Watchful Waiting

Despite the current publicity in the United States about the early detection and treatment of prostate cancer, an argument can be made that many prostate cancers may not have to be treated. This is particularly germane to the geriatric population, especially those 75 and older or those with a life expectancy of less than 10 years. Scandinavian populations that have been managed, in large part, with watchful waiting and no treatment for prostate cancer have shown very good 10-year survival for untreated local prostate cancer.[8, 9] The downside of watchful waiting is the progression of disease to a noncurable state

or possibly premature death. There are no established guidelines for determining who should be encouraged to elect watchful waiting, although all patients should know that it is an option. There is no substitute for good sound medical judgment. The geriatric patient with medical problems that may limit life expectancy to less than 5 or 10 years may benefit from a program of watchful waiting in that by electing no treatment he may "outlive" the prostate tumor—that is, he may die of other causes before the tumor grows to be harmful.

Investigational Treatment Options

There is no ideal therapy for prostate cancer at this time. New modalities are being investigated that may prove to be reasonable treatment options or perhaps preferred treatment options. Cryotherapy is an outpatient therapy that involves temporary transperineal insertion of probes that can freeze the prostate to temperatures that result in tissue necrosis and thus hopefully tumor destruction. Although this technique seems promising, it will take years before studies have accumulated enough follow-up to prove a durable response without recurrence.

ADVANCED CANCER

Prostate cancer that presents in an advanced stage or progresses to an advanced stage may or may not be symptomatic. There is still no known cure for prostate cancer that has metastasized, and the prognosis for locally advanced disease is also poor in terms of hope for cure. Hormonal ablation is the cornerstone of treatment for advanced prostate cancer as it has been for the last 50 years.

Bilateral Orchiectomy

Bilateral orchiectomy can be performed in less than 30 minutes as an outpatient surgical procedure. It results in permanent castrate levels of testosterone. It has been the standard treatment for metastatic prostate cancer for the last five decades. Complications are rare and usually minor. The major side effect is loss of libido and secondary sexual dysfunction, which are side effects of any treatment that results in castrate levels of testosterone.

Diethylstilbestrol

Diethylstilbestrol (DES) is an inexpensive oral estrogen preparation that if taken daily will result in castrate levels of testosterone. It acts by negative feedback to the pituitary-hypothalamic axis by diminishing the release of luteinizing hormone and thus lowering the production of testosterone. Unfortunately, DES, if taken in doses of 3 to 5 mg/day, will increase the risk of cardiovascular disease and stroke. At doses of 1 to 2 mg/day such risks may be lessened, and the medication may still be effective in treating prostate cancer. DES is seldom used today in the United States for reasons that may be more related to medical-legal fears than to actual fear that the medication may not serve the patient well. The medication will probably enjoy renewed popularity in the future as costs become more of an issue in the practice of medicine.

Luteinizing Hormone-Releasing Hormone Agonists

Luteinizing hormone-releasing hormone (LHRH) agonists are now available in sustained release forms that can be given by injection that will last either 1 or 3 months. With sustained levels of such hormonal agonists, the pituitary stops producing luteinizing hormone, and testosterone production from the testis therefore stops. These medications do not carry the risks of vascular disease that were associated with high-dose DES therapy in the past. As such, they have gained popularity because they represent an option other than orchiectomy. Side effects are similar to those of orchiectomy and include hot flashes and sweats associated with androgen withdrawal in addition to loss of libido. A major disadvantage is cost. These drugs are very expensive and are not affordable for most individuals without insurance coverage. Leuprolide acetate (Lupron Depot, TAP Pharmaceuticals) and goserelin acetate (Zoladex, Zeneca, Inc.) are the two preparations available in 1-month and 3-month injection kits.

Antiandrogens

Drugs in this class are not designed to be used alone in the treatment of advanced prostate can-

cer. When combined with either orchiectomy or LHRH agonists they result in so-called total androgen ablation and may prolong life in a patient with advanced prostate cancer. Unfortunately, the survival advantage with total androgen ablation is not understood well enough nor is it long enough to recommend such combined therapy at this time.[10] The cost of these medicines is also quite high and without medical coverage is beyond the reach of most individuals. Flutamide (Eulexin, Schering, Inc.), the first such medicine available, is taken in doses of 250 mg tid, and bicalutamide (Casodex, Zeneca, Inc.), a newer preparation, can be taken as a 50 mg dose once daily. Hepatic dysfunction and gastrointestinal disturbances must be watched for with these medications.

Palliative Intervention

Despite hormonal ablation, many cancers continue to progress or reactivate after an initial remission. If such tumor activity results in local symptoms such as bone pain, palliative measures are available; they include local radiation therapy and estrogen-tagged nuclear medicines, which may result in improvement of symptoms.

References

1. Benign Prostatic Hyperplasia Guideline Panel: Symptom assessment. *In* McConnell JD, Barry MJ, Bruskewitz RC, et al (eds): Benign Prostatic Hyperplasia: Diagnosis and Treatment. Clinical Practice Guideline No. 8. AHCPR Publication No. 94-0582. Rockville, MD, U.S. Department of Health and Human Services, Public Health Service, Agency for Health Care Policy and Research, 1994, pp. 29–34.
2. Steinberg GD, Carter BS, Beaty TH, et al: Family history and the risk of prostate cancer. Prostate 1990;17:337–437.
3. Stoner E: Three-year safety and efficacy data on the use of finasteride in the treatment of benign prostatic hyperplasia. Urology 1994;43(3):284–292.
4. Lepor H, Williford WO, Barry MJ, Brawer MK, et al: The efficacy of terazosin, finasteride, or both in benign prostatic hyperplasia. N Engl J Med 1996;335(8): 533–539.
5. Oesterling JE: Using prostate-specific antigen to eliminate unnecessary diagnostic tests: Significant worldwide economic implications. Urology 1995;46:26–33.
6. Oesterling JE, Jacobsen SJ, Klee GG, et al: Free complexed and total serum prostate specific antigen: The establishment of appropriate reference ranges for their concentrations and ratios. J Urol 1995;154(3): 1090–1095.
7. Gleason DF: Histologic grading and staging of prostatic carcinoma. *In* Tannenbaum M (ed): Urologic Pathology: The Prostate. Philadelphia, Lea & Febiger, 1977, pp. 171–179.
8. Adolfsson J, Ronstrom L, Lowhagen T, et al: Deferred

treatment of clinically localized low grade prostate cancer: The experience from a prospective series at the Karolinska Hospital. J Urol 1994;152:1757–1760.

9. Johansson JE: Watchful waiting for early stage prostate cancer. Urology 1994;43(2):138–142.

10. Prostate Cancer Trialists' Collaborative Group: Maximum androgen blockade in advanced prostate cancer: An overview of 22 randomized trials with 3283 deaths in 5710 patients. Lancet 1995;346(8970): 265–269.

49 Renal and Electrolyte Disorders

Robert D. Lindeman, M.D.

The accuracy and simplicity with which renal clearance measurements can be performed, requiring only timed urine samples and blood samples drawn at the midpoints of these periods, has made the kidney an ideal organ system for the study of changes that occur with aging. Both cross-sectional and longitudinal studies using mean values suggest that a dramatic decrease in kidney function occurs as one ages. One major problem is the need to distinguish between changes related to "normal" aging and changes influenced by disease. For the purposes of discussion, one can separate medical renal diseases in the elderly by anatomic sites of involvement, etiologic agents, or clinical presentations. Each approach has its advantages and disadvantages.

In this chapter, the last approach is used because it best meets the needs of geriatric clinicians who are faced with clinical challenges that require a problem-solving, differential diagnostic approach. After opening discussions of the pathophysiology of the normal aging kidney and the tests available to evaluate kidney function in the elderly, subsequent sections of the chapter deal with the diagnosis and management of acute renal failure, nephrotic syndrome, chronic renal failure, and stone formation, in that order. Urinary tract infections are discussed in Chapter 38.

This approach involves obvious overlaps. For example, diseases affecting the renal vessels (arteriolar nephrosclerosis, occlusive arterial disease including renal artery stenosis due to atherosclerosis, and vasculitis) most often present as chronic renal insufficiency but can present acutely or with hypertension or hematuria as the principal manifestations. Analgesic abuse can produce both acute and chronic renal failure and is therefore discussed under both headings.

In the normal young adult, the renal capacity to regulate fluid and electrolyte balance far exceeds the ordinary demands for conservation and excretion. Even when this capacity is substantially decreased in old age, renal function still allows adequate regulation of the volume and composition of extracellular fluid. Inability to maintain normal extracellular electrolyte concentrations is generally due to extrarenal defects in the regulatory (homeostatic) mechanisms rather than to insufficient renal function. Nevertheless, the subspecialty of nephrology has traditionally dealt with fluid, electrolyte, and acid-base balances, and because these functions involve a number of problem areas that specifically or predominantly affect the elderly, these will be discussed in this chapter.

PATHOPHYSIOLOGY OF THE AGING KIDNEY

Renal function declines after the age of 40 years at a mean rate of 1% per year. These observations, first reported from cross-sectional analyses, were confirmed in a population of normal aging subjects who were followed longitudinally.[1] However, when the same subjects were later restudied by calculating regression equations for each individual, it was found that one third of the subjects showed no decline over periods of up to 23 years.[2] The decrease in mean creatinine clearance, then, occurred primarily in the other two thirds, who showed decreases in renal function, some very appreciable. There has been a growing awareness, confirmed in functional tests of other organ systems, that a decline in function with age is not inevitable (i.e., there is no progressive involutional process whereby kidney function deteriorates with age). The terms successful and usual aging have been used to distinguish between the values seen in some subjects who weather aging well and the mean values obtained in any "normal" aging population. Much of the decrease in the latter is due to the superimposition of asymptomatic or at least undocumented pathology.

Changes in most renal functions (renal blood flow, tubular secretory and reabsorptive maximums, concentrating and diluting abilities, ability to excrete an acid load, etc.) tend to parallel changes in glomerular filtration rates.[3] With age, renal blood flow appears to shift from the cortical to the juxtamedullary nephrons. As cortical glomeruli become obsolete (sclerotic), the vasculature atrophies and disappears. In contrast, as the juxtamedullary glomeruli become obsolete, a shunt forms between the afferent and efferent arterioles so that blood flow is maintained but no glomerular filtrate is generated. The finding that renal blood flow decreases more rapidly than glomerular filtration rate in the elderly appears to be inconsistent with these observations. One possible explanation is that, in the elderly there may be a relative vasoconstriction of the glomerular efferent arteriole as opposed to the afferent arteriole, thereby raising glomerular pressure and filtration. Another potential explanation is that the filtration fraction (glomerular filtration rate/effective renal plasma flow) is higher in the juxtamedullary than in the cortical nephrons, and the elderly lose primarily the latter. Glomerular permeability to albumin, other proteins, and infused substances, such as hemoglobin or dextran, remains unaltered by age.

EVALUATION OF RENAL FUNCTION IN THE ELDERLY

The most important clinical function that requires monitoring with age is the glomerular filtration rate (GFR). The most reproducible clinical measure of GFR is the creatinine clearance. In a study by Rowe and colleagues[1] of the Baltimore Longitudinal Study of Aging population, the mean true creatinine clearance rates fell from 140 mL/minute/1.73 m² at age 25 to 34 years to 97 mL/minute/1.73 m² at age 75 to 84 years.[1] Nevertheless, the mean serum creatinine concentrations rose insignificantly from 0.81 to 0.84 mg/100 mL. This occurs because creatinine production falls at nearly the same rate as the renal clearance of creatinine, reflecting the decrease in body muscle mass that occurs with age. The practical implication of this observation is that the serum creatinine concentration, when used alone in the older patient, must be interpreted with this change in mind when it is used to determine or modify dosages of drugs cleared totally (e.g., aminoglycoside antibiotics) or partially (e.g., digoxin) by the kidney. Also, drugs that compete with the tubular secretion of creatinine (e.g., trimethoprim-sulfamethoxazole, ci-

metidine, and cefoxitin) cause an increase in serum creatinine concentration while not changing the true GFR.

The serum urea nitrogen (SUN) and urea clearance similarly make use of endogenously produced urea as the test substance. Since large amounts of urea may be reabsorbed in the tubule at low flow rates, vigorous hydration must be used to make the clearance results interpretable. Dietary protein intake also affects results appreciably. Therefore, in general, creatinine determinations have largely replaced urea and urea nitrogens in the evaluation of renal function.

A formula derived by Cockcroft and Gault[4] can be used to predict creatinine clearances from serum creatinine concentrations using age and weight for men as follows:

$$\text{Creatinine clearance} = \frac{(140 - \text{age in years}) \times \text{weight (in kg)}}{72 \times \text{serum creatinine (mg/100 mL)}}$$

For females, this value is multiplied times 0.85. This formula has been shown to be unreliable in very old patients, however.

Generally, tests of tubular function add little to one's knowledge of renal functional pathology. Although the response to 12 or more hours of water deprivation can be determined in terms of ability to concentrate the urine, this test creates some risk for older patients by imposing on them a period of dehydration sufficient to expose the kidneys in patients with underlying renal disease to further damage. Most normal older adults should be able to increase urine osmolality to 800 to 900 mOsm/kg H_2O (specific gravity 1.020 to 1.022). Failure to increase urine osmolality much above 300 mOsm/kg H_2O (specific gravity 1.010) implies tubular disease, diabetes insipidus, obstructive uropathy, or advanced renal disease.

Renal disease may present with asymptomatic urinary abnormalities identified with screening urinalysis. Hematuria can be due to renal parenchymal disease, diseases of the collecting systems, or systemic coagulation defects. The presence of red cell casts in a freshly voided urine is consistent only with a glomerular cause. The finding of associated proteinuria or an elevated serum creatinine concentration also suggests renal parenchymal disease.

If the lower urinary tract is thought to be the source of hematuria, a segmental analysis of a voided urine specimen may be helpful. Initial hematuria suggests a urethral source, terminal hematuria suggests a bladder source, and constant hematuria suggests a source in the upper urinary tract. Evaluation of isolated hematuria should include a urine culture, radiologic evaluation (intravenous pyelography [IVP] or sonography) to rule out renal parenchymal masses, and a urologic consultation for cystoscopy. In addition, a platelet count, bleeding time, prothrombin time, and partial thromboplastin time should be obtained to rule out a coagulopathy. In approximately 85% of patients, a cause of bleeding can be found on work-up, with malignancies, most often bladder, hypernephroma, and prostate tumors, accounting for one third of the cases of hematuria.

Normal protein excretion in the elderly does not differ significantly from that in young adults. Significant proteinuria is defined as greater than 150 mg urinary protein excretion per 24 hours. The dipstick is a good screening method for the detection of proteinuria but detects only albumin; light chains, which are present in patients with multiple myeloma, and low-molecular-weight protein (tubular protein) must be detected with the sulfosalicylic acid test. When the proteins excreted in the urine are primarily albumin and higher molecular weight proteins, the pathology is believed to be glomerular in origin. Generally a level of 3 g protein a day is used to separate nephrotic proteinuria from non-nephrotic proteinuria. On microscopic examination of the urine, the finding of pyuria, hematuria, and casts is of some value in determining the cause of the renal disease in the elderly, as it is in younger patients.

A variety of imaging techniques are available to evaluate the genitourinary system in the elderly. Ultrasonography is a noninvasive and safe test that can provide many diagnostic clues, showing kidney size, hydronephrosis, and solid or cystic parenchymal renal masses. Preceding a renal biopsy, an ultrasound examination should be performed to ensure the presence of two normal sized kidneys. An IVP will demonstrate sites of obstruction and other pathology (e.g., papillary necrosis). Elderly patients are placed at risk when undergoing dehydration and thereby can develop contrast media–induced acute renal failure, especially when there is an underlying diagnosis of diabetes mellitus, renal insufficiency, hypertension, or, especially, multiple myeloma.

Computed tomographic (CT) scans, angiography, and magnetic resonance imaging (MRI) are additional procedures available for the evaluation of renal masses, unexplained hematuria, or obstruction. Finally, for patients with suspected primary glomerular disease or unexplained renal failure, a renal biopsy may be indicated after all other available means of establishing a diagnosis have been exhausted.

RENAL DISEASES IN THE ELDERLY

The most common presenting manifestations of renal disease in the elderly, as in younger persons, are acute and chronic renal insufficiency (azotemia), proteinuria (nephrotic and non-nephrotic), and hematuria. Often the definitive diagnostic test is the renal biopsy. Moorthy and Zimmerman[5] reviewed the clinical indications and histologic diagnoses in 115 patients, aged 60 years or more, who underwent renal biopsy. The major clinical presentations were renal insufficiency in 57 patients, nephrotic syndrome in 35 patients, and hematuria with variable amounts of proteinuria in 23 patients. Rapidly progressive (crescentic) glomerulonephritis (19 patients) was the most common cause of renal insufficiency. Membranous glomerulopathy and minimal change lesions were the most commonly observed causes of nephrotic syndrome.

One of the largest series of biopsy (449 cases) and autopsy (51 cases) studies of renal disease in the elderly is that reported from the Armed Forces Institute of Pathology, which reviewed pathologic diagnoses in 500 patients over the age of 60 years (Table 49–1).[6] Although it must be recognized that this study is not an accurate reflection of the true prevalence of renal disease in the elderly because biopsy in diabetics and hypertensives with renal insufficiency often is not done, it does show that the spectrum of renal diseases seen in the elderly is no different from that seen in younger persons; only the frequencies are different.

Acute Renal Failure

In two large European series,[7, 8] 35% of patients with acute renal failure (ARF) were older than 65 and 70 years, respectively. One of these studies[8] indicated that the incidence of ARF was three times more frequent than expected in the elderly (age over 70 years). In another study in which acute glomerulonephritis and acute interstitial nephritis were excluded as causes of ARF, 64% of patients were older than 60 years and 36% were older than 70 years.[9]

Elderly patients have the same spectrum of causes of ARF as younger patients. However, within that spectrum there are some significant differences in the incidence of some causes in the elderly as opposed to the young. Obstructive disease, renal embolization or thrombosis, and hypovolemic postischemic acute tubular necrosis (ATN) were more common causes of ARF in the elderly; acute glomerulonephritis and pigment-induced (myoglobinuric) ATN were more common causes in the young. ARF can be divided into three major categories—specifically, prerenal, renal, and postrenal. The serum urea nitrogen to serum creatinine ratios of prerenal and postrenal ARF tend to run more than 20 to 1,

TABLE 49–1 **DISTRIBUTION OF VARIOUS RENAL DISEASES IN THE ELDERLY (500 BIOPSIES AND AUTOPSIES)**

Primary Glomerulopathies	
Minimal change disease	12.0%
Membranous glomerulopathy	10.2%
Acute postinfectious glomerulonephritis (GN)	2.0%
Other GN (mesangiocapillary, mesangial, focal segmental GN)	6.6%
Total	**30.8%**
Secondary Glomerulonephritis	
Focal proliferating GN (crescentic, vasculitis)	11.8%
Lupus nephritis	2.0%
IgA nephropathy, Henoch-Schönlein's purpura	0.8%
Other immune complex GN	0.8%
Total	**15.4%**
Associated with Systemic Disease	
Diabetic nephropathy	5.6%
Renal amyloidosis	5.8%
Multiple myeloma or cancer	4.0%
Total	**15.4%**
Vascular and Tubulointerstitial Disease	
Arterial and arteriolar nephrosclerosis	8.4%
Drug-related interstitial nephritis	6.6%
Pyelonephritis	3.0%
Acute tubular necrosis or cortical necrosis	5.8%
Total	**23.8%**
Other	
Insufficient tissue	6.0%
Normal, transplant, end-stage renal disease, miscellaneous	8.3%
Total	**14.3%**

Modified from Sabonis SG, Antonovych TT: A study of 500 cases of kidney diseases in the elderly. Geriatr Nephrol Urol 1993;3:15–22.

whereas the ratio in renal disease–associated ARF tends to average 10 to 14 to 1 depending on dietary protein intake.

PRERENAL ACUTE RENAL FAILURE

Prerenal ARF is due to renal hypoperfusion (dehydration, congestive heart failure, sepsis) and is often associated with recovery of renal function after correction of the hemodynamic distur-

bance. It can also occur in patients with excessive protein catabolism (intestinal bleeding, hematoma). Many milder forms of prerenal ARF remain undetected because they are treated with rehydration or with treatment for congestive heart failure or sepsis. Lamiere and associates[7] required a serum creatinine level of 3 mg/100 mL or more before a diagnosis of ARF could be made. In one study in which records of all patients admitted to three acute care geriatric units in England were reviewed, more than half of those with increased urea or creatinine concentrations had prerenal ARF.[10]

The kidney is very sensitive to the action of toxic agents because it receives 25% of the resting cardiac output. It also has a very high capacity for concentrating solutes, so the medullary portion of the kidney is exposed to high concentrations of these toxic compounds. The elderly, because of their age-related, compromised renal function and their use of many prescribed and over-the-counter drugs, are more susceptible to toxic renal injury than the young.

The use of nonsteroidal anti-inflammatory agents (NSAIDs) or angiotensin-converting enzyme (ACE) inhibitors in the elderly is largely responsible for the increasing incidence of iatrogenic hemodynamically mediated ARF in the elderly. The use of NSAIDs increases with age, but renal function impairment increases disproportionately. A number of clinical conditions (e.g., congestive heart failure, decompensated cirrhosis, nephrotic syndrome, and chronic renal failure) require local synthesis of vasodilating prostaglandins to maintain renal perfusion. Introduction of these drugs allows unopposed vasoconstriction to occur, resulting in an acute ischemic renal insult. Other risk factors for NSAID- and ACE inhibitor–induced ARF include underlying renal disease with or without renal insufficiency, hypertension, diabetes mellitus, diuretic therapy, volume depletion, and atherosclerotic cardiovascular disease.

Patients with bilateral renal artery stenosis or severe chronic heart failure may develop ARF when ACE inhibitors are prescribed. In fact, it is not uncommon for physicians to detect bilateral atheromatous renal artery disease in patients with impaired renal function because of an acute deterioration of condition after therapy with ACE inhibitors for hypertension or congestive heart failure is started.

ACUTE TUBULAR NECROSIS

Postischemic acute tubular necrosis (ATN) is the most common type of ATN and is relatively more frequent in the elderly than in younger individuals. Renal hypoperfusion can result from a variety of insults, the most common being septic shock, hypovolemia, hepatobiliary or pancreatic disease, and cardiovascular catastrophes. Many cases start as prerenal ARF that is recognized too late or not at all. Generally, renal hypoperfusion is due to systemic hypotension in a situation in which autoregulatory capacities for preservation of renal blood flow and GFR are either overwhelmed or are interrupted by preexisting renal (vascular) disease or by therapeutic interventions.

The diagnosis of hypovolemia in the elderly is often difficult. There is no reliable laboratory test that can make this diagnosis because vital signs or orthostatic decreases in blood pressure and increases in pulse rate and changes in body weight can be difficult to evaluate. The differentiation between prerenal (often hypovolemic) ARF and established renal ARF (ATN) depends on the analysis of urinary electrolytes and osmolality. The fractional excretion of sodium (FE_{na}), however, is not very reliable in elderly patients.

Antibiotics, especially the aminoglycosides, are the predominant causes of nephrotoxic ATN. The monitoring of serum concentrations of the aminoglycosides has greatly reduced the incidence of ARF due to this cause, but even with careful monitoring some cases still occur. The radiocontrast agents now used in IVP, angiography, and computed tomography are the second most common cause of drug-induced ATN. The principal contrast agents currently in use are the sodium and meglumine salts of diatrizoate, iothalamate, metrizamide, and ioxadate. The incidence of contrast-induced ARF is less than 2% unless risk factors exist, and most cases of ARF from this cause are reversible. Acute renal failure following oral cholecystography or biliary tract visualization with the use of iopanoic acid (Telepaque) is now rare unless excessively high doses are used. Factors that increase risk include age, diabetes mellitus, preexisting renal insufficiency, multiple myeloma, renal hypoperfusion (dehydration), hypertension, and hepatic disease. The risk of contrast-induced ARF in the elderly diabetic with preexisting renal insufficiency approaches 100%, and much of this may be irreversible. Other causes of ATN in the elderly population include heavy metal exposure, cisplatinum therapy, hemoglobinuria, myoglobinuria, and exposure to fluorinated anesthetic agents (Penthrane).

ACUTE INTERSTITIAL NEPHRITIS

Drug-induced acute interstitial nephritis (AIN) has become an increasingly common cause of ARF; AIN may also be seen as a complication of infectious or systemic disease. More than 40 drugs have been implicated as possible etiologic agents, with the penicillins (penicillin G, methicillin, ampicillin, oxacillin, nafcillin), cephalosporins, and NSAIDs being most commonly involved. Methicillin is the most frequently reported penicillin causing ARF; at times nearly 20% of patients treated with this drug develop ARF, perhaps because higher doses are used over a long period in patients with staphylococcal septicemia and endocarditis. Patients with penicillin-associated AIN frequently develop fever, rash, and eosinophilia or eosinophiluria in addition to a nonoliguric progressive azotemia.

The widespread use of NSAIDs has led to many reports of acute to chronic renal failure, especially in the elderly. Patients taking NSAIDs who present with ARF and nephrotic syndrome often have a histologic picture showing a combination of AIN and minimal change disease.

ACUTE GLOMERULONEPHRITIS

Although acute glomerulonephritis (AGN) is generally regarded as a disease of children and young adults, a number of reports in the literature indicate that AGN in the elderly is more common than is generally believed.[11] The essential clinical features (hematuria, proteinuria, sodium and fluid retention, decreased renal function, and hypertension) are no different in the elderly. The diagnosis may be obscured by the presence of preexisting conditions or preconceived ideas about its occurrence in the elderly. Adults frequently have a picture of cardiovascular decompensation that is attributed to underlying atherosclerotic or hypertensive heart disease, and azotemia that is either overlooked or attributed to prerenal causes. The diagnostic red cell casts are often not sought because of a low index of suspicion. Although histologic examination in many of these patients shows a poststreptococcal or postinfectious acute proliferative glomerulonephritis, it may be difficult to distinguish these patients clinically from patients with rapidly progressive (crescentic) glomerulonephritis or glomerulonephritis resulting from a systemic disease (systemic lupus erythematosus, vasculitis, subacute bacterial endocarditis, Henoch-Schönlein's purpura).

POSTRENAL OBSTRUCTION

Postrenal obstruction is an important cause of ARF because it is common and is often treatable. Prostatic hyperplasia is the most frequent cause. Hospitalized elderly patients on bed rest may be unable to generate the necessary pressure to void if they cannot stand. The frequent use of anticholinergic drugs, particularly the tricyclic antidepressants, may potentiate urinary retention.

MANAGEMENT OF ACUTE RENAL FAILURE

The first step in management of patients with acute renal failure is to identify and correct any prerenal or postrenal component. Prerenal azotemia should be suspected whenever the SUN–serum creatinine ratio exceeds 20 to 1, the urine osmolality exceeds 500 mOsm/kg H_2O, the urinary sodium concentration falls below 20 mEq/liter and/or the fractional excretion of sodium (FE_{na}) is less than 1% (this last measurement is the percentage of filtered sodium excreted in the urine). If a diagnosis of prerenal azotemia is made, volume should be replaced with saline, blood, or blood products. If cardiac output is impaired, the patient should be treated with a combination of diuretics, nitrates, inotropic agents (digoxin), and/or afterload-reducing agents (ACE inhibitors) to maximize cardiac output.

Postrenal factors, again if the SUN–serum creatinine ratio exceeds 20 to 1, should be suspected and evaluated by bladder catheterization, renal ultrasound, or nuclide urography. If an obstruction is documented and cannot be relieved by catheterization, cystoscopy with stent placement or percutaneous nephrostomy may be indicated.

Subsequent treatment should focus on maintaining control of uremic symptoms by dialysis and dietary protein restriction (caloric intake must be maintained), maintaining fluid, electrolyte, and acid-base balance, and avoiding and controlling any possible infectious complications. Hemodialysis or peritoneal dialysis should be selected based on institutional capabilities, access availability, and contraindications (e.g., heparinization).

Nephrotic Syndrome

The nephrotic syndrome consists of the urinary excretion of more than 3 g protein per day with other features that are a consequence of this continued protein loss (hypoalbuminemia, hyperlipidemia, edema, and a hypercoagulable state). Hypertension and renal failure are seen in about a third of the patients. The nephrotic syndrome can result from primary glomerular disease or from glomerular disease resulting from exposure to drugs, allergens, infection, neoplastic disease, or multisystem disease. The incidence of ne-

phrotic syndrome is at least as common in the elderly as it is in younger age groups.

Brown[11] reviewed the histopathologic findings in five series with 215 patients over the age of 60 years who presented with nephrotic syndrome. Histopathologic examination showed membranous nephropathy in 38%, minimal change nephropathy in 18%, proliferative glomerulonephritis in 13%, amyloidosis in 15%, and a variety of other lesions in the remaining 17%. The incidence of membranous nephropathy and amyloidosis was higher than it is in younger adults, that of proliferative glomerulonephritis was much lower, and the incidence of minimal change disease was comparable but much lower than it is in children. A subsequent study[12] showed a similar incidence of primary glomerular diseases in individuals older than 60 years compared to young adults, but there was a different distribution of causes. IgA nephritis was seen less frequently, and membranous glomerulopathy and pauci-immune crescentic glomerulonephritis were more frequent. Glomerulopathies resulting from systemic disease are more common in the elderly because there is an increased incidence of such underlying diseases as diabetes mellitus, amyloidosis (dysproteinemias), neoplastic disease, vasculitis, and scleroderma in older people.

MEMBRANOUS NEPHROPATHY

Membranous nephropathy (MN) is consistently the most common cause of nephrotic syndrome in the elderly; at least 85% of patients with MN present with nephrotic proteinuria. The two most common causes of secondary MN are drugs (e.g., NSAIDs) and cancer. Brown[11] reported that 11% of patients with MN had an underlying malignancy.

It remains unclear whether the prognosis of elderly patients with MN is worse than that of younger persons; however, it does appear that older patients are more susceptible to the extrarenal complications of the nephrotic syndrome and its treatment (e.g., cardiovascular, thrombotic, and infectious events).[13] Corticosteroid therapy alone appears to be of little benefit in inducing remission or preventing deterioration of renal function; the combination of an immunosuppressive (e.g., chlorambucil and corticosteroids) appears more likely to be helpful, but side effects of treatment are frequent.

MINIMAL CHANGE NEPHROPATHY

The clinical presentation of minimal change nephropathy (MCN) is similar in old and young (i.e., nephrotic syndrome), but older individuals are much more likely to have nonselective proteinuria, microscopic hematuria, hypertension, and renal insufficiency. While Lorca and Ponticelli,[13] in reviewing 11 series, reported that 80% of patients with MCN responded initially to treatment with corticosteroids or cytotoxic agents, almost a third experienced a relapse, and half then developed renal failure or died. These authors recommended treating the patient initially with corticosteroids followed by a cytotoxic agent in 12 weeks if steroids are not tolerated or are not effective.

FOCAL AND SEGMENTAL GLOMERULOSCLEROSIS

In patients with sclerotic lesions the presence of nephrotic syndrome and the finding of fusion of foot processes on electron microscopy are the most reliable features for a diagnosis of idiopathic focal and segmental glomerulosclerosis. Although some of these patients will respond to prolonged administration of corticosteroid or cytotoxic agents, the risk of side effects generally outweighs the benefits of these agents in the elderly.

RAPIDLY PROGRESSIVE GLOMERULONEPHRITIS

Rapidly progressive glomerulonephritis (RPGN) is the result of a number of diseases of immunologic pathogenesis resulting in a renal lesion characterized by extracapillary proliferation in the glomeruli (crescent formation within Bowman's capsule). These patients often test positive for serum p-antinuclear cytoplasmic antibody (p-ANCA). Keller and colleagues[14] reported a linear increase in the incidence of RPGN with age; over 40% of their patients were older than 60 years. Although they used aggressive corticosteroid-immunosuppressive therapy in their elderly patients and noted better results in maintenance of self-sustaining renal function in treated versus untreated patients, they found that the long-term efficacy of such treatment was limited and the complication rate was high. Initial oliguria was the most significant risk factor for permanent loss of renal function.

NEPHROTIC SYNDROME RESULTING FROM SYSTEMIC DISEASE

Nephritis associated with systemic lupus erythematosus (SLE) can be classified into one of four histologic patterns—mesangial, focal proliferative, diffuse proliferative, or membranous. The diagnosis is established by a positive antinuclear antibody (ANA) titer in the serum or, more specifically, by positive results on the antideoxyribonucleoprotein antibody (anti-DNA) test. Renal involvement appears to be less common in the elderly than in younger populations. The prognosis is determined by both renal and extrarenal involvement. Impressive responses have been reported with either azathioprine or cyclophosphamide combined with prednisone therapy.

Diabetic nephropathy is the most frequent cause of glomerular disease associated with systemic illness in the elderly. The diagnosis can be made clinically from a history of long-standing diabetes, evidence of proteinuria (usually in the nephrotic range), diabetic retinopathy, and hypertension. Once nephrotic proteinuria develops, the disease follows a downhill course (3 to 5 years) ending in dialysis regardless of treatment. Control of blood pressure is important in slowing the rate of deterioration of renal function. The use of ACE inhibitors or angiotensin-II receptor blockade even in normotensive individuals to promote efferent arteriolar vasodilatation and a decrease in glomerular capillary pressure also slows the rate of deterioration of renal function. Tight control of blood glucose, in contrast, does not appear to affect the course of the disease. Vigorous treatment of urinary tract infections and avoidance of analgesics to prevent the development of papillary necrosis are warranted.

Amyloidosis is characterized by deposition of amyloid fibrils in glomerular capillary loops. In primary amyloidosis, these fibrils are light chains that have a composition similar to those of Bence Jones proteins. Patients with plasma cell dyscrasias often have an amyloidosis similar to that seen with primary amyloidosis. Secondary amyloidosis is associated with such chronic inflammatory diseases as rheumatoid arthritis, tuberculosis, chronic bone, lung, or urinary tract infections, and inflammatory bowel disease. The amyloid fibrils, in contrast, are composed of a nonimmunoglobulin protein and are distributed throughout the organ systems in a different pattern from that seen in primary amyloidosis. All nephrotics over the age of 50 years should undergo performance of urine and serum electrophoresis because amyloidosis is a frequent cause of secondary nephrotic syndrome.

Lesions associated with the collagen vascular diseases (e.g., SLE, vasculitis, and Wegener's granulomatosis) respond well to corticosteroid or cytotoxic or immunosuppressant therapy, whereas most other lesions tend to be resistant to treatment. Because of the potential adverse effects of these treatments, renal biopsy is important in determining whether or not therapeutic trials should be initiated in patients in whom the diagnosis is unclear.

Chronic Renal Failure

Chronic renal failure results from irreversible damage to both kidneys from a wide variety of causes. Up to 90% of kidney function may be lost without significant morbidity. The physician's role in these patients is to prevent progression of the renal lesions and worsening of the condition by managing hypertension, infection, obstructive uropathy, heart failure, and dehydration. Some of the more common clinical entities that can cause chronic renal failure without preceding nephrotic syndrome are discussed in the following section.

RENAL VASCULAR DISORDERS

Occlusive arterial disease can cause either acute or chronic renal failure. Renal arterial embolization or thrombosis may occur in patients with acute myocardial infarction, chronic atrial fibrillation, and subacute bacterial endocarditis. Symptoms vary from essentially a slowly progressive, clinically silent event to acute severe flank pain and tenderness, hematuria, hypertension, and fever. Intravenous pyelography or renal scans followed by aortography are used to establish a diagnosis. Anticoagulant therapy may be beneficial; surgery is generally not indicated for embolization but may be helpful in selected patients with renal arterial arteriosclerosis or when an intra-abdominal aortic aneurysm is the underlying cause.

Renal cholesterol embolization may occur spontaneously or in association with aortic surgery or angiography in patients with diffuse atherosclerosis. The clinical course is variable, but in most cases a progressive renal insufficiency develops. A definitive diagnosis is difficult because it requires visualization of cholesterol crystals on biopsy, and other diagnoses are often valid possibilities.

Renal artery stenosis (RAS) is common in the elderly and is usually due to atherosclerosis. Although often totally asymptomatic, it should be considered in the differential diagnosis whenever an older person suddenly develops hypertension, or if a patient with well-controlled hypertension shows an accelerated course, or if an unexplained increase in blood urea nitrogen or serum creatinine occurs, especially after treatment with an ACE inhibitor.

Intravenous pyelography or isotopic renography can be used for screening purposes. A difference in kidney length of 1 cm or more, delayed appearance or disappearance of dye in the involved kidney, or enhanced concentration of dye in the involved kidney should suggest the diagnosis. An acute decrease in renal perfusion of the involved kidney can be produced by any ACE inhibitor in a patient with RAS, and this change can be detected using isotopes or dyes; little decrease in renal perfusion will be observed in kidneys without RAS. The arteriogram is the definitive study and must be done prior to any contemplated surgical repair. Although antihypertensive therapy often results in adequate blood pressure control, surgical correction of the stenosis or angioplasty is indicated if one wishes to avoid loss of renal function in the involved kidney.

ARTERIOLAR NEPHROSCLEROSIS, BENIGN AND MALIGNANT

The small arteries and arterioles of the kidney are usually affected by an elevation in systemic blood pressure. Patients with mild to moderate blood pressure elevation develop a benign arteriolar nephrosclerosis characterized by fibrosis and thickening of the intima of the larger arteries and by patchy hyaline thickening of the afferent arteriolar wall, both resulting in a progressive decrease in luminal size. Chronic renal failure associated with this lesion tends to develop very slowly over a period of years. In hypertensives with diastolic pressures in excess of 130 mmHg an accelerated or malignant phase develops in which afferent arterioles and interlobular arteries show a proliferative endarteritis ("onion skin" appearance of the endothelium) and necrotizing arteriolitis (fibrinoid necrosis of media) along with a glomerulitis with necrosis. Hematuria with red cell casts, albuminuria, and rapid loss of renal function develops.

SYSTEMIC VASCULITIS

This term refers to a heterogeneous group of disorders characterized by inflammation and necrotizing lesions of the blood vessel walls. These may be primary lesions or may be associated with other systemic diseases. Manifestations include fever, weight loss, arthritis, abdominal pain, polyneuritis, myopathy, and cardiac and central nervous system dysfunction. In some instances, these problems can be classified into specific disorders (e.g., periarteritis nodosa or Wegener's granulomatosis). Hematuria with or without red cell casts is an almost universal finding, with proteinuria (nephrotic syndrome) and renal insufficiency variably present. These patients often have a positive serum c–antinuclear cytoplasmic antibody (c-ANCA) pattern.

Classic polyarteritis nodosa (PAN) is a necrotizing vasculitis of the small and medium-sized muscular arteries; aneurysmal dilatations seen in the arteriograms of kidney, liver, and intestine are virtually pathognomonic of PAN. Fever, weight loss, hypertension, gastrointestinal symptoms, weakness, myalgia, angina, and hepatic dysfunction may accompany the renal insufficiency. Biopsy of the involved tissue (kidney, nerve, testicles) reveals a mononuclear fibrinoid necrosis without granuloma that is diagnostic. Treatment with immunosuppressive agents and corticosteroids greatly prolongs survival.

Wegener's granulomatosis is a necrotizing granulomatous vasculitis of the nasopharynx, paranasal sinuses, lungs, and renal glomeruli. In the glomeruli, a focal-segmental fibrinoid necrosis and sclerosis accompanies mesangial and endothelial cell proliferation. Fever, weight loss, weakness, and arthralgias along with upper and lower respiratory symptoms should suggest the diagnosis. Anemia, elevated erythrocyte sedimentation rate, and leukocytosis are usually present. Chest radiograph usually shows nodules or infiltrates. Biopsy of a respiratory tract lesion should provide the diagnosis; a renal biopsy shows only a nonspecific vasculitis. Cyclophosphamide produces long-standing remissions.

POLYCYSTIC RENAL DISEASE

Although the diagnosis of polycystic kidney disease is usually made before the age of 60 years, a few patients are not diagnosed until later in life. A family history is not always present. The presenting symptoms usually are those of renal insufficiency, often with a history of hypertension or hematuria. The enlarged kidneys often are palpable. Microscopic hematuria and mild proteinuria (< 1 g/24 hours) are often present. The diagnosis is made by intravenous pyelography or ultrasonography. Control of hypertension, bleeding, and infection helps to delay the onset of renal insufficiency.

ANALGESIC NEPHROPATHY

The frequency of arthritis and arthralgias in the elderly increases the risk of long-term analgesic use and abuse. Phenacetin is the drug most frequently incriminated, but salicylates, acetaminophen, and NSAIDs also must be considered. These drugs, because they inhibit the action of vasodilatory prostaglandins, leading to oxidative injury of medullary cells, frequently cause chronic interstitial nephritis and ultimately papil-

lary necrosis, leading to renal insufficiency, mild proteinuria, and hypertension, which are often severe. The lesions are dose- and duration-dependent. Therapy consists of discontinuation of all analgesics if possible, control of hypertension, and conservative management of renal insufficiency.

MULTIPLE MYELOMA

Multiple myeloma should be ruled out in any patient with unexplained renal insufficiency. A strong relationship exists between the presence of Bence Jones proteinuria (immunoglobulin light chains) and renal insufficiency. The renal damage may result from tubular obstruction or tubular nephrotoxicity from the light chains. Other causes of renal insufficiency in the patient with multiple myeloma include amyloidosis, hypercalcemia, and urate deposition. Myeloma patients are specifically at risk for renal failure with the use of radiocontrast dyes and antibiotics such as the aminoglycosides.

SCLERODERMA

Elderly patients with other manifestations consistent with scleroderma may develop hypertension, at times malignant, and acute to chronic renal insufficiency. Narrowing of the interlobular arteries without inflammatory infiltrates produces the renin-mediated hypertension. Aggressive antihypertensive therapy, especially with ACE inhibitors, has been reported to slow the progression of this condition.

MANAGEMENT OF CHRONIC RENAL FAILURE

Both the clinical manifestations and the management of chronic renal failure are similar, with only minor exceptions, no matter what disease process caused the initial damage. A low protein intake (40 g protein/day) and control of blood pressure are important in slowing the progression of renal insufficiency. As serum phosphate increases, phosphate-binding antacids (aluminum hydroxide gels such as Amphojel or Basaljel) should be given with meals. If hypocalcemia persists after correction of the hyperphosphatemia, vitamin D or its active metabolite $1,25(OH)_2$ cholecalciferol (calcitriol) should be given to normalize the serum calcium level. Anemia associated with chronic renal failure can be due to iron deficiency, hemolysis, or a deficient erythropoietin concentration. After elimination of the first by evaluation of the serum iron or ferritin level, a decision must be made about when to start treatment with either transfusions of packed red cells or recombinant human erythropoietin. Whereas younger patients often tolerate hematocrit levels of as low as 20% (because of the increase in 2,3-diphosphoglycerate [2,3-DPG] levels, which shifts the oxyhemoglobin affinity curve to promote better tissue oxygenation), the older patient, often because of associated cardiac disease, may need a higher hematocrit to function optimally.

At some point, a decision must be made about whether and when to place the patient on dialysis. Absolute indications for dialysis include hyperkalemia, acidosis, or volume overload that do not respond to medical management, pericarditis, and progressing peripheral neuropathy. There is no absolute level of blood urea nitrogen or serum creatinine concentration above which dialysis should be started. Patients should be started on maintenance dialysis when the more subjective symptoms first occur, most commonly loss of appetite and weight. To qualify for Medicare reimbursement, the creatinine clearance must be below 10 mL/minute using the Cockcroft-Gault formula.[4] This means that elderly individuals with little muscle mass to generate creatinine may require dialysis when the serum creatinine is as low as 5 mg/dL. Diabetics, in general, do better when dialysis is started early.

Elderly patients with end-stage renal disease (ESRD) generally have, in addition to renal disease, other complicating medical illnesses. Because of this, their life expectancy is less than that in younger patients. Despite the lower life expectancy, most nephrologists are willing to offer maintenance dialysis therapy to older patients. Most older patients can be rehabilitated and have a quality of life comparable to that of their age-matched counterparts without ESRD.

Elderly patients with ESRD, like younger patients, have a number of therapeutic options available to them including in-hospital or in-center hemodialysis, home hemodialysis, continuous ambulatory peritoneal dialysis (CAPD), and renal transplantation. If hemodialysis is elected, special care must be taken in the creation of a mode of dialysis access. Generally, construction of an autogenous arteriovenous fistula is the most satisfactory and lasting method, but it may be more difficult to create in elderly patients, especially those with a history of diabetes, arteriosclerosis, vascular accidents, or secondary hyperparathyroidism.

Increasing numbers of patients are electing CAPD as an alternative form of therapy. This mode of treatment allows dialysis to be performed at home, results in better stabilization of serum chemistries, and puts less stress on the cardiovascular system. CAPD also can be selected for patients who are developing arteriovenous access problems. Complications associated with CAPD include peritonitis, catheter exit site infections, pancreatitis, and technical failure.

Although it was formerly believed that older patients were at much greater risk after undergoing transplantation, this has not proved to be the case. One-year graft survival is no worse in older patients than in younger ones. Compared to dialysis, however, 1- and 3-year survival of older transplant patients is substantially better. The general decline in T-cell function with aging may actually facilitate graft survival in the elderly. However, this phenomenon may also predispose the elderly to more infectious complications. Infections, cardiovascular diseases, and stroke continue to be the principal causes of death in older transplant patients.

RENAL CALCULI

Many of the constituents of renal calculi, most notably calcium, are normally present in the urine as supersaturated solutions and are maintained in solution by protective colloids. A delicate balance is maintained, and precipitation results if an infectious nidus or a change in concentration or pH occurs. Calcium phosphate or oxalate becomes insoluble at an alkaline pH; an acid pH favors precipitation of uric acid and cystine. Triple phosphates generally indicate infection with a urea-splitting organism.

Calcium Stones

Identification of calcium on stone analysis should lead one to suspect hypercalciuria as an underlying cause. On a normal diet, approximately 150 mg/day of calcium is excreted by the normal person. More than 250 mg/day is considered hypercalciuric. Most of these patients have an absorptive defect as opposed to a renal defect. Serum calcium, phosphorus, and alkaline phosphatase concentrations can be used to screen for hyperparathyroidism, but hypercalciuria can result from hypercalcemia of any cause. Immobilization, particularly that resulting from paralysis or a fracture with extensive casting, greatly increases urinary calcium excretion (>500 mg/day), which in turn can lead to stone formation. Immobilization is particularly important in elderly patients, in whom there is often an increase in oxalate excretion (related to increased intestinal absorption and dehydration).

Idiopathic hypercalciuria (normal serum calcium level without underlying cause of hypercalciuria) can be treated with a high fluid intake (2 to 3 liters/day), restriction of calcium intake (dairy products), urinary acidification, and thiazides, which decrease urinary calcium excretion. Hypercalcemia is a potential side effect of the last.

Uric Acid

Uric acid stones develop when urinary uric acid exceeds 1000 mg/day or when pH falls to the range of 5.5. Therapy is directed at raising the pH level using an alkali such as potassium citrate. Often calcium oxalate precipitates with the hyperuricosuric stone, so that treatment with a thiazide as well as allopurinol is indicated.

DISTURBANCES IN SODIUM AND WATER BALANCE

Sodium is the primary extracellular cation and is responsible for maintaining the state of hydration outside the cell. The serum sodium concentration is an accurate and precise laboratory determination that can be used to classify disturbed states of sodium balance into hyponatremic, hypernatremic, or normal categories. Water balance is determined by the clinical assessment of extracellular fluid volume (ECFV), which is much more subjective.

Dehydration

Dehydration, by definition, means a decrease in total body water. Dehydration may develop either from a primary loss of water, in which case hypernatremia occurs, or from a loss of salt with obligated water. Patients with the latter condition become volume depleted but maintain normal serum sodium concentrations and osmolalities until the volume depletion becomes sufficient to stimulate antidiuretic hormone release. If fluid is then replaced, water is retained, and hyponatremia develops.

Hypertension and Edema Formation

Acute sodium loading is associated with appropriate enhancement of sodium excretion, but, this is markedly delayed in older people compared with younger ones.[15] The regulation of sodium excretion after a sodium load is complex and depends on arterial pressure, GFR, natriuretic factors (prostaglandins, dopamine, atrial natriuretic peptide, kinins), and antinatriuretic factors (renin-angiotensin-aldosterone system, sympathetic nervous system, renal sodium-potassium-ATPase activity). In older sodium-sensitive subjects, volume is apparently modestly expanded, leading to hypertension and edema formation.

TABLE 49–2 **CAUSES OF HYPONATREMIA**

I. Hyponatremia with contracted extracellular fluid volume (ECFV) (salt depletion with Na+ loss greater than H_2O loss)
   A. Gastrointestinal loss
   B. Renal loss
      1. Adrenal (Addison's disease, hypoaldosteronism)
      2. Renal (renal tubular acidosis, salt wasting)
      3. Diuretic therapy
II. Hyponatremia with normal ECFV
   A. Displacement syndromes (pseudohyponatremia)
      1. Hyperglycemia
      2. Hyperlipidemia
      3. Hyperproteinemia
   B. Syndrome of inappropriate antidiuretic hormone (ADH)
      1. Cerebral (trauma, infection, cerebrovascular accident, tumor)
      2. Tumor (lung, pancreas, breast)
      3. Pulmonary disease
      4. Drugs (sulfonylureas, thiazides, antitumor agents, psychotropics, antidepressants)
      5. Myxedema
      6. Idiopathic
III. Hyponatremia with expanded ECFV (dilutional with H_2O retention more than Na+ retention)
   A. Congestive heart failure
   B. Cirrhosis
   C. Renal disease (nephrotic syndrome, renal failure)
   D. Water intoxication (schizophrenics)

Hyponatremia

A low serum sodium concentration may result from (1) a loss of sodium in excess of osmotically obligated water (primary salt depletion), (2) a retention of water in excess of sodium (dilutional hyponatremia), or (3) a combination of both (syndrome of inappropriate antidiuretic hormone (SIADH) (Table 49–2). Hyponatremia may also result from a displacement of plasma water with large-molecular-weight solute (proteins, lipids) or from the addition of an uncharged solute (glucose, mannitol) to the extracellular fluid.

HYPONATREMIA WITH CONTRACTED EXTRACELLULAR FLUID VOLUME (PRIMARY SALT DEPLETION)

In primary salt depletion, if the urinary sodium concentration is less than 10 mEq/liter, the cause can be decreased salt intake, excessive sweating with replacement of losses by water alone, or gastrointestinal salt losses. If the urinary sodium concentration is greater than 10 mEq/liter, inappropriate renal losses of sodium and water may be due to excessive use of diuretics, adrenal or pituitary insufficiency, or intrinsic renal disease (salt-losing nephritis, renal insufficiency, or renal tubular acidosis). In patients with severe vomiting with metabolic alkalosis and bicarbonaturia, urinary sodium concentrations may be elevated despite hypovolemia and hyponatremia. Elderly subjects are more prone to develop hyponatremia under these conditions because there is a modest reduction in the capacity of the kidney to conserve sodium in normal elderly people subjected to salt depletion,[16] probably at least partly because of a decrease in circulating aldosterone.[17] Another contributing factor may be an increased circulating level of atrial natriuretic peptide (ANP) because the metabolic clearance is prolonged in the elderly.

Treatment of hyponatremia with contracted ECFV generally is accomplished with isotonic saline, although in severe cases hypertonic saline may be used initially. In trying to distinguish primary salt depletion from SIADH, an important clue may be provided by the SUN because this value is elevated in the former but is often subnormal in the latter.

HYPONATREMIA WITH EXPANDED EXTRACELLULAR VOLUME (DILUTIONAL HYPONATREMIA)

Impairment in water excretion occurs in situations in which salt excretion is also severely impaired. Patients with advanced cardiac, hepatic, or renal disease and generalized edema often are placed on diets that restrict salt intake but place no limits on fluid intake. Although total ECFV in such patients usually is increased, the effective blood volume in the arterial vascular system tends to be decreased, thus stimulating receptors in the left atrium and arterial system to initiate retention of salt and water. A decrease in glomerular filtration rate or an increase in sodium reabsorption in the proximal tubule decreases the delivery of salt and water to the distal diluting segment of the nephron. If little salt and water reach the distal nephron, the individual becomes unable to dilute urine much below isotonic concentrations. Because normally the intake of water relative to salt represents a hypotonic solution, this situation results in the development of hyponatremia. Treatment is accomplished with fluid restriction or the use of diuretics active in the loop of Henle (e.g., furosemide, which promotes

excretion of a hypotonic urine even in the presence of ADH).

HYPONATREMIA WITH NORMAL EXTRACELLULAR VOLUME (SYNDROME OF INAPPROPRIATE ANTIDIURETIC HORMONE)

Persistence of circulating ADH is considered inappropriate when neither serum hyperosmolality nor volume depletion is present. In patients with pulmonary disease, there may be decreased blood flow circulating through the lung and impaired filling of the left atrium, resulting in ADH stimulation. Inability to excrete water because of inappropriate levels of ADH in the circulation leads to volume expansion, which, by multiple mechanisms, promotes urinary salt loss. Ultimately, volume returns to normal. SIADH is seen most frequently in patients with oat cell carcinomas of the lung, but it is also seen in other conditions as shown in Table 49–2.

Treatment is accomplished with fluid restriction. If hyponatremia becomes severe, furosemide can be given, replacing salt losses as necessary with normal or hypertonic saline. Rapid correction carries with it some risk, specifically central pontine myelinolysis. Lithium and demeclocycline (Declomycin) also have been used to promote increased water loss (nephrogenic diabetes insipidus).

The serum sodium concentrations in patients with hyperlipidemia and hyperproteinemia are decreased because of the volume actually occupied by the lipids and proteins respectively. If the lipids or proteins are removed from the plasma, the sodium concentration in the remaining plasma water is normal. In patients with hyperglycemia, the cause of hyponatremia is the glucose-related increase in osmolality of the extracellular fluids, resulting in a shift of water from the intracellular to the extracellular fluid compartments. The expansion of ECFV triggers a loss in the urine of excessive fluid along with sodium, bringing ECFV back to normal.

HYPONATREMIA IN THE ELDERLY

Surveys in older persons in both acute and chronic care facilities show a high prevalence of hyponatremia. Kleinfeld and colleagues[18] reported that 36 of 160 chronically ill patients (23%) had a serum sodium concentration of below 132 mEq/liter (mean, 120 mEq/liter). In most, the low serum sodium concentration was not readily explainable except by the presence of debilitating disease and old age.

Other evidence suggests that elderly persons

may be more susceptible to the development of hyponatremia similar to that seen in SIADH than are their younger counterparts. Postoperative hyponatremia and hyponatremia induced by diuretics and sulfonylureas occur almost exclusively in older patients. In one study, older subjects increased serum arginine vasopressin (AVP) concentrations much more after a standardized hypertonic saline infusion (designed to raise serum osmolality to 306 mOsm/liter) than did younger subjects.[19] In contrast, ethanol, which inhibits ADH secretion, produced a more prolonged depression of serum AVP concentrations in young than in older subjects. These two observations suggest an increasing osmoreceptor sensitivity with age.

Following quiet standing, older subjects often failed to increase serum AVP, whereas younger subjects did.[20] This suggests that the vasopressin response to volume-pressure stimuli might be the primary defect in the elderly and the osmotic hyperresponsiveness might be compensatory.

Hypernatremia

An increase in serum sodium concentration usually results from a larger loss of body water than of salt (dehydration), although it also can result from ingestion or administration of sodium (e.g., sodium bicarbonate without sufficient water to provide an isotonic intake). Among elderly patients, hypernatremia is most common in those who are bedridden or restricted and are not provided sufficient drinking water or in those whose sensation of thirst is impaired. A net deficit of water can also be associated with vomiting and diarrhea, diabetes insipidus, an osmotic diuresis (e.g., hyperosmolar nonketotic diabetic acidosis), and hyperpyrexia (excessive sweating).

Older patients appear to be predisposed to the development of hypernatremia (dehydration). Snyder and associates[21] reported that more than 1% of their hospital admissions were patients over the age of 60 years who developed hypernatremia (serum sodium concentration of more than 148 mEq/liter). Surgery, febrile illness, infirmity, and diabetes mellitus accounted for two thirds of their cases. Half developed hypernatremia while in the hospital.

Alterations in thirst perception were studied by Phillips and colleagues[22] in healthy old and young persons. After 24 hours of water deprivation, all subjects were given free access to water. Older subjects showed less thirst and drank less water even though they lost more fluid during the period of water deprivation, and they showed higher plasma sodium concentrations and osmolalities.

The earliest manifestation of hypernatremia is thirst followed by confusion and lethargy and, ultimately, by delirium, stupor, and coma. Because intravascular volume is preserved at the expense of cell water, changes in blood pressure, pulse rate, and skin turgor are not prominent features of hypernatremia.

Once significant hypernatremia develops, parenteral restoration of fluid balance is usually necessary. The amount of water (or dextrose and water) needed can be determined by multiplying the percentage of increase in serum sodium concentration above normal by the total body water (60% of body weight). To prevent a recurrence, a fluid prescription (quantity of fluid to be ingested daily) may be an important component of treatment.

DISTURBANCES IN POTASSIUM BALANCE

Potassium is the primary intracellular cation; less than 2% of total body potassium is found in the extracellular fluid compartment. Thus, the serum potassium concentration may not accurately reflect total body potassium stores. A flux of potassium into cells occurs with cell growth, with intracellular nitrogen and glycogen deposition, and with increases in extracellular pH. Potassium leaves the cell with cell destruction, with intracellular glucose use (assuming that cell uptake of glucose under the influence of insulin is limited), and with decreases in extracellular pH. Because a steep concentration gradient normally is maintained between intracellular and extracellular compartments, the factors affecting this gradient must be kept in mind when evaluating any serum potassium concentration. For example, the diabetic patient with ketoacidosis admitted with a high serum potassium concentration experiences a dramatic decrease in this value with rehydration, correction of the acidosis with bicarbonate, and treatment of the hyperglycemia with insulin as the cation moves intracellularly. Age alone does not appear to affect one's ability to maintain this gradient. However, certain clinical conditions commonly seen in the elderly (e.g., metabolic and respiratory acidosis, congestive heart failure, cirrhosis, and uremia) are accompanied by a decrease in the intracellular to extracellular gradient.

Hypokalemia

The causes of hypokalemia are listed in Table 49-3. Diuretic therapy is probably the most frequent cause of hypokalemia in the elderly. The most frequently overlooked cause, however, is excessive use of enemas and purgatives. Multiple pathophysiologic mechanisms are often impli-

TABLE 49–3   **CAUSES OF HYPOKALEMIA**

I.   Inadequate intake
II. Metabolic alkalosis
III. Gastrointestinal losses
   A. Vomiting (alkalosis)
   B. Diarrhea, fistulas
   C. Excessive use of enemas, purgatives
IV. Renal losses
   A. Diuretic therapy
   B. Adrenal
     1. Cushing's syndrome
       (mineralocorticoid excess)
     2. Hyperaldosteronism (primary,
       secondary)
   C. Renal disease
     1. Renal tubular acidosis (proximal,
       distal)
     2. Salt-wasting renal disease
   D. Drug-induced (e.g., licorice)
   E. Hypomagnesemia

cated in the development of hypokalemia. For example, the person who is vomiting reduces potassium intake and loses small amounts of potassium, but, more important, he loses hydrogen ions, causing a metabolic alkalosis, which shifts potassium intracellularly and increases urinary potassium losses. The contracted intravascular volume increases proximal tubular sodium and bicarbonate reabsorption, which further enhances the metabolic alkalosis and produces a secondary hyperaldosteronism. This in turn increases urinary potassium losses.

Although the normal kidney does not conserve potassium as effectively as sodium, excretion can be reduced to below 20 mEq/day even in the presence of an acidosis or alkalosis. Since little potassium is lost through the gastrointestinal tract, it takes 2 to 3 weeks on a potassium-free diet for a person to develop hypokalemia (potassium <3.0 mEq/liter), provided that other organ systems are functioning normally. The causes of excessive urinary potassium loss can be separated into four categories, specifically: (1) pituitary-adrenal excess, (2) renal abnormalities, (3) drug-induced losses, and (4) idiopathic and miscellaneous causes, as outlined in Table 49–3.

Structural and functional defects associated with potassium deficiency include involvement of the kidney (concentrating defect), myocardium (depressed ST segment, inversion of T waves, accentuated U waves, arrhythmia, potentiation of digitalis toxicity, salt retention, hypotension), muscle (weakness to paralysis, tenderness), gastrointestinal tract (decreased motility), and endocrine-metabolic system (carbohydrate intolerance, growth failure). Depressive reactions

(weakness, lethargy, apathy, fatigue) and acute brain syndromes also have been reported.

Since an alkalosis (chloride depletion) usually accompanies hypokalemia, replacement therapy should be accomplished with potassium chloride rather than with the alkaline salts of potassium. The exception is the patient with renal tubular acidosis. One can question the need for routine replacement potassium therapy in patients receiving diuretics, especially those being treated for hypertension. A great deal of concern and discussion has been generated suggesting that hypokalemia may precipitate cardiac arrhythmias and sudden death in patients receiving diuretics, especially those taking digitalis for cardiac disorders and those with acute myocardial infarction. Controlled trials suggest that treatment with potassium supplementation fails to affect the outcome. A significant incidence of life-threatening hyperkalemia in patients receiving supplements must be weighed against the benefits of supplemental therapy.

Age and azotemia were the two significant risk factors identified in the Boston Collaborative Drug Surveillance Program for the development of hyperkalemia after potassium supplementation.[23] Only 0.8% of patients under age 50 developed hyperkalemia after potassium supplementation; in contrast, the incidence rose from 4.2% to 6.0% with advancing age in patients over age 50. As described earlier, elderly people with both restricted and unrestricted salt intakes, both upright and supine, have a much lower plasma renin activity and urinary aldosterone excretion than do comparable young subjects, which probably explains their inability to excrete excessive potassium in the urine.[17]

Hyperkalemia

Most episodes of hyperkalemia are seen in patients with impaired renal function. However, most patients with chronic renal failure are able to maintain good urine flow rates and do not develop significant hyperkalemia until azotemia becomes life-threatening. Because the distal nephron has such a sizable capacity for secreting potassium, even in patients with advanced renal failure, hyperkalemia develops only when there is some associated contributing factor, such as oliguria (acute renal failure), excessive potassium load (tissue catabolism, exogenous supplements), severe acidosis, administration of a diuretic to block sodium-potassium exchange (triamterene, spironolactone), a deficiency of endogenous steroid (aldosterone, mineralocorticoid), or administration of an NSAID or ACE inhibitor. In older persons, especially diabetics and patients with interstitial nephritis, the renin-aldosterone system often fails, and the patient develops what is often referred to as a type IV renal tubular acidosis (hyperkalemia and mild metabolic acidosis).

The clinical manifestations of hyperkalemia can be very subtle (anxiety, restlessness, apprehension, weakness) and may precede death from cardiac arrhythmia only briefly. Characteristic electrocardiographic changes start with peaking of T waves and are followed by loss of P waves and widening of the QRS complex. Therapy should be started when the serum potassium concentration exceeds 5.5 mEq/liter and becomes a true medical emergency when it exceeds 7.0 mEq/liter. Acute treatment is accomplished with glucose, insulin, and sodium bicarbonate to shift potassium intracellularly, and with calcium and sodium salts, which act as physiologic antagonists. Ion exchange resins (Kayexalate) are used to remove excess potassium from the body and can be given orally or in enema form. To avoid constipation, sorbitol can be given orally. When hyperkalemia is due to a mineralocorticoid deficiency, fludrocortisone (Florinef) can be given.

DISTURBANCES IN ACID-BASE BALANCE

Alterations in acid-base balance are generally described in terms of changes in the carbon dioxide-bicarbonate system because these changes reflect shifts in all other buffer systems in the blood and tissues and can be easily quantified. Most clinical laboratories measure pH and PCO_2 with highly accurate and reproducible electrodes and then extrapolate the bicarbonate concentration from a nomogram.

The body jealously guards pH and maintains it within a narrow normal range. Only small changes in pH (6.9 to 7.7) remain compatible with life. An acidosis results from the introduction of excess acid into the body fluids and an alkalosis from excess loss of acid. The body must cope with two types of acid, specifically carbonic acid derived from the hydration of carbon dioxide, and fixed hydrogen ions. The lungs remove the volatile carbon dioxide generated during metabolism. Retention of carbon dioxide results in an acidosis; excessive loss of carbon dioxide (hyperventilation) results in an alkalosis. The hydrogen ions and associated organic (lactate, beta-hydroxybutyrate) and inorganic (phosphate, sulfate) anions are buffered in body fluids and can be excreted only by the kidney or lost through other fluids (e.g., through the gastrointestinal tract).

Although acid-base parameters remain normal in the elderly under basal conditions, the ability of an older person to correct abnormalities after an acute event is impaired.[24] Although the minimum urinary pH achieved is similar in young and old, older men excrete only about half as much of the acid load over an 8-hour period as do younger men. When one factors net acid excretion by glomerular filtration rate, the excretion rates are comparable, suggesting that the decrease is related to a decreased nephron mass with age. There does appear to be a defect in ammonia excretion in the elderly, even when urinary excretions are factored by glomerular filtration rate, which is balanced by an increase in titratable acid excretion per unit of GFR in the elderly.

Acid-base disturbances can be separated into metabolic acidosis (low pH, PCO_2, bicarbonate), metabolic alkalosis (high pH, PCO_2, bicarbonate), respiratory acidosis (low pH, high PCO_2), and respiratory alkalosis (high pH, low PCO_2). Most primary disturbances are accompanied by a compensatory correction to maintain pH as close to normal as possible. For example, in a person with a metabolic acidosis, one sees a compensatory respiratory alkalosis (hyperventilation).

Metabolic Acidosis

It is useful in any patient with a metabolic acidosis to determine if an "anion gap" exists. Normally, the difference between sodium concentration and the sum of the chloride and bicarbonate concentrations is less than 12 mEq/liter. When the difference is larger, an anion gap exists, indicating excessive accumulation of organic (lactate, beta-hydroxybutyrate, salicylate, formate) or inorganic (phosphate, sulfate) anions. If no anion gap exists, the serum chloride concentration increases as the serum bicarbonate decreases (hyperchloremic acidosis). The causes of metabolic acidosis are listed in Table 49–4.

TABLE 49–4 **CAUSES OF METABOLIC ACIDOSIS**

   I. With anion gap
     A. Azotemic renal failure
     B. Diabetic and starvation ketoacidosis
     C. Methyl alcohol intoxication
     D. Paraldehyde intoxication
     E. Ethylene glycol intoxication
     F. Salicylate intoxication
     G. Lactic acidosis
       1. Circulatory insufficiency and shock
       2. Primary
  II. Without anion gap
     A. Diarrhea and fistula drainage (bicarbonate loss)
     B. NH_4Cl ingestion
     C. Renal tubular acidosis
     D. Ureterosigmoidostomy

Metabolic Alkalosis

A metabolic alkalosis results from an excess intake of alkali (e.g., sodium bicarbonate) or abnormal losses of acid (e.g., pernicious vomiting). Volume contraction (dehydration) produces a metabolic alkalosis by increasing sodium and bicarbonate reabsorption in the proximal tubules and is often seen in patients who are on aggressive diuretic therapy. A metabolic alkalosis also occurs with potassium depletion owing to a shift of acid from the extracellular to the intracellular compartments in exchange for potassium, and an increase in the exchange of hydrogen ion for sodium ion in the distal nephron.

The causes of a metabolic alkalosis can be subdivided on the basis of the amount of chloride in the urine and whether or not the alkalosis can be corrected with chloride administration. Chloride-responsive alkalosis (urine chloride concentration of more than 20 mEq/liter) is generally due to excessive vomiting or administration of diuretics. Chloride-unresponsive alkalosis (urine chloride concentration of less than 20 mEq/liter) is generally due to hypokalemia resulting from mineralocorticoid excess.

Respiratory Acidosis

Respiratory acidosis results from carbon dioxide retention. Pulmonary disease, characterized by impaired ventilation-perfusion dynamics and hypoventilation due to respiratory center pathology or use of respiratory center depressants (e.g., morphine), can usually be implicated. Inhalation of high concentrations of oxygen by patients with chronic pulmonary insufficiency may perpetuate the respiratory acidosis (carbon dioxide retention).

Respiratory Alkalosis

Respiratory alkalosis is produced by hyperventilation and is seen primarily in patients with acute anxiety reactions, central nervous system lesions, and cirrhosis. Anxiety with hyperventilation is common at all ages and produces sensations of dyspnea ("smothering"), numbness and tingling periorally and in the extremities, lightheadedness, and chest pain or discomfort (hyperventilation syndrome).

References

1. Rowe JW, Andres R, Tobin JD, et al: The effect of age on creatinine clearance in men: Cross-sectional and longitudinal study. J Gerontol 1976;31:155–163.
2. Lindeman RD, Tobin JD, Shock NW: Longitudinal studies on the rate of decline in renal function with age. J Am Geriatr Soc 1985;33:278–285.
3. Lindeman RD: Overview: Renal physiology and pathophysiology of aging. Am J Kidney Dis 1990;16:275–282.
4. Cockcroft DW, Gault MH: Prediction of creatinine clearance from serum creatinine. Nephron 1976; 16:31–41.
5. Moorthy AV, Zimmerman SW: Renal disease in the elderly: Clinicopathologic analysis of renal disease in 115 elderly patients. Clin Nephrol 1980;14:223–229.
6. Sabonis SG, Antonovych TT: A study of 500 cases of kidney diseases in the elderly. Geriatr Nephrol Urol 1993;3:15–22.
7. Lamiere N, Verspeelt J, Vanholder R, Ringoir S. A review of the pathophysiology, causes and prognosis of acute renal failure in the elderly. Geriatr Nephrol Urol 1991;1:77–91.
8. Pascual J, Orofino L, Liano F, et al. Incidence and prognosis of acute renal failure in older patients. J Am Geriatr Soc 1990;38:25–30.
9. Bullock ML, Umen AJ, Finkelstein M, Keane WF. The assessment of risk factors in 462 patients with acute renal failure. Am J Kidney Dis 1985;5:97–103.
10. McInnes EG, Levy DW, Chaudhuri MD, Bhan GL: Renal failure in the elderly. Q J Med 1987;243:583–588.
11. Brown WW: Glomerulonephritis in the elderly. *In* Michelis MF, Davis BB, Preuss HG (eds): Geriatric Nephrology. New York, Field, Rich and Associates, 1986, pp. 90–98.
12. Simon P, Charasse C, Autuly V, et al. Primary nephrotic syndrome in the elderly. Contrib Nephrol 1993; 105:161–166.
13. Lorca E, Ponticelli C. Idiopathic nephrotic syndrome in the elderly. Geriatr Nephrol Urol 1995;4:189–195.
14. Keller F, Michaelis C, Buttner P, et al. Risk factors for long-term survival and renal function in 64 patients with rapidly progressive glomerulonephritis. Geriatr Nephrol Urol 1994;4:5–13.
15. Luft FC, Weinberger MH, Fineberg NS, et al. Effect of age on renal sodium homeostasis and its relevance to sodium sensitivity. Am J Med 1987;82(Suppl 1B):9–15.
16. Epstein M, Hollenberg N: Age as a determinant of renal sodium conservation in normal man. J Lab Clin Med 1976;37:411–417.
17. Crane MG, Harris JJ: Effect of aging on renin activity and aldosterone excretion. J Lab Clin Med 1976; 87:947–959.
18. Kleinfeld M, Casimir M, Borra S: Hyponatremia as observed in a chronic disease facility. J Am Geriatric Soc 1979;27:156–161.
19. Helderman JH, Vestal RE, Rowe JW, Shock NS: The response of arginine vasopressin to intravenous ethanol in man: The impact of aging. J Gerontol 1978;33:39–47.
20. Rowe JH, Minaker KL, Sparrow D, Robertson GL: Age-related failure of volume pressure-mediated vasopression release. J Clin Endocrinol 1982; 54:661–664.
21. Snyder NA, Feigal DW, Arieff AI: Hypernatremia in elderly patients. A heterogenous, morbid, and iatrogenic entity. Ann Intern Med 1987;107:309–319.
22. Phillips PA, Rolls BJ, Ledingham JJG, et al: Reduced thirst after water deprivation in healthy elderly men. N Engl J Med 1984;311:753–759.
23. Lawson DH: Adverse reactions to potassium chloride. Q J Med 1974;171:433–440.
24. Adler S, Lindeman RD, Yiengst MJ, et al: Effect of acute acid loading on urinary acid excretion by the aging human kidney. J Lab Clin Med 1986;72:278–289.

50 Endocrine Disorders

Paul J. Davis, M.D.

Faith B. Davis, M.D.

The generalist who manages endocrine problems in elderly patients must distinguish among three clinical states: (1) endocrine function that is altered relative to younger subjects but is an expected consequence of normal aging, (2) altered endocrine function that is secondary to coincident nonendocrine disease but is of no pathologic significance, and (3) authentic endocrinopathy. The patterns of change in endocrine function in the course of normal aging are summarized in Table 50–1. Certain of these changes can affect diagnostic evaluations in important ways—for example, the relative nonresponsiveness of the renin-aldosterone axis in the normal elderly, the increased incidence of the uncomplicated empty sella turcica syndrome in older subjects, and alterations in carbohydrate tolerance. These changes create an impression of endocrine disease and are discussed in subsequent sections of this chapter. There is no unifying physiologic mechanism that explains the alterations in endo-

crine function that accompany normal aging. Some of the changes represent decreased organ function, and others reflect enhanced sensitivity of one or more aspects of an endocrine axis (Table 50–1).

The impact of substantial nonendocrine disease on endocrine physiology in subjects of all ages can also lead to a misimpression of the presence of endocrinopathy. Examples of the effects of nonendocrine disease are the reductions in serum 3,5,3'-L-triiodothyronine (T_3) and thyrotropin (TSH) concentrations in both sexes and the fall in serum testosterone levels in men who have serious systemic diseases such as cancer or heart failure. In elderly patients with multisystem disease, caution must be used in interpreting the results of laboratory tests of endocrine function.

Finally, bona fide endocrinopathies in older patients need not present with the conventional findings observed in younger patients. For example, the presentation of hyperthyroidism or hyperparathyroidism in the elderly may be muted or may be obscured by the coincident presence of unrelated heart, lung, or nervous system disorders whose life-threatening consequences divert the attention of the clinician from the possible presence of endocrine disease.

The epidemiology of the various endocrinopathies is also different in the older patient population (Fig. 50–1). For example, in older subjects, diabetes mellitus is of the noninsulin-dependent or type II variety, and adrenocortical disease is rare. The aggressiveness of endocrine tumors, notably thyroid cancer, is different in elderly patients than in younger ones despite identical histologic findings. The treatment of endocrinopathies may also require modification in the older patient population.

PITUITARY-THYROID FUNCTION

Physiology

Thyroid hormone is a principal regulator of cell and higher organism respiration, and its actions affect virtually all body systems. To understand thyroid function and tests of thyroid function in

TABLE 50–1 PATTERNS OF CHANGE IN ENDOCRINE FUNCTION WITH NORMAL AGING[a]

Change	Example
Endocrine gland failure	Ovary
Reduction in target organ sensitivity	Peripheral tissue response to insulin
	Renal collecting tubule response to AVP[b]
Failure of adaptive response	Renin-aldosterone response to change in posture
	AVP response to change in posture
Heightened sensitivity within endocrine axis	AVP response to increase in plasma osmolality

[a]Examples of endocrine axes in which no physiologically substantive change in function occurs with aging are the pituitary-thyroid and pituitary-adrenal cortex (specifically, cortisol) axes.

[b]AVP, arginine vasopressin (antidiuretic hormone).

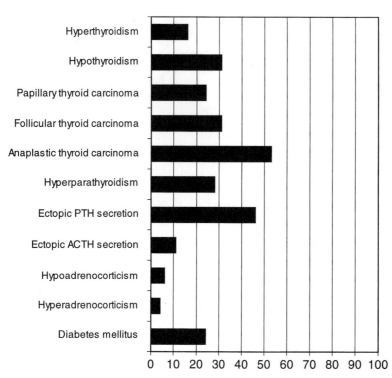

Figure 50–1 Percentage of patients with selected endocrinopathies who are 60 years of age or more.

Percent of patients with each endocrinopathy who are ≥60 years old.

the healthy elderly and to diagnose thyroid disease in aged subjects, it is important to understand the physiology of the pituitary-thyroid gland complex during the life span.

Thyroid hormone circulates in blood as L-thyroxine (T_4, tetraiodothyronine) and 3,5,3′-L-triiodothyronine (T_3). T_4 is released by the thyroid gland under the direction of normal levels of pituitary thyrotropin (TSH), and T_4 in turn regulates TSH secretion by a negative feedback inhibition loop at the pituitary gland. T_3 is derived from T_4 by deiodination (activity of iodothyronine 5′-monodeiodinase) in various organs (e.g., liver and kidney), but it is also released by the thyroid gland when plasma TSH levels increase. T_3 is biologically ten times more active than T_4. Because of its biologic activity, particularly in the elderly, T_3 is not desirable as hormone replacement in hypothyroid patients, and T_4 is prescribed.

When the 5-iodine rather than the 5′-iodine in various organs is removed from T_4, a hormone analog called reverse T_3 (rT_3) is formed; this is a relatively inactive form of the hormone. Intrapituitary conversion of T_4 to T_3 controls TSH secretion by the negative feedback loop. Circulating T_4 and T_3 are bound to plasma proteins, the most important of which is thyroxine-binding globulin (TBG). Less than 0.01% of T_4 is un-

bound by TBG and other proteins, and less than 0.1% of T_3 is unbound; these unbound species of hormone are free T_4 and free T_3 and are the metabolically active forms of the hormone.

Regardless of a patient's age, conventional forms of hyperthyroidism (which is due to excessive production of hormone by the thyroid gland) suppress endogenous TSH levels. Conventional forms of hypothyroidism (which is due to primary failure of the thyroid gland) are associated with increased circulating levels of TSH. In the course of normal aging, serum levels of T_4 and free T_4 do not change, T_3 and free T_3 concentrations decline modestly, and TSH levels remain stable.[1] One can conclude from these observations that the function of the pituitary-thyroid complex is preserved over the life span and that the great majority of healthy elderly, up to centenarian status, have normal results on serum thyroid function tests (concentrations of total and free T_4, total and free T_3, and TSH). However, a few healthy older subjects appear to have an increased sensitivity of the negative feedback loop in that they have somewhat low free T_4 levels, but the serum TSH concentrations do not increase as a result.

The most important feature of thyroid hormone metabolism in the evaluation of elderly patients is the impact of nonthyroidal illness

(NTI) on thyroid function.[1] Many studies of "healthy elderly" in the literature have not rigorously excluded NTI and, as a result, have confused changes due to disease states with those due to normal aging. NTI impairs T_4 to T_3 conversion, leading to very low serum T_3 and free T_3 levels. At the same time, in most clinical situations in which NTI occurs (with the exception of end-stage renal disease), rT_3 formation is enhanced. NTI can promote degradation of TBG and decrease its secretion by the liver, leading to low serum total T_4 concentrations. NTI can be associated with low or high free hormone levels, and pituitary TSH secretion may be suppressed. The suppression can suggest either hyperthyroidism or decreased pituitary function (hypopituitarism). Despite these alterations, most patients with NTI are eumetabolic. It is important to note that significantly reduced caloric intake acutely reproduces some of the changes of NTI (decreased T_3 and increased rT_3; low serum T_4, if the condition is chronic, may result from decreased hepatic synthesis of TBG). Finally, during recovery from NTI, patients may show modest elevations of serum TSH that are consistent with early hypothyroidism but actually represent recovery of the pituitary-thyroid axis from the impact of NTI. The effort to document bona fide thyroid disease in the presence of NTI is thus a complex issue, and the presence or absence of thyroid disease is sometimes documented by laboratory tests only when NTI has resolved.

There is no evidence currently that a decrease in thyroid function contributes to the aging process. There is suggestive evidence that certain tissues, such as the heart and perhaps the pituitary gland, may acquire in some patients heightened sensitivity to thyroid hormone during the life span. The latter statement is based on the appearance of single-organ hyperthyroidism (monosystemic hyperthyroidism) in occasional patients (e.g., those who may present only with myocardial symptoms and signs of thyroid hyperfunction).

It should also be noted that behavioral changes associated with normal aging, such as decreased physical activity and altered bowel function, may be accentuated or mimicked by thyroid disorders. Because thyroid disorders are common, the physician must consider the possible contribution of these diseases in every patient in whom behavioral changes "consistent with normal aging" have occurred.

Clinical Assessment

HYPERTHYROIDISM

The prevalence of hyperthyroidism in the ambulatory urban elderly population is as high as 0.7%.

TABLE 50–2 **CLINICAL FEATURES OF HYPERTHYROIDISM IN THE ELDERLY**

	Frequency (%)
Symptom	
Hyperhidrosis	38
Heat intolerance	63
Weight loss	69
Palpitation	63
Angina pectoris	20
Respiratory symptoms consistent with congestive heart failure	66
Polyphagia	11
Anorexia	36
Increased stool frequency	12
Constipation	26
Tremor or nervousness	55
Sign	
Hyperkinesis	25
Apathy	16
Cachexia or chronically ill appearance	39
Classic skin changes (warm, fine, moist skin)	81
Proptosis	8
Lid-lag	35
Extraocular muscle palsy	22
Impalpable or normal-sized thyroid gland	37
Multinodular thyroid gland	20
Solitary thyroid nodule	21
Diffuse thyroid gland enlargement	22
Atrial fibrillation	39
Supraventricular tachycardia (rate >120 beats/minute)	11
Brisk deep tendon reflexes, shortened relaxation phase of reflexes	26

Modified from Davis PJ, Davis FB: Hyperthyroidism in patients over the age of 60 years. Medicine 1974;53:161–181.

The clinical symptoms and signs found in hyperthyroid older patients are summarized in Table 50–2. The majority of older patients with thyrotoxicosis have classic findings.[2] About 25% of elderly hyperthyroid patients have subtle symptoms or present with authentic thyrotoxicosis in the presence of severe nonthyroidal illness, such as congestive heart failure, systemic infection, or cerebrovascular disease. In such patients, hyperthyroidism may be readily overlooked ("masked" hyperthyroidism). Alternatively, the older subject with thyrotoxicosis may have symptoms and signs limited to a single organ system such as the heart, or may present with phlegmatic or apathetic mien rather than in the hyperkinetic state.

Crescendo angina pectoris may herald the presence of hyperthyroidism, but acute myocardial infarction has occurred relatively infrequently in patients with thyroid hyperfunction and coronary artery disease. Older hyperthyroid patients may experience anorexia rather than increased appetite, and the constellation of anorexia, weight loss, and constipation occurs in as many as 15% of elderly thyrotoxic subjects. New-onset hypertension or exacerbation of previously well-controlled hypertension may occur. The impressively widened pulse pressure observed in younger hyperthyroid patients is less frequently seen in the elderly because the diastolic pressure may not fall in older patients who become thyrotoxic. Demineralizing bone disease may be a presenting sign in elderly patients with hyperthyroidism.

Atrial fibrillation is eight times more frequent in hyperthyroidism in the elderly than in young patients. This arrhythmia usually reverts to a sinus mechanism in the course of treatment of hyperthyroidism in younger people but does so in only 50% of older thyrotoxic patients. Atrial fibrillation may be associated with a slow ventricular response in elderly hyperthyroid patients (ventricular rate of 50 to 60 beats/minute). This atrioventricular conduction block is related to the concomitant presence of atherosclerotic or other disease such as amyloidosis in the cardiac conducting system or to the use of digitalis, or both. The risk of stroke is increased in patients with atrial fibrillation associated with thyrotoxicosis despite the fact that the left atrium may be small and blood flow through the heart may be increased.

Goiter is absent in 40% of older patients with hyperthyroidism.[2] Insistence by the physician on the presence of goiter before obtaining tests of thyroid function will therefore lead to underdiagnosis of hyperthyroidism in the elderly. Hyperthyroidism due to a single thyroid nodule or to multinodular goiter is more common in older subjects than in younger patients, but a third or more of thyrotoxic elderly who have thyroid enlargement have diffusely enlarged (non-nodular) thyroid glands.

Serious endocrine ophthalmopathy is infrequent in older patients. Stare and lid-lag are common in both old and young hyperthyroid subjects. These signs are less specific than proptosis for thyroid disease because they may occur in the presence of chronic congestive heart failure, chronic obstructive pulmonary disease, or renal or liver failure.

In the great majority of older patients with hyperthyroidism, the laboratory profile includes elevations of traditional parameters of thyroid function: serum T_4 and free T_4 concentrations and thyroidal uptake of radioactive iodine. The sensitive sandwich radioimmunoassay (RIA) for TSH in serum—the lower limit of normal of which is 0.2 μU/mL or less—distinguishes between suppressed TSH (characteristic of hyperthyroidism) and low normal levels of the hormone and may be used to screen both young and elderly subjects for the presence of hyperthyroidism. Low normal serum TSH levels do not imply the presence of imminent thyrotoxicosis, but undetectable (suppressed) serum TSH levels are consistent with subclinical hyperthyroidism (see later discussion). Measurement of serum total T_4 and free T_4 by RIA is an alternative method and should be compared within the institution for cost effectiveness relative to TSH assay. Low serum concentrations of TBG due to chronic nonthyroidal illness are associated with low serum T_4 levels. Constitutional (X-linked) increases in TBG are associated with increased circulating concentrations of T_4 in patients without hyperthyroidism. In these states in which TBG is abnormal, serum free T_4 and TSH measurements are within the normal range.

As many as 10% of older patients with thyrotoxicosis have standard thyroid function test results that are misleadingly normal. Some of these patients have T_3 toxicosis, a syndrome in which only serum T_3, measured by radioimmunoassay, is elevated. Serum T_4 and free T_4 concentrations are normal. A few patients may have free T_3 toxicosis with normal results in the remaining serum tests of thyroid function. Finally, an interesting group of patients 65 years of age or older have suppressed serum TSH concentrations but otherwise normal or high normal thyroid function test results (subclinical hyperthyroidism). Some of these patients have chronic or paroxysmal atrial fibrillation[3] or unexplained weight loss and appear to have emerging hyperthyroidism, characterized by a single symptom or a limited number of clinical findings. As mentioned earlier, these patients have hyperthyroidism that appears to represent a condition of heightened sensitivity of a hormone target organ (myocardium) to apparently normal levels of circulating T_4 and T_3. Rarely, younger patients may have hyperthyroidism due to pituitary secretion of excessive amounts of TSH. It is not yet clear whether there is an appreciable risk of this syndrome in elderly patient populations.

No accurate cost-effective tests are available to measure the action of thyroid hormone on its target tissues, such as the heart or nervous system. Measurements of serum cholesterol concentration, alkaline phosphatase activity, and calcium concentration may be abnormal in thyrotoxic pa-

TABLE 50–3 MEDICAL THERAPEUTIC ALTERNATIVES FOR HYPERTHYROIDISM IN THE ELDERLY

Modality	Dosage	Therapeutic Goal	Onset of Clinical Effect
Propylthiouracil[a]	100–300 mg po daily	Inhibition of thyroid hormonogenesis[b]	2–8 weeks
Iodide	1–3 drops saturated solution of potassium iodide (SSKI) po 1–3 times daily[c]	Inhibition of thyroid hormone release Inhibition of thyroid hormonogenesis	Hours
Propranolol[d]	10–40 mg po[e] qid	Suppression of peripheral manifestations of hyperthyroidism	Hours to days

[a]Propylthiouracil (PTU) may be administered as a single daily dose or every 8 hours. While another thioamide drug, methimazole, may be substituted for PTU, methimazole has an increased risk of hepatotoxicity in elderly patients.
[b]PTU also acts to inhibit conversion in extrathyroidal tissues of T_4 to T_3; whether this is a clinically significant action is unclear.
[c]In situations in which oral administration of SSKI is temporarily impractical, iodide may be administered intravenously as NaI, 250- to 500-mg bolus daily.
[d]Caution is advised in treating thyrotoxicosis in patients with congestive heart failure with beta-blocking agents (see text). Beta-blockers other than propranolol may be used to manage peripheral manifestations of hyperthyroidism, particularly tachycardia. Dosage is titrated against heart rate. In the elderly, the short $T_{1/2}$ of propranolol is an advantage. Propranolol also inhibits peripheral conversion of T_4 to T_3, but it is not clear whether this is clinically significant.
[e]When it is temporarily impractical to administer propranolol po, the agent may be given intravenously in 0.5- to 1.0-mg boluses, titrating the dose against heart rate (e.g., maintenance of heart rate at ≤ 120 beats/minute).

tients of any age, but they are not useful in establishing the diagnosis of hyperthyroidism or for monitoring the effects of treatment.

Therapeutic alternatives in the acute management of hyperthyroidism in elderly patients are shown in Table 50–3. Acute management involves control of symptoms of thyroid dysfunction, anticipation of possibly life-endangering complications of thyrotoxicosis, and preparation of the patient for definitive long-term therapy. The latter usually consists of ablation of the thyroid gland with radioactive iodine ($Na^{131}I$).

Thioamide-related suppression of bone marrow granulocyte production is more likely to develop in patients over the age of 40 years than in younger subjects when conventional doses of methimazole (30 mg/day) are exceeded; thus, propylthiouracil is recommended in older patients when a thioamide is required. Patients with subclinical hyperthyroidism who develop atrial fibrillation are candidates for radioablation of the thyroid gland or for a trial of PTU to reduce circulating T_4 and T_3 levels sufficiently to result in detectable serum TSH levels and to determine whether the cardiac findings then subside. Ablative treatment may then be used, and hypothyroidism should be anticipated.

Many of the symptoms of hyperthyroidism in the elderly can be controlled by cautious administration of a beta-adrenergic blocking agent. As little as 40 mg of propranolol daily in four doses of 10 mg each can be effective in controlling

tachycardia in the older thyrotoxic patient, although total daily doses of 80 to 120 mg (1.2 mg/kg body weight/day) are more commonly required. It is critical to recognize that as the patient is rendered euthyroid by the use of radioactive iodide or by thioamide drugs, the dose of beta-blocker that was formerly therapeutic can become toxic. Symptomatic sinus bradycardia may emerge as thyrotoxicosis subsides if relatively high doses of propranolol are continued. Although the most substantial experience with beta-blockade has been accumulated with propranolol, other beta-blockers are effective as well.

It is widely acknowledged that beta-adrenergic blockade may exacerbate congestive heart failure in patients with hyperthyroidism. However, cautious slowing of tachycardia with small doses of a beta-blocker may improve the symptoms of heart failure in hyperthyroid patients by increasing diastolic filling time. We recommend a careful trial of a short-acting beta-blocking agent in elderly patients with hyperthyroidism and ventricular response rates of more than 140 beats/minute. Titration is carried out to achieve a heart rate of 100 to 110 beats/minute. In patients with hyperthyroidism and heart failure who have ventricular rates of less than 140 beats/minute, the authors avoid beta-blockade.

The life-threatening phase of hyperthyroidism—"thyroid storm"—does occur in the elderly. This state is imprecisely defined as "exaggerated symptoms of hyperthyroidism" in association with fever and tachycardia. Sometimes "apathetic thyroid storm" is encountered; this may proceed to coma and death with the manifestation of few signs of thyrotoxicosis except for tachycardia or fever or both. The authors look upon elderly thyrotoxic patients with heart rates of 120 beats/minute or greater, those with a previous history of congestive heart failure unrelated to thyroid disease, and those with significant fever (core temperature higher than 100.6°F) as "pre-storm" patients who should be aggressively managed with nonradioactive iodide administration, thioamide, and propranolol, reserving use of the latter for those with (1) a heart rate greater than 140 beats/minute, or (2) sensorial changes that accompany fever and heart rate greater than 120 beats/minute in patients with suspected or established hyperthyroidism.

The definitive treatment of hyperthyroidism is thyroid gland ablation with $^{131}I^-$. Ablative radioactive iodide therapy should be administered under cover of low-dose beta-blockade or after achievement of eumetabolism with thioamide treatment. This conservative approach—rendering the elderly patient relatively euthyroid with beta-blockade or PTU—minimizes the risk of thyroid storm occurring 7 to 14 days after administration of $^{131}I^-$. The incidence of storm after $^{131}I^-$ is low even without prior conversion of patients to the euthyroid state, but the desirability of avoiding the complication is extraordinarily high. Elderly patients can be treated long-term with PTU should they reject the concept of ablative $^{131}I^-$ therapy. Thyroidectomy is rarely used in older patients for management of hyperthyroidism.

HYPOTHYROIDISM

The prevalence of hypothyroidism in ambulatory urban elderly populations as well as in referral center hospitals is as high as 6%. Because younger patients do not tolerate the major symptom complex of hypothyroidism—lassitude, constipation, ambient cold temperature intolerance, and dry skin—without consulting a physician, moderately advanced and severe hypothyroid states are found almost exclusively in the elderly. Myxedema stupor and coma are rare in patients under the age of 50 years. The subtlety of early hypothyroidism in elderly subjects is easily confused with the progression of "normal aging," and a low diagnostic threshold for the possibility of hypothyroidism should be maintained by the physician in evaluating this age group.

The classic features of hypothyroidism are well known. Several of these should be emphasized

as herald findings of the disease. As many as one third of hypothyroid patients are hypertensive, and one third of these patients can normalize their blood pressure with thyroid hormone replacement therapy alone. Gait disorders, apparently due to cerebellar dysfunction, occur in hypothyroidism, as does a striated muscle myopathy, usually in a proximal muscle distribution. Asymmetrical hypertrophy of the myocardial ventricular septum is an occasional feature of hypothyroidism, and remission of this sign may occur with hormone replacement.

Primary destruction of the thyroid gland, due either to Hashimoto's thyroiditis or to iatrogenic ablation of the previously overactive gland by radioiodide, accounts for 95% of cases of hypothyroidism. The remainder of the hypothyroid patient population have pituitary or hypothalamic-pituitary disease (secondary hypothyroidism). Distinguishing between primary and secondary hypothyroidism is important clinically, as will be discussed in the section on treatment of hypothyroidism. Patients with marginal hypofunction of the thyroid may be acutely hypothyroid when acute systemic nonthyroidal illness supervenes. Unexplained medical deterioration in the condition of elderly patients with appropriately treated severe nonthyroidal illness should cause the physician to consider the possibility that concomitant unappreciated hypothyroidism is present. Reversible sleep apnea syndrome may also be a feature of hypothyroidism.

The diagnosis of primary hypothyroidism in patients of any age is secured with the finding of an elevated serum TSH level and a low serum T_4 concentration. Measurement of the T_4 concentration alone may be misleading because the occurrence of low serum TBG levels is relatively frequent. The free T_4 level has reduced usefulness in patients with hypothyroidism because it is sometimes low normal rather than low. The possibility that TBG content may be contributing to a low serum T_4 level must always be considered and can be excluded by the measurement of serum free T_4 concentration or radioimmunoassay for TBG. Patients with early or subclinical primary hypothyroidism may have an elevated serum TSH and a low normal or even mid-range T_4 level. Excessive stimulation of the thyroid gland in such patients by administration of endogenous TSH is required to maintain the near-euthyroid state. The patient with a low serum T_4 concentration and a low serum TSH level has either hypopituitary (secondary) hypothyroidism or nonthyroidal illness, as discussed earlier under Physiology.

There is no indication for the measurement of serum antithyroid antibody titers in elderly patients with spontaneous hypothyroidism. Although hypothyroidism is presumably autoimmune in origin (end-stage Hashimoto's thyroiditis), antibody levels are infrequently elevated by the time the thyroid gland has been destroyed. The possibility of hypopituitarism can be evaluated by measuring the circulating levels of cortisol and radiographic assessment (by computer-assisted tomography [CT] or magnetic resonance imaging [MRI]) of the sella turcica to look for evidence of a pituitary tumor or the empty sella syndrome. Because the incidence of the empty sella syndrome is appreciable in the elderly, it should be understood that the finding of an enlarged sella does not necessarily imply the presence of a pituitary tumor.

A number of nonthyroidal laboratory test abnormalities can accompany hypothyroidism. These include macrocytic anemia, due either to concomitant pernicious anemia or to erythroid maturation arrest of unknown cause, elevated serum creatine phosphokinase (CPK) activity, hyponatremia, and hyperuricemia. Patients with moderate to severe hypothyroidism may also hypoventilate and retain carbon dioxide. When present, elevated serum CPK activity usually originates in the skeletal muscle (MM isoenzyme), and it tends to be elevated consistently until thyroid hormone replacement therapy is instituted. Increased serum CPK activity in patients with hypothyroidism occasionally includes the myocardial isoenzyme (MB) in the absence of other evidence of myocardial necrosis. Hyponatremia in the hypothyroid population usually reflects decreased renal free water clearance resulting from excessive antidiuretic hormone (ADH, arginine vasopressin [AVP]) of central origin. Thyroid hormone replacement normalizes serum sodium concentration.

Initiation of treatment of primary hypothyroidism in older patients involves oral L-thyroxine (T_4) replacement in graded doses. In many elderly subjects, the concomitant presence of heart disease (usually atherosclerotic disease but occasionally cardiomyopathic on a hypothyroid basis) mandates a conservative incremental approach to hormone replacement. The presence of clinically significant heart disease associated with hypothyroidism is defined as any one or more of the following: cardiomegaly, congestive heart failure, angina pectoris, or a prior history of myocardial infarction or cardiac arrhythmia. Initial hormone therapy in such patients consists of 0.025 mg of T_4 daily. After 2 to 4 weeks, the dose is increased to 0.050 mg of T_4/day, and thereafter the daily dose is raised at 2- to 6-week intervals by 0.025-mg increments until a total daily dose of between 0.075 and 0.150 mg lowers the serum TSH into

the normal range.[4] It is important to avoid full suppression of TSH, since the latter state risks the promotion of metabolic bone disease (osteoporosis) and exacerbation of underlying heart disease.

Metabolic equilibration at a given dose of thyroid hormone may be incomplete for 2 months. Thus, the graded dosage regimen described here is a general recommendation. Once an appropriate reduction in serum TSH level has been achieved, however, adjustments in hormone replacement dose can be considered if symptoms suggestive of hyperthyroidism develop months after an apparently stable dose of T_4 has been achieved. There is no role for the use of T_3 or mixtures of T_4 and T_3 in the management of hypothyroidism in the elderly. A few patients have primary hypothyroidism and primary adrenocortical failure (Schmidt's syndrome) and require chronic replacement therapy for both diseases. It is very rare for hypothyroid elderly patients undergoing oral T_4 replacement therapy to develop *relative* adrenocortical insufficiency, a syndrome of hypotension and mild hyponatremia that requires transient corticosteroid support.

Substantial attention has been focused on the cohort of patients who have minimally elevated or even high normal serum TSH levels, a normal serum T_4 concentration, and few or no symptoms suggestive of hypothyroidism. Hypercholesterolemia may or may not be present. This state has been termed "subclinical hypothyroidism." Patients with these findings are presumed to have mild thyroiditis and defective hormonogenesis that will support normal levels of circulating T_4 when slight increases in endogenous TSH occur compensatorily. Some authorities advocate hormone replacement therapy for patients with this laboratory test profile because subjective improvement may occur in such patients when they are treated. Some cognitive dysfunction in patients in this situation has also been thought to be reversed with hormone replacement. Low-density lipoprotein cholesterol levels may decline. It should be noted that exposure of untreated patients with subclinical hypothyroidism to iodine loads, such as those encountered with amiodarone, radiographic contrast media, or kelp, may precipitate acute hypothyroidism.

The authors view the following findings to be secure indications for T_4 therapy in patients with subclinical hypothyroidism: (1) the presence of goiter; (2) decline of serum T_4 concentration into the lower quartile of the normal range in the context of mildly elevated serum TSH content; or (3) elevated serum antithyroid antibody titers. (Although measurement of antibody titers is not cost-effective in patients with established hypothyroidism, such titers may be useful in subjects with incipient hypothyroidism.) Patients with substantial evidence of heart disease and subclinical hypothyroidism are not candidates for T_4 replacement because the risks outweigh the possible benefits of treatment. If the physician elects not to treat the patient with subclinical hypothyroidism, regular evaluation is indicated to detect the emergence of symptomatic hypothyroidism.

Severe hypothyroidism—myxedema stupor or coma—is a medical emergency and requires treatment with parenteral T_4. The diagnosis is considered when a profound alteration of sensorium is complicated by hypothermia (core body temperature of less than 95°F) or hypotension in a patient with already established or presumptively diagnosed but undertreated primary hypothyroidism. These patients may also have an elevated arterial P_{CO_2} and hypoxemia. Specific management of such patients is beyond the scope of this text but is carried out in the intensive care unit and involves intravenous administration of relatively large doses of T_4 and stress level corticosteroids.

PITUITARY-ADRENAL FUNCTION

Physiology

Basal levels of serum cortisol and the response of cortisol secretion by the adrenal cortex to exogenous adrenocorticotropic hormone (ACTH) are unaffected by normal aging in humans.[5] The provocative stimulus of insulin-induced hypoglycemia and the attendant release of endogenous ACTH by the pituitary gland are also undiminished during the life span. There is an advance in phase in the cortisol circadian rhythm in the elderly (i.e., earlier nadir and peak in diurnal cortisol secretion), but this is thought to be behavioral, reflecting the inverse relationship between age and customary bedtime.

In contrast to cortisol secretion, the sensitivity of aldosterone secretion to the conventional stimuli of sodium restriction and prolonged assumption of the upright posture is diminished in normal elderly subjects. Response of plasma renin levels to the same stimuli is also decreased with normal aging. The physiologic significance, if any, of these changes in control of aldosterone secretion in the course of aging is not clear, although it has been suggested that essential hypertension in the elderly may be associated with retention of the responsiveness of the renin-aldosterone axis observed in younger subjects. Whether stimulation by hyperkalemia of aldosterone release is also diminished in healthy elderly people has not been determined. The diagnosis of hypo-

reninemic hypoaldosteronism as a cause of hyperkalemia should be applied very cautiously in elderly patients because of the diminished sensitivity of the renin-aldosterone axis in the normal elderly population.

Clinical Assessment

HYPOADRENOCORTICISM

The clinical syndrome of adrenocortical hypofunction is unaltered by aging. Because asthenia and easy fatigability may be associated with the stereotype of "normal aging," these symptoms as heralds of hypoadrenocorticism may attract insufficient medical attention in the elderly. Hyponatremic and hyperkalemic syndromes of various causes are relatively common in the older patient. In the majority of elderly patients with hyponatremia, however, euvolemia is present, and hyponatremia reflects impaired free water clearance (syndrome of inappropriate secretion of antidiuretic hormone, SIADH). The situations in which renal free water clearance is decreased include tumoral secretion of arginine vasopressin (AVP, ADH) and administration of a variety of drugs, including diuretics, carbamazepine, chlorpropamide, and antipsychotic medications.

In addition to hypoadrenocorticism, hyperkalemic syndromes in older patients may be related to decreased renal function, excessive use of potassium-sparing diuretics (particularly when oral potassium intake is high, as it is with use of a salt substitute), administration of angiotensin-converting enzyme (ACE) inhibitors, and hypoaldosteronism. The last is rarely encountered as an isolated biochemical abnormality in the adrenal cortex; more commonly it is due to inadequate renin production by the kidney (hyporeninemic hypoaldosteronism). The frequency of hyporeninemic hypoaldosteronism is increased in patients with non-insulin-dependent diabetes mellitus (NIDDM) when modest decreases in glomerular filtration rate have supervened. As pointed out previously, the diagnosis of hyporeninemic hypoaldosteronism is difficult to establish in the elderly because of the physiologic changes in the renin-aldosterone axis that occur in the course of normal aging.

The treatment of adrenocortical insufficiency in the elderly is identical to that in younger patients except that volume and solute replacement in the acutely hypoadrenal elderly patient must be more carefully monitored to avoid overload syndromes. Prescription of mineralocorticoid replacement (in addition to standard glucocorticoid) in older subjects should not be routine; it should be individualized, since excessive mineralocorticoid therapy can promote hypertension and the formation of edema.

HYPERADRENOCORTICISM

Except when caused by ectopic ACTH secretion, hyperadrenocorticism is very uncommon in the elderly. The finding of severe hypokalemia (serum potassium concentration of less than 3.0 mEq/L) is usually related to diuretic administration or gastrointestinal potassium loss, as is seen with laxative abuse. The decreased incidence in the elderly of nonendocrine diseases that require chronic high-dose anti-inflammatory corticosteroid therapy explains the infrequency with which elderly patients are encountered who have iatrogenic Cushing's syndrome. Expected age-related decreases in bone mineral content and in cell-mediated immunity heighten the risks of long-term pharmacologic-dose glucocorticoid therapy in the elderly.

CATECHOLAMINES

Physiology

The ability of the adrenal medulla to release catecholamines remains intact during the life span. The nerve terminals have an apparently heightened capacity to release norepinephrine (NE) into the circulation in aged subjects in response to mental stress. This may represent altered local disposition (decreased reuptake or degradation of NE) rather than a primary increase in production of the neurotransmitter. Whether target tissue responses to epinephrine (adrenal medullary origin) and to NE change with age is not altogether clear. However, increased circulating levels of NE reported in behavioral testing of the elderly do not appear to increase heart rate.

Clinical Assessment

PHEOCHROMOCYTOMA

More than 40% of autopsy-proved pheochromocytomas occurred in patients over age 60 years in one series, and the age-specific incidence of pheochromocytoma was increased.[6] The symptom complex of biologically active pheochromocytomas does not change during the life span, and diagnostic evaluation is similar in young and old subjects.

PARATHYROID GLAND AND VITAMIN D

Physiology

In the course of normal aging, circulating levels of immunoreactive parathyroid hormone (PTH)

increase. The changes are small and have been attributed to the progressive decline in glomerular filtration rate (GFR) that accompanies aging; the mechanism has been postulated to be phosphate retention, hyperphosphatemic depression of serum calcium concentration, and subsequent enhancement of PTH secretion. Recent evidence, however, indicates that the age-dependent rise in serum PTH does not require changes in serum calcium or phosphate levels. The increased serum PTH associated with aging is bioactive and increases the risk of bone demineralization. It has been shown that dietary calcium supplementation in the amount of 1 g of elemental calcium daily can significantly reduce serum PTH levels in older subjects. Small doses of vitamin D_3 (400 IU daily) have been reported to lower serum PTH.

Despite the modest age-related rise in circulating PTH, the PTH-responsive activation of vitamin D—i.e., conversion of liver-source 25-hydroxyvitamin D_3 by the kidney to 1,25-dihydroxyvitamin D_3 (1,25-$[OH]_2D_3$)—is not increased in older subjects. Although studies of vitamin D metabolism in the elderly are flawed by the inclusion of sick or institutionalized patients who are infrequently exposed to sunlight, the conclusion of most studies is that serum levels of vitamin D (including 1,25-$[OH]_2D_3$) in fact decline with age. Progressive modest declines in serum vitamin D concentration contribute to decreased gastrointestinal tract absorption of calcium during the life span.

Osteocalcin is a bone-source noncollagenous protein released into the circulation during bone formation by osteoblasts. In young people, serum osteocalcin levels rise in response to increased circulating PTH concentrations; this response is apparently lost in some, but not all, elderly populations. The osteocalcin response to the administration of 1,25-$(OH)_2D_3$ is intact in older subjects.

Loss of capacity of the parafollicular cells of the thyroid gland to secrete calcitonin in response to hypercalcemia has been observed in the elderly. It is doubtful that decreased responsiveness of the calcitonin axis contributes to bone demineralization, although calcitonin does oppose the action of PTH on bone.

Clinical Assessment

HYPERPARATHYROIDISM AND HYPERCALCEMIA

In practical terms, the extensive differential diagnosis of hypercalcemia is confined to a small group of disease entities in the elderly. These states include hyperparathyroidism, cancer-related hypercalcemia, and drug-induced hypercalcemia. Hypercalcemic states due to sarcoidosis, hyperthyroidism, Addison's disease, and the diuretic phase of postrhabdomyolytic acute renal failure are rarely encountered in the geriatric population. Hypercalcemic states consequent to immobilization of patients with widespread Paget's disease of bone or to the initiation of estrogen therapy in women with breast carcinoma widely metastatic to bone are occasionally seen.

As much as 20% of patients with hyperparathyroidism are over the age of 60 years. The increased frequency with which primary hyperparathyroidism is recognized in older patients is a reflection of the now routine measurement by chemical profiles of serum calcium concentration in inpatients and outpatients who have no symptoms attributable to parathyroid disease. Thiazide diuretic administration promotes hypercalcemia in a small minority of patients; the authors believe that hypercalcemia that develops during thiazide therapy usually represents an unmasking of latent primary hyperparathyroidism. In contrast to thiazides, loop diuretics (furosemide, bumetanide) are calciuretic and thus lower, rather than elevate, serum calcium levels. Lithium administration also elevates serum calcium concentration, apparently by resetting the calcium sensor in the parathyroid glands.

When symptomatic, primary hyperparathyroidism in the elderly is no different from that in younger patients. That is, constipation, increased urinary frequency (due to isosthenuria), urinary tract stone formation, and symptomatic myopathy or arthralgias occur. Except for urinary calculus formation, these findings may be attributed to "normal aging" when patients with unrecognized parathyroid disease are evaluated initially. In asymptomatic patients, mild hyperparathyroidism is regarded as a factor that promotes bone demineralization in both old and young patients.

The diagnosis of primary hyperparathyroidism is based on the presence of elevated immunoreactive PTH levels in serum, together with an increased or high normal serum calcium concentration. If hypercalcemia has a basis other than primary hyperparathyroidism, PTH levels should be low (suppressed). In the presence of humoral hypercalcemia of malignancy (HHM), a PTH-like polypeptide is secreted by a nonparathyroid cancer, particularly squamous cell cancers of lung or head and neck origin. Only a small region of the amino acid sequence of this polypeptide is homologous with that of authentic PTH, but the N-terminal sequence of the molecule is sufficiently similar to mimic a number of the biologic

actions of authentic PTH and sufficient to cross-react partially with antibodies used in the radioimmunoassay for authentic PTH. Improvements in the specificity of the PTH assay allow physicians to identify more often those patients with squamous cell carcinoma, hypercalcemia, and suppressed endogenous (authentic) PTH levels.

Aside from primary hyperparathyroidism and HHM, the major diagnostic considerations in hypercalcemic elderly patients are multiple myeloma, certain nonsquamous cell cancers that promote elevations of serum calcium, such as breast carcinoma metastatic to bone, and iatrogenic causes, such as thiazide and lithium use. Excess amounts of vitamins A and D will induce hypercalcemia, but their abuse is now rare in all age groups.

Therapeutic approaches to hypercalcemia in the elderly are etiology-specific. An issue encountered with some frequency in elderly patients with asymptomatic hyperparathyroidism is when, if ever, to endorse surgical exploration of the neck to remove a parathyroid adenoma or hyperplastic parathyroid glands. The tendency of primary hyperparathyroidism in this age group to be indolent and the presence of concomitant nonendocrine illnesses that heighten the risk of surgery (e.g., chronic obstructive pulmonary disease and cardiac disease) support a decision to withhold surgery if the serum calcium concentration is high-normal or minimally elevated. About 20% of these patients will require parathyroidectomy in 5 to 10 years, usually for relief of worsening hypercalcemia.[7] The authors follow such asymptomatic patients with annual measurements of vertebral trabecular bone mineral content, looking for acceleration of bone mass loss. Monitoring of markers of bone resorption (such as total and free pyridinoline or type I collagen cross-linked N telopeptides has not yet been substantiated in the elderly as a useful approach to the estimation of bone resorption during long-term follow-up of patients with asymptomatic hyperparathyroidism. Persistent serum calcium levels of greater than 11.5 mg/dL (5 mmol/L), accelerated bone demineralization, and an increased rate of decline of GFR are factors indicating a need for parathyroid surgery in patients who have a secure diagnosis of primary hyperparathyroidism.

The hazards of conventional medical management of moderate-to-severe hypercalcemia are increased in older patients. For example, expansion of intravascular volume by saline administration (induction of calcium diuresis) in hypercalcemic patients with impaired left ventricular function may worsen heart failure. Intravenous use of furosemide promotes sodium and calcium diuresis, but concomitant urinary potassium loss may lead to clinically important hypokalemia. In the aged patient with heart disease, treatment of severe hypercalcemia with saline and a loop diuretic requires careful monitoring of intravascular volume.

Attractive alternative management strategies for hypercalcemia in the elderly patient include administration of a bisphosphonate (alendronate, pamidronate, etidronate), calcitonin, or gallium. These agents have modest side effect profiles and do not depend on renal mechanisms for their calcium-lowering effects (although bisphosphonates are excreted by the kidney); they can also be administered without concomitant expansion of intravascular volume. The dosing of these agents is beyond the scope of this text.

Administration of corticosteroids is particularly effective in the management of patients with tumor-related hypercalcemic states in which interleukin-1 beta ("osteclast-activating factor") is produced in excess. When they are effective, corticosteroids usually require several days before they produce a serum calcium-lowering effect.

Chronic management of the elderly patient with hypercalcemia may include the use of a loop diuretic (sodium-calcium diuresis), with frequent monitoring of serum potassium levels, or oral administration of a bisphosphonate. When these strategies are insufficient, oral phosphate (e.g., Neutra-Phos) may be used. Diarrhea is a limiting factor when larger doses of phosphate are required to control hypercalcemia. Chronic corticosteroid administration is an option in patients with hypercalcemic states that have responded to short-term steroid therapy. Successful treatment of the underlying tumor usually removes the mechanism of hypercalcemia and thus the need for specific management of hypercalcemia.

ANTIDIURETIC HORMONE (ARGININE VASOPRESSIN)

Physiology

Normal aging is accompanied by progressive resistance of the renal collecting tubules to AVP. As a result, basal plasma levels of AVP increase slightly during the life span. Central osmoreceptor sensitivity (i.e., the amount of AVP secreted in response to a specific increase in plasma osmolality) is increased in older persons compared with young individuals.

Clinical Assessment

Primary disorders of AVP secretion are uncommon in the older patient population. Management of diabetes insipidus in elderly patients is made difficult by the presence of concomitant nonendocrine disease (particularly heart disease) in which expansion or contraction of intravascular volume is a special risk. Both states can be experienced by patients who incorrectly dose themselves with AVP replacement. Administration of 1-desamino-8-D-arginine vasopressin (DDAVP) is useful in older subjects with central diabetes insipidus because of its short biologic half-life ($T_{1/2}$) and intranasal route of administration. Because it must be administered several times daily, however, noncompliance is encountered in patients with memory loss.

Water intoxication syndromes in older patients result from inappropriate secretion of AVP by nonendocrine cancers (one form of SIADH), from certain endocrine syndromes such as hypothyroidism, and from the administration of a variety of drugs. Most common among the latter are diuretics (which promote saluresis and, more important, decrease free water clearance), carbamazepine, and typical antipsychotic drugs. The first-generation sulfonylurea, chlorpropamide, is a potent inducer of water intoxication but is infrequently used today in the management of diabetes mellitus. (Second-generation sulfonylureas may in fact enhance free water clearance.) A large number of other drugs have been reported to produce hyponatremia but do so infrequently in the general population or rarely in the elderly. Nonsteroidal anti-inflammatory drugs (NSAIDs) decrease free water clearance and may promote modest weight gain (water retention) but rarely lead to water intoxication by themselves. NSAIDs also decrease the diuretic effectiveness of loop diuretics. Additional discussion of water and sodium excretion in the elderly is found in Chapter 49.

ATRIAL NATRIURETIC PEPTIDE

Physiology

Atrial natriuretic peptide (ANP) is a saluretic 28-amino acid molecule that is secreted by the heart in response to intravascular volume expansion. It has a variety of additional effects and its physiologic roles, particularly in the elderly, are not clearly established. Basal levels of plasma ANP are substantially increased in healthy older subjects, and the ANP response to saline infusion is exaggerated in this population. It is possible that these age-dependent changes reflect target tissue insensitivity to the substance and that ANP physiology in the course of normal aging resembles that of AVP.

GROWTH HORMONE

Physiology

Mean basal plasma levels of growth hormone (GH) are similar in healthy young and old subjects, but the normal secretion of GH is phased, and the area under the GH secretory peaks decreases with normal aging.[8] Pituitary secretion of GH in response to provocative stimulation also declines during the life span. Provocative stimuli under controlled diagnostic circumstances are insulin-induced hypoglycemia, intravenous administration of arginine, or intravenous administration of GH-releasing hormone (GHRH). There is evidence that age-dependent attenuation of the GH response to a single dose of GHRH is restored by repetitive treatment with GHRH over a week or more, suggesting that the age-related change in GH release is conditioned by neuroendocrine changes above the pituitary gland. In older women it appears that the decreased responsiveness to single-dose GHRH administration is in part conditioned by the postmenopausal fall in estrogen secretion. The action of GH on its target tissues, such as muscle, bone, and subcutaneous tissue, is mediated by somatomedins, a family of proteins that are growth factors. The basal plasma level of the most important of these factors, insulin-like growth factor 1 (IGF-1), declines with age, and the administration of exogenous GH to elderly subjects normalizes serum IGF-1 levels. The synthesis of an important IGF-binding protein (IGFBP-3) is also GH-dependent; IGFBP-3 levels in blood also fall with normal aging.

The roles of GH in the physiology of the adult and, particularly, the elderly population are not entirely clear, but recent studies suggest that GH participates in maintenance of lean body mass. Two weeks of GH administration increase circulating levels of IGF-1, phosphate, osteocalcin, and 1,25-dihydroxyvitamin D_3. Several months of GH administration to a small group of elderly subjects with lowered serum IGF-1 levels resulted in increased skin thickness and decreased adipose tissue mass. GH also had a modest effect on vertebral bone density. A number of larger long-term studies of GH administration to older patients with decreased IGF-1 levels are in progress. Results of these extensive studies will help to determine whether there are broad therapeutic indications for GH administration in the elderly. There is a possibility that the adverse effects of GH use, such as impaired glucose tolerance, will complicate long-term GH administration.

Clinical Assessment

Disorders of GH secretion are uncommon in the geriatric population. Acromegaly occurring in older people has no features that distinguish it from that in younger individuals. Pituitary deficiency of GH release in the mature adult does not appear to impair the counterregulatory (blood glucose-elevating) response to hypoglycemia. Whether the decreased secretion of GH in the elderly has significant effects on body composition of the elderly population at large, as discussed previously, is speculative.

PROLACTIN

Physiology

Basal levels of serum prolactin (PRL) and the response of PRL secretion to administration of thyrotropin-releasing hormone are not altered in the course of normal aging. The biologic role of PRL in women past reproductive age and in men is unclear.

Clinical Assessment

Abnormalities of PRL secretion in older subjects are uncommon. Hyperprolactinemia may provoke galactorrhea in women of virtually any age. The typical presentation of hyperprolactinemia in premenopausal women is amenorrhea and infertility, abnormalities that are obviously not expressed after the reproductive years. A small minority of breast cancers in women appear to be PRL-dependent, but it is not known whether long-standing hyperprolactinemia in any age group is a risk factor for the induction of breast cancer.

GONADAL FUNCTION

Physiology

The inevitable age-dependent loss of ovarian function in women is of unknown mechanism. The progressive decrease in ovarian secretory capacity is accompanied by increases in circulating levels of gonadotropins (follicle-stimulating hormone [FSH] and luteinizing hormone [LH]) and loss of pulsatile release of gonadotropins by the pituitary gland. Administration of exogenous gonadotropin to menopausal women produces little or no ovarian estrogen response. Adrenocortical secretion of androgens is preserved. During active reproductive life, the functional ovary is a second source of androgens, and, even into the menopause, ovarian androgen secretion persists relative to estrogen production. As a result, the ratio of circulating estrogens to androgens in menopausal women declines as a result of both decreased estrogen secretion and relative sparing of androgen production. Clinical features of the menopause and indications and regimens for hormonal replacement therapy in women are discussed in Chapter 47.

Studies contending that androgen secretion in men falls significantly during the life span usually include data obtained from institutionalized or chronically ill males. Systemic nonendocrine illness depresses the pituitary-gonadal axis in both young and elderly men.[9] When chronically ill subjects are excluded from study, the decline in circulating levels of testosterone with normal aging is detectable but small. On the other hand, serum gonadotropin levels are increased in aging males, even in those whose plasma testosterone concentrations have been stable into the eighth decade of life. This indicates that the response of the testis to gonadotropins indeed declines with aging. The circadian rhythm of serum testosterone levels is diminished in elderly men. Sperm production in older men is decreased despite elevated levels of circulating gonadotropins. None of these data mandate routine testosterone replacement therapy in elderly men.

CARBOHYDRATE METABOLISM AND DIABETES MELLITUS

Physiology

Minimum increases in fasting serum or blood glucose concentration occur with normal aging and probably reflect small changes in non-insulin-mediated glucose disposal (e.g., glucose uptake in insulin-insensitive tissues or uptake in muscle or adipose tissue when circulating levels of insulin are low). In addition, a small decrease in insulin sensitivity occurs by age 45 years in normal subjects. The "dawn phenomenon," a growth hormone-dependent early morning spurt in hepatic glucose output, contributes to fasting hyperglycemia in diabetics but does not occur in healthy elderly subjects. Regardless of age, subjects with fasting serum glucose levels of greater than 140 mg/dL are classified as diabetic.

An extensive literature has documented a decline in carbohydrate tolerance during the life span. Carbohydrate tolerance is measured as the blood glucose response after a standard carbohydrate load. The National Diabetes Data Group excluded age-specific changes in carbohydrate tolerance by defining as "impaired glucose tolerance" those blood glucose concentrations between 140 and 200 mg/dL within 2 hours of administration of a standard oral glucose load.

This performance range encloses the changes in glucose tolerance reported previously as characteristic of normal aging. When followed for 5 years, subjects with "impaired glucose tolerance" may return to normal carbohydrate tolerance, become frankly diabetic, or, in the majority of cases, remain in the impaired glucose tolerance group. The consequences of persistent impaired glucose tolerance — for example, in terms of risk of long-term complications of frank diabetes mellitus—are not yet clear but are one focus of a large current multicenter prospective study.

Hypoglycemia provokes release of counterregulatory hormones (epinephrine, glucagon, cortisol, and GH). Normal aging has little or no impact on the release of catecholamines, glucagon, and cortisol in response to hypoglycemia. Although GH secretion in the presence of hypoglycemia does decline during the life span, the effect of this on the integrity of the counterregulatory (blood glucose elevating) response is not physiologically important.

Clinical Assessment

Diabetes mellitus that begins in middle-age or beyond usually has a clinical pattern that is uncomplicated by a risk of significant ketosis or acidosis. Patients with this pattern are insulinopenic relative to the demands of systemic carbohydrate metabolism but have sufficient residual endogenous insulin secretion to suppress lipolysis and thus prevent ketoacidosis. Such patients may need insulin to control blood glucose levels but do not *depend* on exogenous insulin to suppress lipolysis. This syndrome is termed non-insulin-dependent diabetes mellitus (NIDDM, type II). The prevalence of NIDDM in subjects over age 65 years is as high as 7% to 9%. Patients who are absolutely without endogenous insulin secretion (insulinoprival state) are at risk for ketoacidosis and are said to have insulin-dependent diabetes mellitus (IDDM, type I). Occasionally, type I diabetes mellitus does occur in elderly subjects. Because some type II patients may develop mild starvation ketosis without acidosis when their blood glucose levels are poorly controlled, they may be incorrectly thought to have IDDM.

It is important to appreciate that NIDDM may be iatrogenic. High-dose anti-inflammatory corticosteroid use may induce type II disease, as may thiazide diuretics and furosemide. The diabetogenic effects of thiazides may not be apparent for months or years after their introduction into a therapeutic regimen for hypertension or heart failure. NIDDM in the thiazide-treated patient may occur without an antecedent history of mild or intermittent carbohydrate intolerance.

Obesity (in which insulin resistance appears in the absence of frank diabetes mellitus) and a positive family history for NIDDM are risk factors for the development of thiazide-related hyperglycemia.

The long-term microvascular, macrovascular, renal, and neuropathic complications of diabetes mellitus occur with similar frequency in young and older diabetic patients, given comparable durations of the disease. A number of studies, including the Diabetes Control and Complications Trial (DCCT), have documented the importance of normoglycemia in reducing the risk of complications of diabetes.[10] Participants in these trials have been patients with type I diabetes. A prospective multicenter study of the impact of glycemic control on complications in type II diabetes patients is now under way in the United States.

The therapeutic alternatives that may be considered in managing older diabetic patients include (1) "tight control," based on multiple doses of regular and intermediate-acting insulin or, when oral hypoglycemic therapy is highly effective, on the use of an oral agent; (2) avoidance of substantive hyperglycemia (i.e., blood glucose levels at any period in the day of more than 250 mg/dL, and maintenance of fasting blood glucose levels of below 160 mg/dL through the use of intermediate-acting insulin or an oral agent; (3) dietary restrictions intended to promote weight loss and its attendant improvement in tissue sensitivity to insulin; (4) attenuation of the absorption of dietary glucose postprandially through the use of dietary fiber or acarbose; (5) a permissive approach—applied to asymptomatic hyperglycemic patients—in which control of blood glucose level is not attempted. Combinations of these strategies are of course possible. In all patients in whom euglycemia is the goal, regular measurements by patients of their own blood glucose levels ("home glucose monitoring") is mandatory. When these measurements indicate satisfactory control, the physician should periodically measure glycohemoglobin concentration (hemoglobin A_{1c}) as an index of the accumulated glycemic experience during the preceding 3 to 6 weeks.

A structured approach to management of NIDDM is depicted in Figure 50–2. The NIDDM patient who is 60 to 70 years of age can anticipate 10 to 20 additional years of life unless the complications of diabetes supervene. The authors believe that euglycemia is the goal of therapy in patients with both IDDM and NIDDM and that a permissive approach cannot be justified in any cohort of patients. Weight loss is desirable in all overweight patients. It improves blood pressure control in diabetic patients with concomitant hypertension and reduces mortality risk, at least in individuals who are 30% or more above ideal body weight. Modest weight loss may be achieved by limiting total daily caloric intake to 800 to 1000 kcal and, when it can be safely introduced, regular exercise.

The authors advocate a conventional (nondiabetic) diet in patients with mild type II disease but one that (1) restricts fat intake, particularly saturated fat, (2) is isocaloric from day to day, and (3) contains an adequate amount of fiber. Increased dietary fiber retards glucose absorption and thus may improve glycemic control. In overweight patients, total calorie intake is restricted. Although it is intuitive to restrict simple carbohydrate intake and substitute complex for simple carbohydrates in diabetic diets, the impact of this approach on glycemia may be small. High (complex) carbohydrate diets in patients with mild type II disease paradoxically may improve carbohydrate tolerance compared to carbohydrate restriction. It is for this reason that the authors recommend a conventional diet in these patients. A diabetic diet is advocated in NIDDM patients in whom euglycemia is difficult to achieve.

Multiple-dose insulin therapy is feasible in highly motivated elderly patients. The authors' experience with type II patients indicates that 25% can maintain normal fasting blood glucose levels and normal blood glycohemoglobin concentrations with one or two subcutaneous injections of intermediate-acting and regular insulin daily. A recent study has demonstrated the feasibility of achieving tight control in NIDDM patients with either multiple doses of insulin or insulin taken in conjunction with an oral hypoglycemic agent (glipizide).[11] There is little experience with insulin pumps in this age group because this approach has been almost exclusively applied to type I patients. The risk of hypoglycemia of course exists with tight control, and this risk is heightened in patients with coexisting coronary artery disease, in which tissue ischemia may be intensified by hypoglycemia.

The desirability and convenience of oral hypoglycemic therapy are readily apparent. First-generation sulfonylureas (tolbutamide, chlorpropamide) have disadvantages of ineffectiveness (tolbutamide) or prolonged bioactivity and hypoglycemic risk (chlorpropamide). The latter agent also induces water intoxication and is hepatotoxic. Second-generation sulfonylureas (glyburide, glipizide) have improved side effect profiles and are reasonably effective. The availability of metformin, a biguanide hypoglycemic drug, has considerably improved the effectiveness of oral therapy. Earlier experience with phenformin, a

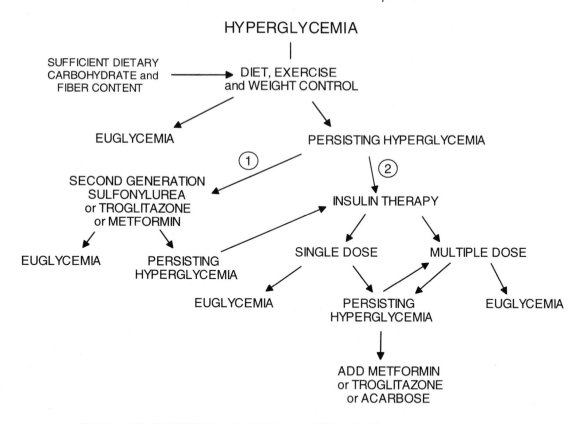

HYPERGLYCEMIA

SUFFICIENT DIETARY
CARBOHYDRATE and ⟶ DIET, EXERCISE
FIBER CONTENT and WEIGHT CONTROL

EUGLYCEMIA PERSISTING HYPERGLYCEMIA

① ②

SECOND GENERATION
SULFONYLUREA INSULIN THERAPY
or TROGLITAZONE
or METFORMIN

EUGLYCEMIA PERSISTING SINGLE DOSE MULTIPLE DOSE
HYPERGLYCEMIA

EUGLYCEMIA PERSISTING EUGLYCEMIA
HYPERGLYCEMIA

ADD METFORMIN
or TROGLITAZONE
or ACARBOSE

GOAL: EUGLYCEMIA, NORMAL GLYCOHEMOGLOBIN LEVEL

Figure 50–2 Treatment options in the management of non-insulin-dependent diabetes mellitus (NIDDM). The choice of oral hypoglycemic therapy (pathway 1) or insulin treatment (pathway 2) depends on multiple factors. Among these are the patient's conviction that he or she can comply with requirements and achieve goals (efficacy), the competence of the patient in administering insulin and monitoring blood sugar levels, the presence of social support, and the degree of hyperglycemia. In pathway 2 note that metformin and acarbose should not be used as combination therapy but are alternative additions to insulin treatment. Acarbose may also be added to oral sulfonylurea (but not metformin) therapy in pathway 1.

biguanide removed from the U.S. marketplace, included episodes of sometimes fatal lactic acidosis. In contrast, metformin has at this point a negligible risk of lactic acidosis. The authors nonetheless counsel avoiding its use in patients who are already at risk for lactic acidosis because of severe peripheral vascular disease (tissue hypoxia or necrosis) until its safety in this situation has been rigorously examined. Patients with renal insufficiency should not be treated with metformin. Metformin is useful as a single-agent oral hypoglycemic therapy and has also been used in combination with insulin or a sulfonylurea to improve glycemic control throughout the day. The incidence of hypoglycemia in patients treated with metformin alone is very low, and it is similarly low when anticipatory reductions in dose of other hypoglycemic medications in complex treatment regimens are made when metformin is introduced.

Thiazolidinediones are oral drugs that improve insulin action at the transcriptional level in insulin-responsive tissues. They do not increase insulin secretion. One member of this class of agents, troglitazone, has been approved for use in type II diabetic patients who require more than 30 U of insulin daily for blood glucose control but continue to have elevated glycohemoglobin levels (insulin-resistant patients). The drug frequently permits a reduction in insulin dosage while improving glycemic control, and NIDDM patients who require insulin may occasionally lose their need for insulin for glycemic control when troglitazone is administered. Although it is approved by the U.S. Food and Drug Administration only for use with insulin, troglitazone is being administered alone by some physicians to manage type II diabetes or in combination with another oral hypoglycemic agent in such patients. Taken alone, it is generally less effective than a sulfonylurea or metformin. Its use with and without insulin is shown in Figure 50–2. Cholestyramine importantly reduces the absorption of troglitazone. The safety of long-term troglitazone administration has not yet been determined.

Acarbose is an oral alpha-glucosidase inhibitor that interferes with the breakdown of both complex dietary carbohydrates and disaccharides. There is little systemic absorption of the drug. It is taken at the beginning of a meal and lowers postprandial glycemia. It may be effective alone and is very effective in combination with sulfonylurea or insulin therapy. It increases the risk of hypoglycemia in such treatment settings, and treatment of hypoglycemia with oral sucrose in these situations may be less effective because sucrose may not be hydrolyzed satisfactorily in the presence of acarbose in the gastrointestinal tract. Other side effects include abdominal cramps and flatulence and, importantly, reduced bioavailability of metformin. Thus, acarbose should probably not be used in combination with this biguanide.

The goals of therapy are (1) freedom from symptoms of hyperglycemia, (2) normal fasting blood glucose levels with minimal risk of hypoglycemia, and (3) glycohemoglobin levels within the normal range. The current therapeutic armamentarium makes these goals more feasible than was the case a decade ago.

As in younger patients, the management of elderly patients with type II diabetes includes systemic surveillance and anticipation of the complications of diabetes mellitus. Surveillance is intended to detect large blood vessel (macrovascular) disease that may be exacerbated by concomitant hyperlipidemia, microvascular disease (retinopathy), neuropathy, and nephropathy. Peripheral neuropathy (polyneuropathy) and large vessel disease of the extremities (peripheral vascular disease) are particularly devastating in the elderly when they lead to limb loss; rehabilitation of older patients who have undergone lower extremity amputation is frequently unsuccessful because of coincident problems, such as dizziness or heart disease, that limit gait reeducation. Good foot care is imperative in all diabetic patients and is usually best provided by a podiatrist.

Extreme loss of glycemic control in NIDDM results in the syndrome of hyperglycemic nonketotic stupor or coma. Acute management of this syndrome is reviewed in standard textbooks of endocrinology. This syndrome has a high mortality rate that in part reflects the presence of nonendocrine disease such as arteriosclerosis and in part the devastating complications of treatment. Such complications include overexpansion of intravascular volume in these previously very hypovolemic patients, precipitous declines in serum potassium levels and in osmolality, and delay in recognition or treatment of precipitating causes of the hyperglycemic state, such as pneumonia or infections of the biliary tree or urinary tract. Some patients may have lactic acidosis caused by infection or tissue ischemia, particularly muscle ischemia.

References

1. Mariotti S, Franceschi C, Cossarizza A, Pinchera A: The aging thyroid. Endocrinol Rev 1995;16:686–715.
2. Davis PJ, Davis FB: Hyperthyroidism in patients over the age of 60 years. Medicine 1974;53:161–181.
3. Sawin CT, Geller A, Wolf PA, et al: Low serum thyrotropin concentrations as a risk factor for atrial fibrillation in older persons. N Engl J Med 1994;331:1249–1252.
4. Davis FB, LaMantia RS, Spaulding SW, Wehmann RE, Davis PJ: Estimation of a physiologic replacement dose of levothyroxine in elderly patients with hypothyroidism. Arch Intern Med 1984;144:1752–1754.
5. Seeman TE, Robbins RJ: Aging and hypothalamic-pituitary-adrenal response to challenge in humans. Endocrinol Rev 1994;15:233–260.
6. St. John Sutton MG, Sheps SG, Lie JT: Prevalence of clinically unsuspected pheochromocytoma. Review of a 50-year autopsy series. Mayo Clin Proc 1981; 56:354–360.
7. Scholz DA, Purnell DC: Asymptomatic primary hyperparathyroidism: 10-year prospective study. Mayo Clin Proc 1981;56:473–478.
8. Corpas E, Harman SM, Blackman MR: Human growth hormone and aging. Endocrinol Rev 1993;14:20–39.
9. Blackman MR, Weintraub BD, Rosen SW, Harman SM: Comparison of the effects of lung cancer, benign lung disease, and normal aging on pituitary-gonadal function in men. J Clin Endocrinol Metab 1988;66:88–95.
10. Diabetes Control and Complications Trial Research Group: The effect of intensive treatment of diabetes on the development and progression of long-term complications in insulin-dependent diabetes mellitus. N Engl J Med 1993;329:977–986.
11. Colwell JA: The feasibility of intensive insulin management in non-insulin-dependent diabetes mellitus. Implications of the Veterans Affairs Cooperative Study on glycemic control and complications in NIDDM. Ann Intern Med 1996;124:131–135.

INDEX

Note: Page numbers in *italics* refer to illustrations; page numbers followed by (t) refer to tables.

ISBN 0-7216-6599-3